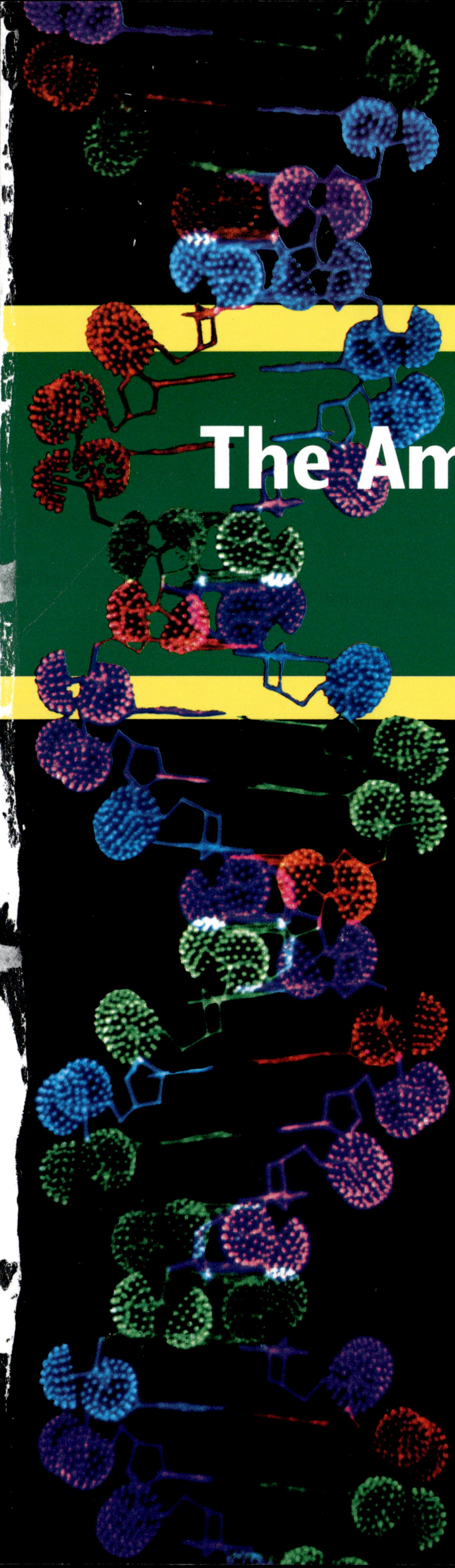

The American Journal of Human Genetics

VOLUME 76 NUMBER 5 MAY 2005

THE AMERICAN SOCIETY OF HUMAN GENETICS

Published for The American Society of Human Genetics
by The University of Chicago Press

DIRECT INQUIRIES AND SUBMISSIONS TO

The American Journal of Human Genetics
Department of Human Genetics
Emory University School of Medicine
615 Michael Street, Room 301
Atlanta, GA 30322-3050

Telephone: (404) 712-9980
Fax: (404) 712-9984
E-mail: ajhg@emory.edu
Web page: http://www.ajhg.org

PAST EDITORS

Subscription orders and correspondence should be addressed to the University of Chicago Press, P.O. Box 37005, Chicago, IL 60637. Checks should be made out to the University of Chicago Press. All orders must be in U.S. currency. Telephone: (8:00 A.M.–5:00 P.M. Central Standard Time, Monday–Friday) U.S. & Canada toll free, (877) 705-1878; Rest of World, (773) 753-3347. Fax: U.S. & Canada toll free, (877) 705-1879; Rest of World, (773) 753-0811. E-mail: subscriptions@press.uchicago.edu; Web site: http://www.journals.uchicago.edu. Remittance for nonmember subscription is payable to the publisher on a calendar-year basis. For domestic nonmember individuals and institutions, the single-copy rate is $88.00 and the calendar-year rate is $995.00; for foreign nonmember individuals and institutions, the single-copy rate is $88.00 (U.S. currency) and the calendar-year rate is $1050.00 (U.S. currency); the calendar-year rate for Canadian citizens, which includes GST, is $1088.65 (U.S. currency). All rates above include International Surface Airlift (ISAL) delivery to addresses outside the U.S. Subscription agent for Japan: Kinokuniya Company, Ltd. Individuals have the option to order directly from the University of Chicago Press.

Memberships.—A membership application and dues schedule appear at the back of each issue of the *Journal.*

The American Journal of Human Genetics (ISSN 0002-9297) is published monthly at 1427 East 60th Street, Chicago, IL 60637. Periodicals postage is paid at Chicago, IL, and at additional mailing offices by the American Society of Human Genetics. All rights reserved.

Postmaster: send address changes to *The American Journal of Human Genetics*, The University of Chicago Press, Journals Division, P.O. Box 37005, Chicago, IL 60637.

The American Journal of Human Genetics

Volume 76 Number 5 May 2005

i **This Month in the *Journal***
Kathryn Garber

Review Article

717 **Autosomal Recessive Primary Microcephaly (MCPH): A Review of Clinical, Molecular, and Evolutionary Findings**
C. Geoffrey Woods, Jacquelyn Bond, and Wolfgang Enard

Articles

729 **Diversity and Function of Mutations in P450 Oxidoreductase in Patients with Antley-Bixler Syndrome and Disordered Steroidogenesis**
Ningwu Huang, Amit V. Pandey, Vishal Agrawal, William Reardon, Pablo D. Lapunzina, David Mowat, Ethylin Wang Jabs, Guy Van Vliet, Joseph Sack, Christa E. Flück, and Walter L. Miller

750 **Exon Array CGH: Detection of Copy-Number Changes at the Resolution of Individual Exons in the Human Genome**
Pawandeep Dhami, Alison J. Coffey, Stephen Abbs, Joris R. Vermeesch, Jan P. Dumanski, Karen J. Woodward, Robert M. Andrews, Cordelia Langford, and David Vetrie

763 **Increased Level of Linkage Disequilibrium in Rural Compared with Urban Communities: A Factor to Consider in Association-Study Design**
Veronique Vitart, Andrew D. Carothers, Caroline Hayward, Peter Teague, Nicholas D. Hastie, Harry Campbell, and Alan F. Wright

773 **Localization of a Type 1 Diabetes Locus in the *IL2RA/CD25* Region by Use of Tag Single-Nucleotide Polymorphisms**
Adrian Vella, Jason D. Cooper, Christopher E. Lowe, Neil Walker, Sarah Nutland, Barry Widmer, Richard Jones, Susan M. Ring, Wendy McArdle, Marcus E. Pembrey, David P. Strachan, David B. Dunger, Rebecca C. J. Twells, David G. Clayton, and John A. Todd

780 **Nonparametric Tests of Association of Multiple Genes with Human Disease**
Daniel J. Schaid, Shannon K. McDonnell, Scott J. Hebbring, Julie M. Cunningham, and Stephen N. Thibodeau

794 **Mutations in *ABCA12* Underlie the Severe Congenital Skin Disease Harlequin Ichthyosis**
David P. Kelsell, Elizabeth E. Norgett, Harriet Unsworth, Muy-Teck Teh, Thomas Cullup, Charles A. Mein, Patricia J. Dopping-Hepenstal, Beverly A. Dale, Gianluca Tadini, Philip Fleckman, Karen G. Stephens, Virginia P. Sybert, Susan B. Mallory, Bernard V. North, David R. Witt, Eli Sprecher, Aileen E. M. Taylor, Andrew Ilchyshyn, Cameron T. Kennedy, Helen Goodyear, Celia Moss, David Paige, John I. Harper, Bryan D. Young, Irene M. Leigh, Robin A. J. Eady, and Edel A. O'Toole

804 **A Novel *STX16* Deletion in Autosomal Dominant Pseudohypoparathyroidism Type Ib Redefines the Boundaries of a *cis*-Acting Imprinting Control Element of *GNAS***
Agnès Linglart, Robert C. Gensure, Robert C. Olney, Harald Jüppner, and Murat Bastepe

815 **Quantitative Founder-Effect Analysis of French Canadian Families Identifies Specific Loci Contributing to Metabolic Phenotypes of Hypertension**
P. Hamet, E. Merlo, O. Šeda, U. Broeckel, J. Tremblay, M. Kaldunski, D. Gaudet, G. Bouchard, B. Deslauriers, F. Gagnon, G. Antoniol, Z. Pausová, M. Labuda, M. Jomphe, F. Gossard, G. Tremblay, R. Kirova, P. Tonellato, S. N. Orlov, J. Pintos, J. Platko, T. J. Hudson, J. D. Rioux, T. A. Kotchen, and A. W. Cowley Jr.

833 **Over- and Underdosage of *SOX3* Is Associated with Infundibular Hypoplasia and Hypopituitarism**
Kathryn S. Woods, Maria Cundall, James Turton, Karine Rizotti, Ameeta Mehta, Rodger Palmer, Jacqueline Wong, W. K. Chong, Mahmoud Al-Zyoud, Maryam El-Ali, Timo Otonkoski, Juan-Pedro Martinez-Barbera, Paul Q. Thomas, Iain C. Robinson, Robin Lovell-Badge, Karen J. Woodward, and Mehul T. Dattani

Reports

850 **Identifying Candidate Hirschsprung Disease–Associated *RET* Variants**
Grzegorz M. Burzynski, Ilja M. Nolte, Agnes Bronda, Krista K. Bos, Jan Osinga, Ivan Plaza Menacho, Bas Twigt, Saskia Maas, Alice S. Brooks, Joke B. G. M. Verheij, Charles H. C. M. Buys, and Robert M. W. Hofstra

859 **Single- and Multilocus Allelic Variants within the $GABA_B$ Receptor Subunit 2 (*GABAB2*) Gene Are Significantly Associated with Nicotine Dependence**
Joke Beuten, Jennie Z. Ma, Thomas J. Payne, Randolph T. Dupont, Karen M. Crews, Grant Somes, Nancy J. Williams, Robert C. Elston, and Ming D. Li

865 **Microduplication and Triplication of 22q11.2: A Highly Variable Syndrome**
Twila M. Yobb, Martin J. Somerville, Lionel Willatt, Helen V. Firth, Karen Harrison, Jennifer MacKenzie, Natasha Gallo, Bernice E. Morrow, Lisa G. Shaffer, Melanie Babcock, Judy Chernos, Francois Bernier, Kathy Sprysak, Jesse Christiansen, Shelagh Haase, Basil Elyas, Margaret Lilley, Steven Bamforth, and Heather E. McDermid

877 **Congenital Diaphragmatic Hernia and Chromosome 15q26: Determination of a Candidate Region by Use of Fluorescent In Situ Hybridization and Array-Based Comparative Genomic Hybridization**
M. Klaassens, M. van Dooren, H. J. Eussen, H. Douben, A. T. den Dekker, C. Lee, P. K. Donahoe, R. J. Galjaard, N. Goemaere, R. R. de Krijger, C. Wouters, J. Wauters, B. A. Oostra, D. Tibboel, and A. de Klein

883 **Saami and Berbers—An Unexpected Mitochondrial DNA Link**
Alessandro Achilli, Chiara Rengo, Vincenza Battaglia, Maria Pala, Anna Olivieri, Simona Fornarino, Chiara Magri, Rosaria Scozzari, Nora Babudri, A. Silvana Santachiara-Benerecetti, Hans-Jürgen Bandelt, Ornella Semino, and Antonio Torroni

887 **A Note on Exact Tests of Hardy-Weinberg Equilibrium**
Janis E. Wigginton, David J. Cutler, and Gonçalo R. Abecasis

894 **The Dual Origin of the Malagasy in Island Southeast Asia and East Africa: Evidence from Maternal and Paternal Lineages**
Matthew E. Hurles, Bryan C. Sykes, Mark A. Jobling, and Peter Forster

902 **The *Epsin 4* Gene on Chromosome 5q, Which Encodes the Clathrin-Associated Protein Enthoprotin, Is Involved in the Genetic Susceptibility to Schizophrenia**
Jonathan Pimm, Andrew McQuillin, Srinivasa Thirumalai, Jacob Lawrence, Digby Quested, Nicholas Bass, Graham Lamb, Helen Moorey, Susmita R. Datta, Gursharan Kalsi, Allison Badacsonyi, Katie Kelly, Jenny Morgan, Bhaskar Punukollu, David Curtis, and Hugh Gurling

Announcements

908 **Employment Opportunities; Conference**

Information for Contributors

This Month in the *Journal*

This month in the *Journal,* Geoff Woods, Jacquie Bond, and Wolfgang Enard discuss primary microcephaly (MCPH). This neurodevelopmental disorder is characterized by a small but architecturally normal brain and nonprogressive mental retardation. Over the past couple of years, four genes involved in MCPH have been identified. The authors present a model that suggests that mutations in these genes lead to MCPH through effects on neurogenic mitosis. Beyond their clinical implications, research results for MCPH have intrigued people interested in evolution, because the *MCPH* genes may have played a role in the dramatic increase in the ratio of brain to body size that developed during human evolution. Woods et al. also describe attempts to examine the selective forces operating on the *MCPH* genes.

Array-CGH at Single-Exon Resolution, *by Dhami et al. (p. 750)*

Dhami et al. developed a method for genomewide analysis of copy-number changes at the resolution of single exons. This array–comparative genome hybridization (array-CGH) method allows the detection of copy-number changes of array elements on the order of hundreds of base pairs in length, which is ~2 orders of magnitude smaller than previous array-CGH methods. Their approach to generating the array uses a modified primer to amplify exonic sequences that can then be attached in a single-stranded fashion to glass slides. The use of single-stranded array elements increases their signal:noise ratio by an average of 1.79-fold. The method is illustrated with an exonic array that represents five disease-related genes: *COL4A5, DMD, PLP1, NF2,* and *PMP22.* DNA samples from 31 patients with known copy-number changes in these genes were used to test the five-gene array. All of the changes were detected, including four that involved only a single exon. The authors are already looking forward to the development of an array that can assess copy-number changes for virtually all exons in the genome, and they propose several potential applications of this technique, including chromatin immunoprecipitation analysis, screens for copy-number polymorphisms, and diagnostics.

LD Extent in Rural Communities, *by Vitart et al. (p. 763)*

I grew up in a small town. Most of the people I grew up with still live there and married other locals. In Atlanta, on the other hand, it's hard to find natives. Vitart et al. wanted to determine whether these rural/urban differences in population stability translate into differences in linkage disequilibrium (LD). They chose Scotland as an example of an outbred European population. Rural, urban, and isolated populations are represented in their sample of >900 people, and inclusion in the study required that all four grandparents came from the same region as the sampled individual. Vitart et al. figured that general differences in population stability between rural and urban populations might translate into differences in LD between the populations. In fact, that holds true; there is greater LD in rural Scottish populations than in urban ones, and isolated island populations have even greater LD. For the design of large sample collections for association studies, the authors think it might be advantageous, in terms of increased study power, to sample within stable rural populations rather than urban populations, as many large-scale studies do.

ABCA12 ***Mutations in Harlequin Ichthyosis,*** *by Kelsell et al. (p. 794)*

Harlequin ichthyosis is a severe congenital skin disorder that is often fatal very soon after birth. In affected babies, the skin is dried out so much that the limbs are held in rigid semiflexion, and the skin forms hard diamond-shaped plaques with cracks between them. There is abnormal keratin structure, keratinocyte differentiation, and lipid transport in the skin of these individuals, but the underlying genetic cause has been a mystery. Kelsell et al. sought the disease gene through a homozygosity approach, using genotypes from a SNP mapping 10K array. A single region, on chromosome 2q35, had a significant amount of homozygosity in five of the six affected individuals examined. Located within that region is *ABCA12,* which encodes an ATP-binding cassette protein that is believed to transport epidermal lipids. Mutations in *ABCA12,* the majority of them truncating, were found in 11 affected individuals. In contrast, missense *ABCA12* mutations have been reported elsewhere in individuals with the less severe but related phenotypes lamellar ichthyosis and nonbullous congenital ichthyosiform erythroderma. In addition to giving insight into this devastating disorder, this work has more practical implications, because it paves the way for prenatal diagnosis for affected families.

0002-9297/2005/7605-0001$15.00

A Novel* STX16 *Deletion Causes PHP-Ib, *by Linglart et al.* (*p. 804*)

GNAS is a complex, imprinted locus associated with pseudohypoparathyroidism (PHP). Through a series of alternative transcripts, it encodes the α-subunit of the stimulatory G protein ($G\alpha_s$), neurosecretory protein 55, the extra large $G\alpha_s$, and some nontranslated RNAs. Some of the transcripts are paternally derived and others are maternal; this is under the control of differentially methylated regions in this locus. Depending on how you look at it, Linglart et al. either simplify or complicate our understanding of this locus with their report of an additional imprinting control element (ICE) associated with *GNAS* that was defined using a family with PHP-Ib. Many families with this disorder carry an identical 3-kb microdeletion, upstream of *GNAS,* that is associated with a methylation defect limited to the *GNAS* exon A/B transcript. The family in this study shares the methylation defect at A/B but did not have the 3-kb deletion. Instead, they have an overlapping 4.4-kb microdeletion within the *STX16* gene. PHP-Ib in this family is not due to loss of *STX16,* because this gene is normally biallelically expressed and therefore not consistent with the maternal inheritance pattern of PHP-Ib. Instead, Linglart et al. propose that the region of overlap of the 3- and 4.4-kb deletions (~1.3 kb) contains a new ICE that is necessary for regulation of methylation at exon A/B.

Exact Tests of Hardy-Weinberg Equilibrium, *by Wigginton et al.* (*p. 887*)

Deviations from Hardy-Weinberg equilibrium (HWE) can indicate several things, including nonrandom mating, genotyping error, population stratification in the sample, and association of an allele with a trait. Most commonly, HWE is tested through a goodness-of-fit χ^2 test. Wigginton et al. show that this test can have inflated type I error rates and can lead to false rejections of HWE. They describe an exact test for HWE and an efficient implementation of this method that is suitable for large-scale data, and they show that it is accurate over many allele frequencies. They test this approach on a set of >18,000 markers from the International HapMap project and find that the exact test—but not the χ^2 test—rejects HWE at the appropriate level. The authors advocate use of the exact test rather than the χ^2 test for tests of HWE.

KATHRYN GARBER
Deputy Editor

Autosomal Recessive Primary Microcephaly (MCPH): A Review of Clinical, Molecular, and Evolutionary Findings

C. Geoffrey Woods,[1] Jacquelyn Bond,[2] and Wolfgang Enard[3]

[1]Department of Medical Genetics, Cambridge Institute for Medical Research, Cambridge, United Kingdom; [2]Molecular Medicine Unit, University of Leeds, Leeds, United Kingdom; and [3]Max Planck Institute for Evolutionary Anthropology, Leipzig, Germany

Autosomal recessive primary microcephaly (MCPH) is a neurodevelopmental disorder. It is characterized by two principal features, microcephaly present at birth and nonprogressive mental retardation. The microcephaly is the consequence of a small but architecturally normal brain, and it is the cerebral cortex that shows the greatest size reduction. There are at least seven MCPH loci, and four of the genes have been identified: *MCPH1,* encoding Microcephalin; *MCPH3,* encoding CDK5RAP2; *MCPH5,* encoding ASPM; and *MCPH6,* encoding CENPJ. These findings are starting to have an impact on the clinical management of families affected with MCPH. Present data suggest that MCPH is the consequence of deficient neurogenesis within the neurogenic epithelium. Evolutionary interest in MCPH has been sparked by the suggestion that changes in the MCPH genes might also be responsible for the increase in brain size during human evolution. Indeed, evolutionary analyses of Microcephalin and ASPM reveal evidence for positive selection during human and great ape evolution. So an understanding of this rare genetic disorder may offer us significant insights into neurogenic mitosis and the evolution of the most striking differences between us and our closest living relatives: brain size and cognitive ability.

Introduction

The aim of this review is to summarize the recent findings in autosomal recessive primary microcephaly (MCPH). First, the clinical features of the disorder are discussed, especially that "microcephaly" is the finding of a reduced head circumference (HC) and that MCPH is but one of many conditions in which the principal features are "microcephaly and mental retardation. Second, we review the molecular genetic findings for the six known recessive loci, for which four of the genes have been discovered. Thirdly, we present the evidence that MCPH is the consequence of deficient mitosis in neural precursors. And finally, we discuss the role that MCPH genes might have played during the evolution of the human brain, which is approximately three times larger than that expected for a primate of our body size.

Clinical Features of MCPH

Microcephaly and HC

The term "microcephaly" refers to a clinical finding: an HC significantly less than expected for an individual's age and sex (Warkany 1981; Aicardi 1998). HC is used as a surrogate measurement of brain size; however, it is only imperfectly correlated with brain volume. Other methods have been used (e.g., volumetric nuclear magnetic resonance [NMR] scanning), but HC remains the common, simple method for evaluating gross brain size (Aicardi 1998), although it needs to be accurately measured and charted relative to age and sex (Nellhaus 1968; Sher and Brown 1975; Babson and Benda 1976; Sells 1977; Gross et al. 1983; Roche et al. 1987). An HC of three standard deviations below the mean (−3 SD) is usually the cut-off for defining microcephaly (Ross and Frias 1977; Baraitser 1990). Importantly, microcephaly is strongly correlated with mental retardation (Warkany 1981; Gross et al. 1983; Dolk 1991). Individuals with an HC of −3 SD and normal intelligence are occasionally reported, but individuals with an HC of −4 SD or less and normal intelligence are very rare (Teebi et al. 1987).

Microcephaly is divided into *primary microcephaly,* which is present at birth, and *secondary microcephaly,* which develops postnatally (Woods 2004). The crucial difference between these groupings is that primary microcephaly is usually a static developmental anomaly, whereas secondary microcephaly indicates a progressive neurodegenerative condition (Qazi and Reed 1973; Opitz and Holt 1992; Dobyns 2002; Rosenberg et al. 2002). There are many nongenetic and genetic causes of "primary microcephaly with mental retardation," such as congenital infection with toxoplasma, maternal alcohol

Received December 3, 2004; accepted for publication February 25, 2005; electronically published March 31, 2005.

Address for correspondence and reprints: Dr. Geoff Woods, Department of Medical Genetics, Cambridge Institute for Medical Research, Wellcome/MRC Building, Addenbrooke's Hospital, Cambridge CB2 2XY, United Kingdom. E-mail: cw347@cam.ac.uk

0002-9297/2005/7605-0002$15.00

overconsumption during pregnancy, and Rubenstein Taybi syndrome, all of which must be excluded before the diagnosis of MCPH is considered (Cowie 1960; Winter and Baraitser 2003).

Definition of MCPH as a Phenotype

"True microcephaly," "microcephaly vera," and "autosomal recessive primary microcephaly" are terms in the literature that were probably all intended to describe the same phenotype. In "true microcephaly," the sloping forehead was a defining feature; however, it is not seen in all cases of MCPH (Bundey 1997; Roberts at al. 2002). Over time, "microcephaly vera" has come to include the condition of any child with congenital microcephaly accompanied by a range of neurological features, and hence it has lost specificity as a diagnosis. This led to the introduction of a new diagnostic label, "autosomal recessive primary microcephaly," shortened to "MCPH" (MIM #251200) (Jackson et al. 1998).

The initial defining clinical features of MCPH in the studies by Jackson et al. (2002) and Roberts et al. (2002) were:

1. Congenital microcephaly at least 4 SD below age and sex means.
2. Mental retardation but no other neurological finding, such as spasticity, seizures, or progressive cognitive decline.
3. Normal height and weight, appearance, and results on chromosome analysis and brain scan.

MCPH is a disorder of fetal brain growth. The timing of the reduction in growth has been elucidated by ultrasound of affected pregnancies. Normal head measurements are found up to 20 wk of gestation, whereas a decreased HC is seen by 32 wk (C.G.W., personal observation). After birth, HC lies between −4 and −12 SD (Roberts et al. 2002). The relative degree of microcephaly does not vary throughout life, and within a family HC usually does not vary by >2 SD between affected individuals (Roberts et al. 2002). NMR and CAT scans of the brain show that MCPH causes a central nervous system of reduced size, with the greatest effect on the cerebral cortex (Bond et al. 2002). MCPH is associated with a simplification of the cerebral cortical gyral pattern and a slight reduction in the volume of the white matter, consistent with the small size of the brain (Barkovich et al. 2001). In general, the architecture of the CNS is normal, with no evidence of a neuronal migration defect (Bond et al. 2002).

Individuals with MCPH are all mentally retarded, but the retardation is usually only of mild to moderate severity (Roberts et al. 2002). There is no evidence of progressive cognitive decline or of any motor deficit. Early milestones such as alertness, smiling to parents, and head control are often normal. Later motor and social milestones are mildly delayed, but speech development is consistently delayed. As teenagers, children with MCPH have good fine motor control, balance, and grace in movements. They achieve well in sports, compared with other mentally retarded children, and often have a "happy affect." Individuals with MCPH tend to be well behaved and are "biddable"—that is, they are compliant with instruction and can be taught skills of daily living, common-sense safety, and some reading and writing (Ross and Frias 1977; Roberts et al. 2002).

Subsequent to MCPH gene discovery, genotype/phenotype studies showed that the original MCPH diagnostic criteria required revision. Whereas the original definition excluded seizures, height reduction, and abnormal cytogenetic findings, these features have now been reported in some cases of MCPH, and the diagnosis of MCPH is no longer excluded by their presence. Specific genotype-phenotype correlations have been made for individuals with *MCPH1* mutations. These individuals may have a reduction in height, although it is not as marked as the degree of microcephaly (Neitzel et al. 2002; Trimborn et al. 2004). In one *MCPH1* family, a small number of periventricular neuronal heterotopias (groups of neurons in an abnormal position within the brain) were found—which is indicative of abnormal neuronal migration (Trimborn et al. 2004). Periventricular neuronal heterotopias were not reported in the original families used to link and identify the *MCPH1* gene, so their relative incidence is unknown (Jackson et al. 2002). *MCPH1* mutations are also consistently associated with an increased proportion of cells with premature chromosome condensation leading to a prophaselike appearance seen on cytogenetic analysis (see below).

The current clinical definition of MCPH is as follows:

1. Congenital microcephaly, with HC at least 4 SD below age and sex means.
2. Mental retardation but no other neurological finding, such as spasticity, or progressive cognitive decline. Fits are unusual but do not exclude the diagnosis.
3. For the majority of people with MCPH, normal height, weight, appearance, chromosome analysis, and brain scan are reported. For people with *MCPH1* mutations, a reduction in height may be found, but the HC will always be significantly more reduced than height; on NMR scan, some *MCPH1* patients show evidence of periventricular neuronal heterotopias suggestive of neuronal migration defects; and cytogenetic analysis may indicate an increased proportion of prophaselike cells.

Incidence of MCPH

Prior to the discovery of MCPH genes, autosomal recessive microcephaly was reported to have an incidence

Table 1

MCPH Loci

Locus	Autosomal Localization	Linkage Reference	Gene	Ethnicity
MCPH1	8p22-pter	Jackson et al. 1998	*Microcephalin*	Northern Pakistani
MCPH2	19q13.1-13.2	Roberts et al. 1999	Unknown	Northern Pakistani and Indian
MCPH3	9q34	Moynihan et al. 2000	*CDK5RAP2*	Northern Pakistani
MCPH4	15q15-q21	Jamieson et al. 1999	Unknown	Moroccan
MCPH5	1q31	Pattison et al. 2000; Jamieson et al. 2000	*ASPM*	Northern Pakistani, Turkish, Jordanian, Dutch, Saudi Arabian, Yemeni, and Indian
MCPH6	13q12.2	Leal et al. 2003	*CENPJ*	Northern Pakistani and Brazilian

NOTE.—The known MCPH loci are listed in chronological order of discovery. For each locus, the autosomal location is given, with the appropriate reference, the name of the gene (if known), and the ethnicities of the individuals in whom a mutation has been reported.

of 1/30,000 in Japan, 1/250,000 in Holland, and 1/2,000,000 in Scotland (Komai et al. 1955; Van den Bosch 1959; Tolmie et al. 1987). More-recent studies have not been performed; however, MCPH seems rarer in whites than in Asian and Arab populations where consanguineous marriage is practiced. Our anecdotal experience in the Yorkshire region of Britain is a white MCPH incidence of 1 per million compared to 1/10,000 in those originating from northern Pakistan. An increased incidence of autosomal recessive diseases in consanguineous populations is expected on theoretical grounds and has been observed (Freire-Maia 1990; Bundey and Alam 1993; Tuncbilek 2001). Given the number of MCPH genes and mutations found in the Pakistani population (see below), the high incidence of MCPH probably reflects the effects of consanguinity and not a founder effect.

Inheritance of Primary Microcephaly

Prior to the discovery of MCPH genes, "true microcephaly" or "microcephaly vera" had been considered to be inherited as an autosomal recessive disorder (Kloepfer et al. 1964; Bundey 1997). This hypothesis was based on the reports of pedigrees with multiple affected siblings but unaffected parents, frequent parental consanguinity, and segregation ratios that suggested a large proportion of primary microcephaly, particularly in consanguineous populations, is caused by recessive genes (Böök et al. 1953; Komai et al. 1955; Van den Bosch 1959; Sujatha et al. 1989). Although the expected recurrence risk for autosomal recessive traits is 1 in 4, the empiric recurrence risk for a nonconsanguineous couple who have had one child with a diagnosis of MCPH has been calculated as 1 in 5 if detailed chromosome studies and neuroimaging yield normal results (Tolmie et al. 1987). It has been suggested that there may be a phenotype in heterozygous carriers of MCPH mutations, because of an increased frequency of intellectual impairment in parents of individuals with recessive microcephaly (Kloepfer et al. 1964; Qazi and Reed 1975). However, this has not been a consistent finding, and this matter awaits reassessment (Van den Bosch 1959; Roberts et al. 2002).

Molecular Genetics of MCPH

Linkage and Heterogeneity

MCPH was expected to exhibit genetic heterogeneity, because of its broad clinical phenotype (Cowie 1960). Six loci have been identified to date (*MCPH1–MCPH6*; see table 1) (Jackson et al. 1998; Jamieson et al. 1999, 2000; Roberts et al. 1999, 2002; Moynihan et al. 2000; Pattison et al. 2000; Leal et al. 2003). Each recessive locus was initially mapped in a large consanguineous family by autozygosity mapping techniques, using panels of ~400 polymorphic autosomal microsatellite markers spread throughout the human genome at a distance of ~12 cM (Lander and Botstein 1987; Mueller and Bishop 1993).

Four of the six loci (*MCPH1–MCPH3* and *MCPH5*) were discovered in families of northern Pakistani origin, with two loci (*MCPH1* and *MCPH3*) remaining exclusive to this population.

MCPH heterogeneity studies have been performed in a northern Pakistani population and *MCPH5* was identified as the most common locus, accounting for linkage of nearly half of the amassed families (24/56 families) (Roberts et al. 2002). *MCPH2* accounted for 10 families (14%); *MCPH1* and *MCPH3* were each associated with two families (4%), whereas *MCPH4* linkage has not been found in the Pakistani population. *MCPH6* had not been identified at the time of the heterogeneity investigation; however, subsequently this locus has been linked to families of northern Pakistani origin (Bond et al. 2005). *MCPH2, MCPH5,* and *MCPH6* are represented in multiple populations (Jamieson et al. 2000; Pattison et al. 2000; Bond et al. 2002, 2003; Leal et al. 2003, Kumar et al. 2004). Further MCPH loci await discovery, as 18/56 northern Pakistani families and

5/9 Indian families show no evidence of linkage to the known loci (Roberts et al. 2002; Kumar et al. 2004).

Genes

Positional cloning strategies have been employed to identify causative genes at four loci (fig. 1 and table 1): *MCPH1* (Jackson et al. 2002), *MCPH5* (Bond et al. 2002), *MCPH3* (Bond et al. 2005), and *MCPH6* (Bond et al. 2005).

MCPH1/Microcephalin.—Using ancestral haplotyping of novel microsatellite markers, Jackson and colleagues further refined the *MCPH1* region from 13 cM to 2.1 Mb before commencing candidate gene sequencing. In two consanguineous families of northern Pakistani origin, a single homozygous 74C→G (S25X) nonsense mutation was identified in the second exon of a 2,505-nucleotide, 14-exon uncharacterized gene named "*Microcephalin*" (Jackson et al. 2002) The mutation segregated correctly within the families and was not present in >200 population-matched control alleles. *Microcephalin* is expressed in fetal brain, fetal liver, and fetal kidney at similar levels and is expressed at low levels in other fetal and adult tissues. Tissue in situ hybridization studies of *Microcephalin* mRNA in mouse fetal sections identified regions of Microcephalin expression in the developing forebrain during the period of neurogenesis.

MCPH5/ASPM.—The most common cause of MCPH is homozygous mutations in the *MCPH5* gene, Abnormal Spindle–like, Microcephaly associated (*Drosophila*) (*ASPM*) (Bond et al. 2002, 2003; Kumar et al. 2004; Pichon et al. 2004; Shen et al., in press). *ASPM* is a large gene with 28 exons and a 10.4-kb ORF, and its name is derived from the *Drosophila* gene *abnormal spindles.* The 24 published *ASPM* mutations comprise nonsense mutations, deletions of 1–7 base pairs, a breakpoint translocation, and intronic splice-donor point mutations (Bond et al. 2002, 2003; Kumar et al. 2004; Pichon et al. 2004). The mutations are distributed throughout the gene and are all predicted to produce truncated protein products ranging in size from 116 amino acids (*R117X*) to 3,357 amino acids (*K3328fsX29*). There is no correlation between the position of the mutation in the gene and the degree of microcephaly or mental retardation (Bond et al. 2002, 2003). This may indicate that the common mechanism of action of *ASPM* mutation is nonsense-mediated decay (Cartegni et al. 2002). Investigation of the fetal expression pattern of *Aspm* mRNA in mouse brain revealed expression at sites of active neurogenesis in the neuroepithelium (Bond et al. 2002). Postnatally, *Aspm* expression decreases with the completion of neurogenesis and upregulation of gliogenesis in the cortex. This expression pattern indicates that Aspm is involved in neuron rather than glia production. Thus, the neuronal reduction associated with MCPH due to *ASPM* mutations is compatible with the expression pattern of *Aspm* in mouse brain.

It has been suggested that a second gene causing MCPH exists at the *MCPH5* locus, as mapping studies in five Jordanian and Dutch families linked the families to the *MCPH5* locus but excluded the genetic region containing *ASPM* (Wallerman et al. 2003). If this is the case, it must be a rare cause of MCPH, since all *MCPH5* linked Pakistani families have mutations in *ASPM* and since *ASPM* mutations in the Dutch and Jordanian populations have been identified (Bond et al. 2002, 2003)

MCPH3/CDK5RAP2.—The *MCPH3* locus was refined from 12 cM to 2.2 Mb by the identification and subsequent microsatellite screening of a second family of northern Pakistani origin that shows linkage and with multiple affected members (Moynihan et al. 2000; Bond et al. 2005). A 34-exon candidate gene, Cyclin Dependent Kinase 5 Regulatory Associated protein 2 (*CDK5RAP2*) was sequenced in the families. A homozygous 243T→A (S81X) nonsense mutation and an intronic mutation 15 bases prior to the normal splice-acceptor sequence IVS26-15A→G (E385fsX4) were identified. Both mutations segregated with the disease within the families and were not present in >380 control alleles. The intronic mutation creates a new, superior splice-acceptor site for exon 27, leading to the translation of 4 amino acids before a termination codon is reached. Gene expression of *Cdk5rap2* in murine sagittal sections was highest in the brain and the spinal cord, particularly in the neuroepithelium of the frontal cortex (Bond et al. 2005).

MCPH6/CENPJ.—The 6-Mb *MCPH6* region was refined by the use of novel polymorphic microsatellite markers that were genotyped in the original Brazilian family used to map the locus and in two additional northern Pakistani multiply-affected consanguineous families (Leal et al. 2003; Bond et al. 2005). This facilitated the reduction of the locus to 3.1 Mb and enabled the selection of a candidate gene, Centromere associated Protein J (*CENPJ*, also known as "*CPAP,*" for centrosomal protein 4.1- associated protein), in which two homozygous mutations were identified: the frameshift mutation 17delC in exon 2 (T6fsX3), in two pedigrees, and the missense mutation 3704A→T in exon 16 (E1235V), in one pedigree. 3704A→T is the only MCPH mutation described to date that is not predicted to result in a protein truncation. The E1235V mutation occurs in a highly conserved Tcp10 binding domain, which is involved in binding to the protein 4.1R-135, but how it leads to a functional null allele is unknown (fig. 1*d*) (Hung et al. 2004).

Mitosis and MCPH

Microcephalin, *Cell Cycle, and DNA Repair.*—The 835-aa *Microcephalin* gene product is predicted to con-

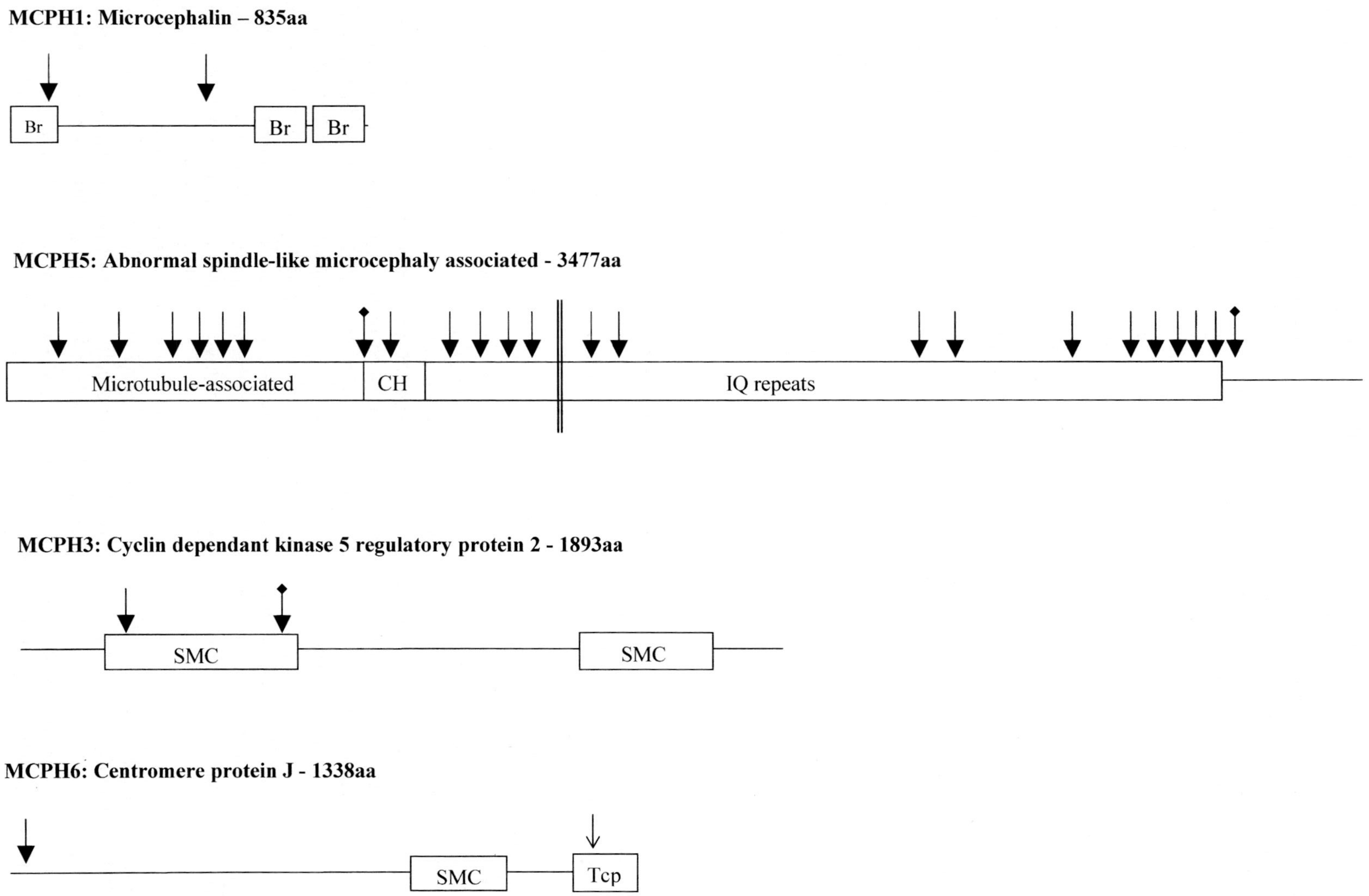

Figure 1 The MCPH proteins, probable functional domains, and sites of mutations. The MCPH loci and protein names are given above a cartoon of the protein. The known or well-predicted domains are shown. Reported mutations are shown at their positions within the gene: nonsense mutations as filled arrows, splicing mutations that lead to premature termination codons as blackened arrows with marked tail, and a missense mutation as an unfilled arrow. Parallel lines indicate the translocation breakpoint in the *ASPM* gene described by Pichon et al. (2004). Each MCPH protein is marked with the known or hypothesized functional domains. Br is a BRCT Breast Cancer Suppressor Protein (BRCA1) carboxy-terminal domain, pfam00533. SMC is a chromosome segregation ATPase domain, COG1196, but all are only possible predictions. CH is calponin homology domain, pfam00307. IQ repeats is an isoleucine-glutamine calmodulin-binding domain, pfam00612. Tcp is a T-complex protein 10 C-terminus domain, pfam07202.

tain three BRCA1 C-terminal domains (BRCT domains), with the S25X protein-truncating mutation occurring in the first of these domains (fig. 1*a*). Other proteins containing BRCT domains have roles in cell-cycle control and DNA repair (Hyton et al. 2000), and a loss of DNA repair genes can lead to apoptosis during neurogenesis (Mochida and Walsh 2001). This led Jackson and colleagues to hypothesize that Microcephalin may have a function in DNA repair or cell-cycle control and that the phenotype of MCPH might result from perturbation of normal cell-cycle regulation in neuronal progenitors (Jackson et al. 2002).

Two potential roles of Microcephalin have emerged, one on the control of cell-cycle timing and the other of DNA repair following ionizing radiation damage (Trimborn et al. 2004; Xu et al. 2004). A novel autosomal recessive disorder was described that was characterized by premature chromosome condensation (PCC) in siblings from a consanguineous family exhibiting microcephaly, growth retardation, and mental retardation (Neitzel et al. 2002). Patient cell preparations exhibited a high proportion of prophaselike cells (7%–17%), signifying early onset of chromosome condensation. The disorder was found to result from a 427insA mutation in *Microcephalin* (Trimborn et al. 2004). *MCPH1* primary microcephaly shares this cellular phenotype of PCC, and it can also be recapitulated by small-interfering-RNA–mediated depletion of Microcephalin (Trimborn et al. 2004). Experimental depletion of Microcephalin also impairs radiation-induced intra-S-phase and G2/M cell-cycle checkpoints by decreasing the levels of BRCA1 and Checkpoint kinase 1 (Xu et al. 2004). MCPH may therefore result from a perturbation of the cell cycle in neurogenesis (Trimborn et al. 2004).

ASPM and the Spindle Pole Body.—Bioinformatics analyses suggest that the 3,477-aa human ASPM protein contains a putative amino terminal microtubule binding domain (Saunders et al. 1997); at least one calponin homology domain; 74 isoleucine-glutamine (IQ) domains, which potentially bind calmodulin (Craig and Norbury 1998; Bond et al. 2002); and a carboxy terminal region of no known function (fig. 1*b*).

Asp, the probable ortholog of ASPM in *Drosophila,* is essential for organization and bundling of microtubules at the spindle poles and has been shown to be necessary for the proper formation of a central mitotic spindle in mitosis and meiosis (Ripoll et al. 1985; Gonzalez et al. 1990; Avides and Glover 1999; Avides et al. 2001; Wakefield et al. 2001; Riparbelli et al. 2001). This role is supported by results from immunofluorescence studies, which have shown wild-type Asp to be distributed throughout the cytoplasm in interphase but to localize to the spindle poles during mitosis when the bipolar spindle is formed (Saunders et al. 1997; Wakefield et al. 2001; Riparbelli et al. 2002). During late anaphase and telophase, when the spindle begins to disassemble, Asp relocates to the minus ends of the central spindle microtubules, where it remains until the central spindle has broken down (Saunders et al. 1997; Avides and Glover 1999; Wakefield et al. 2001).

CDK5RAP2, CENPJ, and the Centrosome.—Human CDK5RAP2 and CENPJ are also centrosomal proteins, being localized to the centrosomes in interphase and to the spindle poles during mitosis (Hung et al. 2000; Bond et al. 2005). The probable *Drosophila* ortholog of CDK5RAP2, centrosomin (cnn), interacts with the gamma tubulin ring complexes within the centrosome, which are responsible for the production of the microtubules forming the mitotic spindle (Li and Kaufman 1996; Megraw et al. 1999; Terada et al. 2003). *Drosophila* cnn mutants exhibit a gross reduction in cell number in the central and peripheral nervous systems (Li and Kaufman 1996). CENPJ is known to interact via a Tcp10 domain with nonerythrocyte 4.1 protein 135 splice variant (4.1R-135) (Hung et al. 2000). CENPJ is associated with the γ-tubulin ring complex (Hung et al. 2004). In vitro evidence suggests that CENPJ might be able to inhibit microtubule nucleation and to depolymerize microtubules (Hung et al. 2004). Therefore, CDK5RAP2 and CENPJ may be involved in the control of the centrosomal production of microtubules during neurogenic mitosis (Bond et al. 2005).

Neurodevelopmental Etiology of MCPH

All data to date suggest that MCPH is a primary disorder of neurogenic mitosis and not one of neural migration, neural apoptosis, or neural function. This is because all four known MCPH genes are expressed in the neuroepithelium, and phenotypic features and brain scans suggest that MCPH patients have a small brain that functions normally for its size.

The majority of neurons in the brain are thought to originate from neuronal progenitors that are the predominant cells in the neuroepithelium, which line the ventricles of the brain (Brand and Rakic 1979). Neural progenitor cells have a specific pattern of mitotic activity that was first delineated in fly neuroblasts: *symmetric* cell divisions, which have mitotic spindles in the plane of the neuroepithelium that yield two neural progenitor cells, or *asymmetric* divisions, which occur when the mitotic spindle is oriented perpendicular to the neuroepithelium, giving rise to one postmitotic neuron and one progenitor cell (Doe and Bowerman 2001; Haydar et al. 2003; Albertson and Doe 2003). Since the timing of these two types of divisions during development is likely to be crucial to the final number of neurons, it has been proposed that changes in its regulation might be responsible for some cortical disorders, like microcephaly (Rakic 1988), and also for differences in brain

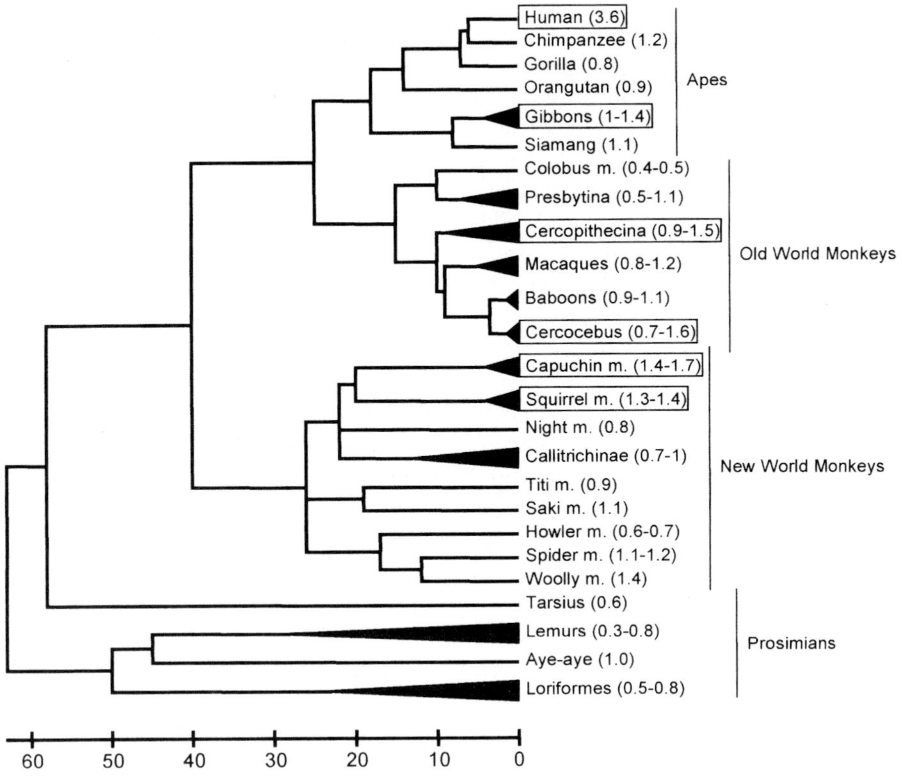

Figure 2 Encephalization in primates. The relative encephalization of various primate species was mapped on a phylogeny of primates (Goodman 1999). Data on brain weight and body weight was taken from Marino (1998) for apes, Old World monkeys, and New World monkeys and from Stephan et al. (1981), as given by Clark et al. (2001), for prosimians. The encephalization quotient (i.e., the ratio of observed brain weight to expected brain weight) is given in parentheses. The range is given when the data from several species are collapsed in the tree. The expected brain weight was calculated from a linear regression on log transformed brain and body weights for the Marino data, excluding humans (brain weight = $10\exp(0.6765 \times \text{body weight} + 2.3406)$). Species showing at least a 1.4-fold–heavier brain than expected for their body weights are marked by rectangles.

size among different species (Rakic 1995). In mammals, it has also been shown experimentally that larger brains can result from increasing the number of neural progenitor symmetric cell divisions (Kornack and Rakic 1998; Chen and Walsh 2003).

The function of MCPH genes during neurogenic mitosis is unknown but is likely to be either (1) controlling the expansion of the neural progenitor pool or (2) involvement in the decision to switch from symmetric to asymmetric cell division. The latter hypothesis is supported by *Drosophila* studies showing that homozygous *asp* mutations result in metaphase arrest during asymmetric cell division in larval brain and that cnn mutants result in deficient asymmetric cell division in the male germ line (Wakefield et al. 2001; Yamashita et al. 2003). The cellular localization of three of the MCPH proteins—CDK5RAP2, ASPM, and CENPJ—is known to be centrosomal during mitosis. This suggests that the centrosome is an organelle of great importance during neurogenic mitosis.

MCPH, Brain Size, and Evolution

Brain size differs among animals mainly because animals come in different sizes. In mammals, >90 % of variation in brain weight can be explained by variation in body weight (Jerison 1973). Outliers from this relationship are of interest and if certain species or groups of species have brain sizes that are larger than expected from their body size (i.e., that are more "encephalized"), this is usually interpreted as an adaptation of these species (Harvey and Krebs 1990). No other species is as encephalized as humans, which have an ~5-fold larger brain than expected for a mammal of their body size and an ~3-fold larger brain than expected for an ape of their body size. But increases in relative brain size have also occurred in many other lineages among primates (see fig. 2 and, e.g., Armstrong 1985; Stephan et al. 1988; Marino 1998). Also notable are dolphins and related whales, which are more encephalized than any primate other than humans (Marino 1998). Fossil evidence suggests that encephalization increased several times during human evolution, starting around 2 million years ago and reaching its current state probably before the lineage leading to modern humans split from that leading to Neanderthals, ~500,000 years ago (McHenry 1994). Interestingly, at least one reduction of relative brain size occurred during the evolution of human species, as well: a recently discovered species, *Homo florensis,* which lived until 18,000 years ago on the Indonesian island Flores, evolved probably from an ancestral *Homo erectus* population but had a relative brain size substantially lower than that in *Homo erectus* (Brown et al. 2004; Morwood et al. 2004).

MCPH is an intriguing disease from an evolutionary standpoint, since it affects specifically the ratio of brain size to body size and since the brain of affected individuals can be of comparable size to that of a chimpanzee or gorilla (Bond et al. 2002; Jackson et al. 2002). Maybe even more intriguing is that MCPH genes—as discussed above—seem to play a role in the mitosis of neuronal precursors and that this is the process that has been hypothesized to be affected during the evolution of larger brains (Rakic 1995). So, from a genetic point of view, MCPH genes are excellent candidate genes for gain-of-function mutations, because they can carry loss-of-function mutations that affect the phenotype of interest. With the discovery of the first two MCPH genes, *Microcephalin* and *ASPM,* it has been possible to study whether there is evidence for adaptive changes in these genes and whether such changes correlate with changes in relative brain size during evolution.

Studying Protein Evolution

When one compares the coding regions of a gene in two species, one can find two types of differences: synonymous differences, which do not change the encoded protein sequence, and nonsynonymous differences, which do. The ratio of synonymous differences to synonymous sites (K_s) and the ratio of nonsynonymous differences to nonsynonymous sites (K_a) can then be calculated and compared (for reviews, see Yang and Bielawski 2000; Hurst 2002; Fay and Wu 2003). If one assumes that differences at synonymous sites do not have any functional consequences (i.e., do not affect the fitness of an organism), K_s can be regarded as an estimate of the neutral mutation rate. So, if mutations at all nonsynonymous sites also have no functional consequence—as is the case in a pseudogene—then K_a should be not different from K_s, and the expected K_a/K_s ratio would be 1. Since often mutations that change the protein sequence have negative consequences, these are not observed as differences between two species and the K_a/K_s ratio is <1. Sometimes, however, mutations at nonsynonymous sites can have advantageous consequences and these are then more likely to be observed between two species. Therefore, a K_a/K_s ratio (significantly) larger than one is interpreted as evidence for positive selection in that gene. Of course, both of these effects can act on a given gene, so that for example K_a/K_s can be smaller than one if only a few nonsynonymous mutations have been positively selected and many nonsynonymous sites are under constraint. Consequently, if K_a/K_s ratios <1 differ (e.g., between two evolutionary lineages), this can be due to a different amount of positive selection or to a different amount of constraint in these two lineages. One possible way to estimate the amount of constraint is to analyze common polymorphisms within a species. If this estimate of K_a/K_s is (significantly) smaller than the K_a/K_s estimate of fixed differences along the species lineage, positive selection can be inferred (McDonald 1991).

Unfortunately, other genetic changes in a gene (such as insertions and deletions, changes in splicing pattern, regulatory changes), can not currently be tested in a similar way, mainly because a neutral mutation rate like K_s is missing for these kinds of changes so that expected values can not rigorously be estimated. Although single adaptive genetic changes can in principle be identified by their signature of selection at closely linked sites within a population, this signature vanishes quickly after the selected site has been fixed in a population, so that for example in humans such a signature is not expected if the fixation of the adaptive mutation is more than 200,000 years ago (Przeworski 2002). The relative brain size of modern humans was probably attained around 500,000 years ago (see above). Therefore, seeking the signature of selection in this way does not seem a very promising method by which to find human-specific adaptive changes related to brain size increase.

Evolutionary Studies of Microcephalin

Two studies have examined the evolution of *MCPH1,* and both find some evidence for positive selection (Evans et al. 2004*a*; Wang and Su 2004). In the study by Wang and Su, a signature of positive selection on the lineage leading from the ancestor of all apes to the ancestor of great apes was found, as well as some signature of positive selection during recent human evolution (i.e., very likely less than half a million years ago). In the study by Evans et al., a signature of positive selection on the lineages leading to the ancestor of Old World Monkeys, apes, great apes, African apes, and finally humans was found. Given the relatively low power to detect positive selection at all, these findings are remarkable. However, their results need to be viewed with caution, as the strongest signatures of selection are detected on lineages, which show no particular evidence for an increase in encephalization, and the human lineage, for which the biggest change in brain size has occurred, does not show a tendency for higher K_a/K_s compared with other lineages. As discussed above, this does not exclude the possibility that some changes in *Microcephalin* might have been positively selected which lead to the human brain increase, but independent evidence for this (e.g., by functional studies) is needed.

Evolutionary Studies of ASPM

The evolution of the ASPM gene in primates and mammals has been examined in three studies (Zhang 2003; Evans et al. 2004*b*; Kouprina et al. 2004). An initial and tempting speculation that the number of IQ repeats (74 in man, 62 in mouse, and 24 in *Drosophila*) could correlate with brain size in animals could not be confirmed, since many mammals have as many IQ repeats as humans and since the difference in IQ length between mouse and human is specific for the lineage leading to mouse (Bond et al. 2002; Zhang 2003). Interestingly, however, the highest K_a/K_s ratio is found on the human lineage, and analyses of polymorphisms among humans suggest that ASPM is currently under a high evolutionary constraint, indicating that human-specific amino acid changes might have been fixed by positive selection. As for Microcephalin, these findings are remarkable in the light of the relatively low power of these tests, and this time the biggest increase in K_a/K_s correlates with the biggest increase in brain size. However, high K_a/K_s values have also been found on other ape lineages, and polymorphisms in gorillas suggest that amino acid changes in ASPM might already have been fixed by positive selection in the ancestors of humans, chimpanzees, and gorillas (Kouprina et al. 2004). Additionally, the high K_a/K_s ratio on the human lineage seems to be caused, to a large extent, by a lower number of fixed synonymous substitutions. This would imply a lower mutation rate on the human lineage, in addition to positive selection. So some aspects of these evolutionary findings do not have a straightforward interpretation for human brain expansion.

Implications of Evolutionary Findings

Although the signatures of positive selection for ASPM and for Microcephalin are not so strong that they clearly implicate a role for these genes in human brain expansion, they have an encouraging tendency. Further evolutionary analyses of other primate or mammalian lineages in which increases in relative brain size occurred (see above) might be fruitful, to clarify how well evolutionary changes in MCPH genes correlate with brain size increase. In addition, the identification of genes that interact with MCPH genes, especially in neuronal progenitor cell mitosis, will lead to further candidates that might be involved in the evolution of brain size increase in humans and other species. It is worth noting that an increase in relative brain size is not the only phenotypic change that occurred during the evolution of the human brain (Preuss 2004) and that recent studies suggest that positive selection might have acted on a considerable number of genes important for brain function and development during human evolution (Dorus et al. 2004). It will be important (and difficult) to find functional model systems in which these kinds of evolutionary hypotheses can be further tested. Transgenic mice could be one such possibility, and, although it is unclear to what extent mice would work as a model system in this respect, it is encouraging that artificial genetic changes can cause a brain size increase in mice (Chenn and Walsh 2002).

Conclusions

Given the many possible causes of microcephaly, the diagnosis of MCPH should only be made after differential diagnoses have been sought and eliminated. With identification of MCPH genes, the following are becoming increasingly available for patients: prenatal diagnosis (to detect a recurrence of the disorder), postnatal diagnosis (to distinguish the disorder from the many differential diagnoses), and carrier testing (in consanguineous families in which the disease is known to occur). There are at least seven genes that can cause this neurodevelopmental disorder; four have been identified, and current evidence suggests that MCPH is probably a primary disorder of neurogenic mitosis. As such, it may have much to teach us about the control of neuron production by neural stem cells and about how this has been modulated by evolution to control the brain sizes of different species.

Acknowledgments

We thank Professor Arthur Boylston, for helpful discussion, and Jeffrey Keen, for first setting our minds thinking about evolution.

Electronic-Database Information

URLs for data presented herein are as follows:

Online Mendelian Inheritance in Man (OMIM), http://www.ncbi.nlm.nih.gov/Omim/ (for MCPH)

pfam, http://pfam.wustl.edu/, and COG, http://www.ncbi.nlm.nih.gov/COG/ (for protein domain identification)

References

Aicardi J (1998) Malformations of the central nervous system. In: Aicardi J (ed) Diseases of the nervous system in childhood, 3rd ed. McKeith Press, London, pp 90–91

Albertson R, Doe CQ (2003) Dlg, Scrib and Lgl regulate neuroblast cell size and mitotic spindle asymmetry. Nat Cell Biol 5:166–170

Armstrong E (1985) Relative brain size in monkeys and prosimians. Am J Phys Anthropol 66:263–273

Avides MC, Glover DM (1999) Abnormal spindle protein, Asp, and the integrity of mitotic centrosomal microtubule organizing centres. Science 283:1733–1735

Avides MC, Tavares A, Glover DM (2001) Polo kinase and Asp are needed to promote the mitotic organizing activity of centrosomes. Nat Cell Biol 3:421–424

Babson SG, Benda GI (1976) Growth graphs for the clinical assessment of infants of varying gestational age. J Pediatr 89:814–820

Baraitser M (1990) Microcephaly. In: The genetics of neurological disorders, Vol. 18, 2nd ed. Oxford Medical Publications, Oxford, pp 26–33

Barkovich AJ, Kuzniecky RI, Dobyns WB (2001) Radiologic classification of malformations of cortical development. Curr Opin Neurol 14:145–149

Bond J, Roberts E, Mochida GH, Hampshire DJ, Scott S, Askham JM, Springell K, Mahadevan M, Crow YJ, Markham AF, Walsh CA, Woods CG (2002) ASPM is a major determinant of cerebral cortical size. Nat Genet 32:316–320

Bond J, Scott S, Hampshire DJ, Springell K, Corry P, Abramowicz MJ, Mochida G, Hennekam RCM, Maher ER, Alswaid A, Jafri H, Rashid Y, Mubaidin A, Walsh C, Roberts E, Woods CG (2003) Protein truncating mutations in *ASPM* cause variable reduction in brain size. Am J Hum Genet 73: 1170–1177

Böök JA, Schut JW, Reed SC (1953) A clinical and genetical study of microcephaly. Am J Ment Defic 57:637–660

Brand S, Rakic P (1979) Genesis of the primate neostriatum: [3H]thymidine autoradiographic analysis of the time of neuron origin in the rhesus monkey. Neuroscience 4:767–778

Brown P, Sutikna T, Morwood MJ, Soejono RP, Jatmiko, Saptomo EW, Due RA (2004) A new small-bodied hominin from the Late Pleistocene of Flores, Indonesia. Nature 431:1055–1061

Bundey S (1997) Abnormal mental development. In: Rimoin DL, Connor JM, Pyeritz RE (eds) Emery and Rimoin's principles and practice of medical genetics, 3rd ed. Churchill Livingstone. New York, p 730

Bundey S, Alam H (1993) A five-year prospective study of the health of children in different ethnic groups, with particular reference to the effect of inbreeding. Eur J Hum Genet 1: 206–219

Cartegni L, Chew SL, Krainer AR (2002) Listening to silence and understanding nonsense: exonic mutations that affect splicing. Nat Rev Genet 3:285–298

Chenn A, Walsh CA (2002) Regulation of cerebral cortical size by control of cell cycle exit in neural precursors. Science 297:365–369

——— (2003) Increased neuronal production, enlarged forebrains and cytoarchitectural distortions in β-catenin overexpressing transgenic mice. Cereb Cortex 13:599–606

Clark DA, Mitra PP, Wang SS (2001) Scalable architecture in mammalian brains. Nature 411:189–193

Cowie V (1960) The genetics and sub-classification of microcephaly. J Ment Defic Res 4:42–47

Craig R, Norbury C (1998) The novel murine calmodulin-binding protein Sha1 disrupts mitotic spindle and replication checkpoint functions in fission yeast. J Cell Sci 111:3609–3619

Dobyns WB (2002) Primary microcephaly: new approaches for an old disorder. Am J Med Genet 112:315–317

Doe CQ, Bowerman B (2001) Asymmetric cell division: fly neuroblast meets worm zygote. Curr Opin Cell Biol 13:68–75

Dolk H (1991) The predictive value of microcephaly during the first year of life for mental retardation at seven years. Dev Med Child Neurol 33:974–983

Dorus S, Vallender EJ, Evans PD, Anderson JR, Gilbert SL, Mahowald M, Wyckoff GJ, Malcom CM Lahn BT (2004) Accelerated evolution of nervous system genes in the origin of *Homo sapiens.* Cell 119:1027–1040

Evans PD, Anderson JR, Vallender EJ, Choi SS, Lahn BT (2004*a*) Reconstructing the evolutionary history of microcephalin, a gene controlling human brain size. Hum Mol Genet 13:1139–1145

Evans PD, Anderson JR, Vallender EJ, Gilbert SL, Malcom CM, Dorus S, Lahn BT (2004*b*) Adaptive evolution of ASPM, a major determinant of cerebral cortical size in humans. Hum Mol Genet 13:489–494

Fay JC, Wu CI (2003) Sequence divergence, functional constraint, and selection in protein evolution. Annu Rev Genomics Hum Genet 4:213–235

Freire-Maia N (1990) Consanguinity marriages in Brazil. Rev Bras Biol 50:863–866

Gonzalez C, Saunders RD, Casal J, Molina I, Carmena M, Ripoll P, Glover DM (1990) Mutations at the asp locus of *Drosophila* lead to multiple free centrosomes in syncytial embryos, but restrict centrosome duplication in larval neuroblasts. J Cell Sci 96:605–616

Goodman M (1999) The genomic record of humankind's evolutionary roots. Am J Hum Genet 64:31–39

Gross SJ, Oehler JM, Eckerman CO (1983) Head growth and developmental outcome in very low birth weight infants. Pediatrics 71:70–75

Harvey PH, Krebs JR (1990) Comparing brains. Science 249: 140–146

Haydar TF, Ang E Jr, Rakic P (2003) Mitotic spindle rotation and mode of cell division in the developing telencephalon. Proc Natl Acad Sci USA 100:2890–2895

Hung LY, Chen H-L, Dhang C-W, Li B-R, Tang TK (2004) Identification of a novel microtubule-destabilizing motif in CPAP that binds to tubulin heterodimers and inhibits microtubule assembly. Mol Biol Cell 15:2697–2706

Hung LY, Tang CJ, Tang TK (2000) Protein 4.1 R-135 interacts with a novel centrosomal protein (CPAP) which is associated with the γ-tubulin complex. Mol Cell Biol 20:7813–7825

Hurst LD (2002) The Ka/Ks ratio: diagnosing the form of sequence evolution. Trends Genet 18:486–487

Huyton T, Bates PA, Zhang X, Sternberg MJ, Freemont PS (2000) The BRCA1 C-terminal domain: structure and function. Mutat Res 460:319–332

Jackson AP, Eastwood H, Bell SM, Adu J, Toomes C, Carr IM, Roberts E, Hampshire DJ, Crow YJ, Mighell AJ, Karbani G, Jafri H, Rashid Y, Mueller RF, Markham AF, Woods CG (2002) Identification of microcephalin, a protein implicated in determining the size of the human brain. Am J Hum Genet 71:136–142

Jackson AP, McHale DP, Campbell DA, Jafri H, Rashid Y, Mannan J, Karbani G, Corry P, Levene MI, Mueller RF, Markham AF, Lench NJ, Woods CG (1998) Primary autosomal recessive microcephaly (MCPH1) maps to chromosome 8p22-pter. Am J Hum Genet 63:541–546

Jamieson CR, Fryns JP, Jacobs J, Matthijs G, Abramowicz MJ (2000) Primary autosomal recessive microcephaly: MCPH5 maps to 1q25-q32. Am J Hum Genet 67:1575–1577

Jamieson CR, Govaerts C, Abramowicz MJ (1999) Primary autosomal recessive microcephaly: homozygosity mapping of MCPH4 to chromosome 15. Am J Hum Genet 65:1465–1469

Jerison HJ (1973) Evolution of the brain and intelligence. Academic Press, New York

Kloepfer HW, Platou RV, Hansche WJ (1964) Manifestations of a recessive gene for microcephaly in a population isolate. J Genet Hum 13:52–59

Komai T, Kishimoto K, Ozaki Y (1955) Genetic study of microcephaly based on Japanese material. Am J Hum Genet 47:51–65

Kornack DR, Rakic P (1998) Changes in cell-cycle kinetics during the development and evolution of primate neocortex. Proc Natl Acad Sci USA 95:1242–1246

Kouprina N, Pavlicek A, Mochida GH, Solomon G, Gersch W, Yoon YH, Collura R, Ruvolo M, Barrett JC, Woods CG, Walsh CA, Jurka J, Larionov V (2004) Accelerated evolution of the ASPM gene controlling brain size begins prior to human brain expansion. PLoS Biol 2:E126

Kumar A, Blanton SH, Babu M, Markandaya M, Girimaji SC (2004) Genetic analysis of primary microcephaly in Indian families: novel ASPM mutations. Clin Genet 66:341–348

Lander ES, Botstein D (1987) Homozygosity mapping: a way to map human recessive traits with the DNA of inbred children. Science 236:1567–1570

Leal GF, Roberts E, Silva EO, Costa SMR, Hampshire DJ, Woods CG (2003) A Brazilian locus for autosomal recessive primary microcephaly maps to 13q12.2. J Med Genet 40: 540–542

Li K, Kaufman TC (1996) The homeotic target gene *centrosomin* encodes an essential centrosomal component. Cell 88: 585–596

Marino L (1998) A comparison of encephalization between odontocete cetaceans and anthropoid primates. Brain Behav Evol 51:230–238

McDonald JH, Kreitman M (1991) Adaptive protein evolution at the Adh locus in *Drosophila*. Nature 351:652–654

McHenry HM (1994) Tempo and mode in human evolution. Proc Natl Acad Sci USA 91:6780–6786

Megraw TL, Li K, Kao L-R, Kaufman TC (1999) The Centrosomin protein is required for centrosome assembly and function during cleavage in *Drosophila*. Development 126: 2829–2839

Mochida GH, Walsh CA (2001) Molecular genetics of human microcephaly. Curr Opin Neurol 14:151–156

Morwood MJ, Soejono RP, Roberts RG, Sutikna T, Turney CS, Westaway KE, Rink WJ, Zhao JX, van den Bergh GD, Due RA, Hobbs DR, Moore MW, Bird MI, Fifield LK (2004) Archaeology and age of a new hominin from Flores in eastern Indonesia. Nature 431:1087–1091

Moynihan L, Jackson AP, Roberts E, Karbani G, Lewis I, Corry P, Turner G, Mueller RF, Lench NJ, Woods CG (2000) A third novel locus for primary autosomal recessive microcephaly maps to chromosome 9q34. Am J Hum Genet 66: 724–727

Mueller RF, Bishop DT (1993) Autozygosity mapping, complex consanguinity, and autosomal recessive disorders. J Med Genet 30:798–799

Neitzel H, Neumann LM, Schindler D, Wirges A, Tonnies H, Trimborn M, Krebsova A, Richter R, Sperling K (2002) Premature chromosome condensation in humans associated with microcephaly and mental retardation: a novel autosomal recessive condition. Am J Hum Genet 70:1015–1022

Nellhaus G (1968) Head circumference from birth to eighteen years: practical composite of international abd interracial graphs. Pediatrics 41:106–114

Opitz JM, Holt MC (1992) Microcephaly: general considerations and aids to nosology. J Craniofac Genet Dev Bio 10: 175–204

Pattison L, Crow YJ, Deeble VJ, Jackson AP, Jafri H, Rashid Y, Roberts E, Woods CG (2000) A fifth locus for primary autosomal recessive microcephaly maps to chromosome 1q31. Am J Hum Genet 67:1578–1580

Pichon B, Vankerckhove S, Bourrouillou G, Duprez L, Abramowicz MJ (2004) A translocation breakpoint disrupts the ASPM gene in a patient with primary microcephaly. Eur J Hum Genet 12:419–421

Preuss TM (2004) What is it like to be a human? In: Gazzaniga MS (ed) The cognitive neurosciences III. MIT Press, Cambridge, MA

Przeworski M (2002) The signature of positive selection at randomly chosen loci. Genetics 160:1179–1189

Qazi QH, Reed TE (1973) A problem in diagnosis of primary versus secondary microcephaly. Clin Genet 4:46–52

——— (1975) A possible major contribution to mental retardation in the general population by the gene for microcephaly. Clin Genet 7:85–90

Rakic P (1988) Specification of cerebral cortical areas. Science 241:170–176

——— (1995) A small step for the cell, a giant leap for mankind: a hypothesis of neocortical expansion during evolution. Trends Neurosci 18:383–388

Riparbelli MG, Callaini G, Glover DM, Avides MdoC (2001) A requirement for the abnormal spindle protein to organise microtubules of the central spindle for cytokinesis in *Drosophila.* J Cell Sci 115:913–922

Ripoll P, Pimpinelli S, Valdivia MM, Avila J (1985) A cell division mutant of *Drosophila* with a functionally abnormal spindle. Cell 41:907–912

Roberts E, Bond J, Springell K, Lizarraga S, Scott S, Higgins J, Hampshire DJ, Morrison E, Leal GF, Silva EO, Costa SM, Karbani G, Rashid Y, Jafri H, Bennett C, Corry P, Walsh CA, Woods CG (2005) A centrosomal mechanism involving CDK5RAP2 and CENPJ controls brain size. Nat Genet 37: 353–355

Roberts E, Hampshire DJ, Springell K, Pattison L, Y Crow, Jafri H, Corry P, Kabani G, Mannon J, Rashid Y, Keen J, Bond J, Woods CG (2002) Autosomal recessive primary microcephaly: an analysis of locus heterogeneity and phenotypic variation. J Med Genet 39:718–721

Roberts E, Jackson AP, Carradice AC, Deeble VJ, Mannan J, Rashid Y, Jafri H, McHale DP, Markham AF, Lench NJ, Woods CG (1999) The second locus for autosomal recessive primary microcephaly (MCPH2) maps to chromosome 19q13.1-13.2. Eur J Hum Genet 7:815–820

Roche AF, Mukherjee D, Guo S, Moore WM (1987) Head circumference reference data: birth to 18 years. Pediatrics 79:706–712

Rosenberg MJ, Agarwala R, Bouffard G, Davis J, Fiermonte G, Hilliard MS, Koch T, Kalikin LM, Makalowska I, Morton DH, Petty EM, Weber JL, Palmieri F, Kelley RI, Schaffer AA, Biesecker LG (2002) Mutant deoxynucleotide carrier is associated with congenital microcephaly. Nat Genet 32:175–179

Ross JJ, Frias JL (1977) Microcephaly. In: Vinken PJ, Bruyn GW (eds) Congenital malformations of the brain and skull, part 1, vol 30. Elsevier Holland Biomedical Press, Amsterdam, pp 507–524

Saunders RD, Avides MC, Howard T, Gonzalez C, Glover DM (1997) The *Drosophila* gene abnormal spindle encodes a novel microtubule-associated protein that associates with the polar regions of the mitotic spindle. J Cell Biol 137:881–890

Sells CJ (1977) Microcephaly in a normal school population. Pediatrics 59:262–265

Shen J, Eyaid W, Mochida GH, Bodell A, Woods CG, Walsh CA (2005) ASPM mutations identified in microcephaly with seizures patients. J Med Genet (in press)

Sher PK, Brown SB (1975) A longitudinal study of head growth in preterm infants. I. Normal rates of head growth. Dev Med Child Neurol 17:705–710

Stephan H, Baron G, Frahm HD (1988) Comparative size of brain and brain components. Comp Primate Biol 4:1–38

Stephan H, Frahm HD, Baron G (1981) New and revised data on volume of brain structures in insectivores and primates. Folia Primatol 35:1–29

Sujatha M, Kumari CK, Murty JS (1989) Segregation frequency in microcephaly. Hum Genet 81:388–390

Teebi AS, Al-Awadi SA, White AG (1987) Autosomal recessive nonsyndromal microcephaly with normal intelligence. Am J Med Genet 26:355–359

Terada Y, Uetake Y, Kuriyama R (2003) Interaction of Aurora-A and centrosomin at the microtubule-nucleating site in *Drosophila* and mammalian cells. J Cell Biol 162:757–763

Tolmie JL, McNay M, Stephenson JBP (1987) Microcephaly: genetic counselling and antenatal diagnosis after the birth of an affected child. Am J Med Genet 27:583–594

Trimborn M, Bell SM, Felix C, Rashid Y, Jafri H, Griffiths PD, Neumann LM, Krebs A, Reis A, Sperling K, Neitzel H, Jackson AP (2004) Mutations in microcephalin cause aberrant regulation of chromosome condensation. Am J Hum Genet 75:261–266

Tuncbilek E (2001) Clinical outcomes of consanguineous marriages in Turkey. Turk J Pediatr 43:277–279

Van den Bosch J (1959) Microcephaly in the Netherlands: a clinical and genetical study. Ann Hum Genet 23:91–116

Wakefield JG, Bonaccorsi S, Gatti M (2001) The *Drosophila* protein asp is involved in microtubule organization during spindle formation and cytokinesis. J Cell Biol 153:637–648

Wallerman O, Van Eeghen A, Ten Kate LP, Wadelius C (2003) Evidence for a second gene for primary microcephaly at MCPH5 on chromosome 1. Hereditas 139:64–67

Wang YQ, Su B (2004) Molecular evolution of microcephalin, a gene determining human brain size. Hum Mol Genet 13:1131–1137

Warkany J (1981) Microcephaly. In: Warkany J, Lemire RJ, Cohen MM (eds) Mental retardation and congenital malformations of the central nervous system. Year Book Medical, Chicago and London, pp 13–40

Winter R, Baraitser M (1998) WBDB: The Winter-Baraitser Dysmorphology Database, version 1. London Medical Databases Ltd, London

Woods CG (2004) Human microcephaly. Curr Opin Neurobiol 14:112–117

Xu X, Lee J, Stern DF (2004) Microcephalin is a DNA damage response protein involved in regulation of CHK1 and BRCA1. J Biol Chem 279:34091–34094

Yamashita YM, Jones DL, Fuller MT (2003) Orientation of asymmetric stem cell division by the APC tumor suppressor and centrosome. Science 301:1547–1550

Yang Z, Bielawski JP (2000) Statistical methods for detecting molecular adaptation. Trends Ecol Evol 15:496–503

Zhang J (2003) Evolution of the human ASPM gene, a major determinant of brain size. Genetics 165:2063–2070

Diversity and Function of Mutations in P450 Oxidoreductase in Patients with Antley-Bixler Syndrome and Disordered Steroidogenesis

Ningwu Huang,[1] Amit V. Pandey,[1] Vishal Agrawal,[1] William Reardon,[2] Pablo D. Lapunzina,[3] David Mowat,[4] Ethylin Wang Jabs,[5] Guy Van Vliet,[6] Joseph Sack,[7] Christa E. Flück,[8] and Walter L. Miller[1]

[1]Department of Pediatrics, University of California, San Francisco; [2]Department of Clinical Genetics, Our Lady's Hospital for Sick Children, Dublin, Ireland; [3]Department of Medical Genetics, Hospital Universitario La Paz, Madrid, Spain; [4]Department of Medical Genetics, Sydney Children's Hospital, Sydney, Australia; [5]Department of Pediatrics, Medicine, and Surgery, Johns Hopkins University, Baltimore; [6]Department of Pediatrics, University of Montreal, Montreal, Canada; [7]Department of Pediatrics, Tel Aviv University, Tel Aviv, Israel; and [8]Pediatric Endocrinology, University Children's Hospital, Bern, Switzerland

P450 oxidoreductase (POR) is the obligatory flavoprotein intermediate that transfers electrons from reduced nicotinamide adenine dinucleotide phosphate (NADPH) to all microsomal cytochrome P450 enzymes. Although mouse *Por* gene ablation causes embryonic lethality, *POR* missense mutations cause disordered steroidogenesis, ambiguous genitalia, and Antley-Bixler syndrome (ABS), which has also been attributed to fibroblast growth factor receptor 2 (*FGFR2*) mutations. We sequenced the *POR* gene and *FGFR2* exons 8 and 10 in 32 individuals with ABS and/or hormonal findings that suggested POR deficiency. *POR* and *FGFR2* mutations segregated completely. Fifteen patients carried *POR* mutations on both alleles, 4 carried mutations on only one allele, 10 carried *FGFR2* or *FGFR3* mutations, and 3 patients carried no mutations. The 34 affected *POR* alleles included 10 with A287P (all from whites) and 7 with R457H (four Japanese, one African, two whites); 17 of the 34 alleles carried 16 "private" mutations, including 9 missense and 7 frameshift mutations. These 11 missense mutations, plus 10 others found in databases or reported elsewhere, were recreated by site-directed mutagenesis and were assessed by four assays: reduction of cytochrome c, oxidation of NADPH, support of 17α-hydroxylase activity, and support of 17,20 lyase using human P450c17. Assays that were based on cytochrome c, which is not a physiologic substrate for POR, correlated poorly with clinical phenotype, but assays that were based on POR's support of catalysis by P450c17—the enzyme most closely associated with the hormonal phenotype—provided an excellent genotype/phenotype correlation. Our large survey of patients with ABS shows that individuals with an ABS-like phenotype and normal steroidogenesis have *FGFR* mutations, whereas those with ambiguous genitalia and disordered steroidogenesis should be recognized as having a distinct new disease: POR deficiency.

Introduction

P450 oxidoreductase (POR) is the single flavoprotein that transfers electrons from reduced nicotinamide adenine dinucleotide phosphate (NADPH) to all microsomal (type 2) cytochrome P450 enzymes. The human genome contains 57 genes for cytochrome P450 enzymes, of which 50 encode microsomal P450s, including 15 genes encoding hepatic drug-metabolizing P450s; 20 genes encoding P450s involved in the biosynthesis of cholesterol, steroid hormones, fatty acids, and eicosanoids; and 15 genes encoding "orphan" P450 enzymes whose catalytic roles are unclear (Guengerich 2004). As all of these microsomal enzymes require POR for catalysis, one would predict that disruption of POR would have devastating consequences. Not surprisingly, *Por* knockout mice are embryonic lethal (Shen et al. 2002; Otto et al. 2003), apparently due to disruption of extrahepatic P450 enzymes, as liver-specific knockout of *Por* yields phenotypically and reproductively normal mice that accumulate hepatic lipids and have a remarkably diminished capacity for hepatic drug metabolism (Gu et al. 2003; Henderson et al. 2003). Similarly, globally hypomorphic *Por* mice also have reduced hepatic drug metabolism (Wu et al. 2005).

Despite the dire consequences in *Por* knockout mice, we have recently identified five missense mutations and a splicing mutation in the *POR* genes of four patients who had hormonal evidence for partial, combined deficiencies of two steroidogenic microsomal P450 enzymes: P450c17, which catalyzes steroid 17α-hydroxylation and 17,20 lyase activity, and P450c21, which

Received November 10, 2004; accepted for publication February 4, 2005; electronically published March 25, 2005.

Address for correspondence and reprints: Dr. Walter L. Miller, Department of Pediatrics, Building MR4, Room 209, University of California, San Francisco, 1466 Fourth Avenue, San Francisco, CA 94143-0978. E-mail: wlmlab@itsa.ucsf.edu

0002-9297/2005/7605-0003$15.00

catalyzes steroid 21-hydroxylase activity (Flück et al. 2004). Combined deficiency of these enzymes was first reported in 1985 (Peterson et al. 1985), and we had suggested that mutation of *POR* might explain the hormonal phenotype (Miller 1986). However, the involvement of *POR* with so many P450 enzymes, the lack of a published *POR* gene sequence, and the severity of the *Por* knockout mouse phenotype had dissuaded investigators from pursuing *POR* as a candidate gene (Miller 2004). Three of the four index cases also had the Antley-Bixler skeletal malformation syndrome (ABS [MIM 207401]), which is characterized by craniosynostosis, radioulnar or radiohumeral synostosis, bowed femora, and other bony deformities (Antley and Bixler 1975; DeLozier et al. 1980; Hassell and Butler 1994; Crisponi et al. 1997).

Work in the 1990s showed that four phenotypically related craniosynostosis syndromes—Apert, Crouzon, Jackson-Weiss, and Pfeiffer syndromes—were caused by mutations in the gene for fibroblast growth factor receptor 2 (*FGFR2*) (Jabs et al. 1994; Muenke et al. 1994; Reardon et al. 1994; Gorry et al. 1995; Park et al. 1995*a*, 1995*b*; Schell et al. 1995; Wilkie et al. 1995; Meyers et al. 1996) and that the same *FGFR2* missense mutation, S351C, could be found in Crouzon and Pfeiffer syndromes (Pulleyn et al. 1996; Gripp et al. 1998; Okajima et al. 1999), suggesting that each eponymic syndrome is a phenotypic variant of a single genetic disorder. The heterozygous gain-of-function mutation C342Y is sufficient to cause craniosynostosis and skeletal abnormalities in knock-in mice (Eswarakumar et al. 2004), consistent with the dominant inheritance of these craniosynostosis syndromes. *FGFR2* mutations were also reported in patients with ABS without genital ambiguity or other evidence of disordered steroidogenesis (Chun et al. 1998; Reardon et al. 2000). However, *FGFR2* mutations were not found in a series of patients with ABS who had evidence of disordered steroidogenesis (Reardon et al. 2000), and *FGFR1* and *FGFR3* mutations were not found in a similar patient (Roth et al. 2000). We (Flück et al. 2004)—and subsequently others (Adachi et al. 2004; Arlt et al. 2004; Fukami et al. 2005)—have found *POR* mutations in all examined patients who had the ABS phenotype with evidence of abnormal steroidogenesis, indicating that what has been termed "ABS" is, in fact, two distinct disorders, as was first suggested by Reardon and Winter (Reardon et al. 2000). Thus, ABS without disordered steroidogenesis is a variant of the autosomal dominant group of craniosynostosis syndromes caused by mutant FGF receptors, usually FGFR2, and ABS with disordered steroidogenesis is a novel autosomal recessive disorder caused by mutations in *POR*.

We have now examined the *POR* genes in 32 additional patients, including 31 patients in whom ABS was initially diagnosed, and in another 6 patients with the Beare-Stevenson craniosynostosis syndrome, which can be associated with genital anomalies. Fifteen of the 19 patients having abnormal genitalia and disordered steroidogenesis were homozygotes or apparent compound heterozygotes for *POR* mutations that destroyed or dramatically inhibited POR activity; only one mutant allele was identified in the other 4 patients. Of the 12 patients with normal genitalia and normal steroidogenesis diagnosed as having ABS, 9 carried *FGFR2* or *FGFR3* mutations and none carried *POR* mutations on both alleles. These data are consistent with the emerging view that patients with ABS fall into two distinct groups that should now be categorized as two distinct diseases (Miller 2004).

Subjects and Methods

Clinical Material

Samples 1–32 were from patients identified by various medical geneticists as having ABS on the basis of dysmorphic features or identified by pediatric endocrinologists as having combined 17α-hydroxylase and 21-hydroxylase deficiencies. All samples were collected in accordance with local institutional review board or medical ethics committee guidelines. Not all clinical data are available for all subjects. Exons 8 and 10 of *FGFR2* were sequenced in all patients; only the *FGFR* sequencing in addition to exons 8 and 10 of *FGFR2* is specifically mentioned below. The available clinical histories and hormonal data are summarized below, and the available dysmorphological data are summarized in table 1; craniosynostosis and radioulnar or radiohumeral synostosis were confirmed radiographically.

Patient 1 (IRL1), who has been described recently (Hurley et al. 2004), was born at 38 wk, weighed 2.98 kg, and had a head circumference of 31 cm, with midface hypoplasia. He had fused lambdoid and sagittal sutures, radiohumeral synostosis, and femoral bowing. He was 46,XY, with a stable 8;12 translocation that was also seen in the father. The phallus was small, and the labioscrotal folds were fused. At age 2 wk, the patient had low serum cortisol (2.3 μg/dl), but it rose normally to 16.5 μg/dl after stimulation with adrenocorticotropic hormone (ACTH [corticotropin]). ACTH was normal, at 28 pg/ml. At age 2 wk, the patient had normal values for androstenedione (1.2–2.5 nmol/L), dehydroepiandrosterone sulfate (DHEAS) (0.1 μmol/L), and testosterone (1.8 nmol/L). Urinary steroids included decreased amounts of C19 steroid sulfates and increased C21 steroids. No mutations were found in exons 7 and 10 of *FGFR3*, but the patient was heterozygous for the *FGFR1* mutation I300T. This mutation has been reported in a single case of trigonocephaly (Kress et al. 2000).

Table 1

Physical Findings in Patients

Patient No.	Patient ID	Dysmorphologic Feature: Craniosynostosis	Brachycephaly	RH/RU[a] Synostosis	Femoral Bowing	Femoral Fractures	Midface Hypoplasia	Proptosis	Rocker-Bottom Feet	Arachnodactyly	Camptodactyly	Choanal Stenosis/ Atresia	Abnormal Steroids	Abnormal Genitalia
1	IRL1	Y	N	Y	Y	N	Y	Y	N	N	N		Y	Y
2	AUS2	Y	Y	Y	N	N	Y	Y	Y	Y	Y	Y	Y	Y
3	PL1	Y	N	Y	N	N	Y	N	N	N	Y		Y	Y
4	CF1	Y		Y			Y						Y	
5	337	Y		Y	Y					Y				Y
6	259	Y		Y	Y					Y				
7	699	Y		Y	Y					Y				
8	JPSZ	Y	Y	Y	Y	N	Y	Y	N	Y		Y		Y
9	JPSS	Y		Y					Y	Y		Y		Y
10	JPSB	Y	Y	Y	Y	Y		Y		Y		Y		Y
11	MC25	Y	Y	Y	Y	N	Y	Y	Y	Y	Y	Y		Y
12[b]	07942	Y	Y	Y	Y		Y	Y	Y	Y				
13[b]	50081	Y		Y	Y								Y	
14[b]	11314	Y	Y	Y	N	Y	Y	N	N	N	N	N		
15[b]	14506	Y	Y	Y	Y	Y	Y	Y		N	N	Y		
16[b]	14683	Y	Y	Y	Y	N	Y	Y				Y	Y	Y
17[b]	15441	Y	Y	Y	Y	N	Y	Y			Y	Y		
18[b]	16666	Y	Y	Y	Y		Y	Y				Y		
19[b]	20554	Y	Y	Y			Y	Y						
20[b]	24019	Y	Y	Y	Y								Y	Y
21[b]	07862	Y	Y	Y	Y	N	Y	Y				Y		
22[b]	24872	Y	Y	N	N	N	Y	Y				N	Y	
23[b]	14837	Y	Y		N	N		Y			Y	Y		
24	56661	Y	Y	Y		Y	Y	Y				Y		
25	JPAS	Y		Y	Y	Y		Y	Y	Y				
26	1110	Y										Y		
27	1115		N	N			Y	Y				Y		
28	1323	Y					Y	Y				Y		
29	1434	Y		Y	N		Y	Y		N	N	Y		
30	2430		Y	N			Y	Y				Y		
31	STJ1	Y	Y	Y	Y	N	Y	Y	N	N	N	Y	Y	Y
32	ISRL1	N	N		N	N	N	N	N	N	N	N	Y	Y

Note.—“Y” (yes) means the patient had this finding; “N” (no) means the patient did not have the finding. Blank cells indicate that the case reports did not mention whether the patient had this finding.

[a] RH = radiohumeral; RU = radioulnar.

[b] These patients were described by Reardon et al. (2000). Patient 12 is MF; patient 13 is RS; patient 14 is DW; patient 15 is HD; patient 16 is SP; patient 17 is MN; patient 18 is NC; patient 19 is ID; patient 20 is JH; patient 21 is KM; patient 22 is BW; patient 23 is MR.

Patient 2 (AUS2), a 46,XY male, was delivered at 37 wk by emergency cesarean section for abruptio placenta. Height, weight, and head circumference were at the 50th percentile for gestational age. There was proptosis, brachycephaly, frontal and temporal bossing, and ridging of the posterior sutures, but the metopic, sagittal, and coronal sutures were open. There was limitation of supination and elbow extension but no radiologically apparent synostosis. There also was camptodactyly, arachnodactyly, rocker-bottom feet, choanal stenosis, several hemivertebrae, bronchomalacia, and an absent auditory meatus and absent ossicular chain on one side. There was a horseshoe kidney, micropenis, hooded prepuce, hypospadias, chordee, bilaterally descended testes, and anteriorly placed anus. At age 1 year, the patient had normal cortisol (594 nmol/L), but ACTH was elevated (137 pg/ml; normal [nl] <50 pg/ml). Progesterone (143 nmol/L; nl <1.6 nmol/L) and 17-hydroxyprogesterone (17OHP) (71.6 nmol/L; nl <3 nmol/L) were elevated and were hyperresponsive to stimulation with ACTH, whereas DHEA (0.31 nmol/L; nl >0.7 nmol/L) and androstenedione (0.3 nmol/L; nl >0.4 nmol/L) were low and were unresponsive to ACTH. Sequencing of exons 7, 8, and 10 of *FGFR1, FGFR2,* and *FGFR3* was normal.

Patient 3 (PL1), born at 38 wk with severe oligohydramnios, had a large forehead, hypertelorism, abnormal ears, conductive hearing loss, craniosynostosis requiring ventriculoperitoneal shunting, radiohumeroulnar synostosis, and camptodactyly. He was 46,XY, with micropenis, hypospadias, and bilateral cryptorchidism. The 17OHP on newborn screening was 120 nmol/L at age 3 d and 193 nmol/L at age 5 d (nl <10 nmol/L) and was 3,780 μg/dl by radioimmunoassay at age 12 d (nl <200 μg/dl). These 17OHP data led to a presumptive diagnosis of congenital adrenal hyperplasia due to 21-hydroxylase deficiency (despite the genital findings), but sequencing of the *CYP21* gene was normal. The patient was treated with replacement doses of glucocorticoids and mineralocorticoids but died of "septic shock" at another hospital at age 3 years; no hormonal evaluation was done at that time.

Patient 4 (CF1) was a 38-wk-old, 46,XY, SRY-positive phenotypic female who weighed 2,055 g at birth. ABS was diagnosed at birth on the basis of craniosynostosis, radiohumeral synostosis with shortened humeri, midface hypoplasia, a narrow thoracic cage with pectus excavatum, and an absent corpus callosum (all confirmed by radiographic studies). She had normal female external genitalia; ultrasonography showed no uterus or ovaries, small adrenals, and normal kidneys; and a radiographic contrast study confirmed the presence of a blind vaginal pouch. She had profound respiratory distress and frequent apneic episodes and died at age 3 wk. A limited hormonal evaluation included a Müllerian inhibiting substance of 34.9 pmol/L (normal for a female but indicating Sertoli cell failure in a male); slightly elevated aldosterone (126 ng/dl; nl <100 ng/dl); high 11-deoxycortisol (6271 ng/dl; nl <150 ng/dl); and normal plasma renin content (27 ng/L), ACTH (26 pg/ml), cortisol (205 nmol/L), 17OHP (1.4 nmol/L), DHEA (25 nmol/L), DHEAS (8.9 μmol/L), and androstenedione (5.4 nmol/L). The mother also had two spontaneous abortions, and a maternal uncle died soon after birth with ambiguous genitalia, but no hormonal testing was done, and no samples are available for DNA sequencing.

Patient 5 (337) was a phenotypically female infant with cloverleaf skull, craniosynostosis, bowed femora, radiohumeral synostosis, and arachnodactyly, who also had an imperforate anus, clitoromegaly, hypoplastic labia majora, and fused labia minora; a karyotype was not done. Although these findings suggest hyperandrogenism, no hormonal studies were done. She died at age 4 years from pneumonia, complicated by severe kyphoscoliosis. Sequencing of all *FGFR2* exons was normal.

Patient 6 (259), a boy born to parents from Senegal, had craniosynostosis, cloverleaf skull, radiohumeral synostosis, bowed femora, arachnodactyly, and micropenis. No hormonal data are available. He is now 9 years old and has severe kyphoscoliosis. Sequencing of all *FGFR2* exons was normal.

Patient 7 (699) was the product of a therapeutic abortion performed at 22 wk gestation because of ultrasonographic detection of craniosynostosis, bilateral radiohumeral synostosis, bowing of long bones, and arachnodactyly. Karyotype was 46,XY, and the external genitalia were normal. Amniotic fluid steroids were not measured, but, because of the suspicion of ABS, gas chromatographic analysis of liver tissue was performed and showed "substantially increased" lanosterol and dihydrolanosterol.

Patient 8 (JPSZ) had craniosynostosis, bowed femora, elbow synostosis, Arnold-Chiari malformation, scrotal hypoplasia, and a "small" penis. No steroids were measured other than normal total serum cholesterol.

Patients 9 (JPSS) and 10 (JPSB) were siblings. Both had craniosynostosis and elbow synostosis. Patient 9 had bowed femurs and fractures; this information is not known for patient 10. Patient 9 was said to have an undescribed genital anomaly, and patient 10 had undescended testes. No other data are available.

Patient 11 (MC25), who has been described elsewhere (Hassell and Butler 1994), was small for gestational age and had brachycephaly, midface hypoplasia, proptosis, radiohumeral synostosis, bowed femora, and choanal atresia or stenosis. She was 46,XX, with clitoromegaly, no vaginal orifice, and a vesicovaginal fistula. No hormonal data are available.

Patients 12–23 were described elsewhere (Reardon et al. 2000) (see table 1). Patients 17, 18, and 22 were

Table 2

Oligonucleotide Primers for PCR, Sequencing, and Site-Directed Mutagenesis

The table is available in its entirety in the online edition of *The American Journal of Human Genetics.*

46,XY; the others were 46,XX. Patient 12 was originally described by DeLozier et al. (1980); genital anomalies were not described. At age 18 years, patient 12 had normal excretion of urinary free cortisol (67 μg/24 h), 17-hydroxycorticosteriods (7.5 mg/24 h), and 17-ketosteroids (8.5 mg/24 h). Patient 13 had low excretion of free cortisol (3.7 μg/24 h), 17-hydroxycorticosteroids (0.2 mg/24 h), and 17-ketosteroids (1.9 mg/24 h). Patient 16, illustrated in figure 1 of Reardon et al. (2000), had genital ambiguity (clitoromegaly and hooded prepuce), fused labia, elevated 17OHP (42.8 nmol/L; nl <12 nmol/L), and a cortisol of 220 nmol/L (nl 80–800), which rose to 534 nmol/L in response to ACTH. Patient 20, initially described by Kumar and Masel (1997), reportedly had an "abnormal steroid profile," which was not described further, and had a urogenital sinus, vestigial uterus, and a posteriorly placed septated vagina. For patient 22, gas chromatographic analysis of urinary steroids at age 18 mo showed elevated excretion of 11β-hydroxyandrosterone plus 17-hydroxypregnanolone (80 μg; nl <50 μg), pregnanetriol (60 μg; nl <50 μg), tetrahydrocortisone (320 μg; nl 50–250 μg), allotetrahydrocortisol (380 μg; nl 20–300 μg), α-cortolone (380 μg; nl <50 μg), α-cortol (120 μg; nl <20 μg), and β-cortolone plus β-cortol (80 μg; nl <50 μg).

Patient 24 (56661) had craniosynostosis with cloverleaf skull, brachycephaly, midface hypoplasia, elbow synostosis, bilateral choanal atresia, proptosis, femoral fractures, and only 11 pairs of ribs. The corpus callosum was "small," and the cerebral gyri were "abnormal." A randomly obtained cortisol in infancy was 3.9 μg/dl, but an ACTH test was not done; hence, this value is not informative.

Patients 25–30 initially had a clinical diagnosis of ABS, which has been reconsidered in some cases. None of these patients had genital malformations or known disorders of steroidogenesis. Patient 25 (JPAS), a 46,XY male with unilateral agenesis of one adrenal, kidney, ureter, testis, and spermatic cord, had a classic ABS phenotype (table 1), but sequencing of all exons of *FGFR2* was normal. Gas chromatographic analysis of urinary steroids at age 4 years showed normal 24-h excretions of tetrahydrocortisone (690 μg), tetrahydrocortisol (240 μg), allotetrahydrocortisol (180 μg), α-cortolone (260 μg), α-cortol (110 μg), and β-cortolone plus β-cortol (240 μg). Patient 26 (1110) had a family history of unspecified renal disease. Patients 28 (1323) and 29 (1434), reported as cases 1 and 2 by Okajima et al. (1999), are both heterozygous for *FGFR2* mutation S351C. Patient 28 had a 2.5-cm phallus, contractures of the elbows and knees without synostosis and Peters anomaly, and was subsequently considered to have Pfeiffer syndrome. Patient 29 had radioulnar—but not radiohumeral—synostosis, knee contractures without synostosis and Peters anomaly, and was subsequently considered to have Crouzon syndrome. Patient 30 (2430) developed acanthosis nigricans 4–5 years after the initial diagnosis of ABS and was then considered to have Crouzonodermoskeletal syndrome; the patient was found to be heterozygous for *FGFR3* mutation A391E.

Patient 31 (STJ1), a 46,XY male identified as having ABS at birth, had craniosynostosis, brachycephaly, radioulnar synostosis, femoral bowing, midface hypoplasia, and bilateral choanal stenosis. There was no genital ambiguity, but the patient had microphallus and bilaterally descended testes. At age 9 mo, an afternoon 17OHP was 360 nmol/L (nl <2 nmol/L at this age), but 8 A.M. values for cortisol (371 nmol/L), androstenedione (1.7 nmol/L), DHEAS (0.33 μmol/L), testosterone (<0.17 nmol/L), and aldosterone (2.8 nmol/L) were all normal for the patient's age. The elevated 17OHP in the presence of normally low C19 steroids suggested combined partial deficiencies of P450c17 and P450c21. At age 32 mo, the 17OHP remained greatly elevated (72.6 nmol/L).

Patient 32 (ISRL1), who has been described elsewhere (Augarten et al. 1992), was the 46,XY, 2,620-g, 48-cm product of a 38-wk pregnancy; the patient had no dysmorphic features suggestive of ABS but had a 1-cm microphallus, a bifid scrotum, glandular hypospadias, and bilaterally palpable testes. He had some limitation of elbow extension attributed to arthrogryposis; X-rays of the elbow joints were not done. Hormonal stimulation of the adrenal with ACTH and of the testes with human chorionic gonadotropin showed a pattern consistent with partial deficiencies of the activities of both P450c17 and P450c21 (Augarten et al. 1992). He entered puberty spontaneously but had hypergonadotropic hypogonadism and required ongoing supplementation with testosterone. He is now 22 years old and has required no glucocorticoid, mineralocorticoid, or salt supplementation.

Patients 33–38 had Beare-Stevenson syndrome, which can result in skeletal and genital anomalies (Przylepa et al. 1996). Patients 33, 36, and 37 had rugated labia majora; patient 36 had hypoplastic labia majora. Patients 35, 36, 37, and 38 had anteriorly placed anus. No endocrine data are available for these patients.

PCR and Sequencing

Specific primers in the intronic regions flanking the 15 exons of *POR* were designed on the basis of National Center for Biotechnology Information (NCBI) sequences

Table 3

Primers for PCR and Sequencing, and Product Sizes of POR Amplicons

The table is available in its entirety in the online edition of *The American Journal of Human Genetics.*

GI 4508114 and GI 11181841 (see table 2). These primers amplified each exon with at least 100 bases of flanking intronic DNA; the sizes of the PCR products are listed in table 3. Genomic DNA samples (10 ng) were used as templates for PCR amplification in a 5-μl or 10-μl reaction. PCR amplification of exons 1, 2, 3, 5, 7, and 8–9 was performed using AmpliTaq Gold (Applied Biosystems) under high touchdown cycling conditions, starting at 95°C for 5 min, followed by 14 touchdown cycles of 94°C for 20 s, 65°C–58.5°C for 20 s (the annealing temperature for each subsequent cycle was decreased by 0.5°C), and 72°C for 1 min. This was followed by 35 cycles of PCR amplification at 94°C for 20 s, at 58°C for 20 s, and at 72°C for 1 min; the final extension was held at 72°C for 10 min, followed by 4°C to stop the reaction. PCR amplification of exons 3, 6, and 10–11 was performed using Platinum Taq (Invitrogen), and amplification of exons 12–15 was performed using Platinum Taq with N,N,N-trimethylglycine (betain) (Invitrogen) at 95°C for 1 min, followed by 14 touchdown cycles, 35 cycles of PCR amplification, and a 10-min final extension at 72°C, as described above. When updated databases revealed SNPs in the sites recognized by some primers, additional primers were designed (see table 2) and used as described for exons 12–15. *FGFR2* exons 8 and 10 were sequenced as described elsewhere (Meyers et al. 1996), and *FGFR2* exon 11 was sequenced in the patients with Beare-Stevenson syndrome, as described by Przylepa et al. (1996). The PCR products were subjected to automated direct sequencing with the use of the primers listed in table 2. All cycling for PCR and sequencing was performed on ABI GeneAmp PCR System 9700 thermocyclers. The sequencing was performed with ABI BigDye terminator, version 3.1, and was displayed on ABI 3730 × 1 DNA Analyzer. Genomic DNA from four normal males and four normal females was used as a reference. Mutations were analyzed with Mutation Surveyor 2.02 (see the Softgenetics Web site). All identified mutations were confirmed by forward and reverse sequencing. Nucleotide mutations are numbered in accordance with the NCBI reference sequence NM_000941.1, and protein sequence mutations are numbered in accordance with the NCBI reference sequence NP_000932.1.

Sequence Analysis and Molecular Modeling of Human POR

The POR sequences from human, rat, *Xenopus, Drosophila,* and yeast were aligned with ClustalW (Thompson et al. 1994), and sequences were displayed and edited using GeneDoc. Molecular modeling of human POR was performed by MODELLER (Sali and Blundell 1993; Fiser et al. 2000), which uses satisfaction of spatial restraints for comparative modeling of proteins. The model was based on the X-ray crystal structure of rat POR (Wang et al. 1997), which shares 94% sequence identity with human POR. Energy minimizations were performed with GROMOS96 (see the GROMOS Home Page), and the model was examined and edited using DeepView (Guex and Peitsch 1997) and POVRAY (see the Persistence of Vision Raytracer Web site).

Expression of Wild-Type and Mutant POR in Bacteria

Human *POR* cDNA lacking codons for 27 N-terminal residues (Dierks et al. 1998) was subcloned into pET22b for bacterial expression. Mutant cDNA expression vectors were generated by PCR-based, site-directed mutagenesis with the use of the primers shown in table 2. The resulting mutated plasmids were selected by digestion with *Dpn*I and were propagated in *Escherichia coli* DH5α. All *POR* mutations were confirmed by direct sequencing.

E. coli BL21DE3(pLysS) transformed with pET22b were grown in terrific broth (Dierks et al. 1998) supplemented with 40 μM $FeCl_3$, 4 μM $ZnCl_2$, 2 μM $CoCl_2$, 2 μM Na_2MoO_4, 2 μM $CaCl_2$, 2 μM $CuCl_2$, 2 μM H_3BO_3, 10% (v/v) potassium phosphate solution (0.17 M KH_2PO_4, 0.72 M K_2HPO_4 pH 7.4), 0.5 mg/ml riboflavin, 50 μg/ml ampicillin, and 34 μg/ml chloramphenicol at room temperature to an optical density (OD) 600 nm of 0.4 and were induced with 0.4 mM isopropyl-1-thio-β-D-galactopyranoside (IPTG) overnight. The bacteria were washed with PBS and were resuspended in 100 mM Tris-acetate (pH 7.6), 0.5 M sucrose, and 1 mM EDTA. The bacteria were treated with lysozyme (0.5 mg/ml) and EDTA (0.1 mM [pH 8.0]) to generate spheroplasts. The spheroplasts were pelleted by centrifugation (5,000 × *g* for 15 min); were resuspended in 100 mM potassium phosphate (pH 7.6), 6 mM MgOAc, 0.1 mM DTT, 20% (v/v) glycerol, 0.2 mM PMSF, and 0.1 mM DNase I; and were disrupted by sonication (30-s on/off cycles for 15 min at 40% power). The lysate was cleared of cellular debris by centrifugation at 12,000 × *g* for 5 min, and then the membranes in the supernatant were pelleted at 150,000 × *g* for 45 min at 4°C. Membranes were resuspended in 50 mM Tris-HCl (pH 8.0), 1 mM EDTA, and 20% (v/v) glycerol; were stored at −70°C; and were used as a source of POR.

Purification and Quantitation of Wild-Type and Mutant POR

Bacterial membranes containing POR were solubilized by stirring for 2 h at 4°C in 20 mM potassium phosphate (pH 7.6) containing 20% glycerol, 0.1 mM EDTA, 1 mM PMSF, 1 mg/L pepstatin, 10 mg/L leupeptin, 0.2% sodium cholate, and 0.2% Triton X-100 (Calbiochem). Insoluble material was removed by centrifugation at 100,000 × *g* for 1 h, and the supernatant was loaded on a 2′,5′-ADP-Sepharose column (Sigma) equilibrated with 20 mM potassium phosphate (pH 7.6) containing 20% glycerol, 0.1 mM EDTA, and 0.2% sodium cholate. The column was first washed with 5 vol of this buffer; then with 5 vol of 100 mM potassium phosphate (pH 7.6) containing 20% glycerol, 0.1 mM EDTA, 0.2% sodium cholate, and 250 mM sodium chloride; and finally with 5 vol of 20 mM potassium phosphate (pH 7.6) containing 20% glycerol, 0.1 mM EDTA, 0.2% sodium cholate, and 2 mM adenosine. POR was eluted with 20 mM potassium phosphate (pH 7.6) containing 20% glycerol, 0.1 mM EDTA, 0.2% sodium cholate, and 5 mM 2′-AMP. The cholate and 2′-AMP were removed from POR preparations by dialysis against 20 mM potassium phosphate (pH 7.6) containing 10% glycerol.

The mutant POR proteins were quantitated by western blotting by comparison with a standard curve of purified wild-type POR protein. Wild-type POR protein was quantitated by Bradford assay, and the purity of the POR preparation was confirmed by SDS-PAGE (fig. 1). The standard curve, using different amounts of wild-type POR protein, and the membrane preparations from bacteria expressing various POR mutants were separated by SDS-PAGE, transferred on polyvinyldifluoride (PVDF) membranes, and probed with a rabbit polyclonal antibody against wild-type human POR (Stressgen) at a dilution of 1:1,000. The blot was developed with a chemiluminescence-based detection reagent (Pierce) by employing goat anti-rabbit antibody, coupled with horseradish peroxidase. Signals were detected on a STORM 860 phosphorimager, operating in blue fluorescence mode, and were quantitated with ImageQuant software. All POR levels were normalized against wild-type POR.

Expression of Human P450c17 in Yeast

Yeast strain W(B), which lacks the endogenous yeast *Cpr1* gene (Pompon et al. 1995), was propagated and transiently transfected with pYeSF2 expressing human P450c17, as described (Auchus et al. 1998). Yeast microsomes were prepared as described (Auchus et al. 1998), microsomal proteins were quantitated colorimetrically (protein Assay Dye Reagent [Bio-Rad]), and

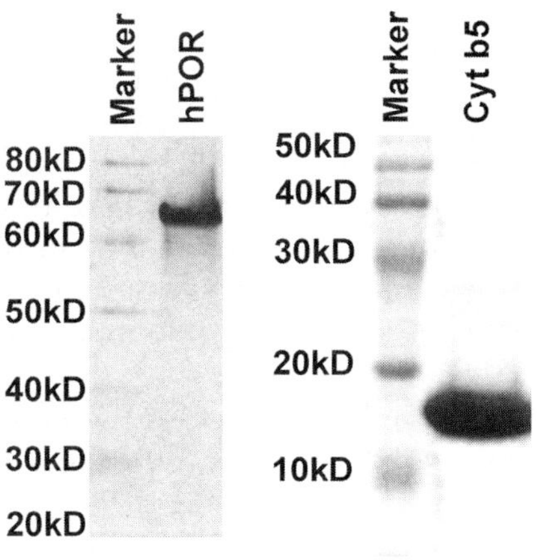

Figure 1 Purification of POR and cytochrome b_5. *Left panel,* 10% SDS-polyacrylamide gel showing purified preparations of wild-type POR used for quantitation and normalization of POR mutants; *right panel,* 12% SDS-polyacrylamide gel showing purified cytochrome b_5 used in assays of the 17,20 lyase reaction. Both gels were purposely overloaded to permit identification of trace contamination. The gels were stained with Coomassie Brilliant Blue.

P450 content was measured spectroscopically (Omura and Sato 1964).

POR Assays Based on Cytochrome c

The ability of bacterially expressed POR to reduce cytochrome c or to oxidize NADPH was measured, using a method based on that of Lu et al. (1969), by quantitating the change in A550 when oxidized cytochrome c is reduced (extinction coefficient of 21.1 mM^{-1}) (Van and Slater 1962). The assay system contained an NADPH regeneration system, consisting of 0.1M Tris-HCl (pH 7.8), 2 mM glucose-6-phoshate (Sigma), and 3 U glucose-6-phosphate dehydrogenase (Sigma) in a 1-ml volume. The cytochrome c concentration was 40 μM when NADPH was the variable substrate, and the NADPH concentration was 5 μM when cytochrome c was the variable substrate. Assays were performed with 15–20 μg of bacterial membranes containing 5 pmol of POR, as assessed in comparison to bacterially expressed wild-type POR, as described above. A550 was monitored against time, and velocities were expressed as (nmol reduced cytochrome c) · $(\text{nmol POR})^{-1}$ · (min^{-1}). Data were analyzed using LEONORA (Cornish-Bowden 1995) (see the Centre National de la Recherche Scientifique Marseilles Group in Enzyme Kinetics and Control Analysis Web site).

POR Assays Based on P450c17

The various POR missense mutants all expressed at similar levels. The ability of bacterially expressed POR to support 17α-hydroxylase and 17,20 lyase activities of P450c17 was then assayed using human P450c17 expressed in yeast. Yeast membrane fractions containing 10 pmol of P450c17 were combined with bacterial membranes containing 20 pmol POR by emulsifying with 20 μg phosphatidylcholine in 100 mM potassium phosphate, 6 mM potassium acetate, 10 mM $MgCl_2$, 1 mM reduced glutathione, 20% glycerol, 3 U glucose-6-phosphate dehydrogenase, 0.1 mM glucose-6-phosphate, and radiolabeled substrate for 20 min at 25°C in a total volume of 200 μl. For the 17α-hydroxylase reaction, the substrate was ^{14}C progesterone; for the 17,20 lyase reaction, the substrate was ^{3}H 17α-hydroxypregnenolone (17OH Preg), with 50 pmol cytochrome b_5 (added to facilitate the lyase reaction allosterically) (Auchus et al. 1998). The reactions were started by adding 20 μl 10 mM NADPH; reactions were incubated at 37°C for various lengths of time and were stopped by adding ethyl acetate:iso-octane (3:1) to extract the steroids. Steroids from different reactions were spotted on silica gel 60 F-254 thin-layer chromatography (TLC) plates (Merck) and were developed with ethyl acetate:chloroform (3:1) (Lin et al. 1991). Steroids were quantified by phosphorimaging for P450c17/POR assays, and kinetic behavior was approximated as a Michaelis-Menten system. Curve fitting and calculations of maximum velocity (V_{max}) and apparent Michaelis constant (K_m) values were performed using LEONORA (Cornish-Bowden 1995).

Expression and Purification of Cytochrome b_5

For use in the 17,20 lyase assays, human cytochrome b_5 was prepared in *E. coli* strain BL21(DE3) transformed with plasmid pLW01b5 containing human cytochrome b_5 cDNA and was selected over several cycles, as described (Miroux and Walker 1996). A single colony of transformed *E. coli* was inoculated into Luria-Bertani (LB) medium containing 100 μg/ml carbenicillin, grown to an OD 600 nm of 0.5–0.7, and IPTG was added to a final concentration of 0.4 mM. Cell density was measured every 30 min; when the OD 600 nm started to rise again (90–180 min after induction), 100 μl of cells diluted at a ratio of 1:50 were plated on LB agar plates containing 100 μg/ml carbenicillin and 0.4 mM IPTG and were allowed to grow overnight at 37°C. A single colony was grown the next day, and the process of induction and selection with carbenicillin and IPTG was repeated three more times. After four cycles of selection, the *E. coli* were transformed with plasmid pLysS/RARE, which encodes lysozyme and six rare tRNAs that assist the expression of mammalian proteins by complementing the codon bias of *E. coli*. The resultant *E. coli* A11(DE3) pLysS/RARE cells were used for expression of cytochrome b_5. Expression and purification was performed as described (Mulrooney and Waskell 2000), and purity was assessed by SDS-PAGE (fig. 1).

Results

Anatomic Phenotype

A summary of the dysmorphologic features in our patients is presented in table 1. The most consistent features were radiographically demonstrated craniosynostosis, either radioulnar or radiohumeral synostosis, and femoral bowing. Other features generally associated with ABS (brachycephaly, femoral fractures, midface hypoplasia, proptosis choanal atresia, arachnodactyly, camptodactyly, and rocker-bottom feet) were also reported in several patients, and some patients also had conductive hearing loss. A comparison of these clinical findings and the mutation analyses (table 4) shows that, aside from the genital anomalies attributable to disordered steroidogenesis, no morphologic feature distinguished patients with *POR* mutations from those with *FGFR* mutations.

Hormonal Phenotype

Clear hormonal and genital data are not available for all patients, since most were not seen by a pediatric endocrinologist. Where data are available, a pattern emerges that closely resembles the pattern originally described by Peterson et al. (1985), as well as that described in our previous study (Flück et al. 2004). In all patients in whom it was measured, 17OHP was markedly elevated and was hyperresponsive to stimulation with ACTH, as is typical of defects in steroid 21-hydroxylase (P450c21) (Miller 1994). Basal values for cortisol and other steroids tended to be normal, but such values are not truly informative in the absence of stimulation with ACTH. Despite the elevated values for 17OHP, values for C19 steroids were normal or low, indicating a relatively greater deficiency in the 17,20 lyase activity of P450c17 (Geller et al. 1997). There was no clear evidence of any patient suffering a life-threatening adrenal crisis from glucocorticoid and mineralocorticoid deficiency, but there also was no hormonal evaluation of the several individuals who died in childhood. The possibility of life-threatening adrenal insufficiency remains a concern.

DNA Sequencing

Exons 8 and 10 of *FGFR2* are the most frequent sites of mutation in the various craniosynostosis syndromes; these exons were sequenced in all patients. In patients 5, 6, and 26, all exons of *FGFR2* were sequenced. Excluding patients 33–38 with Beare-Stevenson syndrome, *FGFR2* mutation S351C was found in five patients, other *FGFR2* mutations (C342S, C342R, and P276V) were found in three other patients, and one patient carried the *FGFR3* mutation A391E (table 4). None of these

Table 4

Summary of Genetic Findings

Patient No.	Patient ID	Mutation (Parental Ethnicity) at Allele 1	Mutation (Parental Ethnicity) at Allele 2	*FGFR2* (Exons 8 and 10)
1	IRL1	G539R (Irish)	Frame 1 (white)	*FGFR1* I300T
2	AUS2	F646del (Laotian)	A287P (white)	nl
3	PL1	A287P (white)	Frame 2 (Moroccan)	nl (all *FGFR2*)
4	CF1	M263V (white)	Not found (white)	nl
5	337	A287P (French)	Not found (French)	nl (all *FGFR2*)
6	259	R457H (Senegalese)	Not found (Senegalese)	nl (all *FGFR2*)
7	699	Q153R (Algerian)	Q153R (Algerian)	nl
8	JPSZ	R457H (Japanese)	R457H (Japanese)	nl
9	JPSS	R457H (Japanese)	Y459H (Japanese)	nl
10	JPSB	R457H (Japanese)	Y459H (Japanese)	nl
11	MC25	A287P (white)	Frame 3 (Hispanic)	nl
12	09742	A287P (white)	A287P (white)	nl
13	50081	A287P (white)	Frame 4 (white)	nl
14	11314	None found (British)	None found (British)	*FGFR2* C342S
15	14506	None found (British)	None found (British)	*FGFR2* S351C
16	14683	A287P (British)	None found (British)	nl
17	15441	None found (Pakistani)	None found (Pakistani)	*FGFR2* C342R
18	16666	None found (white)	None found (white)	*FGFR2* S351C
19	20554	None found	None found	*FGFR2* S351C
20	24019	R457H (British)	Frame 6 (British)	nl
21	07862	None found (British)	None found (British)	nl
22	24872	A287P (British)	Frame 7 (British)	nl
23	14837	None found (Hispanic)	None found (Hispanic)	*FGFR2* F276V
24	56661	A287P (white)	R616X (white)	nl
25	JPAS	None found (Japanese)	None found (Japanese)	All *FGFR2* nl
26	1110	None found (Arab)	None found	nl
27	1115	None found (white)	None found (white)	nl
28	1323	None found (Black)	None found (Black)	*FGFR2* S351C
29	1434	None found (Black)	None found (Black)	*FGFR2* S351C
30	2430	None found (Hispanic)	None found	*FGFR3* A391E
31	STJ1	L565P (white)	R457H (white)	nl
32	ISRL1	T142A (Iraqi)	Frame 5 (Yemeni)	nl
33	MC15	None found (white)	None found (white)	*FGFR2* Y375C
34	1095	None found (Hispanic)	None found	nl
35	1603	None found (Vietnamese)	None found (Vietnamese)	*FGFR2* S372C
36	1771	None found (black)	None found (black)	*FGFR2* Y375C
37	2353	A115V (white)	None found	*FGFR2* Y375C
38	1156	None found	None found	nl

NOTE.—Frameshift mutations (base numbers refer to the ORF, with A of the first ATG as base 1): frame 1, 580-581insTACGTGGACAAGC; frame 2, 1551-1552ins TGCCCATGTTCGTGCGC; frame 3, 1619-1620insCCTTCAAGGCCACCACGCCTGTCATCATGATGGGCCCCGGCACCGG-GGT; frame 4, 1621-1622insC; frame 5, 1348-1349ins GAGC; frame 6, IVS6-2A→T; and frame 7, IVS7+(2-3)insT.

individuals with *FGFR2* or *FGFR3* mutations carried a mutation in *POR*. Patient 1 carried the *FGFR1* mutation I300T and was also a compound heterozygote for two *POR* mutations.

For the *POR* gene, all 15 exons and at least 50 bases of each intron lying adjacent to the exons were sequenced on both strands in all samples. Additional primers were used at primer sites where the University of California Santa Cruz (UCSC) Genome Browser identified polymorphisms. Allele assignments of identified mutations were made by sequencing parental DNA when such samples were available. SNPs permitted the identification of two alleles in most cases; however, we can not rule out hemizygosity in patients 4–8 and 12 (table 4). The sequencing results are shown in figure 2, and the allele assignments and the available data on ethnic origins are summarized in table 4. The numbering of the nucleotides is based on the NCBI human *POR* cDNA sequence NM_000941.1; the ORF with A of the first ATG is base 1. The corresponding amino acid numbers in the protein are based on the NCBI POR protein reference sequence NP_000932.1. These sequences correspond to the full-length, 680-aa human POR sequence. Some other investigators (Adachi et al. 2004; Arlt et al.

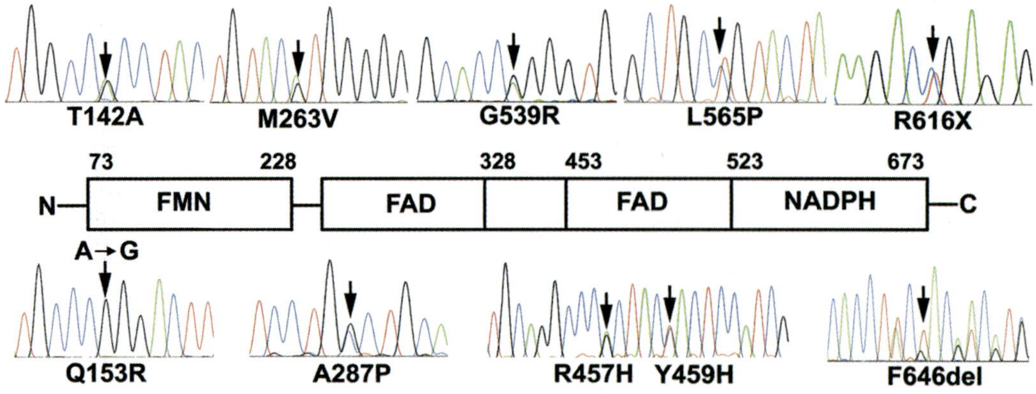

Figure 2 Sequences of *POR* mutations. The mutants shown are from the patients in the present study who had disordered steroidogenesis. Each mutant is shown as a heterozygote in association with a wild-type allele, except for Q153R, which was only seen in a homozygously affected patient. The mutated nucleotides, indicated by arrows, are 424A→G, causing T142A; 458A→G, causing Q153R; 787A→G, causing M263V; 859G→C, causing A287P; 1370G→A, causing R457H; 1375T→C, causing Y459H; 1615G→A, causing G539R; 1694T→C, causing L565P; 1845C→T, causing R616X; and 1937-1939delTCT, causing F646del. The location of each mutation is shown on a linear diagram of the POR protein, as described by Wang et al. (1997), which illustrates the crystallographically inferred boundaries of the functional domains of POR.

2004) have used NCBI sequence P16435, which is derived from the SwissProt database and indicates that human POR contains 677 residues (as does rat POR), but the older SwissProt database misses the Met-Ile-Asn sequence that precedes the Met in position 4 (corresponding to rat position 1).

POR mutations were found in 19 of the 32 patients with ABS (patients 33–38 are excluded because they had Beare-Stevenson syndrome). Mutations were found on only one allele in four samples (patients 4, 5, 6, and 16). The other 15 patients carrying *POR* mutations included 3 in whom the mutation was homozygous, 4 proven compound heterozygotes in whom allele assignments were made by sequencing parental DNA, and 8 probable compound heterozygotes in whom two heterozygous mutations were found but allele assignments could not be done because parental samples were not available. The 34 affected alleles included 5 unique frameshift mutations, 2 splice-site mutations, 26 missense mutations, and 1 premature stop codon near the carboxyl-terminus of the encoded POR protein. The five frameshift mutations ("Frames 1–5" in table 4) grossly disrupted the flavin mononucleotide (FMN)- and NADPH-binding sites of *POR,* and four of them (Frames 1, 2, 4, and 5) also caused premature stop codons upstream from residue 616, where the spontaneously occurring nonsense mutation R616X was devoid of activity (described below). The two intronic mutations, termed "Frame 6" and "Frame 7" (table 4), disrupted the canonical splice-acceptor or -donor sites; the splice-site recognition programs FSPLICE (see the Softberry Web site) and NNSplice (see the Berkeley *Drosophila* Genome Project Web site) indicate that each is very likely to disrupt splicing. Thus, the mutations termed "Frames 1–7" were not tested in vitro. Most missense mutations were found once, but A287P was found on 10 alleles, and R457H was found on 7 alleles. Thus, these two missense mutations accounted for 17 of 34 (50%) of the identified *POR* missense mutations.

A287P and R457H Mutations

The A287P mutation was found only in samples from subjects described as "white," "Caucasian," or "European." This same mutation was also found on two of eight alleles in our initial study (Flück et al. 2004) and on one of four alleles in a subsequent study (Arlt et al. 2004), all in individuals of European heritage. Thus, A287P is a frequent mutation causing POR deficiency in this group. The nucleotide change 859G→C, which is responsible for all identified cases of A287P, lies in exon 8, changing the sequence from ↓(N)$_{12}$GCTGC to (N)$_{12}$CCTGC, destroying the site recognized by restriction endonuclease *Bbv*I. We amplified exons 8 and 9 in a single PCR using primers OR-8-9F and OR-8-9R (table 3), yielding a product of 613 bp. Digestion of this PCR product with *Bbv*I yields four fragments of 250 bp, 167 bp, 101 bp, and 95 bp in the wild type but yields only three fragments of 262 bp, 250 bp, and 101 bp in the mutant.

The R457H mutation was found in four of eight alleles from Japanese patients. This mutation destroyed *Bsa*XI and *Tst*I sites, but these enzymes recognize degenerate 33–37 base sequences and cut both strands twice; hence, this approach did not yield a reliable diagnostic tactic. R457H was also found on 1 of 2 Japanese alleles in our initial study (Flück et al. 2004) and on 2 of 4 alleles (Adachi et al. 2004) and 10 of 16 alleles (Fukami et al. 2005) in two recent studies of Japanese patients. However, other ethnic groups may also carry the R457H mutation. The samples from patient 6, whose parents are from Senegal; patient 21, from the United Kingdom; and patient 31, whose parents are both French Canadian, were heterozygous for the same 1370G→A mutation causing the R457H missense mutation. In addition, Arlt et al. (2004) found R457H in a Polish patient. Thus, R457H is strongly—but not uniquely—associated with patients of Japanese heritage.

Mutations and Polymorphisms

Our previous study described the enzymology of the five missense mutations (A287P, R457H, V492E, C569Y, and V608F) identified in our initial four patients (Flück et al. 2004). The present series adds the mutants or polymorphisms A115V, T142A, Q153R, M263V, Y459H, A503V, G539R, L565P, R616X, V631I, and F646del. In addition, we found the mutants or polymorphisms P228L, R316W, G413S, and G504R by searching a publicly available sequence database (see the BioVentures Web site), and the missense mutation Y181D was reported in another study (Arlt et al. 2004) but was not characterized in a P450 assay. The incidences of these alleles and their ethnic distributions are not yet available in the NCBI, HapMap (see the International HapMap Project Web site), or UCSC Genome Browser databases, although these are being updated regularly. As discussed below, the changes that were found in the patients disrupted steroidogenesis and hence appear to be mutations, whereas the changes that were found in databases had lesser (but variable) effects and hence appear to be polymorphisms. In the discussion of the enzymology below, all of these amino acid changes are referred to as "mutations."

Enzymology of the Amino Acid Replacement Mutations

To understand the enzymatic consequences of each amino acid replacement mutation, we built a computer graphic model of the human POR that was based on the crystallographically determined structure of rat POR, which is 94% identical to human POR (Wang et al. 1997). The model of human POR was energetically favorable (total free energy was −33,952 kJ/mol for the human POR model, compared with −27,850 kJ/mol for the rat POR structure) and closely resembled the rat POR structure, as expected (fig. 3). In general, the missense mutations found in patients with ABS mapped to functionally important domains of POR, and the apparent polymorphisms mapped to less crucial regions. Therefore, to assess the enzymatic consequences of each missense mutant, we built bacterial expression vectors for each and characterized their activities in four assays.

From the time of the initial identification and isolation of POR (Lu et al. 1969), the standard POR assay has been the reduction of cytochrome c, which is easily assayed as change in absorption at 550 nm. To perform this assay and also to measure NADPH oxidation, we expressed human POR mutants in bacteria in a form lacking 27 amino-terminal residues (N-27 POR) (Dierks et al. 1998), which is similar to N-24 rat POR, as human POR has a 3-aa amino-terminal extension, compared with rodent POR (NCBI accession numbers NC_000007, NM_000941.1, and NP_000932.1). This form of POR remains associated with membranes, as does wild-type POR, and it is distinct from the soluble N-49 POR used by Arlt et al. (2004). Table 5 shows the K_m, V_{max}, and V_{max}/K_m (an estimate of catalytic efficiency) for the capacity of the wild type and the 21 missense mutants of POR to catalyze the reduction of cytochrome c and the oxidation of NADPH. We have previously measured these variables for wild-type POR and for the A287P, R457H, V492E, C569Y, and V608F mutants (Flück et al. 2004); in each case, the values in table 5 are within 20% of the previously measured values. An examination of the V_{max}/K_m values, shown as percentages of the wild-type values, reveals that there is a very broad range of enzymatic impairment and that there is generally good agreement between the two assays. P228L, R316W, G413S, A503V, and G504R, which were polymorphisms identified from databases, retained 47%–100% of wild-type activity in both assays, but the apparent polymorphism A115V, found in a patient with Beare-Stevenson syndrome with an *FGFR2* mutation, had 41%–63% of wild-type activity in the cytochrome c assays (but 70%–80% of wild-type activity in P450c17 assays [table 6]); M263V and V631I, found as heterozygotes during the sequencing of other individuals, had 23%–76% of wild-type activity (table 5).

However, cytochrome c is a soluble protein and is not a physiologic substrate for normal, membrane-bound POR (Lu et al. 1969). Therefore, we supplemented this classic assay with direct assays of the capacity of POR mutants to support catalysis by a cytochrome P450 enzyme. We previously reported assays of POR activity that were based on its ability to support catalysis by P450c17 with the use of doubly transformed yeast (Flück et al. 2004). In this system, a yeast strain lacking the gene for yeast POR was transiently transfected with vectors expressing human P450c17 and POR (Auchus et al. 1998). This system was originally developed to assay P450c17 activities: the transfected human POR was abundant and not limiting, and the amount of P450c17 was measured by difference spectra, yielding reproducible measures of P450c17 enzymology (Auchus et al. 1998; Arlt et al. 2001), but the ratio of P450c17

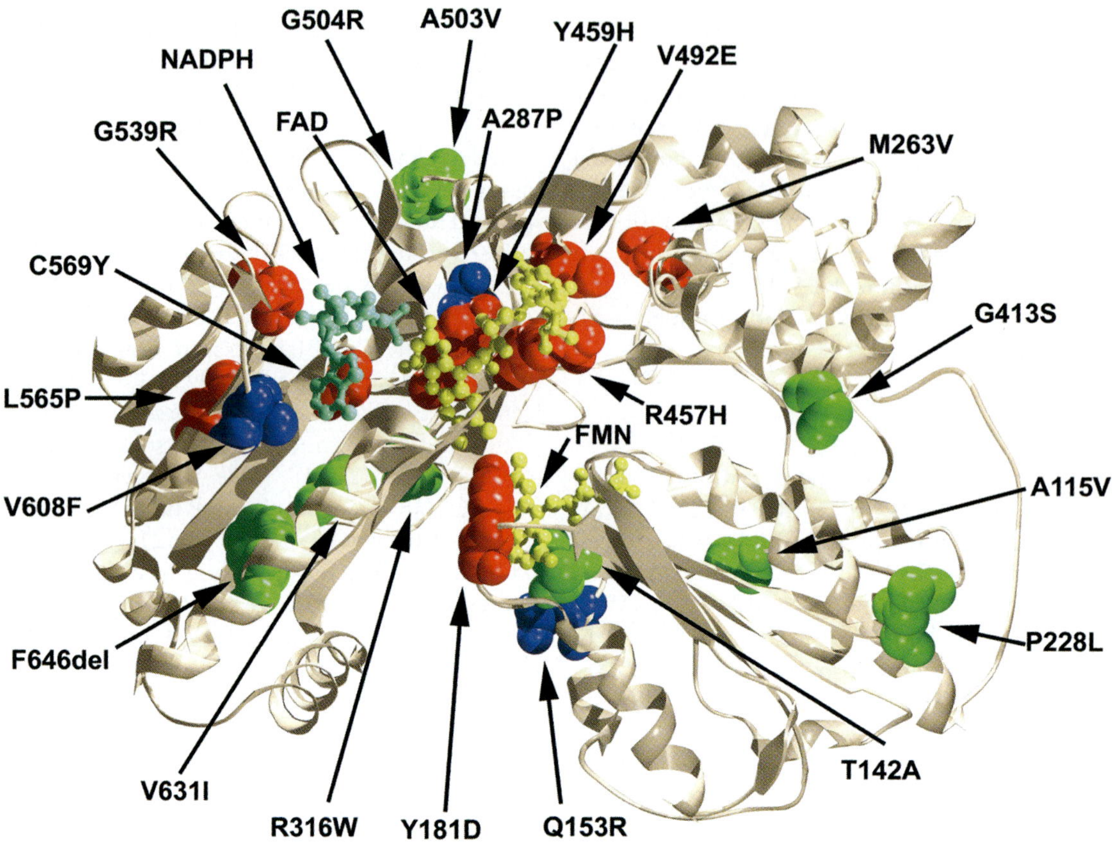

Figure 3 Model of human POR, showing the location of the mutants. The model is based on the X-ray crystal structure of rat POR and was created using the programs DeepView and POVRAY (see the Persistence of Vision Raytracer Web site). The α-carbon backbone is shown as a narrow ribbon, permitting visualization of buried residues. The missense residues identified by sequencing are depicted by charged packed sphere images. Mutations retaining >50% of activity are shown in green, those retaining 25%–50% are shown in blue, and those retaining <25% are shown in red. Ball-and-stick models are used to represent the FMN (*yellow*), FAD (*yellow*) and NADPH (*cyan*) moieties.

to POR could not be measured or chosen precisely. However, when POR is limiting, the 17,20 lyase activity of P450c17 is sensitive to changes in the molar ratio of POR to P450c17 (Yanagibashi and Hall 1986; Lin et al. 1993). Therefore, we have developed a modification of this assay using microsomes containing human P450c17 expressed in yeast, as before, combined with a membrane fraction containing human N-27 POR expressed in *E. coli* (fig. 1). Each component is prepared and assayed separately before mixing, so the P450c17:POR ratio can be set, improving reproducibility and consistency. As the 17,20 lyase activity of P450c17 is facilitated by the allosteric action of cytochrome b_5 (Auchus et al. 1998), we also prepared cytochrome b_5 in bacteria, to add in support of the lyase reactions (fig. 1). Adding exogenous phosphatidylcholine fostered association of the yeast and bacterial membranes, permitting association of the catalytic components. In this system, POR remains intimately associated with the endoplasmic reticulum and, thus, has a physiologically relevant membrane insertion. As defective androgen synthesis is a hallmark of the patients with POR deficiency and as the 17,20 lyase activity of human P450c17 is exquisitely sensitive to the topology of its interactions with POR (Geller et al. 1997; Auchus and Miller 1999; Geller et al. 1999), we assayed the capacity of the POR mutants to support the 17α-hydroxylase and 17,20 lyase activities of human P450c17.

Table 6 shows the K_m, V_{max}, and V_{max}/K_m for the 17α-hydroxylase and 17,20 lyase activities of P450c17 when catalysis is supported by either wild-type POR or each of the missense mutants. We previously measured these values for the A287P, R457H, V492E, C569Y, and V608F mutants (Flück et al. 2004). Those prior data are in excellent agreement with the data in table 6, except for C569Y, which has lower activity in the present study. The polymorphic A115V, P228L, R316W, G413S, A503V, and G504R variants retained 41%–141% of wild-type activity. The V608F mutant, which had 3%–8% of wild-type activity in the cytochrome c assays, had

Table 5

Kinetics of POR Variants Using Cytochrome c as Substrate

	VALUE OF VARIABLE ± SD FOR							
	Cytochrome c				NADPH			
POR VARIANT	K_m	V_{max}	V_{max}/K_m (% of Wild Type)	K_{cat}	K_m	V_{max}	V_{max}/K_m (% of Wild Type)	K_{cat}
Wild type	1.4 ± .3	91.2 ± 5.1	65.1 (100)	388	.22 ± .05	68.4 ± 2.9	310 (100)	292
A115V	2.0 ± .4	82.5 ± 4.3	41.2 (63)	350	.29 ± .04	37.2 ± 5.9	128 (41)	158
T142A	1.6 ± .2	51.3 ± 6.3	32.1 (49)	218	.23 ± .03	41.7 ± 4.6	161 (52)	178
Q153R	3.7 ± .4	21.4 ± 5.7	5.7 (9)	90	1.2 ± .09	43.2 ± 3.1	36 (11)	184
Y181D	>50	...	...	...	>50	...	...	...
P228L	1.4 ± .3	69.2 ± 5.2	49.4 (75)	294	.24 ± .06	53.7 ± 3.8	224 (72)	229
M263V	1.9 ± .2	94.5 ± 3.7	49.7 (76)	402	.39 ± .07	69.1 ± 2.4	177 (57)	294
A287P	5.9 ± .8	37.3 ± 6.4	6.3 (9)	158	.71 ± .10	35.1 ± 4.3	49 (16)	150
R316W	1.9 ± .4	75.9 ± 8.3	39.9 (61)	322	.29 ± .07	69.3 ± 9.7	238 (77)	294
G413S	1.3 ± .2	64.5 ± 7.9	49.6 (76)	274	.20 ± .05	61.7 ± 2.1	309 (100)	262
R457H	17.2 ± 2.5	7.5 ± 2.1	.43 (.7)	32	>50	...	...	...
Y459H	22.9 ± 6.6	6.1 ± .7	.26 (.4)	26	>50	...	...	...
V492E	29.7 ± 5.1	6.8 ± 1.1	.22 (.3)	28	>50	...	...	...
A503V	1.8 ± .2	81.3 ± 6.6	45.2 (69)	344	.21 ± .06	55.7 ± 1.9	265 (86)	238
G504R	2.1 ± .2	72.9 ± 4.1	34.7 (53)	312	.35 ± .06	51.2 ± 3.9	146 (47)	218
G539R	6.3 ± 1.2	37.8 ± 6.7	6.0 (9)	160	18.3 ± 2.1	9.3 ± 1.2	.5 (.2)	40
L565P	2.8 ± .6	26.2 ± 3.2	9.3 (14)	112	5.3 ± 1.6	23.8 ± 2.3	4.5 (1.4)	102
C569Y	5.8 ± .2	24.3 ± 2.7	4.1 (6)	104	1.8 ± .43	12.1 ± .7	7 (2)	52
V608F	5.2 ± 1.3	26.3 ± 5.2	5.1 (8)	112	3.3 ± .7	32.7 ± .6	10 (3)	140
R616X	>50	...	...	...	>50	...	...	...
V631I	1.6 ± .4	77.3 ± 8.6	48.3 (74)	328	.47 ± .06	32.8 ± 5.3	70 (23)	140
F646del	3.9 ± .7	90.7 ± 5.7	23.3 (36)	384	.21 ± .13	61.2 ± 8.5	291 (94)	260

NOTE.—K_m values are in μM (cytochrome c or NADPH); V_{max} values are in nmol of cytochrome c reduced/mg POR protein/min. K_{cat} values were calculated on the basis of the molar content of POR, and, hence, the values are in min^{-1}. POR content of each membrane preparation was measured, and all samples were normalized against wild-type POR.

57%–80% of wild-type activity in the P450c17 assays. Other, lesser, differences can be seen by comparing tables 5 and 6.

Careful comparison of the enzymatic data with the clinical data show that the P450c17 assays provide a much better correlation between genotype and phenotype. Patient 1 was a compound heterozygote for a null (frameshift) mutation and the novel missense mutation G539R. This mutant retained 46% of the 17α-hydroxylase activity but only 8% of the 17,20 lyase activity. Consistent with this, the patient was able to synthesize cortisol adequately (17α-hydroxylase activity) but had poor production of sex steroids (17,20 lyase activity). Patients 2 and 3 were compound heterozygotes, each carrying the previously described A287P mutation on one allele but carrying very different mutations on the other allele. Patient 2 carried F646del, which retained normal hydroxylase activity and about half of normal 17,20 lyase activity, whereas patient 3 carried a null (frameshift) mutation on the second allele. Consistent with this, the hormonal and anatomic phenotype in patient 2 was less severe, with no genital ambiguity and normal cortisol (17α-hydroxylase activity) but with clear evidence of decreased 17,20 lyase activity (elevated 17OHP, low DHEA, and androstenedione). By contrast, patient 3 had moderately severe genital ambiguity, early evidence of disordered steroidogenesis, and a more severe skeletal phenotype. A close correlation between assays of the 17,20 lyase activity of P450c17 and the genital phenotype is to be expected, as 17,20 lyase activity is required for the production of all sex steroids and because the 17,20 lyase activity is much more sensitive than the 17α-hydroxylase activity of P450c17 to minor disturbances in the interactions between P450c17 and POR (Geller et al. 1997, 1999; Auchus and Miller 1999).

Discussion

Assessment of POR Activity

In the present study, we assayed POR activity both by the conventional cytochrome c assays (reduction of cytochrome c and oxidation of NADPH) and by a direct measure of POR-supported catalysis by a microsomal cytochrome P450 enzyme. For this purpose, we used steroidogenic P450c17, as its 17,20 lyase activity is very sensitive to the amount of POR available (Yanagibashi and Hall 1986; Lin et al. 1993) and to the qualitative nature of the interaction between P450c17 and POR (Zhang et al. 1995; Geller et al. 1997, 1999; Auchus et

Table 6

Kinetics of P450c17 Activities Supported by POR Variants

POR Variant	17α-Hydroxylase K_m	17α-Hydroxylase V_{max}	17α-Hydroxylase V_{max}/K_m (% of Wild Type)	17α-Hydroxylase K_{cat}	17,20 Lyase K_m	17,20 Lyase V_{max}	17,20 Lyase V_{max}/K_m (% of Wild Type)	17,20 Lyase K_{cat}
Wild type	4.3 ± .09	.149 ± .021	.035 (100)	.67	.93 ± .18	.059 ± .014	.063 (100)	.27
A115V	3.5 ± .05	.097 ± .013	.028 (80)	.43	.71 ± .11	.032 ± .006	.045 (71)	.14
T142A	5.1 ± .07	.106 ± .019	.021 (60)	.48	.86 ± .15	.029 ± .009	.034 (54)	.13
Q153R	3.7 ± .09	.039 ± .017	.011 (31)	.18	.97 ± .20	.017 ± .007	.017 (27)	.08
Y181D	>50	...	...	...	>50	...	...	...
P228L	3.7 ± .06	.131 ± .013	.035 (100)	.59	1.54 ± .21	.041 ± .005	.026 (41)	.18
M263V	7.2 ± 1.7	.025 ± .011	.003 (9)	.11	1.17 ± .13	.009 ± .003	.008 (13)	.04
A287P	3.5 ± 1.0	.049 ± .010	.014 (40)	.22	1.34 ± .09	.018 ± .002	.013 (21)	.08
R316W	3.1 ± .04	.104 ± .017	.033 (94)	.47	.87 ± .18	.078 ± .003	.089 (141)	.35
G413S	5.9 ± 1.1	.172 ± .015	.029 (83)	.77	1.28 ± .15	.089 ± .011	.069 (110)	.40
R457H	5.1 ± 1.2	.008 ± .003	.001 (3)	.04	...	...	...	...
Y459H	6.5 ± 1.1	.027 ± .009	.004 (11)	.12	...	...	...	...
V492E	7.7 ± 1.5	.011 ± .004	.001 (3)	.05	...	...	...	...
A503V	5.5 ± .03	.110 ± .018	.021 (60)	.50	1.04 ± .09	.037 ± .006	.035 (56)	.17
G504R	3.9 ± .07	.124 ± .020	.032 (91)	.56	.85 ± .12	.056 ± .009	.065 (103)	.25
G539R	4.5 ± 1.0	.073 ± .006	.016 (46)	.33	1.95 ± .27	.009 ± .002	.005 (8)	.04
L565P	5.9 ± .65	.067 ± .008	.011 (32)	.30	1.39 ± .16	.017 ± .005	.0120 (19)	.08
C569Y	9.3 ± 1.9	.094 ± .009	.010 (28)	.42	1.22 ± .15	.010 ± .012	.008 (13)	.05
V608F	3.5 ± .04	.099 ± .014	.028 (80)	.45	1.03 ± .17	.037 ± .012	.036 (57)	.17
R616X	4.7 ± .07	.008 ± .003	.002 (6)	.04	...	...	...	...
V631I	4.3 ± .06	.077 ± .008	.018 (51)	.34	1.32 ± .22	.033 ± .009	.025 (40)	.15
F646del	3.5 ± .07	.118 ± .011	.034 (97)	.53	1.77 ± .27	.051 ± .006	.029 (46)	.23

NOTE.—K_m values are in μM progesterone for 17α-hydroxylase and μM 17OH-pregnenolone for 17,20 lyase. V_{max} values are in pmol/μg P450c17/min. K_{cat} values were calculated on the basis of the molar content of P450c17, and, hence, the values are in min^{-1}. POR content of each membrane preparation was measured, and all samples were normalized against wild-type POR.

al. 1998; Auchus and Miller 1999; Pandey et al. 2003). Our previous studies of POR mutations (Flück et al. 2004) used a yeast system in which endogenous yeast POR is absent and human P450c17 and human POR are expressed in yeast from transiently transfected plasmids (Auchus et al. 1998). This system works well, but it does not permit direct assessment of the amount of POR present, and each transfection must be tediously assayed for P450c17 content to calculate meaningful enzymatic parameters. In the present study, we modified this system by using yeast-expressed human P450c17, combined in vitro with human N-27 POR, prepared from *E. coli*. By comparing the enzymatic parameters (K_m and V_{max}) obtained for the wild type and for five different POR missense mutants (A287P, R457H, V492E, C569Y, and V608F) assessed in the double-transfected yeast system (Flück et al. 2004) with those obtained with the in vitro fused-membrane system (present study), we see that both systems give similar values for K_m and that the present system yields slightly lower values for V_{max}. Because the present system permits quantitation of all relevant variables, we consider these values to be a more reliable approximation of actual POR activity. Nevertheless, actual activity in vivo may vary as a result of other unknown intracellular factors.

The surface of the electron-donating (FMN) domain of POR is characterized by acidic residues (Shen and Kasper 1995; Estabrook et al. 1996; Wang et al. 1997), whereas the redox-partner-binding site of microsomal P450 enzymes is typically characterized by basic residues (Hasemann et al. 1995; Fisher et al. 1996; Geller et al. 1997; Auchus and Miller 1999; Kondo et al. 1999; Davydov et al. 2000). Thus, electrostatic interactions between oppositely charged residues are obviously important in governing the association of POR with a P450 enzyme. Consistent with this, mutation of arginine residues in the POR-binding site of P450c17 selectively ablates 17,20 lyase activity (Geller et al. 1997, 1999), and chemical modification of acidic residues in the FMN site of POR similarly reduces the activity of P450 (Nadler and Strobel 1988, 1991; Shen and Kasper 1995). In addition, hydrophobic interactions between POR and P450 also play a role (Strobel et al. 1989). The activities assessed in different studies are a function of the specific P450 enzyme used as the readout of the POR activity and are also a function of the form of POR used. Both the full-length POR used in our previous studies (Flück et al. 2004) and the N-27 human POR used here remain associated with membranes and are able to support the reduction of a cytochrome P450. By contrast, when rat

POR or human POR is rendered wholly soluble by deleting 54 N-terminal residues, it can still reduce cytochrome c (which is not a physiological substrate for POR), but it cannot reduce P450 (Lu et al. 1969; Roman et al. 2003). Human, rat, and *Xenopus* PORs have a long hydrophobic domain following the strongly basic sequence RKKK (residues 48–51) that resembles a transmembrane domain (von Heijne 1984), but this sequence is not found in *Drosophila* or yeast POR (fig. 4). Thus, reliable measurements of POR activity require the use of a membrane-bound form of POR and a sensitive P450-based enzymatic readout.

Structure/Function Correlation of POR Mutants

The mutations examined in this study provide reasonable scanning mutagenesis of POR. Human POR shares highly conserved binding domains for FMN, FAD, and NADPH with the PORs of other species (fig. 4), and the FAD- and NADPH-binding domains are also similar to the FAD- and NADPH-binding domains of ferredoxin reductase (Hanukoglu and Gutfinger 1989; Karplus et al. 1991) and nitric oxide synthase (Bredt et al. 1991). By analogy with the crystallographically determined structure of rat POR (Wang et al. 1997), residues 143–147 and 173–185 of human POR participate in binding the isoalloxazine ring of FMN, with the side chain of Y181 stabilizing the interaction with the flavin. Replacing the rat POR residue Y178 (human Y181) with Asp eliminated 99% of its activity to reduce cytochrome c (Shen et al. 1989), and the corresponding human Y181D mutation caused ABS (Arlt et al. 2004) and reduced activities toward cytochrome c (table 5) and P450c17 (table 6) to undetectable levels. The mutation Q153R, which is near the FMN-binding site, reduced POR activity to ~30% (table 5). The highly conserved domain that interacts with and donates electrons to the cytochrome P450 comprises residues 194–231, especially residues 178–185 and 210–214 (DDDGN) (Wang et al. 1997) (fig. 4). We found no mutations in this domain; the closest mutations were M263V, which lost ~90% of activity, and A287P, the mutation commonly found in patients of European ancestry, which lost 60%–80% of activity (table 6). The RY sequence of residues 316–317 is conserved from yeast to human POR, suggesting an important function (fig. 4), yet the nonconservative mutant R316W was found as a polymorphism in a database and retained normal activity, as did the conservative polymorphism G413S (table 6). Thus, the activities of each mutant or polymorphism must be tested experimentally to determine the degree of impairment.

The FAD-binding domain (residues 453–495) is highly conserved, and the sequence RYYSI (457–461) is invariant among human, rat, *Xenopus, Drosophila,* and yeast POR (fig. 4). X-ray crystallography shows that rat R454 (human R457) forms a hydrogen bond with the pyrophosphate group of FAD and that rat Y456 (human Y459) contacts the FAD isoalloxazine ring and hydrogen bonds with the ribityl 3′-hydroxyl group (Wang et al. 1997; Shen and Kasper 2000). Mutation of each of these residues caused ABS and ablated virtually all measurable activity. Similar results were obtained when these mutations were studied in rat POR (Shen and Kasper 1996, 2000; Shen et al. 1999). Residues 491–497, which lie in helix N, form hydrogen bonds with the FAD pyrophosphate (Wang et al. 1997). The mutation V492E is predicted to disrupt this hydrogen bonding; this mutation causes ABS and is virtually devoid of activity. By contrast, the conservative change A503V and the nonconservative change G504R lie in an unstructured loop, were identified as polymorphisms, and retain >50% activity (table 6).

The NADPH-binding domain comprising the carboxy-terminus of the protein is highly conserved (fig. 4)—especially the sequence GTGVAP (residues 537–542), which contains the consensus GXG sequence typical of $NADP^+$-binding proteins (Hanukoglu and Gutfinger 1989; Scrutton et al. 1990). The mutation G539R lost >90% activity in the 17,20 lyase assay but retained 46% activity in the 17α-hydroxylase assay, indicating that the mutant could still bind some NADPH. Consistent with this, the cytochrome c assays showed that the greatest effect was on NADPH oxidation, for which the K_m value was increased ~100-fold (table 5). Studies in which C569 of human POR was alkylated with iodoacetic acid eliminated activity, implicating a role for cysteine in the binding of NADPH to human POR (Haniu et al. 1989), but mutagenesis of the corresponding C566 to S in rat POR suggested that this residue was not essential, despite a 4.6-fold higher K_m value for NADPH (Shen et al. 1991); alkylation of pig POR did not change activity (Haniu et al. 1984). The mutation C569Y in human POR, which we previously found in a patient with disordered steroidogenesis but without ABS (Flück et al. 2004), also had a high K_m value for NADPH (table 5) but retained 13% of 17,20 lyase activity and 28% of 17α-hydroxylase activity (table 6). The C569Y mutation was found as a compound heterozygote with V608F (Flück et al. 2004), which retained 57% of 17,20 lyase activity and 80% of 17α-hydroxylase activity, thus explaining that individual's hormonal profile, which resembled isolated 17,20 lyase deficiency. The crystallographic data indicated that rat W677 (human W679) directly participates in interactions with both FMN and NADPH, suggesting that any carboxy-terminal truncation will have severe consequences. Consistent with this, the premature chain truncation mutant R616X was devoid of activity. The mutations A115V and V631I were detected as heterozygotes only in individuals with normal steroidogenesis,

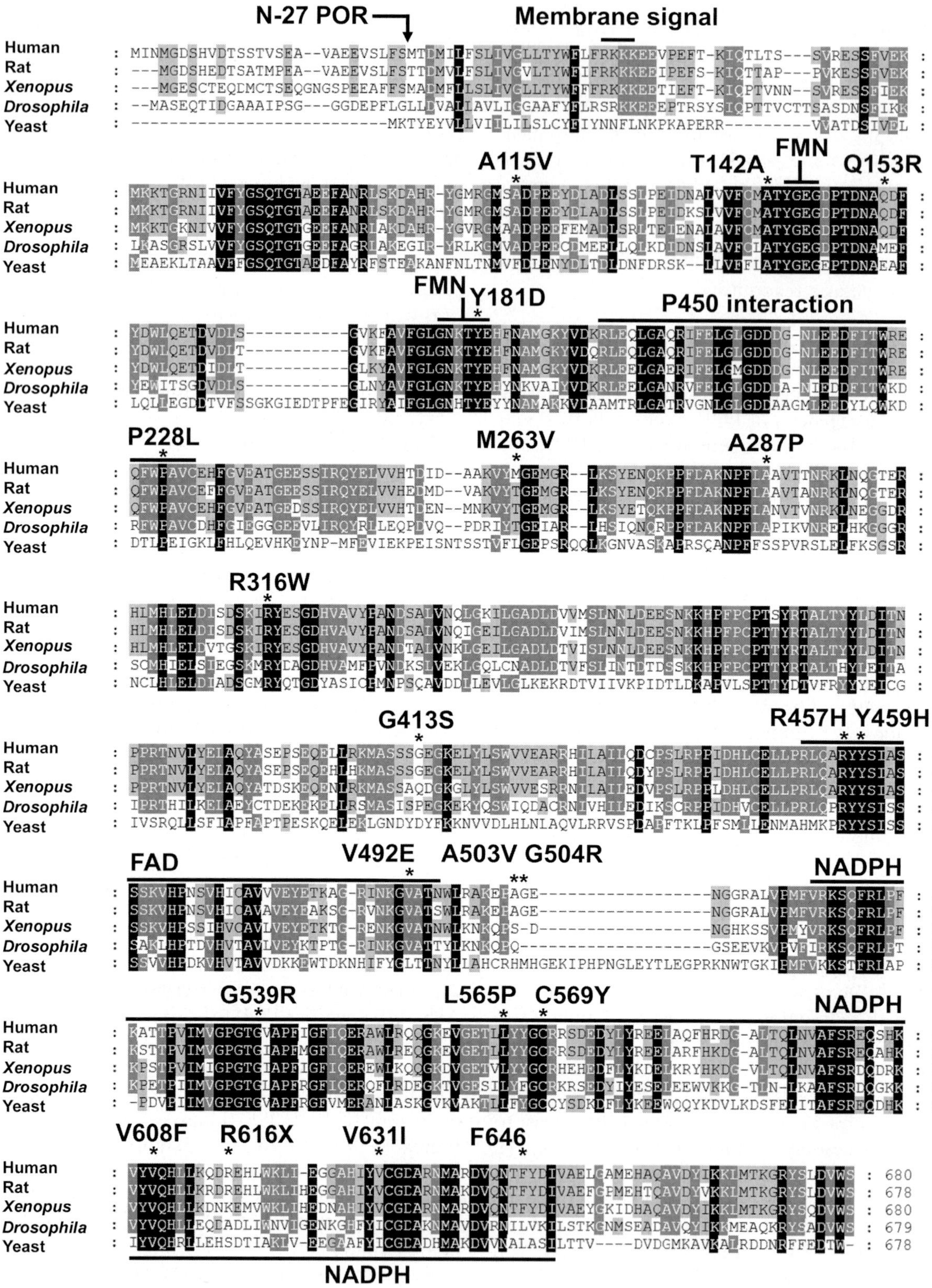

Figure 4 Amino acid sequence alignment of POR from five species. The protein sequences used are those of human (NCBI accession number NP_000932.1), rat (NCBI accession number NP_113764.1), *Xenopus* (NCBI accession number AAH59318.1), yeast (NCBI accession number NP_596046.1) and *Drosophila* (NCBI accession number NP_477158.1). Alignments were made with ClustalW and are displayed with GeneDoc. Residues that are identical in all species (when the residue exists) are highlighted in black, those identical in four of five species are shown in dark gray, and those identical in three of five species are shown in light gray. Amino acid numbers are shown at the right. Note that the human POR sequence has a three-residue amino-terminal extension. The functional domains and individual residues discussed in the text are shown above the human sequence. The location of the truncation used to create the N-27 POR used in the functional assays is shown.

and hence they may be polymorphisms. A115V is a conservative change in a region without apparent function, and it retained full activity with P450c17 (table 6). Although the conservative mutant V631I lies in a highly conserved segment of the NADPH-binding domain, it retained normal activity in the cytochrome c assays (table 5) and 40%–50% of activity in the P450c17 assays. Finally, the in-frame deletion of F646, a residue for which the crystal structure of rat POR does not ascribe a specific function, had no effect on 17α-hydroxylase activity but caused a 54% reduction in 17,20 lyase activity. As POR must interact with all 50 human microsomal P450 enzymes and as the stereochemistry of those interactions with different P450 enzymes will vary with the geometry of the redox-partner-binding site of P450, it is clear that no assay that is based on a single P450 enzyme will reliably forecast all the consequences of a specific POR mutant.

Nosology of ABS and POR Deficiency

ABS was initially described as a skeletal malformation syndrome (Antley and Bixler 1975; DeLozier et al. 1980; Hassell and Butler 1994); descriptions of genital ambiguity were added later, as a finding described in about half of these patients (Crisponi et al. 1997). In contrast to the autosomal dominant craniosynostosis syndromes caused by *FGFR* mutations, reports of ABS in siblings and in children of consanguineous parents have suggested autosomal recessive inheritance (Reardon et al. 2000). The finding of mutations in receptors for fibroblast growth factors, especially FGFR2, in other craniosynostosis syndromes led to the successful search for *FGFR2* mutations in some patients with ABS. These eponymic syndromes resulting from *FGFR2* mutations may be regarded as presenting variants of a single disease, as single genotypes often give somewhat varied phenotypes. Reardon et al. (2000) called attention to ambiguous genitalia and/or disordered sterol metabolism as the major feature that appeared to distinguish patients with ABS resulting from *FGFR2* mutations from patients with ABS who lacked *FGFR2* mutations. We recently reported that three such patients, plus another patient without ABS, carried autosomal recessive mutations in *POR,* and we provided biochemical and enzymologic support for this observation (Flück et al. 2004). We have now confirmed and expanded that original study by sequencing *POR* in 32 patients, including 12 of the 16 patients studied by Reardon et al. (2000). Reardon et al. (2000) had suggested that ABS with abnormal genitalia was digenic, resulting from mutations in an *FGFR2* gene plus a mutation elsewhere. Although we failed to find mutations in 3 of the 32 patients, we found complete genetic segregation of *POR* and *FGFR* mutations in patients with the ABS phenotype. Thus, digenic inheritance appears to be most unlikely, but it cannot be completely excluded, as not all *FGFR* exons were sequenced.

Patients with ABS with disordered steroidogenesis have been born to mothers who became virilized during gestation and, hence, were thought to have luteomas of pregnancy (Roth et al. 2000; Warmann et al. 2000); it is more likely that these cases reflect feto-placental hyperandrogenism resulting from decreased activity of POR-dependent aromatase (P450aro), which converts androgens to estrogens, as described in our initial study (Flück et al. 2004). Alternatively, it has been suggested that increased androgen synthesis through an alternative "backdoor" pathway (Auchus 2004) may result in the virilization of mothers carrying a POR-deficient fetus (Arlt et al. 2004), but definitive data are lacking. It is noteworthy that, aside from the genital ambiguity, no dysmorphologic feature distinguishes ABS secondary to *FGFR2* mutations from ABS secondary to *POR* mutations; thus, this distinction requires careful hormonal evaluation of adrenal steroidogenesis.

Thus, we propose that the term "ABS" be reserved for those patients with the skeletal dysmorphologic findings initially reported by Antley and Bixler (1975) but who have normal genitalia and normal steroidogenesis, and that patients with the skeletal dysmorphologic phenotype plus evidence of disordered steroidogenesis be referred to as having "POR deficiency." It is clinically important to view patients with *POR* mutations as having a disease that is distinctly different from the disease caused by *FGFR* mutations. Not only are the genes and patterns of inheritance different (dominant *FGFR* mutations vs. recessive *POR* mutations), but the patients are also vulnerable to different risk factors and require different management and different teams of physicians. Several of the patients with *POR* mutations died unexpectedly without clear explanation, and Reardon et al. (2000) noted that several patients required steroid hormone supplementation. Now that the steroidogenic defect is understood, it is apparent that patients with *POR* mutations may be at risk for adrenal insufficiency and Addisonian crisis, especially at times of severe febrile illness or major surgery. Thus, any patient thought to have ABS should be evaluated by a pediatric endocrinologist for the ability to mount an adequate cortisol response to stress, as well as for the adrenal and gonadal pattern of synthesis of C21 and C19 steroids.

The mechanism(s) by which POR deficiency causes a skeletal disorder resembling ABS remains unclear. Substantial speculation has centered on cholesterol, as some disorders of cholesterol biosynthesis include disorders of skeletal development (Herman 2003). Cholesterol biosynthesis requires two POR-dependent enzymes: squalene epoxidase, a non-P450 enzyme (Ono and Bloch 1975), and lanosterol demethylase (CYP51). Furthermore, cholesterol is required for C-terminal modification of hedgehog proteins, which play multiple roles in morphogenesis (Mann and Beachy 2004). Clinical reports have associated ABS with maternal ingestion of fluconazole, an antifungal agent that acts by preferentially inhibiting yeast CYP51 (Pursley et al. 1996; Aleck and Bartley 1997). Lymphoblastoid cells from a patient having ABS and ambiguous genitalia accumulated lanosterol and dihydrolanosterol, consistent with a lesion in CYP51, but the *CYP51* gene was normal (Kelley et al. 2002). We subsequently found that this individual was homozygous for the *POR* mutation A287P (Flück et al. 2004). Although fluconazole should not inhibit human CYP51, the absence of POR-dependent hepatic enzymes that normally metabolize fluconazole might permit fetal concentrations to rise substantially. However, liver-specific knockout of *Por* yields morphologically normal mice (Henderson et al. 2003; Wu et al. 2003), whereas the global *Por*-knockout mouse is embryonic lethal (Shen et al. 2002; Otto et al. 2003). Thus, the absence of a hepatic P450 activity appears to be unrelated to the dysmorphology of POR deficiency in mouse. Similarly, Otto et al. (2003) suggested that the phenotype might be associated with decreased activity of CYP26, which degrades retinoids; decreasing the retinoic acid in the diets of pregnant mice carrying *Por*-knockout fetuses partially ameliorated the phenotype. However, as CYP26 is also a hepatic enzyme, the answer would appear to lie elsewhere. We speculate that the dysmorphology in POR deficiency is associated with a decrease in one of the numerous extrahepatic enzymes that require electron transfer from POR.

Acknowledgments

This study is dedicated to the memory of Professor Robin M. Winter, who played a central role in associating *FGFR* mutations and craniosynostosis syndromes. This work was supported by the National Institutes of Health (NIH) Mentored Investigator Grant KO1 DK02939 (to N.H.) and by NIH grants RO1 DK37922, RO1 HD41958, and RO1 GM73020 (to W.L.M.). E.W.J. was supported by NIH grants P60 DE013078 and M01 RR00052. We thank Dr. Jacky Bonaventure and Dr. Martine LeMerrer (Hôpital Necker, Paris), Dr. Marie Gonzalez (Hôpital St. Antoine, Paris), and Dr. Kazuki Okajima (Case Western Reserve University, Cleveland), for contributing DNA samples and clinical information; Dr. Richard Kelly, for growing lymphoblastoid cell lines from several patients; Ms. Izabella Damm, for excellent technical assistance; and all the patients and families who participated in this study.

Electronic-Database Information

Accession numbers and URLs for data presented herein are as follows:

Berkeley *Drosophila* Genome Project, http://www.fruitfly.org/seq_tools/splice.html (for the program NNSplice)
BioVentures, http://www.bioventures.com/products/dmg/por/ (for *POR* gene polymorphism data)
Centre National de la Recherche Scientifique Marseilles Group in Enzyme Kinetics and Control Analysis, http://bip.cnrs-mrs.fr/bip10/homepage.htm (for the program LEONORA)
ClustalW, http://www.ebi.ac.uk/clustalw/index.html
DeepView, http://www.expasy.org/spdbv/
GeneDoc, http://www.psc.edu/biomed/genedoc
GROMOS Home Page, http://igc.ethz.ch/gromos/ (for the program GROMOS96)
International HapMap Project, http://www.hapmap.org/cgi-perl/gbrowse/gbrowse/hapmap
MODELLER, http://salilab.org/modeller/modeller.html
National Center for Biotechnology Information (NCBI), http://www.ncbi.nlm.nih.gov/ (for human *POR* gene sequence [accession number NC_000007], human *POR* cDNA sequence [accession number NM_000941.1], human POR protein sequence [accession number NP_000932.1], rat POR protein sequence [accession number NP_113764.1], *Xenopus* POR protein sequence [accession number AAH59318.1], yeast POR protein sequence [accession number NP_596046.1], *Drosophila* POR protein sequence [accession number NP_477158.1], mRNA, and SNPs)
Online Mendelian Inheritance in Man (OMIM), http://www.ncbi.nlm.nih.gov/Omim/ (for ABS)
Persistence of Vision Raytracer, http://www.povray.org/ (for the program POVRAY)
Softberry, http://www.softberry.com/berry.phtml?topic=fsplice&group=programs&subgroup=gfind (for the program FSPLICE)
Softgenetics, http://www.softgenetics.com (for the program Mutation Surveyor)
University of California Santa Cruz (UCSC) Genome Browser, http://genome.ucsc.edu/ (for SNP information)

References

Adachi M, Tachibana K, Asakura Y, Yamamoto T, Hanaki K, Oka A (2004) Compound heterozygous mutations of cytochrome P450 oxidoreductase gene (POR) in two patients with Antley-Bixler syndrome. Am J Med Genet A 128A: 333–339
Aleck KA, Bartley DL (1997) Multiple malformation syndrome following fluconazole use in pregnancy: report of an additional patient. Am J Med Genet 72:253–256
Antley R, Bixler D (1975) Trapezoidocephaly, midfacial hypoplasia and cartilage abnormalities with multiple synostoses and skeletal fractures. Birth Defects Orig Artic Ser 11: 397–401
Arlt W, Auchus RJ, Miller WL (2001) Thiazolidinediones but not metformin directly inhibit the steroidogenic enzymes P450c17 and 3β-hydroxysteroid dehydrogenase. J Biol Chem 276:16767–16771
Arlt W, Walker EA, Draper N, Ivison HE, Ride JP, Hammer F, Chalder SM, Borucka-Mankiewicz M, Hauffa BP, Malunowicz EM, Stewart PM, Shackleton CH (2004) Congenital adrenal hyperplasia caused by mutant P450 oxidoreductase and human androgen synthesis: analytical study. Lancet 363: 2128–2135
Auchus RJ (2004) The backdoor pathway to dihydrotestosterone. Trends Endocrinol Metab 15:432–438

Auchus RJ, Lee TC, Miller WL (1998) Cytochrome b5 augments the 17,20-lyase activity of human P450c17 without direct electron transfer. J Biol Chem 273:3158–3165

Auchus RJ, Miller WL (1999) Molecular modeling of human P450c17 (17α-hydroxylase/17,20-lyase): insights into reaction mechanisms and effects of mutations. Mol Endocrinol 13:1169–1182

Augarten A, Pariente C, Gazit E, Chayen R, Goldfarb H, Sack J (1992) Ambiguous genitalia due to partial activity of cytochromes P450c17 and P450c21. J Steroid Biochem Mol Biol 41:37–41

Bredt DS, Hwang PM, Glatt CE, Lowenstein C, Reed RR, Snyder SH (1991) Cloned and expressed nitric oxide synthase structurally resembles cytochrome P-450 reductase. Nature 351:714–718

Chun K, Siegel-Bartelt J, Chitayat D, Phillips J, Ray PN (1998) FGFR2 mutation associated with clinical manifestations consistent with Antley-Bixler syndrome. Am J Med Genet 77:219–224

Cornish-Bowden A (1995) Analysis of enzyme kinetic data. Oxford University Press, Oxford, United Kingdom

Crisponi G, Porcu C, Piu ME (1997) Antley-Bixler syndrome: case report and review of the literature. Clin Dysmorphol 6:61–68

Davydov DR, Kariakin AA, Petushkova NA, Peterson JA (2000) Association of cytochromes P450 with their reductases: opposite sign of the electrostatic interactions in P450BM-3 as compared with the microsomal 2B4 system. Biochemistry 39:6489–6497

DeLozier CD, Antley RM, Williams R, Green N, Heller RM, Bixler D, Engel E (1980) The syndrome of multisynostotic osteodysgenesis with long-bone fractures. Am J Med Genet 7:391–403

Dierks EA, Davis SC, Ortiz de Montellano PR (1998) Glu-320 and Asp-323 are determinants of the CYP4A1 hydroxylation regiospecificity and resistance to inactivation by 1-aminobenzotriazole. Biochemistry 37:1839–1847

Estabrook RW, Shet MS, Fisher CW, Jenkins CM, Waterman MR (1996) The interaction of NADPH-P450 reductase with P450: an electrochemical study of the role of the flavin mononucleotide-binding domain. Arch Biochem Biophys 333:308–315

Eswarakumar VP, Horowitz MC, Locklin R, Morriss-Kay GM, Lonai P (2004) A gain-of-function mutation of Fgfr2c demonstrates the roles of this receptor variant in osteogenesis. Proc Natl Acad Sci USA 101:12555–12560

Fiser A, Do RK, Sali A (2000) Modeling of loops in protein structures. Protein Sci 9:1753–1773

Fisher CW, Shet MS, Estabrook RW (1996) Construction of plasmids and expression in *Escherichia coli* of enzymatically active fusion proteins containing the heme-domain of a P450 linked to NADPH-P450 reductase. Methods Enzymol 272:15–25

Flück CE, Tajima T, Pandey AV, Arlt W, Okuhara K, Verge CF, Jabs EW, Mendonca BB, Fujieda K, Miller WL (2004) Mutant P450 oxidoreductase causes disordered steroidogenesis with and without Antley-Bixler syndrome. Nat Genet 36:228–230

Fukami M, Horikawa R, Nagai T, Tanaka T, Naiki Y, Sato N, Okuyama T, Nakai H, Soneda S, Tachibana K, Matsuo N, Sato S, Homma K, Nishimura G, Hasegawa T, Ogata T (2005) Cytochrome P450 oxidoreductase gene mutations and Antley-Bixler syndrome with abnormal genitalia and/or impaired steroidogenesis: molecular and clinical studies in 10 patients. J Clin Endocrinol Metab 90:414–426

Geller DH, Auchus RJ, Mendonca BB, Miller WL (1997) The genetic and functional basis of isolated 17,20-lyase deficiency. Nat Genet 17:201–205

Geller DH, Auchus RJ, Miller WL (1999) P450c17 mutations R347H and R358Q selectively disrupt 17,20-lyase activity by disrupting interactions with P450 oxidoreductase and cytochrome b5. Mol Endocrinol 13:167–175

Gorry MC, Preston RA, White GJ, Zhang Y, Singhal VK, Losken HW, Parker MG, Nwokoro NA, Post JC, Ehrlich GD (1995) Crouzon syndrome: mutations in two spliceoforms of FGFR2 and a common point mutation shared with Jackson-Weiss syndrome. Hum Mol Genet 4:1387–1390

Gripp KW, Stolle CA, McDonald-McGinn DM, Markowitz RI, Bartlett SP, Katowitz JA, Muenke M, Zackai EH (1998) Phenotype of the fibroblast growth factor receptor 2 Ser351Cys mutation: Pfeiffer syndrome type III. Am J Med Genet 78:356–360

Gu J, Weng Y, Zhang QY, Cui H, Behr M, Wu L, Yang W, Zhang L, Ding X (2003) Liver-specific deletion of the NADPH-cytochrome P450 reductase gene: impact on plasma cholesterol homeostasis and the function and regulation of microsomal cytochrome P450 and heme oxygenase. J Biol Chem 278:25895–25901

Guengerich FP (2004) Cytochrome P450: what have we learned and what are the future issues? Drug Metab Rev 36:159–197

Guex N, Peitsch MC (1997) SWISS-MODEL and the Swiss-PdbViewer: an environment for comparative protein modeling. Electrophoresis 18:2714–2723

Haniu M, Iyanagi T, Legesse K, Shively JE (1984) Structural analysis of NADPH-cytochrome P-450 reductase from porcine hepatic microsomes: sequences of proteolytic fragments, cysteine-containing peptides, and a NADPH-protected cysteine peptide. J Biol Chem 259:13703–13711

Haniu M, McManus ME, Birkett DJ, Lee TD, Shively JE (1989) Structural and functional analysis of NADPH-cytochrome P-450 reductase from human liver: complete sequence of human enzyme and NADPH-binding sites. Biochemistry 28:8639–8645

Hanukoglu I, Gutfinger T (1989) cDNA sequence of adrenodoxin reductase: identification of NADP-binding sites in oxidoreductases. Eur J Biochem 180:479–484

Hasemann CA, Kurumbail RG, Boddupalli SS, Peterson JA, Deisenhofer J (1995) Structure and function of cytochromes P450: a comparative analysis of three crystal structures. Structure 3:41–62

Hassell S, Butler MG (1994) Antley-Bixler syndrome: report of a patient and review of literature. Clin Genet 46:372–376

Henderson CJ, Otto DM, Carrie D, Magnuson MA, McLaren AW, Rosewell I, Wolf CR (2003) Inactivation of the hepatic cytochrome P450 system by conditional deletion of hepatic cytochrome P450 reductase. J Biol Chem 278:13480–13486

Herman GE (2003) Disorders of cholesterol biosynthesis: prototypic metabolic malformation syndromes. Hum Mol Genet 12:R75–R88

Hurley ME, White MJ, Green AJ, Kelleher J (2004) Antley-

Bixler syndrome with radioulnar synostosis. Pediatr Radiol 34:148–151

Jabs EW, Li X, Scott AF, Meyers G, Chen W, Eccles M, Mao JI, Charnas LR, Jackson CE, Jaye M (1994) Jackson-Weiss and Crouzon syndromes are allelic with mutations in fibroblast growth factor receptor 2. Nat Genet 8:275–279

Karplus PA, Daniels MJ, Herriott JR (1991) Atomic structure of ferredoxin-NADP+ reductase: prototype for a structurally novel flavoenzyme family. Science 251:60–66

Kelley RI, Kratz LE, Glaser RL, Netzloff ML, Wolf LM, Jabs EW (2002) Abnormal sterol metabolism in a patient with Antley-Bixler syndrome and ambiguous genitalia. Am J Med Genet 110:95–102

Kondo S, Sakaki T, Ohkawa H, Inouye K (1999) Electrostatic interaction between cytochrome P450 and NADPH-P450 reductase: comparison of mixed and fused systems consisting of rat cytochrome P450 1A1 and yeast NADPH-P450 reductase. Biochem Biophys Res Commun 257:273–278

Kress W, Petersen B, Collmann H, Grimm T (2000) An unusual FGFR1 mutation (fibroblast growth factor receptor 1 mutation) in a girl with non-syndromic trigonocephaly. Cytogenet Cell Genet 91:138–140

Kumar D, Masel JP (1997) A new multiple malformation syndrome of Mullerian dysgenesis and conductive hearing loss with facial hypoplasia, bilateral forearm deformity, brachydactyly, spinal stenosis and scoliosis. Clin Genet 52:30–36

Lin D, Black SM, Nagahama Y, Miller WL (1993) Steroid 17α-hydroxylase and 17,20-lyase activities of P450c17: contributions of serine106 and P450 reductase. Endocrinology 132:2498–2506

Lin D, Harikrishna JA, Moore CCD, Jones KL, Miller WL (1991) Missense mutation serine106 proline causes 17 α-hydroxylase deficiency. J Biol Chem 266:15992–15998

Lu AY, Junk KW, Coon MJ (1969) Resolution of the cytochrome P-450-containing ω-hydroxylation system of liver microsomes into three components. J Biol Chem 244:3714–3721

Mann RK, Beachy PA (2004) Novel lipid modifications of secreted protein signals. Annu Rev Biochem 73:891–923

Meyers GA, Day D, Goldberg R, Daentl DL, Przylepa KA, Abrams LJ, Graham JM Jr, Feingold M, Moeschler JB, Rawnsley E, Scott AF, Jabs EW (1996) FGFR2 exon IIIa and IIIc mutations in Crouzon, Jackson-Weiss, and Pfeiffer syndromes: evidence for missense changes, insertions, and a deletion due to alternative RNA splicing. Am J Hum Genet 58:491–498

Miller WL (1986) Congenital adrenal hyperplasia. N Engl J Med 314:1321–1322

——— (1994) Clinical review 54: genetics, diagnosis, and management of 21-hydroxylase deficiency. J Clin Endocrinol Metab 78:241–246

——— (2004) P450 oxidoreductase deficiency: a new disorder of steroidogenesis with multiple clinical manifestations. Trends Endocrinol Metab 15:311–315

Miroux B, Walker JE (1996) Over-production of proteins in *Escherichia coli:* mutant hosts that allow synthesis of some membrane proteins and globular proteins at high levels. J Mol Biol 260:289–298

Muenke M, Schell U, Hehr A, Robin NH, Losken HW, Schinzel A, Pulleyn LJ, Rutland P, Reardon W, Malcolm S, Winter RM (1994) A common mutation in the fibroblast growth factor receptor 1 gene in Pfeiffer syndrome. Nat Genet 8:269–274

Mulrooney SB, Waskell L (2000) High-level expression in *Escherichia coli* and purification of the membrane-bound form of cytochrome b(5). Protein Expr Purif 19:173–178

Nadler SG, Strobel HW (1988) Role of electrostatic interactions in the reaction of NADPH-cytochrome P-450 reductase with cytochromes P-450. Arch Biochem Biophys 261:418–429

——— (1991) Identification and characterization of an NADPH-cytochrome P450 reductase derived peptide involved in binding to cytochrome P450. Arch Biochem Biophys 290:277–284

Okajima K, Robinson LK, Hart MA, Abuelo DN, Cowan LS, Hasegawa T, Maumenee IH, Jabs EW (1999) Ocular anterior chamber dysgenesis in craniosynostosis syndromes with a fibroblast growth factor receptor 2 mutation. Am J Med Genet 85:160–170

Omura T, Sato R (1964) The carbon monoxide-binding pigment of liver microsomes. I. Evidence for its hemoprotein nature. J Biol Chem 239:2370–2378

Ono T, Bloch K (1975) Solubilization and partial characterization of rat liver squalene epoxidase. J Biol Chem 250:1571–1579

Otto DM, Henderson CJ, Carrie D, Davey M, Gundersen TE, Blomhoff R, Adams RH, Tickle C, Wolf CR (2003) Identification of novel roles of the cytochrome P450 system in early embryogenesis: effects on vasculogenesis and retinoic acid homeostasis. Mol Cell Biol 23:6103–6116

Pandey AV, Mellon SH, Miller WL (2003) Protein phosphatase 2A and phosphoprotein SET regulate androgen production by P450c17. J Biol Chem 278:2837–2844

Park WJ, Meyers GA, Li X, Theda C, Day D, Orlow SJ, Jones MC, Jabs EW (1995*a*) Novel FGFR2 mutations in Crouzon and Jackson-Weiss syndromes show allelic heterogeneity and phenotypic variability. Hum Mol Genet 4:1229–1233

Park WJ, Theda C, Maestri NE, Meyers GA, Fryburg JS, Dufresne C, Cohen MM Jr, Jabs EW (1995*b*) Analysis of phenotypic features and FGFR2 mutations in Apert syndrome. Am J Hum Genet 57:321–328

Peterson RE, Imperato-McGinley J, Gautier T, Shackleton CHL (1985) Male pseudohermaphroditism due to multiple defects in steroid-biosynthetic microsomal mixed-function oxidases: a new variant of congenital adrenal hyperplasia. N Engl J Med 313:1182–1191

Pompon D, Perret A, Bellamine A, Laine R, Gautier JC, Urban P (1995) Genetically engineered yeast cells and their applications. Toxicol Lett 82–83:815–822

Przylepa KA, Paznekas W, Zhang M, Golabi M, Bias W, Bamshad MJ, Carey JC, Hall BD, Stevenson R, Orlow S, Cohen MM Jr, Jabs EW (1996) Fibroblast growth factor receptor 2 mutations in Beare-Stevenson cutis gyrata syndrome. Nat Genet 13:492–494

Pulleyn LJ, Reardon W, Wilkes D, Rutland P, Jones BM, Hayward R, Hall CM, Brueton L, Chun N, Lammer E, Malcolm S, Winter RM (1996) Spectrum of craniosynostosis phenotypes associated with novel mutations at the fibroblast growth factor receptor 2 locus. Eur J Hum Genet 4:283–291

Pursley TJ, Blomquist IK, Abraham J, Andersen HF, Bartley JA (1996) Fluconazole-induced congenital anomalies in three infants. Clin Infect Dis 22:336–340

Reardon W, Smith A, Honour JW, Hindmarsh P, Das D,

Rumsby G, Nelson I, Malcolm S, Ades L, Sillence D, Kumar D, DeLozier-Blanchet C, McKee S, Kelly T, McKeehan WL, Baraitser M, Winter RM (2000) Evidence for digenic inheritance in some cases of Antley-Bixler syndrome? J Med Genet 37:26–32

Reardon W, Winter RM, Rutland P, Pulleyn LJ, Jones BM, Malcolm S (1994) Mutations in the fibroblast growth factor receptor 2 gene cause Crouzon syndrome. Nat Genet 8:98–103

Roman LJ, McLain J, Masters BSS (2003) Chimeric enzymes of cytochrome P450 oxidoreductase and neuronal nitric-oxide synthase reductase domain reveal structural and functional differences. J Biol Chem 278:25700–25707

Roth C, Hinney B, Peter M, Steinberger D, Lakomek M (2000) Features of Antley-Bixler syndrome in an infant born to a mother with pregnancy luteoma. Eur J Pediatr 159:189–192

Sali A, Blundell TL (1993) Comparative protein modelling by satisfaction of spatial restraints. J Mol Biol 234:779–815

Schell U, Hehr A, Feldman GJ, Robin NH, Zackai EH, de Die-Smulders C, Viskochil DH, Stewart JM, Wolff G, Ohashi H, Price RA, Cohen MM, Muenke M (1995) Mutations in FGFR1 and FGFR2 cause familial and sporadic Pfeiffer syndrome. Hum Mol Genet 4:323–328

Scrutton NS, Berry A, Perham RN (1990) Redesign of the coenzyme specificity of a dehydrogenase by protein engineering. Nature 343:38–43

Shen AL, Christensen MJ, Kasper CB (1991) NADPH-cytochrome P-450 oxidoreductase: the role of cysteine 566 in catalysis and cofactor binding. J Biol Chem 266:19976–19980

Shen AL, Kasper CB (1995) Role of acidic residues in the interaction of NADPH-cytochrome P450 oxidoreductase with cytochrome P450 and cytochrome c. J Biol Chem 270:27475–27480

——— (1996) Role of Ser457 of NADPH-cytochrome P450 oxidoreductase in catalysis and control of FAD oxidation-reduction potential. Biochemistry 35:9451–9459

——— (2000) Differential contributions of NADPH-cytochrome P450 oxidoreductase FAD binding site residues to flavin binding and catalysis. J Biol Chem 275:41087–41091

Shen AL, O'Leary KA, Kasper CB (2002) Association of multiple developmental defects and embryonic lethality with loss of microsomal NADPH-cytochrome P450 oxidoreductase. J Biol Chem 277:6536–6541

Shen AL, Porter TD, Wilson TE, Kasper CB (1989) Structural analysis of the FMN binding domain of NADPH-cytochrome P-450 oxidoreductase by site-directed mutagenesis. J Biol Chem 264:7584–7589

Shen AL, Sem DS, Kasper CB (1999) Mechanistic studies on the reductive half-reaction of NADPH-cytochrome P450 oxidoreductase. J Biol Chem 274:5391–5398

Strobel HW, Nadler SG, Nelson DR (1989) Cytochrome P-450: cytochrome P-450 reductase interactions. Drug Metab Rev 20:519–533

Thompson JD, Higgins DG, Gibson TJ (1994) CLUSTAL W: improving the sensitivity of progressive multiple sequence alignment through sequence weighting, position-specific gap penalties and weight matrix choice. Nucleic Acids Res 22:4673–4680

Van GB, Slater EC (1962) The extinction coefficient of cytochrome c. Biochim Biophys Acta 58:593–595

von Heijne G (1984) Analysis of the distribution of charged residues in the N-terminal region of signal sequences: implications for protein export in prokaryotic and eukaryotic cells. EMBO J 3:2315–2318

Wang M, Roberts DL, Paschke R, Shea TM, Masters BSS, Kim JJ (1997) Three-dimensional structure of NADPH-cytochrome P450 reductase: prototype for FMN- and FAD-containing enzymes. Proc Natl Acad Sci USA 94:8411–8416

Warmann S, Roth C, Glüer S, Fuchs J (2000) Congenital adrenal hyperplasia associated with maternal pregnancy luteoma and the Antley-Bixler syndrome. J Pediatr Surg 35:528–530

Wilkie AO, Slaney SF, Oldridge M, Poole MD, Ashworth GJ, Hockley AD, Hayward RD, David DJ, Pulleyn LJ, Rutland P, Malcolm S, Winter RM, Reardon W (1995) Apert syndrome results from localized mutations of FGFR2 and is allelic with Crouzon syndrome. Nat Genet 9:165–172

Wu L, Gu J, Cui H, Zhang QY, Behr M, Fang C, Weng Y, Kluetzman K, Swiatek PJ, Yang W, Kaminsky L, Ding X (2005) Transgenic mice with a hypomorphic NADPH-cytochrome P450 reductase gene: effects on development, reproduction, and microsomal cytochrome P450. J Pharmacol Exp Ther 312:35–43

Wu L, Gu J, Weng Y, Kluetzman K, Swiatek P, Behr M, Zhang QY, Zhuo X, Xie Q, Ding X (2003) Conditional knockout of the mouse NADPH-cytochrome P450 reductase gene. Genesis 36:177–181

Yanagibashi K, Hall PF (1986) Role of electron transport in the regulation of the lyase activity of C21 side-chain cleavage P-450 from porcine adrenal and testicular microsomes. J Biol Chem 261:8429–8433

Zhang LH, Rodriguez H, Ohno S, Miller WL (1995) Serine phosphorylation of human P450c17 increases 17,20-lyase activity: implications for adrenarche and the polycystic ovary syndrome. Proc Natl Acad Sci USA 92:10619–10623

Exon Array CGH: Detection of Copy-Number Changes at the Resolution of Individual Exons in the Human Genome

Pawandeep Dhami,[1] Alison J. Coffey,[1] Stephen Abbs,[3] Joris R. Vermeesch,[5] Jan P. Dumanski,[6] Karen J. Woodward,[4] Robert M. Andrews,[2] Cordelia Langford,[2] and David Vetrie[1]

[1]Human Genetics and [2]Microarray Facility, The Wellcome Trust Sanger Institute, Wellcome Trust Genome Campus, Hinxton, United Kingdom; [3]DNA Laboratory, Genetics Centre, Guy's and St. Thomas's National Health Service Foundation Trust, and [4]Clinical and Molecular Genetics, Institute of Child Health, London; [5]Center for Human Genetics and Department of Ophthalmology, University of Leuven, Leuven, Belgium; and [6]Department of Genetics and Pathology, Rudbeck Laboratory, Uppsala University, Uppsala, Sweden

The development of high-throughput screening methods such as array-based comparative genome hybridization (array CGH) allows screening of the human genome for copy-number changes. Current array CGH strategies have limits of resolution that make detection of small (less than a few tens of kilobases) gains or losses of genomic DNA difficult to identify. We report here a significant improvement in the resolution of array CGH, with the development of an array platform that utilizes single-stranded DNA array elements to accurately measure copy-number changes of individual exons in the human genome. Using this technology, we screened 31 patient samples across an array containing a total of 162 exons for five disease genes and detected copy-number changes, ranging from whole-gene deletions and duplications to single-exon deletions and duplications, in 100% of the cases. Our data demonstrate that it is possible to screen the human genome for copy-number changes with array CGH at a resolution that is 2 orders of magnitude higher than that previously reported.

Introduction

The extent to which genomic copy-number polymorphisms (CNPs) contribute to human genetic diversity is not known. Recent studies have demonstrated the presence of CNPs, a proportion of which encompass genes, in the genomes of normal individuals (Iafrate et al. 2004; Sebat et al. 2004). This suggests that these variants may be important in our understanding of phenotypic variation or may predispose to or directly cause disease. On the basis of current knowledge, ~5%–6% of gene mutations that are causative of inherited disorders are copy-number changes defined as gross deletions or duplications (Armour et al. 2002), although this frequency may represent an underestimate. These disease-causing copy-number changes can range in size from 100 bp to several megabases and can encompass as little as a single exon and as much as entire genes or several genes.

The ability to detect CNPs and pathogenic chromosomal imbalances has been dramatically improved through the use of array-based comparative genome hybridization (array CGH) (Solinas-Toldo et al. 1997; Pinkel et al. 1998). Array CGH offers high sensitivity and dynamic range to quantitatively measure from single copy-number losses or gains to high copy-number amplifications, as well as sufficient resolution and scalability for complete genomewide scans (Snijders et al. 2001; Fiegler et al. 2003; Vissers et al. 2003; Iafrate et al. 2004; Inazawa et al. 2004; Ishkanian et al. 2004). Currently, the most robust array CGH approaches utilize large genomic clone inserts as array elements but have a maximum resolution of ~40–50 kb (Albertson and Pinkel 2003; Snijders et al. 2003; Mantripragada et al. 2004*a*). The use of oligonucleotides (Lucito et al. 2000, 2003; Bignell et al. 2004; Carvalho et al. 2004; Sebat et al. 2004), cDNA clones (Pollack et al. 1999, 2002; Heiskanen et al. 2000), or sequence-defined PCR products (Mantripragada et al. 2003, 2004*b*) for array CGH allow this resolution to be theoretically increased solely on the basis of the size of the genomic region covered by the array element. However, because of limitations of the technologies, the effective resolution for these methods is no greater than 15–30 kb, since they rely on averaging measurements taken from multiple array elements, pooling PCR products to be spotted as single array elements, or reducing the complexity of the human genome to detect and quantitate copy-number changes. Therefore, it has not yet been demonstrated that array elements covering small regions of the genome can deliver substantially higher resolution than that of large

Received December 7, 2004; accepted for publication February 9, 2005; electronically published March 8, 2005.

Address for correspondence and reprints: Dr. David Vetrie, Human Genetics, Wellcome Trust Sanger Institute, Wellcome Trust Genome Campus, Hinxton, Cambridgeshire CB10 1SA, United Kingdom. E-mail: vt1@sanger.ac.uk

0002-9297/2005/7605-0004$15.00

genomic clone array CGH to identify small genomic deletions and duplications (100 bp to 15 kb).

The ability to detect copy-number changes encompassing such small regions of the genome has thus far been achievable only by using other types of molecular assays. Apart from the more traditional approaches of Southern analysis, FISH, and quantitative PCR (Armour et al. 2002), more-recent approaches have included the development of multiplex amplifiable probe hybridization (MAPH) (Armour et al. 2000; Sellner and Taylor 2004) and the multiplex ligation-dependent probe amplification (MLPA) (Schouten et al. 2002; Sellner and Taylor 2004). For MAPH and MLPA, the resolution is at the level of individual exons, and they are becoming widely used as research and diagnostic tools, with very high reliability for identifying and quantitating copy-number changes in human disease genes (White et al. 2002, 2003, 2004; Akrami et al. 2003; Sellner and Taylor 2004). However, because both methods rely on multiplexing, the number of measurements obtainable from a single assay is limited. Therefore, the development of approaches that provide robust measurement precision of copy-number changes, scalability, and very high resolution have thus far been unavailable in the field of human molecular genetics.

We describe here an array CGH–based approach that addresses all of these issues for the analysis of copy-number changes in the human genome. We have developed an array platform that allows single strands of DNA derived from double-stranded PCR products to be retained on the surface of a slide through the use of 5′-aminolink chemistry. This platform improves the signal:noise ratio, such that it is possible to detect individual exons in the human genome and to quantify their copy number accurately. We refer to this method as "exon array CGH." To demonstrate the utility of the approach, we constructed an array containing 162 exons that collectively span five human genes (*COL4A5* [MIM 303630], *DMD* [MIM 300377], *NF2* [MIM 607379], *PLP1* [MIM 300401], and *PMP22* [MIM 601097]) involved in inherited genetic disorders (see table 1). We have analyzed a series of 31 DNA samples from patients affected with these disorders and have characterized copy-number changes that have been validated with other molecular methods for all 31 samples. Our method is 2 orders of magnitude more sensitive than other forms of array CGH and provides resolution and accuracy that are similar to other current methods of screening genes for copy-number changes at the level of the exon. Since exon array CGH is completely scalable, this new molecular tool will provide the means for researchers to screen the human genome at high resolution to identify and annotate novel CNPs and causative mutations in normal and disease states, respectively, as well as to facilitate array-based applications to study other aspects of genome biology.

Material and Methods

PCR Amplification and Microarray Fabrication

Primers pairs for exons of the *COL4A5, DMD, NF2, PLP1,* and *PMP22* genes (table 2); for amplicons covering the 3′ UTRs of genes on chromosome 22 (normalization controls); and for other amplicons used here were obtained from primer sets published elsewhere (Strautnieks et al. 1992; Plant et al. 1999; Leiden University Medical Center Web site) or were designed using the relevant genomic sequence and the Primer3 software and Web site (Rozen and Skaletsky 2000; Whitehead Institute). All amplicons used in the present study were repeat free. When possible, primer pairs were designed or obtained for each exon and, ideally, were located in the upstream and downstream intronic sequences flanking the exon. In a few instances, however, primers were designed within the exonic sequence. When two adjacent exons were separated only by a very small intron, a single pair of primers was designed to contain both exons. Primer pairs and all amplicons sequences were compared with the entire human genome sequence by use of e-PCR (Schuler 1997) and BLASTN to identify any potential cross-reacting DNA sequences. In cases in which the PCR product for a given exon did not accurately or reproducibly report copy-number values, additional PCR assays were designed and tested on the array.

To generate arrays containing single-stranded array elements, all PCR products used in the present study were prepared as follows. To the 5′ end of the forward primer of each pair was added an 8-bp universal sequence (5′-TGACCATG-3′). These primer pairs (final concentration 0.5 μM) were used to amplify exon-containing PCR products in a 20-μl final volume first-round PCR containing 50 mM KCl, 5 mM Tris HCl (pH 8.5), 2.5 mM $MgCl_2$, 10 mM dNTPs (Pharmacia), 0.625 U *Taq* polymerase (Perkin Elmer–Cetus), and 50 ng of human genomic DNA. Thermocycling was optimized for each primer pair by use of an annealing temperature of 50°C–60°C (cycling conditions available on request). PCR products from these reactions were diluted 1:1000 and were used in second-round reactions containing the 5′-(C6) amino-modified universal primer 5′-GCTGAACAGCTATGACCATG-3′ (Eurogentec) and the reverse gene-specific primer of each set. Reaction conditions were the same as those in the first round, except the reaction volume was 60 μl. For the comparison of single- versus double-stranded DNA array elements, the universal linker was also added to the 5′ end of the reverse gene-specific primer. This allowed a 5′-aminolink to be

Table 1

Human Disease Genes Represented on the Exon Array

Gene	Chromosomal Location	Genomic Size (kb)	No. of Exons[a]	Disease	Frequency in Population	Pathogenic Copy-Number Changes[b]	Technical Consideration
DMD	Xp21.1	2,400	79 (+1)	Duchenne muscular dystrophy (DMD [MIM 310200])/Becker muscular dystrophy (MIM 300376)	1/3,500[c]	60–70[d]	Complex gene for diagnostic screening
NF2	22q12	95	17	Neurofibromatosis type 2 (NF2 [MIM 101000])	1/40,000[e]	20–30[e]	High repeat content results in quantitation issues for array CGH[f]
COL4A5	Xq22.3	257.6	51 (+2)	Alports syndrome (AS [MIM 301050])	1/5,000[g]	10–15[h]	Specificity issues, since it is a member of a six-gene triple helical collagen family
PMP22	17p12	35.6	5	Charcot-Marie Tooth type 1 disease (CMT1A [MIM 118220]); hereditary neuropathy with liability to pressure palsy (HNPP [MIM 162500])	10/100,000–40/100,000[i]	70 dupl (for CMT1A); 84 del (for HNPP)[j]	
PLP1	Xq22.2	15.8	7	Pelizaeus-Merzbacher disease (PMD [MIM 312080])	Extremely rare[k]	60–70[l]	

NOTE.—Genomic characteristics and clinical/technical relevance for inclusion on the array of the five human disease genes are shown.

[a] The number of exons shown in parentheses represents alternative exons found in some transcripts that were included as array elements.

[b] As a percentage of all mutations.

[c] DMD is the most common inherited neuromuscular disorder (Worton and Thompson 1988).

[d] Den Dunnen et al. 1989; Gillard et al. 1989.

[e] Bruder et al. 2001.

[f] Mantripragada et al. 2003.

[g] Atkin et al. 1988.

[h] Lemmink et al. 1997; Plant et al. 1999.

[i] Rautenstrauss et al. 2000.

[j] Nelis et al. 1996.

[k] Heim et al. 1997.

[l] Sistermans et al. 1998; Mimault et al. 1999.

Table 2

Primer Pairs Used to Amplify Exons for Array CGH

The table is available in its entirety in the online edition of *The American Journal of Human Genetics.*

incorporated on either the forward or the reverse strand in second-round reactions.

To prepare second-round PCR products for arraying, spotting buffer was added at final concentrations of 0.25 M sodium phosphate buffer pH 8.5 and 0.00025% sarkosyl (BDH Laboratory Supplies). The PCR products were then filtered through multiscreen-GV 96-well filter plates (Millipore), were aliquoted into 384-well plates (Genetix), and were arrayed onto Codelink slides (Amersham) in quadruplicate in a 16-block format by use of a Microgrid II arrayer (Biorobotics/Genomic Solutions). Slides were processed to generate single-stranded array elements, as described on the Sanger Institute microarray Web pages, and were stored at room temperature until hybridized.

Patient and Control DNA Samples

Thirty-one patient samples were obtained from a number of laboratories; all samples had been screened for mutations in the relevant disease gene at accredited diagnostic laboratories. Samples from patients with mutations in the *COL4A5*, *DMD*, and *PMP22* genes were obtained from the Southeast Thames Regional Genetics Centre (at King's, Guy's, and St. Thomas's Hospitals, London). These samples were all made anonymous for inclusion in this study. DNA samples from patients with *NF2* mutations were obtained from the Department of Genetics and Pathology at Uppsala University. DNA samples from patients with mutations in the *PLP1* gene were obtained from the Institute of Child Health (London); additional patients with mutations in the *PMP22* gene were obtained from the Center for Human Genetics (Leuven). Control DNA was obtained from archives of normal male and female DNA housed at the Sanger Institute (Cambridge). DNA was extracted using a variety of standard methods (salt/chloroform, phenol, commercial kits, etc.) from either peripheral blood or cultured cell lines. Aliquots of patient and control DNA samples were quantitated using a fluorometer (TD-360 [Turner]), were sonicated to an average size of ~10 kb by use of a water-bath sonicator (VirSonic 300 [Virtis]), and were visualized by agarose-gel electrophoresis. Female and male pool DNA samples that were used as reference DNA controls were derived by combining equal amounts of peripheral blood DNA from five females and five males, respectively. Male (XY) and female (XX) lymphoblastoid cell lines were also used as controls in the validation experiments. None of the control samples had mutations in the genes analyzed in this study.

Fluorescent DNA Labeling, Microarray Hybridization, and Data Analysis

Fluorescent-labeled DNA samples were prepared using a modified Bioprime labeling kit (Invitrogen) in 100-μl reaction volumes containing 600 ng genomic DNA, dNTPs (0.2 mM dATP, 0.2 mM dTTP, 0.2 mM dGTP, and 0.05 mM dCTP), and 0.04 mM Cy5/Cy3 dCTP (GE Healthcare). Reference control samples were labeled with Cy3, and test samples were labeled with Cy5. Labeling reactions were purified using Micro-spin G50 columns (Pharmacia-Amersham) in accordance with the manufacturer's instructions. Reference and test samples were combined and precipitated with 3 M sodium acetate (pH 5.2) in 2.5 volumes of ethanol with 90 μg human C_0t DNA (Invitrogen). The DNA pellet was resuspended in hybridization buffer containing 50% deionized formamide, 10% dextran sulphate, 10 mM Tris-HCl (pH 7.4), 2 × SSC, 0.1% Tween-20, and 300 μg yeast tRNA (Invitrogen). Similarly, the prehybridization mixture was prepared by precipitating 400 μg herring sperm DNA (Sigma) and 67.5 μg human C_0t DNA with 3 M sodium acetate (pH 5.2) and 2.5 volumes of ethanol; this DNA pellet was resuspended in the same hybridization buffer but with no yeast tRNA included.

Microarrays were prehybridized, hybridized, and washed using methods described elsewhere (Fiegler et al. 2003). Microarrays were scanned using a ScanArray 4000 confocal laser-based scanner (Perkin Elmer). Mean spot intensities from images were quantified using QuantArray or ScanArray Express (Perkin Elmer) with background subtraction. Mean ratios and SDs for all exon PCR products in quadruplicate were calculated, and the mean exon ratios were normalized to the chromosome 22 control element mean ratios for each of the 16 blocks independently to within 2% of the theoretical value (1.00 ± 0.02). Ratios were obtained for each exon independently, except in the cases in which more than one exon was contained in a single PCR product. Furthermore, there was no averaging of copy-number data for exons found in different PCR products. Although some exons were represented by more than one PCR product, the data from only the array element that most accurately reported copy number (i.e., that behaved closest to the theoretical values) were retained in the final data set for each sample in all but two instances—for the *PMP22* gene, the data from two PCR products representing exon 1 were pooled to derive a mean exon 1 ratio for both products. Similarly, this procedure was also performed for *PMP22* exon 5. To visualize the data, the final data set of mean ratios was plotted on a histogram for each exon or exon pair of *COL4A5*, *DMD*,

NF2, *PLP1*, and *PMP22*. Microarray experiments with control samples and patient samples were performed—multiple times, in some cases—to determine the reproducibility of the method. However, the derived mean-ratio data were determined for each hybridization experiment rather than from pooling of data from multiple experiments. For single- versus double-stranded DNA comparisons, mean intensities of quadruplicate spots were calculated with background subtraction in a single channel.

Results

Single-Stranded Technology Allows Detection of Exon-Sized Array Elements

One of the main considerations for array CGH is related to the complexity of the genome, as well as how this complexity is reflected in the signal measurements from which the copy-number changes are derived. Given that a typical exon in the human genome (median and mean sizes of 133 bp and 262 bp, respectively) represents a segment of genomic DNA found at a level of 1–2 in 4×10^7 sequence equivalents in the diploid human genome, it was necessary to address how to detect such a sequence at this level without reducing genome complexity or compromising the accuracy of the measurements. To this end, we developed an array system that allows single strands of DNA derived from double-stranded PCR products to be retained on the surface of the microarray slide. By incorporating a 5′-aminolink modification onto the end of one strand of a double-stranded DNA molecule during PCR, it is possible to covalently attach this strand to the surface of the slide, and the unmodified strand can be removed (fig. 1). Since single-stranded array elements cannot reanneal to form duplex molecules, we anticipated an increase in the signal:noise ratio in array CGH experiments, since there would be more single-stranded DNA on the surface of the slide capable of hybridizing with labeled sample. We demonstrated increased signal:noise measurements for single-stranded array elements (fig. 1). Test arrays were printed with array elements on which 5′-aminolink modifications were incorporated on either one or both strands. For a series of genomic array elements of 200–400 bp in size that we tested in hybridizations with fluorescently labeled human genomic DNA, single-stranded elements provided an increased signal:noise ratio, with a range of 1.16–2.51-fold increase, depending on the array element. On average, this translated into a 1.79-fold increase in the signal:noise ratio. We had previously demonstrated a similar increase in the signal:noise ratio for cDNA expression analysis (C.L. and D.V., unpublished data). Thus, this array platform facilitated increased signal:noise ratios and thereby provided evidence that we could improve the signal sufficiently to detect human genomic DNA sequences at the resolution of single exons.

Assessing the Performance of DNA Elements on Exon Arrays

We generated an exon array that included a set of array elements designed for every exon of five genes. The five genes included on this array were chosen to assess technical aspects of the technology and to demonstrate its clinical relevance (table 1) (Atkin et al. 1988; Worton and Thompson 1988; Den Dunnen et al. 1989; Gillard et al. 1989; Nelis et al. 1996; Heim et al. 1997; Lemmink et al. 1997; Sistermans et al. 1998; Mimault et al. 1999; Plant et al. 1999; Rautenstrauss et al. 2000; Bruder et al. 2001). These were the X-linked genes *COL4A5*, *DMD*, and *PLP1* and the autosomal genes *NF2* and *PMP22*. Mutations and/or copy-number changes in these five genes result in human inherited disorders. For the 162 exons of these genes, 158 array elements were initially designed and spotted on our arrays. We included a second array element for each of 18 exons that we chose at random to help assess sequence context on reporting accuracy, which brought the total number of array elements for these genes to 176. From the 3′ UTRs of genes on chromosome 22, 360 repeat-free amplicons were also spotted on these arrays and were used as normalization controls. These controls were, on average, of a size similar to that of the exon elements. We performed a series of validation experiments of male (XY) versus female (XX), and female (XX) versus female (XX) competitive hybridizations across a series of five batches of array printed at different times, with elements printed in quadruplicate, to assess the performance of the exon array in measuring copy-number changes. From the initial minimal set of 158 array elements, 135 (85.4%) reported copy-number measurements that were within 0.15 copy-number units of the theoretical values. The second array element for each of the 18 exons that had two different elements on the array showed a similar success rate (16 [88.9%] of 18). To obtain accurate copy-number measurements for all remaining exons in the five genes, we designed and tested a second element for each of 23 exons, 2 of which required a third iteration of design. These redesigned elements replaced the original elements for those exons in all subsequent analyses. In total, we analyzed 201 array elements, 174 (86.6%) of which reported accurate copy-number measurements and had a size range of 139–571 bp. On the basis of these experiments, we demonstrated that we could obtain accurate copy-number measurements for ~85% of the exons in our study by designing a single array element and for 100% of all exons by designing a second or, in a small minority of cases, a third array element. Typical examples of the quality of the data that we obtained from

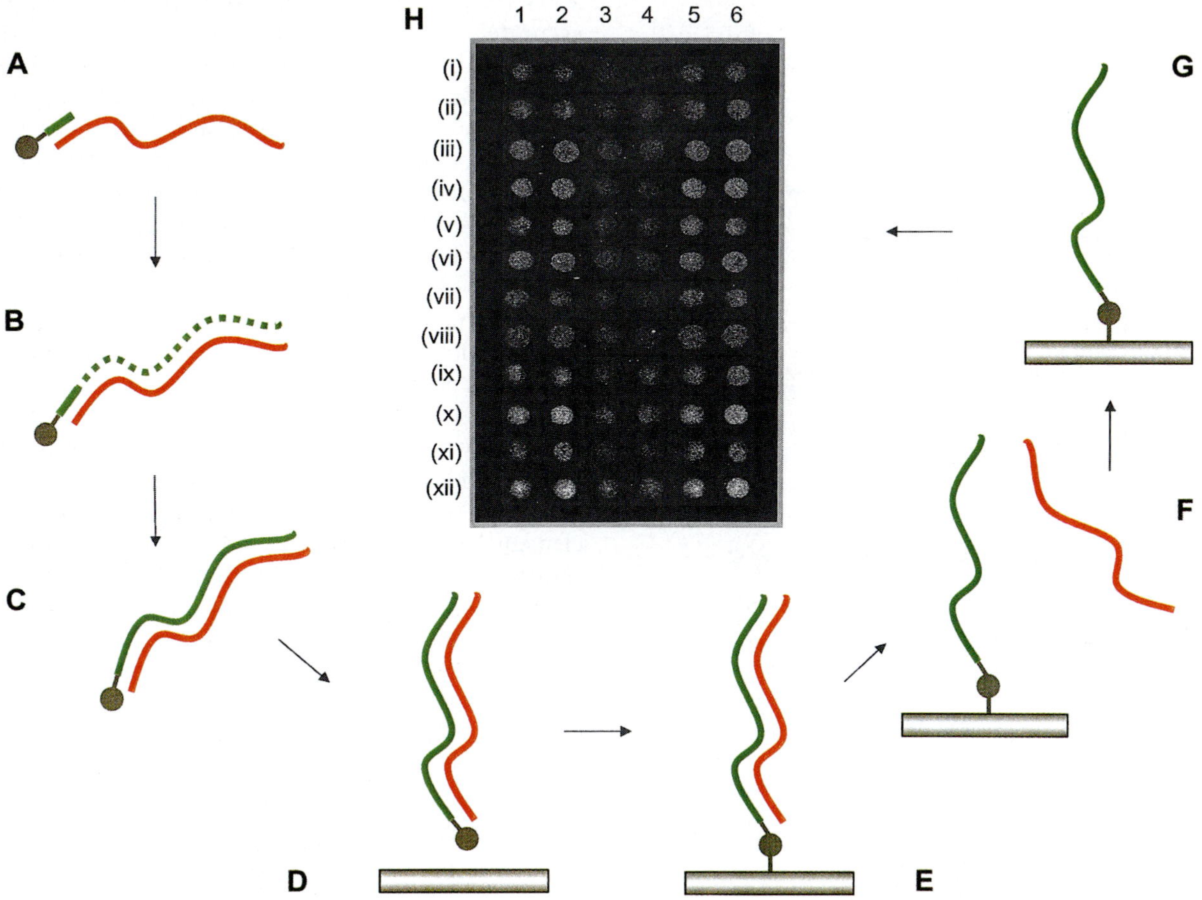

Figure 1 Development of single-stranded array platform for exon array CGH. Schematic diagram shows the approach adopted to make single-stranded PCR products with the increased sensitivity on the array platform described in this article. *A*, Oligonucleotide containing a 5′-C6-aminolink modification (*gray ball*) used as a primer (*short green bar*) on a genomic DNA or PCR template strand (*red wavy line*) in a PCR reaction. *B* and *C*, Synthesized double-stranded PCR product containing the 5′-aminolink modification on one strand only. Newly synthesized strand containing the 5′-aminolink modification is shown as a green dotted/solid line. *D*, PCR product spotted onto the microarray slide. *E*, Covalent attachment to the surface formed through the 5′-aminolink modification by subjecting the slide to high humidity. *F*, Removal of reverse strand that is not covalently attached to the surface of the slide by use of physical and chemical denaturation. *G*, The resultant single-stranded array element. *H*, Microarray image (*gray scale*) showing the results of fluorescently labeled genomic DNA hybridized to test arrays containing single-stranded and double-stranded PCR products for a series of genomic array elements ("i–xii") spotted in duplicate. Single-stranded elements for either one strand (5′-aminolink on forward strand [*lanes 1* and *2*]) or the other strand (5′-aminolink on the reverse strand [*lanes 5* and *6*]) or for double-stranded elements (5′-aminolinks on both strands [*lanes 3* and *4*]) were prepared on the test array. Single-stranded elements gave a higher signal for all genomic products (see the "Results" section).

these validation experiments for array elements covering all 162 exons of the five genes are shown in figure 2. The three X-linked genes (*DMD, PLP1,* and *COL4A5*) showed easily discernible single copy-number differences in XX versus XY validation experiments, when compared with the two autosomal genes (*PMP22* and *NF2*) (fig. 2*A*). XX versus XX validation experiments also showed the expected copy-number equivalence for all genes (fig. 2*B*).

Across the validation experiments, signal:noise ratios varied from hybridization to hybridization, which we attributed to variations in cyanine dye quality, DNA quality, labeling efficiencies, array batch, and other technical considerations. However, whereas signal:noise ratio did not appear to dramatically affect the range of mean copy-number values for each exon spotted in quadruplicate, the accuracy of the measurements was noticeably improved as the signal:noise ratio increased (fig. 2*C*). SDs in the quadruplicate measurements made for each exon showed a strong negative correlation with signal:noise ratio ($r = -0.97$). This would suggest that the single-stranded array platform we have developed not only helps to improve signal:noise ratio, but, as a consequence, also reduces measurement error. More importantly, our data also demonstrate that even exons that exhibit an extremely low signal:noise ratio on our

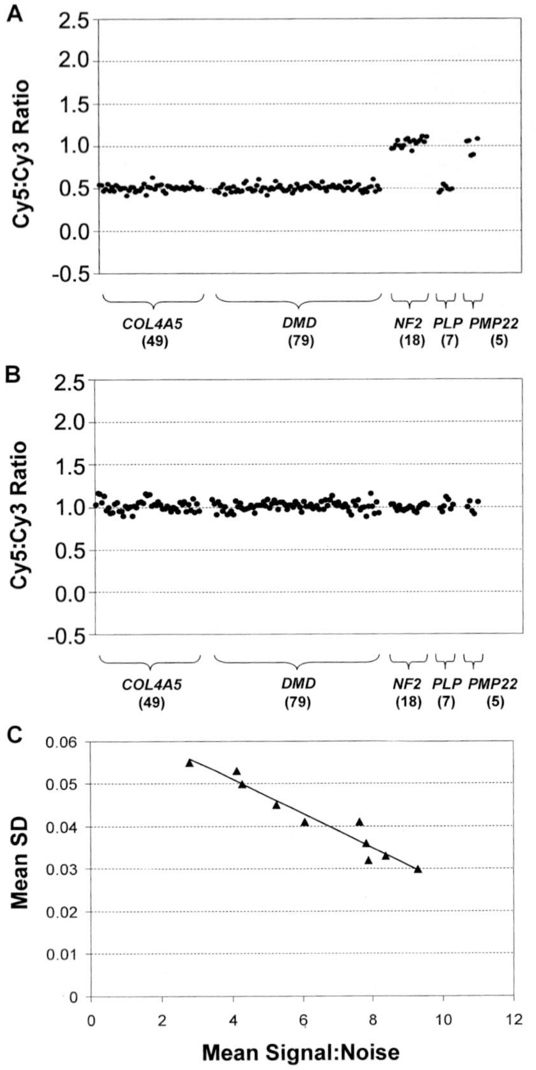

Figure 2 Validation experiments for exon arrays. *A*, Fluorescently labeled DNA derived from genomic DNA from a single male (Cy5) hybridized on the exon array with that derived from five females (used as a pool) (Cy3). The plot shows the Cy5 channel:Cy3 channel ratios obtained for exons (represented as black dots) for *COL4A5*, *DMD*, *NF2*, *PLP1*, and *PMP22*. Each exon is plotted as a function of its position 5′→3′ for each gene. The number of exon array elements assayed for each gene is shown in parentheses below the gene name. Exons for the three X-linked genes and the two autosomal genes showed ratios centered around the theoretical values of 0.5 and 1, respectively. *B*, Fluorescently labeled DNA derived from genomic DNA from a single female (Cy5) hybridized on the exon array with that derived from the female pool (Cy3). The plot shows the ratios obtained for each exon, as described above (*A*), centered around the theoretical value of 1. *C*, The effect of signal:noise ratio on measurement error determined, using exon arrays, in 10 male versus female-pool validation experiments. The plot shows the relationship between mean signal:noise and mean SD. Both means were derived as the mean of all mean quadruplicate element measurements per experiment. The black triangles represent each of the 10 male/female validation experiments. The correlation coefficient (r) between mean SD and mean signal:noise was −0.97.

array (i.e., in the range of 1–1.5) could be quantitated accurately.

We studied further the performance of our single-stranded array elements to identify other features that may contribute to reporting accuracy in array CGH experiments. Using regression analysis on data obtained from all 201 exon array elements, we found no strong correlations between the accuracy of copy-number measurements and inherent features of the array elements, such as G+C content, length, melting temperature, secondary structure, similarity to other genomic sequences, and distance from upstream or downstream repeat sequences in genomic DNA. However, given that we could obtain accurate copy-number measurements for some exons only by redesigning array elements, sequence context is likely to contribute in some way to reporting accuracy. We also assessed whether the location of an element on the array affected reporting accuracy, by spotting independent preparations of 12 of the array elements in alternative locations on the array. All 12 of these array elements reported accurate copy-number measurements irrespective of their array coordinate. This evidence, together with the rest of our empirical data, demonstrates that, although it is unclear which factors may influence the performance of DNA elements on our exon array, this platform is robust within a variety of sequence contexts and technical constraints.

Detection of Copy-Number Changes in Patient Material

We further tested the performance of the exon array and its potential application as a research and diagnostic tool by detecting copy-number changes in DNA samples from patients with inherited disorders. Thirty-one patient DNA samples (from 24 males and 7 females) were collected that all had known pathogenic copy-number changes in one of the five disease genes represented on the array. We were able to determine copy-number changes in all 31 DNA samples and with equal efficacy in affected males, affected females, and nonsymptomatic carrier females (for X-linked disorders). All of these results were in agreement with the molecular data determined elsewhere for these patients (Ellis and Malcolm 1994; Harding et al. 1995; Woodward et al. 1998, 2000; Bruder et al. 2001; Buckley et al. 2002; Mantripragada et al. 2003; S.A., unpublished data; J.R.V., unpublished data) or as part of the present study. Our results are summarized in table 3 and figure 3. In total, we detected copy-number changes (either a gain or loss) in patient samples for 121 of the 158 array elements containing exons that were present on the array. The demonstrated copy-number changes included 10 whole-gene deletions (fig. 3*A*), 8 whole-gene duplications (fig. 3*B*), 2 whole-gene triplications (fig. 3*C* and 3*D*), 3 partial-gene du-

Table 3

Copy-Number Changes Detected in 31 Patient Samples

Sample	Patient Reference	Sex	Gene Affected	Mutation
1	JP[a,b,c]	Male	*NF2*	Whole-gene deletion
2	p7[a,b]	Male	*NF2*	Whole-gene deletion
3	p130[b]	Male	*NF2*	Deletion (exons 13–15)
4	EA01(241397)	Male	*PMP22*	Whole-gene deletion
5	EA02(260055)	Female	*PMP22*	Whole-gene deletion
6	EA03(218861)	Male	*PMP22*	Whole-gene deletion
7	EA04(268266)	Male	*PMP22*	Whole-gene deletion
8	EA05(251650)	Male	*PMP22*	Whole-gene deletion
9	EA06(263902)	Female	*PMP22*	Whole-gene duplication
10	EA07(221358)	Male	*PMP22*	Whole-gene duplication
11	EA08(138116)	Male	*PMP22*	Whole-gene duplication
12	EA09(231345)	Male	*PMP22*	Whole-gene duplication
13	EA10(271065)	Male	*PMP22*	Whole-gene duplication
14	EA11	Male	*COL4A5*	Whole-gene deletion
15	EA12	Male	*DMD*	Deletion (exon 51)
16	EA13	Male	*DMD*	Deletion (exon 44)
17	EA14	Male	*DMD*	Deletion (exons 3–7)
18	EA15	Female	*PMP22*	Whole-gene deletion
19	EA16	Male	*PMP22*	Whole-gene deletion
20	EA17	Male	*DMD*	Deletion (exons 45–52)
21	EA18	Female	*DMD*	Deletion (exons 45–48)
22	EA19	Male	*DMD*	Duplication (exon 2)
23	EA20	Female	*DMD*	Deletion (exons 17–48)
24	EA21	Male	*DMD*	Deletion (exons 45–50)
25	EA22	Male	*DMD*	Duplication (exons 2–7)
26	EA23	Male	*DMD*	Duplication (exon 3)
27	DH/PMD2-1[d,e,f]	Male	*PLP1*	Whole-gene triplication
28	PMD2-2[d,e,f]	Female	*PLP1*	Whole-gene triplication
29	NO/PMD9-1[d,f]	Male	*PLP1*	Whole-gene duplication
30	PMD4-2[f]	Female	*PLP1*	Whole-gene duplication
31	PMD4-1[f]	Male	*PLP1*	Whole-gene duplication

NOTE.—Copy-number changes in a collection of 31 patient samples found using the exon array described in the present study. Where relevant, patient references have been included from other published studies.

[a] Mantripragada et al. 2003.
[b] Bruder et al. 2001.
[c] Buckley et al. 2002.
[d] Ellis and Malcolm 1994; Woodward et al. 1998.
[e] Harding et al. 1995.
[f] Woodward et al. 2000.

plications (fig. 3*E*), and 8 partial-gene deletions (fig. 3*F*, 3*G*, and 3*H*).

In the DNA sample of one patient (patient EA11), in which the entire *COL4A5* gene was deleted, we detected a copy-number measurement in *COL4A5* exon 1 (0.26) that did not suggest a complete absence of this exon (theoretical value of 0). The PCR product for this exon showed an 86% sequence similarity across 212 bp to a sequence on the short arm of chromosome X. This was the highest degree of sequence similarity found for any of the elements on the exon array. Therefore, although exon 1 was completely deleted in patient EA11 (as confirmed by PCR), the cross-hybridizing X-linked sequence was being reported by the exon 1 array element.

Of the 11 partial-gene duplications/deletions, 4 involved only a single exon, 1 of which was a single-copy number gain of *DMD* exon 2 (fig. 3*E*). The array element for *DMD* exon 2 displayed the lowest signal:noise ratio across all array CGH experiments performed for the present study. This not only helps demonstrate the sensitivity of the array system and our ability to quantitate weak signals, but it also shows the utility of the array for accurate prediction of copy-number changes involving only *DMD* exon 2; a single-exon duplication of exon 2 is the most frequently occurring *DMD* mutation, according to one study that used the MAPH assay (White et al. 2002), but is also one of the most difficult to determine using hybridization-based approaches, because it is highly AT rich (PCR product is 73.4% AT rich) (White et al. 2002).

Discussion

We report here an array CGH platform that can measure copy-number changes accurately at the resolution of sin-

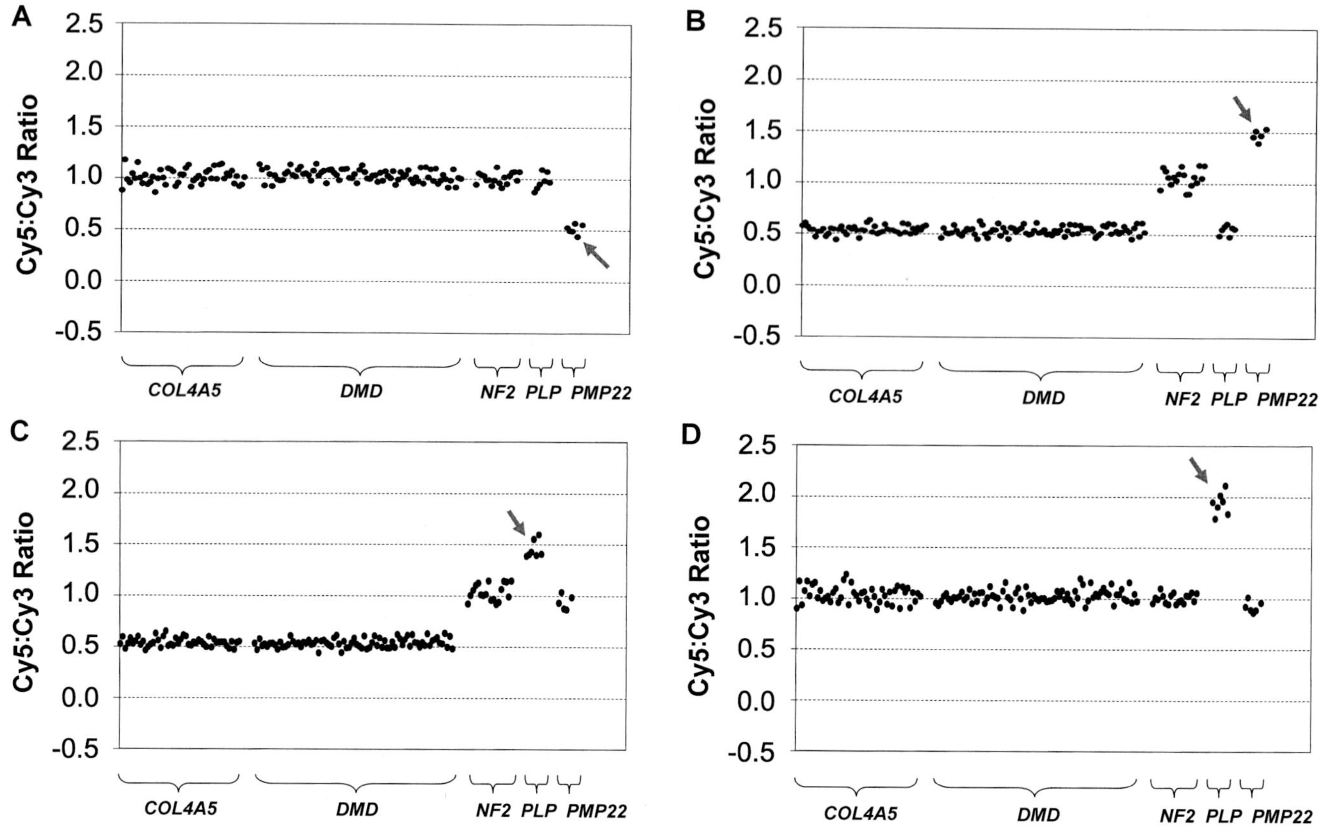

Figure 3 Exon copy-number changes in medically relevant disease genes. Representative results of exon array CGH for patient DNA samples hybridized against a female pool that demonstrates the variety of copy-number changes detected in the present study. All patient samples were fluorescently labeled using Cy5, and all control female-pool samples were fluorescently labeled using Cy3. The features of the plots are as described for figure 2. The gray arrows highlight the copy-number changes. *A,* Female patient—EA02(260055)—with HNPP showing a deletion of the entire *PMP22* gene. *B,* Male patient—EA07(221358)—with CMT1 showing a duplication of the entire *PMP22* gene. *C,* Male patient (DH/PMD2–1) with PMD showing a triplication of the entire *PLP1* gene. *D,* Female PMD carrier (PMD2–2, mother of patient in panel C) showing a triplication of the entire *PLP1* gene. *E,* Male patient (EA19) with DMD showing a duplication of exon 2 in the *DMD* gene. *F,* Male patient (p130) with NF2 showing a deletion of exons 13–15 of the *NF2* gene. *G,* Male patient (EA14) with DMD showing a deletion of exons 3–7 of the *DMD* gene. Panel also shows the confirmatory PCR results; lanes are numbered according to the exons assayed and size markers ("M"), in base pairs, shown at the left of the gel image. *H,* Male patient (EA12) with DMD showing the deletion of exon 51 of the *DMD* gene. Confirmatory PCR is also shown with lanes numbered according to the exons assayed and size markers ("M"), in base pairs, shown at the left.

gle exons. By developing an array system that results in single-stranded DNA elements being bound to the surface of a slide, we have demonstrated an improved signal:noise ratio that facilitates the accuracy in copy-number measurements for array elements in the size range of 139–571 bp. We have further shown that constitutionally inherited copy-number changes, as either deletions or duplications, were detected in 100% of patient samples analyzed on an exon array containing array elements for 162 exons from five disease genes. The results described here represent the first time, to our knowledge, that array CGH has been shown to perform robustly at the resolution of single exons. This represents an increase in array CGH resolution that is 2 orders of magnitude higher than has been reported elsewhere.

Our study provides compelling empirical evidence that it will be possible to obtain accurate copy-number measurements for virtually all exons in the genome, with ~85% of exons requiring that a single-array element be designed and tested and the remainder requiring that additional array elements be validated in an iterative process. Indeed, in the present study, we were able to design array elements for 161 (99.4%) of 162 exons that faithfully reported copy number in validation experiments and in the analysis of patient samples. For the one remaining exon, similarity with a cross-hybridizing genomic sequence was an issue, which suggests that this and possibly other sequence-based factors may affect the performance of array elements for other exons in the genome. What these factors are remains unclear.

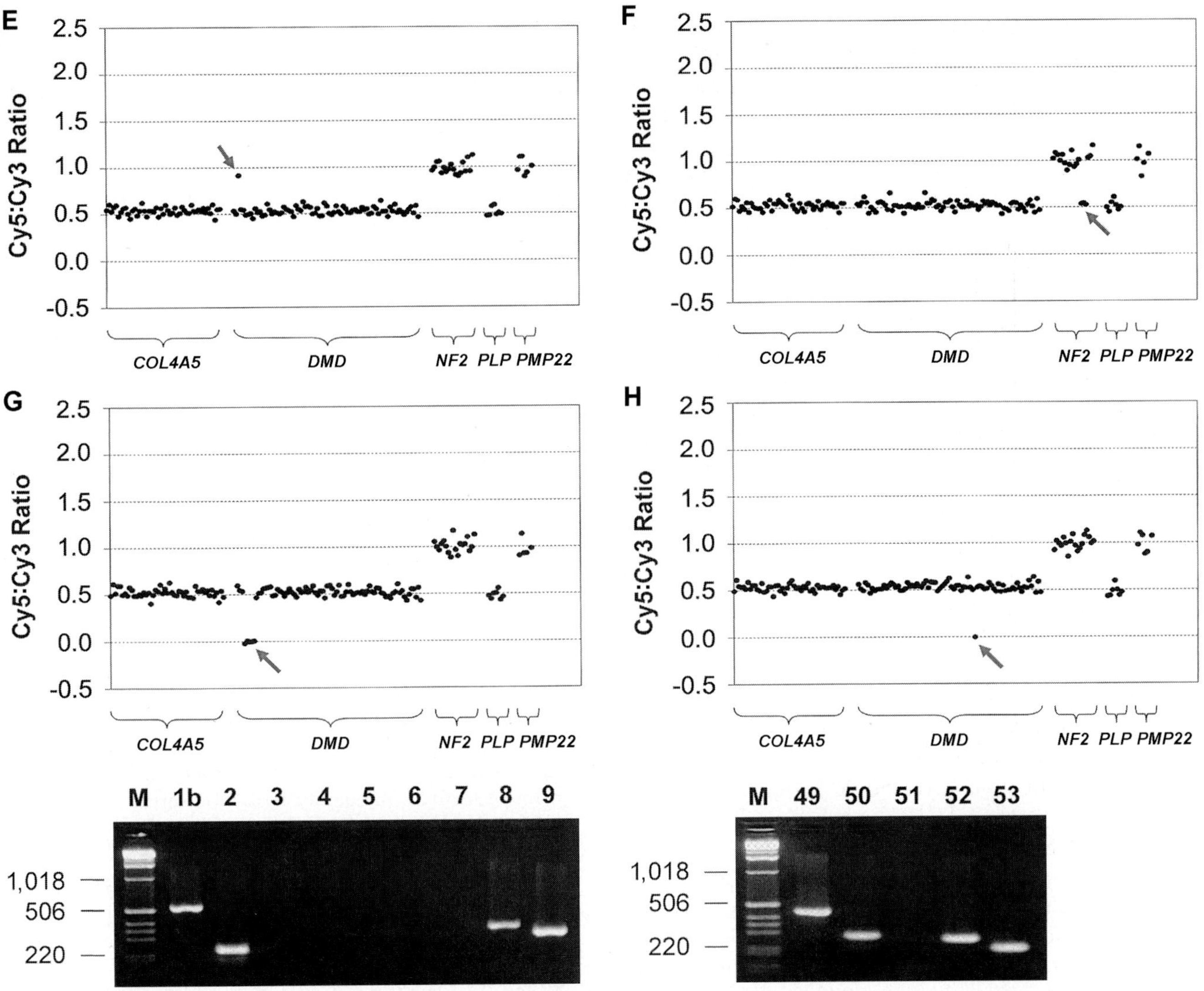

In some instances, it may be necessary to use "surrogate" exons—that is, array elements designed for sequences that lie adjacent to exons and that may perform more robustly in array CGH. Averaging measurements from multiple array elements may also provide the means to improve quantitative measurements for other exons.

The applications of this technology are numerous. Since our arrays are both scalable and sensitive at the resolution of single exons, they fill a technological gap between the high-throughput technologies (e.g., array CGH by use of BAC arrays) and the high-resolution but less scalable assays (e.g., *MAPH* and *MLPA*). Therefore, the development of this technology opens the way for identifying copy-number changes at high resolution in both normal and disease states, as a research or diagnostic tool, and in both large-scale and small-scale studies.

The construction of a genomewide exon array would represent an important achievement for the analysis of DNA-copy number in the human genome. To maintain single-exon resolution for genomewide screening, such an array would require at least one array element for each of the ~245,000 exons that have been annotated in the human genome. On the basis of the data presented here, that would require the design and testing of 280,000–300,000 exon-specific primer pairs and their conversion to array elements to obtain a quantitative working assay for every exon. Furthermore, on the basis of current spotting technologies, multiple microarray slides would be required to spot the entire set of exons, resulting in increased costs per genome assayed. Although this may appear to represent an enormous undertaking, it must be balanced against the tremendous value that such an array set could contribute to human genetics—it would allow the identification and annotation of CNPs and mutations, in normal individuals and in disease, that have previously been undiscovered because of limitations in the resolution of other array CGH technologies.

In more focused approaches, exon arrays would also facilitate positional cloning strategies of novel disease genes in well-characterized patient collections. Given that we have shown here a direct application of this technology to identify copy-number changes in patient material for several single-gene disorders, its use as a diagnostic tool for known disease genes is evident. Furthermore, it should be possible to screen many genes in an exon array CGH format to quickly elucidate copy-number changes for some categories of disease phenotypes that are difficult to distinguish clinically. Exon array CGH could also be applied to cancer genetics. Given that there are several hundreds of genes that have been shown to be mutated in cancer (Futreal et al. 2004), this set serves as an excellent starting point for the construction of cancer-specific exon arrays.

It will also be possible to use our array system at this level of resolution to answer other questions about genome biology, with the one obvious application being chromatin immunoprecipitation (ChIP)-on-chip (Ren et al. 2002; Weinmann et al. 2002). Given the quantifiable signal:noise ratios we have shown here, obtaining detailed maps of protein-binding sites, histone modifications, and other features, such as origins of replications and matrix attachment regions, should also be possible with genomic tiling-path arrays or intergenic arrays at high resolution. This type of approach for identifying transcription-factor binding sites onto human chromosomal regions (Horak et al. 2002) and whole chromosomal tiling paths (Martone et al. 2003; Cawley et al. 2004; Euskirchen et al. 2004) has already been described, although the proportions of sites identified that are false-positive results or false-negative results are not yet known. In particular, our array system is well suited to identify low-affinity DNA-protein interactions that give relatively poor enrichments in ChIP and small quantifiable copy-number increases on arrays. We are currently extending our work in this area by generating high-resolution genomic tiling arrays for regions of interest in the human genome.

Acknowledgments

The authors thank Nigel Carter, Heike Fiegler, and Philippa Carr, for assistance with initial hybridizations; Hazel Arbury and Ruth Bennett, for generating male and female control DNA; David Beare, for designing the primers for the chromosome 22 control elements; and David Bentley, for his critical reading of the manuscript. This work was supported by the Wellcome Trust.

Electronic-Database Information

The URLs for data presented herein are as follows:

Leiden University Medical Center, http://www.dmd.nl

Online Mendelian Inheritance in Man (OMIM), http://www.ncbi.nlm.nih.gov/Omim/ (for *COL4A5, DMD, NF2, PLP1, PMP22,* DMD, Becker muscular dystrophy, NF2, AS, CMT1A, HNPP, and PMD)

Sanger Institute, http://www.sanger.ac.uk/Projects/Microarrays/arraylab/methods.shtml

Whitehead Institute, http://frodo.wi.mit.edu/cgi-bin/primer3/primer3_www.cgi (for Primer3)

References

Akrami SM, Rowland JS, Taylor GR, Armour JA (2003) Diagnosis of gene dosage alterations at the PMP22 gene using MAPH. J Med Genet 40:e123

Albertson DG, Pinkel D (2003) Genomic microarrays in human genetic disease and cancer. Hum Mol Genet Spec 2 12:R145–R152

Armour JA, Barton DE, Cockburn DJ, Taylor GR (2002) The detection of large deletions or duplications in genomic DNA. Hum Mutat 20:325–337

Armour JA, Sismani C, Patsalis PC, Cross G (2000) Measurement of locus copy number by hybridisation with amplifiable probes. Nucleic Acids Res 28:605–609

Atkin CL, Hasstedt SJ, Menlove L, Cannon L, Kirschner N, Schwartz C, Nguyen K, Skolnick M (1988) Mapping of Alport syndrome to the long arm of the X chromosome. Am J Hum Genet 42:249–255

Bignell GR, Huang J, Greshock J, Watt S, Butler A, West S, Grigorova M, Jones KW, Wei W, Stratton MR, Futreal PA, Weber B, Shapero MH, Wooster R (2004) High-resolution analysis of DNA copy number using oligonucleotide microarrays. Genome Res 14:287–295

Bruder CE, Hirvela C, Tapia-Paez I, Fransson I, Segraves R, Hamilton G, Zhang XX, et al (2001) High resolution deletion analysis of constitutional DNA from neurofibromatosis type 2 (NF2) patients using microarray-CGH. Hum Mol Genet 10:271–282

Buckley PG, Mantripragada KK, Benetkiewicz M, Tapia-Paez I, Diaz de Ståhl T, Rosenquist M, Ali H, et al (2002) A full-coverage, high-resolution human chromosome 22 genomic microarray for clinical and research applications. Hum Mol Genet 11:3221–3229

Carvalho B, Ouwerkerk E, Meijer GA, Ylstra B (2004) High resolution microarray comparative genomic hybridisation analysis using spotted oligonucleotides. J Clin Pathol 57:644–646

Cawley S, Bekiranov S, Ng HH, Kapranov P, Sekinger EA, Kampa D, Piccolboni A, Sementchenko V, Cheng J, Williams AJ, Wheeler R, Wong B, Drenkow J, Yamanaka M, Patel S, Brubaker S, Tammana H, Helt G, Struhl K, Gingeras TR (2004) Unbiased mapping of transcription factor binding

sites along human chromosomes 21 and 22 points to widespread regulation of noncoding RNAs. Cell 116:499–509
Den Dunnen JT, Grootscholten PM, Bakker E, Blonden LAJ, Ginjaar HB, Wapenaar MC, van Paassen HMB, van Broeckhoven C, Pearson PL, van Ommen GJB (1989) Topography of the Duchenne muscular dystrophy (DMD) gene: FIGE and cDNA analysis of 194 cases reveals 115 deletions and 13 duplications. Am J Hum Genet 45:835–847
Ellis D, Malcolm S (1994) Proteolipid protein gene dosage effect in Pelizaeus-Merzbacher disease. Nat Genet 6:333–334
Euskirchen G, Royce TE, Bertone P, Martone R, Rinn JL, Nelson FK, Sayward F, Luscombe NM, Miller P, Gerstein M, Weissman S, Snyder M (2004) CREB binds to multiple loci on human chromosome 22. Mol Cell Biol 24:3804–3814
Fiegler H, Carr P, Douglas EJ, Burford DC, Hunt S, Scott CE, Smith J, Vetrie D, Gorman P, Tomlinson IP, Carter NP (2003) DNA microarrays for comparative genomic hybridization based on DOP-PCR amplification of BAC and PAC clones. Genes Chromosomes Cancer 36:361–374
Futreal PA, Coin L, Marshall M, Down T, Hubbard T, Wooster R, Rahman N, Stratton MR (2004) A census of human cancer genes. Nat Rev Cancer 4:177–183
Gillard EF, Chamberlain JS, Murphy EG, Duff CL, Smith B, Burghes AHM, Thompson MW, Sutherland J, Oss I, Bodrug SE, Klamut HJ, Ray PN, Worton RG (1989) Molecular and phenotypic analysis of patients with deletions within the deletion-rich region of the Duchenne muscular dystrophy (*DMD*) gene. Am J Hum Genet 45:507–520
Harding B, Ellis D, Malcolm S (1995) A case of Pelizaeus-Merzbacher disease showing increased dosage of the proteolipid protein gene. Neuropathol Appl Neurobiol 21:111–115
Heim P, Claussen M, Hoffmann B, Conzelmann E, Gartner J, Harzer K, Hunneman DH, Kohler W, Kurlemann G, Kohlschutter A (1997) Leukodystrophy incidence in Germany. Am J Med Genet 71:475–478
Heiskanen MA, Bittner ML, Chen Y, Khan J, Adler KE, Trent JM, Meltzer PS (2000) Detection of gene amplification by genomic hybridization to cDNA microarrays. Cancer Res 60: 799–802
Horak CE, Mahajan MC, Luscombe NM, Gerstein M, Weissman SM, Snyder M (2002) GATA-1 binding sites mapped in the β-globin locus by using mammalian chIp-chip analysis. Proc Natl Acad Sci USA 99:2924–2929
Iafrate AJ, Feuk L, Rivera MN, Listewnik ML, Donahoe PK, Qi Y, Scherer SW, Lee C (2004) Detection of large-scale variation in the human genome. Nat Genet 36:949–951
Inazawa J, Inoue J, Imoto I (2004) Comparative genomic hybridization (CGH)-arrays pave the way for identification of novel cancer-related genes. Cancer Sci 95:559–563
Ishkanian AS, Malloff CA, Watson SK, DeLeeuw RJ, Chi B, Coe BP, Snijders A, Albertson DG, Pinkel D, Marra MA, Ling V, MacAulay C, Lam WL (2004) A tiling resolution DNA microarray with complete coverage of the human genome. Nat Genet 36:299–303
Lemmink HH, Schroder CH, Monnens LA, Smeets HJ (1997) The clinical spectrum of type IV collagen mutations. Hum Mutat 9:477–499
Lucito R, Healy J, Alexander J, Reiner A, Esposito D, Chi M, Rodgers L, Brady A, Sebat J, Troge J, West JA, Rostan S, Nguyen KC, Powers S, Ye KQ, Olshen A, Venkatraman E, Norton L, Wigler M (2003) Representational oligonucleotide microarray analysis: a high-resolution method to detect genome copy number variation. Genome Res 13:2291–2305
Lucito R, West J, Reiner A, Alexander J, Esposito D, Mishra B, Powers S, Norton L, Wigler M (2000) Detecting gene copy number fluctuations in tumor cells by microarray analysis of genomic representations. Genome Res 10:1726–1736
Mantripragada KK, Buckley PG, Diaz de Ståhl T, Dumanski JP (2004*a*) Genomic microarrays in the spotlight. Trends Genet 20:87–94
Mantripragada KK, Buckley PG, Jarbo C, Menzel U, Dumanski JP (2003) Development of NF2 gene specific, strictly sequence defined diagnostic microarray for deletion detection. J Mol Med 81:443–451
Mantripragada KK, Tapia-Paez I, Blennow E, Nilsson P, Wedell A, Dumanski JP (2004*b*) DNA copy-number analysis of the 22q11 deletion-syndrome region using array-CGH with genomic and PCR-based targets. Int J Mol Med 13:273–279
Martone R, Euskirchen G, Bertone P, Hartman S, Royce TE, Luscombe NM, Rinn JL, Nelson FK, Miller P, Gerstein M, Weissman S, Snyder M (2003) Distribution of NF-κB-binding sites across human chromosome 22. Proc Natl Acad Sci USA 100:12247–12252
Mimault C, Giraud G, Courtois V, Cailloux F, Boire JY, Dastugue B, Boespflug-Tanguy O, and the Clinical European Network on Brain Dysmyelinating Disease (1999) Proteolipoprotein gene analysis in 82 patients with sporadic Pelizaeus-Merzbacher disease: duplications, the major cause of the disease, originate more frequently in male germ cells, but point mutations do not. Am J Hum Genet 65:360–369
Nelis E, Van Broeckhoven C, De Jonghe P, Lofgren A, Vandenberghe A, Latour P, Le Guern E, Brice A, Mostacciuolo ML, Schiavon F, Palau F, Bort S, Upadhyaya M, Rocchi M, Archidiacono N, Mandich P, Bellone E, Silander K, Savontaus ML, Navon R, Goldberg-Stern H, Estivill X, Volpini V, Friedl W, Gal A (1996) Estimation of the mutation frequencies in Charcot-Marie-Tooth disease type 1 and hereditary neuropathy with liability to pressure palsies: a European collaborative study. Eur J Hum Genet 4:25–33
Pinkel D, Segraves R, Sudar D, Clark S, Poole I, Kowbel D, Collins C, Kuo WL, Chen C, Zhai Y, Dairkee SH, Ljung BM, Gray JW, Albertson DG (1998) High resolution analysis of DNA copy number variation using comparative genomic hybridization to microarrays. Nat Genet 20:207–211
Plant KE, Green PM, Vetrie D, Flinter FA (1999) Detection of mutations in COL4A5 in patients with Alport syndrome. Hum Mutat 13:124–132
Pollack JR, Perou CM, Alizadeh AA, Eisen MB, Pergamenschikov A, Williams CF, Jeffrey SS, Botstein D, Brown PO (1999) Genome-wide analysis of DNA copy-number changes using cDNA microarrays. Nat Genet 23:41–46
Pollack JR, Sorlie T, Perou CM, Rees CA, Jeffrey SS, Lonning PE, Tibshirani R, Botstein D, Borresen-Dale AL, Brown PO (2002) Microarray analysis reveals a major direct role of DNA copy number alteration in the transcriptional program of human breast tumors. Proc Natl Acad Sci USA 99:12963–12968
Rautenstrauss B, Lupski, J, Timmerman V (2000) Draft best practice guidelines for molecular analysis of hereditary motor and sensory neuropathies. European Molecular Genetics

Quality Network (http://www.emqn.org/Assets/uploadpdfs/HMSN.pdf) (accessed March 1, 2005)

Ren B, Cam H, Takahashi Y, Volkert T, Terragni J, Young RA, Dynlacht BD (2002) E2F integrates cell cycle progression with DNA repair, replication, and G(2)/M checkpoints. Genes Dev 16:245–256

Rozen S, Skaletsky H (2000) Primer3 on the WWW for general users and for biologist programmers. Methods Mol Biol 132: 365–386

Schouten JP, McElgunn CJ, Waaijer R, Zwijnenburg D, Diepvens F, Pals G (2002) Relative quantification of 40 nucleic acid sequences by multiplex ligation-dependent probe amplification. Nucleic Acids Res 30:e57

Schuler GD (1997) Sequence mapping by electronic PCR. Genome Res 7:541–550

Sebat J, Lakshmi B, Troge J, Alexander J, Young J, Lundin P, Maner S, Massa H, Walker M, Chi M, Navin N, Lucito R, Healy J, Hicks J, Ye K, Reiner A, Gilliam TC, Trask B, Patterson N, Zetterberg A, Wigler M (2004) Large-scale copy number polymorphism in the human genome. Science 305: 525–528

Sellner LN, Taylor GR (2004) MLPA and MAPH: new techniques for detection of gene deletions. Hum Mutat 23:413–419

Sistermans EA, de Coo RF, De Wijs IJ, Van Oost BA (1998) Duplication of the proteolipid protein gene is the major cause of Pelizaeus-Merzbacher disease. Neurology 50:1749–1754

Snijders AM, Nowak N, Segraves R, Blackwood S, Brown N, Conroy J, Hamilton G, Hindle AK, Huey B, Kimura K, Law S, Myambo K, Palmer J, Ylstra B, Yue JP, Gray JW, Jain AN, Pinkel D, Albertson DG (2001) Assembly of microarrays for genome-wide measurement of DNA copy number. Nat Genet 29:263–264

Snijders AM, Pinkel D, Albertson DG (2003) Current status and future prospects of array-based comparative genomic hybridisation. Brief Funct Genomic Proteomic 2:37–45

Solinas-Toldo S, Lampel S, Stilgenbauer S, Nickolenko J, Benner A, Dohner H, Cremer T, Lichter P (1997) Matrix-based comparative genomic hybridization: biochips to screen for genomic imbalances. Genes Chromosomes Cancer 20:399–407

Strautnieks S, Rutland P, Winter RM, Baraitser M, Malcolm S (1992) Pelizaeus-Merzbacher disease: detection of mutations Thr^{181}→Pro and Leu^{223}→Pro in the proteolipid protein gene, and prenatal diagnosis. Am J Hum Genet 51:871–878

Vissers LELM, de Vries BBA, Osoegawa K, Janssen IM, Feuth T, Choy CO, Straatman H, van der Vliet W, Huys EHLPG, van Rijk A, Smeets D, van Ravenswaaij-Arts CMA, Knoers NV, van der Burgt I, de Jong PJ, Brunner HG, van Kessel AG, Schoenmakers EFPM, Veltman JA (2003) Array-based comparative genomic hybridization for the genomewide detection of submicroscopic chromosomal abnormalities. Am J Hum Genet 73:1261–1270

Weinmann AS, Yan PS, Oberley MJ, Huang TH, Farnham PJ (2002) Isolating human transcription factor targets by coupling chromatin immunoprecipitation and CpG island microarray analysis. Genes Dev 16:235–244

White S, Kalf M, Liu Q, Villerius M, Engelsma D, Kriek M, Vollebregt E, Bakker B, van Ommen G-JB, Breuning MH, den Dunnen JT (2002) Comprehensive detection of genomic duplications and deletions in the *DMD* gene, by use of multiplex amplifiable probe hybridization. Am J Hum Genet 71: 365–374

White SJ, Sterrenburg E, van Ommen GJ, den Dunnen JT, Breuning MH (2003) An alternative to FISH: detecting deletion and duplication carriers within 24 hours. J Med Genet 40:e113

White SJ, Vink GR, Kriek M, Wuyts W, Schouten J, Bakker B, Breuning MH, den Dunnen JT (2004) Two-color multiplex ligation-dependent probe amplification: detecting genomic rearrangements in hereditary multiple exostoses. Hum Mutat 24:86–92

Woodward K, Kendall E, Vetrie D, Malcolm S (1998) Pelizaeus-Merzbacher disease: identification of Xq22 proteolipid-protein duplications and characterization of breakpoints by interphase FISH. Am J Hum Genet 63:207–217

Woodward K, Kirtland K, Dlouhy S, Raskind W, Bird T, Malcolm S, Abeliovich D (2000) X inactivation phenotype in carriers of Pelizaeus-Merzbacher disease: skewed in carriers of a duplication and random in carriers of point mutations. Eur J Hum Genet 8:449–454

Worton RG, Thompson MW (1988) Genetics of Duchenne muscular dystrophy. Annu Rev Genet 22:601–629

Increased Level of Linkage Disequilibrium in Rural Compared with Urban Communities: A Factor to Consider in Association-Study Design

Veronique Vitart,[1] Andrew D. Carothers,[1] Caroline Hayward,[1] Peter Teague,[1] Nicholas D. Hastie,[1] Harry Campbell,[2] and Alan F. Wright[1]

[1]Medical Research Council Human Genetics Unit, Western General Hospital, and [2]Department of Public Health Sciences, University of Edinburgh Medical School, Edinburgh

Few studies have investigated genetic differentiation within nonisolate European populations, despite the initiation of large national sample collections such as U.K. Biobank. Here, we used short tandem repeat markers to explore fine-scale genetic structure and to examine the extent of linkage disequilibrium (LD) within national subpopulations. We studied 955 unrelated individuals of local ancestry from nine Scottish rural regions and the urban center of Edinburgh, as well as 96 unrelated individuals from the general U.K. population. Despite little overall differentiation on the basis of allele frequencies, there were clear differences among subpopulations in the extent of pairwise LD, measured between a subset of X-linked markers, that reflected presumed differences in the depths of the underlying genealogies within these subpopulations. Therefore, there are strategic advantages in studying rural subpopulations, in terms of increased power and reduced cost, that are lost by sampling across regions or within urban populations. Similar rural-urban contrasts are likely to exist in many other populations with stable rural subpopulations, which could influence the design of genetic association studies and national biobank data collections.

Introduction

The genetic characterization of sampled populations is a critical step in the design and interpretation of complex disease–mapping studies. One aspect that has recently been emphasized is the impact of population stratification on association studies, since even low-level differentiation (e.g., between European populations with F_{ST} close to 1%) can lead to false-positive results and failure to detect genuine association in large-scale studies (Freedman et al. 2004; Marchini et al. 2004). Few studies have investigated the level of genetic differentiation within typical outbred Western populations, despite the initiation of national sample collections, such as U.K. Biobank, that will be used for large-scale genetic association studies. We therefore set out to explore the level of genetic differentiation within the Scottish population of 5 million people, which, in most respects, is representative of the wider U.K. population, in that it contains large urban and smaller rural subpopulations but includes a number of geographically isolated island communities in which greater differentiation might be expected. The proportion of large Western populations living in rural versus urban communities within Europe and North America varies from 21% (United States) to 33% (Canada), with both England/Wales (28%) and Scotland (32%) lying in the middle of the range. Rural populations are typically more stable and homogeneous than the dense urban populations that constitute the population majority. This raises the question whether there are genetically detectable rural-urban differences that might influence association-study design.

The origin of the earliest Scottish inhabitants is unknown, but those of 1,500–2,500 years ago may have been of P-Celtic origin, similar to that of inhabitants of parts of Wales and Brittany. After that, there was a succession of both peaceful and hostile incomers, including Romans, Irish Q-Celts, Vikings, Anglo-Saxons, Normans, and Flemish, all of whom mixed with local populations to varying degrees in each region. Clear regional patterns reflecting some of these historical events have been preserved in the present day distribution of Y-chromosome haplogroup lineages (Capelli et al. 2003), and the Viking legacy has been especially well studied (Helgason et al. 2000; Wilson et al. 2001; Capelli et al. 2003). However, Y chromosomes capture only a small fraction of the overall ancestry, and it is not clear whether these patterns are typical of the rest of the genome. Mainland Scotland also displays discontinuity with regard to ABO blood-group distributions, with uniformity in southern and eastern Scotland, whereas northern and western Scotland show much higher O and lower A group frequencies (Brown 1965; Mourant

Received November 22, 2004; accepted for publication February 21, 2005; electronically published March 24, 2005.

Address for correspondence and reprints: Dr. Veronique Vitart, Medical Research Council Human Genetics Unit, Western General Hospital, Crewe Road, Edinburgh EH4 2XU, United Kingdom. E-mail: v.vitart@hgu.mrc.ac.uk

0002-9297/2005/7605-0005$15.00

Table 1

Response Results from the Scottish Survey

Subpopulation and GP	Response Rate (%)	Percentage of Local Respondents
Grampian:		
Turriff	32	42
Edinburgh:		
Portobello	18	12
Restalrig	23	25
Lewis:		
Lochs	33	62
Orkney:		
Stromness	34	43
Galloway:		
Castle Douglas	28	20
Shetland:		
Mid Yell	30	60
Wester Ross/Skye:		
Aultbea	35	16
Portree	27	32
Borders:		
Selkirk	30	14
Melrose	26	18
Angus:		
Alyth	28	18
Kirriemuir	13	28
Argyll:		
Lochgilphead	24	10
Campbeltown	19	59

[a] "Local Respondents" was defined in the present study as those whose four grandparents were born or had lived in the region sampled.

et al. 1976). In the northeast, a locally high group-B frequency has been associated with fishing communities and is thought to reflect a Norse component (Brown 1965; Mourant et al. 1976).

Subjects and Methods

Our study was designed to maximize the detection of genetic discontinuities within Scotland. Hence, the population-sampling scheme was based on local ancestry to reflect an older and more extreme level of differentiation prior to the recent breakdown of traditional subpopulations. Participants were selected at random from local primary care centers (general practice [GP]) and were recruited by questionnaire as being "of local ancestry." The requirement was that all four grandparents had been born in or had lived in the region sampled. Data was discarded from the study for individuals whose known relatives were already included. Close degrees of relatedness were sought in participant questionnaires and were further checked at the GP after recruitment. All participants gave informed consent for providing mouthwash-extracted DNA, and the study received ethical approval from regional research ethics committees. Two GPs within an area were approached, when necessary, to recruit ~100 suitable participants per region. Ten Scottish regions were sampled: three island regions, Lewis/Harris (GP: Lochs), Orkney (GP: Stromness), and Shetland (GP: Mid Yell); one urban, Edinburgh (two GPs: Portobello and Restalrig); six rural regions, Wester Ross (GP: Aultbea)/Skye (GP: Portree), Grampian (rural Aberdeenshire) (GP: Turriff), Borders (two GPs: Melrose and Selkirk), Angus (two GPs: Alyth and Kirriemuir), Argyll (two GPs: Lochgilpead and Campbeltown), and Dumfries and Galloway (GP: Castle Douglas) (fig. 1). Additionally, for comparison, we used the control plate HRC-1 (human random control) (European Collection of Cell Cultures) of extracted DNA from lymphoblastoid cell lines from 96 unrelated whites whose grandparents were born in the United Kingdom or Ireland.

Results

Population Differentiation

The proportion of "locals" among contacted residents varied widely across regions (table 1) and reflected expectations based on social and demographic knowledge. The lowest proportion of locals (15%) was found in places of greater migratory flow—the urban center Edinburgh and the Borders region neighboring England—and the highest (60%) was found in the islands of Shetland and Lewis, which have undergone constant population decline since the end of the 19th century, with very little immigration (apart from a recent oil industry–related influx into Shetland, which did not contribute to the gene pool investigated).

Table 2

Population Substructure: Comparison of Wright's F_{IS} Statistics for Population Samples

	Findings for Loci That are					
	X Linked			Autosomal		
Population	N[a]	F_{IS}	95% CI	N[a]	F_{IS}	95% CI
Grampian	46	.086[b]	.025–.126	87	.096[b]	.051–.120
Edinburgh	63	.046	.001–.064	119	.013	.011–.029
Lewis	68	.027	−.029–.055	122	.052[b]	.027–.082
Orkney	57	.064	.001–.103	101	.067[b]	.030–.096
Galloway	50	.082[b]	.016–.130	99	.037	.001–.055
Shetland	38	.061	.007–.095	78	.039	.007–.061
Wester Ross/Skye	38	.012	−.049–.041	92	.027	.010–.058
Borders	50	.046	−.015–.071	86	.007	.023–.032
Angus	45	.074[b]	.006–.114	77	.061[b]	.019–.082
Argyll	64	.072[b]	.024–.105	94	.042	.001–.074
United Kingdom	49	.035	−.013–.063	NP	NP	NP

NOTE.—The F_{IS} statistic, a measure of departure from random mating within a population, is used to classify the table. Sixteen unlinked autosomal microsatellite loci and 15 X-linked microsatellite loci with an interlocus distance of at least 5 cM were tested. The multilocus estimates of Wright's fixation indexes, F_{IS}, were computed following the guidelines of Weir and Cockerham (1984), by use of the Genetix software, with the whole data set for autosomal markers and the female-only data set for the X-linked markers. Significant departure from the null hypothesis of equilibrium was tested after 3,200 permutations. After performing 100 bootstrap samples, 95% CIs for the F_{IS}-statistic values were estimated. NP = not performed.

[a] N = number of diploid individuals.

[b] Significance at the 1% level.

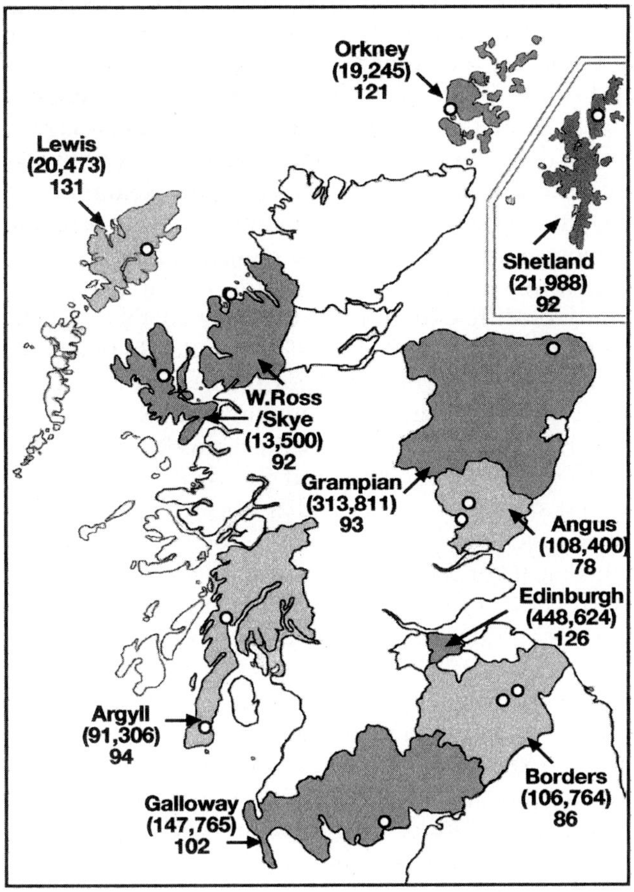

Figure 1 Map of the 10 sampled Scottish regions. For each region, the 2001 census size is indicated in parentheses, and the number of local residents recruited is indicated below the census number. Apart from Edinburgh, all recruitment locations are indicated by an open circle. "Lewis" = Lewis and Harris, "Galloway" = Dumfries and Galloway.

We set out to study if these differences in population stability translated into detectable genetic differentiation. We used STR markers, which have relatively high mutation rates, so that patterns of variation reflect more recent divergence. The whole Scottish sample of 955 individuals was typed for 16 unlinked autosomal STR markers (*D20S119, D21S266, D20S107, D19S902, D20S186, D22S420, D22S280, D19S216, D22S423, D19S884, D21S1252, D22S539, D22S274, D6S393, D4S1530,* and *D3S1537*) and for 34 X-linked STR markers (*DXS1060, DXS8051, DXS1226, DXS1214, sWXD2451, DXS1068, DXS8014, DXS8113, DXS1058, DXS8015, DXS8042, DXS1368, DXS993, DXS8012, DXS1201, DXS8085, DXS7, MAOB, DXS991, DXS983, DXS1165, DXS8092, DXS8037, DXS56, DXS1225, DXS8082, DXS995, DXS990, DXS1106, DXS8055, DXS1001, DXS1047, DXS1227,* and *DXS8043*). (Raw data can be found at the authors' Web site.) Only a subset of 15 "unlinked" X-linked markers was used to study differentiation, corresponding to the markers that are at least 5 cM apart. The overall sample displayed a highly significant excess of homozygous genotypes compared with expectation under random mating, whereas most regions taken singly did not (table 2), which suggests the presence of genetic structure within Scotland. Wright's fixation index F_{IT}, which measures the global heterozygote deficit, was 0.045 (95% CI 0.035–0.057) for autosomal markers and 0.059 (95% CI: 0.042–0.078) for X-linked data (519 females). Only the regions of Angus and especially Grampian showed a large excess of homozygous genotypes that was consistent in both marker sets, which suggests residual substructure in these two regions (table 2).

Population differentiation was highly significant when we tested for equal allelic distributions across the overall Scottish sample with an exact test (Raymond and Rousset 1995), both for autosomal and X-linked marker sets.

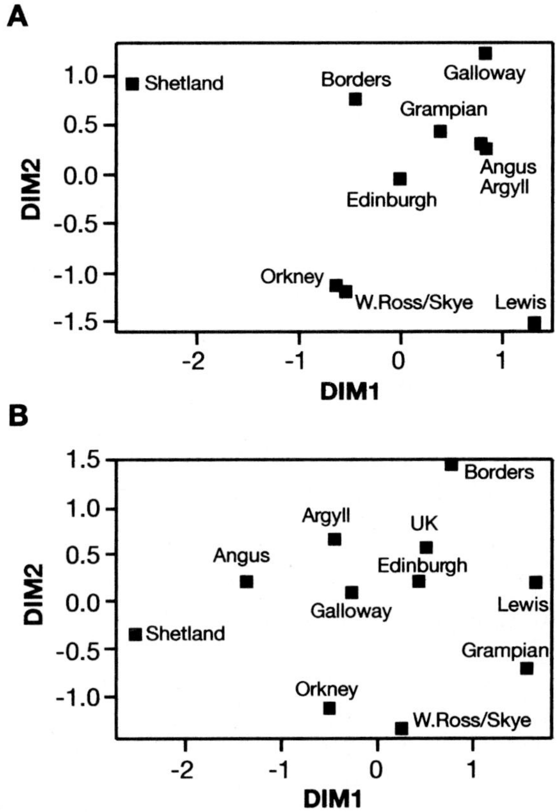

Figure 2 Representation, in two-dimensional space, of genetic distances between subpopulations, on the basis of allele frequencies at 16 autosomal (*A*) and at 15 X-linked (*B*) STR markers. Nei's unbiased genetic distances (Nei 1978) were computed using the Genetix software and were represented in two-dimensional space by use of multidimensional scaling analysis (Kruskal and Wish 1977) with the SPSS software package. The average proportion of variance of the disparities in the initial distance matrix in the two-dimensional plots are 94% (*A*) and 92% (*B*).

Likewise, the variance-based measure of differentiation, F_{ST}, indicated a low but highly significant level of differentiation overall, with an estimated F_{ST} value of 0.0025 (95% CI 0.0014–0.0039) for the autosomal marker set and 0.0034 (95% CI 0.0012–0.0057) for the X-linked set. However, pairwise comparisons among populations indicated that it is the island populations that accounted for most of the differentiation signal (table 3). The highest pairwise F_{ST} measure, observed for the Lewis-Shetland comparison, reached 1% for the X-linked marker set. Mainland Scottish populations were undifferentiated with respect to autosomal marker frequencies. With the X-linked marker set, a slightly higher level of differentiation was uncovered, as expected, since it represents a smaller gene pool (and hence is more prone to genetic drift). When X-linked STRs were used, Grampian was significantly distinct from Angus and Argyll, as was the United Kingdom from Angus. Global F_{ST} estimates for the mainland Scottish subpopulations (i.e., removal of Lewis, Orkney, Shetland, and Wester Ross/Skye) were 0.0004 (95% CI −0.00036 to 0.0012) for the autosomal markers and 0.00154 (95% CI −0.00071 to 0.00415) for the X-linked set, and none was significantly different from zero at the 5% level after a permutation test. Representation in two-dimensional space of the genetic distances derived from STR allele frequencies by use of multidimensional scaling summarized the amount of differentiation among populations when all data were considered simultaneously (fig. 2). Therefore, even with a sampling scheme that is based on local ancestry and that uses STR markers, the differences among Scottish subpopulations (and U.K.-Scottish subpopulations [table 3]) are low, with corresponding pairwise F_{ST} under 1%. Likewise, attempts failed to assign individuals to distinct source populations solely on the basis of multilocus data (16 autosomal plus 34 X-linked markers, 15 of which are "unlinked"). Attempts were performed using the model-based clustering approach implemented in the STRUCTURE program (Pritchard et al. 2000). Our results suggest that gene flow has homogenized most of the historical differences among the regions investigated. Within mainland Scotland, gross stratification was ruled out by the analysis. Our study design does not have the power to detect the very low level of differentiation that may exist within mainland Scotland (more markers and/or more individuals would be required to reach significance); however, our study informs on the likely magnitude of differentiation on the basis of the F_{ST} value obtained; that is, 0.0004 (95% CI −0.00036 to 0.0012) for the autosomal markers. For this reason, association studies aimed at finding common variants of small or moderate effect should not be negatively impacted by stratification in the mainland Scottish population for modest sample size, and studies can be guided by published simulations (Helgason et al. 2005) on the required adjustment for large sample size (>500 cases and >500 controls). It is likely that, at a finer scale, heterogeneity remains, as suggested by the high F_{IS} values for Grampian. Brown (1965), in her survey of blood-group distributions in the north of Scotland, noted local heterogeneity between inland and coastal distributions, which may be explained by their contrasting histories of emigration from inland areas, after the introduction of large-scale sheep farming (the Highland Clearances), compared with more static fishing communities on the coast.

Linkage Disequilibrium

To further the analysis, we next examined the extent of linkage disequilibrium (LD) between pairs of markers that were based on the analysis of 34 X-linked markers, which included 8 markers on Xq13-21 and 15 on Xp21-11 regions, thus covering, at higher density, both a region of low average recombination rate (on Xq13-21; 0.25

Table 3

Pairwise Subpopulation Differentiation

	Grampian	Edinburgh	Lewis	Orkney	Galloway	Shetland	Wester Ross/ Skye	Borders	Angus	Argyll	United Kingdom
Grampian		.0017	***.0041***[a]	.0037	.0027	***.0125***[b]	−.0003	.0035	***.0096***[b]	***.0051***[a]	.0026
Edinburgh	−.0002		.0022	***.0041***[a]	−.0018	***.0082***[b]	−.0002	.0011	.0004	.0004	−.0005
Lewis	***.0033***[b]	***.0032***[b]		***.0049***[b]	.0021	***.0124***[b]	***.0053***[a]	***.004***[a]	***.0083***[b]	***.0053***[b]	.0016
Orkney	***.0029***[a]	.0005	***.0026***[b]		−.0001	.0035	−.0036	***.0086***[b]	.0024	.002	.0025
Galloway	.0011	.0008	***.0045***[b]	***.0046***[b]		.0021	.0011	−.0001	.0018	−.0009	−.0030
Shetland	***.0051***[b]	***.0044***[b]	***.0073***[b]	***.0042***[b]	***.0069***[b]		***.0099***[b]	***.0109***[b]	.0017	***.0056***[a]	***.0086***[b]
Wester Ross/Skye	***.003***[a]	−.0002	***.0039***[b]	.002	***.0042***[b]	***.0057***[b]		***.0069***[b]	.0039	.0029	.0037
Borders	.0013	.0002	***.0044***[b]	***.0033***[a]	.0014	***.004***[b]	***.0023***[a]		.004	.0002	−.0027
Angus	.0001	−.0004	***.0032***[b]	***.0026***[a]	.0003	***.0062***[b]	***.0028***[a]	−.002		.0014	***.0048***[a]
Argyll	.0016	.0008	***.0034***[b]	***.0024***[a]	.0018	***.0059***[b]	***.003***[b]	−.0004	0		.0015

NOTE.—Pairwise F_{ST} estimates based on allele frequencies of 16 unlinked autosomal STRs (*below diagonal*) and 15 unlinked X-linked STRs (*above diagonal*) are used to classify the table. The levels of statistical significance were tested by performing 1,600 permutations with the Genetix software. Statistically significant results are shown in bold italics.

[a] Significance at 5% level.

[b] Significance at 1% level.

The figure is available in its entirety in the online edition of *The American Journal of Human Genetics.*

Figure 3 Comparison of LD decay across populations by model fitting. The figure legend is available in its entirety in the online edition of the *American Journal of Human Genetics.*

cM/Mb) and a region of high recombination rate (on Xp21-11; 1.8 cM/Mb). Xq13-21 has been used extensively to explore population-specific differences in LD (Laan and Pääbo 1997; Zavattari et al. 2000; Angius et al. 2002; Katoh et al. 2002; Latini et al. 2004). Clear signals of increased pairwise LD by use of markers in this region have been consistently found in populations in which the demographic histories were favorable to building LD (Zavattari et al. 2000; Angius et al. 2002; Kaessmann et al. 2002; Katoh et al. 2002; Latini et al. 2004).

To perform interpopulation comparisons with a standardized metric, we introduced an empirical measure of LD between pairs of multiallelic markers, denoted as "*W*," based on a normalized transformation of the standard χ^2 statistic. Compared with the frequently used LD measure *D*′ (Hedrick 1987), of which the distributional properties are unknown, we found, in independent data sets, that *W* was less sensitive to factors such as sample size and allele numbers and that it provided a better fit than did *D*′ to the decline of LD with interlocus distance (authors' unpublished data). We developed this measure rather than using the association metric that others introduced for a similar purpose (Collins et al. 2001), since this latter measure (swept radius) is better suited for diallelic markers and requires collapsing of nonassociated alleles to reduce the loci, in a biased way, to diallelic systems. All the genotypic data were used (i.e., haplotypes in males and diplotypes in females). For haplotype data, a statistical χ^2 can be derived from a $k \times l$ contingency table, where the entry in the *i*th row and *j*th column corresponds to the number of $A_i B_j$ haplotypes. χ^2 is then defined as the standard contingency table statistic for tests of the null hypothesis of no association between loci *A* and *B*, which is distributed under the null hypothesis as χ^2 with $(k-1)(l-1)$ df. With genotype data, the haplotype frequencies must be estimated, and we obtained the relevant statistic in the present study by taking the difference between 2 × the log likelihood for a fully saturated model (i.e., the assumption of random mating but not linkage equilibrium, with $k \times l - 1$ df) and for a model that has the assumption of random mating and linkage equilibrium (with $k + l - 2$ df). With random mating and under the null hypothesis of linkage equilibrium, the difference is distributed as χ^2, with $(k-1)(l-1)$ df. The χ^2 measures were determined, respectively, using the programs ldmax and haploxt from the GOLD suite (Abecasis and Cookson 2000) with a pooling threshold set at 7%, and their values were summed in a combined χ^2. To reduce the dependence of χ^2 on the degrees of freedom, it was transformed to an approximate standard normal deviate, *W*, by

$$W = \left(\frac{9\nu}{2}\right)^{\frac{1}{2}}\left[\left(\frac{X^2}{\nu}\right)^{\frac{1}{3}} - 1 + \frac{2}{9\nu}\right],$$

where ν denotes degrees of freedom (Wilson and Hilferty 1931) and where $\nu = \nu_1 + \nu_2$ (i.e., from haplotypic and diplotypic data). We supposed that the LD measure, *W*, is related to the genetic-distance measure, *x*, by the linear form, $W = \alpha + \beta f(x;\gamma) + \varepsilon$, where α and β are parameters to be estimated, ε is a random variable normally distributed with mean 0 and unknown variance σ^2, *x* is the genetic-map distance (in cM), and the link function *f* is characterized by a single parameter γ, such that $f(x=\gamma;\gamma) = \frac{1}{2}$, $f(x=0;\gamma) = 1$, and $f(x=\infty;\gamma) = 0$. Hence, γ can be interpreted as the distance (in cM) at which the expected LD is equal to half the difference between its maximum ($\alpha + \beta$, at $x = 0$) and minimum (α, at $x = \infty$) expected values (γ is referred to as the LD–half distance [distance at which LD decays to half the difference between its maximum and minimum value]). This parameter γ provides a measure of the strength of LD. The link function

$$f = \frac{1}{1 + \frac{x}{\gamma}}$$

was fitted. Maximum-likelihood estimates were obtained for α, β, and γ, and the goodness of fit was assessed using the deviance (−2 × the log-likelihood ratio), with 2 df (see fig. 3 for illustration of the linear model fitting). Most of the weight is given by the short intermarker distances (<1.5 cM), to which marker pairs on Xq13-11 and Xp21-11 contribute equally but disproportionately compared with the other X-linked markers. The marker pair *DXS1225-DXS8082* was removed as being atypical (i.e., in strong LD in all populations examined worldwide). The Scottish subpopulations displayed a 270-fold range of LD–half distances (however, with large associated CIs), from low values in the general U.K. population (0.003 cM) and urban Edinburgh (0.01cM) to increased values in mainland rural subpopulations—Galloway (0.026 cM), Argyll (0.059 cM), Angus (0.14 cM), Borders (0.18 cM), and Grampian (0.21 cM)—and highest levels in the island populations of Shetland (0.22 cM), Orkney (0.29 cM), Wester Ross/Skye (0.29 cM), and Lewis (0.8 cM) (fig. 4). The lower and upper support intervals (which correspond to a 90% CI) for Lewis are

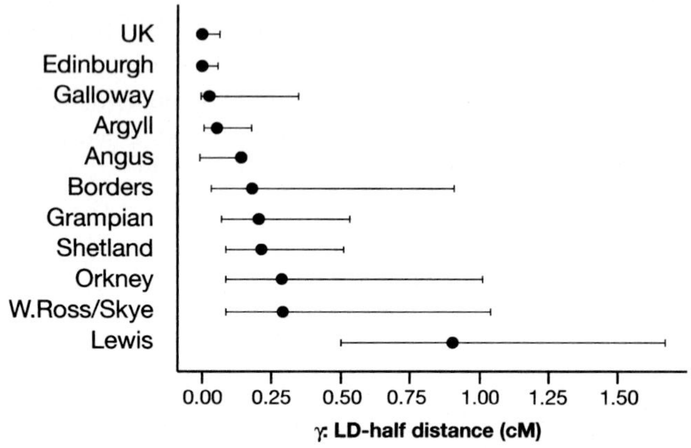

Figure 4 LD decay in 10 Scottish subpopulations and unrelated U.K. subjects, on the basis of 34 X-linked STR markers. Maximum-likelihood estimates of LD–half distance are indicated by a blackened circle. Subpopulations are ordered by increasing values of these estimates. Upper and lower support limits were defined by values of the likelihood equal to 26% of the maximum (equivalent to a 90% CI for estimates with a normally distributed error). The Angus sample size was low ($n = 78$) and had missing data, so that the upper bound for its half-distance decay is high (2.5 cM).

0.5–1.7 cM, compared with 0–0.07 cM for the general U.K. and urban Edinburgh populations, which represents a difference of at least 8-fold. A similar continuum in the extent of LD among the populations studied was obtained when analyzing the subset of male haplotypes (i.e., with no inference bias) on Xq13-21, by use of a different measure of disequilibrium (an exact test) for comparison with published data sets (tables 4 and 5).

To evaluate the effect of sampling between rather than within subpopulations on the extent of LD, 15 randomized samples of size 100 were created by bootstrap sampling across mainland rural areas, in accordance with their census size. The average LD–half distance obtained was 0.089 cM (90% CI 0.061–0.129), which indicates reduced LD compared with four of the rural subpopulations taken singly (0.14, 0.18, 0.21, and 0.29 cM). Similarly, sampling within all of mainland Scotland, including the urban center of Edinburgh, a scheme similar to the U.K. Biobank design, led to an even smaller LD–half distance of 0.062cM (90% CI 0.044–0.088).

These conclusions are based on the analysis of STR markers that span only two regions of the X chromosome—for which LD extent has been shown to be generally greater than for autosomes (Taillon-Miller et al. 2004)—as expected, since their effective population size is three-quarters that of the autosomes. The LD–half distance is thus likely to be scaled down for autosomal STRs, and more so for SNPs, which have lower mutation rates, so that the detection of differences between populations with SNPs would require considerably more markers to be typed. The X-linked STR markers therefore provide sensitive measures of differentiation with efficient detection and quantification of population differences arising from demographic and other factors. Demographic factors act globally across the genome, whereas local factors such as recombination rates and selection may be region specific. There is no evidence, to date, that these two investigated chromosomal regions have been subject to significant selection. In two previous studies, these X-chromosome regions displayed extended LD in isolated populations compared with nonisolate populations, which was also observed in autosomal regions (Zavattari et al. 2000; Kaessmann et al. 2002). Critically, the power to detect association declines exponentially rather than linearly as the extent of LD falls toward zero (Blangero 2004), which suggests that even a small increase in the extent of LD could increase power and reduce cost by more than an order of magnitude.

Genetic Complexity

The extent of LD between marker loci reflects the amount of historical recombination and past effective population size (N_e), so that, for a given genomic region, LD can differ dramatically between populations with different demographic histories (Pritchard and Przeworski 2001). We aimed to explore the level of LD between X-chromosomal STRs in relation to the predicted effective population size, N_e. N_e reflects the number of ancestors who have contributed to the gene pool. The more N_e is reduced, the greater the effect of genetic drift and the greater the genealogical relationship within a sample, which, in turn, can result in increased LD. Therefore, for Xp21-11 and Xq13-21, female haplotypes were inferred using the Bayesian statistical method implemented in PHASE (v2.0.2) on the basis of the coalescent model (Stephens et al. 2001). The algorithm that integrates recombination in the simulations (Li and Stephens 2003) was run independently five times, and the run with the best average goodness of fit to the approximate coalescent model was kept. Point estimates of the population average recombination parameter $3N_er$ were obtained by taking the median value among 1,000 sampled from the corresponding posterior distribution, as implemented in PHASE (v2.0.2). The values shown in table 6 display a ranking similar to that obtained for the extent of LD, which is especially clear for the more recombinogenic chromosomal region (i.e., Xp21-11) data, from high values in the urban and U.K. samples to intermediate values in the Scottish mainland regions to low values in the

Table 4

Comparison of Pairwise LD at Xq13-21 for Male Haplotypes with Representative Published Data Sets

The table is available in its entirety in the online edition of *The American Journal of Human Genetics.*

Table 5

Pairwise Significance of LD, for All Pairs of STR Loci Studied at Xq13-21 in Male Haplotypes

The table is available in its entirety in the online edition of *The American Journal of Human Genetics.*

islands. The differences between subpopulations, within each chromosomal region, can be attributed to differences in effective population size (N_e). Although the posterior distributions of the recombination parameters overlap, there is a clear trend toward a reduction in N_e in Orkney, Lewis, Shetland, and Wester Ross/Skye compared with U.K. or Edinburgh (in the range of 2–5-fold), which implies a less complex gene pool (table 6). This was noticeable by the reduction in computation time when running the PHASE-implemented algorithm for the island subpopulations. Within each subpopulation, the estimates obtained in the two investigated chromosomal regions were significantly correlated (Spearman's rank correlation 63%; $P = .02$), and the difference between Xq13-21 and Xp21-11 average recombination estimates are in agreement with pedigree-based estimates (6-fold [Kong et al. 2002]), suggesting that the coalescence-based algorithm performed well.

The observed increase in LD seen in rural subpopulations is also mirrored by the haplotype-diversity data. Table 7 shows haplotypes for six STRs on Xq13-21 that span 0.85 cM, together with a subset of three STR haplotypes. For six-locus haplotypes, the highest haplotype diversity was found in Edinburgh (98% of haplotypes were different) and the U.K. (96%), and the lowest diversity was found in Orkney (76%), Shetland (76%), and Lewis (64%). Gene diversity, a measure based on allele frequency, was estimated for Xq13-21 markers and was very similar across regions, although it tended to be lower for the Lewis subpopulation (table 7).

Discussion

The Scottish island populations represent both unusually stable and older populations whose declining numbers—due to past bottlenecks, large-scale emigration, and little immigration—may have contributed to the creation of LD as a result of genetic drift and endogamous mating. Clear evidence of a reduced female gene pool had been reported in the Western Isles and Orkney, on the basis of the low mtDNA diversity in the region (Helgason et al. 2001). These populations may be suitable for the drift-mapping strategy (Terwilliger et al. 1998), as proposed for mapping genetic factors that influence complex disease. In our study, the island of Lewis appeared to be the most extreme with regard to the extent of LD, in agreement with a previous report showing high differentiation, compared with Ireland and mainland Scotland, on the basis of serum protein polymorphisms (Clegg et al. 1985).

Interestingly, despite little differentiation based on allele-frequency distributions, evidence for population structure was also detectable in mainland rural subpopulations (e.g., Galloway, Grampian, and Argyll), which showed levels of LD intermediate between the urban/general U.K. and island samples. This intermediate extent of LD is likely to reflect increased sharing of ancestral chromosomal segments. Because of their larger size compared with that of the islands (fig. 1), these subpopulations (91,000–314,000) represent a valuable resource for conducting large-scale genetic-association studies, especially when a high percentage of the population is "local"—such as in Grampian (42% local), which is comparable in population size to Iceland. Variable levels of LD among populations that are not differentiated by allele-frequency distributions have been observed in at least one other study. Although differentiation, as estimated by pairwise F_{ST}, was not significant

Table 6

Median Population Recombination-Rate Estimates

Population	$3N_er$ (N_e) for Loci on	
	Xp21-11[a]	Xq13-21[b]
Shetland	21×10^{-6} (1,400)	3.4×10^{-6} (435)
Lewis	21×10^{-6} (1,400)	6.1×10^{-6} (782)
Orkney	44×10^{-6} (2,933)	8.7×10^{-6} (1,115)
Galloway	44×10^{-6} (2,933)	15.8×10^{-6} (2,025)
Wester Ross/Skye	46×10^{-6} (3,067)	6.5×10^{-6} (833)
Argyll	46×10^{-6} (3,067)	7.5×10^{-6} (961)
Grampian	60×10^{-6} (4,000)	14.3×10^{-6} (1,833)
Angus	77×10^{-6} (5,133)	18.0×10^{-6} (2,031)
United Kingdom	94×10^{-6} (6,267)	11.7×10^{-6} (1,500)
Edinburgh	94×10^{-6} (6,267)	29.0×10^{-6} (3,718)
Borders	100×10^{-6} (6,667)	14.1×10^{-6} (1,808)

NOTE.—Subpopulations are shown in increasing order, by values of their adjusted recombination rate based on Xp21-11 data. Estimates of the population-adjusted recombination rates, $3N_er$, were obtained after haplotype inference from female genotypes by use of the coalescent model implemented in PHASE v2.0.2. The algorithm was run independently five times, and the run with the best average goodness of fit to the approximate coalescent model was kept. Within each run, the number of iterations of the final step (i.e., all loci considered) was increased by a factor of 10, compared with the default setting, to obtain better estimates. The median of 1,000 values sampled from the posterior distribution was taken as point estimate for each population-adjusted recombination rate. The units of r are per meiosis and per base pair.

[a] Within Xp21-11, 13 Xp11 markers (*DXS1068, DXS8014, DXS8113, DXS1058, DXS8015, DXS8042, DXS1368, DXS993, DXS8012, DXS1201, DXS8085, DXS7,* and *MAOB*), spanning 4.7 Mb (7 cM), were used.

[b] Within Xq13-21, all eight markers (*DXS983, DXS1165, DXS8092, DXS8037, DXS56, DXS1225, DXS8082,* and *DXS995*) were used, spanning 13 Mb (3.36 cM). Estimates of the subpopulation effective size were calculated from the average map-based estimate of recombination rates.

Table 7

Gene and Haplotype Diversity of a Subset of Six Xq13-21 Markers

	Findings for Haplotype Set				Gene diversity (No. of Alleles) for Haplotype[b]							
	DXS8092-DXS8037-DXS56-DXS1225-DXS8082-DXS995		*DXS56-DXS1225-DXS8082*									
Population[a]	N^c	k^d (%)	N^c	k^d (%)	*DXS983*	*DXS1165*	*DXS8092*	*DXS8037*	*DXS56*	*DXS1225*	*DXS8082*	*DXS995*
Lewis	101	65 (64)	169	37 (22)	.64 (5)	.67 (8)	.83 (11)	.68 (10)	.74 (10)	.74 (11)	.73 (10)	.57 (5)
Shetland	58	44 (76)	87	32 (37)	.62 (6)	.67 (10)	.85 (11)	.71 (7)	.76 (8)	.74 (10)	.74 (8)	.61 (6)
Orkney	73	56 (76)	99	38 (38)	.63 (9)	.68 (10)	.85 (13)	.69 (8)	.79 (10)	.73 (12)	.71 (9)	.59 (5)
Argyll	58	48 (83)	102	42 (41)	.59 (5)	.66 (10)	.84 (11)	.68 (8)	.77 (8)	.75 (10)	.77 (9)	.67 (5)
Grampian	49	41 (84)	72	36 (50)	.66 (6)	.68 (9)	.86 (13)	.71 (8)	.78 (9)	.76 (11)	.68 (9)	.52 (7)
Wester Ross/Skye	61	53 (87)	97	40 (41)	.64 (5)	.68 (9)	.85 (12)	.73 (9)	.74 (9)	.74 (11)	.73 (9)	.63 (6)
Borders	46	42 (91)	90	37 (41)	.65 (8)	.73 (6)	.86 (12)	.73 (10)	.75 (8)	.76 (11)	.76 (9)	.57 (6)
Galloway	56	51 (91)	94	47 (50)	.69 (7)	.67 (11)	.88 (12)	.66 (8)	.80 (8)	.75 (10)	.78 (10)	.61 (5)
Angus	34	32 (94)	56	25 (45)	.69 (6)	.69 (9)	.87 (14)	.68 (7)	.79 (8)	.74 (11)	.74 (9)	.66 (6)
United Kingdom	53	51 (96)	101	46 (46)	.70 (7)	.67 (11)	.87 (13)	.66 (9)	.78 (8)	.77 (11)	.75 (10)	.59 (6)
Edinburgh	40	39 (97.5)	87	40 (57)	.68 (8)	.74 (11)	.86 (14)	.70 (10)	.79 (8)	.76 (12)	.77 (10)	.54 (6)

NOTE.—Allele frequencies for each microsatellite locus were estimated using Genepop software. Nei's average heterozygosity, or gene diversity, was calculated as 1 − the sum of the squared allele frequencies.

[a] Subpopulations are shown in increasing order, by values of the six-loci haplotype diversity.

[b] Gene diversity is based on whole data set.

[c] N = number of complete (i.e., without missing data) Xq13-21 six- or three-locus haplotypes from the male data set and inferred from the female data set. (For the inferred haplotype at each locus, the genotypes with phase certainty under 80% were discarded.)

[d] k = number of distinct haplotypes.

between the Saami and the Finnish populations when SNP data from ACE, β-globin, LPL, and MX were combined, these populations showed very different levels of LD (Kaessmann et al. 2002). The extent of LD appears to be more sensitive to factors such as reduction in effective population size and/or levels of endogamy than to measures of differentiation based on allele-frequency distributions (e.g., F_{ST}).

Finally, it is clear that the advantages of sampling within rural subpopulations, such as for reduced haplotype diversity and increased extent of LD for association mapping, are diminished by sampling across multiple regions or from within large urban populations. An increasing number of national genetic databases are being set up to exploit the biomedical opportunities offered by dense, high-throughput SNP genotyping in the context of association studies. The U.K. Biobank study is the largest of such studies to date, which proposes recruitment of 500,000 individuals from across the United Kingdom, including 80,000 from Scotland. Recruitment strategies for such large-scale studies tend to be representative of the population as a whole and therefore underrepresent rural populations. The higher haplotype diversity and low levels of LD within urban samples may make whole-genome scans prohibitively expensive and either increase the cost or reduce the power of more-focused genotyping studies. The major value of such national collections may therefore be not in the discovery of new genetic associations but in the further characterization of known ones. There is a strong case for additional biobanks of individuals recruited from large, stable rural subpopulations, which have the potential for providing increased power and efficiency to detect new genetic variants influencing biomedical traits.

Acknowledgments

The authors are indebted to the participants who allowed use of their DNA for this study and to the general practitioners who agreed to take part in the study. We thank Yoshiro Shibasaki, for help in making early contacts; Pauline McDonald and Lindsey Walls, for their secretarial help in the recruitment phase; Susan Fitzsimmon and Isla Campbell, for help in genotyping; and Douglas Stuart, for figure reproduction. This research received support from the U.K. Medical Research Council (MRC). V.V. holds an MRC Special Training Fellowship in Bioinformatics.

Electronic-Database Information

The URLs for data presented herein are as follows:

Authors' Web site, http://www.hgu.mrc.ac.uk/Rawdata/AJHG76/Vitart/ (for the authors' raw data)
Genepop, http://wbiomed.curtin.edu.au/genepop/
Genetix, http://www.univ-montp2.fr/~genetix/genetix/genetix.htm
GOLD, http://www.well.ox.ac.uk/asthma/GOLD/
PHASE, http://www.stat.washington.edu/stephens/software.html

References

Abecasis GR, Cookson WO (2000) GOLD—graphical overview of linkage disequilibrium. Bioinformatics 16:182–183

Angius A, Bebbere D, Petretto E, Falchi M, Forabosco P, Maestrale B, Casu G, Persico I, Melis PM, Pirastu M (2002) Not all isolates are equal: linkage disequilibrium analysis on Xq13.3 reveals different patterns in Sardinian sub-populations. Hum Genet 111:9–15

Blangero J (2004) Localization and identification of human quantitative trait loci: king harvest has surely come. Curr Op Genet Dev 14:233–240

Brown ES (1965) Distribution of ABO and Rhesus (D) blood groups in the North of Scotland. Heredity 20:289–303

Capelli C, Redhead N, Abernethy JK, Gratrix F, Wilson JF, Moen T, Hervig T, Richards M, Stumpf MP, Underhill PA, Bradshaw P, Shaha A, Thomas MG, Bradman N, Goldstein DB (2003) A Y chromosome census of the British Isles. Curr Biol 13:979–984

Clegg EJ, Tills D, Warlow A, Wilkinson J, Marin A (1985) Blood group variation in the Isle of Lewis. Ann Hum Biol 12:345–361

Collins A, Ennis S, Taillon-Miller P, Kwok PY, Morton NE (2001) Allelic association with SNPs: metrics, populations, and the linkage disequilibrium map. Hum Mutat 17:255–262

Freedman ML, Reich D, Penney KL, McDonald GJ, Mignault AA, Patterson N, Gabriel SB, Topol EJ, Smoller JW, Pato CN, Pato MT, Petryshen TL, Kolonel LN, Lander ES, Sklar P, Henderson B, Hirschhorn JN, Altshuler D (2004) Assessing the impact of population stratification on genetic association studies. Nat Genet 36:388–393

Hedrick PW (1987) Gametic disequilibrium measures: proceed with caution. Genetics 117:331–341

Helgason A, Hickey E, Goodacre S, Bosnes V, Stefánsson K, Ward R, Sykes B (2001) mtDNA and the islands of the North Atlantic: estimating the proportions of Norse and Gaelic ancestry. Am J Hum Genet 68:723–737

Helgason A, Sigurðardóttir S, Nicholson J, Sykes B, Hill EW, Bradley DG, Bosnes V, Gulcher JR, Ward R, Stefánsson K (2000) Estimating Scandinavian and Gaelic ancestry in the male settlers of Iceland. Am J Hum Genet 67:697–717

Helgason A, Yngvadottir B, Hrafnkelsson B, Gulcher J, Stefánsson K (2005) An Icelandic example of the impact of population structure on association studies. Nat Genet 37:90–95

Kaessmann H, Zöllner S, Gustafsson AC, Wiebe V, Laan M, Lundeberg J, Uhlén M, Pääbo S (2002) Extensive linkage disequilibrium in small human populations in Eurasia. Am J Hum Genet 70:673–685

Katoh T, Mano S, Ikuta T, Munkhbat B, Tounai K, Ando H, Munkhtuvshin N, Imanishi T, Inoko H, Tamiya G (2002) Genetic isolates in East Asia: a study of linkage disequilibrium in the X chromosome. Am J Hum Genet 71:395–400

Kong A, Gudbjartsson DF, Sainz J, Jonsdottir GM, Gudjonsson SA, Richardsson B, Sigurdardottir S, Barnard J, Hallbeck B, Masson G, Shlien A, Palsson ST, Frigge ML, Thorgeirsson TE, Gulcher JR, Stefansson K (2002) A high-resolution recombination map of the human genome. Nat Genet 31:241–247

Kruskal JB, Wish M (1977) Multidimensional scaling. Sage Publications, Beverly Hills

Laan M, Pääbo S (1997) Demographic history and linkage disequilibrium in human populations. Nat Genet 17:435–438

Latini V, Sole G, Doratiotto S, Poddie D, Memmi M, Varesi L, Vona G, Cao A, Ristaldi MS (2004) Genetic isolates in Corsica (France): linkage disequilibrium extension analysis on the Xq13 region. Eur J Hum Genet 12:613–619

Li N, Stephens M (2003) Modeling linkage disequilibrium and identifying recombination hotspots using single-nucleotide polymorphism data. Genetics 165:2213–2233

Marchini J, Cardon LR, Phillips MS, Donnelly P (2004) The effects of human population structure on large genetic association studies. Nat Genet 36:512–517

Mourant AE, Kopéc AC, Domaniewska-Sobczak K (1976) The distribution of the human blood groups and other polymorphisms. Oxford University Press, London

Nei M (1978) Estimation of average heterozygosity and genetic distance from a small number of individuals. Genetics 89: 583–590

Pritchard JK, Przeworski M (2001) Linkage disequilibrium in humans: models and data. Am J Hum Genet 69:1–14

Pritchard JK, Stephens M, Donnelly P (2000) Inference of population structure using multilocus genotype data. Genetics 155: 945–959

Raymond M, Rousset F (1995) An exact test for population differentiation. Evolution 49:1280–1283

Stephens M, Smith NJ, Donnelly P (2001) A new statistical method for haplotype reconstruction from population data. Am J Hum Genet 68:978–989

Taillon-Miller P, Saccone SF, Saccone NL, Duan S, Kloss EF, Lovins EG, Donaldson R, Phong A, Ha C, Flagstad L, Miller S, Drendel A, Lind D, Miller RD, Rice JP, Kwok PY (2004) Linkage disequilibrium maps constructed with common SNPs are useful for first-pass disease association screens. Genomics 84:899–912

Terwilliger JD, Zollner S, Laan M, Paabo S (1998) Mapping genes through the use of linkage disequilibrium generated by genetic drift: "drift mapping" in small populations with no demographic expansion. Hum Heredity 48:138–154

Weir BS, Cockerham CC (1984) Estimating F-statistics for the analysis of population structure. Evolution 38:1358–1370

Wilson EB, Hilferty MM (1931) The distribution of chi-square. Proc Natl Acad Sci USA 17:694

Wilson JF, Weiss DA, Richards M, Thomas MG, Bradman N, Goldstein DB (2001) Genetic evidence for different male and female roles during cultural transitions in the British Isles. Proc Natl Acad Sci USA 98:5078–5083

Zavattari P, Deidda E, Whalen M, Lampis R, Mulargia A, Loddo M, Eaves I, Mastio G, Todd JA, Cucca F (2000) Major factors influencing linkage disequilibrium by analysis of different chromosome regions in distinct populations: demography, chromosome recombination frequency and selection. Hum Mol Genet 9:2947–2957

Am. J. Hum. Genet. 76:773–779, 2005

Localization of a Type 1 Diabetes Locus in the *IL2RA/CD25* Region by Use of Tag Single-Nucleotide Polymorphisms

Adrian Vella,[1] Jason D. Cooper,[1] Christopher E. Lowe,[1] Neil Walker,[1] Sarah Nutland,[1] Barry Widmer,[2] Richard Jones,[3] Susan M. Ring,[3] Wendy McArdle,[3] Marcus E. Pembrey,[3,4] David P. Strachan,[5] David B. Dunger,[2] Rebecca C. J. Twells,[1] David G. Clayton,[1] and John A. Todd[1]

[1]Juvenile Diabetes Research Foundation/Wellcome Trust Diabetes and Inflammation Laboratory, Cambridge Institute for Medical Research, and [2]Department of Paediatrics, Addenbrooke's Hospital, University of Cambridge, Cambridge, United Kingdom; [3]Department of Community-Based Medicine, Bristol University, Bristol, United Kingdom; and [4]Clinical and Molecular Genetics Unit, Institute of Child Health, University College London, and [5]Department of Community Health Sciences, St. George's Hospital Medical School, London

As part of an ongoing search for genes associated with type 1 diabetes (T1D), a common autoimmune disease, we tested the biological candidate gene *IL2RA* (*CD25*), which encodes a subunit (IL-2Rα) of the high-affinity interleukin-2 (IL-2) receptor complex. We employed a tag single-nucleotide polymorphism (tag SNP) approach in large T1D sample collections consisting of 7,457 cases and controls and 725 multiplex families. Tag SNPs were analyzed using a multilocus test to provide a regional test for association. We found strong statistical evidence in the case-control collection ($P = 6.5 \times 10^{-8}$) for a T1D locus in the *CD25* region of chromosome 10p15 and replicated the association in the family collection ($P = 7.3 \times 10^{-3}$; combined $P = 1.3 \times 10^{-10}$). These results illustrate the utility of tag SNPs in a chromosome-regional test of disease association and justify future fine mapping of the causal variant in the region.

Introduction

Despite hundreds of association studies, few have been consistently replicated (Dahlman et al. 2002; Hirschhorn et al. 2003; Ioannidis et al. 2003; Lohmueller et al. 2003). In type 1 diabetes (T1D [MIM 222100]), only four loci have been identified and successfully replicated: the HLA class II genes on chromosome 6p21 (Cucca et al. 2001), the insulin gene (*INS*) on chromosome 11p15 (Bell et al. 1984; Barratt et al. 2004), the CTLA-4 gene on chromosome 2q33 (Nisticó et al. 1996; Ueda et al. 2003), and the recently associated PTPN22 gene on chromosome 1p13 (Bottini et al. 2004; Smyth et al. 2004). It is now generally accepted that large numbers of individuals and more stringent criteria for interpreting association studies are required to ensure reliable detection of association (Dahlman et al. 2002; Ioannidis et al. 2003; Lohmueller et al. 2003; Thomas and Clayton 2004; Wacholder et al. 2004; Freimer and Sabatti 2004; Smyth et al. 2005; Wang et al. 2005).

Most cases of T1D result from immune-mediated destruction of the insulin-producing β cells of the pancreas in an inflammatory process that involves many cell types of the immune system, including T lymphocytes. The four identified T1D loci underpin these known features of the disease, since they are all involved in T cell development (for *INS*, in terms of thymic tolerance of the insulin molecule), activation, expansion, and regulation (Todd and Wicker 2001; Ueda et al. 2003; Anjos and Polychronakos 2004). As part of an ongoing search for genes associated with T1D, we tested the biological candidate gene *CD25* (MIM 147730). In common with the T1D loci identified elsewhere, *CD25* is central to immune regulation. *CD25* expression on regulatory T cells is essential for their function in suppressing T cell immune responses and autoimmune disease (Salomon et al. 2000; Malek and Bayer 2004; Viglietta et al. 2004). Additionally, in humans, a rare mutation of *CD25* caused severe autoimmune disease (Sharfe et al. 1997).

We adopted a linkage disequilibrium (LD)-mapping approach to test for an association between T1D and the *CD25* region, using tag SNPs (Johnson et al. 2001; Chapman et al. 2003; Clayton et al. 2004) in large case-control and family collections. Elsewhere, we have shown that the use of tag SNPs can reduce genotyping costs by approximately two-thirds (Chapman et al. 2003; Clayton et al. 2004; Lowe et al. 2004).

Received December 13, 2004; accepted for publication February 21, 2005; electronically published March 17, 2005.

Address for correspondence and reprints: Prof. John A. Todd, Juvenile Diabetes Research Foundation/Wellcome Trust Diabetes and Inflammation Laboratory, University of Cambridge, Cambridge Institute for Medical Research, Wellcome Trust/Medical Research Council Building, Addenbrooke's Hospital, Hills Road, Cambridge, CB2 2XY, United Kingdom. E-mail: john.todd@cimr.cam.ac.uk

0002-9297/2005/7605-0006$15.00

Subjects and Methods

Subjects

The resequencing panel consisted of 32 CEPH individuals (Utah residents with ancestry from northern and western Europe) (Fondation Jean Dausset–CEPH).

The 3,527 cases were recruited as part of the United Kingdom Genetic Resource Investigating Diabetes (U.K. GRID) study, which is a joint project between the University of Cambridge Department of Paediatrics and the Department Medical Genetics at the Cambridge Institute for Medical Research and is funded by the Juvenile Diabetes Research Foundation and the Wellcome Trust. The eventual aim of the project is to collect 8,000 cases with T1D for comparison with 8,000 controls from the 1958 British Birth Cohort (1958 BBC), to allow well-powered genetic association studies. The 1958 BBC is an ongoing follow-up of all persons born in Great Britain during one week in 1958 (National Child Development Study), including a recent biomedical assessment during 2002–2004 at which blood samples and informed consent were obtained for creation of a genetic resource. All cases were white, and at least 97% of the controls were of white ethnicity.

All families were of white European descent and were composed of two parents and at least one affected child. The population studied consisted of 472 multiplex families from the Diabetes United Kingdom Warren collection and 268 multiplex families from the (U.S.) Human Biological Data Interchange. The characteristics and inclusion criteria for each family collection have been described elsewhere (Vella et al. 2004), and these and reference to the case-control samples can be obtained from the Juvenile Diabetes Research Foundation/Wellcome Trust Web site. All DNA samples were collected with approval of the relevant research ethics committees, and written informed consent was obtained from the participants.

Identifying Polymorphisms

To identify polymorphisms in the CD25 gene, the exons, exon/intron boundaries, and up to 3 kb of 3′ and 5′ flanking sequence were resequenced in DNA samples from 32 CEPH DNA samples by use of nested PCR products; we also sequenced the regions −9,000 to −8,000, −4,000 to −3,000, and +3,000 to +4,000 bases, numbered relative to the transcription start site, to encompass the CD28 response element (CD28rE), the Positive Regulatory Region (PRR) III, and PRR IV, respectively (Toledano et al. 1990; Kim and Leonard 2002). In total, 15 kb was sequenced from the *CD25* region, spanning ~60 kb. The sequencing reactions were performed using the Applied Biosystems (ABI) BigDye (version 3.1) chemistry, and the sequences were analyzed using an ABI 3700 capillary sequencer. Analysis of the sequence traces was performed using the Staden package (Bonfield et al. 1998) and was double scored by a second operator. All sequence information and primer locations are provided at the T1DBase Web site.

Tag SNPs

As described elsewhere (Chapman et al. 2003; Clayton et al. 2004), we used the resequencing genotype data to investigate the ability of smaller subsets of SNPs to predict the genotypes of the remainder. Predictive performance was assessed using a locus R^2 measure (coefficient of determination), which measures the ability to predict each known SNP genotype by linear regression on the tag SNP genotypes (Chapman et al. 2003). We considered only SNPs with a minor-allele frequency (MAF) $\geqslant 5\%$ and required that the subset of tag SNPs predict the remaining SNPs with a minimum R^2 of 0.8.

We selected an optimal set of tag SNPs, using a mixture of step-up, step-down, and exhaustive subset search algorithms. Since the exhaustive subset search procedure can be slow, we initially identified a set of tag SNPs selected by both step-up and step-down searches, and we determined the best additional set of tag SNPs by exhaustive subset search of the remaining SNPs (Lowe et al. 2004). The programs for the selection and analysis of tag SNPs are implemented in STATA and can be downloaded from D.G.C.'s Web site.

Genotyping

Tag SNPs were genotyped using either Taqman (Applied Biosystems) or Invader (Third Wave Technologies) technologies on a British case-control collection (3,527 cases and 3,930 controls), in accordance with the manufacturers' protocols. All genotyping data were double scored to minimize error.

Multilocus Test for Association

Chapman et al. (2003) suggested the use of a multivariate test statistic in the analysis of a tagged region. Essentially, the test contrasts the profile of tag SNP allele frequencies between cases and controls by use of Hotelling's T^2 test (Xiong et al. 2002; Chapman et al. 2003; Fan and Knapp 2003). The test does not assume Hardy-Weinberg equilibrium in cases and controls; since no imputation of haplotype phase is required, variance and covariances of genotypes are estimated empirically. In the analysis of the case-control collection, the multilocus test was stratified by broad geographical region within Great Britain to exclude the possibility of confounding by geography. For each of 12 regions, we computed the vector of contrasts between case and control allele frequencies. The final test was based on a weighted sum of these contrast vectors, with weights inversely proportional to variance. This procedure is a multivariate generali-

Table 1

Polymorphisms Identified in *CD25*

The table is available in its entirety in the online edition of *The American Journal of Human Genetics.*

zation of standard methods for control of confounding in epidemiological studies (Breslow and Day 1980; Clayton and Hills 1993).

In the analysis of the family collection, parent-child trios were analyzed by a very closely related procedure. Each trio contributed a vector of transmitted allele pairs and a vector of untransmitted allele pairs. These can be thought of as "cases" and matched "pseudocontrols," respectively. Each pair was then scored 0, 1, or 2, and the case and control profiles were compared using a paired Hotelling's T^2 test (Chapman et al. 2003).

These tests are most powerful when the effect of the causal variant is codominant. A recessive mode of inheritance results in reduced heterozygosity at the causal locus, but this may be reflected only weakly at any one tag SNP. Chapman et al. (2003) suggested a method for incorporation of this information into the multilocus test, but we did not judge it to be necessary in our study.

The evidence from case-control and family collections was combined in the same manner as was used to amalgamate the evidence from different geographical regions in the analysis of the case-control collection; a vector of contrasts comparing case and control allele frequencies for the set of tag SNPs was contributed from both studies, and a weighted mean of this vector was computed and tested against 0 (appendix A).

Imputation of Missing Tag SNP Genotypes

The multilocus test takes account of correlations between genotype for different tags and, therefore, requires that a complete set of scores be entered for each subject. Even a modest genotyping failure rate can result in a substantial attrition of subjects for such "complete case" analyses and substantial loss of power. We have avoided this by imputation of missing values.

Imputation of missing genotypes was performed using linear regression; that is, the missing tag SNP, $t_i (i = 1,2,\ldots,n)$, genotypes (scored 0, 1, or 2) were predicted from the regression of t_i on the set of complete tag SNP genotypes, excluding t_i. Clayton et al. (2004) justify this procedure for high-LD regions. Imputation was performed under the null hypothesis so that, for the same genotypes at observed loci, a missing locus would be assigned the same score whether the subject were a case or a control. The effect of this is to shrink case-control differences toward zero, but, since their variances and covariances are estimated empirically, the size of the test is preserved.

We evaluated the effect of imputation on type 1 error rates and on power in a simulation study. A number of scenarios, defined by the number of tag SNPs (maximum 20) and the percentage of missing at-random tag SNP genotypes (5% or 10%), in both case-control samples (1,000 cases and 1,000 controls) and families (1,000 parent-child trios), were considered. The effect of imputation on type 1 error rates in data generated under the null hypothesis of no association was evaluated on the basis of how often the null hypothesis was rejected when a significance test with a critical P value of P_1 was applied. The null hypothesis should be rejected with probability P_1. The power, with and without the imputation of missing tag SNP genotypes, was evaluated on the basis of how often the null hypothesis was rejected when applied to data generated under the alternative hypothesis.

Results

The resequencing of *CD25* for 32 CEPH individuals identified 55 polymorphisms (table 1), 54 of which were SNPs; 13 of these SNPs were novel when compared with dbSNP build 123, and 1 polymorphism, *ss35031434,* was a novel G insertion/deletion. Sixteen SNPs had an MAF <5% and were consequently not included in the tag SNP selection. From the 39 common SNPs (MAF $\geqslant$5%), 20 tag SNPs were selected and genotyped in the case-control collection (table 2). All tag SNP genotypes in cases and controls were in Hardy-Weinberg equilibrium.

The multilocus test P value for the case-control collection was 6.5×10^{-8} (3,521 case and 3,930 control genotypes; $F_{20,7419} = 3.7$). The multilocus test was stratified by 12 broad geographic regions, to minimize any confounding due to variation in allele frequencies across Great Britain (see the "Subjects and Methods" section) (unstratified P value was 1.4×10^{-8}).

We proceeded to genotype the tag SNPs in a large family collection (472 British and 268 U.S. multiplex families with T1D). tag SNP genotypes in parents and affected offspring were all in Hardy-Weinberg equilibrium. We replicated the association in the family collection, with a multilocus test P value of 7.3×10^{-3} (parent-child trio genotypes = 1,378; $\chi^2_{20} = 38.7$) (table 3), thus providing independent evidence of an association between T1D and *CD25*. Figure 1 shows the striking agreement between the odds ratios and the relative risks (transmission ratios) for the minor alleles of the tag SNPs genotyped in the case-control and family collections. Consequently, when results from both studies were combined, the multilocus test (Smyth et al. 2004)

Table 2

Summary of Tag SNPs for the Case-Control Collection

The table is available in its entirety in the online edition of *The American Journal of Human Genetics.*

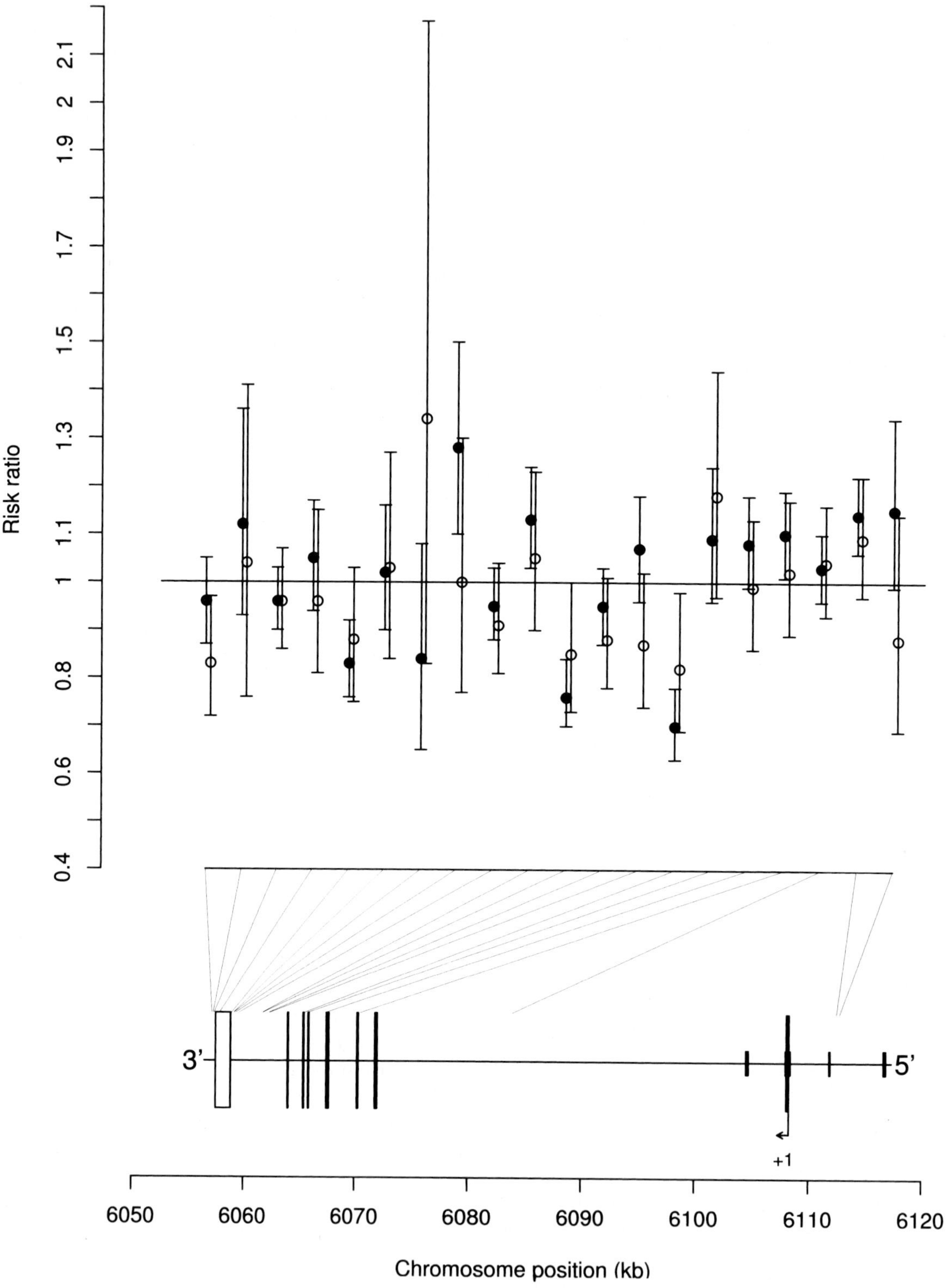

Figure 1 *Upper panel,* Odds ratios and transmission ratios for the minor allele of *CD25* tag SNPs genotyped in the case-control (*filled circles*) and family (*open circles*) collections, respectively. Vertical lines indicate 95% CIs. *Lower panel,* Chromosome position of *CD25* tag SNPs. Open long rectangle indicates UTR, filled long rectangles indicate exons, filled short rectangles indicate regulatory regions, and the arrow labeled "+1" indicates the transcript start site. A version of this figure can be viewed at the T1DBase Web site.

Table 3

Summary of Tag SNPs for the Family Collection

The table is available in its entirety in the online edition of *The American Journal of Human Genetics.*

(appendix A) provided strong statistical support for a T1D locus in the *CD25* region of chromosome 10p15.1 ($\chi^2_{20} = 88.6$; $P = 1.3 \times 10^{-10}$). There was no suggestion of reduced heterozygosity in cases or affected offspring, an indication of recessive inheritance.

Simulations of data generated under the null hypothesis indicated that imputation did not affect type 1 error rates; that is, the null hypothesis was rejected with probability P_1 when a significance test with a critical P value of P_1 was applied. For example, the null hypothesis was rejected in 483, 102, and 9 of 10,000 simulations of 1,000 cases and 1,000 controls genotyped in 20 tag SNPs, with 5% of tag SNP genotypes missing at critical P values of 0.05, 0.01, and 0.001, respectively. Simulations also indicated that imputation partially recaptures the loss of power incurred by restricting the analysis to subjects with a complete set of tag SNP genotypes (table 4). For example, if a genomic region has 20 tag SNPs that are genotyped in 1,000 cases and 1,000 controls with 5% of tag SNP genotypes missing at random, by imputing missing genotypes, power to detect a causal variant with an odds ratio of 1.5 (causal allele frequency of 0.35 in controls) at a significance level of $P = .05$ increases from 46.5% to 96.0% in 1,000 simulations. In the equivalent exercise in families (1,000 parent-child trios), power increases from 12.9% to 99.1%. Imputation is particularly important for parent-child trios and for candidate genes with a relatively large number of tag SNPs, since, in those cases, restriction of the analysis to complete cases is particularly damaging. The multilocus test P values for the case-control and family collections without imputation were 2.1×10^{-6} (2,812 case and 2,981 control genotypes; $F_{20,5761} = 3.2$) and .052 (parent-child trio genotypes = 558; $\chi^2_{20} = 31.2$), respectively.

Discussion

In the present study, we have assessed only the polymorphisms located in or close to exons and known regulatory regions, as well as up to 3 kb of 3′ and 5′ flanking sequence. Since we have found strong statistical evidence for a T1D locus in the *CD25* region, we have now started to resequence an extended and, where possible, contiguous *CD25* chromosome region of ∼190 kb including *CD25* to identify potential causal variants. Fine mapping of an extended region is required, since the *CD25* tag SNPs could be in LD with a causal variant beyond *CD25*. For example, *IL15RA*, a strong functional candidate (Fehniger and Caligiuri 2001), is ∼30 kb from the 3′ flanking sequence of *CD25*.

Since the causal variant(s) in the *CD25* region remains unknown, to replicate the association with T1D reported in the present study, a tag SNP approach would be required, genotyping either the same or a new set of tag SNPs. A new selection could be required—when the population in a subsequent study has a different pattern of LD in the *CD25* region, for instance. The temptation to ignore the foundations of the reported association, the set of tag SNPs, and the pattern of LD behind their

Table 4

Effect of Imputation on Power of a Simulated Case-Control Study and of a Family Study

No. of Tag SNPs and *P*	Percentage of Tag SNP Genotypes Missing at Random							
	In Case-Control Study with				In Family Study with			
	No Imputation		Imputation		No Imputation		Imputation	
	5%	10%	5%	10%	5%	10%	5%	10%
4:								
.05	99.9	98.8	100.0	99.8	97.3	78.6	99.8	99.9
.01	98.6	95.4	99.6	99.3	90.8	62.5	98.7	97.8
.001	94.3	84.8	98.1	96.6	75.2	35.3	95.5	92.0
12:								
.05	89.7	57.5	99.7	99.5	38.9	3.3	99.3	98.6
.01	74.2	33.2	97.8	97.3	19.0	.1	95.8	93.6
.001	48.7	13.1	92.4	91.0	3.3	.0	85.1	79.7
20:								
.05	46.5	16.9	96.0	94.7	12.9	.0	99.1	97.7
.01	24.1	5.2	88.1	85.3	2.1	.0	95.3	92.4
.001	7.9	.6	67.7	65.2	.1	.0	80.9	78.0

NOTE.—Power was estimated from 1,000 simulations of each type of study (1,000 each, cases, controls, and parent-child trios). The causal variant had an OR of 1.5 and a causal-allele frequency of ∼35% in controls and parents.

selection and to genotype only the most-associated tag SNP may well lead to false-negative results, since the power of the present study is based on the complete set of tag SNPs.

Acknowledgments

We gratefully acknowledge the participation of all patients with T1D, their family members, and control individuals. We thank Helen Rance, Tasneem Hassanali, Jayne Hutchings, Gillian Coleman, Sarah Field, Trupti Mistry, Kirsi Bourget, Sally Clayton, Matthew Hardy, Jennifer Keylock, Pamela Lauder, Meeta Maisuria, William Meadows, Meera Sebastian, and Sarah Wood, for preparing DNA samples; the Avon Longitudinal Study of Parents and Children Laboratory in Bristol, for preparing DNA samples; Luc Smink, Oliver Burren, and Alex Lam, for bioinformatic support. We acknowledge use of DNA from the 1958 BBC collection, funded by Medical Research Council grant G0000934 and Wellcome Trust grant 068545/Z/02. We acknowledge Diabetes UK and the Human Biological Data Interchange, for multiplex family collections, and the Wellcome Trust, the Juvenile Diabetes Research Foundation, Diabetes UK, and the Medical Research Council, for financial support. A.V. is a Mayo Foundation Scholar, and D.G.C. is a Juvenile Diabetes Research Foundation/Wellcome Trust Principal Research Fellow.

Appendix A

In an earlier study (Smyth et al. 2004), we used and defined a score test to combine single-locus tests from family- and population-based studies; in the present article, we used a multivariate version of that test. Chapman et al. (2003) defined the multilocus test as a multivariate score test, $T^2 = \mathbf{U}^T\mathbf{V}^\theta\mathbf{U}$, where $\mathbf{U}$ is a score vector—with one element for each tag SNP, contrasting allele frequencies in cases and controls or, in family studies, frequencies of transmitted and untransmitted alleles. $\mathbf{V}$ is the estimated variance of the score statistic, and θ denotes a generalized inverse. The test statistic is asymptotically distributed as χ^2, with degrees of freedom equal to the rank of $\mathbf{V}$, which is equal to the number of tag SNPs. When combining results from family- and population-based studies, we first calculate the $\mathbf{U}$ vector and $\mathbf{V}$ matrix for each study. We then calculate an overall $\mathbf{U}$ and $\mathbf{V}$ by summation of the contributions from each study—$\mathbf{U} = \mathbf{U}_1 + \mathbf{U}_2$ and $\mathbf{V} = \mathbf{V}_1 + \mathbf{V}_2$—and calculate the T^2 test statistic as before.

Electronic-Database Information

The URLs for data presented herein are as follows:

dbSNP Home Page, http://www.ncbi.nlm.nih.gov/SNP/index.html

D.G.C.'s Web site, http://www-gene.cimr.cam.ac.uk/clayton/software/ (for the programs used for the selection and analysis of tag SNPs)

Fondation Jean Dausset–CEPH, http://www.cephb.fr/ (for information about the individuals used in the sequencing panel)

Juvenile Diabetes Research Foundation/Wellcome Trust, http://www-gene.cimr.cam.ac.uk/todd/dna-refs.shtml (for references to DNA collections used at the Juvenile Diabetes Research Foundation/Wellcome Trust Diabetes and Inflammation Laboratory)

National Center for Biotechnology Information (NCBI), http://www.ncbi.nlm.nih.gov/

National Child Development Study, http://www.cls.ioe.ac.uk/Cohort/Ncds/mainncds.htm (for information about the control collection)

Online Mendelian Inheritance in Man (OMIM), http://www.ncbi.nlm.nih.gov/Omim/ (for T1D and *CD25*)

STATA, http://www.stata.com (for statistical software used)

T1DBase, http://www.t1dbase.org/cgi-bin/welcome.cgi (for further information about the *CD25* region)

U.K. GRID, http://www-gene.cimr.cam.ac.uk/ucdr/grid.shtml (for information about the case collection)

References

Anjos S, Polychronakos C (2004) Mechanisms of genetic susceptibility to type I diabetes: beyond HLA. Mol Genet Metab 81:187–195

Barratt BJ, Payne F, Lowe CE, Hermann R, Healy BC, Harold D, Concannon P, Gharani N, McCarthy MI, Olavesen MG, McCormack R, Guja C, Ionescu-Tirgoviste C, Undlien DE, Ronningen KS, Gillespie KM, Tuomilehto-Wolf E, Tuomilehto J, Bennett ST, Clayton DG, Cordell HJ, Todd JA (2004) Remapping the insulin gene/*IDDM2* locus in type 1 diabetes. Diabetes 53:1884–1889

Bell GI, Horita S, Karam JH (1984) A polymorphic locus near the human insulin gene is associated with insulin-dependent diabetes mellitus. Diabetes 33:176–183

Bonfield JK, Rada C, Staden R (1998) Automated detection of point mutations using fluorescent sequence trace subtraction. Nucleic Acids Res 26:3404–3409

Bottini N, Musumeci L, Alonso A, Rahmouni S, Nika K, Rostamkhani M, MacMurray J, Meloni GF, Lucarelli P, Pellecchia M, Eisenbarth GS, Comings D, Mustelin T (2004) A functional variant of lymphoid tyrosine phosphatase is associated with type I diabetes. Nat Genet 36:337–338

Breslow NE, Day NE (1980) Statistical methods in cancer research: volume 1—the analysis of case-control studies. IARC Scientific Publications, Lyon

Chapman JM, Cooper JD, Todd JA, Clayton D (2003) Detecting disease associations due to linkage disequilibrium using haplotype tags: a class of tests and the determinants of statistical power. Hum Hered 56:18–31

Clayton D, Chapman J, Cooper J (2004) Use of unphased multilocus genotype data in indirect association studies. Genet Epidemiol 27:415–428

Clayton D, Hills M (1993) Statistical models in epidemiology. Oxford Science Publications, Oxford, United Kingdom

Cucca F, Lampis R, Congia M, Angius E, Nutland S, Bain SC, Barnett AH, Todd JA (2001) A correlation between the relative predisposition of MHC class II alleles to type 1 diabetes and the structure of their proteins. Hum Mol Genet 10:2025–2037

Dahlman I, Eaves IA, Kosoy R, Morrison VA, Heward J, Gough SC, Allahabadia A, Franklyn JA, Tuomilehto J, Tuomilehto-Wolf E, Cucca F, Guja C, Ionescu-Tirgoviste C, Stevens H, Carr P, Nutland S, McKinney P, Shield JP, Wang W, Cordell HJ, Walker N, Todd JA, Concannon P (2002) Parameters for reliable results in genetic association studies in common disease. Nat Genet 30:149–150

Fan R, Knapp M (2003) Genome association studies of complex diseases by case-control designs. Am J Hum Genet 72: 850–868

Fehniger TA, Caligiuri MA (2001) Interleukin 15: biology and relevance to human disease. Blood 97:14–32

Freimer N, Sabatti C (2004) The use of pedigree, sib-pair and association studies of common diseases for genetic mapping and epidemiology. Nat Genet 36:1045–1051

Hirschhorn JN (2003) Genetic epidemiology of type 1 diabetes. Pediatr Diabetes 4:87–100

Ioannidis JPA, Trikalinos TA, Ntzani EE, Contopoulos-Ioannidis DG (2003) Genetic associations in large versus small studies: an empirical assessment. Lancet 361:567–571

Johnson GCL, Esposito L, Barratt BJ, Smith AN, Heward J, Di Genova G, Ueda H, Cordell HJ, Eaves IA, Dudbridge F, Twells RCJ, Payne F, Hughes W, Nutland S, Stevens H, Carr P, Tuomilehto-Wolf E, Tuomilehto J, Gough SCL, Clayton DG, Todd JA (2001) Haplotype tagging for the identification of common disease genes. Nat Genet 29:233–237

Kim HP, Leonard WJ (2002) The basis for TCR-mediated regulation of the IL-2 receptor α chain gene: role of widely separated regulatory elements. EMBO J 21:3051–3059

Lohmueller KE, Pearce CL, Pike M, Lander ES, Hirschhorn (2003) Meta-analysis of genetic association studies supports a contribution of common variants to susceptibility to common disease. Nat Genet 33:177–182

Lowe CE, Cooper JD, Chapman JM, Barratt BJ, Twells RCJ, Green EA, Savage DA, Guja C, Ionescu-Tîrovişte C, Tuomilehto-Wolf E, Tuomilehto J, Todd JA, Clayton DG (2004) Cost-effective analysis of candidate genes using htSNPs: a staged approach. Genes Immun 5:301–305

Malek TR, Bayer AL (2004) Tolerance, not immunity, crucially depends on IL-2. Nat Rev Immunol 4:665–674

Nisticó L, Buzzetti R, Pritchard LE, Van der Auwera B, Giovannini C, Bosi E, Larrad MT, Rios MS, Chow CC, Cockram CS, Jacobs K, Mijovic C, Bain SC, Barnett AH, Vandewalle CL, Schuit F, Gorus FK, Tosi R, Pozzilli P, Todd JA (1996) The CTLA-4 gene region of chromosome 2q33 is linked to, and associated with, type 1 diabetes. Hum Mol Genet 5:1075–1080

Salomon B, Lenschow DJ, Rhee L, Ashourian N, Singh B, Sharpe A, Bluestone JA (2000) B7/CD28 costimulation is essential for the homeostasis of the CD4+CD25+ immunoregulatory T cells that control autoimmune diabetes. Immunity 12:431–440

Sharfe N, Dadi HK, Shahar M, Roifman CM (1997) Human immune disorder arising from mutation of the α chain of the interleukin-2 receptor. Proc Natl Acad Sci USA 94:3168–3171

Smyth D, Cooper JD, Collins JE, Heward JM, Franklyn JA, Howson JM, Vella A, Nutland S, Rance HE, Maier L, Barratt BJ, Guja C, Ionescu-Tirgoviste C, Savage DA, Dunger DB, Widmer B, Strachan DP, Ring SM, Walker N, Clayton DG, Twells RC, Gough SC, Todd JA (2004) Replication of an association between the lymphoid tyrosine phosphatase locus (*LYP/PTPN22*) with type 1 diabetes, and evidence for its role as a general autoimmunity locus. Diabetes 53:3020–3023

Smyth D, Howson JM, Lowe CE, Walker N, Lam AC, Nutland S, Hutchings J, Tuomilehto-Wolf E, Tuomilehto J, Guja C, Ionescu-Tirgoviste C, Undlien DE, Ronningen KS, Savage DA, Dunger DB, Twells RC, McArdle W, Strachan DP, Todd JA (2005) Assessing the validity of the association between the SUMO4 M55V variant and risk of type 1 diabetes. Nat Genet 37:110–111

Thomas DC, Clayton DG (2004) Betting odds and genetic associations. J Natl Cancer Inst 96:421–423

Todd JA, Wicker LS (2001) Genetic protection from the inflammatory disease type 1 diabetes in humans and animal models. Immunity 15:387–395

Toledano MB, Roman DG, Halden NF, Lin BB, Leonard WJ (1990) The same target sequences are differentially important for activation of the interleukin 2 receptor α-chain gene in two distinct T-cell lines. Proc Natl Acad Sci USA 87:1830–1834

Ueda H, Howson JM, Esposito L, Heward J, Snook H, Chamberlain G, Rainbow DB, et al (2003) Association of the T-cell regulatory gene *CTLA4* with susceptibility to autoimmune disease. Nature 423:506–511

Vella A, Howson JM, Barratt BJ, Twells RC, Rance HE, Nutland S, Tuomilehto-Wolf E, Tuomilehto J, Undlien DE, Ronningen KS, Guja C, Ionescu-Tirgoviste C, Savage DA, Todd JA (2004) Lack of association of the Ala(45)Thr polymorphism and other common variants of the NeuroD gene with type 1 diabetes. Diabetes 53:1158–1161

Viglietta V, Baecher-Allan C, Weiner HL, Hafler DA (2004) Loss of functional suppression by CD4+CD25+ regulatory T cells in patients with multiple sclerosis. J Exp Med 199: 971–979

Wacholder S, Chanock S, Garcia-Closas M, El Ghormli L, Rothman N (2004) Assessing the probability of false-positive reports in molecular epidemiology studies. J Natl Cancer Inst 96:434–442

Wang WYS, Barratt BJ, Clayton DG, Todd JA (2005) Genome-wide association studies: theoretical and practical concerns. Nat Rev Genet 6:109–118

Xiong M, Zhao J, Boerwinkle E (2002) Generalized T^2 test for genome association studies. Am J Hum Genet 70:1257–1268

Am. J. Hum. Genet. 76:780–793, 2005

Nonparametric Tests of Association of Multiple Genes with Human Disease

Daniel J. Schaid,[1] Shannon K. McDonnell,[1] Scott J. Hebbring,[2] Julie M. Cunningham,[2] and Stephen N. Thibodeau[2]

Departments of [1]Health Sciences Research and [2]Laboratory Medicine and Pathology, Mayo Clinic College of Medicine, Rochester, MN

The genetic basis of many common human diseases is expected to be highly heterogeneous, with multiple causative loci and multiple alleles at some of the causative loci. Analyzing the association of disease with one genetic marker at a time can have weak power, because of relatively small genetic effects and the need to correct for multiple testing. Testing the simultaneous effects of multiple markers by multivariate statistics might improve power, but they too will not be very powerful when there are many markers, because of the many degrees of freedom. To overcome some of the limitations of current statistical methods for case-control studies of candidate genes, we develop a new class of nonparametric statistics that can simultaneously test the association of multiple markers with disease, with only a single degree of freedom. Our approach, which is based on *U*-statistics, first measures a score over all markers for pairs of subjects and then compares the averages of these scores between cases and controls. Genetic scoring for a pair of subjects is measured by a "kernel" function, which we allow to be fairly general. However, we provide guidelines on how to choose a kernel for different types of genetic effects. Our global statistic has the advantage of having only one degree of freedom and achieves its greatest power advantage when the contrasts of average genotype scores between cases and controls are in the same direction across multiple markers. Simulations illustrate that our proposed methods have the anticipated type I–error rate and that they can be more powerful than standard methods. Application of our methods to a study of candidate genes for prostate cancer illustrates their potential merits, and offers guidelines for interpretation.

Introduction

The genetic basis of common human diseases is widely studied by evaluating the association of genetic variants with disease status, as in candidate-gene case-control studies. The power of this approach depends on the effect size of the disease locus (typically considered in terms of an odds ratio), the frequency of the disease allele(s), the frequency of the marker allele(s), and the magnitude of linkage disequilibrium between the marker and disease loci (Zondervan and Cardon 2004). Although there is debate on whether common diseases are caused by many rare mutations (Pritchard and Cox 2002) or a few common genetic variants (Reich and Lander 2001), it is clear that allelic heterogeneity will dilute power to detect genetic associations (Slager et al. 2000). Furthermore, when multiple genes are functionally related—for instance, when their products are related through a cascade of enzymatic reactions—mutations at any of several genes could lead to disease. Also, it may not be unusual for genes in a functional pathway to have complex interactions, given evidence of feedback loops and compensatory enzymatic activities among the protein products of biosynthesis pathways.

Received September 7, 2004; accepted for publication February 21, 2005; electronically published March 22, 2005.

Address for correspondence and reprints: Dr. Daniel J. Schaid, Department of Health Sciences Research, Harwick 7, Mayo Clinic, 200 First Street SW, Rochester, MN 55905. E-mail: schaid@mayo.edu

0002-9297/2005/7605-0007$15.00

Standard methods to evaluate the association of multiple markers with disease status are based on either single-marker analyses or multimarker multivariate analyses. For single-marker analyses of diallelic markers, it is common to compare the allele frequencies of each marker between cases and controls by use of Armitage's test for trend (Sasieni 1997) and to adjust for multiple testing by use of either the Bonferroni correction or a permutation *P* value for the most extreme statistic. This approach is likely to be most powerful if there is only a single marker strongly associated with disease. For multimarker multivariate analyses, one can use logistic regression to test simultaneously the main effects (and possibly interactions) of multiple markers. For each marker, a covariate can be created, such as the number of rare alleles at each marker. When this type of coding is used in logistic regression, the resulting score statistic for each marker is Armitage's test for trend, so simultaneously testing multiple marker loci by this type of coding and using the score statistic from logistic regression is a multivariate version of Armitage's score statistic. For K markers, each coded into covariates, the resulting score statistic has a χ^2 distribution with K degrees of freedom. This statistic is equivalent to the multivariate Hotelling's T^2 statistic proposed by Fan and Knapp (2003). Although this approach can be more powerful than testing each marker separately (Longmate 2001), it still suffers from weak power because of the large number of degrees of freedom. When evaluating the association of multiple genes with disease status, the power to detect associations can be weak when the effects of individual genes are weak and when correcting for multiple testing.

An alternative approach to evaluate the association of multiple genes with disease status might be to model all the complex interrelationships of genes, say within a common pathway, and how they relate to disease. This parametric method, however, would lead to models with too many parameters, possibly causing multicollinearity and model instability. Although Bayesian modeling of metabolic pathways with case-control data has achieved some level of success (Conti et al. 2003), it is difficult to evaluate whether complex models are overfitted to the data.

To improve power over that of standard methods, we propose a class of nonparametric statistics that combines information across all genetic markers, resulting in a global statistic that has a standard normal distribution. We expect that this approach would be sensitive to situations in which multiple genes influence the disease but the effect of each individual gene is weak. Our nonparametric methods are based on U-statistics, which are used to measure an average genetic score between pairs of subjects. Intuitively, we expect that any two subjects with similar disease status should also have similar genetic scores if any of the markers are associated with the disease. Hence, we measure the average genetic score for all pairs of cases and compare this to the average genetic score for all pairs of controls.

In the "Statistical Methods" section below, we describe the intuition and derivation of our methods, showing their generality, as well as important special cases. We illustrate how power can be computed, and we use this to show how to determine an optimal genotype score. To illustrate the properties of our methods, we perform simulations. We also apply our methods to a study of candidate genes for prostate cancer, to illustrate their utility and interpretation.

Statistical Methods

To compare the distribution of all marker genotypes between cases and controls, we first compute the scores for all possible pairs of subjects within each of the case and control groups. We then contrast the average scores between cases and controls by use of a global statistic with one degree of freedom instead of the implicit many degrees of freedom when many markers are analyzed.

U-Statistics for Within-Group Genotype Scores

First, consider a measure of genotype score within a single group of n subjects. Let $\mathbf{g}_i$ denote a vector of measured genotypes at K markers for subject i, with element $g_{i,k}$ the kth genotype. To measure the score of all genotypes for subjects i and j, we use a symmetric kernel, denoted as $h(\mathbf{g}_i,\mathbf{g}_j)$. A general U-statistic that measures the average score across all pairs of subjects is

$$U_{\text{global}} = \frac{\sum_{i<j} h(\mathbf{g}_i,\mathbf{g}_j)}{\binom{n}{2}} . \quad (1)$$

Hence, no matter how many markers are measured, the global U-statistic uses a kernel function to reduce the arrays of genetic markers for pairs of subjects into a single score, which then are averaged across all possible pairs. Although a wide variety of kernels can be considered, we shall consider primarily kernels that are additive across all K markers, so that $h(\mathbf{g}_i,\mathbf{g}_j) = \sum_k h(g_{i,k},g_{j,k})$. In general, the kernel can differ across markers, which might be desirable if we knew that some markers are likely to have dominant effects and others recessive effects. However, we assume that the same kernel is used for all markers, to simplify our presentation. Additive kernels are attractive because they make it easy to account for missing genotypes, weighted sums can be created, and they can be computed rapidly. For example, a weighted sum kernel in equation (1) results in

$$\begin{aligned} U_{\text{global}} &= \frac{\sum_{i<j}\sum_k w_k h(g_{i,k},g_{j,k})}{\binom{n}{2}} \\ &= \sum_k w_k \frac{\sum_{i<j} h(g_{i,k},g_{j,k})}{\binom{n}{2}} \\ &= \sum_k w_k U_k , \end{aligned}$$

emphasizing that U_{global} is a weighted sum of marker-specific U-statistics. Let $\mathbf{U}$ denote the vector of marker-specific U-statistics. We shall contrast the vector $\mathbf{U}$ between cases and controls and average this contrast across all markers. First, however, we need to consider the variance matrix for the vector $\mathbf{U}$, because this variance matrix will be used to create optimal weights for averaging across the markers.

We assume that subjects are independent of each other,

but genetic markers can be correlated due to linkage disequilibrium, or perhaps natural selection. To determine the asymptotic covariance matrix of **U**, we use standard results on U-statistics (Hoeffding 1948, Serfling 1980). For now assume that there is no missing data. Let $h_1(g_{i,k}) = E[h(g_{i,k},G_{j,k})]$, where lowercase g is fixed and uppercase G is random. In other words, one of the random genotypes is integrated out of the bivariate kernel h to create the marginal function h_1. Then, the asymptotic covariances can be expressed as

$$\mathrm{Cov}\,(\sqrt{n}U_k,\sqrt{n}U_l) = 4\sigma_{k,l}\ , \tag{2}$$

where $\sigma_{k,l} = \mathrm{Cov}\,[h_1(G_{i,k}),h_1(G_{i,l})]$. To apply this general expression, we need to account for missing data (i.e., to allow n to vary over the different markers), and we need a way to determine $\sigma_{k,l}$ for a specified kernel.

We shall first illustrate the derivation of $\mathrm{Var}\,(\sqrt{n_k}U_k)$, where n_k denotes the number of subjects without missing data for marker k. To determine $\sigma_{k,k} = \mathrm{Var}\,[h_1(G_{i,k})]$, let $P(g_k)$ denote the probability of genotype g_k. The term $h_1(g_{i,k})$ can then be expressed as

$$h_1(g_{i,k}) = \sum_{G_k} h(g_{i,k},G_k)P(G_k)\ .$$

By using the genotype probabilities again, the expected value of $h_1(G_{i,k})$ can be easily derived according to

$$\mu_k = \sum_{G_k} h_1(G_k)P(G_k) \tag{3}$$

and its variance according to

$$\sigma_{k,k} = \sum_{G_k} h_1(G_k)^2P(G_k) - \mu_k^2\ . \tag{4}$$

Then, $\mathrm{Var}\,(\sqrt{n_k}U_k) = 4\sigma_{k,k}$.

Now consider $\mathrm{Cov}\,(\sqrt{n_k}U_k,\sqrt{n_l}U_l)$. This covariance depends on the number of subjects that contribute to both U_k and U_l; let $n_{k,l}$ be this number. Then, allowing for missing data,

$$\mathrm{Cov}\,(\sqrt{n_k}U_k,\sqrt{n_l}U_l) = \frac{4\sigma_{k,l}n_{k,l}\sqrt{n_kn_l}}{(n_kn_l)}\ .$$

Note that this expression reduces to expression (2) when there is no missing data (e.g., $n_k = n_l = n_{k,l}$). To determine $\sigma_{k,l}$, we reduce the sample to those $n_{k,l}$ subjects with complete data for both markers, and compute the expected value of $h_1(G_{i,k})h_1(G_{i,l})$,

$$\mu_{k,l} = \sum_{G_k}\sum_{G_l} h_1(G_k)h_1(G_l)P(g_k,g_l)\ , \tag{5}$$

where $P(g_k,g_l)$ is the joint probability of genotypes at both markers. This is then used to compute

$$\sigma_{k,l} = \mu_{k,l} - \mu_k\mu_l\ . \tag{6}$$

Computational Issues

The computations of the U_k statistics and their covariances are very time-consuming when summing over all pairs of subjects. The most efficient computational method is to weight the kernel scores by the counts of distinguishable genotypes. Let x_s denote the number of subjects with the sth genotype category ($s = 1,\dots,S$). Then, U_k can be expressed as

$$U_k = \frac{\sum_{i<j} h_k(g_{i,k},g_{j,k})}{\binom{n}{2}}$$

$$= \frac{1}{\binom{n}{2}}\left[\sum_{s=1}^{S}\binom{x_s}{2}h(g_s,g_s) + \frac{1}{2}\sum_{s\neq t} x_sx_th(g_s,g_t)\right]$$

$$= \sum_{s=1}^{S}\frac{x_s(x_s-1)}{n(n-1)}h(g_s,g_s)$$

$$+2\sum_{s<t}\frac{x_sx_t}{n(n-1)}h(g_s,g_t)\ . \tag{7}$$

The term $\frac{1}{2}$ in equation (7) is needed because the sum over $s \neq t$ gives a double count. Derivations of other types of U-statistics for genetic studies have emphasized this way of computing U-statistics (Kowalski 2001; Kowalski et al. 2002; Tzeng et al. 2003*a*, 2003*b*), and in fact often rely on $U = \mathbf{P}'\mathbf{H}\mathbf{P} + O(1/n)$, where $\mathbf{P}$ is the vector of relative frequencies of the categories (genotypes, in our situation) and $\mathbf{H}$ is a symmetric matrix of corresponding kernel scores (Tzeng 2003).

To compute $\mathrm{Var}\,(\sqrt{n_k}U_k)$, we use the estimate $\widehat{P(g_s)} = x_s/n$ to compute μ_k (eq. 3) and $\sigma_{k,k}$ (eq. 4). To compute $\mathrm{Cov}\,(\sqrt{n_k}U_k,\sqrt{n_l}U_l)$, we subset to those subjects not missing data at both markers, create a contingency table of genotype counts for $g_k \times g_l$, with cell counts x_{g_k,g_l}, and use estimate $\widehat{P(g_k,g_l)} = x_{g_k,g_l}/n_{k,l}$ in equation (5) to compute $\sigma_{k,l}$.

Contrast of Case with Control Genotype Scores

To compare the vector of within-group scores for cases with that for controls, we use the contrast vector

$$\delta = \mathbf{U}_d - \mathbf{U}_c\ ,$$

where the subscripts d and c denote the diseased cases and controls, respectively. Under the null hypothesis of no differences between cases and controls, standard results for U-statistics imply that δ has a multivariate normal distribution with mean zero and covariance matrix V_o, which has elements

$$V_{o,k,l} = \begin{cases} \dfrac{4\sigma_{o,k,k}}{n_{d,k}} + \dfrac{4\sigma_{o,k,k}}{n_{c,k}} & \text{if } k = l \\ \dfrac{4\sigma_{o,k,l}n_{d,k,l}}{n_{d,k}n_{d,l}} + \dfrac{4\sigma_{o,k,l}n_{c,k,l}}{n_{c,k}n_{c,l}} & \text{if } k \neq l \end{cases} ,$$

where $\sigma_{o,k,l}$ is computed under the null hypothesis. This is accomplished by pooling cases and controls to compute estimates $\widehat{P(g_s)}$ and $\widehat{P(g_k, g_l)}$ and then using these to estimate $\sigma_{o,k,l}$, as described above in the "Computational Issues" section.

To construct a statistic that is sensitive to alternatives for which all elements of δ are in the same direction (i.e., all positive or all negative), we use a weighted sum of the elements of δ. To choose the weight vector **w**, we use the generalized least squares procedure, which provides the best (i.e., smallest variance) linear unbiased estimator (BLUE) and corresponding optimal test statistic. In this case, the weight w_k is proportional to the kth row total of V_o^{-1}. That is,

$$w_k = (\mathbf{1}'V_o^{-1}\mathbf{1})^{-1}(\mathbf{1}'V_o^{-1})_k ,$$

where **1** is a vector of ones. Hence, the global statistic is

$$Z_{\text{global}} = \frac{\mathbf{w}'\delta}{\sqrt{\mathbf{w}'V_o\mathbf{w}}} ,$$

and Z_{global} has an asymptotic standard normal distribution.

Choice of Kernel for Genotype Scores

A challenging aspect of our proposed methods is the choice of a kernel that is powerful for a wide range of genetic effects. An intuitive choice is to simply count the number of alleles that match between a pair of subjects; we call this the "allele-match" kernel. This type of similarity measure has been used for linkage statistics, such as the affected-pedigree member linkage statistic (Weeks and Lange 1988), and to evaluate the association of haplotypes with disease (Tzeng et al. 2003*b*). This similarity kernel counts the number of matches among the four comparisons between the two alleles of subject i and the two alleles of subject j, and it can be expressed as

$$\begin{aligned} h(g_i = a_1/a_2, g_j = a_3/a_4) &= I[a_1 = a_3] + I[a_1 = a_4] \\ &\quad + I[a_2 = a_3] + I[a_2 = a_4] , \end{aligned}$$

where $I[\ldots]$ is the indicator function having a value of 1 or 0 according to whether its argument is true or false. This kernel ranges from 0, for no matches, to 4, when a pair of subjects have the same homozygous genotype. On the surface, this similarity kernel is appealing, because one could easily extend it to multiple alleles and multiple markers (summing the allele-match scores across markers). However, further consideration shows that it can have undesirable properties when summing across markers and contrasting between cases and controls. The main issue is that the expected value of this allele-match kernel is symmetric about its minimum value, which occurs when all alleles at a marker have the same frequency. For example, consider a diallelic marker, with one of the alleles having frequency p. Under the assumption of Hardy Weinberg proportions for the genotypes, the expected value of the allele-match kernel is $\mu_{\text{allele match}} = 4 - 8p(1 - p)$. This expectation is illustrated in figure 1, which shows that it is symmetric around 0.5. In this figure, we also plot solid vertical lines for cases and broken vertical lines for controls, for hy-

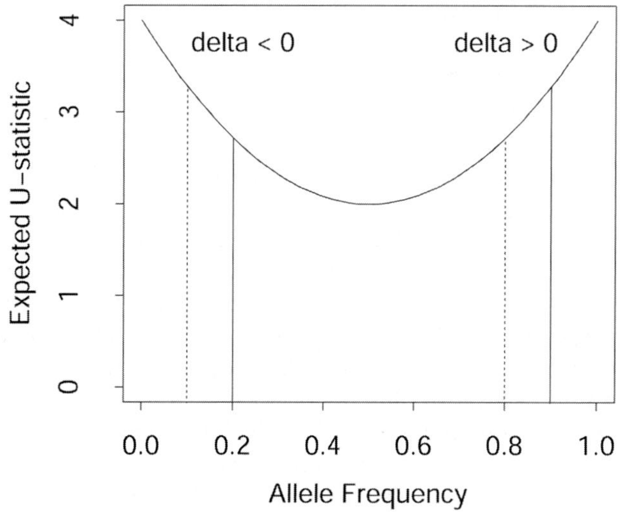

Figure 1 Expected value of U-statistic, μ, for the allele-match kernel versus allele frequency (under the assumption of Hardy-Weinberg proportions of genotypes). For hypothetical allele frequencies, the vertical solid lines represent cases and the vertical broken lines represent controls, illustrating that differences in expected kernels (delta) between cases and controls can change sign according to whether allele frequencies are less than or greater than 0.5.

Table 1

Examples of Kernels for Genotypes g_i and g_j

g_i	g_j: a/a	a/b	b/b
	Allele Match		
a/a	4	2	0
a/b	2	2	2
b/b	0	2	4
	Linear Dosage		
a/a	0	1	2
a/b	1	2	3
b/b	2	3	4
	Dominant		
a/a	0	1	1
a/b	1	2	2
b/b	1	2	2
	Recessive		
a/a	0	0	1
a/b	0	0	1
b/b	1	1	2
	Quadratic		
a/a	2	3	5
a/b	3	4	6
b/b	5	6	8

pothetical allele frequencies such that cases have higher allele frequencies than controls. These vertical lines illustrate that when allele frequencies are <0.5, the difference in the mean scores between cases and controls ("delta" in fig. 1) will be negative. In contrast, when allele frequencies are >0.5, the delta will be positive. Summing over these two hypothetical markers is equivalent to summing over deltas of opposite signs and hence eliminates any potential signal for the association. It can be shown that a similar problem exists when there are more than two alleles at a marker, with the expected kernel score having its minimum value when alleles are equally frequent. That is, similarity is smallest when genotypes have the greatest amount of variability, which occurs when alleles are equally frequent. Hence, comparing average similarities between cases and controls will be influenced by how much the allele frequencies depart from equality within a group, potentially eliminating a signal when summing these allele-match kernels across markers.

Because of the problems with the allele-match kernel, we consider an alternative approach. One can score each subject's genotype separately, by a dosage function $d(g)$, and then sum these dosage functions for a pair of subjects to create a kernel, $h(g_i,g_j) = d(g_i) + d(g_j)$. For example, for diallelic markers, one can count the number of alleles of a specific type, such as the more rare allele, to create the linear dosage score $d(g) = 0,1,2$. This "linear-dosage" kernel, along with the above allele-match kernel, and a few other kernels based on the sum of other dosage functions, are illustrated in table 1. Before we describe how to determine an optimal kernel for a specified genetic effect, we show in the next section that the "sum-dosage" kernel, $h(g_i,g_j) = d(g_i) + d(g_j)$, with an arbitrary dosage score $d(g)$, leads to a U-statistic that is equivalent to Armitage's trend statistic for proportions. This relationship provides an intuitive guide on the choice of kernels.

Relationship of Contrast of Within-Group U-Statistics with Armitage's Test for Trend.—Armitage's test for trend in proportions is frequently used to compare the genotype frequencies between cases and controls. For diallelic markers, the 2 × 3 table for affection status by genotype category can be arranged as in table 2. Armitage's trend statistic measures a trend in proportions, weighted by a general measure of exposure dosage, d_i. Armitage's trend statistic can be expressed as $Z_{\text{Arm}} = T/\sqrt{\text{Var}(T)}$, where

$$T = \sum_i d_i\left(\frac{S}{N}r_i - \frac{R}{N}s_i\right) ,$$

$$\text{Var}(T) = RS\frac{N\sum_i d_i^2 n_i - \left(\sum_i d_i n_i\right)^2}{N^3} ,$$

and summations are over all possible genotypes. The statistic Z_{Arm} has an approximate standard normal distribution.

A common way to score the genotypes is to let $d_i = 0,1,2$, according to the count of the number of rare b alleles. For this type of scoring, Z^2_{Arm} reduces to Pearson's χ^2 statistic for the 2 × 2 table that compares allele counts between cases and controls when the genotypes are in Hardy-Weinberg proportions (Devlin and Roeder 1999), yet the Z_{Arm} statistic is robust to departures from Hardy-Weinberg proportions (Sasieni 1997). Furthermore, Z^2_{Arm} is the score statistic from logistic regression, when the independent covariate for the genotypes is coded as 0, 1, or 2 for the number of copies of allele b. The power of Armitage's statistic depends on how close the chosen scoring of genotypes matches the true genetic effect (Slager and Schaid 2001). For example, if allele b is dominant, then the most powerful scoring is $d = 0,1,1$ for genotypes a/a , a/b, and b/b. For a recessive

Table 2

Contingency Table for Computing Armitage's Test for Trend

	a/a	a/b	b/b	Total
Cases	r_0	r_1	r_2	R
Controls	s_0	s_1	s_2	S
Total	n_0	n_1	n_2	N

effect of allele b, the corresponding scoring should be $d = 0,0,1$. For an additive effect on the log odds ratio, the most powerful scoring is linear, $d_i = 0,1,2$.

When there are only two alleles at a marker, it can be shown that Armitage's trend test is a special case of our δ contrast statistic that contrasts the within-group U-statistic for cases with that for controls when a particular kernel is used. Let $d(g_i)$ denote the dosage scoring of genotype g_i for Armitage's trend test. Then, if the kernel is defined to be the sum of these genotype dosage scores, $h(g_i,g_j) = d(g_i) + d(g_j)$, it can be shown that the numerator of Armitage's trend test, T, and $\delta = U_d - U_c$ have the relationship $T = \delta C$, where $C = RS/(2N)$. Furthermore, $\mathrm{Var}(T) = \mathrm{Var}(\delta)C^2$, so that the standardized statistics are equivalent. This equivalence allows us to determine the most powerful kernels for the U-statistics, by first choosing $d(g)$ for a specified genetic effect and then converting this to a sum kernel.

Kernels that Maximize Power.—Power depends on the choice of kernel, as well as the distribution of genotypes for cases and controls. Let Q_0, Q_1, and Q_2 denote the genotype probabilities for the controls having genotypes a/a, a/b, and b/b, respectively. Let P_0, P_1, and P_2 denote the corresponding genotype probabilities for the cases. These probabilities correspond to the layout of table 2. The probabilities for the cases can be expressed in terms of odds ratios and the genotype probabilities for the controls. Let ψ_1 and ψ_2 denote the odds ratios for genotypes a/b and b/b, relative to genotype a/a. Then,

$$P_1 = \frac{\psi_1 Q_1}{Q_0 + \psi_1 Q_1 + \psi_2 Q_2} ,$$

$$P_2 = \frac{\psi_2 Q_2}{Q_0 + \psi_1 Q_1 + \psi_2 Q_2} ,$$

and, of course, $P_0 = 1 - P_1 - P_2$. When the appropriate genotype probabilities are used, the expected value of δ is $\mu_d - \mu_c$, where μ is the expected value of the U-statistic, as illustrated in equation (3), evaluated with either the case or control genotype probabilities. The variance term, σ^2, is computed according to equation (4). Because the variance term is computed under the null hypothesis by pooling cases and controls, we use the average of the genotype probabilities for cases and controls (e.g., $[P + Q]/2$ for equal numbers of cases and controls) in the variance formula. Under the assumption that the number of cases, n, is equal to the number of controls, the power for a one-sided test ($\delta > 0$) is $1 - \Phi(z_\beta)$, where Φ is the cumulative distribution function for a standard normal distribution,

$$z_\beta = z_\alpha - \sqrt{n}\frac{\delta}{\sqrt{8\sigma^2}} ,$$

and z_α is the $(1 - \alpha)$ quantile of the standard normal distribution. It is clear from the above expression that power is maximized by maximizing δ/σ. For a given distribution of genotypes for controls and specified genotype odds ratios, the goal is to determine which values of the kernel maximize δ/σ. We accomplish this by using the simplex method (Press et al. 1992). This method is used to find parameters that minimize a general function; in our case, we minimize $-(\delta/\sigma)^2$. Because multiple solutions give the same minimum and, hence, the same power, we restricted the kernels to be nondecreasing as genotype similarity increases. That is, for kernels displayed as in table 1, we require that the elements within a row do not decrease as we read from left to right, and elements within a column do not decrease as we read from top to bottom. We applied this approach to a variety of genetic models, including rare and common alleles (i.e., those with disease allele frequencies equal to 0.05 or 0.25, respectively), and dominant, recessive, or multiplicative effects of the disease allele. These effects were modeled by the odds ratios, with dominant having $\psi_1 = \psi_2 = \psi$, recessive having $\psi_1 = 1, \psi_2 = \psi$, and multiplicative having $\psi_2 = \psi_1^2$, with $\psi_1 = \psi$, and ψ having a value of either 2 or 4. In all cases, we could not find kernels with greater power than those predicted by the corresponding "sum" kernels, as outlined in the previous section.

To illustrate the relative efficiency of the different sum kernels for different genetic models, we present in table

Table 3

Relative Efficiency of Different Kernels for Different Genetic Effects

	Relative Efficiency for Kernel[a]			
Model, ψ, and P	Dominant	Recessive	Linear Dosage	Quadratic
Dominant:				
$\psi = 2$:				
.05	1	.15	.99	.95
.25	1	.27	.91	.79
$\psi = 4$:				
.05	1	.14	.99	.95
.25	1	.25	.9	.76
Recessive:				
$\psi = 2$:				
.05	.19	1	.37	.52
.25	.35	1	.7	.85
$\psi = 4$:				
.05	.24	1	.46	.62
.25	.41	1	.77	.89
Multiplicative:				
$\psi = 2$:				
.05	.99	.35	1	.98
.25	.91	.69	1	.96
$\psi = 4$:				
.05	1	.4	1	.95
.25	.89	.76	1	.96

[a] Relative efficiency is the ratio of noncentrality parameters, where a noncentrality parameter for a specified kernel is δ/σ.

3 the relative efficiencies of a variety of kernels. The kernels "dominant," "recessive," and "linear" are based on the dosage functions $d(g)$ defined in the previous section. The "quadratic" kernel is based on $d(g) = 1,2,4$. The relative efficiencies in table 3 are presented such that the kernel with greatest power has a value of 1. The interpretation of a less-efficient kernel is that the sample size would need to be increased by $1/e$, where e is the relative efficiency in table 3. The results in table 3 illustrate that when a recessive kernel is used for a dominant effect, there is a large loss in efficiency, and vice versa. The linear kernel performs best for multiplicative models (i.e., log-additive effects) and performs well for dominant effects but poorly for recessive effects. Although the quadratic kernel is not the most efficient for any of the presented models, it is fairly robust, performing reasonably well for most genetic models, except for rare recessive effects. This suggests that the quadratic kernel may be a reasonable choice when the true underlying genetic effect is unknown—a frequent situation.

Although not immediately obvious, the allele-match kernel and the linear-dosage kernel give the same statistic for a diallelic marker, except that the sign of the statistics can differ, depending on the allele frequencies for cases and controls. This follows from the symmetry in figure 1 for the allele-match kernel, whereas the linear-dosage kernel has expected value $\mu_{\text{linear dosage}} = 4p$, which is a straight line with slope 4, and so avoids the complications when adding contrasts between cases and controls across markers. Without showing all the detailed algebraic derivations, it can be shown that the ratio of δ/σ for the allele-match kernel over that for the linear-dosage kernel is equal to -1 if $(p_d + p_c) < 1$ and is equal to $+1$ if $(p_d + p_c) > 1$, where p_d and p_c are the frequencies of one of the alleles for the cases and controls. In figure 2, we plot δ/σ for both kernels, for $p_c = p_d - 0.05$. This illustrates that the absolute magnitudes of the statistics are equal, yet different in sign, when the allele frequencies for cases and controls are both <0.5. This again emphasizes caution when the allele-match kernel is being used for multiple markers.

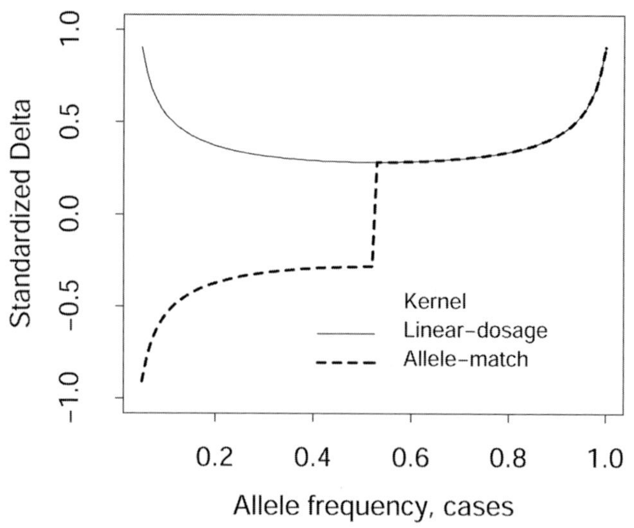

Figure 2 Standardized δ/σ for the allele-match and linear-dosage kernels, under the assumption that the allele frequency for controls is $p_d - 0.05$, where p_d is the allele frequency for cases (X-axis).

Simulations

A series of simulations were used to evaluate the type I error rates and the power of our proposed Z_{global} statistic, relative to the power of the maximum of the single-marker tests with Bonferroni correction for multiple testing (denoted as "*max-single*"), and the power of Hotelling's T^2 multimarker multivariate statistic (denoted as "*multimarker*"). The genotypes for 10 independent markers were simulated, and, of these 10, the number of markers associated with disease ranged from 0 (to evaluate the type I error rate) to 10. The frequency of the high-risk allele, for all markers, was set to either 0.05 or 0.10 (denoted in our tables as "MAF," for "minor allele frequency"). Hardy-Weinberg proportions were used to generate the genotypes for the controls, and the genotypes for cases were generated by assuming that the high-risk allele had a multiplicative effect on the odds ratio. The effect per allele was set at either 1.25 or 1.5. The total sample size was set to either 500 or 1,000 individuals, of which half were cases and half were controls. Two-sided tests were used, and all simulations were based on 1,000 replicates.

The type I error rates for all three of the test statistics, calculated using a variety of kernels for Z_{global}, are presented in table 4. Almost all type I error rates for Z_{global} and *multimarker* are within the 95% CIs for the nominal error rates ($\alpha = 0.01$, 95% CI 0.004–0.016; $\alpha = 0.05$, 95% CI 0.036–0.064), suggesting that the normal distribution is adequate for the null distribution of Z_{global} and that the χ^2 distribution is adequate for *multimarker*. For the *max-single* statistic, the type I error rates are also adequate, except for the recessive kernel, which was overly conservative (most likely because of the sparseness of homozygotes for the more rare allele).

The power of the linear kernel for Z_{global}, the *max-single* statistic, and the *multimarker* statistic, with a type I error rate of 0.05, are presented in figure 3 for high-risk allele frequencies of 0.05 and in figure 4 for high-risk allele frequencies of 0.10. The X-axis presents the number of high-risk markers, ranging from 0 to 10. These figures illustrate that, as the number of high-risk markers increases, there is a gain in power of the Z_{global} statistic over the *max-single* and *multimarker* statistics, and that the gain is greatest when the effect size of the high-risk allele is not large (odds ratio per allele

Table 4

Type I Error Rates for *max-single, multimarker,* and Z_{global} Statistics

α, Kernel, MAF, and N	Type I Error Rate for		
	max-single	*multimarker*	Z_{global}
α = .01:			
Linear dosage:			
MAF = .05:			
500	.005	.007	.008
N = 1,000	.009	.008	.01
MAF = .10:			
N = 500	.011	.01	.009
N = 1,000	.013	.013	.01
Quadratic:			
MAF = .05:			
N = 500	.002	.008	.021
N = 1,000	.01	.011	.018
MAF = .10:			
N = 500	.009	.009	.014
N = 1,000	.003	.009	.008
Dominant:			
MAF = .05:			
N = 500	.005	.007	.009
N = 1,000	.009	.01	.012
MAF = .10:			
N = 500	.009	.008	.018
N = 1,000	.006	.008	.008
Recessive:			
MAF = .05:			
N = 500	0	.009	.005
N = 1,000	0	.011	.006
MAF = .10:			
N = 500	0	.005	.003
N = 1,000	0	.012	.007
α = .05:			
Linear:			
MAF = .05:			
N = 500	.034	.042	.041
N = 1,000	.051	.057	.055
MAF = .10:			
N = 500	.056	.058	.042
N = 1,000	.053	.061	.06
Quadratic:			
MAF = .05:			
N = 500	.05	.055	.048
N = 1,000	.047	.046	.047
MAF = .10:			
N = 500	.041	.039	.055
N = 1,000	.054	.05	.061
Dominant:			
MAF = .05:			
N = 500	.053	.054	.048
N = 1,000	.038	.047	.038
MAF = .10:			
N = 500	.048	.038	.06
N = 1,000	.047	.043	.046
Recessive:			
MAF = .05:			
N = 500	0	.056	.034
N = 1,000	0	.046	.031
MAF = .10:			
N = 500	0	.042	.056
N = 1,000	.017	.051	.062

of 1.25 in the figures). The benefit of using the Z_{global} statistic seemed to occur when there were >3 high-risk markers among the set of 10 markers in these simulations. In contrast, when there were only one or two high-risk markers, the *max-single* and *multimarker* statistics had greater power than the Z_{global} statistic. This was most accentuated when both the allele effect size and the sample size were large (see lower right panel of fig. 4).

Although our simulation results show the potential gain in power provided by the Z_{global} statistic, our simulations are somewhat unrealistic, assuming no interactions among the high-risk markers. Simulating true biological mechanisms is also unrealistic, given our limited knowledge of underlying genes influencing complex disease. So, to evaluate how our methods behave in the presence of interactions, we consider two extreme scenarios. For the 10 markers, there are 45 possible pairwise interactions. In the first scenario, we simulate from a logistic model that has no main effects, but all 45 pairwise interactions contribute to the logistic regression model according to $x_k x_l \beta$, where x_l and x_l are the linear dosage scores for the rare alleles at markers k and l, and β is the log odds ratio for the interaction effect; we allow the interaction odds ratio to be either 1.1. or 1.25. In the second scenario, we also assume no main effects, but 22 of the interactions have positive values of β and 23 have negative ones. That is, half the interactions increase disease risk, and the other half decrease disease risk. The results from these simulations are presented in table 5. When all interactions are positive, the Z_{global} statistic has a substantial power advantage over the other methods. This is likely because all methods are picking up some signal from the main effects of each marker (main effects and pairwise interactions are correlated), but the signal of each main effect is weak, so the weighted average over all markers strengthens the signal. In contrast, the model with half-positive and half-negative interactions creates main effects that have opposite signs, so that the weighted average for Z_{global} is near zero. Note that *max-single* and *multimarker* also have weak power for this interaction model.

Application to Prostate Cancer Candidate Genes

To evaluate common genetic polymorphisms for genes that are likely to be associated with prostate cancer, we measured common variations of single nucleotide polymorphisms (SNPs), chosen such that the minor allele frequency was expected to be at least 5%, in order to have adequate power to detect moderate associations. A total of 499 cases and 493 controls were recruited. We have focused on two biologic pathways: (1) 17 SNPs for genes that encode enzymes in the androgen metabolic pathway and (2) 17 SNPs for genes that encode enzymes

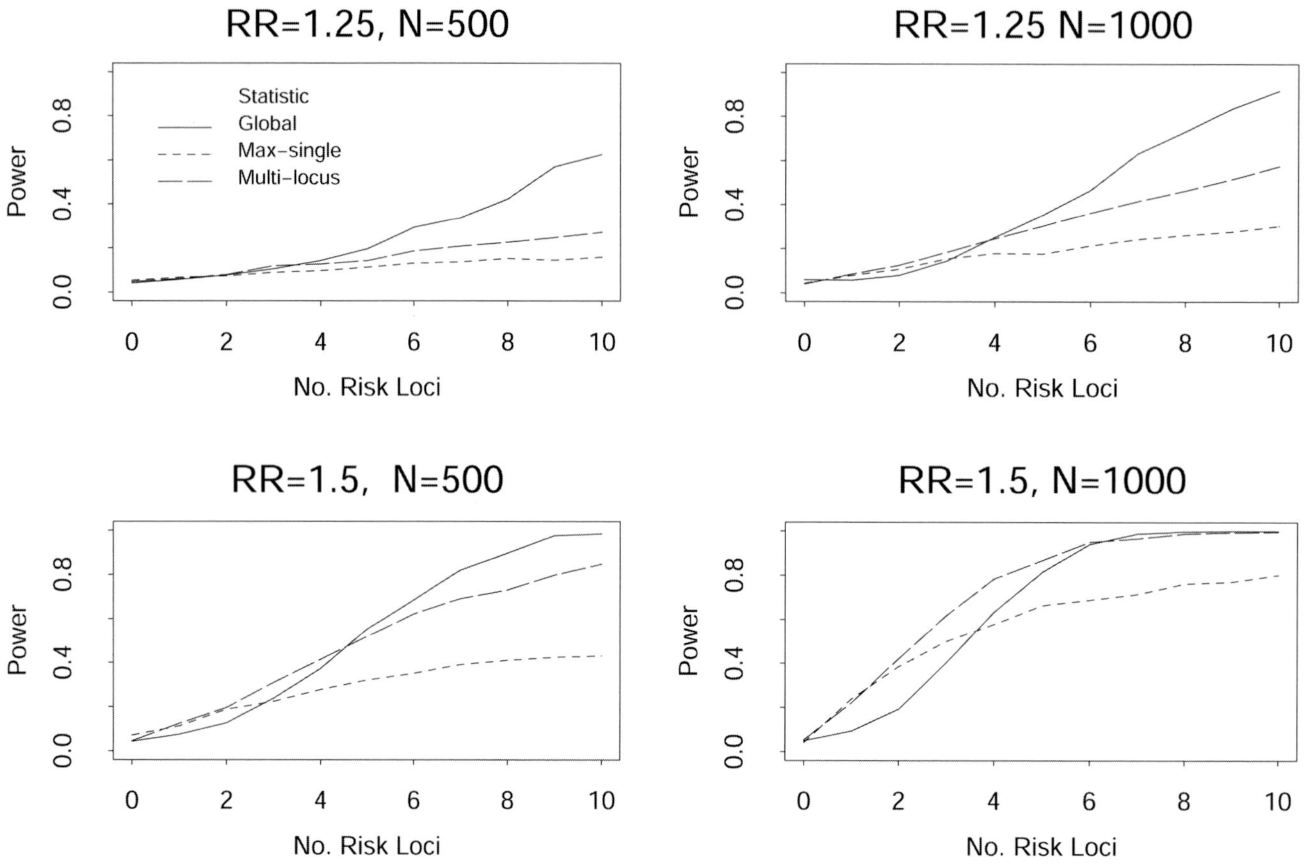

Figure 3 Power from simulated data with the number of high-risk markers ranging from 0 to 10 among 10 markers, with a minor allele frequency of 0.05 for each marker.

involved in the estrogen metabolic pathway (authors' unpublished data). These two pathways are presented in figure 5. The 34 SNPs are identified by numbers within boxes, with their corresponding gene labels. Note that some genes have multiple SNPs measured; these were at different sites within the gene, at positions where prior reports suggested that variants might be associated with the risk of prostate cancer. This figure also illustrates that these two pathways have some biological links, although we analyze them separately.

The association of all SNPs within a pathway with prostate cancer status was evaluated with the global statistic Z_{global}, using different types of kernels. The results of these global tests are presented in table 6. No tests for the androgen pathway SNPs showed statistically significant associations. For the estrogen pathway SNPs, the quadratic kernel resulted in a statistically significant association ($P = .028$), and the linear kernel was marginally significant ($P = .074$).

Although our proposed methods control the overall type I error rate, interpretation of a significant global test can be difficult. To evaluate which markers "explain" the significance of the global test, we performed a stepwise procedure. Intuitively, we expect that removal of the markers that explain the statistical significance of the global test should result in nonsignificance of the remaining markers. However, because the statistical tests can be correlated, we account for this by conditioning on the removed markers when evaluating the markers that are kept. Furthermore, because the global statistic is computed under the null hypothesis, all computations of the stepwise adjusted statistics are also computed under the null hypothesis, to evaluate which markers are the most influential. To start, the marker with the smallest single-marker P value is removed, and a global test for the remaining markers is performed, adjusted for the removed marker. To determine the next marker to remove, we create a test statistic for each of the kept markers, with each statistic adjusted for the set of removed markers, and then remove the marker that has the smallest P value. After a marker is removed, a global test is performed for the kept markers, adjusted for all of the removed markers. This process is continued until the global adjusted test is no longer significant. To illustrate this adjustment procedure, partition the δ vector into the markers kept and removed, $\delta = (\delta_k, \delta_r)$, where the subscripts k and r denote "kept" and "removed," respectively. Partition the null variance matrix accordingly, into submatrices $V_{k,k}$, $V_{k,r}$, and $V_{r,r}$. From multivariate normal theory, under the null hypothesis, the distribution of δ_k conditional on δ_r is multivariate normal with mean vector

$$\mu_{k.r} = \mathbf{V}_{k,r}\mathbf{V}_{r,r}^{-1}\delta_r$$

and variance matrix

$$\mathbf{V}_{k.r} = \mathbf{V}_{k,k} - \mathbf{V}_{k,r}\mathbf{V}_{r,r}^{-1}\mathbf{V}_{k,r}' \ .$$

We use the adjusted covariance matrix $\mathbf{V}_{k.r}$ to define the weight vector $\mathbf{w}_{k.r}$, to compute the global statistic for the kept markers, adjusted for all the removed markers,

Table 5

Simulated Power for Pairwise Interaction Models

Model, MAF, and Odds Ratio	Simulated Power for		
	max-single	*multimarker*	Z_{global}
All positive:			
MAF = .05:			
1.1	.054	.022	.104
1.25	.104	.050	.522
MAF = .10:			
1.1	.135	.73	.503
1.25	.614	.595	.998
Half positive:			
MAF = .05:			
1.1	.044	.014	.049
1.25	.070	.027	.060
MAF = .10:			
1.1	.077	.045	.052
1.25	.265	.194	.062

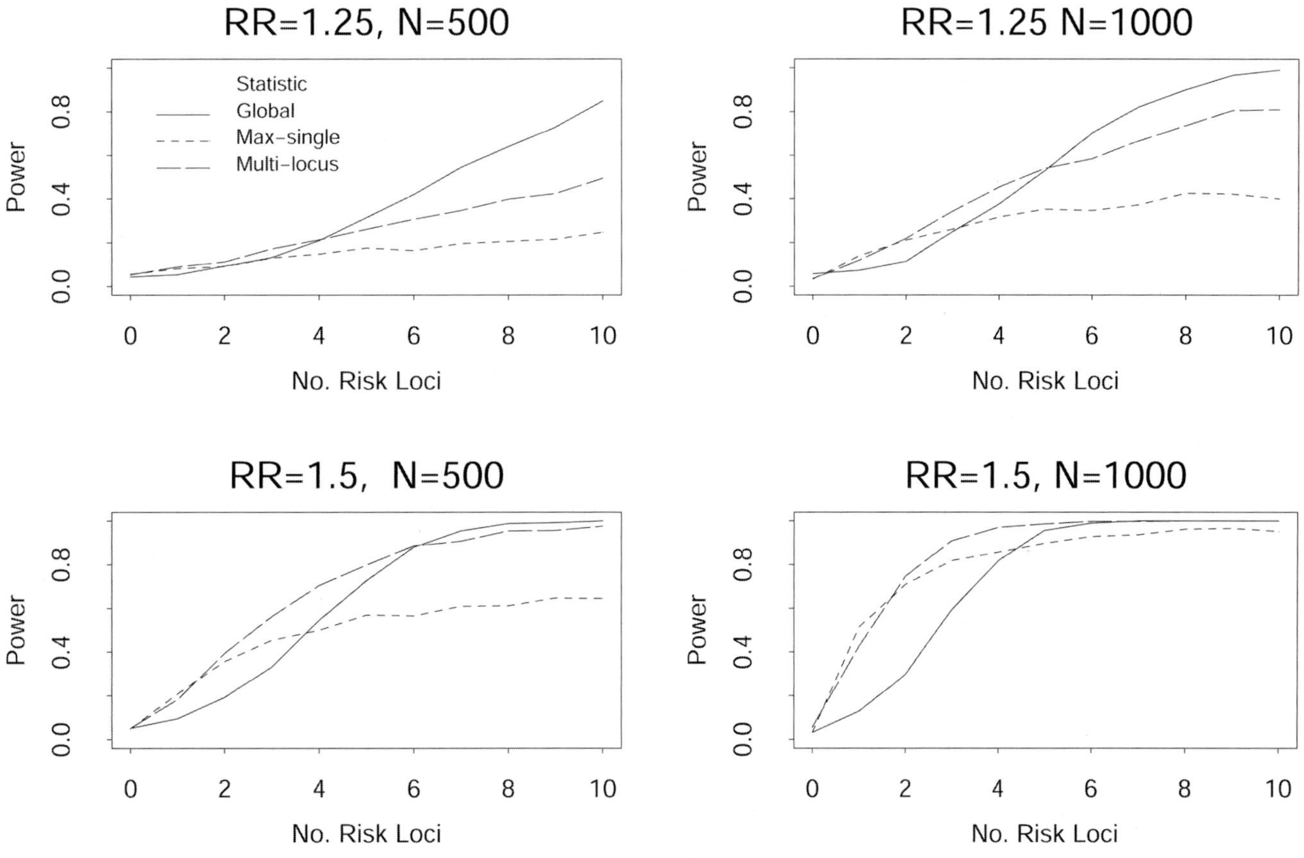

Figure 4 Power from simulated data with the number of high-risk markers ranging from 0 to 10 among 10 markers, with a minor allele frequency of 0.10 for each marker.

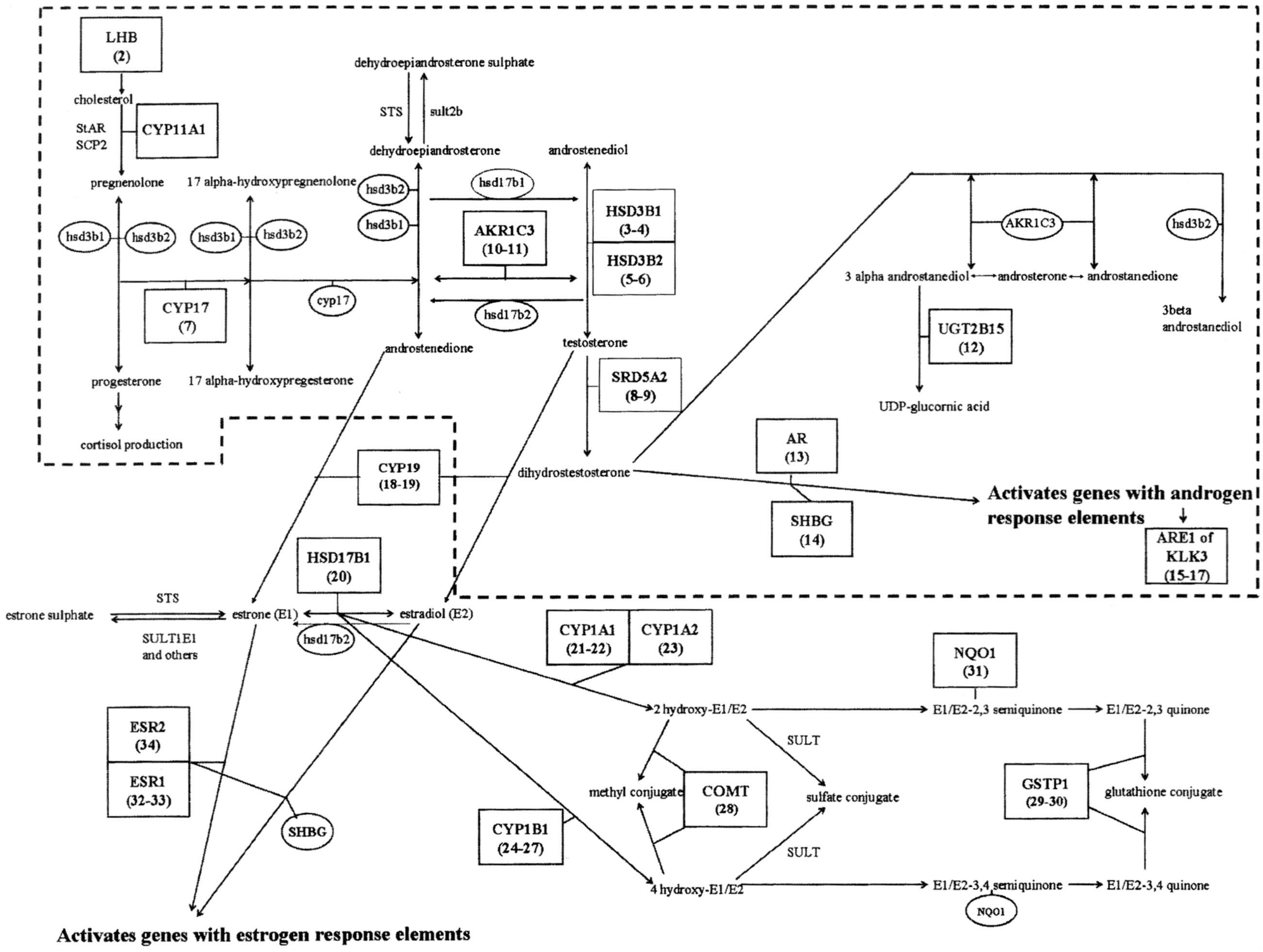
LHB
(2)
cholesterol
StAR
SCP2
CYP11A1
pregnenolone
17 alpha-hydroxypregnenolone
hsd3b1
hsd3b2
CYP17
(7)
cyp17
progesterone
17 alpha-hydroxypregesterone
cortisol production
dehydroepiandrosterone sulphate
STS
sult2b
dehydroepiandrosterone
androstenediol
hsd17b1
AKR1C3
(10-11)
hsd17b2
HSD3B1
(3-4)
HSD3B2
(5-6)
androstenedione
testosterone
SRD5A2
(8-9)
CYP19
(18-19)
dihydrostestosterone
AKR1C3
hsd3b2
3 alpha androstanediol
androsterone
androstanedione
3beta
androstanediol
UGT2B15
(12)
UDP-glucornic acid
AR
(13)
SHBG
(14)
Activates genes with androgen
response elements
ARE1 of
KLK3
(15-17)
HSD17B1
(20)
STS
estrone sulphate
estrone (E1)
estradiol (E2)
SULT1E1
and others
hsd17b2
CYP1A1
(21-22)
CYP1A2
(23)
NQO1
(31)
2 hydroxy-E1/E2
E1/E2-2,3 semiquinone
E1/E2-2,3 quinone
SULT
ESR2
(34)
ESR1
(32-33)
SHBG
methyl conjugate
COMT
(28)
sulfate conjugate
GSTP1
(29-30)
glutathione conjugate
CYP1B1
(24-27)
SULT
4 hydroxy-E1/E2
E1/E2-3,4 semiquinone
E1/E2-3,4 quinone
NQO1
Activates genes with estrogen response elements

$$Z_{\text{global adjusted}} = \frac{\mathbf{w}_{k.r}'(\delta_k - \mu_{k.r})}{\sqrt{\mathbf{w}_{k.r}'\mathbf{V}_{k.r}\mathbf{w}_{k.r}}} \; .$$

To determine the next marker to remove, adjusted for all markers removed at prior steps, we use the statistic for the ith single marker, adjusted for the previously removed markers,

$$Z_i = \frac{(\delta_{k,i} - \mu_{k.r,i})}{\sqrt{\mathbf{V}_{k.r,i,i}}} \; .$$

Both the single-marker–adjusted and global-adjusted statistics have an asymptotic standard normal distribution.

The results from the first three steps of removing "explanatory" SNPs are presented in table 7, for the linear and quadratic kernels. The global statistics are adjusted for the all the previously removed SNPs. For comparison, we also present the marginal single-marker P values, not adjusted for other SNPs and not adjusted for multiple testing. The Bonferroni correction would require the marginal single-marker P values to be <0.0029 to achieve statistical significance, which none of our SNPs achieved. In contrast, the global test for the quadratic kernel, at step 0, demonstrates statistical significance, emphasizing the benefit of our global test. On the basis of the quadratic kernel, it appears that the SNPs HSD17B1 and NQ01 have the most influence on the global test, since conditioning on these two SNPs, the global test has a P value of 0.111; the SNP CYP1A1 may also have some influence, although the statistical evidence is weaker. Similar evidence, although not as dramatic, is provided by the linear kernel.

Discussion

Common diseases are expected to be controlled by complex genetic mechanisms, with small-to-moderate effect sizes per gene, because of natural selection having removed those genes with large effects. Given the large body of evidence indicating that metabolic pathways are likely to play a major role in complex diseases and that these types of pathways have complex interactions and feedback loops, it would not be surprising to find that multiple genes within a biologic pathway are associated with disease, complicated by both allelic and locus heterogeneity. Recognizing that testing the association of disease with one marker at a time can have weak power due to small genetic effects and the need to correct for multiple testing, we have proposed a class of U-statistics that combine information from multiple genetic markers. This combined statistic achieves its greatest power when the contrasts of the within-group genetic scores between cases and controls are in the same direction across multiple markers.

The *multimarker* Hotelling's T^2 statistic is limiting, because it does not allow for missing genotypes at some markers and does not combine information across markers into a single-df statistic, which would have less power than our proposed methods when the effects of genotypes are in the same direction across markers. Hence, an advantage of our approach is that it provides a mechanism to handle missing data while combining results from multiple markers.

Another advantage of our methods is the general framework to consider alternative types of kernels. The allele-match kernel has intuitive appeal but can be limiting, because it is influenced by how much allele frequencies differ from equality within a group—which, in turn, can cause contrasts between cases and controls to differ in sign across markers. Further work is needed to evaluate the best kernels when there are multiple alleles per marker. To provide guidance on the choice of kernel, we have illustrated how to compute the power for a given type of kernel and a specified genetic effect size (e.g., in terms of control genotype frequencies and genotype odds ratios). Our numerical comparisons suggest that the quadratic kernel is fairly robust, in the sense that it does not lose as much power as other kernels, despite not giving the greatest power.

All of our proposed kernels are additive across markers. The benefit of an additive kernel is that it can easily handle missing marker data, which is a common occurrence. Furthermore, weighted averages can be easily computed, where the weights are data driven, with the optimal weights determined by BLUEs. This strategy has been used elsewhere in genetics, such as in the use of

Table 6

Global Tests of Association of All SNPs within a Pathway with Prostate Cancer Status

	Global P for Kernel			
Pathway	Linear Dosage	Quadratic	Dominant	Recessive
Androgen	.590	.706	.395	.958
Estrogen	.074	.028	.281	.654

Figure 5 Candidate genes that are involved with the metabolism of androgen and estrogen. The androgen portion of the pathway is within the broken line, and the estrogen pathway is outside of the broken line, at the bottom of the figure. The measured SNPs are indicated within boxes, with their corresponding genes labeled and the SNPs numbered below each gene. Other genes and enzymes that are part of the pathway are also illustrated, emphasizing that the measured SNPs are for genes whose products act at different steps of androgen and estrogen biosynthesis.

Table 7

Global Tests Adjusted for SNPs Removed Sequentially, as well as Marginal *P* Values for Single-Marker Tests (Not Adjusted for Multiple Testing)

		P Value			
		Global		Single Marker	
Step	SNP Removed	Linear Dosage	Quadratic	Linear Dosage	Quadratic
0	None	.074	.028		
1	HSD17B1 (20)	.143	.053	.018	.034
2	NQ01 (31)	.252	.111	.048	.049
3	CYP1A1 (21)	.510	.339	.140	.123

generalized least squares to derive BLUEs of allele frequencies from pedigree data (McPeek et al. 2004). Weighted global statistics have been also used to derive optimal nonparametric statistics to compare two treatment groups over multiple endpoints (O'Brien 1984; Wei and Johnson 1985). Further work is warranted to determine if more powerful kernels can be found, such as kernels that are nonlinear over the genetic markers. For example, kernels that increase exponentially with the number of rare variants across multiple markers might be more sensitive to situations in which multiple rare variants are required for disease, suggesting higher-order interactions among markers.

A potential advantage of our approach is that linkage disequilibrium among markers is implicitly accounted for by the covariance matrix of the **U** vectors. This allows our methods to be used in evaluating the association of multiple markers within a candidate gene with disease. A potential limitation is that we do not evaluate the association of haplotypes (i.e., particular combinations of alleles on a chromosome) with disease, as others have proposed (Tzeng et al. 2003*b*). However, carefully selected SNPs that "tag" a haplotype can reduce the number of SNPs that are required to be genotyped, and analyzing these types of markers jointly—yet without regard to haplotype phase—can increase the power over haplotype analyses, because of the reduced degrees of freedom for joint marker analyses relative to the many degrees of freedom for haplotype analyses (Chapman et al. 2003). If all contrasts of marker scores between cases and controls are in the same direction, then our global statistic with 1 df will have even greater power, as is demonstrated by our simulations.

Our simulations suggest that the global statistic maintains the appropriate type I error rate and that the power of the global statistic is greater than both single-marker and multimarker tests when there are more than just a few associated genetic markers. Application to our prostate cancer study illustrates the potential gain of our global test by providing significant results that would not be found significant by use of single-marker tests with Bonferroni correction. However, this example also illustrates that, once found, a significant global test can be difficult to interpret, because it is not immediately clear which markers are driving the statistical significance. To guide our interpretation, we used a stepwise removal of the markers that had the smallest single-marker *P* value, with recomputation of an adjusted global test after each marker was removed. This process helped to identify a few markers that seemed to contribute the most to the global test. Further work regarding the statistical properties of the proposed stepwise procedure might be beneficial, since many stepwise selection procedures are known to have some difficulties identifying the most important subsets. Cross validation, to determine the ability to replicate the most important subset of explanatory markers, may offer guidance.

In summary, we have proposed a novel class of *U*-statistics that provide a simultaneous test of association of multiple genetic markers with disease. Our approach is quite general, allowing a wide variety of kernels to be used. Simulations demonstrate that our approach can be more powerful than standard methods, and application to our prostate cancer study illustrates the potential merits of our statistics, as well as their interpretations.

Software

Software that implements the methods described in this manuscript is written in the S programming language as a package called *multigene,* which runs in both S-PLUS and R computing environments. The package will be available from our Web site (http://mayoresearch.mayo.edu/mayo/research/biostat/schaid.cfm) and, for R users, from the Comprehensive R Archive Network site (http://cran.us.r-project.org).

Acknowledgments

This research was supported by United States Public Health Services, National Institutes of Health (contract grant numbers GM65450, CA91956, and CA89600).

References

Chapman JM, Cooper JD, Todd JA, Clayton DG (2003) Detecting disease associations due to linkage disequilibrium using haplotype tags: a class of tests and the determinants of statistical power. Hum Hered 56:18–31

Conti DV, Cortessis V, Molitor J, Thomas DC (2003) Bayesian modeling of complex metabolic pathways. Hum Hered 56: 83–93

Devlin B, Roeder K (1999) Genomic control for association studies. Biometrics 55:997–1004

Fan R, Knapp M (2003) Genome association studies of complex diseases by case-control designs. Am J Hum Genet 72: 850–868

Hoeffding W (1948) A class of statistics with asymptotically normal distribution. Ann Math Statist 22:165–179

Kowalski J (2001) A nonparametric approach to translating gene region heterogeneity associated with phenotype into location heterogeneity. Bioinformatics 17:775–790

Kowalski J, Pagano M, DeGruttola V (2002). A nonparametric test of gene region heterogeneity associated with phenotype. Am J Stat Assoc 97:398–408

Longmate JA (2001) Complexity and power in case-control association studies. Am J Hum Genet 68:1229–1237

McPeek MS, Wu X, Ober C (2004) Best linear unbiased allele-frequency estimation in complex pedigrees. Biometrics 60: 359–367

O'Brien PC (1984) Procedures for comparing samples with multiple endpoints. Biometrics 40:1079–1087

Press WH, Teukolsky SA, Vetterling WT, Flannery BP (1992) Numerical recipes in C. Cambridge University Press, Cambridge, United Kingdom

Pritchard JK, Cox NJ (2002) The allelic architecture of human disease genes: common disease-common variant…or not? Hum Mol Genet 11:2417–2423

Reich DE, Lander ES (2001) On the allelic spectrum of human disease. Trends Genet 17:502–510

Sasieni PD (1997) From genotypes to genes: doubling the sample size. Biometrics 53:1253–1261

Serfling RJ (1980) Approximation theorems of mathematical statistics. John Wiley and Sons, New York

Slager SL, Huang J, Vieland VJ (2000) Effect of allelic heterogeneity on the power of the transmission disequilibrium test. Genet Epidemiol 18:143–156

Slager S, Schaid D (2001) Case-control studies of genetic markers: Power and sample size approximations for Armitage's test for trend. Hum Hered 52:149–153

Tzeng J-Y (2003) Identification of mutations affecting liability to complex disease by the analysis of haplotypes. PhD thesis, Carnegie Mellon University, Pittsburgh

Tzeng J-Y, Byerley W, Devlin B, Roeder K, Wasserman L (2003*a*) Outlier detection and false discovery rates for whole-genome DNA matching. Am J Stat Assoc 98:236–246

Tzeng J-Y, Devlin B, Wasserman L, Roeder K (2003*b*) On the identification of disease mutations by the analysis of haplotype similarity and goodness of fit. Am J Hum Genet 72: 891–902

Weeks DE, Lange K (1988) The affected-pedigree-member method of linkage analysis. Am J Med Genet 42:315–326

Wei LJ, Johnson WE (1985) Combining dependent tests with incomplete repeated measurements. Biometrika 72:359–364

Zondervan KT, Cardon LR (2004) The complex interplay among factors that influence allelic association. Nat Rev Genet 5:89–100

Mutations in *ABCA12* Underlie the Severe Congenital Skin Disease Harlequin Ichthyosis

David P. Kelsell,[1] Elizabeth E. Norgett,[1] Harriet Unsworth,[1] Muy-Teck Teh,[1] Thomas Cullup,[2] Charles A. Mein,[2] Patricia J. Dopping-Hepenstal,[5] Beverly A. Dale,[8,9,10] Gianluca Tadini,[13] Philip Fleckman,[10] Karen G. Stephens,[11] Virginia P. Sybert,[10,12] Susan B. Mallory,[14] Bernard V. North,[3] David R. Witt,[15] Eli Sprecher,[16] Aileen E. M. Taylor,[17] Andrew Ilchyshyn,[18] Cameron T. Kennedy,[19] Helen Goodyear,[20] Celia Moss,[21] David Paige,[6] John I. Harper,[7] Bryan D. Young,[4] Irene M. Leigh,[1] Robin A. J. Eady,[5] and Edel A. O'Toole[1]

[1]Centre for Cutaneous Research, Institute of Cell and Molecular Science, [2]Genome Centre, William Harvey Research Institute, [3]Academic Department of Psychiatry, and [4]Molecular Oncology Unit, Institute of Cancer, Barts and the London School of Medicine and Dentistry, Queen Mary, University of London, [5]Genetic Skin Disease Group, Division of Skin Sciences, Guy's, King's, and St. Thomas' School of Medicine, St. Thomas' Hospital, [6]Department of Dermatology, Royal London Hospital, and [7]Department of Paediatric Dermatology, Great Ormond Street Hospital for Children, London; Departments of [8]Oral Biology, [9]Biochemistry, [10]Medicine/Dermatology, and [11]Laboratory Medicine, University of Washington, and [12]Department of Dermatology, Group Health Permanente, Seattle; [13]Institute of Dermatological Sciences, University of Milan, Milan; [14]Division of Dermatology, Department of Internal Medicine, Washington University School of Medicine, St. Louis; [15]Genetics Department, Kaiser Permanente, San Jose, CA; [16]Department of Dermatology and Laboratory of Molecular Dermatology, Rambam Medical Center, Haifa; [17]Department of Dermatology, Royal Victoria Infirmary, Newcastle upon Tyne, United Kingdom; [18]Department of Dermatology, Walsgrave Hospital, Coventry, United Kingdom; [19]Department of Dermatology, Southmead Hospital, Bristol, United Kingdom; and [20]Department of Paediatrics, Birmingham Heartlands Hospital, and [21]Department of Dermatology, Birmingham Children's Hospital, Birmingham, United Kingdom

Harlequin ichthyosis (HI) is the most severe and frequently lethal form of recessive congenital ichthyosis. Although defects in lipid transport, protein phosphatase activity, and differentiation have been described, the genetic basis underlying the clinical and cellular phenotypes of HI has yet to be determined. By use of single-nucleotide–polymorphism chip technology and homozygosity mapping, a common region of homozygosity was observed in five patients with HI in the chromosomal region 2q35. Sequencing of the *ABCA12* gene, which maps within the minimal region defined by homozygosity mapping, revealed disease-associated mutations, including large intragenic deletions and frameshift deletions in 11 of the 12 screened individuals with HI. Since HI epidermis displays abnormal lamellar granule formation, ABCA12 may play a critical role in the formation of lamellar granules and the discharge of lipids into the intercellular spaces, which would explain the epidermal barrier defect seen in this disorder. This finding paves the way for early prenatal diagnosis. In addition, functional studies of ABCA12 will lead to a better understanding of epidermal differentiation and barrier formation.

Introduction

Harlequin ichthyosis (HI [MIM 242500]) is a very severe and usually lethal skin disorder of unknown cause (Hsu et al. 1989; Moreau et al. 1999; Sarkar et al. 2000). HI is also known as "harlequin fetus" because of the tendency for affected babies to be born prematurely. The neonate is covered in a thick "coat of armor" that severely restricts movement (Hsu et al. 1989; Dahlstrom et al. 1995; Sarkar et al. 2000). The skin dries out to form hard diamond-shaped plaques separated by fissures, resembling "armor plating." The normal facial features are severely affected, with distortion of the lips (eclabion), eyelids (ectropion), ears, and nostrils. Historically, an HI-affected neonate would usually die within 2 d of birth because of feeding problems, bacterial infection, and/or respiratory distress. However, a number of patients have survived because of the wider availability of neonatal intensive care and likely benefits from oral retinoids (Hsu et al. 1989; Moreau et al. 1999; Elias et al. 2000; Sarkar et al. 2000). In survivors, the disease comes to resemble severe nonbullous congenital ichthyosiform erythroderma (NBCIE) (Haftek et al. 1996; Choate et al. 1998). The skin barrier remains severely compromised, which leads to increased transepidermal water loss, impaired thermal regulation, and increased risk of secondary infection (Moskowitz et al. 2004).

HI occurs in both sexes and in many ethnic groups. Autosomal recessive (AR) inheritance of HI has been

Received January 4, 2005; accepted for publication February 21, 2005; electronically published March 8, 2005.

Address for correspondence and reprints: Prof. David P. Kelsell, Centre for Cutaneous Research, Institute of Cell and Molecular Science, Barts and the London School of Medicine and Dentistry, 2 Newark Street, London E1 2AT, United Kingdom. E-mail: d.p.kelsell@qmul.ac.uk

0002-9297/2005/7605-0008$15.00

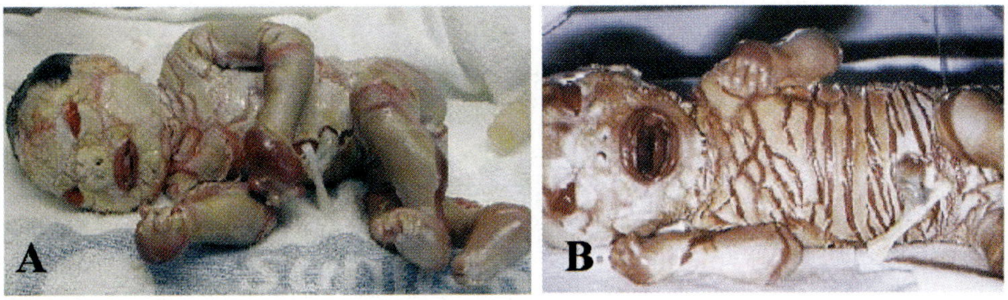

Figure 1 Typical clinical presentation of HI at birth

inferred, but, in a large number of cases, the inheritance pattern cannot be ascertained, and the disorder could be due to a new dominant mutation. It has been subdivided into three types based on the expression of keratin 16 and profilaggrin and the appearance of keratohyalin granules (Dale et al. 1990). Studies have also reported abnormalities in the localization of epidermal lipids and have highlighted the abnormal ultrastructure of epidermal lamellar granules in HI that are associated with the absence of extracellular lamellar structures in all three subtypes (Dale et al. 1990; Akiyama et al. 1996, 1997, 1998). The nuclei of the keratinocytes also show abnormalities, since they appear to become flattened early on in differentiation (in the lower cell layers), but some are retained even as the cornified layer is sloughed off. This parakeratosis along with hyperkeratosis and hypergranulosis (retention of keratohyalin granules in the stratum granulosum) is a characteristic phenotype of the epidermis of neonates with HI (Buxman et al. 1979; Hsu et al. 1989). This may suggest that the process of terminal differentiation is not completed in HI-affected skin. Alterations in calcium-mediated signaling and protein phosphatase activity have also been reported in HI keratinocytes (Kam et al. 1997; Michel et al. 1999). Plausible candidate genes underlying these diverse cellular phenotypes in HI have included *filaggrin, claudins, PP2A,* and *calpain 1* (Kam et al. 1997; Michel et al. 1999).

Mutations in the genes encoding transglutaminase-1 (*TGM1* [MIM 190195]), ichthyin, 4 lipoxygenase 3 (*ALOXE3* [MIM 607206]), and 12(R)-lipoxygenase (*ALOX12B* [MIM 603741]) have all been shown to underlie both NBCIE and lamellar ichthyosis (LI) (Huber et al. 1995; Jobard et al. 2002; Lefevre et al. 2004). Recently, missense mutations in the gene encoding the adenosine triphosphate (ATP)-binding cassette (ABC [GenBank accession number NM_173076]) transporter protein ABCA12 (MIM 607800) have also been shown to cause LI (Lefevre et al. 2003). Unlike the other AR forms of ichthyosis, the genetic basis of HI has not been elucidated.

In the present study, we have used SNP-array technology to localize the HI gene, on the basis of the principle of homozygosity mapping. This identified a major locus for HI on chromosome 2q35 and subsequent disruptive mutations in the *ABCA12* gene in 11 of the 12 analyzed patients with HI. Most of the mutations identified would result in a severely truncated protein. This genetic study immediately establishes the means for early prenatal DNA diagnosis of HI and provides a molecular clue toward understanding the numerous biological abnormalities of epidermal differentiation in HI-affected skin.

Material and Methods

Clinical

Twelve families, from diverse ethnic backgrounds, with individuals affected with HI were included in the present genetic study—three from the United States, seven from Great Britain, and two from Italy. Ethical approval was obtained from the local research ethics committees. The clinical phenotype was verified as HI by at least two clinicians; the typical clinical presentation at birth is shown in figure 1. A summary of the clinical details is shown in table 1. The control population was of mixed ethnicity and consisted of 60 unrelated individuals.

SNP-Array Analysis

A SNP GeneChip Mapping 10K (Affymetrix) array analysis was performed on affected individuals from six families. Two of these families were consanguineous, with AR inheritance of HI. Patient DNA samples were processed in accordance with the standard GeneChip Mapping 10K *Xba* Assay protocol. Briefly, 350 ng of DNA was digested with *Xba*I and ligation to the *Xba*I adaptor prior to PCR amplification by use of AmpliTaq Gold with Buffer II (Applied Biosystems). For each DNA sample, four 100-μl PCRs were set up to obtain sufficient purified PCR product (20 μg), by use of Ultrafree-MC filtration column (Millipore), for subsequent fragmenta-

Table 1

Clinical Details of Patients with HI

Patient	Ethnicity	Gestation (wk)	Birth Weight (g)	Treatment: Retinoid (Dose [mg/kg/d])	Treatment: Begun at Age (d)	Outcome	Other Problems
49	British Bangladeshi	35	2,500	Acitretin (1)	2	SIE, now aged 2.5 years[a]	Pseudomonal SI, FTT, gastrostomy
6	British Pakistani	34	1,750	Etretinate (1.15)	2	SIE, now aged 20 years[b]	Anemia ectropion (surgery)
7	Bangladeshi	38	2,800	Acitretin	NA	SIE, now aged 14 years[c]	FTT, limb deformity
55	British Indian	36	2,600	Acitretin (.75)	4	SIE, now aged 8 years[b]	Neonatal sepsis (SA), hypernatremia, ectropion
40	Italian	40	3,200	Acitretin (1)	3	SIE, now aged 6 years[a]	Neonatal sepsis (CA), ectropion surgery, limb strictures
44	Italian	36	2,000	Acitretin (1)	7	SIE, now aged 6 years[a]	Nystagmus, PDA, neonatal sepsis
63	British Pakistani	36	2,600	Acitretin (.5)	4	SIE, now aged 2 years[b]	Nystagmus, MDD, cataracts, FTT
50	British white	36	2,300	Acitretin (1)	3	SIE, now aged 4 years[b]	Neonatal mild hypothermia
955-01	African-American	36	2,355	Isotretinoin (1)	7	Died at age 6 mo	Septicemia
915-06	Iranian	36	2,980	Isotretinoin (2)	19	Died at age 4 mo	Septicemia (SA)
928-01	Native American	40	NA	Not given		Died at age 1.5 d	Respiratory failure
69	British Pakistani	36	2,820	Not given		Died at age 3 d	Gram-negative sepsis

NOTE.—CA = *Candida albicans*; FTT = failure to thrive; MDD = motor developmental delay; NA = information not available; PDA = patent ductus arteriosus; SA = *Staphylococcus aureus*; SI = skin infection; SIE = severe ichthyosiform erythroderma.

[a] Remains on retinoids.

[b] Now off retinoids.

[c] Intermittent courses of retinoids.

tion with DNase I. Fragmentation was visualized by 4% agarose-gel electrophoresis to confirm the production of 50–100-bp PCR fragments prior to 3′ labeling with biotin and hybridization to the SNP array. Hybridized arrays were processed with an Affymetrix Fluidics Station 450, and fluorescence signals were detected using the Affymetrix GeneChip Scanner 3000. Raw SNP call data were exported to Microsoft Excel for analysis. The average call rate (expressed as a percentage) ± SEM for the six patients was 97.62% ± 0.41%.

Microsatellite and Linkage Analysis

Data from SNP chips revealed an overlapping region of homozygosity, in five of the six affected individuals, at a position on chromosome 2. Microsatellite markers mapping to this region were used to confirm and refine the minimal region of homozygosity. DNA from patient blood samples was first amplified with the microsatellite markers *D2S325* (chromosome 2q33.3) and *D2S126* (chromosome 2q36.1) from the Applied Biosystems Linkage Mapping Set. Sample DNA was amplified with these primers at 5 μM for 30 cycles at 55°C, by use of Amplitaq Gold PCR Mastermix (Applied Biosystems). *D2S128* (chromosome 2q34) and *D2S1345* (chromosome 2q34) were selected from the University of California–Santa Cruz (UCSC) Genome Bioinformatics database, and PCR was performed using Bioline Biotaq DNA Polymerase, Bioline PCR buffer, 60 nM $MgCl_2$, and 20 pM of each primer, with a final reaction volume of 20 μl. Fluorescent-tagged PCR products were analyzed using the ABI 3700 capillary sequencer. Haplotypes were constructed from the microsatellite data of affected individuals and unaffected siblings. Linkage analysis was performed using the Genehunter program (Kruglyak et al. 1996).

Sequence Analysis of ABCA12

Primer design and PCR conditions were the same as those described elsewhere (Lefevre et al. 2003), with the exception that a 15-μl reaction volume was used. The PCR products covering each of the 53 exons and respective intron boundaries were purified using ExoSAP-IT (Amersham Pharmacia Biotech) and were sequenced on either the forward or reverse strand, by use of ABI BigDye Terminator reagents (Applied Biosystems) and an ABI 3700 sequencer (sequencing reaction conditions: 5 μl of purified product, 1 μl of BigDye Terminator v.1.1, 3 μl of Better Buffer [Microzone], 1 μl water; annealing temperature of 60°C). Sequence analysis was performed using Phred, Phrap, and Consed, and variants were detected using reference sequences taken from the Ensembl Genome Browser (Ewing and Green 1998; Ewing et al. 1998; Gordon et al. 1998). Likely disease-associated mutations were screened in a total of 120 control chromosomes—either by direct sequencing or by RFLP analysis if the mutation altered a restriction site.

Results

Genetic Mapping

From the SNP-array analysis, only one region of the genome, 2q35, was found to have large blocks of homozygosity in common for five of the six affected individuals assessed by means of this methodology (fig. 2). This common interval was calculated to be a genetic distance of ~1.5 Mb. To support linkage of HI to 2q35, microsatellite markers that map to this region were identified using the UCSC Genome Browser. The microsatellite genotype data are consistent with a recessive mode of inheritance of HI and linkage of the disease gene to 2q35 in the largest consanguineous family with HI (fig. 3*A*). Linkage analysis was performed for this family, but the size of the family prohibited the calculation of a statistically significant LOD score (data not shown). This highlights the usefulness of the SNP array for homozygosity mapping in diseases not applicable to classic genetic linkage studies. Affected individuals from families in which the mode of inheritance is unknown were also genotyped with these microsatellite markers. Of the 12 affected individuals analyzed in the present study, 11 were homozygous for one or more of the markers analyzed in the 2q35 region (fig. 3*B*).

Candidate-Gene Analysis

Six genes were identifiable, from the UCSC Genome Browser, that map within the minimal region, including *BARD1,* which interacts with the breast-ovarian cancer–associated protein BRCA1; *ATIC,* in which mutations are the cause of a purine biosynthesis disorder (AICA-ribosuria [MIM 608688]); *Fibronectin 1,* which is involved in cell adhesion and migration; the *FLJ10116* gene, which encodes a protein of unknown biological function; and the *PECR* gene, which encodes a peroxisomal trans 2-enoyl CoA reductase. The gene *ABCA12,* which encodes the ABC transporter protein, also maps within the minimal homozygous region on chromosome 2q35. Missense mutations in this gene have recently been shown to underlie the less severe ichthyotic disorders LI and NBCIE (Lefevre et al. 2003). Since the transport of extracellular epidermal lipids is abnormal in HI (Dale et al. 1990) and a defect in epidermal lipid metabolism has been suggested in the pathogenesis of the disease (Buxman et al. 1979), *ABCA12* could be a plausible candidate gene on the basis of chromosome position and function. The 53 coding exons of the *ABCA12* gene were individually amplified by PCR and were sequenced for 12 patients. Mutations in *ABCA12* were detected in 11

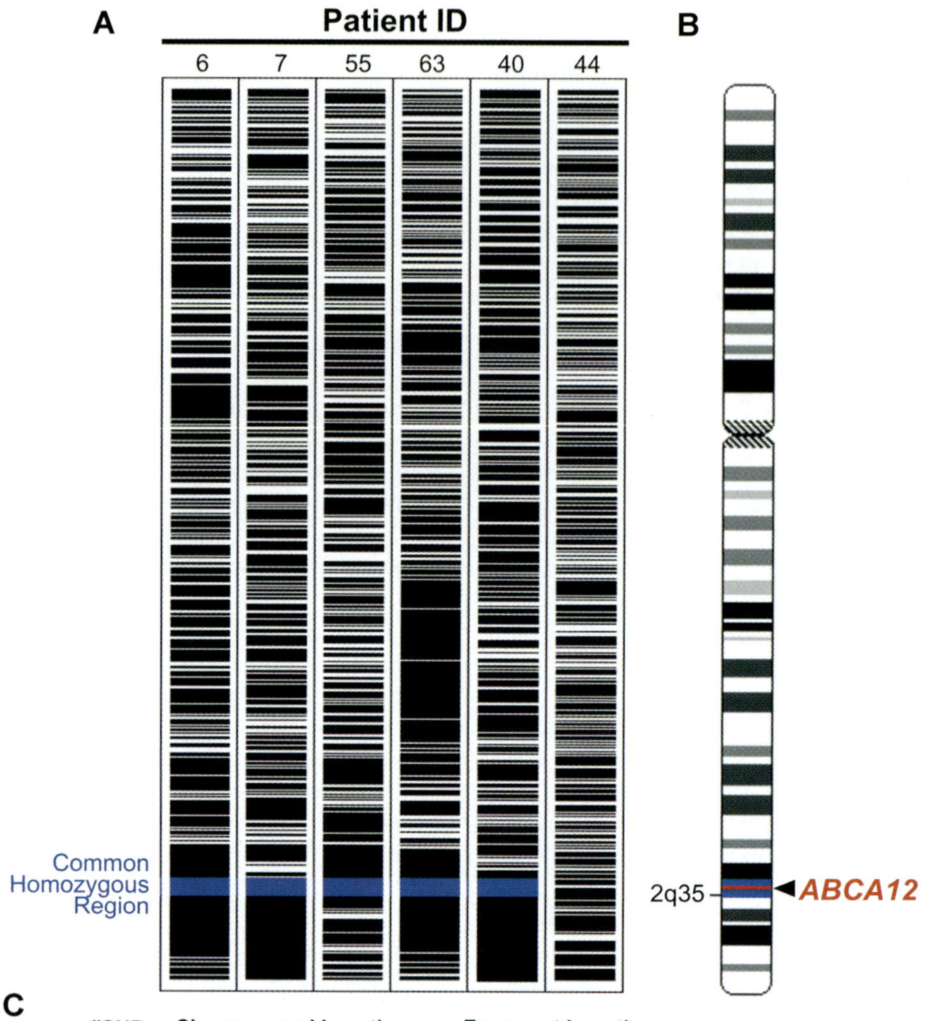

C

ID	#SNP Block	Chromosomal Location of Homozygous Blocks	Fragment Length (b)	Fragment Length (Mb)
6	98	205,575,039-228,043,462	22,468,423	22.5
7	87	215,298,287-239,656,540	24,358,253	24.4
55	59	206,829,958-220,974,685	14,144,727	14.1
63	98	207,811,086-229,706,887	21,895,801	21.9
40	100	212,265,353-238,925,942	26,660,589	26.7
44	15	222,894,585-225,898,656	3,004,071	3.0

Common Homozygous Region*: 215,298,287-216,798,076 (8 SNPs; ~1.5 Mb)

*ABCA12: (215,621,773-215,828,657)

Figure 2 Localization of the HI gene to chromosome 2q35 by use of SNP-array mapping. *A*, Homozygous SNP profiles of chromosome 2 in six patients with HI. Black bars indicate homozygous SNP call data. Blue bars indicate the minimal common region of homozygous SNPs in patients 1–5, a genetic distance of ~1.5 Mb. *B*, Ideogram of chromosome 2 showing the position of *ABCA12* (*red bar*), located within the minimal common region of homozygous SNPs (*blue*) identified in panel A. *C*, The genetic interval of the homozygous SNP "blocks" in each patient with HI, with clear indication that the *ABCA12* gene maps within the common homozygous region for five of the six patients.

of the 12 patients (fig. 4). This indicates that *ABCA12* mutations are a major genetic cause of HI. The majority of the mutations were predicted to result in a truncated protein; indeed, in one patient (40), the last 25 exons were homozygously deleted. Four patients all harbored the same homozygous frameshift mutation and, on the basis of haplotype analysis (see fig. 3*B*) and their shared ethnicity, it is likely to be the same founder mutation in at least three of the four patients. In individual 955–01, a homozygous missense substitution (W198C) in exon 6 was identified in addition to the more disruptive homozygous nonsense substitution in exon 44. The latter sequence change is more likely to be associated with HI. Unlike the other individuals with HI in the mutation study who were homozygous for a specific *ABCA12* mutation, individual 44 was a compound heterozygote for two different *ABCA12* mutations. Both SNP and microsatellite genotypes were heterozygous in the chromo-

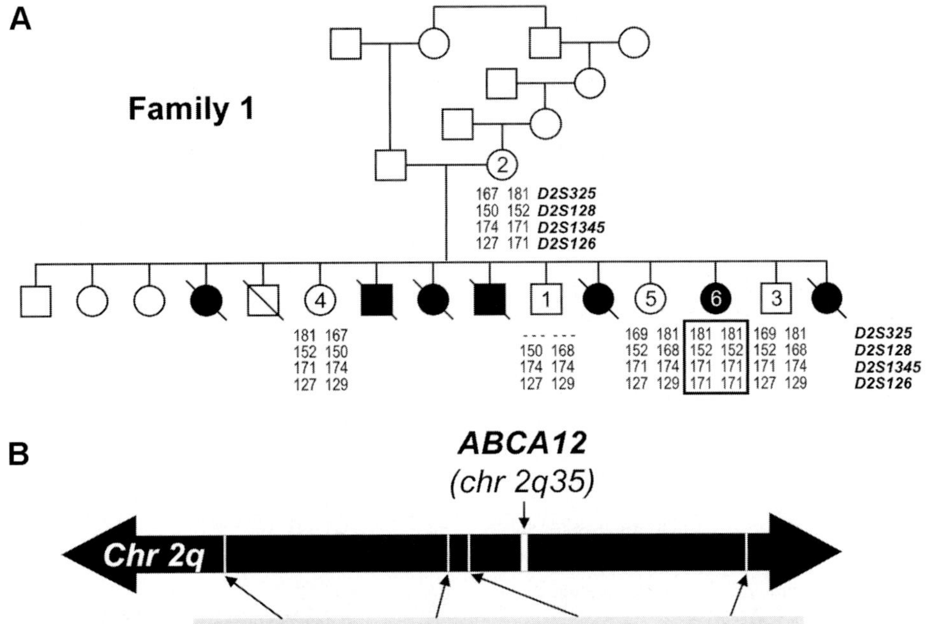

Marker (chr location)	D2S325 (chr 2q33.3)	D2S128 (chr 2q34)	D2S1345 (chr 2q34)	D2S126 (chr 2q36.1)
Affected Patient ID				
6	**181 181**	**152 152**	**171 171**	**171 171**
69	--- ---	**152 152**	**171 171**	--- ---
55	**159 159**	**152 152**	**171 171**	--- ---
63	--- ---	150 152	171 168	**141 141**
7	**169 169**	**160 160**	174 177	**141 141**
40	169 173	148 150	--- ---	**127 127**
49	**161 161**	**160 160**	**174 174**	**139 139**
50	--- ---	154 158	**174 174**	--- ---
915-06	**177 177**	148 150	**168 168**	**126 126**
955-01	**169 169**	**143 143**	**174 174**	**138 138**
928-01	**169 169**	152 154	**177 177**	**138 138**
44	183 179	156 158	174 177	139 141

Figure 3 Analysis of microsatellite markers flanking the *ABCA12* gene. *A,* Segregation of microsatellite markers flanking *ABCA12* at chromosome 2q35 in a family with HI. Only affected individual 6 is homozygous at this region of chromosome 2. Note that the majority of siblings with HI are deceased. *B,* Haplotype analysis of individuals with HI. Microsatellite markers map around the *ABCA12* gene locus (215, 621, 772–215, 828, 657) at chromosome 2q35. Several patients are homozygous for the markers *D2S325* (208, 096, 142–208, 096, 490), *D2S128* (214, 917, 811–214, 918, 065), *D2S1345* (214, 991, 103–214, 991, 425), and *D2S126* (221, 842, 419–221, 842, 782). The genome positions (Mb) for *ABCA12* and microsatellite markers on chromosome 2 are shown in parentheses.

somal region harboring the *ABCA12* locus in this patient. In only one patient (50) with HI was there no *ABCA12* mutation detected. None of the mutations were detected in the control population.

Discussion

The ABC superfamily is a large family of transmembrane proteins involved in transport of substrates across both the plasma membrane and intracellular membranes. Mutations in ABC genes cause diverse diseases, including cystic fibrosis, X-linked adrenoleukodystrophy, Tangier disease, pseudoxanthoma elasticum, and Dubin-Johnson syndrome (Stefkova et al. 2004). In the present article, we report, we believe for the first time, that mutations in the *ABCA12* gene, a member of the ABCA subfamily, cause HI. Genetic studies of this disorder have been hampered by the fact that families with more than one affected child are rare. Families with only one affected individual are unsuitable for genetic linkage studies be-

A

Patient	Mutation type	Resultant change	Exon	Mutation
49	Exon deletion	Truncated protein	23	Homozygous exon deletion
6	Frameshift	Truncated protein	49	7541delC/7541delC TACAGAACAAATGTTC[C]GTCATCCTCACATCTC
7	Frameshift	Truncated protein	42	6378delGC/6378delGC TCAATTGGTATCATT[GC]GATTTTCAAATTACC
55	Frameshift	Truncated protein	49	7541delC/7541delC TACAGAACAAATGTTC[C]GTCATCCTCACATCTC
40	Exon deletion	Truncated protein	28-53	Homozygous deletion from exon 28 to 53
44	Frameshift/amino acid change	Truncated protein/Reduced protein function	33/47	5229delA AAAGAGTCACAAAAAA[A]TAGTGCTATGAGTC D2363N ATTCCAGAAAAG[G]ATATTAAAGAAACTGTTC
63	Frameshift	Truncated protein	49	7541delC/7541delC TACAGAACAAATGTTC[C]GTCATCCTCACATCTC
50	None found			
955-01	Nonsense substitution	Truncated protein	44	R2203* CATGTTTTTTTCCTTG[C/T]GACTCTTAATCAACGA
915-06	Base change at splice junction	Unknown, possible splice variants	42	TGTATCTCTCCTACTTCTCCTGTTTGG[g/t]taagctgc (lower case are intronic)
928-01	Nonsense substitution	Truncated protein	34	W1742* CCACACCCGCAGGAACT[G/A]GAAAGGTCTCATT
69	Frameshift	Truncated protein	49	7541delC/7541delC TACAGAACAAATGTTC[C]GTCATCCTCACATCTC

B

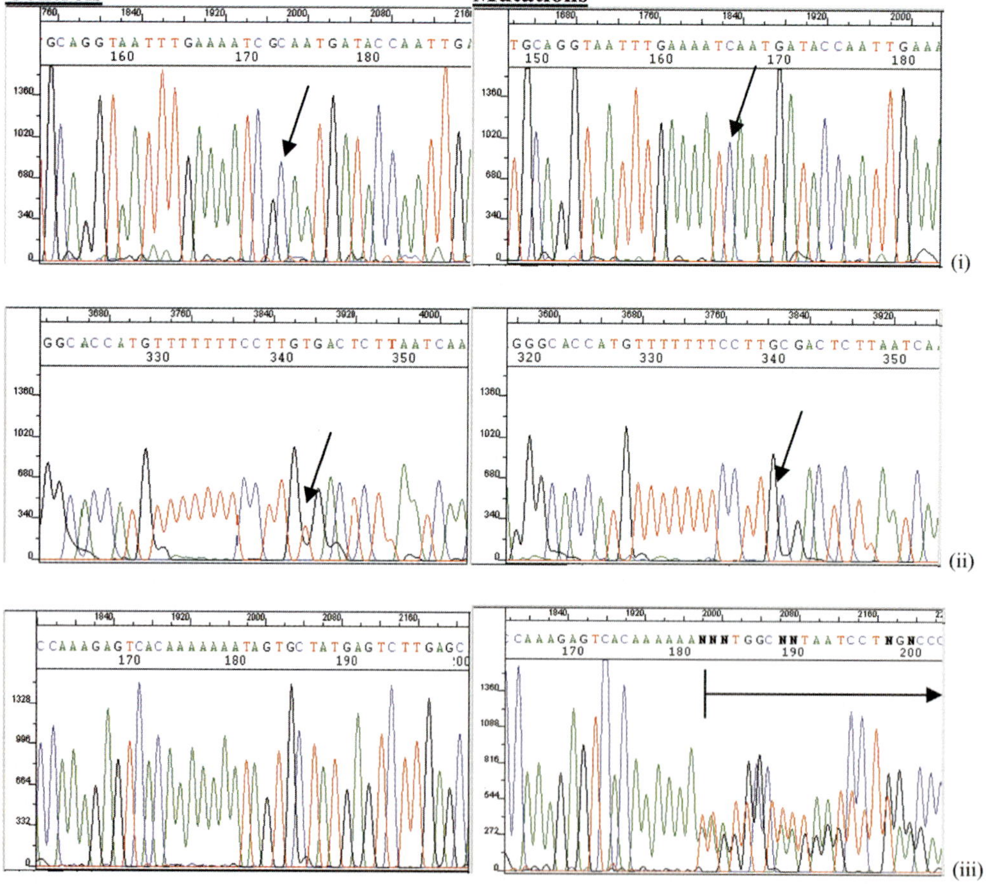

Figure 4 Mutation analysis of the *ABCA12* gene in patients with HI. *A*, Table summarizing mutation analysis. An asterisk (*) indicates a sequence change to a stop codon. *B*, *i*, Chromatogram showing homozygous GC deletion in exon 42 of patient 7. *ii*, Chromatogram showing homozygous T→C substitution in exon 44 in patient 955-01. *iii*, Chromatogram showing heterozygous A deletion in exon 33 of patient 44.

cause of (1) the difficulties in determining whether the disease has been inherited in an AR mode or is due to a new dominant mutation and (2) the low statistical power for linkage analysis. An additional complicating factor is the possibility of genetic heterogeneity.

The results of the Affymetrix 10K SNP-array genome scan of five unrelated patients with HI showed suggestive linkage to a region on chromosome 2q35 on the basis of having a large homozygous SNP haplotype "block" in common, a genetic distance of ~1.5 Mb. Microsatellite markers from this region were identified from the UCSC Genome Browser, and subsequent genotypes were consistent with a locus for HI on 2q35 on the basis of homozygosity at that locus in 11 of the 12 patients with HI described in this study. The *ABCA12* gene encoding an ABC transporter protein that is postulated to be involved in the transport of epidermal lipids is localized within the chromosomal region encompassed by these microsatellite markers. This was regarded as an excellent candidate gene to underlie the HI phenotype, since abnormal or absent epidermal lipids in HI skin have been described. Mutation analysis revealed that 11 of the 12 analyzed patients with HI had a disease-associated mutation in the *ABCA12* gene. The majority of the mutations were predicted to lead to a severely truncated protein, with the exception of a missense substitution and a splice-site mutation. In contrast, the *ABCA12* mutations in LI/NCBIE were all missense and were restricted to within the ATP-binding domain of the protein. Thus, the mutations in HI are likely to disrupt other aspects of *ABCA12* function and may provide the molecular reason behind the severity of HI compared with the milder skin conditions LI and NCBIE. Further mutation studies are in progress to identify the molecular spectra of mutations in a larger panel of patients with HI, including those subcategorized into the different types of HI (Dale et al. 1990). The data in the present article reveal that *ABCA12* mutations are the major cause of HI.

In normal epidermis, the cytoplasm of cells of the upper spinous and granular cell layers contain small granules, 100–300 nm in size, known as "Odland bodies" (Odland 1960); lamellar granules; lamellar bodies; or membrane-coating granules. These move toward the cell membrane as they enter the granular cell layer. They discharge their lipid components and proteases into the intercellular space and play important roles in barrier function, desquamation, and intercellular cohesion within the stratum corneum (Menon et al. 1992; Elias et al. 2000). Lipid delivery to lamellar bodies has also been shown to be required for subsequent delivery of protein to the organelle (Rassner et al. 1999). The defect in *ABCA12* in HI may explain the observed abnormalities in the lamellar granules, possibly associated with severely compromised skin-barrier function. This is analogous to the situation in lung in which surfactant is stored in lamellar bodies in alveolar type II cells. Mutations in *ABCA3* cause fatal surfactant deficiency in newborns, with markedly abnormal lamellar bodies observed ultrastructurally (Shulenin et al. 2004). The lamellar bodies in epidermis also contain beta-defensin, a microbicidal peptide that is also found in the intercellular space, which suggests that it might be discharged with lipid components of the lamellar body (Oren et al. 2003). The defect in epidermal barrier and the loss of beta-defensin may also result in increased susceptibility to infection. Additionally, mutations in two other genes of the ABCA family cause disorders of lipid transport. The *ABCA1* gene is mutated in Tangier disease and in the less severe, heterozygous, familial hypoalphalipoproteinemia as well as in premature atherosclerosis, the resultant disorder dependent on the site of the mutation (Brooks-Wilson et al. 1999; Rust et al. 1999; Clee et al. 2000). The *ABCA4* gene is mutated in patients with Stargardt disease, in some patients with AR retinitis pigmentosa, and in patients with AR cone-rod dystrophy (Stefkova et al. 2004). Our observation that mutations in the *ABCA12* gene cause HI is analogous to other systemic disorders of lipid transport. In addition, like *ABCA1* and *ABCA4*, the site and type of mutation in the *ABCA12* gene determine the severity of the condition, with the more disruptive genetic lesions, such as deletion or frameshift mutations, causing HI.

Prenatal screening tests for HI historically involved invasive procedures, such as fetoscopically and ultrasonographically guided fetal-skin biopsies that reveal key ultrastructural features, such as multivesicular lamellar granules in affected fetuses at 20–24 wk of gestation (Elias et al. 1980; Suzumori and Kanzaki 1991). Similar morphological changes have been described in amniotic fluid cells at 17 wk of gestation (Akiyama et al. 1994). Other methods that have been used in recent years for the prenatal diagnosis of HI are three-dimensional and four-dimensional real-time sonography (Vohra et al. 2003). A major translational benefit of our present findings is that DNA-based analysis should now be possible, which paves the way for earlier (i.e., first trimester) prenatal testing that is more reliable and conclusive than the other non-DNA–based prenatal screening techniques.

In summary, we have applied the rapid SNP-array genotyping technology to identify, by homozygosity mapping, *ABCA12* mutations as the major underlying genetic cause of the devastating skin disease HI. Previously, this disease had proved difficult to map by classic linkage analysis because of the limited size of pedigrees. The association of *ABCA12* mutations with HI will facilitate prenatal DNA diagnosis of this life-threatening disorder as well as the possibility of preimplantation genetic testing. In addition, results of the present study suggest a major role for ABCA12 in lipid transport, barrier formation, and keratinocyte differentiation. The increased understanding of the biological role of ABCA12 in HI may lead to the development of targeted therapy to lessen the burden of this disease for both surviving children with HI and their parents.

Acknowledgments

The authors acknowledge the patients and their families who have contributed to the study. In addition, we acknowledge the contributions of Drs. Nick Lench and Sarah Hatsell during the early stages of our genetic studies of HI; Tracy Chaplin, who runs the SNP Array facility at Queen Mary; and Drs. Sandra Charles-Holmes (Coventry), Vinnie Biggs (Holyoke, MA), Michael Heffernan (St. Louis), and Richard Mupanemunda (Birmingham), for assistance with the clinical aspects of this study. We also acknowledge the major contribution of Dr. Karen Holbrook (Columbus, OH) to our understanding of the pathogenesis of HI. Funding was from the Wellcome Trust (to R.A.J.E.), a Wellcome Trust Prize Studentship (to E.E.N.), United States Public Health Service grant 2P01 AR 21557 (to P.F.), the Odland Endowed Research Fund (to P.F.), and the Barts and The London Charitable Foundation (to B.D.Y.).

Electronic-Database Information

The accession number and URLs for data presented herein are as follows:

Ensembl Genome Browser, http://www.ensembl.org/

GenBank, http://www.ncbi.nlm.nih.gov/Genbank/ (for ABC [accession number NM_173076])

Online Mendelian Inheritance in Man (OMIM), http://www.ncbi.nlm.nih.gov/Omim/ (for HI, *TGM1, ALOXE3, ALOX12B,* ABCA12, and AICA-ribosuria)

UCSC Genome Bioinformatics, http://www.genome.ucsc.edu/ (for the Human Genome working draft of chromosome 2)

References

Akiyama M, Dale BA, Smith LT, Shimizu H, Holbrook KA (1998) Regional difference in expression of characteristic abnormality of harlequin ichthyosis in affected fetuses. Prenat Diagn 18:425–436

Akiyama M, Kim DK, Main DM, Otto CE, Holbrook KA (1994) Characteristic morphologic abnormality of harlequin ichthyosis detected in amniotic fluid cells. J Invest Dermatol 102:210–213

Akiyama M, Shimizu H, Yoneda K, Nishikawa T (1997) Collodion baby: ultrastructure and distribution of cornified cell envelope proteins and keratins. Dermatology 195:164–168

Akiyama M, Yoneda K, Kim SY, Koyama H, Shimizu H (1996) Cornified cell envelope proteins and keratins are normally distributed in harlequin ichthyosis. J Cutan Pathol 23:571–575

Brooks-Wilson A, Marcil M, Clee SM, Zhang LH, Roomp K, van Dam M, Yu L, et al (1999) Mutations in ABC1 in Tangier disease and familial high-density lipoprotein deficiency. Nat Genet 22:336–345

Buxman MM, Goodkin PE, Fahreenback WH (1979) Harlequin icthyosis with epidermal lipid abnormality. Arch Dermatol 115:189–193

Choate KA, Williams ML, Elias PM, Khavari PA (1998) Transglutaminase 1 expression in a patient with features of harlequin ichthyosis: case report. J Am Acad Dermatol 38:325–329

Clee SM, Kastelein JJ, van Dam M, Marcil M, Roomp K, Zwarts KY, Collins JA, Roelants R, Tamasawa N, Stulc T, Suda T, Ceska R, Boucher B, Rondeau C, DeSouich C, Brooks-Wilson A, Molhuizen HO, Frohlich J, Genest J Jr, Hayden MR (2000) Age and residual cholesterol efflux affect HDL cholesterol levels and coronary artery disease in ABCA1 heterozygotes. J Clin Invest 106:1263–1270

Dahlstrom JE, McDonald T, Maxwell L, Jain S (1995) Harlequin ichthyosis—a case report. Pathology 27:289–292

Dale BA, Holbrook KA, Fleckman P, Kimball JR, Brumbaugh S, Sybert VP (1990) Heterogeneity in harlequin icthyosis, an inborn error of epidermal keratinisation: variable morphology and structural protein expression and a defect in lamellar granules. J Invest Dermatol 94:6–18

Elias PM, Fartasch M, Crumrine D, Behne M, Uchida Y, Holleran WM (2000) Origin of the corneocyte lipid envelope (CLE): observations in harlequin ichthyosis and cultured human keratinocytes. J Invest Dermatol 115:765–769

Elias S, Mazur M, Sabbagha R, Esterly NB, Simpson JL (1980) Prenatal diagnosis of harlequin ichthyosis. Clin Genet 17:275–280

Ewing B, Green P (1998) Base-calling of automated sequencer traces using Phred. II. Error probabilities. Genome Res 8:186–194

Ewing B, Hillier L, Wendl MC, Green P (1998) Base-calling of automated sequencer traces using Phred. I. Accuracy assessment. Genome Res 8:175–185

Gordon D, Abajian C, Green P (1998) Consed: a graphical tool for sequence finishing. Genome Res 8:195–202

Haftek M, Cambazard F, Dhouailly D, Reano A, Simon M, Lachaux A, Serre G, Claudy A, Schmitt D (1996) A longitudinal study of a harlequin infant presenting clinically as non-bullous congenital ichthyosiform erythroderma. Br J Dermatol 135:448–453

Hsu WY, Chen JY, Lin WL, Tsay CH (1989) [Harlequin fetus: a case report.] Zhonghua Yi Xue Za Zhi (Taipei) 43:63–66

Huber M, Rettler I, Bernasconi K, Frenk E, Lavrijsen SP, Ponec M, Bon A, Lautenschlager S, Schorderet DF, Hohl D (1995) Mutations of keratinocyte transglutaminase in lamellar ichthyosis. Science 267:525–528

Jobard F, Lefevre C, Karaduman A, Blanchet-Bardon C, Emre S, Weissenbach J, Ozguc M, Lathrop M, Prud'homme JF, Fischer J (2002) Lipoxygenase-3 (ALOXE3) and 12(R)-lipoxygenase (ALOX12B) are mutated in non-bullous congenital ichthyosiform erythroderma (NCIE) linked to chromosome 17p13.1. Hum Mol Genet 11:107–113

Kam E, Nirunsuksiri W, Hager B, Fleckman P, Dale BA (1997) Protein phosphatase activity in human keratinocytes cultured from normal epidermis and epidermis from patients with harlequin ichthyosis. Br J Dermatol 137:874–882

Kruglyak L, Daly MJ, Reeve-Daly MP, Lander ES (1996) Parametric and nonparametric linkage analysis: a unified multipoint approach. Am J Hum Genet 58:1347–1363

Lefevre C, Audebert S, Jobard F, Bouadjar B, Lakhdar H, Boughdene-Stambouli O, Blanchet-Bardon C, Heilig R, Foglio M, Weissenbach J, Lathrop M, Prud'homme JF, Fischer J (2003) Mutations in the transporter ABCA12 are associated with lamellar ichthyosis type 2. Hum Mol Genet 12: 2369–2378

Lefevre C, Bouadjar B, Karaduman A, Jobard F, Saker S, Ozguc M, Lathrop M, Prud'homme JF, Fischer J (2004) Mutations in ichthyin a new gene on chromosome 5q33 in a new form of autosomal recessive congenital ichthyosis. Hum Mol Genet 13:2473–2482

Menon GK, Ghadially R, Williams ML, Elias PM (1992) Lamellar bodies as delivery systems of hydrolytic enzymes: implications for normal and abnormal desquamation. Br J Dermatol 126:337–345

Michel M, Fleckman P, Smith LT, Dale BA (1999) The calcium-activated neutral protease calpain I is present in normal foetal skin and is decreased in neonatal harlequin ichthyosis. Br J Dermatol 141:1017–1026

Moreau S, Salame E, Goullet de Rugy M, Delmas P (1999) Harlequin fetus: a case report. Surg Radiol Anat 21:215–216

Moskowitz DG, Fowler AJ, Heyman MB, Cohen SP, Crumrine D, Elias PM, Williams ML (2004) Pathophysiologic basis for growth failure in children with ichthyosis: an evaluation of cutaneous ultrastructure, epidermal permeability barrier function, and energy expenditure. J Pediatr 145:82–92

Odland GF (1960) A submicroscopic granular component in human epidermis. J Invest Dermatol 34:11–15

Oren A, Ganz T, Liu L, Meerloo T (2003) In human epidermis, β-defensin 2 is packaged in lamellar bodies. Exp Mol Pathol 74:180–182

Rassner U, Feingold KR, Crumrine DA, Elias PM (1999) Coordinate assembly of lipids and enzyme proteins into epidermal lamellar bodies. Tissue Cell 31:489–498

Rust S, Rosier M, Funke H, Real J, Amoura Z, Piette JC, Deleuze JF, Brewer HB, Duverger N, Denefle P, Assmann G (1999) Tangier disease is caused by mutations in the gene encoding ATP-binding cassette transporter 1. Nat Genet 22: 352–355

Sarkar R, Sharma RC, Sethi S, Basu S, Das R, Mendiratta V, Sardana K, Kakar N (2000) Three unusual siblings with harlequin icthyosis in an Indian family. J Dermatol 27:609–611

Shulenin S, Nogee LM, Annilo T, Wert SE, Whitsett JA, Dean M (2004) ABCA3 gene mutations in newborns with fatal surfactant deficiency. N Engl J Med 350:1296–1303

Stefkova J, Poledne R, Hubacek JA (2004) ATP-binding cassette (ABC) transporters in human metabolism and diseases. Physiol Res 53:235–243

Suzumori K, Kanzaki T (1991) Prenatal diagnosis of harlequin ichthyosis by fetal skin biopsy: report of two cases. Prenat Diagn 11:451–457

Vohra N, Rochelson B, Smith-Levitin M (2003) Three-dimensional sonographic findings in congenital (harlequin) ichthyosis. J Ultrasound Med 22:737–739

Am. J. Hum. Genet. 76:804–814, 2005

A Novel *STX16* Deletion in Autosomal Dominant Pseudohypoparathyroidism Type Ib Redefines the Boundaries of a *cis*-Acting Imprinting Control Element of *GNAS*

Agnès Linglart,[1] Robert C. Gensure,[3] Robert C. Olney,[4] Harald Jüppner,[1,2] and Murat Bastepe[1]

[1]Endocrine Unit, Department of Medicine, and [2]Pediatric Nephrology Unit, MassGeneral Hospital *for* Children, Massachusetts General Hospital and Harvard Medical School, Boston; [3]Department of Pediatrics, Tulane University School of Medicine, New Orleans; and [4]Nemours Children's Clinic and Mayo Medical School, Jacksonville, FL

A unique heterozygous 3-kb microdeletion within *STX16*, a closely linked gene centromeric of *GNAS*, was previously identified in multiple unrelated kindreds as a cause of autosomal dominant pseudohypoparathyroidism type Ib (AD-PHP-Ib). We now report a novel heterozygous 4.4-kb microdeletion in a large kindred with AD-PHP-Ib. Affected individuals from this kindred share an epigenetic defect that is indistinguishable from that observed in patients with AD-PHP-Ib who carry the 3-kb microdeletion in the *STX16* region (i.e., an isolated loss of methylation at *GNAS* exon A/B). The novel 4.4-kb microdeletion overlaps with the previously identified deletion by 1,286 bp and, similar to the latter deletion, removes several exons of *STX16* (encoding syntaxin-16). Because these microdeletions lead to AD-PHP-Ib only after maternal transmission, we analyzed expression of this gene in lymphoblastoid cells of affected individuals with the 3-kb or the 4.4-kb microdeletion, an individual with a NESP55 deletion, and a healthy control. We found that *STX16* mRNA was expressed in all cases from both parental alleles. Thus, *STX16* is apparently not imprinted, and a loss-of-function mutation in one allele is therefore unlikely to be responsible for this disorder. Instead, the region of overlap between the two microdeletions likely harbors a *cis*-acting imprinting control element that is necessary for establishing and/or maintaining methylation at *GNAS* exon A/B, thus allowing normal Gα_s expression in the proximal renal tubules. In the presence of either of the two microdeletions, parathyroid hormone resistance appears to develop over time, as documented in an affected individual who was diagnosed at birth with the 4.4-kb deletion of *STX16* and who had normal serum parathyroid hormone levels until the age of 21 mo.

Introduction

GNAS is a complex imprinted locus that yields—in addition to the α-subunit of the stimulatory G protein (Gα_s)—multiple alternative transcripts (fig. 1). These transcripts encode extra-large Gα_s (XLα_s) (Kehlenbach et al. 1994; Hayward et al. 1998*a*; Peters et al. 1999) or neurosecretory protein 55 (NESP55) (Ischia et al. 1997; Hayward et al. 1998*b*; Peters et al. 1999), or they lead to presumably nontranslated RNAs, such as the A/B transcript (also referred to as "1A" or "1′") (Ishikawa et al. 1990; Swaroop et al. 1991; Liu et al. 2000*b*) and the antisense (AS) transcript (referred to as "*Nespas*" in mouse) (Hayward and Bonthron 2000; Liu et al. 2000*b*; Wroe et al. 2000). NESP55, XLα_s, and A/B differ from Gα_s only by their first exons, whereas AS transcripts consist of entirely distinct exons. AS, XLα_s, and A/B are paternally derived transcripts, whereas NESP55 is a maternally derived transcript. Consistent with their monoallelic expression, the promoters of these imprinted transcripts are located within differentially methylated regions (DMRs) (fig. 1). In contrast, the promoter that gives rise to Gα_s is not methylated, and, accordingly, expression of Gα_s occurs in most tissues from both parental *GNAS* alleles (Campbell et al. 1994; Hayward et al. 1998*a*, 1998*b*; Zheng et al. 2001). In some tissues (including proximal renal tubules, pituitary, gonads, and thyroid), however, Gα_s transcripts are predominantly derived from the maternal allele (Hayward et al. 1998*a*, 2001; Yu et al. 1998; Li et al. 2000; Mantovani et al. 2002).

Pseudohypoparathyroidism (PHP) is a disorder characterized by hypocalcemia, hyperphosphatemia, and parathyroid hormone (PTH) levels that are elevated as a result of end-organ resistance to this hormone. One of the two main subtypes of PHP, PHP type Ia (PHP-Ia [MIM 103580]), is caused by heterozygous maternally inherited loss-of-function mutations in *GNAS* exons 1–13, which encode Gα_s. In addition to PTH resistance, affected individuals typically show clinical abnormali-

Received December 30, 2004; accepted for publication February 23, 2005; electronically published March 30, 2005.

Address for correspondence and reprints: Dr. Murat Bastepe, Endocrine Unit, Massachusetts General Hospital, 50 Blossom Street, WEL 5, Boston, MA 02114. E-mail: bastepe@helix.mgh.harvard.edu

0002-9297/2005/7605-0009$15.00

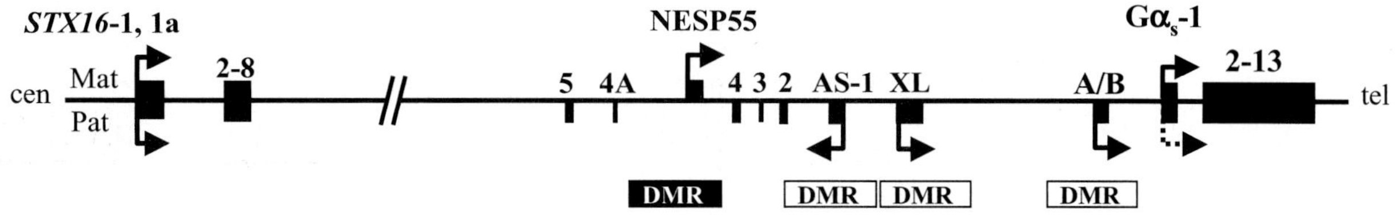

Figure 1 Schematic representation of the human *STX16* and *GNAS* loci (not to scale). Exons are depicted as blackened boxes; arrows indicate direction (sense, antisense) and allelic origin (Mat = maternal [*above the line*]; Pat = paternal [*below the line*]) of transcription. Note that $G\alpha_s$ is transcribed from both alleles in most tissues (Campbell et al. 1994; Hayward et al. 1998*a*, 1998*b*; Zheng et al. 2001) and that the paternal allele is silenced (*dotted arrow*) in some tissues, including kidney, adipose tissue, and pituitary (Hayward et al. 1998*a*, 2001; Yu et al. 1998; Li et al. 2000; Mantovani et al. 2002). Paternal and maternal DMRs are indicated by blackened and unblackened rectangles, respectively.

ties referred to as "Albright hereditary osteodystrophy" (AHO) and resistance toward several additional hormones, including thyroid-stimulating hormone (TSH) and gonadotropins. When inherited paternally, $G\alpha_s$ loss-of-function mutations are associated with AHO alone, in the absence of hormonal resistance—a variant termed "pseudopseudohypoparathyroidism" (PPHP) (Weinstein et al. 2001; Levine 2002). The other main form of PHP, PHP type Ib (PHP-Ib [MIM 603233]), differs from PHP-Ia and PPHP, in that PHP-Ib patients do not have the AHO phenotype (Weinstein et al. 2001). Furthermore, hormone resistance in PHP-Ib appears to be limited to the renal actions of PTH, although resistance to TSH is also seen occasionally (Bastepe et al. 2001*a*, 2001*b*; Liu et al. 2003).

The autosomal dominant variant of PHP-Ib (AD-PHP-Ib) has been linked to a region of chromosome 20q13.3 that comprises the *GNAS* locus, and, similar to PHP-Ia, this disorder is maternally transmitted (Jüppner et al. 1998). Most individuals affected by AD-PHP-Ib show a methylation defect that is limited to *GNAS* exon A/B, whereas most apparently sporadic cases of the disease display abnormal methylation at other *GNAS* DMRs as well (Liu et al. 2000*a*, 2005; Bastepe et al. 2001*b*, 2003). An identical 3-kb microdeletion located ~220 kb upstream of *GNAS* has been identified in all affected members and obligate carriers of 14 unrelated families with AD-PHP-Ib and in two apparently sporadic cases (Bastepe et al. 2003). All affected individuals share the same epigenetic defect at exon A/B and lack methylation abnormalities at the other DMRs of *GNAS*. The 3-kb microdeletion lies between two direct repeats and removes intronic as well as exonic sequences of the gene encoding syntaxin-16 (*STX16*). Consistent with the imprinted inheritance pattern of the disease, transmission of the microdeletion from a female obligate carrier causes PTH resistance, whereas transmission of the same mutation from a male obligate carrier results in normal PTH responsiveness (Bastepe et al. 2003). Recently, additional patients with PHP-Ib and with the isolated *GNAS* exon A/B methylation defect have been reported to carry the same 3-kb microdeletion (Liu et al. 2005; Mahmud et al. 2005), thereby strengthening the likely causative association between the exon A/B methylation defect and this deletion.

In one family with AD-PHP-Ib (kindred W), the 3-kb microdeletion was not found, despite a loss of methylation at *GNAS* exon A/B alone in the affected individuals (Bastepe et al. 2001*b*, 2003), suggesting the presence of another mutation in the *STX16* region. We thus searched, in this family, for mutations within *STX16* and identified a novel microdeletion in all affected members and unaffected carriers.

Subjects and Methods

Kindred W and Methylation Analysis of GNAS *Exon A/B*

The pedigree (kindred W) and the clinical and laboratory data of most members of this family have been described elsewhere (Bastepe et al. 2001*b*) (see also fig. 2*A*). Genomic DNA was isolated from blood leukocytes of all family members, and a lymphoblastoid cell line was established for patient W-III/3 (Harvard-Partners Center for Genetics and Genomics Biosample Services Facility). Written informed consent was obtained from all investigated individuals (Massachusetts General Hospital institutional review board [#2001p-000648]).

Since 2001, when this family was first reported (Bastepe et al. 2001*b*), two children have been born: W-III/12 (born to W-II/9) and W-III/13 (born to W-II/10). Genomic DNA was extracted from cord blood of both children. Methylation of *GNAS* exon A/B was assessed by nucleotide sequence analysis of PCR-amplified bisulfite-treated genomic DNA and by Southern blot analysis with the use of *Eag*I (methylation sensitive) and *Eco*RV (methylation insensitive) (New England Biolabs), as described elsewhere (Jüppner et al. 1998; Bastepe et al. 2001*b*, 2003). Total serum calcium, phosphorus, intact PTH (Nichols Institute), and TSH were measured

A

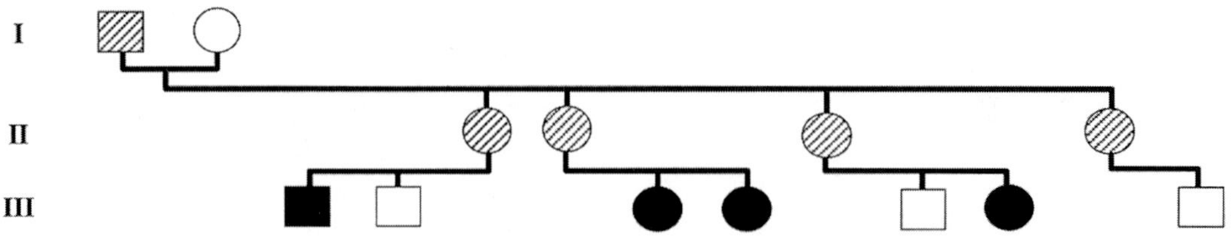

	1		2		3		4		5		6		7		8		9		11		12		10		13	
907-rep2	2	6	2	2	2	6	2	2	2	6	2	6	6	6	6	6	2	2	2	2	2	2	2	6	2	2
rs6100157	T	-	C	T			C	T	C	-	C	-	C	-	C	-	-	T			T	-	T	-	T	T
rs6100158	T	T	C	T	T	T	C	T	C	T	C	T	C	T	C	T	T	T	T	T	T	T	T	T	T	T
261P9-CA1	7	5	9	7	3	5	9	3	9	5	9	5	1	5	1	5	5	7	7	7	7	5	7	5	7	7
806M20-CA	9	1	1	3	1	1	1	1	1	1	1	1	9	1	9	1	1	3	7	3	7	1	3	1	9	3
AFM248tf5	2	1	2	2	2	1	2	3	2	1	2	1	2	1	2	1	1	2	2	2	2	1	2	1		
543J19-TTA	8	1	8	1	4	1	8	1	8	1	8	1	1	1	1	1	1	1	4	1	4	1	1	1	4	1
D20S171	5	11	5	5	7	11	5	7	5	11	5	11	11	11	11	11	11	5	9	5	9	11	5	11	1	5

B

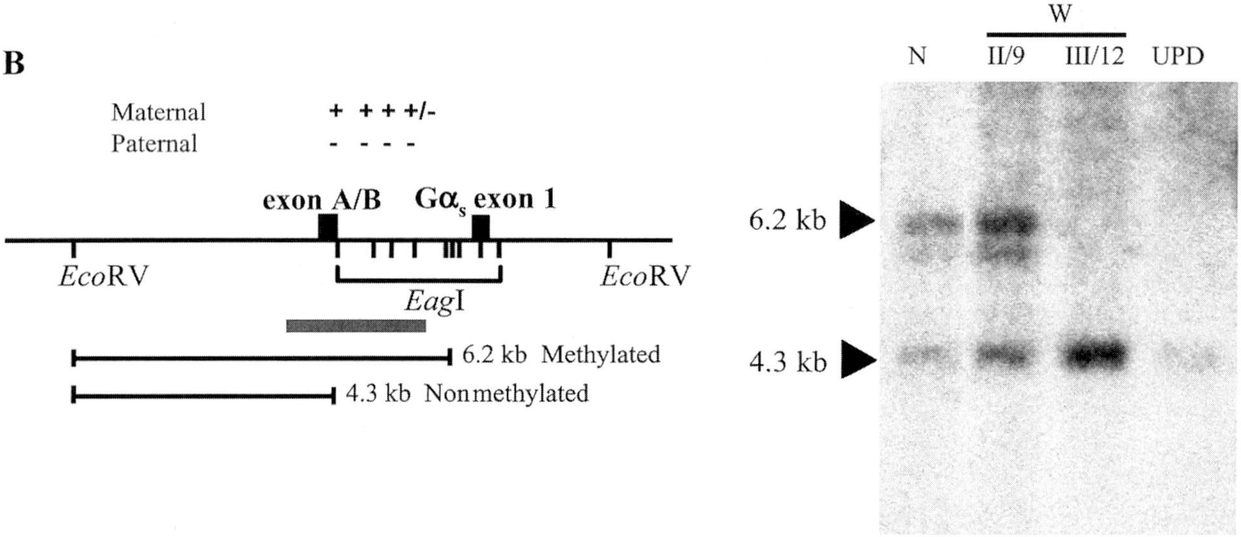

Figure 2 *A,* Evidence of allelic loss within the *STX16* locus in the obligate carriers W-II/5 and W-II/6. All the affected individuals (*blackened symbols*) as well as the obligate carriers (*striped symbols*) share the same disease-associated haplotype (*gray columns*) at 20q13.3; note that not all investigated markers are shown. A recombination event occurred in individual W-II/9 between markers *907-rep2* and *261P9-CA1* and was transmitted to her affected daughter, W-III/12, thus reducing the critical interval likely containing the genetic lesion that causes AD-PHP-Ib. Evidence of allelic loss was found at SNP *rs6100157* (*bold typeface*) in obligate carriers W-II/5 and W-II/6. *B,* Loss of methylation at *GNAS* exon A/B in the newborn W-III/12. The methylation status of *GNAS* exon A/B was assessed by Southern blot analysis of cord blood DNA from patient W-III/12 and of genomic DNA from her unaffected mother (W-II/9), an individual with paternal uniparental isodisomy of chromosome 20q ("UPD") (Bastepe et al. 2001*a*), and a healthy control individual ("N"). These samples were digested with a methylation-sensitive (*Eag*I) and a methylation-insensitive (*Eco*RV) restriction endonuclease, as described elsewhere (Bastepe et al. 2001*b*). Locations of restriction sites and their methylation status ("+" = methylated; "−" = nonmethylated), the predicted fragments, and the probe (*gray bar*) are shown in the left panel. Affected individuals (UPD and W-III/12) show loss of methylation at exon A/B, whereas unaffected individuals (N and W-II/9) have one methylated and one nonmethylated allele. Fragment sizes are indicated by arrowheads. Note that the faint hybridizing band below the 6.2-kb band reflects partial methylation ("+/−") and, hence, incomplete digestion at one of the *Eag*I sites between exon A/B and $G\alpha_s$ exon 1.

in patient W-III/12 shortly after birth and subsequently at regular intervals.

Analysis of Microsatellite Markers and SNPs

Microsatellite markers *D20S102, D20S25, D20S86, D20S164, 907-Rep2, 907-Rep4, 261P9-CA1, 806M20-CA, AFM248tf5, GNAS, 543J19-TTA, D20S171, st-AFMa202yb9,* and *D20S93* were analyzed as described elsewhere (Bastepe et al. 2003). SNPs *rs6100157, rs2296524,* and *rs6100158*—which correspond to nucleotides 3959, 4712, and 5326, respectively, of AL139349—were analyzed by nucleotide sequence anal-

Table 1

Sequences of the Primers Used in the Present Study

The table is available in its entirety in the online edition of *The American Journal of Human Genetics.*

ysis after PCR amplification, which was performed using conditions and primers reported elsewhere (table 1) (Jüppner et al. 1998; Bastepe et al. 2001*b*, 2003).

Southern Blot and PCR Analysis for Detection of the Deletion

For Southern blot analysis, genomic DNA (5 μg) was digested with *Afl*II, *Bcl*I, or *Bgl*II (New England Biolabs). After separation on a 0.8% agarose gel, DNA fragments were transferred onto a nitrocellulose filter and were hybridized with a ^{32}P-radiolabeled probe (nucleotides 8299–9921 of AL139349), which was generated by PCR; primers are listed in table 1.

PCR amplification of genomic DNA across the predicted deletion was performed using primers 5.9 kb apart from each other (primers A and B) (table 1) and the Expand Long-Template PCR System with Buffer 3 (Roche Molecular Biochemicals). The cycling conditions were an initial 94°C for 3 min; 10 cycles of 94°C for 10 s, 58°C for 30 s, and 68°C for 5 min; 25 cycles of 94°C for 10 s, 58°C for 30 s, and 68°C for 5 min, with an additional 20 s at 68°C after each cycle; and 1 final cycle at 72°C for 10 min. These conditions yielded a 5.9-kb amplicon, which was not consistently amplified in all samples. The same conditions also yielded an ~1.5-kb amplicon in affected individuals and obligate carriers, which was gel purified and submitted for nucleotide sequence analysis (Massachusetts General Hospital DNA Core Facility).

For multiplex PCR, two pairs of primers (C and D, E and F) were designed, to amplify small fragments across each boundary of the deletion (table 1). Both pairs were used for simultaneous PCR amplification of three different fragments: a 616-bp fragment (primers C and D) and a 252-bp fragment (primers E and F), derived from the centromeric and telomeric ends of the deleted region, respectively, as well as a 4.8-kb fragment (primers C and F), derived from the wild-type allele. As a result of its large size, however, the latter fragment could not be effectively amplified each time.

Analyzing STX16 *Transcripts*

Total RNA was extracted from lymphoblastoid cells derived from the affected individuals W-III/3, F-III/37, C-II/1, as well as a healthy control individual (Harvard-Partners Center for Genetics and Genomics Biosample Services Facility). Subject F-III/37 carries the previously described 3-kb deletion (Bastepe et al. 2003). Subject C-II/1 has methylation abnormalities at all *GNAS* DMRs and has been recently shown to carry a novel microdeletion involving exon NESP55 and antisense exons 3 and 4 (Bastepe et al. 2005). Consistent with the conclusion that the *STX16* region is intact, subject C-II/1 was furthermore shown to be heterozygous at SNPs *rs6100157* and *rs2296524,* which are located within the centromeric repeat and *STX16* exon 4, respectively. STX16 mRNAs were amplified by RT-PCR. One microgram of lymphoblast-derived total RNA was reverse transcribed using Superscript II (Invitrogen) and oligo (dT) primers, in accordance with manufacturer recommendations; the same reactions, without reverse transcriptase, served as negative controls. PCR was then performed using 1 μl of 1:10 dilution of the reverse-transcription mixture, a forward primer located in exon 1 (primer G), and a reverse primer located in exon 8 (primer H) in a total reaction volume of 50 μl (table 1 and fig. 3). The amplification conditions were an initial 94°C for 2 min; 31 cycles of denaturation at 95°C for 30 s, annealing at 61°C for 30 s, and extension at 72°C for 1 min; and 1 final cycle of extension at 72°C for 10 min. Amplicons were separated on a 2% agarose gel, were purified, and were submitted for nucleotide sequence analysis (Massachusetts General Hospital DNA Core Facility), as described elsewhere (Bastepe et al. 2001*b*). To determine the allelic origin of the STX16 transcripts in the healthy control individual and in subject C-II/1, total RNA was amplified by RT-PCR as described above, and the polymorphic nucleotide at position 527 of STX16 isoform B was analyzed by direct sequence analysis of the amplicon; this corresponds to SNP *rs2296524* (table 1).

Results

Loss of Exon A/B Methylation and Development of PTH Resistance

We have reported elsewhere that affected members of kindred W show a loss of exon A/B methylation without additional epigenetic defects of *GNAS* (Bastepe et al. 2003). Nucleotide sequence analysis of PCR-amplified bisulfite-treated cord blood DNA from the newborn W-III/13 showed a normal methylation pattern at *GNAS* exon A/B (data not shown). Accordingly, haplotype analysis across the *GNAS* region revealed that this individual had inherited the grandmaternal haplotype, which is not associated with disease (fig. 2*A*) (Bastepe et al. 2001*b*). Thus, two independent approaches indicated that subject W-III/13 would not be affected with AD-PHP-Ib. In contrast, Southern blot analysis of cord blood DNA from his cousin, W-III/12, performed using the restriction endonucleases *Eco*RV and *Eag*I, showed loss of methylation at *GNAS* exon A/B (fig. 2*B*), and

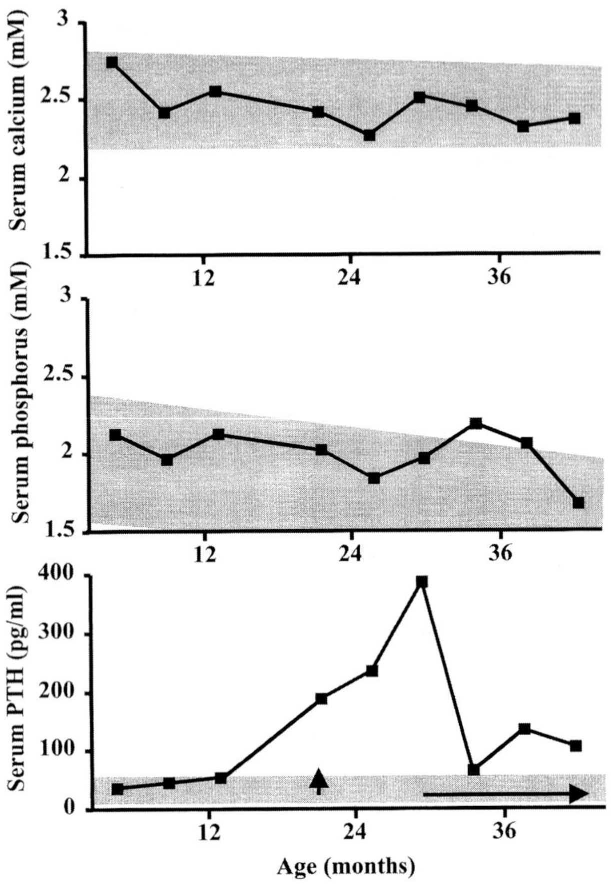

Figure 3 Delayed onset of PTH resistance in patient W-III/12. Serum calcium, phosphorus, and PTH levels were measured during follow-up visits of the patient—in whom loss of methylation at *GNAS* exon A/B was identified at birth—and the 4.4-kb deletion was discovered subsequently. Normal ranges are indicated by gray shading. Treatment with an active vitamin D analog (Rocaltrol) was first started at age 21 mo (*vertical arrow*). However, the parents discontinued the treatment shortly thereafter, and continuous treatment was not resumed until the child was 30 mo old (*horizontal arrow*).

haplotype analysis revealed inheritance of the disease-associated grandpaternal haplotype (fig. 2*A*). She was therefore predicted to develop PTH resistance, which was subsequently documented (see below). Because patient W-III/12 was found to be affected, the maximum LOD score increased from 2.03 (Bastepe et al. 2001*b*) to 2.43 for genetic linkage to 20q13.3 (*D20S171* [$\theta = 0$]), increasing the likelihood that the defect leading to AD-PHP-Ib in this family also resides close to the *GNAS* locus.

Birth weight and height of patient W-III/12 were 4.2 kg (95th percentile [North American reference chart]) and 53 cm (95th percentile), respectively. Her weight, height, and BMI remained above the 95th percentile during infancy and early childhood. Except for being overweight, she had no features suggestive of AHO. PTH resistance was absent at birth but developed by age 21 mo, when serum PTH levels were first noted to be above the normal range (188 pg/ml; normal range 10–65 pg/ml). Both total serum calcium and phosphorous concentrations remained within normal range during this period, although serum phosphorus was close to the upper limit (fig. 3). Because of the genetic findings and the elevation in PTH concentration, treatment with an active vitamin D analog (Rocaltrol) and calcium supplements was first initiated at age 21 mo. However, the parents discontinued these medications shortly thereafter, and it was not until the child was 30 mo old that uninterrupted treatment was started. By that time, the PTH concentration had increased to 386 pg/ml. In addition, mild TSH resistance was suspected at age 30 mo because of elevated TSH (14.5 mUI/l; normal range 0.5–5 mUI/l), normal free T4 (0.9 ng/dl; normal range 0.7–1.7 ng/dl), and undetectable serum anti-thyroglobulin and anti-thioperoxidase antibodies. L-thyroxine treatment was then started, and the TSH level dropped to the normal range (2.89 mUI/l at 41 mo).

Identification of a Novel Deletion within the STX16 *Region*

All affected individuals of kindred W (W-III/3, W-III/7, W-III/8, and W-III/12) showed a loss of methylation at *GNAS* exon A/B, without methylation abnormalities involving the NESP55, XL, or AS DMRs (fig. 2*B* and Bastepe et al. [2001*b*]). Nevertheless, unlike many other kindreds with AD-PHP-Ib with the same epigenetic defect, the previously described 3-kb deletion (nucleotides 3786–6764 of AL139349) could not be found in this kindred. In fact, all affected individuals and obligate carriers were heterozygous at microsatellite marker *261P9-CA1,* and some of them, furthermore, were heterozygous at SNP *rs6100158* (figs. 2*A* and 4*A*). In addition, PCR analysis across the 3-kb deletion, performed using previously established primers and conditions (Bastepe et al. 2003), revealed no evidence of a smaller deletion within this region.

Analysis of additional polymorphisms centromeric of the heterozygous SNP *rs6100158* revealed allelic loss at SNP *rs6100157* for the obligate carriers W-II/5 and W-II/6, indicating the presence of a deletion comprising this region (figs. 2*A* and 4*A*). This deletion was confirmed by Southern blot analysis of genomic DNA from individual W-II/5 and her unaffected child W-III/4, performed using restriction enzymes *Afl*II, *Bcl*I, or *Bgl*II (fig. 4*B*). The probe, located telomeric of SNP *rs6100158,* detected wild-type hybridizing fragments of 7.9 kb, 9.8 kb, and 9.2 kb in both samples. In addition, however, hybridizing *Afl*II, *Bcl*I, and *Bgl*II fragments of ~6.8 kb, 11.1 kb, and 7 kb were detected, respectively, in the DNA sample from individual W-II/5 but not in the DNA

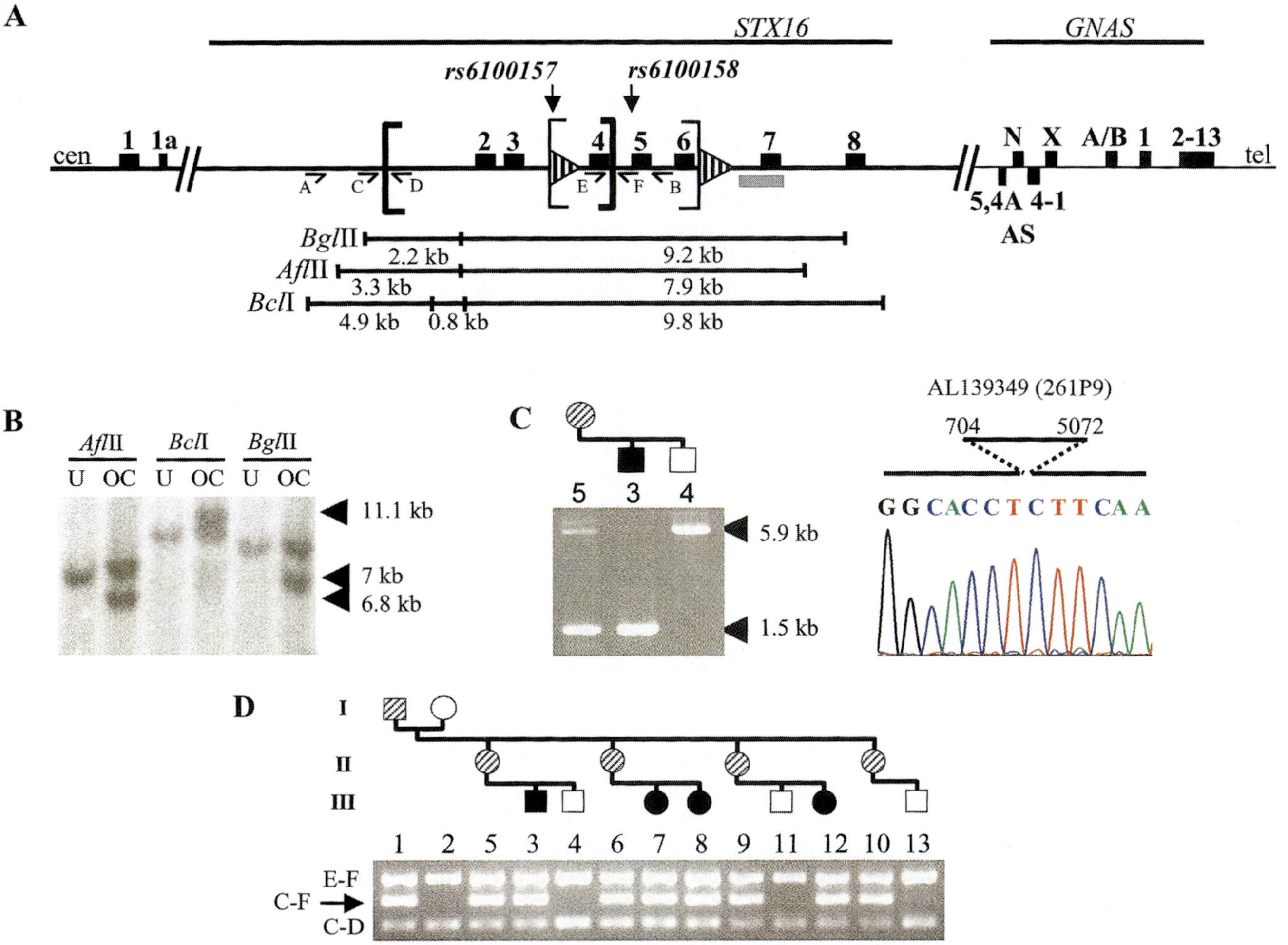

Figure 4 Identification of a novel 4.4-kb deletion in kindred W. *A*, Simplified map of the 20q13.3 region and the localization of the two known microdeletions. Sequence of the depicted region is included in AL050327 (clone 907D15) and AL139349 (clone 261P9). Exons are depicted as blackened rectangles, and direct repeats are shown as striped arrowheads. The 3-kb and 4.4-kb deleted regions lie between the thin and thick brackets, respectively. The locations of recognition sites for the restriction endonucleases used in the Southern blot analysis are shown under the gene map. The location of the 1.6-kb probe is marked by the gray bar, and primers A, B, C, D, E, and F, which were used for PCR analyses, are indicated by arrowed lines; cen = centromeric; tel = telomeric; N = NESP55; AS = antisense; X = $XL\alpha_s$; A/B = exon A/B. *B*, Southern blot analysis of genomic DNA from an unaffected ("U") subject, W-III/4, and an obligate carrier ("OC"), W-II/5, which was digested with three different restriction endonucleases (*Afl*II, *Bcl*I, and *Bgl*II). Hybridization with the 1.6-kb ^{32}P-labeled probe (nucleotides 8299–9921 of AL139349) showed the expected wild-type bands of 7.9 kb, 9.8 kb, and 9.2 kb, respectively. Additional bands (*arrowheads*) in the obligate carrier (6.8 kb, 11.1 kb, and 7 kb, respectively) are compatible with a 4.4-kb deletion removing one *Afl*II site, two *Bcl*I sites, and one *Bgl*II site—all of which are centromeric of *STX16* exon 2. *C*, Confirmation and exact localization of the deletion by PCR. Amplification across the predicted location of the deletion, performed using one pair of primers (A [forward] and B [reverse]), yielded a 5.9-kb wild-type fragment in the unaffected subject, the affected individual, and the obligate carrier; both the affected individual and the obligate carrier also showed a shorter fragment (of 1.5 kb). Direct nucleotide sequence analysis of the short amplicon revealed the lack of 4,368 bp extending from nucleotide 704 to nucleotide 5072 of AL139349. *D*, Amplification of the *STX16* region with four different primers, located at nucleotides 404 (primer C [forward]), 1020 (primer D [reverse]), 4938 (primer E [forward]), and 5190 (primer F [reverse]) of AL139349. The sizes of expected wild-type PCR products are 616 bp (primers C and D), 252 bp (primers E and F), and 4.8 kb (primers C and F [not shown]). Obligate carriers and affected individuals show an additional 422-bp amplicon (*arrow* [primers C and F]). Results are shown for each individual in the family (blackened symbols represent affected individuals, striped symbols represent obligate carriers, and unblackened symbols represent unaffected individuals).

sample from individual W-III/4. The sizes of these additional bands were compatible with an ~4.4-kb deletion that removed one centromeric *Afl*II site, two *Bcl*I sites, and one *Bgl*II site.

To determine the exact location of the deletion, we performed a series of PCRs with the use of primers that were predicted to amplify a region of the mutant allele spanning the deletion breakpoint. One set of primers (primers A and B) amplified a single product of ~5.9 kb from genomic DNA of the unaffected individual W-III/4, whereas the same primers produced an additional smaller amplicon of ~1.5 kb from DNA of the affected individual W-III/3 and unaffected carrier W-II/5 (fig. 4*A* and 4*C*). The difference between the lengths of the small and the large amplicons was consistent with a 4.4-kb deletion, suggesting that the small amplicon was derived from the mutant allele. Direct nucleotide sequence analysis of this mutant fragment showed that the deletion occurred between nucleotides 704 and 5072 of AL139349, thus eliminating exons 2–4 of *STX16* (fig. 4*C*). The presence of this deletion was also confirmed in the remaining affected individuals or unaffected carriers by multiplex PCR, performed using primers designed to amplify across the deleted region and across the predicted boundaries. All affected individuals and obligate carriers of kindred W showed—in addition to the wild-type products of 616 bp (primers C and D) and 252 bp (primers E and F)—a 422-bp product amplified across the deletion breakpoints (primers C and F) (fig. 4*A* and 4*D*). In contrast, genomic DNA from the healthy individuals generated only the two wild-type fragments; note that the 4.8-kb product derived from the wild-type allele (primers C and F) could not be routinely amplified, because of its size (data not shown).

Biallelic Expression of STX16

Although the identified deletion removes coding exons from the gene *STX16*, a loss-of-function mutation in one *STX16* allele could not directly explain the imprinted AD-PHP-Ib phenotype unless *STX16* itself is an imprinted gene. We therefore examined allelic expression of *STX16* in total RNA extracted from lymphoblastoid cells of a healthy control individual and of three AD-PHP-Ib individuals carrying different mutations. *STX16* normally gives rise to at least three differently spliced mRNA transcripts: STX16A, STX16B, and STX16C (AL050327 and AL139349 [fig. 5*A*]). RT-PCR amplification of total RNA from both the control individual and subject C-II/1 (deletion of the NESP55 DMR [Bastepe et al. 2005]), performed using primers G and H, yielded products of 861 bp and 802 bp, corresponding to isoform B of STX16 and its splice variant (which is missing the alternatively spliced exon 4), respectively (fig. 5*B*). Subsequent nucleotide sequence analysis of the 861-bp products revealed heterozygosity at position 527 of STX16 isoform B located within exon 4 (SNP *rs2296524* [fig. 5*C*]), indicating that both parental alleles were transcribed and amplified. Furthermore, RT-PCR performed using lymphoblast-derived total RNA of the affected individual W-III/3 (4.4-kb *STX16* deletion) showed amplicons from the wild-type splice variants of STX16 isoform B, as well as a shorter amplicon of 449 bp (fig. 5*A* and 5*B*). Direct sequence analysis of this short product confirmed the absence of nucleotides derived from *STX16* exons 2, 3, and 4. Likewise, transcripts amplified by RT-PCR from individual F-III/37 (3-kb *STX16* deletion) included, in addition to the wild-type splice variants of STX16 isoform B, a shortened transcript represented by an amplicon of 462 bp (fig. 5*A* and 5*B*). Nucleotide sequence analysis of this shorter product confirmed the deletion of exons 4, 5, and 6. Together, these findings suggested that both parental *STX16* alleles are transcribed in lymphoblastoid cells and that the identified deletions do not appear to alter this biallelic expression. We also searched the EST database and identified two ESTs (CN348556 and CN417685) matching the *STX16* exon 8 sequence that were derived from the same cDNA library yet differed by one nucleotide (position 937 of STX16 isoform B; position 11538 of AL139349). Since this nucleotide change was also seen in several other ESTs from the database, it indicated its polymorphic nature rather than a sequence error. This finding strongly suggested that STX16 mRNAs were amplified from both parental alleles in that particular library as well.

Discussion

We report a novel *STX16* microdeletion of 4.4 kb in all affected individuals and obligate carriers of a large kindred with AD-PHP-Ib. This 4.4-kb microdeletion was present in the unaffected mothers of the affected individuals ($n = 4$) and in the father of these obligate carriers (figs. 2 and 4). This mode of inheritance is concordant with the paternal imprinting of the disease in this and other families with AD-PHP-Ib. The 4.4-kb microdeletion is the first *STX16* mutation identified in patients with AD-PHP-Ib that differs from the 3-kb microdeletion present in multiple unrelated kindreds with this disorder (Bastepe et al. 2003; Liu et al. 2005; Mahmud et al. 2005). Our findings thus provide further evidence supporting the conclusion that *STX16* harbors an important element involved in the pathogenesis of PHP-Ib. As the two deletions overlap by 1,286 bp, it is likely that this element is contained in this overlap region. Thus far, of the 31 unrelated individuals with PHP-Ib that we have investigated, 18 (58%) carry a deletion within *STX16* (Bastepe et al. 2003; Mahmud et al. 2005). Recently, the 3-kb deletion has also been found

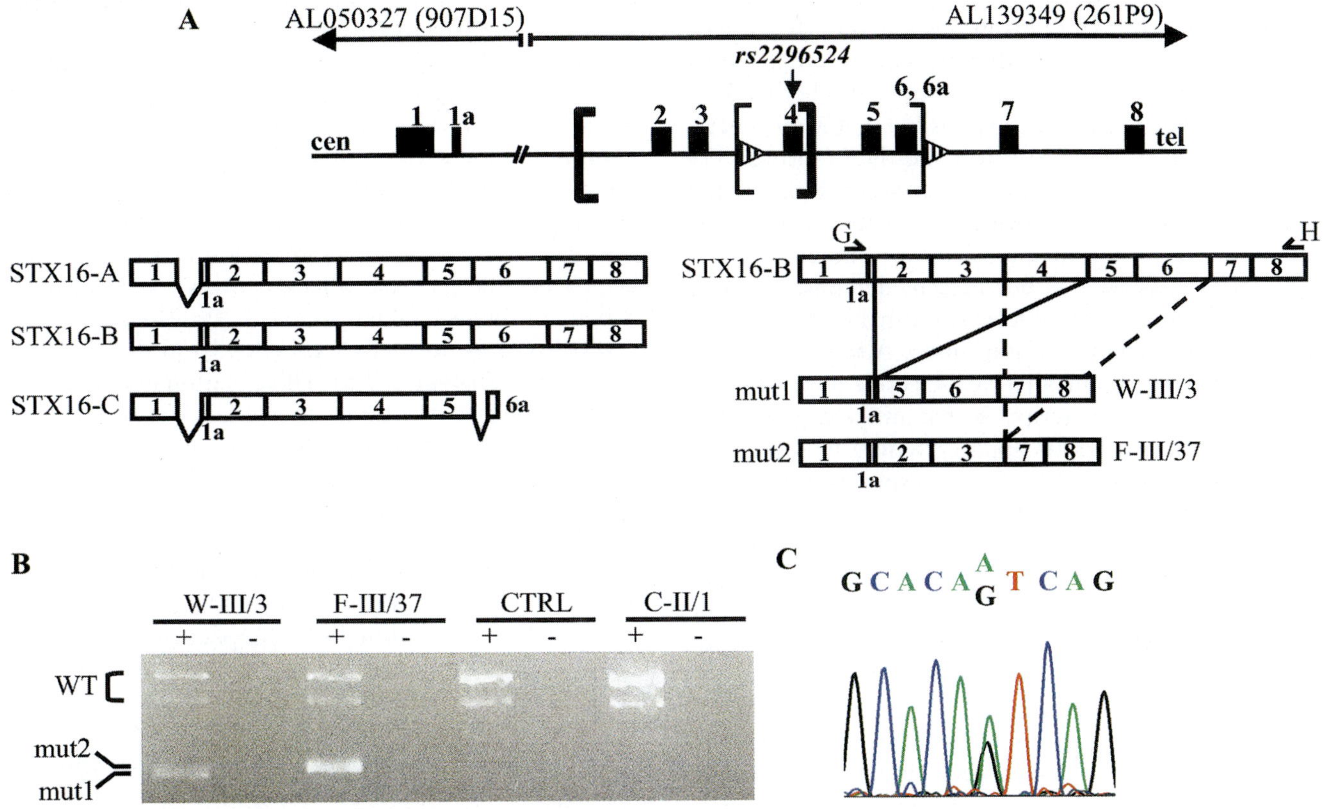

Figure 5 Biallelic expression of *STX16*. *A*, *STX16* gives rise to at least three distinct transcripts (*left*). Isoform A (915 bp) differs from isoform B (965 bp) by a shorter sequence derived from exon 1, whereas isoform C (422 bp) comprises this short exon 1 sequence as well as exons 2–5 and terminates with exon 6a. In addition, exon 4 is alternatively spliced in each isoform, leading to a total of at least six variants. Wild-type STX16 isoform B and the transcripts derived from individuals W-III/3 and F-III/37 ("mut1" and "mut2," respectively) are depicted (*right*). The 4.4-kb deletion (*thick brackets*) removes exons 2–4; the 3-kb deletion (*thin brackets*) removes exons 4–6. Exons are depicted as blackened boxes, and direct repeats are shown as striped arrowheads. Primers G and H are represented as arrowed lines; cen = centromeric; tel = telomeric. *B*, RT-PCR analysis of STX16 transcripts in total RNA of immortalized lymphocytes from a healthy control individual (CTRL) and the following individuals with AD-PHP-Ib: W-III/3 (present study), F-III/37 (carrying the 3-kb deletion in *STX16* region [Bastepe et al. 2003]), and C-II/1 (carrying a deletion affecting NESP55 but not the *STX16* region [Bastepe et al. 2005]). Reactions were performed with ("+") or without ("−") reverse transcriptase, as described in the "Subjects and Methods" section. Products derived from the mutant alleles ("mut1" and "mut2") and from the wild-type alleles ("WT") are indicated. Note that the wild-type products represent STX16 isoform B with or without sequences derived from exon 4. *C*, Direct nucleotide sequence of STX16 isoform B amplified from RNA of a healthy control individual shows heterozygosity at the polymorphic nucleotide 527, corresponding to SNP *rs2296524*.

in 5 of 20 unrelated individuals with PHP-Ib (Liu et al. 2005). Thus, mutations in this region are frequently the cause of PHP-Ib. Affected individuals who carry the 3-kb and 4.4-kb microdeletions exhibit loss of methylation only at *GNAS* exon A/B; the methylation pattern is not altered at other *GNAS* DMRs. Conversely, individuals with PHP-Ib who lack such *STX16* deletions display methylation abnormalities at all *GNAS* DMRs (Bastepe et al. 2003; Liu et al. 2005). On the basis of these findings, we conclude that PHP-Ib comprises at least two distinct conditions sharing the same clinical phenotype: one is associated with the loss of exon A/B methylation alone—and, in most of the cases, with a heterozygous microdeletion in the *STX16* region—and the other is associated with methylation abnormalities at all *GNAS* DMRs, including the DMR at exon A/B. In two unrelated kindreds with AD-PHP-Ib with broad methylation defects of *GNAS*, we have recently identified deletions affecting the NESP55 DMR (Bastepe et al. 2005), and it remains to be determined whether the sporadic cases with this epigenotype also carry an as-yet-undefined microdeletion within or close to this region.

Deletion of *STX16* exons 2–4, caused by the mutation presented in the present study, results in a frameshift and a premature termination codon following 20 new amino acids, whereas deletion of *STX16* exons 4–6, caused by the previously described 3-kb microdeletion (Bastepe et al. 2003), maintains the ORF. Thus, the syntaxin-16 proteins generated by the 4.4-kb or 3-kb deleted alleles either are shortened by 276 amino acids at the carboxyl-terminus or have a deletion of 133 amino acids in the midportion, respectively. Because of these severe alterations, both products are predicted to be nonfunctional, raising the question of whether syntaxin-16 deficiency may be responsible for the epigenetic abnormality at *GNAS* exon A/B and the resulting PTH resistance. However, this possibility seems unlikely for two reasons. First, the previously reported lack of differential methylation at the *STX16* promoter (Bastepe et al. 2003)—as well as our present demonstration of biallelic expression of STX16 isoform B—strongly argues that this gene is not imprinted. Although not entirely ruled out by our analysis, selective imprinting of the other STX16 transcripts seems unlikely, given that all the known transcripts apparently use the same promoter. This lack of parental origin–specific STX16 expression is inconsistent with the imprinted mode of inheritance in kindreds with AD-PHP-Ib. Second, PTH resistance can develop despite the presence of two intact copies of *STX16*, as shown in a case of paternal uniparental isodisomy of chromosome 20q (Bastepe et al. 2001*a*). On the other hand, maternal inheritance of *STX16* mutations is associated with loss of methylation at maternal *GNAS* exon A/B, and it is therefore more likely that these deletions disrupt a *cis*-acting imprinting control element (ICE) necessary for the methylation imprint at exon A/B.

The novel 4.4-kb microdeletion overlaps with the former 3-kb deletion and therefore reduces the size of the critical region containing the putative ICE for *GNAS* exon A/B to 1,286 bp. This region encompasses the centromeric direct repeat, and the flanking telomeric sequence of 896 bp, which includes exon 4 of *STX16* and intronic sequences of 244 bp and 344 bp on the centromeric and telomeric side, respectively. We could not identify, within the 1,286-bp overlapping region, sequences or elements homologous to those previously identified in other ICEs. For example, microdeletions at the ICE of the *IGF2/H19* locus abolish two CTCF binding sites required for the *H19* DMR and thus result in the Beckwith-Wiedemann syndrome (Sparago et al. 2004). Sequence analysis of the overlapping region encompassing exon 4 of *STX16* did not reveal such known CTCF sites. Another feature of ICEs is that they are mostly located within CpG-rich sequences; in addition, they display differential methylation (Spahn and Barlow 2003). Although the overlapping region includes a 140-bp CpG-rich sequence within exon 4 (nucleotides 4572–4711 of AL139349), we have shown elsewhere that this region is not differentially methylated (Bastepe et al. 2003). It is therefore possible that the mechanisms governing the function of the identified ICE are different from those of most other ICEs in the genome (Spahn and Barlow 2003). Further investigations are necessary to identify the specific features required for the proper activity of the putative ICE.

Two candidate ICEs have been previously identified in the mouse *Gnas* cluster: one comprising exon 1A (homolog of human A/B) and the other comprising the *Gnasxl* (homolog of human XLα_s) and *Nespas* promoters (Liu et al. 2000*b*; Coombes et al. 2003). Mice with a paternal ablation of exon 1A exhibit loss of Gα_s silencing in *cis*, leading to expression of the Gα_s transcript from the paternal allele in brown fat and renal proximal tubules (Williamson et al. 2004)—two tissues in which Gα_s is normally expressed from the maternal allele alone (Yu et al. 1998). This ablation does not alter the imprinting of the other alternative transcripts, and it therefore appears that a *cis*-acting element at exon 1A specifically regulates Gα_s expression in brown fat, kidney, and perhaps other tissues. Findings in patients with PHP-Ib indicate that this element allows active transcription from the Gα_s promoter in the kidney only when it is methylated (Liu et al. 2000*a*; Bastepe et al. 2001*b*). However, although the impact of this element is confined to certain tissues, its methylation on the maternal *GNAS* allele appears to be ubiquitous (Liu et al. 2000*b*). Our findings in patients with AD-PHP-Ib provide evidence of another *cis*-acting element within the overlapping region encompassing *STX16* exon 4. The latter appears to specifically control the methylation of *GNAS* exon A/B and, thus, of the *cis*-acting element regulating the tissue- and parent-specific expression of Gα_s. Deletion of this putative *STX16* ICE results in a switch from a maternal to a paternal epigenotype at exon A/B, thereby causing derepression of maternal A/B transcription. Because the epigenetic changes associated with the deletion of this putative element have been identified in lymphocytes, its impact seems ubiquitous rather than restricted to kidney and brown fat. In addition to this putative ICE that controls methylation on a restricted area of *GNAS* (i.e., exon A/B), the identification of deletions of the NESP55 DMR in two unrelated families with AD-PHP-Ib has recently provided evidence of an additional ICE that is involved in methylation of the entire *GNAS* cluster (Bastepe et al. 2005). Thus, in humans, maternal methylation at *GNAS* exon A/B (and, hence, Gα_s transcription) requires at least two ICEs: one at the *STX16* locus, which affects exon A/B, and the other at the NESP55 DMR, which affects all the maternally methylated promoters within the *GNAS* cluster.

Genetic analysis of cord blood (i.e., exon A/B methylation analysis and multiplex PCR) was particularly useful, allowing us to rule out the diagnosis of AD-PHP-Ib in one newborn and to establish the diagnosis in another. The child with the genetic diagnosis of AD-PHP-Ib was subsequently monitored with respect to development of PTH resistance, and treatment eventually was started to prevent hypocalcemia and to avoid long-term elevation of serum PTH; the latter can lead to increased bone resorption, resulting from the apparent absence of PTH resistance in this tissue. The observed delay in the onset of PTH resistance in this patient is consistent with past studies of individuals affected with PHP-Ib (Marguet et al. 1997; Bastepe et al. 2001*b*) and was also noted in patients with loss-of-function mutations of Gα_s (i.e., PHP-Ia) (Weinstein et al. 2001). PTH signaling through the PTH/PTHrP receptor, therefore, seems intact in the renal proximal tubule during the early postnatal period and infancy. One could hypothesize that Gα_s is biallelically expressed in this tissue during this specific period of development. Consistent with this hypothesis, biallelic expression of Gα_s has been shown by RT-PCR in whole kidneys and renal cortices from mouse and human fetuses (Hayward et al. 1998*a*; Zheng et al. 2001). However, these findings—which contradict those showing the exclusive maternal expression of Gα_s in renal cortices of adult mice (Yu et al. 1998)—do not rule out the possibility that Gα_s expression is monoallelic in renal proximal tubules of fetal or newborn kidney, especially considering that proximal tubules constitute a small portion of the entire kidney. Thus, there may be alternative possibilities to explain the delay in the onset of PTH resistance. One of those possible explanations may involve XLα_s, the paternally expressed variant of Gα_s. XLα_s is expressed in multiple fetal and adult tissues (Kehlenbach et al. 1994; Pasolli et al. 2000), including murine kidney at postnatal day 4 (Plagge et al. 2004). Furthermore, on the basis of data from transfected cells lacking endogenous Gα_s and XLα_s, XLα_s is capable of functionally coupling to the PTH/PTHrP receptor (Bastepe et al. 2002). It is thus possible that PTH actions during early postnatal period are mediated through XLα_s.

In conclusion, in the present study, we have (1) identified a novel deletion in the *STX16* locus as a cause of AD-PHP-Ib and therefore established a strong association between a unique epigenotype (i.e., loss of A/B methylation alone) and a genotype (i.e., microdeletion involving *STX16*), (2) refined the boundaries of a putative *cis*-acting ICE crucial for the establishment/maintenance of methylation at *GNAS* exon A/B, (3) demonstrated biallelic expression of STX16 mRNAs in lymphoblastoid cells, and (4) established a molecular diagnosis that was based on cord blood DNA in a patient, which helped in the subsequent clinical management of that patient.

Acknowledgments

This work was supported by grants from National Institutes of Health National Institute of Diabetes and Digestive and Kidney Diseases (RO1 46718-10 [to H.J.] and KO1 DK-062973-01 [to M.B.]) and by a Research Fellowship Grant from the European Society for Paediatric Endocrinology (to A.L.).

Electronic-Database Information

The URL for data presented herein is as follows:

Online Mendelian Inheritance in Man (OMIM), http://www.ncbi.nlm.nih.gov/Omim/

References

Bastepe M, Fröhlich LF, Hendy GN, Indridason OS, Josse RG, Koshiyama H, Korkko J, Nakamoto JM, Rosenbloom AL, Slyper AH, Sugimoto T, Tsatsoulis A, Crawford JD, Jüppner H (2003) Autosomal dominant pseudohypoparathyroidism type Ib is associated with a heterozygous microdeletion that likely disrupts a putative imprinting control element of *GNAS*. J Clin Invest 112:1255–1263

Bastepe M, Fröhlich LF, Linglart A, Abu-Zahra HS, Tojo K, Ward LM, Jüppner H (2005) Deletion of the NESP55 differentially methylated region causes loss of maternal *GNAS* imprints and pseudohypoparathyroidism type Ib. Nat Genet 37:25–27

Bastepe M, Gunes Y, Perez-Villamil B, Hunzelman J, Weinstein LS, Jüppner H (2002) Receptor-mediated adenylyl cyclase activation through XLαs, the extra-large variant of the stimulatory G protein α-subunit. Mol Endocrinol 16:1912–1919

Bastepe M, Lane AH, Jüppner H (2001*a*) Paternal uniparental isodisomy of chromosome 20q—and the resulting changes in *GNAS1* methylation—as a plausible cause of pseudohypoparathyroidism. Am J Hum Genet 68:1283–1289

Bastepe M, Pincus JE, Sugimoto T, Tojo K, Kanatani M, Azuma Y, Kruse K, Rosenbloom AL, Koshiyama H, Jüppner H (2001*b*) Positional dissociation between the genetic mutation responsible for pseudohypoparathyroidism type Ib and the associated methylation defect at exon A/B: evidence for a long-range regulatory element within the imprinted *GNAS1* locus. Hum Mol Genet 10:1231–1241

Campbell R, Gosden CM, Bonthron DT (1994) Parental origin of transcription from the human *GNAS1* gene. J Med Genet 31:607–614

Coombes C, Arnaud P, Gordon E, Dean W, Coar EA, Williamson CM, Feil R, Peters J, Kelsey G (2003) Epigenetic properties and identification of an imprint mark in the Nesp-Gnasxl domain of the mouse *Gnas* imprinted locus. Mol Cell Biol 23:5475–5488

Hayward B, Barlier A, Korbonits M, Grossman A, Jacquet P, Enjalbert A, Bonthron D (2001) Imprinting of the $G_s\alpha$ gene *GNAS1* in the pathogenesis of acromegaly. J Clin Invest 107: R31–R36

Hayward B, Bonthron D (2000) An imprinted antisense transcript at the human *GNAS1* locus. Hum Mol Genet 9:835–841

Hayward B, Kamiya M, Strain L, Moran V, Campbell R, Hayashizaki Y, Bonthron DT (1998*a*) The human *GNAS1* gene is imprinted and encodes distinct paternally and biallelically expressed G proteins. Proc Natl Acad Sci USA 95:10038–10043

Hayward BE, Moran V, Strain L, Bonthron DT (1998*b*) Bidirectional imprinting of a single gene: *GNAS1* encodes maternally, paternally, and biallelically derived proteins. Proc Natl Acad Sci USA 95:15475–15480

Ischia R, Lovisetti-Scamihorn P, Hogue-Angeletti R, Wolkersdorfer M, Winkler H, Fischer-Colbrie R (1997) Molecular cloning and characterization of NESP55, a novel chromogranin-like precursor of a peptide with 5-HT1B receptor antagonist activity. J Biol Chem 272:11657–11662

Ishikawa Y, Bianchi C, Nadal-Ginard B, Homcy CJ (1990) Alternative promoter and 5′ exon generate a novel $G_s\alpha$ mRNA. J Biol Chem 265:8458–8462

Jüppner H, Schipani E, Bastepe M, Cole DEC, Lawson ML, Mannstadt M, Hendy GN, Plotkin H, Koshiyama H, Koh T, Crawford JD, Olsen BR, Vikkula M (1998) The gene responsible for pseudohypoparathyroidism type Ib is paternally imprinted and maps in four unrelated kindreds to chromosome 20q13.3. Proc Natl Acad Sci USA 95:11798–11803

Kehlenbach RH, Matthey J, Huttner WB (1994) XLαs is a new type of G protein. Nature 372:804–809 (erratum 375: 253)

Levine MA (2002) Pseudohypoparathyroidism. In: Bilezikian JP, Raisz LG, Rodan GA (eds) Principles of bone biology. Vol 2. Academic Press, New York, pp 1137–1163

Li T, Vu TH, Zeng ZL, Nguyen BT, Hayward BE, Bonthron DT, Hu JF, Hoffman AR (2000) Tissue-specific expression of antisense and sense transcripts at the imprinted *Gnas* locus. Genomics 69:295–304

Liu J, Erlichman B, Weinstein LS (2003) The stimulatory G protein α-subunit Gsα is imprinted in human thyroid glands: implications for thyroid function in pseudohypoparathyroidism types Ia and Ib. J Clin Endocrinol Metab 88:4336–4341

Liu J, Litman D, Rosenberg M, Yu S, Biesecker L, Weinstein L (2000*a*) A *GNAS1* imprinting defect in pseudohypoparathyroidism type Ib. J Clin Invest 106:1167–1174

Liu J, Nealon JG, Weinstein LS (2005) Distinct patterns of abnormal *GNAS* imprinting in familial and sporadic pseudohypoparathyroidism type Ib. Hum Mol Genet 14:95–102

Liu J, Yu S, Litman D, Chen W, Weinstein L (2000*b*) Identification of a methylation imprint mark within the mouse *gnas* locus. Mol Cell Biol 20:5808–5817

Mahmud FH, Linglart A, Bastepe M, Jüppner H, Lteif AN (2005) Molecular diagnosis of pseudohypoparathyroidism type Ib in a family with presumed paroxysmal dyskinesia. Pediatrics 115:e242–e244

Mantovani G, Ballare E, Giammona E, Beck-Peccoz P, Spada A (2002) The Gsα gene: predominant maternal origin of transcription in human thyroid gland and gonads. J Clin Endocrinol Metab 87:4736–4740

Marguet C, Mallet E, Basuyau JP, Martin D, Leroy M, Brunelle P (1997) Clinical and biological heterogeneity in pseudohypoparathyroidism syndrome: results of a multicenter study. Horm Res 48:120–130

Pasolli H, Klemke M, Kehlenbach R, Wang Y, Huttner W (2000) Characterization of the extra-large G protein α-subunit XLαs. I. Tissue distribution and subcellular localization. J Biol Chem 275:33622–33632

Peters J, Wroe SF, Wells CA, Miller HJ, Bodle D, Beechey CV, Williamson CM, Kelsey G (1999) A cluster of oppositely imprinted transcripts at the *Gnas* locus in the distal imprinting region of mouse chromosome 2. Proc Natl Acad Sci USA 96: 3830–3835

Plagge A, Gordon E, Dean W, Boiani R, Cinti S, Peters J, Kelsey G (2004) The imprinted signaling protein XLαs is required for postnatal adaptation to feeding. Nat Genet 36:818–826

Spahn L, Barlow DP (2003) An ICE pattern crystallizes. Nat Genet 35:11–12

Sparago A, Cerrato F, Vernucci M, Ferrero GB, Silengo MC, Riccio A (2004) Microdeletions in the human H19 DMR result in loss of *IGF2* imprinting and Beckwith-Wiedemann syndrome. Nat Genet 36:958–960

Swaroop A, Agarwal N, Gruen JR, Bick D, Weissman SM (1991) Differential expression of novel Gsα signal transduction protein cDNA species. Nucleic Acids Res 19:4725–4729

Weinstein LS, Yu S, Warner DR, Liu J (2001) Endocrine manifestations of stimulatory G protein α-subunit mutations and the role of genomic imprinting. Endocr Rev 22:675–705

Williamson CM, Ball ST, Nottingham WT, Skinner JA, Plagge A, Turner MD, Powles N, Hough T, Papworth D, Fraser WD, Maconochie M, Peters J (2004) A cis-acting control region is required exclusively for the tissue-specific imprinting of *Gnas*. Nat Genet 36:894–899

Wroe SF, Kelsey G, Skinner JA, Bodle D, Ball ST, Beechey CV, Peters J, Williamson CM (2000) An imprinted transcript, antisense to Nesp, adds complexity to the cluster of imprinted genes at the mouse *Gnas* locus. Proc Natl Acad Sci USA 97: 3342–3346

Yu S, Yu D, Lee E, Eckhaus M, Lee R, Corria Z, Accili D, Westphal H, Weinstein LS (1998) Variable and tissue-specific hormone resistance in heterotrimeric G_s protein α-subunit ($G_s\alpha$) knockout mice is due to tissue-specific imprinting of the $G_s\alpha$ gene. Proc Natl Acad Sci USA 95:8715–8720

Zheng H, Radeva G, McCann JA, Hendy GN, Goodyer CG (2001) Gαs transcripts are biallelically expressed in the human kidney cortex: implications for pseudohypoparathyroidism type Ib. J Clin Endocrinol Metab 86:4627–4629

Am. J. Hum. Genet. 76:815–832, 2005

Quantitative Founder-Effect Analysis of French Canadian Families Identifies Specific Loci Contributing to Metabolic Phenotypes of Hypertension

P. Hamet,[1] E. Merlo,[2] O. Šeda,[1] U. Broeckel,[4] J. Tremblay,[1] M. Kaldunski,[4] D. Gaudet,[5] G. Bouchard,[6] B. Deslauriers,[1] F. Gagnon,[7] G. Antoniol,[8] Z. Pausová,[1] M. Labuda,[1] M. Jomphe,[6] F. Gossard,[1] G. Tremblay,[5] R. Kirova,[4] P. Tonellato,[4] S. N. Orlov,[1] J. Pintos,[1] J. Platko,[9] T. J. Hudson,[3] J. D. Rioux,[9] T. A. Kotchen,[4] and A. W. Cowley Jr.[4]

[1]Centre hospitalier de l'Université de Montréal, [2]École Polytechnique de Montréal, and [3]McGill University and Genome Quebec Innovation Centre, Montreal; [4]Medical College of Wisconsin, Milwaukee; [5]Complexe Hospitalier de la Sagamie and [6]Université du Québec à Chicoutimi, Chicoutimi, Quebec; [7]University of Ottawa, Ottawa, Ontario; [8]University of Sannio, Benevento, Italy; and [9]The Broad Institute, Cambridge, MA

The Saguenay–Lac St-Jean population of Quebec is relatively isolated and has genealogical records dating to the 17th-century French founders. In 120 extended families with at least one sib pair affected with early-onset hypertension and/or dyslipidemia, we analyzed the genetic determinants of hypertension and related cardiovascular and metabolic conditions. Variance-components linkage analysis revealed 46 loci after 100,000 permutations. The most prominent clusters of overlapping quantitative-trait loci were on chromosomes 1 and 3, a finding supported by principal-components and bivariate analyses. These genetic determinants were further tested by classifying families by use of LOD score density analysis for each measured phenotype at every 5 cM. Our study showed the founder effect over several generations and classes of living individuals. This quantitative genealogical approach supports the notion of the ancestral causality of traits uniquely present and inherited in distinct family classes. With the founder effect, traits determined within population subsets are measurably and quantitatively transmitted through generational lineage, with a precise component contributing to phenotypic variance. These methods should accelerate the uncovering of causal haplotypes in complex diseases such as hypertension and metabolic syndrome.

Introduction

Hypertension, present in 10%–35% of humans, is one of the principal risk factors for cardiovascular disease in the United States, Canada, and other industrialized nations (Franklin et al. 2001; Joffres et al. 2001). Together with obesity and dyslipidemia, it represents a significant proportion of the global and regional burden of diseases (Ezzati et al. 2002). These three entities are frequently present together and are cardinal features of the metabolic syndrome (Reaven 2004). The absence of such phenotypes is associated with longevity in the offspring of centenarians (Atzmon et al. 2004). With the impending pandemic of obesity, the increasing prevalence of these conditions will contribute to the worldwide prominence of cardiovascular mortality by 2020 (Groop and Orho-Melander 2001). The etiologies of these entities are usually multifactorial and the result of polygenic interactions with the environment (Hamet et al. 1998; Pausova et al. 1999). Although effective treatments are available for hypertension and dyslipidemia (Turnbull and Blood Pressure Lowering Treatment Trialists' Collaboration 2003), they do not address the potential causal concomitance of presentation that may, by itself, provide novel therapeutic and preventive targets.

Since tools for the resolution of polygenic diseases are now available (Lander and Schork 1994; Doris 2002), several studies have reported genomewide scans for hypertension (Caulfield et al. 2003; Jacobs et al. 2003; James et al. 2003; Ranade et al. 2003; von Wowern et al. 2003), obesity, and dyslipidemia (Loos et al. 2003; Stein et al. 2003; Tang et al. 2003; Langefeld et al. 2004; Ueno et al. 2004), adding to a much earlier and more complete resolution of the monogenic forms of hypertension (Lifton et al. 2001). However, the results have usually been limited to a few QTLs with marginally significant LOD scores and a modest contribution to overall trait variance (Samani 2003)—even the results from a recent meta-analysis of 6,245 relatives from four multicenter networks of the Family Blood Pressure Program (Province et al. 2003). The most common limiting factors include genetic and environmental heterogeneity, which lead to decreased statistical power (Glazier et al. 2002). The present study proposes an integrative ap-

Received October 5, 2004; accepted for publication March 4, 2005; electronically published March 30, 2005.

Address for correspondence and reprints: Dr. Pavel Hamet, Laboratory of Molecular Medicine, Centre de recherche, CHUM–Hôtel-Dieu, 3850 Saint Urbain Street, Montréal, Québec H2W 1T7, Canada. E-mail: pavel.hamet@umontreal.ca

0002-9297/2005/7605-0010$15.00

proach to the resolution of complex traits. We chose hypertension and dyslipidemia as the ascertainment criteria. Furthermore, we conducted our studies on French Canadians who represent a homogeneous population who had large families until the 1940s and who, more importantly, have computerized genealogical records dating to the original 17th-century settlers (Bouchard et al. 1989; Heyer and Tremblay 1995). With a method similar to our physiological genomics strategy that was applied to a human cohort of African Americans (Kotchen et al. 2002) and to rodent models (Stoll et al. 2001), we have used an integrated multisystem phenotyping protocol to ascertain the characteristics of cardiovascular, renal, metabolic, and anthropometric features, under stringent standard operating procedures.

We report that QTLs for several components of the metabolic syndrome are clustering within the same genomic regions. By extending sequential oligogenic linkage analysis routine (SOLAR)–corrected LOD (LOD_{cor}) scores through density analysis, we were able to define sets of families with distinct contributions to several traits. A novel layered-founder approach strongly underlined the finding of ancestral causality by the demonstration of founder separability. These observations permit us to propose a "quantitative founder effect" in complex diseases.

Methods and Procedures

Family Cohort

Families were recruited from a relatively genetically differentiated population in the Saguenay–Lac St-Jean (SLSJ) area of the Canadian province of Quebec. Families were ascertained by the presence of at least one sib pair with hypertension and dyslipidemia. Sibship sizes ranged from 2 to 11 persons (mean 3.9; median 3). The affected sib pair–inclusion criteria were essential hypertension (systolic blood pressure [SBP] >140 mmHg and/or diastolic blood pressure [DBP] >90 mmHg on two occasions or the use of antihypertensive medication), dyslipidemia (plasma cholesterol ⩾5.2 mmol/liter and/or HDL cholesterol ⩽0.9 mmol/liter or the use of lipid-lowering medication), BMI <35 kg/m^2, age 18–55 years, and Catholic French Canadian origin. Exclusion criteria included secondary hypertension, DBP >110 mmHg and the use of medication, diabetes mellitus, renal or liver dysfunction, malignancy, pregnancy, and substance abuse. Once the affected sib pairs were selected, all first- and second-degree relatives aged >18 years were invited to participate in the study, independent of health status. The recruited population included 120 families (mean size 7.3 persons; median size 5 persons), comprising 897 subjects and 1,617 sib pairs (259 concordant-affected, 556 discordant, and 802 nonaffected sib pairs).

Family structure was tested for consistency by calculating the probabilities of relatedness on the basis of the genotype data (M. J. Daly, personal communication). Because of the results of paternity analysis, two subjects were removed prior to linkage analysis. The SOLAR software package (version 1.7.3) was used to calculate multipoint identity by descent (MIBD) for all subjects. Errors detected by SOLAR were resolved by a review of the genotypes of subjects and/or pedigrees, after which 14 genotypes from 10 subjects were removed because of genotype data inconsistency (mostly due to mistyping). Pedigree and subject genotype reviews continued in an iterative process until MIBDs were calculated with no error messages.

The study was approved by the ethics committees at Complexe Hospitalier de la Sagamie (Chicoutimi, Quebec), Université du Québec à Chicoutimi, and the Centre hospitalier de l'Université de Montréal.

Phenotyping

All phenotyping was performed by trained personnel who followed standard operating procedures (Kotchen et al. 2000, 2002; Pausova et al. 2000, 2002). Restricted phenotyping on day 0 included taking blood samples for DNA extraction and measuring plasma lipid, fasting glucose, uric acid, sitting blood pressure (BP), and bioimpedance (RJL System) to determine water distribution and body fat mass. Anthropometric data included 3 global measures of obesity—BMI and percentage body fat (%body fat) derived from skinfolds and from bioimpedance—and 11 regional measures: 6 trunk and extremity circumferences and 5 skinfolds. Subjects without any contraindications were invited for extensive phenotyping and had their antihypertensive drugs withdrawn for 1 wk and lipid-lowering agents withdrawn for 1 mo. From 499 hypertensive subjects studied, 388 were receiving medication, which was stopped for the purposes of full phenotyping in 135 hypertensive subjects. Full phenotyping was performed for a total of 294 normotensive and hypertensive individuals.

On day 1 of extensive phenotyping, an intravenous catheter was inserted. Fasting samples were taken for the measurement of lipid, glucose, and insulin concentrations. A postural test was conducted for 60 min in the supine position followed by 10 min standing and 20 min sitting, while cardiac functions (by impedance plethysmography [SORBA Medical System]) and BP (Dynamap, Johnson and Johnson Medical) were monitored. Both impedance and BP were then measured after mental stress of mathematical tests (McAdoo et al. 1990). Insulin sensitivity was tested with Bergman's minimal model, and insulin sensitivity and glucose effectiveness were quantified as described elsewhere (Steil et al. 1993). At the end of day 1, 24-h BP monitoring was initiated.

On day 2, BP, renal blood flow by p-aminohippuric acid clearance, and glomerular filtration rate by inulin clearance were measured at baseline and after stepwise norepinephrine infusion of 0.01–0.05 μg/kg/min (Kotchen et al. 2000). Patients received a water load of 15 ml/kg plus normal saline intravenously over a 6-h period. Plasma arginine-vasopressin, atrial natriuretic factor, cyclic nucleotide (cGMP and cAMP) concentrations, and renin activity were quantified at baseline and after fluid challenge. Cardiac echographic measurements were taken on a different day.

Among all phenotypes, those that were measured and analyzed included 3 anthropometric, 3 plasma, 37 BP, 12 time-series BP, 14 cardiac (cardiac output and index), 46 impedance plethysmography, 6 echocardiography, 19 heart rate, 32 neuroendocrine, 22 renal, and 28 plethysmography-related measures. Each phenotype was tested for normality of distribution by kurtosis and skewness and by the Kolmogorov-Smirnov test. When kurtosis was >2, values were normalized by simple function transformation (i.e., transformed by log, square root, or power) (Blangero et al. 2001) and were further analyzed to decrease the likelihood of false-positive errors (e.g., by variance-components, covariance, principal-components, and bivariate analyses). Power transformation was the first choice for any phenotype containing negative numbers (e.g., delta-calculated values). All three transformations were tested, and we used the one that achieved normality without excessive loss of data points. As in the analyses by Allison et al. (1999), we accepted, on rare occasions, slight deviations from normality if it could be assumed that they would not affect the LOD score substantially. Most importantly, however, we ran 100,000 simulations to correct for such deviations from normality and to test the robustness of our results. This method is considered to be one of the best ways to deal with normality issues. When more than two groups were compared, one- or two-way analysis of variance was applied post hoc using the Tukey honest significance difference test for specific pairs of variables. The null hypothesis was rejected whenever *P* was <.05. Phenotype analysis screened for general covariates, including sex, age, and BMI, with stepwise removal of each covariate to test its significance.

Genotyping

DNA samples from the first 500 recruited subjects originating from 97 families were genotyped at the Broad Institute (formerly the Whitehead Institute for Biomedical Research/MIT Center for Genome Research), by use of 377 microsatellite markers, with a modified version of the Cooperative Human Linkage Center Screening Set (version 6.0) that included Genethon markers for an average of 9.1-cM coverage of the entire human genome. Details of the genotyping system can be found elsewhere (Rioux et al. 1998). Additional markers (Genethon) at a 5-cM density were used on chromosome (chr) 1q and chr 3q in a total of 810 subjects. Post hoc analysis determined a genotyping error rate of ~0.016%.

Components of Total Variance

We estimated the individual contribution of QTLs to the trait variance. Other modeled effects included residual effects (including environmental effects) and the effects of the covariates age and sex. For these analyses, we used extended families (i.e., those not split into sib pairs). We performed oligogenic segregation analyses based on reversible-jump Bayesian Markov Chain–Monte Carlo (MCMC) methods and implemented in the computer program Loki, version 2.4.5 (available at the Pangaea Web site), as described elsewhere (Heath 1997; Daw et al. 1999; Gagnon et al. 2003).

These MCMC methods estimate model parameters, including the number of QTLs and their contribution to the trait variance, given the assigned prior distributions for each parameter in the model and the current states of all other model parameters. We applied Poisson prior distribution with a mean of 1 for the number of QTLs. We investigated several values for the prior variance of genotype effects. The choice of the best value for the genotype effects was based on the guidelines proposed by Wijsman (2002). For these analyses, posterior parameter estimates were based on average values of 501,000 iterations of this process, with every second iteration saved for computation. The first 1,000 iterations were discarded to allow for initial burn-in of the MCMC process. Several runs were performed, and the results from one representative run for each trait are presented in this article. Since the Bayesian MCMC methods were not based on a hypothesis-testing framework, *P* values could not be estimated.

Permutation Analysis

To test for LOD robustness, a simulation method for permutation analysis was implemented with SOLAR (Blangero et al. 2001). LOD adjustment was computed with the LOD_{adj} command, which runs a simulation of the distribution of LOD scores that can be expected under the null hypothesis of no linkage. We ran 100,000 trials, and, in each trial, a fully informative marker, completely unlinked to the trait, was simulated and the trait linkage was tested. Under the assumption of multivariate normality, the theoretical null distribution is well known. The LOD_{adj} command regresses the observed LOD scores on the LOD scores expected for a multivariate normal trait. The inverse of the slope of the

The figure is available in its entirety in the online edition of *The American Journal of Human Genetics.*

Figure 1 Example of a LOD score density plot. Three regions can be observed in the density function. The figure legend is available in its entirety in the online edition of *The American Journal of Human Genetics.*

regression line is the LOD adjustment. Adjusted LOD scores are reported here.

Principal-Components and Bivariate Analyses

Principal-components analysis (PCA) is a multivariate statistical method that allows the formulation of quantitatively informative linear combinations of correlated phenotypes by maximizing phenotypic or familial variance—and thus reducing the number of tests performed—by exploring only the proper linear combinations in further variance-components analyses. It is extremely effective for correlated phenotypes regulated by a common locus, and it increases the power significantly. Hence, PCA is applied to maximize the total variance. Eigen pairs of the covariance matrix accounting for 95% of the variance formed the principal components.

Both bivariate analysis and PCA can increase the power of analysis in a case of phenotypes with small or negatively correlated environmental factors and with strong genetic correlation. Although bivariate analysis explicitly models the cross correlation matrix, it also adds more parameters into the model and makes the computations extensive. On the other hand, PCA reduces the number of tests by providing linear combinations of maximum variance for further analysis. Hence, both methods can make valuable contributions.

LOD Score Density Analysis

Density functions are the integral or discrete sum of other function values over a ranked set of function arguments. A discrete example of density δ over function f is

$$f: N \rightarrow R$$

$$\delta: N \rightarrow R$$

$$\delta(x) = \sum_{v \leqslant x} f(v) \ ,$$

where x and v are the integer arguments of functions δ and f, N is the set of integer numbers, and R is the set of real numbers.

LOD score density can be computed on the basis of the LOD score contribution ($\mathrm{LOD_C}$) of individual pedigrees, which are families in this case, as follows:

$$\delta(\mathrm{FAM}_i) = \sum_{\mathrm{FAM}_j/\mathrm{FAM}_j \preccurlyeq \mathrm{FAM}_i} \mathrm{LOD_C}(\mathrm{FAM}_j) \ ,$$

where

$$(\mathrm{FAM}_j \preccurlyeq \mathrm{FAM}_i) \Leftrightarrow$$

$$[\mathrm{LOD_C}(\mathrm{FAM}_j) > \mathrm{LOD_C}(\mathrm{FAM}_i)] \vee$$

$$([\mathrm{LOD_C}(\mathrm{FAM}_j) = \mathrm{LOD_C}(\mathrm{FAM}_i)] \wedge [j \leqslant i])$$

and where $\vee$ is the logic "OR" operator, $\wedge$ is the logic "AND" operator, and i and j are family identifiers.

In other words, LOD score density δ is computed for families ranked by decreasing values of LOD score contribution, $\mathrm{LOD_C}$, as supplied by SOLAR from FAM_i through FAM_j. In the case of equal LOD contribution, the identifiers of families are arbitrarily considered for the purposes of ordering. In this context, density can also be interpreted as an incremental LOD score computation, in which families are incrementally added to the population in decreasing order of LOD score contribution.

An example of a LOD score density plot is reported in figure 1. LOD density represents the LOD score values that would be obtained if the population were restricted to families for which the density is computed. In figure 1, we can observe three regions in the density function: an initial region in which the LOD score increases as families are added to the population, a somehow stable region in which adding families does not significantly change the LOD value, and a final region in which adding families decreases the LOD score. We name the families belonging to these three regions "contributing" families (CF), "noncontributing" families (NCF), and "anticontributing" families (ACF), respectively. The families belonging to these regions can be used to assess whether they can be statistically distinguished by certain phenotypes and markers.

Quantitative Founder Effect

A population is considered subject to a founder effect when a few ancestors from a set F of founders account for most of the genetic contribution to a set S of descendants. In this context, founders can be ranked on the basis of their nonuniform genetic contribution, from the highest to the lowest contributions.

An example of the genetic contribution of founders appears in figure 2*A*, whereas figure 2*B* reveals the constant genetic contribution for the contrasting hypothesis of a uniform contribution of founders. The density δ of genetic contributions is shown in figure 2*C* for a pop-

The figure is available in its entirety in the online edition of *The American Journal of Human Genetics*.

Figure 2 Graphs of genetic contribution and density of genetic contribution. The figure legend is available in its entirety in the online edition of *The American Journal of Human Genetics*.

ulation subject to the founder effect, whereas figure 2*D* displays the density in the case of uniform distribution. In this context, density can also be interpreted as an incremental genetic contribution computation when founders are incrementally considered in decreasing order of genetic contribution.

Qualitatively, a more convex shape of genetic contribution density indicates that a smaller group of founders contributes to most of the genetic pool of a population. Extreme diagrams of genetic contribution density are single-founder diagrams, which result in a horizontal line corresponding to total genetic contribution gc_T, and uniform-founder diagrams, which are depicted as a diagonal line from 0 to gc_T. Usual cases produce convex diagrams between the two extremes.

Quantitatively, the shape of genetic contribution density function δ can be expressed by its average value

$$\bar{\delta} = \frac{1}{n} \times \sum_{i=1}^{n} \delta_i ,$$

where n is the number of density values. When the number of founders n is large enough, $\bar{\delta}$ varies approximately between $gc_T/2$ and gc_T, corresponding to the cases of uniform- and single-founder contributions, respectively. In rigorous language, uniform genetic distribution density is a ladder function with steps of $1/n \times gc_T$, whose average value is discussed in more detail in appendix A (online only).

We call founder-effect measure fe the normalized difference between $\bar{\delta}$ and the average uniform contribution density, as described more precisely in appendix A (online only). The founder-effect measure varies between 0 and 1, and it is equal to 0 when the founders' genetic contributions are exactly uniformly distributed, whereas it is equal to 1 when only one founder contributes to the genetic pool.

The founder-effect measure gives an indication of the polarization and concentration of the genetic contribution from a limited number of founders. It can be used to study, in absolute terms, genetic transmission in different genealogies, or, within the same genealogy, it can compare different subpopulations with respect to the same set of founders or compare different sets of founders with respect to the same subpopulation.

Layered Founders: Ancestral Separability Method

The genetic pool of the SLSJ population included in our analysis reflects its demographic history. It was shaped by its very early founders, starting in 1675 in the Charlevoix settlement and followed by migration to the SLSJ region. Until 1870, >80% of the SLSJ population came from Charlevoix, and 70% were descendants of the first three migration waves (Labuda et al. 1996). The rapid growth of the population was the result of the very large family sizes in each generation. The contribution of the later migration waves to the genetic pool diminished significantly with each generation. Such population characteristics led us to use a "genealogical graph" in which edge direction represents generational steps. We developed the layered-founder approach to overcome distortions discussed by E. Merlo, B. Deslauriers, G. Antoniol, P. L. Brunelle, M. Jomphe, G. Bouchard, O. Seda, U. Broeckel, A. W. Cowley Jr., J. Tremblay, and P. Hamet (unpublished data). Founders who share a common distance from today's individuals constitute a layer within the geometric analogy to the concept. The first layer is the set of parents of the studied individuals, the second is that of grandparents, and so on, until the beginning of the colony. Two ancestors v_i and v_j belong to the same layer L_k if they are at the same distance k from today's population, as follows:

$$v_i, v_j \in L_k \leftrightarrow \text{distance}(v_i) = \text{distance}(v_j) = k .$$

In a given genealogy, several layers of founders can be identified, depending on the different k values of distance from today's individuals. Since the number of generations between an ancient founder and today's population may vary, it is possible that the maximum number of generations and the maximum number of computed layers do not coincide. Furthermore, layers also depend on the definition of distance. In work by E. Merlo, B. Deslauriers, G. Antoniol, P. L. Brunelle, M. Jomphe, G. Bouchard, O. Seda, U. Broeckel, A.W. Cowley Jr., J. Tremblay, and P. Hamet (unpublished data), several definitions of distances and layers are presented, evaluated, and discussed. The definition used in the present article is constrained average distance layered founders. Founders are specific to the class to which their genetic contribution is higher. For example, we can determine the set of founders from a layer L_k whose identical-by-descent probability p to CF is higher than their p to ACF by using a maximum-likelihood classification scheme, and we label them as "CF-specific" founders. Similarly, we can compute the mutually exclusive set of founders specific to ACF. In conceptual terms,

$$p(f/\text{CF}) > p(f/\text{ACF}) \rightarrow f \in \{\text{CF-specific founders}\} .$$

Technically, the previous equation has to be further detailed, as presented in work by E. Merlo, B. Deslauriers, G. Antoniol, P. L. Brunelle, M. Jomphe, G. Bouchard, O. Seda, U. Broeckel, A.W. Cowley Jr., J. Tremblay, and P. Hamet (unpublished data). Although, in absolute terms, specific founders genetically contribute to one class of descendants more than to another, the difference of contributions may be irrelevant. Indeed, there are few founders for whom the gene-transmission probability to both classes is identical. Thus, a new measure called "separability" has been introduced to capture the relevance of the difference in gene-transmission probability. In conceptual terms,

$$\text{separability} = \frac{1}{2}\left(\frac{1}{n}\sum_{i=1}^{n}[gc(f_i/\text{CF}) - gc(f_i/\text{ACF})] + \frac{1}{m}\sum_{j=1}^{m}[gc(f_j/\text{ACF}) - gc(f_j/\text{CF})]\right) ,$$

where n founders f_i in layer L_k are specific to CF and m founders f_i are specific to ACF. Separability can be thought of as the average difference in genetic contribution observed for the two sets of founders specific to either CF or ACF classes. Again, the previous equation has to be further detailed, as presented in work by E. Merlo, B. Deslauriers, G. Antoniol, P. L. Brunelle, M. Jomphe, G. Bouchard, O. Seda, U. Broeckel, A.W. Cowley Jr., J. Tremblay, and P. Hamet (unpublished data). The separability and specificity of layered founders with respect to distinct classes of families in the current generation are illustrated schematically in figure 3.

Results

General Characteristics of Subjects

BP, anthropometric, and selected metabolic data validated in 810 subjects at the time of analysis are reported in table 1, which also identifies traits that are highly significantly different between hypertensive and normotensive subjects of both sexes. These involve BP, as expected, and several anthropometric parameters, including %body fat, particularly as derived from impedance measurements. Noticeably, %body fat determined by impedance correlated significantly with %body fat calculated by skinfolds ($r = 0.70$; $P < .001$), whereas the difference between normotensive and hypertensive subjects was better captured by impedance.

Table 1 also reports familial correlations and estimates of apparent heritability (h^2) calculated by the FCOR program of the SAGE statistical package. Significant correlations within sib pairs ($h^2 = 2xr$ and $r > 0.25$; therefore, $h^2 > 50\%$) were found for SBP, DBP, and heart

The figure is available in its entirety in the online edition of *The American Journal of Human Genetics.*

Figure 3 Schematic illustration of separability and specificity of layered founders with respect to distinct classes of families in the current generation.

rate only in normotensive individuals of both sexes. It must be noted, however, that apparent heritability estimates for BP were much higher for hypertensive subjects ($n = 174$) after the withdrawal of antihypertensive medications, increasing in males from $r = 0.03$ to $r = 0.29$ for SBP and from $r = 0.01$ to $r = 0.22$ for DBP and in females from $r = 0.04$ to $r = 0.35$ for SBP and from $r = 0.14$ to $r = 0.37$ for DBP, regardless of whether the analysis included those who were never treated for hypertension ($n = 293$). As reported elsewhere, anthropometric measures, particularly those related to higher %body fat, exhibited higher heritability percentages in hypertensive than in normotensive subjects (Pausova et al. 2001). This was also evident for heritability estimates of serum glycerol levels (table 1).

Partitioning of Variance

To evaluate the feasibility of detecting and mapping QTLs underlying the hemodynamic, anthropometric, and metabolic traits presented in table 1, we targeted the traits with high heritability by estimating the number of large QTLs and their relative contributions to the variance for traits (table 2).

Estimates of variance contribution for the effects modeled (table 2) showed evidence of at least one major QTL with individual contribution in the range of 18% to >41% for several traits. There was also evidence of a second QTL with a large effect, up to ~25% contribution, for some of these traits. Subscapular skinfolds presented evidence of the highest genetic contribution, with at least three QTLs, each with an individual contribution >20%. Our results also suggest a large contribution (~18%) of age to the variance of SBP but not DBP, which is compatible with the well-known continuous increase in SBP with aging, in contrast to DBP, which reaches a plateau and then declines after age 55 years, as seen in this population and in a population study of 27,000 Canadians (Joffres et al. 2001), with findings similar to data from the Framingham Heart Study (Franklin 2004) and National Health and Nutrition Examination Survey III (Burt et al. 1995). Age was found to contribute, to a large extent, to the variance of %body fat measured by impedance. On the other hand, the covariate sex explained 12%–24% of the variance of waist circumference, LDL levels, and %body fat. These results thus confirmed that age and sex are

Table 1

Biological Characteristics and Familial Correlations of Phenotypes, by Patient Sex and BP Status

	Males						Females					
	With HBP (n = 205[b])			Without HBP (n = 166[c])			With HBP (n = 262[d])			Without HBP (n = 177[e])		
Characteristic[a]	Mean	SE	r	Mean	SE	r	Mean	SE	r	Mean	SE	r
Age (years)	***51.53***	.83		***45.30***	1.07		***57.37***	.74		***42.92***	1.05	
SBP (mmHg)	***142.0***	1.6	.03	***121.9***	1.0	.29	***144.2***	1.4	.04	***113.7***	1.0	.13
DBP (mmHg)	***90.6***	.8	.01	***78.6***	.7	.33	***84.8***	.7	.14	***73.5***	.7	.24
Heart rate (beats/min)	70.7	1.1	.07	67.6	1.0	.55	73.6	.9	.00	72.7	.8	.53
Height (cm)	***171.0***	.5	.56	***173.5***	.5	.68	***157.6***	.4	.46	***160.3***	.5	.47
Weight (kg)	82.4	1.0	.28	79.2	1.2	.31	***68.4***	.9	.16	***63.5***	1.0	.27
BMI (kg/m^2)	***28.1***	.3	.11	***26.3***	.4	.18	***27.5***	.4	.23	***24.8***	.4	.19
Waist-to-hip ratio	***.984***	.005	.26	***.946***	.005	.06	***.849***	.005	.23	***.809***	.007	.19
Waist circumference (cm)	***99.4***	.8	.25	***92.92***	.88	.20	***87.67***	.93	.17	***80.10***	1.01	.10
Hip circumference (cm)	***100.7***	.5	.23	***98.00***	.50	.26	***103.1***	.7	.10	***99.3***	.7	.14
Thigh circumference (cm):												
Proximal	58.2	.4	.28	57.20	.50	.27	58.8	.4	.10	59.0	.5	.28
Mid	43.4	.4	.27	52.60	.50	.23	52.8	.4	.04	52.4	.5	.30
Distal	40.9	.3	.20	39.90	.30	.25	40.6	.3	.07	39.9	.3	.38
Skinfold (mm):												
Biceps	16.82	.96	.37	16.61	.98	.12	23.81	.84	.12	22.13	1.08	.07
Triceps	23.57	.94	.17	23.14	1.06	.07	34.25	.81	.29	30.22	.96	.10
Subscapular	25.81	.78	.15	22.81	.84	.15	28.22	.86	.40	24.24	1.03	.11
Suprailiac	24.90	.94	.41	21.81	1.02	.03	27.11	.74	.29	23.72	1.09	.08
Thigh	24.45	1.08	.35	26.84	1.27	.12	43.27	.89	.08	39.25	1.06	.05
Body fat (%):												
Calculated	25.98	.39	.09	24.96	.49	.15	***39.03***	.42	.31	***36.30***	.61	.12
Derived	***24.58***	.56	.44	***21.16***	.69	.38	***37.39***	.77	.22	***30.35***	.82	.00
Cholesterol (mmol/liter):												
Total	5.53	.09	.06	5.57	.09	.18	***5.75***	.08	.19	***5.24***	.08	.23
HDL	1.16	.03	.32	1.20	.02	.43	1.50	.03	.19	1.54	.03	.00
LDL	3.34	.07	.42	3.60	.09	.37	3.31	.07	.16	3.12	.07	.00
Triglycerides (mmol/liter)	2.40	.15	.12	1.86	.10	.21	***1.98***	.07	.25	***1.29***	.06	.29
Glucose (mmol/liter)	***5.79***	.12	.00	***5.29***	.07	.45	***5.40***	.07	.19	***4.97***	.08	.04
Creatinine (μmol/liter)	91.7	2.0	.13	85.9	.9	.03	70.8	1.1	.03	68.2	.9	.18
Uric acid (μmol/liter):												
Plasma	***356.5***	5.6	.17	***331.8***	4.6	.25	***295.2***	4.6	.21	***245.9***	3.8	.29
Urinary	3.04	.22	.05	2.38	.30	.24	***2.72***	.27	.72	***1.85***	.19	.51
Glycerol (mmol/liter)	.105	.028	.96	.053	.004	.04	***.099***	.004	.44	***.080***	.003	.18
Reactance (Ω):												
Ecw	567.0	5.2	.07	582.2	5.5	.27	677.4	6.5	.39	701.3	7.2	.41
Icw	1,027.2	14.4	.03	1,037.1	15.5	.38	1,407.4	20.5	.23	1,429.2	22.9	.46
Insulin (pmol/liter)	134.7	7.1	.11	114.5	4.6	.32	112.9	3.3	.04	103.4	2.6	.31
Arg-vaso (pg/ml)[f]	4.45	.17	.33	4.56	.19	.53	4.55	.16	.22	4.94	.17	.02
Renin, supine (ng/ml/h)[f]	1.23	.11	.61	1.77	.17	.31	1.25	.13	.17	1.35	.10	.41

Note.—Values in bold italics indicate $P \leq .001$ between groups with and groups without high blood pressure (HBP); underlined values indicate correlation ≥0.25 (i.e., $h^2 > 50\%$). Familial correlation r was calculated with FCOR software.

[a] Arg-vaso = arginine-vasopressin; Ecw = extracellular water; Icw = intracellular water.

[b] Maximum no. of sib pairs generated = 145.

[c] Maximum no. of sib pairs generated = 77.

[d] Maximum no. of sib pairs generated = 234.

[e] Maximum no. of sib pairs generated = 85.

[f] Measured in extensive phenotyping only.

Table 2

Partitioning of Variance of a Set of Hemodynamic, Anthropometric, and Metabolic Traits

Source of Variance	Percentage of Total Variance (Square Root of Variance) Attributed to Modeled Effects: Residual	Age	Sex	Total Genetic Variance	QTLs[a]: First	Second	Other	Absolute Total Variance
SBP (mmHg)	44.2 (176.78)	18.3 (73.03)	.7 (2.97)	36.8 (147.10)	20.8 (83.07)	11.9 (47.44)	4.1 (16.59)	399.88
DBP (mmHg)	66.7 (85.30)	.8 (1.07)	5.1 (6.45)	27.4 (35.08)	18.0 (23.05)	6.7 (8.59)	2.7 (3.44)	127.90
Weight (kg)[b]	22.1 (53.38)	3.8 (9.26)	3.8 (9.20)	42.2 (101.89)	25.4 (61.20)	10.1 (24.45)	6.7 (16.24)	241.30
BMI (kg/m^2)	37.6 (9.61)	1.0 (.25)	2.2 (.55)	59.2 (15.10)	31.5 (8.04)	16.3 (4.15)	11.4 (2.91)	25.50
Waist circumference (cm)	42.1 (91.63)	3.2 (7.02)	19.0 (41.24)	35.7 (77.52)	23.4 (50.63)	9.7 (21.09)	2.6 (5.80)	217.41
Skinfold subscapular (mm)	12.1 (16.24)	.5 (.69)	.3 (.37)	87.1 (116.85)	41.2 (55.32)	25.1 (33.69)	20.8 (27.84)	134.15
HDL cholesterol[c] (mmol/liter)	55.8 (.019)	.8 (.000)	11.8 (.004)	31.6 (.011)	21.8 (.008)	8.1 (.003)	1.7 (.00)	.0343
LDL cholesterol (mmol/liter)	48.9 (.513)	2.1 (.022)	1.1 (.012)	47.9 (.501)	20.1 (.211)	14.0 (.147)	13.8 (.143)	1.05
24-h urinary uric acid[d] (μmol/liter)	60.9 (.086)	1.7 (.002)	1.9 (.003)	35.5 (.050)	31.9 (.045)	3.0 (.004)	.6 (.001)	.142
Body fat by impedance (%)	22.2 (26.85)	18.9 (22.90)	23.6 (28.53)	35.3 (42.72)	20.6 (24.90)	10.2 (12.29)	4.5 (5.53)	121.00

[a] Ranked in order of variance contribution.
[b] Height was added as a covariate in the analysis. The contribution of height to the variance of weight was 28.1% (67.57 kg).
[c] Values are $\log_{10}$ HDL.
[d] Values are the square root of 24-h urinary uric acid.

important covariates for cardiovascular-related phenotypes and that a sizable sexual dimorphism has to be considered for several of these traits. The results presented in table 2 also confirmed the oligogenic and multifactorial nature of these traits, as demonstrated by the relatively large contribution of both genetic (from a few QTLs) and environmental (residual) factors to the variance. For example, the percentage of residual contribution to the variance of LDL levels was about the same as the genetic contribution—that is, ~48%.

BMI is the most often studied phenotype in the search for genes underlying obesity-related traits. However, this trait is a compound phenotype and, therefore, is unlikely to provide accurate estimates. In addition to BMI, we also analyzed weight and modeled height in the segregation analysis. As expected, this strategy provided lower estimates for residual variance. Most of the variance of weight (78%) could thus be explained by the effects modeled for QTLs, age, sex, and height. The contribution of height to the variance of weight was ~30%. The genetic contribution for BMI was ~60% compared with ~40% for weight adjusted for height, suggesting that part of the genetic variance of BMI is due to the genetic contribution of height. As defined in this data set, the phenotypes of glucose and insulin plasma levels did not show evidence for a genetic contribution (data not reported).

Genomewide Linkage

The oligogenic character of most traits under study was also evident from genomewide linkage analysis. Whereas a total of 46 LOD scores >1.9 were detected for the 213 BP, anthropometric, and metabolic traits analyzed, several of them were found in QTL clusters, particularly on chr 1, chr 3, chr 16, and chr 19 (fig. 4 and table 3). These clusters were analyzed further (see fig. 5 for chr 1, fig. 6 for chr 3, fig. 7 for chr 16, and fig. 8 for chr 19). A QTL cluster was defined as a chromosomal region in which at least one trait had a LOD score >2.0 and two additional traits with LOD scores >1.5 followed a similar pattern of linkage. When these conditions were reached, we further analyzed additional dependent and independent traits within the same chromosomal region. On chr 1, the highest LOD scores were reached for thigh circumferences (LOD of 3.8 between markers *D1S1677* and *D1S2878*) and BMI (LOD of 3.4 at *D1S2762* at 175–180 cM). Among the metabolic components, fasting insulin levels peaked at the same location, with a LOD of 2.7 at marker *D1S1679*. Other metabolic features, such as apolipoprotein A (apoA), apoB, leptin, and cAMP levels, were also observed in this region. Several skinfold phenotypes were localized at a somewhat more telomeric location (210–215 cM): subscapular (LOD of 3.6 between *D1S1660* and *D1S2622*) and biceps (LOD of 3.4 at *D1S2816*), as were global obesity measures: %body fat by skinfolds (LOD of 3.1 at *D1S2757*), closely followed by %body fat by impedance (LOD of 2.9 between *D1S238* and *D1S3468*). At an even further telomeric location (~230 cM), several DBP traits clustered, including a peak of average DBP with a LOD of 2.1 at *D1S2141* (fig. 6).

A second major cluster was detected on chr 3 at 170–180 cM. A LOD of 2.6 was obtained for average DBP (between *D3S1763* and *D3S3053*). The narrow peak reflected higher power, because phenotyping was conducted in all subjects, whereas other traits required the extensive phenotyping protocol described in the "Methods and Procedures" section (Kotchen et al. 2000). Thus, asleep DBP (determined by 24-h ambulatory BP monitoring [ABPM]) reached a LOD of 2.0 between *D3S1746* and *D3S1763*, pre–math stress DBP LOD was 1.9 at *D3S3053*, 24-h awake DBP LOD was 1.5 at

D3S1763, and average supine DBP LOD was 1.4 at *D3S3053*, whereas plasma renin while standing LOD was 1.4 (between *D3S3053* and *D3S2427*). Clearly, the strength of these observations resided in the fact that they all appeared in a common, relatively narrow chromosomal segment in spite of having been measured under largely different physiological conditions.

PCA and Bivariate Data Analyses

In analyzing the findings of this study, we were faced with multivariate data recorded from extensive phenotyping. One of the approaches to deciphering the genetic architecture of these multivariable phenotypes (Ghosh and Majumder 2001) is PCA and bivariate analyses of the results, as illustrated in figure 9. For the multiple phenotypes present in the QTL clusters on chr 1 (fig. 5) and chr 3 (fig. 6), PCA was done with the correlation matrix of the phenotypes that were available on >500 subjects. For the PCA for chr 1, we included phenotypes mapping to the region with significant or suggestive LOD scores (BMI; %body fat, determined by bioimpedance; biceps, subscapular, suprailiac, and triceps skinfolds; and circumferences of proximal, middle, and distal thigh). The correlation between principal component factors and initial phenotypes was computed first, and then linkage analysis was performed for both factors, with principal component factor 1 mapping to our initial linkage region on chr 1 with a LOD score of 4.9 at position 212 cM (fig. 9*A* shows a LOD plot for all included phenotypes and factor 1). Bivariate analysis, including that of BMI and glucose insulin, exceeded a LOD of 5 at 175 cM on chr 1. For chr 3, in 130 subjects not receiving medication, bivariate analysis of DBP measured before the mathematical test and average asleep DBP derived from 24-h ABPM, we found a LOD significantly higher than that for both univariate analyses (LOD of 4.4), peaking at 173 cM. The same was true for the results of bivariate analysis on chr 1, in which combined BMI and insulin traits yielded a LOD of 5.1 at 173 cM.

Table 3

Chromosomal Positions, Phenotypes, and Maximum LOD Scores

The table is available in its entirety in the online edition of *The American Journal of Human Genetics*.

Classification of Families on the Basis of Their LOD Score Contributions

In complex traits, it is well known that clinical as well as genetic heterogeneity greatly hampers the uncovering of causal genomic factors. In our study population, in spite of its relative homogeneity, genetic heterogeneity was still clearly present. Although a heterogeneity-corrected LOD_{cor} obtained by SOLAR has the capacity to assess oligogenic traits, we sought additional tools to reduce the impact of locus heterogeneity. We initially deployed the LOD_{cor} obtained by SOLAR and then ranked the families by density, as described in the "Methods and Procedures" section. This approach allowed the ranking of families into CF, NCF, and ACF classes (il-

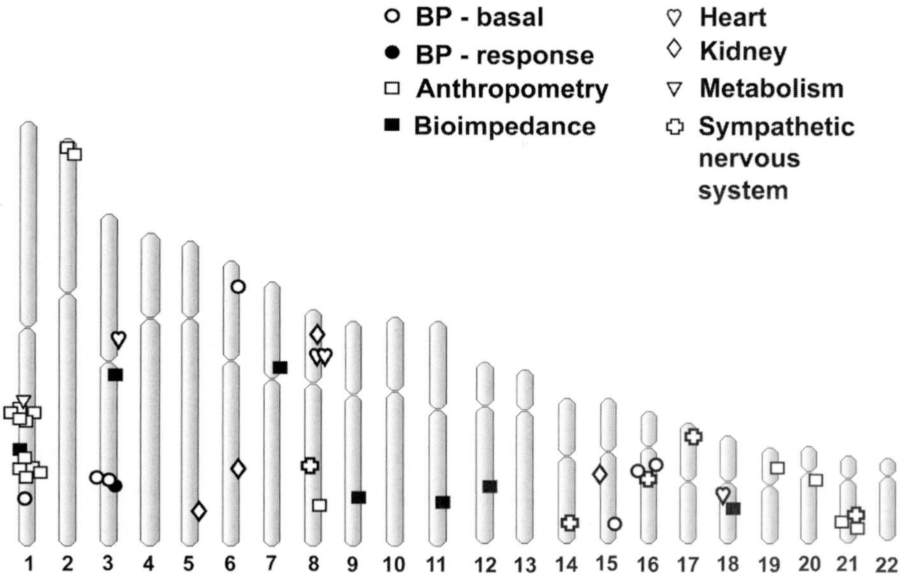

Figure 4 Total-genome view of quantitative-trait linkage analysis by use of SOLAR in French Canadian families with hypertension and/or dyslipidemia. Phenotypes with a LOD score >1.9 after 100,000 permutations are shown. For more details, see table 3.

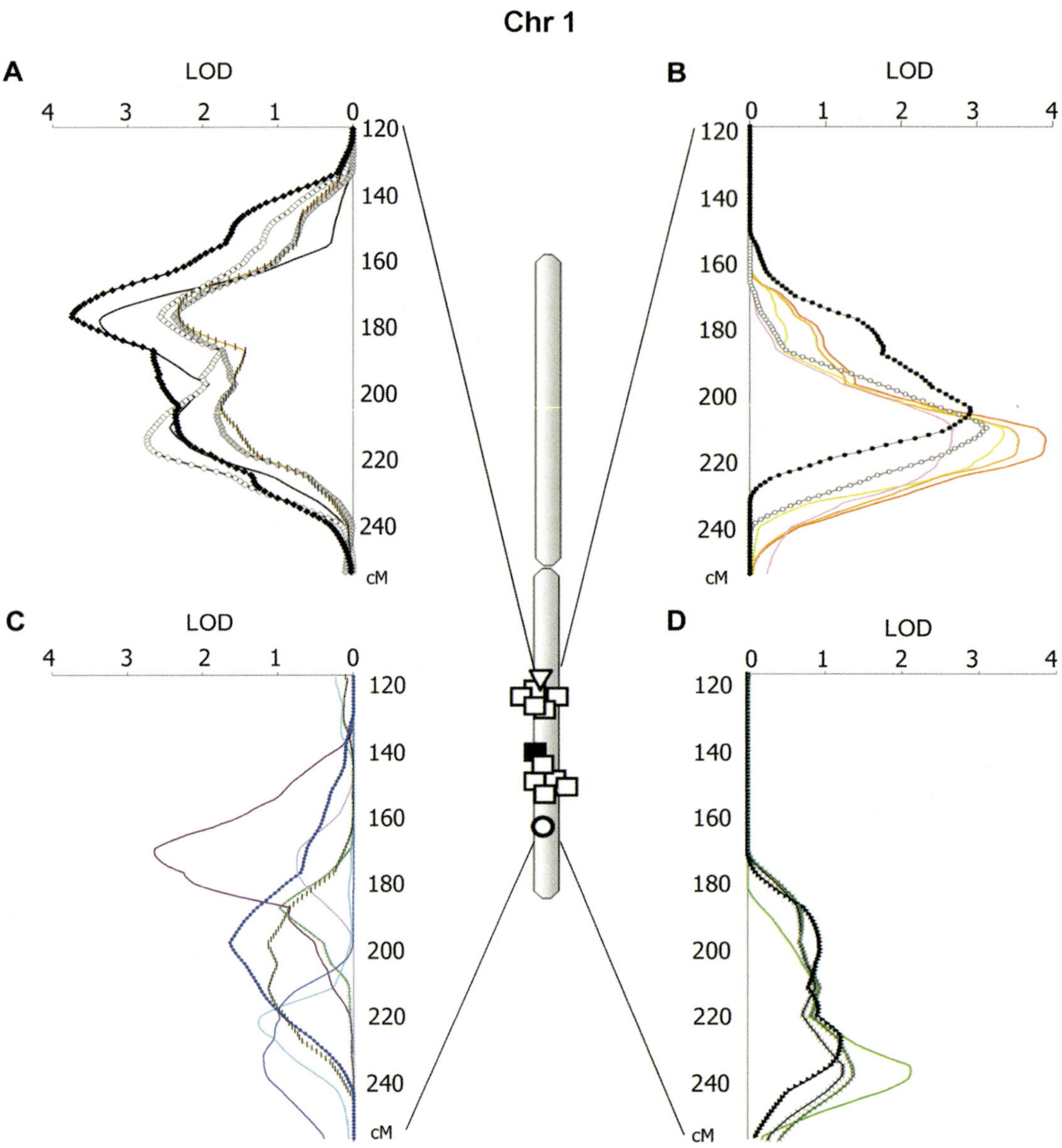

Figure 5 Clusters of phenotypes illustrated by LOD curves for significant and suggestive QTLs on chr 1. *A* and *B*, Obesity-related anthropometric phenotypes. *A*, BMI (*black line*) and circumferences of thigh proximal (*blackened diamonds*), thigh midway (*gray diamonds*), thigh distal (*unblackened diamonds*), and upper arm (*orange line with black dashes*). *B*, Skinfolds: suprailiac (*red line*), subscapular (*orange line*), biceps (*yellow line*), and triceps (*pink line*); and %body fat by impedance (*blackened circles*) and by skinfolds (*unblackened circles*). *C*, Metabolic phenotypes: insulin (*dark purple line*), renin (*blue line*), leptin (*blue circles*), apoB (*yellow line with black dashes*), arginine-vasopressin (*turquoise line*), apoA (*green line*), and cAMP 24-h excretion (*light purple line*). *D*, BP-related phenotypes: average DBP (*green line*), awake DBP (*green line with asterisks* [*]), post–math stress DBP (*blackened triangles*), and mean awake BP (*black line with asterisks* [*]).

lustrated in fig. 1), providing the possibility of uncovering loci contributing to a trait variance that would have been missed by SOLAR analysis. Indeed, our method is novel and was not previously published. To evaluate the significance of the increase in LOD scores from the baseline of 0.49 at this locus, we estimated the probability of obtaining a LOD score of 5.82 by a random selection of families. An empirical *P* value was computed by performing two kinds of permutation tests. In one test, the random variable is the set of CF, so we compare 10,000 random sets of 25 families to see how many times the subset generates a multipoint LOD score at least as high as the maximum subset LOD score found for CF. The *P* value is calculated on the basis of the proportion of 10,000 random sets of families that gave such a maximum subset LOD score. The highest LOD score generated by this method was 3.97 (mean 0.23; SD 0.35) with a corresponding *P* value <.0001. In the

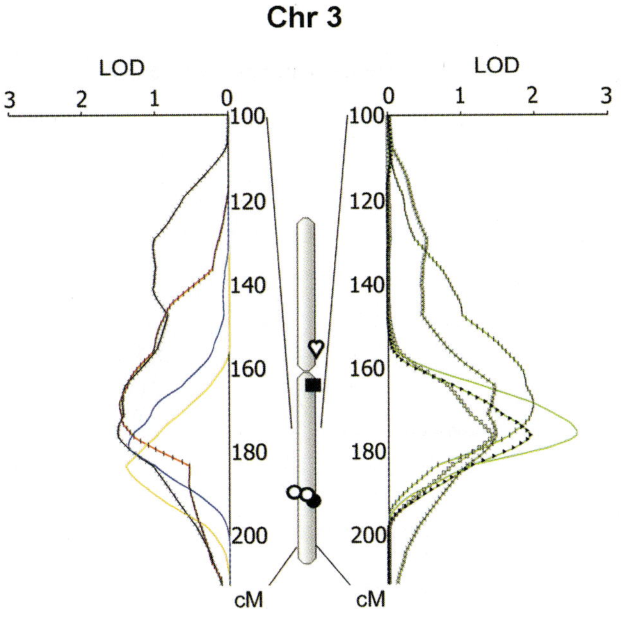

Figure 6 Clusters of phenotypes illustrated by LOD curves for significant and suggestive QTLs on chr 3. *Left panel,* Sodium (*yellow line*), renin (*blue line*), mean awake BP (*black line*), and asleep SBP (*red line with dashes*). *Right panel,* DBP phenotypes: average (*green line*), awake (*green line with asterisks* [*]), sleep (*green line with dashes*), supine (*green line with squares*), and pre–math stress (*green line with blackened triangles*).

other test, we randomly ordered all the families and, beginning with the first-ranked family, we repeatedly considered larger subsets (e.g., 1, 1_2, 1_2_3, ...) and computed the multipoint LOD score by adding the remaining families in order, one by one, until all families were included. The highest LOD score obtained was retained. The above operation was repeated 10,000 times, and the highest LOD score generated was 4.42 (mean 0.88; SD 0.44); thus, the P value was <.0001.

Twenty-thousand LOD score density analysis runs were performed for the entire chr 1 specific to the cluster illustrated in fig. 5, to ascertain the maximized LOD score for BP. Although many metabolic traits were observed in this cluster, only a modest contribution of BP at the more telomeric position was found (fig. 5*D*). Multipoint maximization selection indeed uncovered a robust LOD score for SBP on chr 1 within the metabolic cluster component. As seen in figure 10, whereas SOLAR analysis of recumbent SBP gave a LOD of 0.5 at the locus 195 cM on chr 1, 23 CF reached a LOD of 5.7, and 21 ACF had a LOD of 0. This difference in LOD scores translated into a 10-mmHg recumbent SBP phenotypic gradient between CF and ACF (P = .007, with age and sex as covariates).

Similar multipoint maximization selection was performed for DBP on chr 3. Whereas the DBP QTL at 180 cM on chr 3, in the entire population, peaked at a LOD of 1.2, analysis of 15 CF increased the LOD to 2.9, and 15 ACF had a LOD of 0, accounting for the 5.5-mmHg DBP gradient between CF and ACF (P = .0003). Further analysis indicated that 22% of individuals from seven CF overlapped between the two loci, giving a Jacquard coefficient of 22% and, in fact, that only five ACF overlapped between loci on chr 2, yielding a Jacquard coefficient of 16%. The Jacquard coefficient is defined as $J_c = |CF \cap ACF|/|CF \cup ACF|$—that is, J_c is the ratio of the cardinality of the union to that of the intersection between CF and ACF. Phenotypic analysis of these CF and ACF classes demonstrated that CF sharing maximized LOD scores on chr 1 and chr 3 and that CF families, though bearing similar BP values to those of ACF families, exhibited more obesity features, including BMIs of 28 versus 24 (P = .0005), waist circumferences of 93 versus 78 (P = .002), supscapular skinfolds of 29 versus 21 (P = .003), and %body fat of 26 versus 18 (P = .01) for CF versus ACF classes. A feature of metabolic syndrome was thus apparent in 37% of CF and 9.6% of ACF classes.

Ancestral Separability of Families: The Layered-Founders Approach

At this point in our study, we sought further evidence for shared genetic determinants in the familial classes described above. The eventual ancestral relatedness of these families should constitute such an ascertainment. One of the advantages of studying the French Canadian population of the SLSJ region resides in the richness and completeness of the genealogical data collected since the beginning of the colony in 1608 and computerized in the BALSAC population register (Bouchard et al. 1989). We have used these genealogical data up to the depth of 17 generations over 14 layers of founders (see the "Methods and Procedures" section) to analyze the genetic effect of ancestors in CF and ACF classes of living subjects. The founder-effect measures vary from 0.6 to 0.7 at the most recent layer and from 0.8 to 0.9 at the oldest layer. These figures indicate that the polarization of genetic contribution is more pronounced at distant generations and is more diluted (although still relevant) at recent generations. Figure 11 illustrates that the ancestors of family classes contributing to BP QTLs on either chr 1 or chr 3 displayed a specificity >90% within the 3–4 most recent layers, and, even for the oldest lay-

The figure is available in its entirety in the online edition of *The American Journal of Human Genetics.*

Figure 7 Clusters of phenotypes illustrated by LOD curves for significant and suggestive QTLs on chr 16.

The figure is available in its entirety in the online edition of *The American Journal of Human Genetics.*

Figure 8 Clusters of phenotypes illustrated by LOD curves for significant and suggestive QTLs on chr 19.

ers, the expected drop maintained specificity between ~55% and 85%. By observing founder-effect and specificity measures, one can note that these measures are conceptually and experimentally distinct. In recent layers, we discovered higher specificity and lower polarization, which indicates that genes are transmitted through paths that intersect less than in older layers (higher specificity), whereas the amount of contributions is more similar among recent founders than among older founders (lower polarization). A unique contribution to each family class exceeded 90% for the three most recent layers, and it was still 20%–30% of the most distant ancestors (fig. 11*A* and 11*C*). Figure 11*B* and 11*D* depicts the separability of classes of founders, which is the average differential contribution of separable founders to family classes and which is >80% for the 3–4 most recent layers, remaining at ~40% for the most distant founders. Separability indicates that, for recent generations, the genetic contributions of specific founders to CF and to ACF differ by >80%, on average. For older generations, such genetic contributions differ by >40%, on average, which is still a wide gap in genetic contribution. We then proceeded "back to the future" to regroup the living descendants from the unique ancestors of CF and ACF classes of chr 1 multipoint maximized LOD at 195 cM. Within our cohort of 120 families, after eliminating families with shared ancestral contributions to individuals of both CF or ACF, we identified 25 families with 224 members with unique ancestors of the CF class (streaming out from 66 genotyped subjects) and 26 families with 213 members (62 genotyped individuals) for the ACF class. The SBP was 10 mmHg higher in CF descendants than in ACF descendants ($P = .0009$). These results permit the ascertainment of relevance of family classes sharing both ancestor classes and relevant phenotypes initially determined by their maximized linkage at a specific locus.

Discussion

The oligogenic and epistatic character of complex diseases makes the search for their genetic determinants a challenging task (Lander and Schork 1994; Hamet et al. 1998; Doris 2002; Glazier et al. 2002; Samani 2003). One of the approaches that has had some success is to study relatively isolated human populations, such as the Hutterites from South Dakota (Newman et al. 2003);

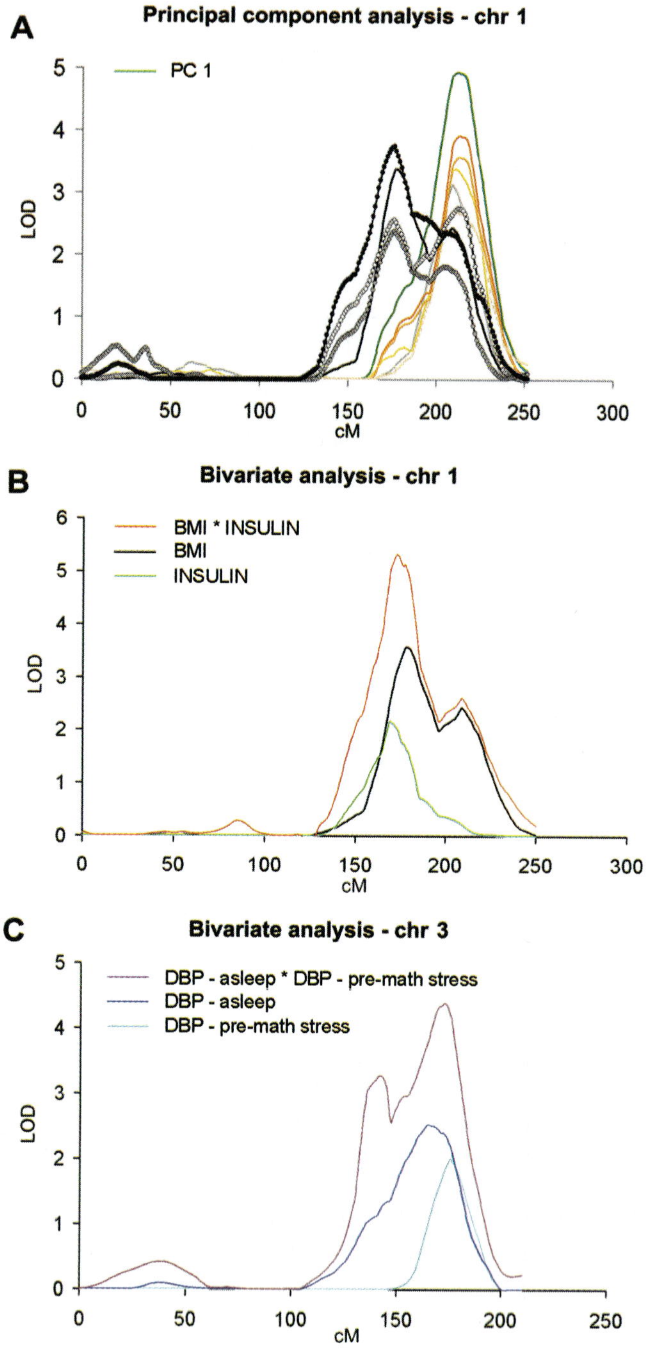

Figure 9 PCA and bivariate analyses of traits linked to chr 1 and chr 3. *A*, Linkage of principal component 1 (PC 1) (*green line*) on chr 1, including BMI; %body fat (determined by bioimpedance); skinfolds: biceps, subscapular, suprailiac, and triceps; and circumferences of proximal, middle, and distal thigh (for details on individual linkage results, see fig. 5). *B* and *C*, Bivariate analyses for chr 1 and chr 3. *B*, Univariate analyses of BMI (*black line*) and fasting insulin (*green line*) and bivariate analysis (*red line*). *C*, Univariate analyses of pre–math stress DBP (*light blue line*) and mean asleep DBP measured by 24-h ABPM (*dark blue line*) and bivariate analysis (*purple line*).

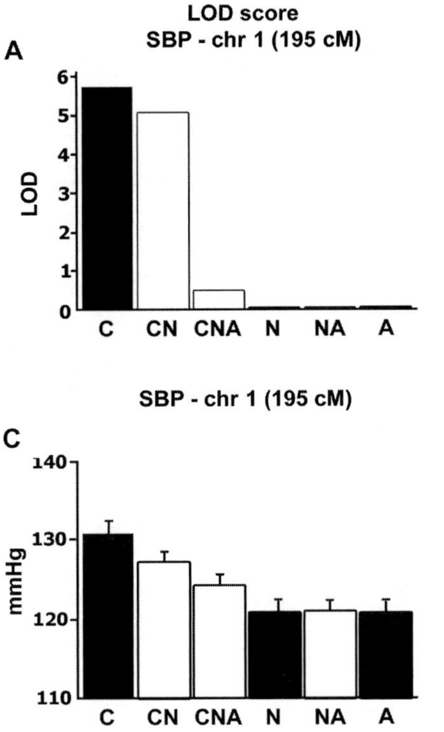

Figure 10 Approximate gradient-driven LOD score density maximization. *A*, LOD scores at 195 cM on chr 1 for the SBP trait in families classified by LOD score contribution. *B*, LOD scores at 180 cM on chr 3 for the average supine DBP trait in family classes. C, Family averages of SBP in family classes at 195 cM on chr 1. *D*, Family averages of supine DBP in family classes at 180 cM on chr 3. C = contributing families; N = noncontributing families; A = anticontributing families. Letter combinations reflect the joining of families in the different groups (e.g., CNA = contributing, noncontributing, and anticontributing families combined).

the Finnish subpopulation from Koilliskaira, relatively isolated since the sixteenth century (Woolley et al. 2002); the Icelandic population analyzed by deCODE (Helgadottir et al. 2004); and the French Canadian population investigated in the present study (Bouchard et al. 1989), or to study populations of Mormons from Salt Lake City because of their unifying religious, nutritional, and genetic characteristics (Jeunemaître et al. 1992; O'Brien et al. 1994; Scriver 2001). These populations offer several advantages over the general population, including the more uniform environment of their living conditions; better mapping opportunities because of the longer linkage disequilibrium intervals, as estimated by the genetic clock (Labuda et al. 1997); and, most importantly, access to their genealogical records (Peltonen et al. 2000). The design and analyses performed in the present investigation were aimed at addressing several of the issues that often cause failure to identify genetic factors responsible for the phenotypic variation of complex traits (Rice et al. 2000; Glazier et al. 2002; Samani 2003). We have applied an extensive phenotyping protocol (Kotchen et al. 2000, 2002; Pausova et al. 2000) to a relatively homogeneous population, which led to the highest number of loci contributing to cardiovascular-related and metabolic traits reported to date. Selection of the proband sib pair, on the basis of the presence of hypertension and dyslipidemia (25% of subjects included in the present study exhibited metabolic syndrome features based on ATPIII criteria), permitted us to map several components of the metabolic syndrome, particularly on chr 1 and chr 3. The application of a battery of classic and more-novel statistical analytical tools, including Bayesian MCMC–based oligogenic segregation analysis, as well as bivariate analysis and PCA, resulted in the identification of highly significant linkage groups for several phenotypes. Bivariate analysis and PCA were performed only for traits that mapped at the same location and showed significant or suggestive linkage in a single-trait analysis, since one can assume that these traits might have a common genetic component and/or a common gene influencing the traits jointly. In view of the extensive phenotyping, we first assessed the feasibility of detecting and localizing QTLs that underlie the collected phenotypes, by use of Bayesian MCMC segregation analysis. This analysis suggested the presence of QTLs with a large effect for several phenotypes (table 2). As highlighted by Beaumont and Rannala (2004), Bayesian methods such as those used for our

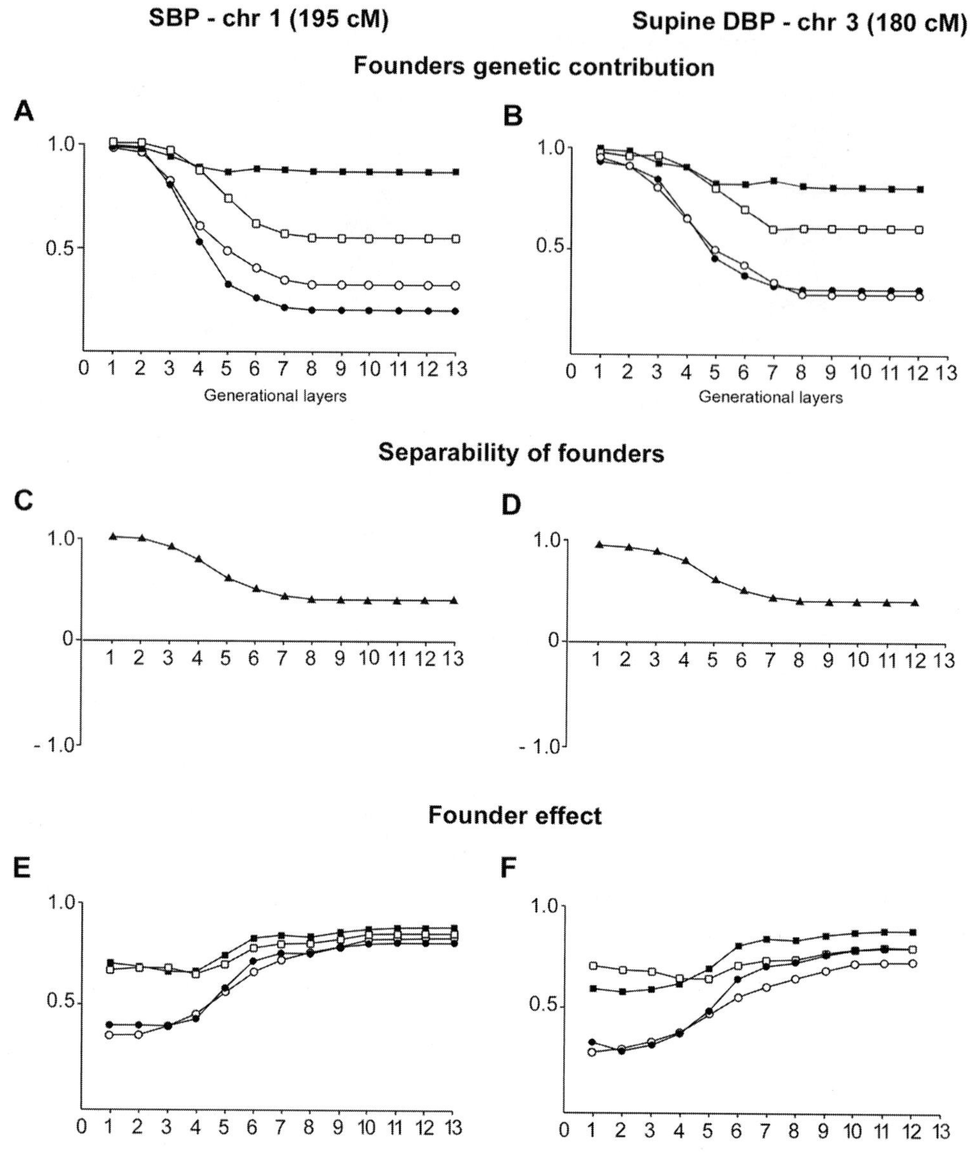

Figure 11 *A* and *B*, Founders' specific (*squares*) and unique (*circles*) genetic contributions to family classes, which are either contributing (*blackened squares and circles*) or anticontributing (*unblackened squares and circles*) to the LOD score. *C* and *D*, Overall separability of CF versus ACF over 14 generational layers at the corresponding loci. *E* and *F*, Founder effect (*squares*) and specific normalized founder effect (*circles*) in CF (*blackened squares and circles*) and ACF (*unblackened squares and circles*). *A–C*, SBP trait at 195 cM on chr 1. *C–E*, Average supine DBP trait at 180 cM on chr 3.

segregation analysis have numerous advantages over classic approaches, and one can foresee their use in an increasing number of areas of genetic analysis. Our subsequent linkage analysis and the identification of significant and suggestive QTLs further support these findings. Although it has been initially suggested that variance-components linkage analysis allows for the estimation of locus-specific variance, on the basis of simulation studies, this is considered imprecise, and therefore we report only LOD scores, to avoid a large upward bias in the estimation of locus-specific effects, with regard to the comments by Göring et al. (2001) and Siegmund (2002). Thus, Bayesian segregation analysis allowed orientation toward phenotypes that exhibited (1) a significant genetic contribution and (2) a restricted number of major loci (see table 2). LOD score density analysis permitted the separation of family groups underlying the phenotypic gradient, exemplified in figure 10 and further confirmed by the genealogical studies discussed below.

In the French Canadian population, the most prominent clusters of QTLs for hemodynamic, anthropometric, and metabolic phenotypes were found on chr 1 and chr 3. Two clusters regrouping >20 QTLs peaked at 175 cM and 210 cM on chr 1, respectively, corresponding to QTLs already identified in diverse ethnic groups, including our hypertensive African American sib pairs (Kotchen et al. 2002), and in studies of the genetics of the metabolic syndrome (Langefeld et al. 2004) and type 2 diabetes (Hanson et al. 1998). One of the strengths of the current investigation is the robustness and comprehensiveness of the phenotyping, since, for any given attribute of the metabolic syndrome, a whole battery of endophenotypes was recorded (e.g., for obesity, three different global phenotypes—BMI and %body fat by impedance and by skinfold—and nine regional obesity measures were all significantly linked to the two subregions of the chr 1 cluster).

Although a BP QTL has been reported elsewhere in Finnish twins (Perola et al. 2000), the mapping of eight BP phenotypes (in addition to renin levels and urinary sodium excretion) at 150–200 cM on chr 3 in the current study enriched our understanding of the contribution of this segment of chr 3 by the fact that a shared QTL was obtained for BP values determined under a variety of physiological conditions, such as wakefulness, sleep, before and after stress, or time-series averaged for longer periods of time. Interestingly, BP QTLs colocalized with renin and sodium QTLs on chr 3, suggesting common pathways for these traits, whereas anthropometric traits colocalized with insulin levels on chr 1. The notion of shared pathways was supported by the results of PCA and bivariate analyses (see fig. 9).

The evidence of linkage, even if reaching significant levels (i.e., LOD of 3.9 for subscapular skinfold on chr 1) and even if corroborated by several independently assessed traits, is not definitive proof of the presence of genetic determinants underlying the observed trait variance. We thus used a novel method of classifying families on the basis of LOD score density analysis, which enabled us to identify families that are likely to harbor susceptible/causal haplotypes. This method is somewhat reminiscent of another approach to decreasing heterogeneity, developed recently by Hauser et al. (2004*a*, 2004*b*), that ranks phenotypes prior to LOD computation. This stratification by phenotypes allowed those investigators to uncover, among others, a QTL for macular degeneration, specifically in hypertensive subjects. It is of interest that we have also observed a significant BP cluster on chr 16 (see fig. 7). Nevertheless, our method of "ranking" is aimed at decreasing heterogeneity at the family level by ranking their LOD score contribution. We believe that both methods will have a specific use in dissecting complex traits.

The completeness of the genealogical data of the ancestors of currently living families in the SLSJ area (Bouchard et al. 1989; Heyer and Tremblay 1995) and the concept of layered founders (E. Merlo, B. Deslauriers, G. Antoniol, P. L. Brunelle, M. Jomphe, G. Bouchard, O. Seda, U. Broeckel, A. W. Cowley Jr., J. Tremblay, and P. Hamet, unpublished data) permitted us to evaluate the extent of shared familial contribution within ancestral lineage. Classes of CF, impacting QTL LOD scores and thus sharing a specific locus, presented a phenotypic gradient, compared with classes of ACF (fig. 10). Families sharing maximized LOD on chr 1 and chr 3 shared obesity/metabolic phenotypes. We then analyzed family classes for their ancestral separability. Indeed, as illustrated in figure 11, we found significant separability of founders between these contrasting family classes, even to the depth of 14 layers (17 generations). Moreover, families contributing to the linkage of metabolic syndrome–related phenotypes on chr 1 were largely distinct from families whose BP determinants resided on chr 3. These distinctions would have been missed if heterogeneity had not been reduced by regrouping the families into specific classes. The last step included the reverse path from unique ancestors to their living descendants. Indeed, thus regrouped, families initially selected along maximized LOD and phenotypic gradient, then separated for uniquely contributing ancestors, bear significant differences in both SBP and DBP in living descendents.

The term "founder effect" is usually applied to Mendelian diseases in expanding, isolated populations. The effect is due to an increase in the frequency of certain alleles, causing a phenotype with relatively little clinical variation. In French Canadians of the SLSJ area, this has been the case for some monogenic dominant and recessive disorders (Scriver 2001). In complex disorders, the situation is a Gordian knot, but certain allele frequencies still may change if, by chance, they were over- or underrepresented among the first settlers who most impacted the population gene pool. It has been estimated that ~70% of today's SLSJ population gene pool has descended from the first three migration waves (Labuda et al. 1996). The changes in common allele frequencies are proportional to those in the outbred population and are thus much less drastic for common than for rare variants. The observation of ancestry sharing, in families contributing to QTLs on chr 1 (for example), corroborate well with the expected overrepresentation of some alleles at certain loci—in this case, cardiovascular susceptibility variants. The chr 1q region is one of the most commonly reported in the literature as being linked with cardiovascular diseases and likely carrying multiple genes with multiple variants, increased in frequency by the stochastic process in the SLSJ region.

The founder effect in our study has been observed over several generations and classes of living individuals. Our quantitative genealogical approach supports the notion of the ancestral causality of traits uniquely present and inherited in distinct family classes. We propose the "quantitative founder effect" in which a trait determined within population subsets is measurably and quantitatively transmitted throughout generational lineage, contributing to a precise component of phenotypic variance.

We believe that the application of these methods, which are particularly relevant for relatively homogeneous populations, enriched by the presence of well-documented genealogical records, will accelerate the uncovering of causal haplotypes (Daly et al. 2001) in diseases as complex as hypertension and the metabolic syndrome.

Acknowledgments

We thank the members of participating families from the SLSJ region of Quebec. Our gratitude is expressed to Eric Lander for his significant input in the inception of this study and his encouragement throughout its pursuit. We acknowledge the generous participation of research nurses Danielle Deguise, Line Julien, Marie-Renée Guertin, and Sylvie Blaquière in Montreal and Nicole Baribeau and Jacinthe Tremblay in Chicoutimi; bioinformaticians Manon Bernard, Pierre-Luc Brunelle, Alexandru Gurau, Zhitao Wang, Qunli Cheng, and Xin Feng; technicians Gilles Corbeil, Carole Long, and Suzanne Cossette; and clinicians G. Tremblay and P. Larochelle. We also acknowledge discussion with and advice from Howard Jacob, Damian Labuda, Vladimir Kren, Clarence E. Grim, Nicholas Schork, Jane M. Kotchen, and Yulin Sun; the secretarial help of Ginette Dignard; and the editorial assistance of Ovid Da Silva. This work was supported by funds from the National Institutes of Health Specialized Center of Research, Canadian Institutes of Health Research (CIHR) (Cardiogene Consortium and MT-14654), the Heart and Stroke Foundation of Canada, Tailored Advanced Collaborative Training in Cardiovascular Science of the CIHR, and Valorisation-Recherche Québec.

Electronic-Database Information

The URL for data presented herein is as follows:

Pangaea, http://www.stat.washington.edu/thompson/Genepi/pangaea.shtml

References

Allison DB, Neale MC, Zannolli R, Schork NJ, Amos CI, Blangero J (1999) Testing the robustness of the likelihood-ratio test in a variance-component quantitative-trait loci–mapping procedure. Am J Hum Genet 65:531–544

Atzmon G, Schechter C, Greiner W, Davidson D, Rennert G, Barzilai N (2004) Clinical phenotype of families with longevity. J Am Geriatr Soc 52:274–277

Beaumont MA, Rannala B (2004) The Bayesian revolution in genetics. Nat Rev Genet 5:251–261

Blangero J, Williams JT, Almasy L (2001) Variance component methods for detecting complex trait loci. Adv Genet 42:151–181

Bouchard G, Roy R, Casgrain B, Hubert M (1989) [Population files and database management: the BALSAC database and the INGRES/INGRID system]. Hist Mes 4:39–57

Burt VL, Culter JA, Higgins M, Horan MJ, Labarthe D, Whelton P, Brown C, Roccella EJ (1995) Trends in the prevalence, awareness, treatment, and control of hypertension in the adult US population: data from the health examination surveys, 1960 to 1991. Hypertension 26:60–69

Caulfield M, Munroe P, Pembroke J, Samani N, Dominiczak A, Brown M, Benjamin N, Webster J, Ratcliffe P, O'Shea S, Papp J, Taylor E, Dobson R, Knight J, Newhouse S, Hooper J, Lee W, Brain N, Clayton D, Lathrop GM, Farrall M, Connell J (2003) Genome-wide mapping of human loci for essential hypertension. Lancet 361:2118–2123

Daly MJ, Rioux JD, Schaffner SF, Hudson TJ, Lander ES (2001) High-resolution haplotype structure in the human genome. Nat Genet 29:229–232

Daw EW, Heath SC, Wijsman EM (1999) Multipoint oligogenic analysis of age-at-onset data with applications to Alzheimer disease pedigrees. Am J Hum Genet 64:839–851

Doris PA (2002) Hypertension genetics, single nucleotide polymorphisms, and the common disease: common variant hypothesis. Hypertension 39:323–331

Ezzati M, Lopez AD, Rodgers A, Vander HS, Murray CJ (2002) Selected major risk factors and global and regional burden of disease. Lancet 360:1347–1360

Franklin SS (2004) Systolic blood pressure: it's time to take control. Am J Hypertens 17:49S–54S

Franklin SS, Jacobs MJ, Wong ND, L'Italien GJ, Lapuerta P (2001) Predominance of isolated systolic hypertension among middle-aged and elderly US hypertensives: analysis based on National Health and Nutrition Examination Survey (NHANES) III. Hypertension 37:869–874

Gagnon F, Jarvik GP, Motulsky AG, Deeb SS, Brunzell JD, Wijsman EM (2003) Evidence of linkage of HDL level variation to APOC3 in two samples with different ascertainment. Hum Genet 113:522–533

Ghosh S, Majumder PP (2001) Deciphering the genetic architecture of a multivariate phenotype. Adv Genet 42:323–347

Glazier AM, Nadeau JH, Aitman TJ (2002) Finding genes that underlie complex traits. Science 298:2345–2349

Göring HH, Terwilliger JD, Blangero J (2001) Large upward bias in estimation of locus-specific effects from genomewide scans. Am J Hum Genet 69:1357–1369

Groop L, Orho-Melander M (2001) The dysmetabolic syndrome. J Intern Med 250:105–120

Hamet P, Pausova Z, Adarichev S, Adaricheva K, Tremblay J (1998) Hypertension: genes and environment. J Hypertens 16:397–418

Hanson RL, Ehm MG, Pettitt DJ, Prochazka M, Thompson DB, Timberlake D, Foroud T, Kobes S, Baier L, Burns DK, Almasy L, Blangero J, Garvey WT, Bennett PH, Knowler WC (1998) Autosomal genomic scan for loci linked to type II diabetes mellitus and body-mass index in Pima Indians. Am J Hum Genet 63:1130–1138

Hauser ER, Crossman DC, Granger CB, Haines JL, Jones CJ,

Mooser V, McAdam B, et al (2004*a*) A genomewide scan for early-onset coronary artery disease in 438 families: the GENECARD Study. Am J Hum Genet 75:436–447

Hauser ER, Watanabe RM, Duren WL, Bass MP, Langefeld CD, Boehnke M (2004*b*) Ordered subset analysis in genetic linkage mapping of complex traits. Genet Epidemiol 27:53–63

Heath SC (1997) Markov chain Monte Carlo segregation and linkage analysis for oligogenic models. Am J Hum Genet 61:748–760

Helgadottir A, Manolescu A, Thorleifsson G, Gretarsdottir S, Jonsdottir H, Thorsteinsdottir U, Samani NJ, et al (2004) The gene encoding 5-lipoxygenase activating protein confers risk of myocardial infarction and stroke. Nat Genet 36:233–239

Heyer E, Tremblay M (1995) Variability of the genetic contribution of Quebec population founders associated to some deleterious genes. Am J Hum Genet 56:970–978

Jacobs KB, Gray-McGuire C, Cartier KC, Elston RC (2003) Genome-wide linkage scan for genes affecting longitudinal trends in systolic blood pressure. BMC Genet 4:S82

James K, Weitzel LR, Engelman CD, Zerbe G, Norris JM (2003) Genome scan linkage results for longitudinal systolic blood pressure phenotypes in subjects from the Framington Heart Study. BMC Genet 4:S83

Jeunemaître X, Soubrier F, Kotelevtsev YV, Lifton RP, Williams CS, Charru A, Hunt SC, Hopkins PN, Williams RR, Lalouel JM, Corvol P (1992) Molecular basis of human hypertension: role of angiotensinogen. Cell 71:169–180

Joffres MR, Hamet P, Maclean DR, L'Italien GJ, Fodor G (2001) Distribution of blood pressure and hypertension in Canada and the United States. Am J Hypertens 14:1099–1105

Kotchen TA, Broeckel U, Grim CE, Hamet P, Jacob H, Kaldunski ML, Kotchen JM, Schork NJ, Tonellato PJ, Cowley AW Jr (2002) Identification of hypertension-related QTLs in African American sib pairs. Hypertension 40:634–639

Kotchen TA, Kotchen JM, Grim CE, George V, Kaldunski ML, Cowley AW, Hamet P, Chelius TH (2000) Genetic determinants of hypertension: identification of candidate phenotypes. Hypertension 36:7–13

Labuda M, Labuda D, Korab-Laskowska M, Cole DEC, Zietkiewicz E, Weissenbach J, Popowska E, Pronicka E, Root AW, Glorieux FH (1996) Linkage disequilibrium analysis in young populations: pseudo–vitamin D–deficiency rickets and the founder effect in French Canadians. Am J Hum Genet 59:633–643

Labuda D, Zietkiewicz E, Labuda M (1997) The genetic clock and the age of the founder effect in growing populations: a lesson from French Canadians and Ashkenazim. Am J Hum Genet 61:768–771

Lander ES, Schork NJ (1994) Genetic dissection of complex traits. Science 265:2037–2048

Langefeld CD, Wagenknecht LE, Rotter JI, Williams AH, Hokanson JE, Saad MF, Bowden DW, Haffner S, Norris JM, Rich SS, Mitchell BD (2004) Linkage of the metabolic syndrome to 1q23-q31 in Hispanic families: the Insulin Resistance Atherosclerosis Study Family Study. Diabetes 53:1170–1174

Lifton RP, Gharavi AG, Geller DS (2001) Molecular mechanisms of human hypertension. Cell 104:545–556

Loos RJ, Katzmarzyk PT, Rao DC, Rice T, Leon AS, Skinner JS, Wilmore JH, Rankinen T, Bouchard C (2003) Genome-wide linkage scan for the metabolic syndrome in the HERITAGE Family Study. J Clin Endocrinol Metab 88:5935–5943

McAdoo WG, Weinberger MH, Miller JZ, Fineberg NS, Grim CE (1990) Race and gender influence hemodynamic responses to psychological and physical stimuli. J Hypertens 8:961–967

Newman DL, Abney M, Dytch H, Parry R, McPeek MS, Ober C (2003) Major loci influencing serum triglyceride levels on 2q14 and 9p21 localized by homozygosity-by-descent mapping in a large Hutterite pedigree. Hum Mol Genet 12:137–144

O'Brien E, Kerber RA, Jorde LB, Rogers AR (1994) Founder effect: assessment of variation in genetic contributions among founders. Hum Biol 66:185–204

Pausova Z, Deslauriers B, Gaudet D, Tremblay J, Kotchen TA, Larochelle P, Cowley AW, Hamet P (2000) Role of tumor necrosis factor-α gene locus in obesity and obesity-associated hypertension in French Canadians. Hypertension 36:14–19

Pausova Z, Gossard F, Gaudet D, Tremblay J, Kotchen TA, Cowley AW, Hamet P (2001) Heritability estimates of obesity measures in siblings with and without hypertension. Hypertension 38:41–47

Pausova Z, Jomphe M, Houde L, Vezina H, Orlov SN, Gossard F, Gaudet D, Tremblay J, Kotchen TA, Cowley AW, Bouchard G, Hamet P (2002) A genealogical study of essential hypertension with and without obesity in French Canadians. Obes Res 10:463–470

Pausova Z, Tremblay J, Hamet P (1999) Gene-environment interactions in hypertension. Curr Hypertens Rep 1:42–50

Peltonen L, Palotie A, Lange K (2000) Use of population isolates for mapping complex traits. Nat Rev Genet 1:182–190

Perola M, Kainulainen K, Pajukanta P, Terwilliger JD, Hiekkalinna T, Ellonen P, Kaprio J, Koskenvuo M, Kontula K, Peltonen L (2000) Genome-wide scan of predisposing loci for increased diastolic blood pressure in Finnish siblings. J Hypertens 18:1579–1585

Province MA, Kardia SL, Ranade K, Rao DC, Thiel BA, Cooper RS, Risch N, Turner ST, Cox DR, Hunt SC, Weder AB, Boerwinkle E (2003) A meta-analysis of genome-wide linkage scans for hypertension: the National Heart, Lung and Blood Institute Family Blood Pressure Program. Am J Hypertens 16:144–147

Ranade K, Hinds D, Hsiung CA, Chuang LM, Chang MS, Chen YT, Pesich R, Hebert J, Chen YD, Dzau V, Olshen R, Curb D, Botstein D, Cox DR, Risch N (2003) A genome scan for hypertension susceptibility loci in populations of Chinese and Japanese origins. Am J Hypertens 16:158–162

Reaven GM (2004) Insulin resistance, cardiovascular disease, and the metabolic syndrome: how well do the emperor's clothes fit? Diabetes Care 27:1011–1012

Rice T, Rankinen T, Province MA, Chagnon YC, Perusse L, Borecki IB, Bouchard C, Rao DC (2000) Genome-wide linkage analysis of systolic and diastolic blood pressure: the Quebec Family Study. Circulation 102:1956–1963

Rioux JD, Stone VA, Daly MJ, Cargill M, Green T, Nguyen H, Nutman T, Zimmerman PA, Tucker MA, Hudson T, Goldstein AM, Lander E, Lin AY (1998) Familial eosinophilia maps to the cytokine gene cluster on human chromosomal region 5q31-q33. Am J Hum Genet 63:1086–1094

Samani NJ (2003) Genome scans for hypertension and blood pressure regulation. Am J Hypertens 16:167–171

Scriver CR (2001) Human genetics: lessons from Quebec populations. Annu Rev Genomics Hum Genet 2:69–101

Siegmund D (2002) Upward bias in estimation of genetic effects. Am J Hum Genet 71:1183–1188

Steil GM, Volund A, Kahn SE, Bergman RN (1993) Reduced sample number for calculation of insulin sensitivity and glucose effectiveness from the minimal model. Diabetes 42: 250–256

Stein CM, Song Y, Elston RC, Jun G, Tiwari HK, Iyengar SK (2003) Structural equation model-based genome scan for the metabolic syndrome. BMC Genet 4:S99

Stoll M, Cowley AW Jr, Tonellato PJ, Greene AS, Kaldunski ML, Roman RJ, Dumas P, Schork NJ, Wang Z, Jacob HJ (2001) A genomic-systems biology map for cardiovascular function. Science 294:1723–1726

Tang W, Miller MB, Rich SS, North KE, Pankow JS, Borecki IB, Myers RH, Hopkins PN, Leppert M, Arnett DK (2003) Linkage analysis of a composite factor for the multiple metabolic syndrome: the National Heart, Lung, and Blood Institute Family Heart Study. Diabetes 52:2840–2847

Turnbull F, Blood Pressure Lowering Treatment Trialists' Collaboration (2003) Effects of different blood-pressure-lowering regimens on major cardiovascular events: results of prospectively-designed overviews of randomised trials. Lancet 362:1527–1535

Ueno T, Tremblay J, Kunes J, Zicha J, Dobesova Z, Pausova Z, Deng AY, Sun YL, Jacob HJ, Hamet P (2004) Rat model of familial combined hyperlipidemia as a result of comparative mapping. Physiol Genomics 17:38–47

von Wowern F, Bengtsson K, Lindgren CM, Orho-Melander M, Fyhrquist F, Lindblad U, Rastam L, Forsblom C, Kanninen T, Almgren P, Burri P, Katzman P, Groop L, Hulthen UL, Melander O (2003) A genome wide scan for early onset primary hypertension in Scandinavians. Hum Mol Genet 12: 2077–2081

Wijsman EM (2002) Joint linkage and segregation analysis using Markov chain Monte Carlo methods. Methods Mol Biol 195:139–161

Woolley N, Holopainen P, Ollikainen V, Mustalahti K, Maki M, Kere J, Partanen J (2002) A new locus for coeliac disease mapped to chromosome 15 in a population isolate. Hum Genet 111:40–45

Am. J. Hum. Genet. 76:833–849, 2005

Over- and Underdosage of *SOX3* Is Associated with Infundibular Hypoplasia and Hypopituitarism

Kathryn S. Woods,[1] Maria Cundall,[2] James Turton,[1] Karine Rizotti,[4] Ameeta Mehta,[1] Rodger Palmer,[6] Jacqueline Wong,[8] W. K. Chong,[7] Mahmoud Al-Zyoud,[9] Maryam El-Ali,[9] Timo Otonkoski,[10] Juan-Pedro Martinez-Barbera,[3] Paul Q. Thomas,[8] Iain C. Robinson,[5] Robin Lovell-Badge,[4] Karen J. Woodward,[2] and Mehul T. Dattani[1]

[1]London Centre for Paediatric Endocrinology, Biochemistry, Endocrinology, and Metabolism Unit, [2]Clinical and Molecular Genetics Unit, and [3]Neural Development Unit, Institute of Child Health, University College London, Divisions of [4]Developmental Genetics and [5]Molecular Neuroendocrinology, MRC National Institute for Medical Research, and [6]North-East London Regional Cytogenetics Laboratory and [7]Department of Neuroradiology, Great Ormond Street Hospital for Children NHS Trust, London; [8]Murdoch Children's Research Institute, Royal Children's Hospital, Melbourne; [9]Department of Paediatric Endocrinology, Hamad Medical Corporation, Doha, Qatar; and [10]Hospital for Children and Adolescents, University of Helsinki, Helsinki

Duplications of Xq26-27 have been implicated in the etiology of X-linked hypopituitarism associated with mental retardation (MR). Additionally, an expansion of a polyalanine tract (by 11 alanines) within the transcription factor *SOX3* (Xq27.1) has been reported in patients with growth hormone deficiency and variable learning difficulties. We report a submicroscopic duplication of Xq27.1, the smallest reported to date (685.6 kb), in two siblings with variable hypopituitarism, callosal abnormalities, anterior pituitary hypoplasia (APH), an ectopic posterior pituitary (EPP), and an absent infundibulum. This duplication contains *SOX3* and sequences corresponding to two transcripts of unknown function; only *Sox3* is expressed in the infundibulum in mice. Next, we identified a novel seven-alanine expansion within a polyalanine tract in *SOX3* in a family with panhypopituitarism in three male siblings with an absent infundibulum, severe APH, and EPP. This mutation led to reduced transcriptional activity, with impaired nuclear localization of the mutant protein. We also identified a novel polymorphism (A43T) in *SOX3* in another child with hypopituitarism. In contrast to findings in previous studies, there was no evidence of MR or learning difficulties in our patients. We conclude that both over- and underdosage of *SOX3* are associated with similar phenotypes, consisting of infundibular hypoplasia and hypopituitarism but not necessarily MR.

Introduction

The pituitary gland consists of anterior, intermediate, and posterior lobes and is a central regulator of growth, metabolism, and development. Its complex functions are coordinated by signals from the hypothalamus that regulate the release of six different hormones secreted by five different cell types in the anterior pituitary. Each cell type is defined by the hormone that is secreted: corticotropes (adrenocorticotrophic hormone [ACTH]), thyrotropes (thyroid-stimulating hormone [TSH]), gonadotropes (luteinizing hormone [LH] and follicle-stimulating hormone [FSH]), somatotropes (growth hormone [GH]), and lactotropes (prolactin) (Dasen and Rosenfeld 2001). The posterior lobe consists primarily of axon-terminal projections from two populations of hypothalamic neuroendocrine neurons, and it secretes vasopressin and oxytocin.

The origins of the anterior and posterior lobes of the pituitary gland are embryologically distinct. Rathke's pouch, the primordial anterior pituitary, arises from the oral ectoderm, whereas the posterior lobe derives from the neural ectoderm of the diencephalon. The apposition of Rathke's pouch and the region of the diencephalon that later develops into the hypothalamus is maintained throughout the early stages of pituitary organogenesis (Takuma et al. 1998) and appears to be critical for normal anterior pituitary development. A number of gene products (Fgf8, Bmp4, and Nkx2.1 [Lazzaro et al. 1991; Ericson et al. 1998; Takuma et al. 1998]) that are expressed in the neural ectoderm but not in Rathke's pouch are thought to play a significant role in normal anterior pituitary development, as illustrated by the phenotype of mouse mutants that are null or hypomorphic for these alleles. These molecules are thought to activate or repress key regulatory genes encoding transcription factors, such as *Hesx1*, *Lhx3*, and *Lhx4*, within the developing Rathke's pouch, and these factors are es-

Received January 19, 2005; accepted for publication March 9, 2005; electronically published March 30, 2005.

Address for correspondence and reprints: Dr. Mehul T. Dattani, London Centre for Paediatric Endocrinology, Biochemistry, Endocrinology, and Metabolism Unit, Institute of Child Health and Great Ormond Street Children's Hospital, 30 Guilford Street, London, WC1N 1EH, United Kingdom. E-mail: mdattani@ich.ucl.ac.uk

0002-9297/2005/7605-0011$15.00

sential for subsequent development of the pituitary (Takuma et al. 1998; Dasen and Rosenfeld 2001).

Failure of normal pituitary development results in congenital hypopituitarism, a condition that is associated with considerable morbidity and occasional mortality if undiagnosed or inadequately treated. Mutations within a number of transcriptional factors have been associated with hypopituitarism in humans, either in isolation or combined with other manifestations, such as optic nerve hypoplasia or a short stiff neck. These genes, mutations of which may be inherited in an autosomal recessive or dominant manner, include *POU1F1* (MIM 173110) (Pfaffle et al. 1992; Radovick et al. 1992), *PROP1* (MIM 601538) (Wu et al. 1998), *HESX1* (MIM 601802) (Dattani et al. 1998), *LHX3* (MIM 600577) (Netchine et al. 2000), and *LHX4* (MIM 602146) (Machinis et al. 2001).

A number of pedigrees with X-linked hypopituitarism and variable degrees of learning difficulty have recently been described. Duplications at Xq26-27 have been described in many of these pedigrees (Hamel et al. 1996; Lagerstrom-Fermer et al. 1997; Hol et al. 2000; Solomon et al. 2002), which together define a 3.9-Mb critical region between Xq26.1 and Xq27.3 (mental retardation, X-linked, with isolated growth hormone deficiency [MIM 300123]) (Solomon et al. 2004). This duplicated region contains 18 annotated transcripts, including well-characterized genes, ESTs, and predicted exon sequences. One of these, the developmental transcriptional factor *SOX3* (MIM 313430), is a good candidate, given that it is expressed in the developing infundibulum in mice, and overexpression in other tissues results in a hypoplastic phenotype in fish (Koster et al. 2000).

SOX3 is a single-exon gene located on the X chromosome in all mammals. It contains an HMG box and is believed to be the gene from which the testis-determining gene *SRY* evolved. On the basis of sequence homology, *SOX3* is closely related to *SOX1* and *SOX2* (MIM 184429), and the products of all three genes belong to the SOXB1 subfamily and are expressed throughout the developing CNS (Collignon et al. 1996). The three genes encoding members of the SOXB1 family are expressed in neuroepithelial progenitor and stem cells from the earliest stages, and there is considerable overlap in their expression patterns.

Recently, an in-frame duplication within *SOX3* that results in an expansion of a polyalanine (PA) tract by 11 alanine residues was described in a pedigree characterized by mental retardation (MR) and short stature due to GH deficiency (Laumonnier et al. 2002). PA expansions have been described in a number of genes associated with diverse human phenotypes (Brown and Brown 2004). These include *FOXL2* (MIM 605597) (Crisponi et al. 2001), *HOXA13* (MIM 142959) (Goodman et al. 2000), *HOXD13* (MIM 142989) (Muragaki et al. 1996), *PABPN1* (MIM 602279) (Brais et al. 1998), *RUNX2* (MIM 600211) (Otto et al. 2002), *ZIC2* (MIM 603073) (Brown et al. 2001), *ARX* (MIM 300382) (Bienvenu et al. 2002; Stromme et al. 2002), and *PHOX2* (MIM 603851) (Nakano et al. 2001). The functional consequences of such expansions are unclear and could be associated with either gain or loss of function. It has been suggested that causative alanine tract expansions within the polyadenine-binding protein nuclear 1 (PABPN1) protein may lead to protein aggregation, with resulting insoluble inclusions and consequent cell death (Brown and Brown 2004), whereas PA expansions within HOXD13 are associated with a shift in localization from the nucleus to the cytoplasm, where the mutant protein forms large amorphous aggregates (Albrecht et al. 2004). Similar cytoplasmic mislocalization was observed in the 11-alanine expansion in SOX3 that was reported by Laumonnier et al. (Laumonnier et al. 2002; Albrecht et al. 2004), although the effects of this expansion on transcription are unknown.

Together, these data suggest that the dosage of *SOX3* could be critical for normal hypothalamopituitary development and that both overdosage (by duplication) and underdosage (by PA tract expansion) could cause hypopituitarism. We therefore sought additional examples of over- and underdosage of *SOX3* among patients with hypopituitarism who were recruited from national and international centers. We now report a submicroscopic duplication at Xq27.1 in association with variable hypopituitarism in two siblings. This duplication spans 685.6 kb and is the smallest described to date, containing only *SOX3* and two other transcripts of unknown function, of which only murine *Sox3* is expressed in the infundibulum. These data strongly implicate *SOX3* duplication as the cause of the hypopituitary phenotype. We have also identified, in three brothers with panhypopituitarism, a novel PA expansion (from 15 to 22 alanine residues) within *SOX3*. We show here that the seven-alanine expansion is associated with loss of transcriptional activation, possibly as a result of its impaired cellular localization. We have also identified a novel polymorphism (A43T) in *SOX3* in a child with hypopituitarism associated with an unusual abnormality of the corpus callosum. In contrast to findings in previous studies (Hamel et al. 1996; Lagerstrom-Fermer et al. 1997; Hol et al. 2000; Laumonnier et al. 2002; Solomon et al. 2002, 2004), there was no evidence of MR or learning difficulties in any of our patients. Both the duplication and the PA expansion mutations in *SOX3* are associated with anterior pituitary hypoplasia (APH), an absent infundibulum, and an ectopic/undescended posterior pituitary. Our data suggest that *SOX3* expression is critical for normal development of the hypothalamopituitary axis in humans, that both over- and underdosage of *SOX3* give rise to a similar phenotype of infundibular hypoplasia and hypopituitarism, and that neither over- nor underdosage of *SOX3* is obligately associated with MR in X-linked hypopituitarism.

Material and Methods

Patient Recruitment

Patients with congenital hypothalamopituitary disorders were recruited into the study from both national and international pediatric and adult endocrinology centers from 1998 through 2004. A total of 76 male probands were screened for mutations within *SOX3,* and 19 were tested for a duplication by interphase FISH. Approval was obtained from the Institute of Child Health/Great Ormond Street Hospital for Children Joint Research and Ethics Committee. Prior to collection of samples and genomic analysis, informed written consent was obtained from the parents and, where applicable, the patients.

Clinical Evaluation

Clinical details were obtained for all patients recruited into the study. These included birth details, perinatal complications, history of consanguinity, family history, and parental heights, as well as the results of standard dynamic tests of pituitary function and magnetic resonance imaging (MRI). For those patients recruited from centers where hormonal assays were performed using different commercial radioimmunoassay kits, normal values for each center were taken into account for the diagnosis of hormone deficiencies.

Interphase FISH for Detection and Characterization of SOX3 *Duplication*

Nineteen individuals (14 sporadic cases and 5 familial cases with presumed X-linked inheritance) with variable degrees of hypopituitarism were screened for duplication of the *SOX3* locus by interphase FISH, performed using a human genomic BAC clone (bA51C14) containing the *SOX3* gene. A control probe was hybridized on a separate slide for each individual, with the use of either another genomic clone from Xq27 or one mapping to Xq22. In many cases, the mother of the affected male was also screened for the presence of possible duplications involving *SOX3*. FISH was performed on cultured lymphocyte nuclei that were isolated from peripheral blood samples by use of standard protocols. The BAC, PAC, or cosmid clones were labeled with Spectrum Green dUTP by nick translation, performed using a Nick Translation kit (Vysis), and this was used in conjunction with a Spectrum Orange–labeled X centromere probe (Vysis). Interphase FISH was performed as described elsewhere, and hybridization signals in >100 nuclei were scored for each slide (Woodward et al. 2003).

Clones around the *SOX3* gene at Xq27.1 (bA197K18, bA35F15, bA364B14, bA189F12, bA359I11, dJ595A18, dJ177G6, and bA338I3) were selected for mapping duplication breakpoints. The clones, which were obtained from the Wellcome Trust Sanger Institute, mapped between positions 137.4 Mb and 138.7 Mb on the X chromosome (Ensembl Genome Browser [NCBI build 34 human genome assembly]).

Genotyping Studies

Polymorphic microsatellite markers mapping near *SOX3* (*DXS1232, DXS8013,* and *DXS984*) and elsewhere on the X chromosome (*DXS6807, DXS9895, DXS6800, DXS1191, DXS8075, DXS6797, DXS8045, DXS1212,* and *DXS1200*) were amplified using fluorescently labeled primers in a standard PCR mix. Cycling conditions were 95°C for 5 min; 30 cycles of 95°C for 45 s, 55°C for 30 s, and 72°C for 45 s; and holding at 72°C for 10 min. Completed reactions were diluted and electrophoresed using an ABI 377 sequencer along with a GeneScan 500 TAMRA size standard (Applied Biosystems) and were analyzed using Genotyper software (Applied Biosystems).

Universal Primer Quantitative Fluorescent Multiplex PCR (UPQFM-PCR)

UPQFM-PCR was performed using primers across the region (see table 1); the method used for UPQFM-PCR was based on that described by Heath et al. (2000). The primary reaction was a standard PCR mix, in a volume of 10 μl, modified only with respect to the concentration of primer (1 pmol, 2 pmol, or 4 pmol of each primer). Up to six pairs of tagged primers were used in each reaction, including two control primer pairs: a primer pair that amplified exon 6 of *PLP1,* which lies on the X chromosome, and one from the *CFTR* locus on chromosome 7. Cycling conditions were 95°C hot start for 15 min; 10 cycles of 94°C for 30 s, 56°C for 45 s, and 72°C for 45 s; and holding at 72°C for 10 min. Secondary PCRs were performed in a total volume of 20 μl, which was seeded with 2 μl of the primary reaction as a template; again, a standard PCR mix was used, with 20 pmol of each universal primer. Cycling conditions were identical to the primary reaction, except that 20 cycles were used. From each completed UPQFM-PCR, 1 μl was electrophoresed on an ABI 377 automatic sequencer (as described above). Dosage of the sequence amplified by each primer pair was calculated from the ratio obtained by dividing the ratio of the fluorescent

Table 1

Primers Used for UPQFM-PCR

The table is available in its entirety in the online edition of *The American Journal of Human Genetics.*

signal from each primer pair to that of each control primer by the same ratio in a group of normal, sex-matched controls.

PCR to Amplify Duplication Breakpoint Junction

Long-range PCR was performed using oligonucleotide primers with a length generally between 25 and 30 nucleotides; the primers were designed using Primer 3 to be near the breakpoint regions mapped by FISH and UPQFM-PCR. A 25-μl standard reaction mix with the following modifications was used: 280 mM dNTPs, 5 μl Q solution (Qiagen), 0.5 μl (0.2 U) diluted ProofStart enzyme (Qiagen) (2 U diluted in 9.2 μl 1 × ProofStart PCR buffer [Qiagen]), and 2.5 U HotStar*Taq* (Qiagen). Cycling conditions were as follows: a 95°C hot start for 15 min; 40 cycles of 95°C for 15 s, 65°C for 30 s, and 68°C for 10 min; and elongation at 68°C for 10 min.

RT-PCR

Ten micrograms of human brain RNA (6–12 wk gestation [ViroGen]) were treated with 1 U DNase I (Invitrogen), in accordance with the manufacturers' recommendations. One hundred pmol random nonamers and oligo d(T) were added to 10 μg RNA, and reverse transcription was performed using Superscript II reverse transcriptase (Invitrogen), followed by incubation with 4 U RNase H (Invitrogen) at 37°C for 30 min. PCR was then performed under standard conditions with the use of oligonucleotide primers specific to *SOX3* (*SOX3*-3F and *SOX3*-3R in Xiang et al. [2000]) and to the Ensembl-annotated genes *ENST00000343662* (RT-1F and RT-1R) and *000329997* (RT-3F and RT-3R). cDNA was also amplified using primers from the *HPRENST00T* gene (HPRT-F and HPRT-R) to check for genomic DNA contamination.

RT-PCR and in situ hybridization analysis of the *ENSMUSG00000036258* and *Sox3* genes was performed as described elsewhere (Solomon et al. 2004). Primers for the following genes were used: *ENSMUSG00000036258* (forward: 5′-catcattcgtcgggaagacctc-3′; reverse: 5′-ccattcggttacgcttgtgc-3′) and *GAPDH* (forward: 5′-cttgctcagtgtccttgctg-3′; reverse: 5′-acccagaagactgtggatgg-3′).

PCR and Automated Sequencing Analysis of DNA

SOX3 is a single-exon gene with a high GC content. Various primer pairs spanning the exon were designed, and different combinations were used for PCR (see table 1) (Xiang et al. 2000). Because of the high GC content of the gene, modified PCR conditions were used; 1 M betaine was included in the PCR mix. An initial denaturation step of 98°C for 15 min was used, followed by the addition of *Taq* enzyme. A standard PCR protocol was then used: 94°C for 4 min; 35 cycles of 94°C for 1 min, 68°C for 30 s, and 72°C for 30 s; and a final extension of 72°C for 10 min. PCR products were treated with shrimp alkaline phosphatase and exonuclease I (PCR Product Presequencing kit [Amersham Biosciences]) prior to sequencing with the ABI Prism BigDye Terminator kit, version 3.1 (Applied Biosystems). The sequencing protocol for *SOX3* was also modified; 1 M betaine was again included in the reaction mix, and an initial denaturation step of 98°C for 15 min was used prior to the addition of the BigDye mix (i.e., BigDye enzyme mix plus dilution buffer) to the PCR products. Sequencing conditions were as follows: 35 cycles of 95°C for 10 s, 62°C for 20 s, and 68°C for 4 min. Sequencing of the duplication breakpoint was performed using a standard sequencing protocol with BigDye version 3.1. The products were directly sequenced using a MegaBace Sequencer (Amersham Biosciences) and were analyzed using Sequencer software (Gene Codes). The sequences that were obtained were compared with the reference sequence (GenBank accession number X71135).

Plasmid Constructs

Since *SOX3* is a single-exon gene, it was possible to amplify the entire gene from both unaffected (wild type) and affected ($A_{(7)}$240∧241 ins) individuals and to clone the wild-type and mutated cDNAs for functional studies. To generate protein for electrophoretic mobility shift assay (EMSA) experiments, *SOX3* cDNAs (*SOX3* and *SOX3*($A_{(7)}$*240∧241 ins*)) were subcloned into the expression vector pCMV/SV-Flag, downstream of the T7 promoter. For the transfection and cell localization experiments, Gal4-SOX3 fusion proteins (Gal4-SOX3 and Gal4-SOX3($A_{(7)}$240∧241 ins)) were constructed as described elsewhere for HESX1 (Brickman et al. 2000, 2001). A reporter construct containing SOX binding sites within the *Hesx1* promoter sequence (Eroshkin et al. 2002), upstream of the firefly luciferase gene, was used in the transcriptional assays. A 570-bp PCR fragment upstream of the initiation ATG was cloned into the pGL3-basic vector (Promega). Primers were 5′-ggcggtaccctgcgttttcattgacaacg-3′ and 5′-ggccctcgagtcttctgggtcgtacagcg-3′. The reporter construct containing reiterated Gal4 binding sites upstream of the SV40 promoter has been described elsewhere (Brickman et al. 2001).

Cell Culture and Transfections

CHO cells were cultured in Dulbecco modified Eagle medium, supplemented with 10% fetal calf serum (FCS) and 2 mM L-glutamine. Transient transfection assays were performed using lipofectamine (Invitrogen), in accordance with the manufacturer's protocol (with modifications). Transfections were performed on three separate occasions, each in triplicate.

Table 2

Endocrine Phenotypes of Patients with *SOX3* Mutation, Duplication, and Polymorphism

Pedigree (Nationality) and Patient	Age at Presentation (years)	Height SDS at Presentation	Weight SDS at Presentation	Concentration of GH (ng/ml)	FT4 (ng/dl)	TSH (μU/ml)	Prolactin (ng/ml)	Peak Cortisol (μg/dl)	Peak LH (IU/liter)	Peak FSH (IU/liter)
A (Finnish):										
1	7.0	−2.8	−.9	1.0	1.0	2.8	6.2	33.7	5.0	4.5
2	.2	−3.8	−1.5	1.3	.6	.01	5.5	2.5	.8	.5
B (Qatari):										
1	3.0	−2.5	NA	1.7	.5	.08	NA	2.0	U	U
2	4.5	−2.5	NA	.7	.7	3.3	7.3	3.9	.5	.5
3	2.7	−1.3	+.7	.7	.5	2.8	NA	3.2	1	<1
C (Ghanaian):										
1	0	NA	−.9	2.2	.7	4.7	34.8	1.8	1.1	.6

Note.—NA = not available; U = undetectable. Normal ranges: peak GH >6.7 ng/ml, FT4 0.9–1.9 ng/dl, TSH 0.5–6.0 μU/ml, peak cortisol >19.8 μg/dl, and prolactin 5–25 ng/ml.

Cell Localization Studies

Cells ($n = 2 \times 10^4$) were seeded into each chamber of a four-chamber tissue culture plate. The DNA concentration of the transfected Gal4-*SOX3* plasmids varied as indicated in the figure legends, but the total amount of DNA transfected per well was normalized to 200 ng by adding the appropriate amount of empty expression vector. Cells were incubated with transfection media (DNA + OptiMem) for ∼15 h and then were refed with normal growth media. Cells were fixed 36 h after transfection in 4% paraformaldehyde. After fixation of the cells, slides were blocked with 10% FCS and then were incubated with an α-Gal4 antibody (Santa Cruz [1:250]) or anti-chick SOX3 antibody (1:500) (a gift from T. Edlund) for 1 h. The slides were washed and incubated with an α-rabbit secondary antibody (Alexa 488 donkey α-rabbit [Molecular Probes]) (1:1,000) for 1 h. Nuclear counterstaining was performed with Vectashield containing 4′,6-diamidino-2-phenylindole dihydrochloride (DAPI) (Vector Laboratories). Immunostaining was then visualized on a Zeiss Axioskop 2 Plus microscope, and images were captured using a Zeiss Axiocam camera.

Dual Luciferase Transfection Experiments

In brief, 1×10^5 cells were seeded into each well of a 12-well plate 24 h prior to transfection with 75 ng of pRL-SV40 *Renilla* luciferase vector (Promega), to control for transfection efficiency, and 100 ng of the appropriate firefly luciferase reporter. The DNA concentrations of the other transfected plasmids varied as indicated in the figure legends, but the total amount of transfected DNA was normalized to 1.2 μg by addition of the appropriate amount of empty expression vector. Cells were incubated with transfection media (DNA + OptiMem) for ∼15 h and then were refed with normal growth media. Cells were collected 24 h later and assayed for luciferase activity following the Dual Luciferase protocol (Promega).

Purification of Recombinant Proteins and Gel Shift Assays

SOX3 proteins were expressed using the TNT Quick Coupled Transcription/Translation System (Promega). EMSAs were performed as described elsewhere (Brickman et al. 1999, 2000), with the use of a consensus binding sequence for SOX proteins present in the mouse *Hesx1* promoter region (Eroshkin et al. 2002) and equivalent amounts of in vitro translated protein. The *SOX3* probe was obtained by annealing the primers 5′-agctcaaacaaata*aacaatt*aactc-3′ and 5′-gtcagagtta*attgtt*tatttgtttg-3′ (italics represent the SOX binding sequence). The annealed probe was radioactively labeled using Ready-To-Go DNA Labeling Beads (−dCTP) (Amersham Biosciences) with ^{32}P dCTP (Amersham Biosciences).

Results

Family A: Overdosage of SOX3

Patient 1.—The first patient presented at age 7 years with a height of 107.6 cm (−2.8 SD score [SDS]), weight of 20.5 kg (−0.9 SDS), and history of hypoglycemia and hyponatremia at birth. The midparental height was 179 cm (+0.2 SDS), with a maternal height of 168 cm (+0.7 SDS). A diagnosis of GH insufficiency was made on the basis of combined insulin/arginine provocation testing (table 2), and the patient was treated with recombinant human GH (rhGH). His FT4 concentrations have ranged from 0.5 ng/dl to 1.0 ng/dl, with normal FT3 concentrations, a basal serum TSH concentration of 2.8 μU/ml, and a peak TSH concentration of 13.9 μU/ml in response to TRH. The variable FT4 concentrations to date may indicate the possibility of evolving TSH deficiency. His serum prolactin and cortisol concentrations were normal. He progressed through puberty spontaneously. His current height is 171 cm (−0.7 SDS) at age 17 years. MRI revealed a hypoplastic anterior pituitary, with hypoplasia of the lower half of the infundibulum and a partially descended posterior pituitary at the tip of the infundibulum. A cyst was noted within the splenium of the corpus callosum, and the septum pellucidum was normal (fig. 1 [*family A, panel a*]). His psychomotor development is normal.

Patient 2.—The half brother of patient 1 presented at age 2 mo (height 54.2 cm [−3.8 SDS]; weight 5.1 kg [−1.5 SDS]) with a history of neonatal hypoglycemia and was found to have severe cortisol, TSH, GH, and gonadotrophin deficiency (table 2). He had hypoplastic genitalia, with both testes palpable high in the inguinal canal and a micropenis. He was treated with thyroxine, rhGH, and hydrocortisone. He is currently 2.5 years old, with a height of 94 cm (+0.6 SDS) and weight of 14.5 kg (+0.4 SDS). MRI revealed hypoplasia of the anterior pituitary, absence of the infundibulum, and an ectopic/undescended posterior pituitary. The corpus callosum was normal (fig. 1 [*family A, panel b*]). He has normal psychomotor development but has been noted to be hyperactive.

Family B: Underdosage of SOX3

Patient 1.—Patient 1 is currently 17 years old. He was born to first-degree consanguineous Qatari parents, and he first presented with short stature (height 83 cm [−2.5 SDS]) at age 3 years. His heterozygous mother is of normal height. General examination revealed two small testes lying in the scrotum. He had elevated fasting triglycerides, and clonidine and L-dopa stimulation revealed low peak GH concentrations (peak GH 1.7 ng/ml and 1.9 ng/ml, respectively) (table 2). The patient showed an excellent response to treatment with rhGH, with a height velocity increasing from 4 cm/year pre-GH to 11 cm/year with rhGH treatment. A CT scan was reported as being normal. A trial period of suspended rhGH treatment was associated with a marked reduction in the patient's height velocity to 1 cm/year. rhGH treatment was therefore recommenced. Although the initial total thyroxine concentration was normal, repeat investigations at age 6.2 years confirmed secondary TSH deficiency (free T4 0.5 ng/dl; TSH 0.08 μU/ml). At age 15 years, he was noted to be prepubertal, with small testes and undetectable concentrations of LH and FSH. Treatment with a depot preparation of testosterone (Sustanon) was therefore commenced. The patient also complained of weakness and was found to have a stimulated serum cortisol concentration of 2.0 μg/dl, confirming ACTH deficiency. Hydrocortisone treatment was therefore commenced. He is currently being treated with Sustanon, rhGH, thyroxine, and hydrocortisone. His cur-

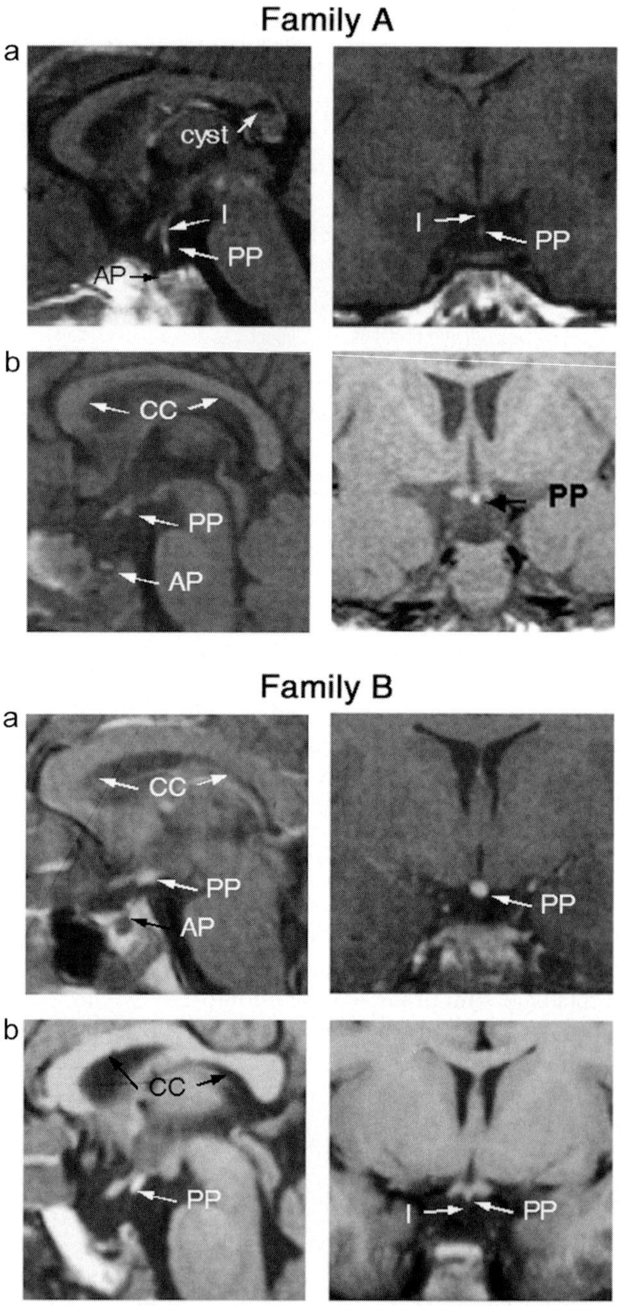

Figure 1 *Family A,* MRI scans in patients with *SOX3* duplication. Coronal and sagittal MRI scans of patient 1 (*panel a*) and patient 2 (*panel b*) from family A, showing APH ("AP"), partial hypoplasia of the infundibulum ("I") in patient 1 (absent in patient 2), and an undescended/ectopic posterior pituitary ("PP") (partial in patient 1). Note the cyst in the corpus callosum identified in patient 1. *Family B,* MRI scans in patients with PA expansion in *SOX3.* Coronal and sagittal MRI scans of patient 2 (*panel a*) and patient 3 (*panel b*) from family B, showing APH ("AP"), hypoplasia of the infundibulum ("I"), and an undescended/ectopic posterior pituitary ("PP").

rent height is 162.5 cm (−1.9 SDS), and his weight is 66.5 kg (+0.2 SDS). His neurodevelopment is normal.

Patient 2.—Patient 2 is currently 15 years old. He presented at age 4.5 years with a height SDS of −2.5 and a poor growth velocity of 4 cm/year. He had a micropenis, with bilaterally undescended testes. Investigations (including a clonidine provocation test) at age 6 years revealed GH deficiency (peak GH 0.7 ng/ml; IGF-1 undetectable), cortisol deficiency (peak cortisol on provocation 3.9 μg/dl), hypothyroidism (FT4 0.7 ng/dl; basal TSH 3.3 μU/ml; peak TSH in response to TRH provocation 24.8 μU/ml [120 min]), and a normal serum prolactin concentration (7.3 ng/ml) (table 2). A 3-mo course of Sustanon led to an increase in the size of the phallus. MRI identified a severely attenuated anterior pituitary gland in the sella turcica, a hypoplastic infundibulum, and an undescended/ectopic posterior pituitary at the level of the third ventricle. The rest of the intracranial structures, including the optic pathways, were normal (fig. 1 [*family B, panel a*]). Treatment with rhGH, hydrocortisone, and thyroxine was commenced. Puberty was induced with Sustanon at age 13.5 years, when the basal and peak serum gonadotrophins following LH-releasing hormone stimulation were <0.5 IU/liter. He has normal neurodevelopment to date, with good school progress. His current height is 159 cm (−1.2 SDS), and his weight is 61.4 kg (+0.6 SDS).

Patient 3.—Patient 3 is currently 13 years old. He was first seen at age 2.7 years, with short stature (height 88.5 cm [−1.3 SDS]; weight 15.2 kg [+0.7 SDS]), micropenis, and undescended testes. Investigations revealed a free T4 concentration of 0.5 ng/dl (normal 0.6–1.9), TSH concentration of 2.8 μU/ml, LH concentration of 1.0 IU/liter, FSH concentration of <1.0 IU/liter, and a low IGF-1 concentration (table 2). Treatment with thyroxine was commenced. Subsequent clonidine provocation testing revealed a peak GH concentration of 0.7 ng/dl, with a stimulated cortisol concentration of 3.2 μg/dl. rhGH and hydrocortisone replacement was commenced. Although the testes descended into the scrotum in response to 3 wk of human chorionic gonadotrophin, the testosterone response was poor (from <0.1 ng/ml to 0.6 ng/ml). His height SDS and weight SDS are currently −0.1 and +1.5, respectively. Pubertal induction was required, and the patient is currently also receiving Sustanon. MRI revealed a small anterior pituitary gland in a small pituitary fossa. The infundibulum was difficult to visualize, since it was severely attenuated, with an ectopic/undescended posterior pituitary (fig. 1 [*family B, panel b*]).

Another male sibling presented at age 9 years with deficiencies of GH (peak GH 2.8 ng/ml on clonidine provocation) and, possibly, gonadotrophin (basal and peak serum LH and FSH <0.5 IU/liter). He has normal serum thyroxine (free T4 1.0 ng/dl), prolactin (8.7 ng/ml), and basal cortisol (12.1 μg/dl) concentrations. Currently, he is 12.5 years old, with a height of 138 cm (−1.8 SDS) and weight of 59.8 kg (+1.9 SDS). MRI revealed APH, an absent infundibulum, and an undescended/ectopic posterior pituitary gland. DNA from this child is unavailable.

Overdosage of SOX3

Identification of a novel SOX3 *duplication.*—A duplication including *SOX3* was found in one family from Finland, with two half brothers affected with differing degrees of hypopituitarism (fig. 2*a*, 2*b*, 2*e*, and 2*g*). Their mother is a carrier of the duplication (fig. 2*c*) and is phenotypically unaffected, with a height of 168 cm; the maternal grandmother does not carry the duplication (fig. 2*d*).

Characterization of duplication.—The size of the duplication was mapped using genomic clones mapping close to *SOX3* (fig. 2*e*). This mapped the extent of the duplication proximal to *SOX3* to between two adjacent genomic clones, ∼500 kb distant from *SOX3*, and the distal end of the duplication mapped within a clone adjacent to bA51C14. Refinement of the location of the two duplication breakpoints was performed by UPQFM-PCR, with the use of unique tagged primer pairs close to the breakpoint regions, as mapped by interphase FISH (fig. 2*e*). We have deduced the size of the duplication from the position of the breakpoints, under the assumption that there are no further deletions/duplications associated with the rearrangement. Long-range PCR amplification across the breakpoint junction was performed using oligonucleotide primers designed within the breakpoint regions, because dual-color interphase FISH, performed using two probes within the duplication, indicated a tandem head-to-tail rearrangement (data not shown). One primer pair combination (35F15R71430 and 595a18F114741), with each oligonucleotide mapping to one end of the duplicated region, amplified a 4–5 kb product from genomic DNA from the members of the family known to carry the duplication, confirming that the duplication rearrangement was in tandem. No amplification was observed with this combination of primers in DNA from normal individuals or the grandmother, who did not carry the duplication.

The use of primers 595A18F116286 and 35F15R-68658 to sequence the breakpoint in both directions from genomic DNA from one of the affected males revealed no homology between the two sequences at either end of the duplication. Four nucleotides (CTCA) were inserted at the breakpoint, consistent with a duplication mechanism involving nonhomologous end joining (Lieber et al. 2003) (fig. 2*f*). The breakpoint at the proximal end of the duplication was located within an AluJb repeat from genomic clone bA35F15, and the distal break-

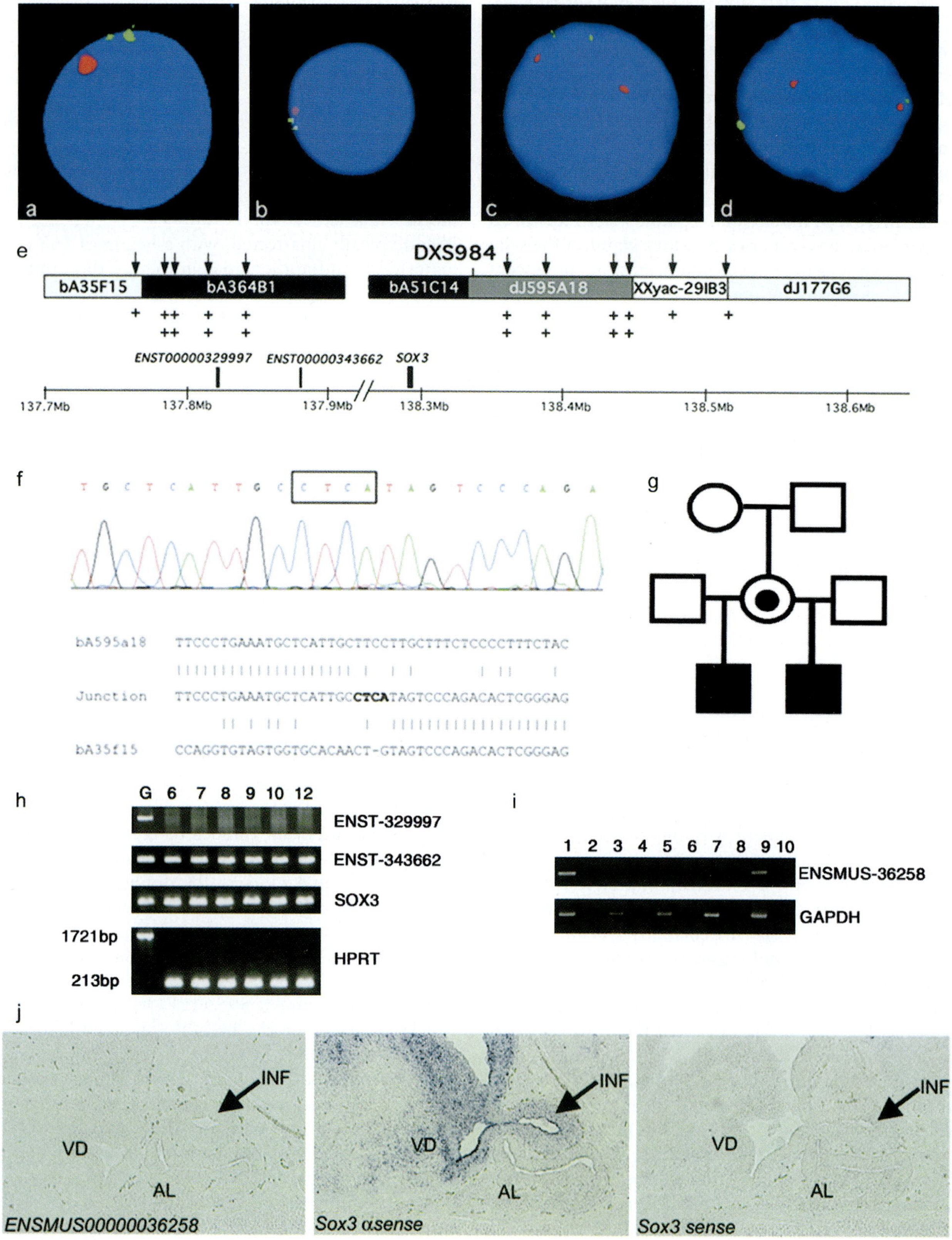
a
b
c
d
e
DXS984
bA35F15
bA364B1
bA51C14
dJ595A18
XXyac-29IB3
dJ177G6
ENST00000329997
ENST00000343662
SOX3
137.7Mb
137.8Mb
137.9Mb
138.3Mb
138.4Mb
138.5Mb
138.6Mb
f
T G C T C A T T G C C T C A T A G T C C C A G A
bA595a18 TTCCCTGAAATGCTCATTGCTTCCTTGCTTTCTCCCCTTTCTAC
Junction TTCCCTGAAATGCTCATTGCCTCATAGTCCCAGACACTCGGGAG
bA35f15 CCAGGTGTAGTGGTGCACAACT-GTAGTCCCAGACACTCGGGAG
g
h
G 6 7 8 9 10 12
ENST-329997
ENST-343662
SOX3
1721bp
213bp
HPRT
i
1 2 3 4 5 6 7 8 9 10
ENSMUS-36258
GAPDH
j
INF
VD
AL
ENSMUS00000036258
Sox3 αsense
Sox3 sense

point was within a unique sequence in genomic clone bA595A18.

The tandem duplication in this family is the smallest described to date (685.6 kb in length). Microsatellite markers on the X chromosome were genotyped to determine the origin of the duplication in the family. Three microsatellites mapping within the duplicated region were typed, but only one, *DXS984* (fig. 2*e*), was informative. Both affected males shared the same allele at this locus, which was inherited from the maternal grandfather (data not shown). No skewing of X inactivation was observed (using a method that is based on differential methylation of *Hpa*II restriction sites near a polymorphic CAG repeat in the androgen receptor gene) in DNA extracted from peripheral blood obtained from the mother, who carried the duplication (data not shown) (Allen et al. 1992).

Expression studies suggest that SOX3 *duplication is associated with an infundibular phenotype.*—The expression of the three genes mapping within the duplicated interval (*SOX3* and two Ensembl-predicted genes, *ENST00000343662* and *ENSG00000329997*) was investigated by RT-PCR. *SOX3* and *ENST00000343662* (a novel coding sequence predicted to contain a proline-rich domain) could be amplified from total human fetal brain RNA (6–12 wk gestation [fig. 2*h*]). However, with the use of E14.5 murine infundibulum, Sox3—but no *ENSG00000343662*-related product (*ENSMUSG00000036258*)—could be amplified (fig. 2*i*). The third predicted human transcript, *ENST00000329997*, was not amplified from human fetal brain (fig. 2*h*). This transcript contains a putative RNA-binding domain with homology to the heterogeneous nuclear ribonucleoprotein family, but it has no murine orthologue, and its biological role remains unclear. Given the above data, and given that murine *Sox3* is expressed within the infundibulum whereas *ENSMUSG00000036258* is not (fig. 2*j*), we suggest that the phenotype in the patients with the 685.6-kb duplication is most likely due to overdosage of *SOX3*.

Underdosage of SOX3

Identification of a novel PA expansion in SOX3.—We next investigated the role of possible loss of *SOX3* function by screening for mutations in *SOX3* in a cohort of 76 patients with variable hypopituitarism. Thirteen cases were assigned as familial (more than one case in each family), whereas 63 cases were assigned as sporadic. The coding region, as well as 145 bp upstream and 121 bp downstream, was sequenced. An expansion by seven alanines of the first PA tract was identified in a consanguineous family (family B) with four affected males ($A_{(7)}240\wedge241$ ins), with the insertion occurring between nucleotides 720 and 721 (the A of the ATG is designated "1") (fig. 3*a* and 3*b*). The mother of these four children was heterozygous for this mutation and did not exhibit significantly skewed X inactivation in DNA extracted from peripheral blood, as observed in family A (data not shown).

SOX3 *Polymorphism*

We identified a novel missense change (c.127 G→A [p.A43T]) in a child originally from Ghana, with spo-

Figure 2 Duplication of *SOX3* in family A. *a–d*, Representative interphase nuclei from four members of the family (older sibling [*a*], younger half brother [*b*], mother [*c*], and maternal grandmother [*d*]), with bA51C14 shown in green and the X centromere shown in red. *e*, Data used to map the extent of the duplication. Clones from the *SOX3* genomic region are shown along with position (in Mb) on the X chromosome (NCBI build 34 assembly of the human genome). The clones duplicated by interphase FISH are blackened, those not duplicated are shaded light gray, and the clone containing the breakpoint is shaded dark gray; unknown duplication status is indicated by the unblackened area. The positions of genes within the duplicated region are designated by blackened boxes above the scale bar. The positions of UPQFM-PCR primer pairs are designated by vertical arrows above the contig. Two plus signs underneath a primer pair indicate that dosage quotients for this primer pair were consistent with a duplication; one plus sign shows that this region had a normal copy number. The position of the informative polymorphic marker, *DXS984*, is also shown. *f*, Electropherogram showing sequence from the duplication breakpoint in family A. The four nucleotides not present in either the proximal or the distal normal sequence are boxed above the electropherogram. Underneath, a ClustalW alignment of the normal distal (bA595A18), normal proximal (bA35F15), and junction sequence is shown, demonstrating that there is no homology at the proximal and distal ends of the duplication. *g*, Pedigree of family A. *h*, RT-PCR for the three genes within the duplication, performed using human brain mRNA at 6, 7, 8, 9, 10, and 12 wk of gestation. Genomic DNA was included as a positive control. Transcripts were present for *SOX3* and a novel gene (Ensembl *ENST00000343662*). The larger 1,721-bp product was not amplified from the brain RNA, showing that there was no genomic DNA contamination. *i*, RT-PCR analysis for *ENSMUSG00000036258* (murine homologue of *ENSG00000343662*), showing expression in the mouse embryo at 14.5 days postcoitum (dpc). Expression was not detected in the hypothalamic/pituitary region, the pituitary progenitor cell line aT1-1, or the adult pituitary. No amplification was evident in the −RT controls, indicating that the cDNA was not contaminated with genomic DNA. *Lane 1,* 14.5–dpc embryo +RT; *lane 2,* 14.5-dpc embryo −RT; *lane 3,* 14.5-dpc hypothalamus/pituitary +RT; *lane 4,* 14.5-dpc hypothalamus/pituitary −RT; *lane 5,* aT1-1 +RT; *lane 6,* aT1-1 −RT; *lane 7,* adult pituitary +RT; *lane 8,* adult pituitary −RT; *lane 9,* genomic DNA as template; *lane 10,* water as a blank. *j,* In situ analysis of the *ENSMUSG00000036258* and *Sox3* genes in the developing murine hypothalamus, infundibulum, and pituitary. No expression of *ENSMUSG00000036258* was detected (*left panel*). *Sox3* is expressed in the infundibulum (*arrow*) and ventral diencephalon but not in the presumptive anterior pituitary (*middle panel*). No staining was observed using the *Sox3* sense control probe (*right panel*). INF = infundibulum; VD = ventral diencephalon; AL = anterior lobe.

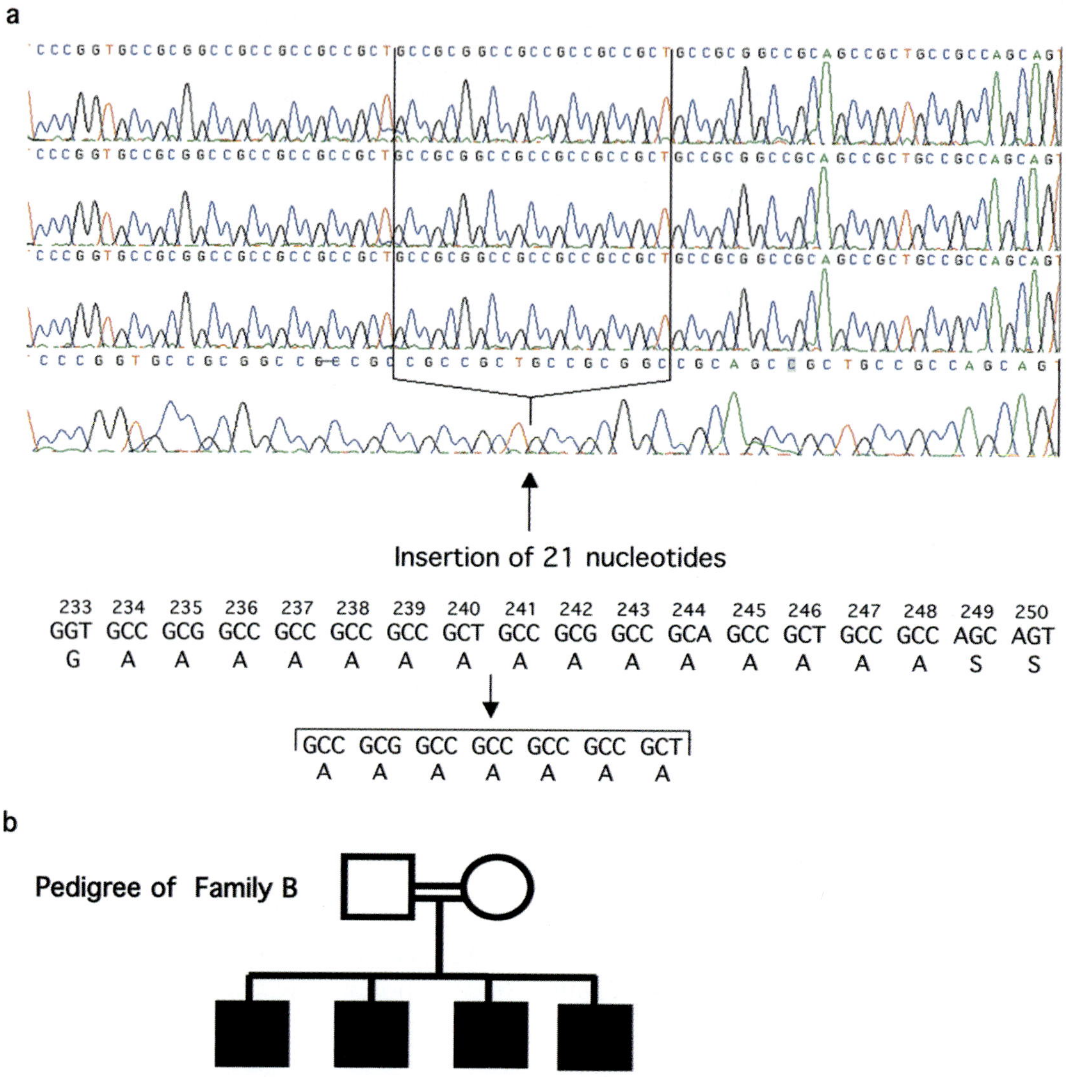

Figure 3 *a*, Protein and genomic sequence showing a PA expansion within *SOX3*. PA expansion (from 15 to 22 alanine residues) in three brothers (*top three electropherograms*) born to a consanguineous union (family B), compared with the normal wild-type sequence (*bottom electropherogram*). *b*, Family tree of a pedigree with a mutation ($A_{(7)}240\wedge241$ ins) within *SOX3*.

radic combined pituitary hormone deficiency (CPHD) (tables 2 and 3). Although this change was not identified in 92 white controls (46 male and 46 female) or in 72 other patients with hypopituitarism, it was identified in a heterozygous state in 3 of 19 normal controls from an Afro-Caribbean background. We therefore conclude that this change is in fact a common Afro-Caribbean polymorphism. A polymorphism was also identified within the first PA tract, as has been described elsewhere (732 A→C) (Raverot et al. 2004). We identified no further changes and found no other expansions in the first PA tract in an additional 72 male patients with hypopituitarism. Previous data have shown no mutations within *SOX3* in 56 patients with idiopathic oligo-/azoospermia and infertility (Raverot et al. 2004); 15 patients with X-linked MR and two Australian families with hypopituitarism (Laumonnier et al. 2002); 8 patients with 46,XX sex reversal and 25 patients with 46,XY gonadal dysgenesis (Lim et al. 2000); and 10 patients with X-linked Rett syndrome (Xiang et al. 2000). Additionally, Laumonnier et al. (2002) sequenced the PA tract in question in 600 normal chromosomes and found no changes.

The Novel PA Expansion within SOX3($A_{(7)}240\wedge241$ ins) Is Associated with Loss of Function

Reporter assays.—To characterize the properties of wild-type and mutant SOX3 proteins, we used the firefly luciferase gene downstream of the proximal promoter of *Hesx1* to make a reporter construct, since this gene

Table 3

Summary of Neuroradiological Findings in Patients with *SOX3* Mutations, Duplications, and Polymorphisms

Pedigree (Nationality) and Patient	Neuroradiological Finding in				
	Anterior Pituitary	Posterior Pituitary	Infundibulum	Corpus Callosum	Septum Pellucidum
A (Finnish):					
1	Hypoplastic	Partially descended	Partial hypoplasia	Cyst	Normal
2	Hypoplastic	Undescended	Absent	Normal	Normal
B (Qatari):					
1	NA	NA	NA	NA	NA
2	Hypoplastic	Undescended	Hypoplastic	Normal	Normal
3	Hypoplastic	Undescended	Hypoplastic	Normal	Normal
C (Ghanaian):					
1	Hypoplastic	Undescended	Absent	Hypoplastic	Normal

Note.—NA = not available.

contains purported binding sites for SOX proteins. In figure 4*a*, increasing amounts of wild-type SOX3 activated the *Hesx1* reporter up to 6-fold in a dose-dependent manner. With the mutated *SOX3* construct, the maximal activation achieved was 3-fold, suggesting that expansion of the PA tract reduced the efficacy of SOX3 in this assay.

This result could be due to the inability of the protein to bind to DNA, or it could be due to an alteration in some other function of the protein (e.g., nuclear localization). To test this, Gal4-SOX3 constructs were cotransfected with a reporter construct containing reiterated Gal4 binding sites (upstream activation sequence [UAS]) upstream of an SV40 promoter driving a luciferase reporter. As shown in figure 4*b*, the loss of activation of the firefly luciferase gene observed with the mutant *SOX3* construct did not appear to reflect direct DNA binding—a finding that supports data from EMSAs that use a consensus binding site for SOX3 (fig. 4*c*). On the other hand, the p.A43T missense sequence variant identified in family C activated transcription and bound to DNA in a manner that was similar to wild-type SOX3 (data not shown), supporting the hypothesis that this change reflects a polymorphic variant.

Cell localization.—Given the hypothesis that nucleocytoplasmic shuttling plays a key role in the function of SOX proteins (Smith and Koopman 2004), we studied the cellular localization of wild-type and mutant SOX3 proteins. First, fusion proteins, with enhanced green fluorescent protein (EGFP) added N- or C-terminal to wild-type or mutant SOX3, were expressed in Chinese hamster ovary (CHO) cells. These showed fluorescence evenly distributed throughout the cell, regardless of the position of the EGFP, with both constructs over a wide range of plasmid concentrations (data not shown).

However, since addition of EGFP could itself cause mislocalization of SOX3 proteins, the experiments were repeated using the wild-type and mutant SOX3/GAL4 fusion constructs, and the transfected, fixed cells were immunostained with antibodies to SOX3 or to the Gal4 DNA-binding domain (fig. 4*d*). These results showed a distinct difference in cellular localization between the wild-type and mutant SOX3 proteins. Wild-type SOX3/Gal4 was predominantly localized to the nucleus of the cell, as would be expected of a transcription factor, although some protein is also present in the cytoplasm. The mutant SOX3/Gal4 protein was largely excluded from the nucleus, although some residual staining was found within the nucleus.

Discussion

Congenital pituitary hormone deficiencies occur in ~1 in 4,000 births. Of these, isolated GH deficiency is the commonest phenotype, followed by CPHD and septo-optic dysplasia. To date, a number of genetic abnormalities have been described in association with these disorders (Dattani and Robinson 2000; Cohen and Radovick 2002). X-linked hypopituitarism is a rare and variable condition. Recent studies have implicated duplications at Xq26-27 in the etiology of this form of hypopituitarism. Solomon et al. (2004) recently narrowed the critical region to a 3.9-Mb interval at Xq27 that contains 18 annotated transcripts. We have now refined the critical interval to a 685.6-kb region in a pedigree in which two half brothers manifest evidence of hypopituitarism. Within this region are three transcripts: *SOX3* and two other transcripts. *ENST0000032997* is not expressed in human fetal brain and does not have a murine homologue. *ENSG00000343662* is expressed in the human fetal brain, but the murine orthologue (*ENSMUSG-00000036258*) is not expressed in the infundibulum. On the other hand, murine *Sox3* is expressed in the infundibulum (Solomon et al. 2004). Hence, our data support the notion that *SOX3* duplication is implicated in the etiology of X-linked hypopituitarism. The first child (patient 1, family A) manifested GH deficiency, with borderline low FT4 concentrations, whereas the second

a

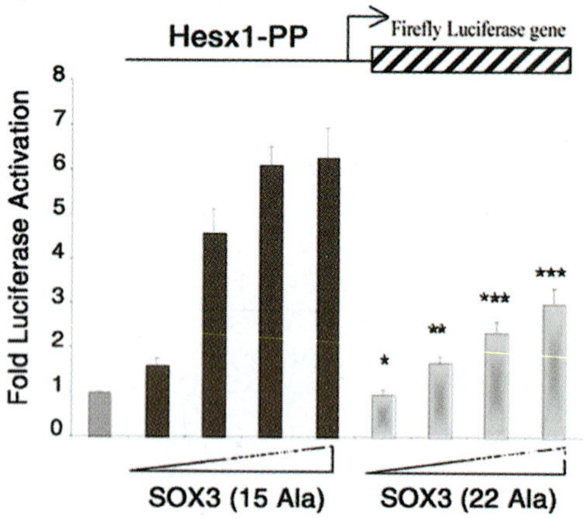
Hesx1-PP
Firefly Luciferase gene
Fold Luciferase Activation
8
7
6
5
4
3
2
1
0
*
**
***
***
SOX3 (15 Ala)
SOX3 (22 Ala)

b

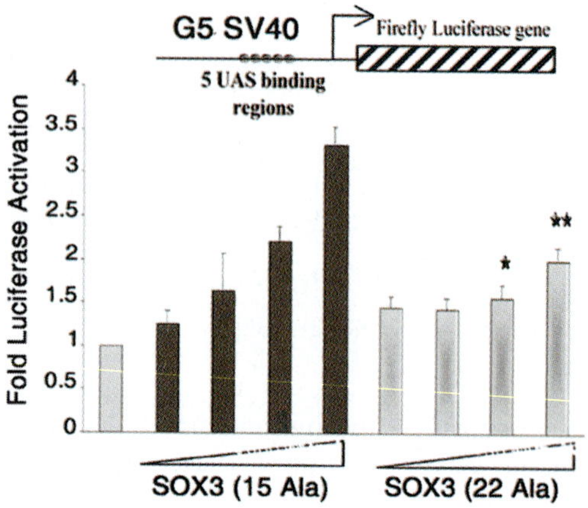
G5 SV40
Firefly Luciferase gene
5 UAS binding regions
Fold Luciferase Activation
4
3.5
3
2.5
2
1.5
1
0.5
0
*
**
SOX3 (15 Ala)
SOX3 (22 Ala)

c

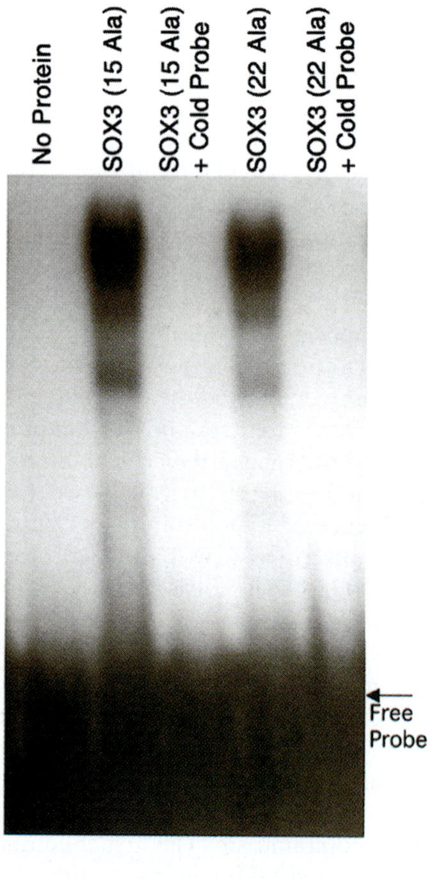
No Protein
SOX3 (15 Ala)
SOX3 (15 Ala) + Cold Probe
SOX3 (22 Ala)
SOX3 (22 Ala) + Cold Probe
Free Probe

d

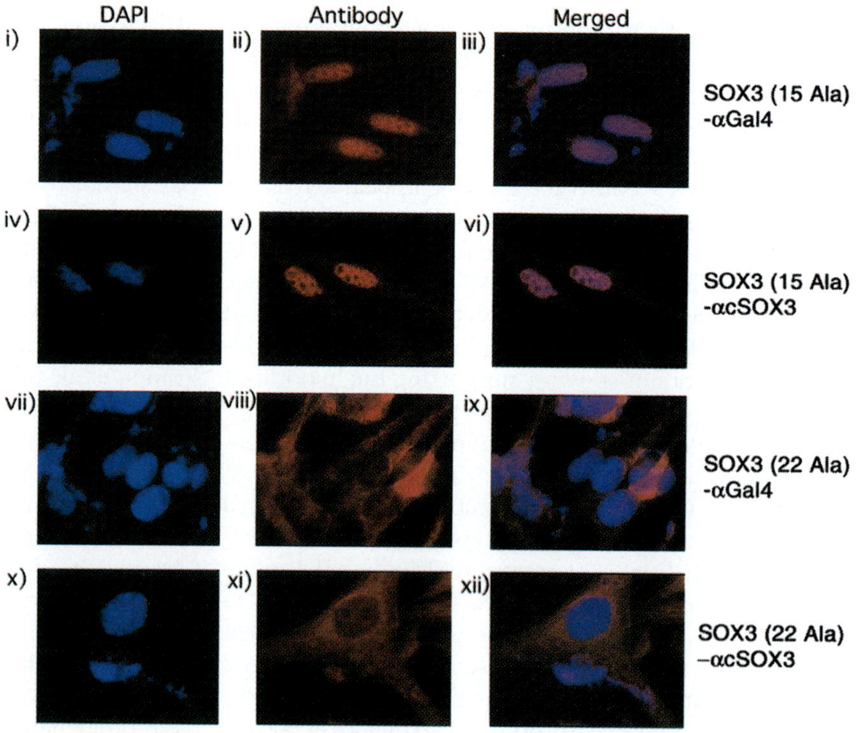
DAPI
Antibody
Merged
i)
ii)
iii)
SOX3 (15 Ala) -αGal4
iv)
v)
vi)
SOX3 (15 Ala) -αcSOX3
vii)
viii)
ix)
SOX3 (22 Ala) -αGal4
x)
xi)
xii)
SOX3 (22 Ala) -αcSOX3

sibling (patient 2, family A) manifested a more severe CPHD phenotype. In keeping with the more severe phenotype in patient 2, the infundibulum was absent in this sibling, whereas that of his half brother, patient 1, was present but was hypoplastic in the distal portion. However, the corpus callosum in patient 1 was abnormal, whereas that in the second sibling was normal, suggesting that *SOX3* is variably implicated in the development of the midline forebrain structures. This variability in phenotype between the two half brothers may reflect differences in genetic background from their different fathers. Their mother, who is a carrier of the duplication, did not manifest an abnormal phenotype. The allele on which the duplication is present was inherited from the maternal grandfather, suggesting either that the duplication was inherited from him, in which case he would have been expected to have an abnormal phenotype, or that it arose de novo in the mother. There was no evidence of skewed X inactivation in DNA extracted from peripheral blood in the mother, but, given that *SOX3* is not expressed in lymphocytes, these data are not surprising and do not exclude the possibility of locally skewed X inactivation (e.g., within the brain and infundibulum).

We have also identified, in three brothers from a consanguineous pedigree, a novel PA expansion within *SOX3* that increases the size of a PA tract from 15 to 22 alanine residues. The phenotype was similar in all three siblings with profound and complete panhypopituitarism in association with APH, an absent or hypoplastic infundibulum, and an ectopic/undescended posterior pituitary. A fourth sibling had GH and possible gonadotrophin deficiencies, but with similar neuroradiological findings. Although DNA was unavailable for genetic testing, it is highly likely that this fourth child also harbored the PA expansion in *SOX3*. The similarity in phenotype may reflect the relative genetic homogeneity of the consanguineous union of their parents.

We have shown that SOX3 can act as an activator of transcription and that the PA expansion was functionally associated with impairment—but not complete loss—of transcriptional activation in this assay. The PA expansion did not appear to affect DNA binding but did lead to impairment of nuclear localization. Thus, the residual transcriptional activity and, hence, partial loss of function might potentially be explained by the presence of some residual SOX3 protein within the nucleus. Our data suggesting that the PA expansion is associated with loss, rather than gain, of function are consistent with those of Albrecht et al. (2004), who have recently shown that PA expansions within Hoxd13 that are associated with synpolydactyly result in a shift in the localization of Hoxd13 from the nucleus to the cytoplasm, where it forms large amorphous aggregates. They suggested that this cytoplasmic aggregation is influenced by the length of the repeat, the level of expression, and the efficacy of degradation by the proteosome. Similar findings have recently been obtained for the previously published PA expansion within SOX3, which resulted in the expansion of the same alanine tract from 15 to 26 alanine residues (Albrecht et al. 2004). The longer PA expansion in this pedigree (Laumonnier et al. 2002) appears to be associated with a more severe phenotype, in that the affected members of the family manifested MR and mild craniofacial abnormalities, in addition to GH deficiency. In contrast, in the present study, the pituitary phenotype is more severe in patients with the shorter PA tract, and none of our patients manifested evidence of MR or learning difficulties. Hence, the relationship between the length of the PA tract and the phenotype remains far from clear, and the brain and infundibulum could be differentially affected, reflecting differences in the relative contributions of the three SOXB1 genes in the two tissues.

The most significant conclusion we draw from these

Figure 4 *a,* Impaired activation of Gal4-SOX3($A_{(7)}$240∧241 ins) (labeled "SOX3 (22 ala)") at SOX binding sites. Increasing concentrations of Gal4-SOX3 (labeled "SOX3 (15 ala)") and Gal4-SOX3($A_{(7)}$240∧241 ins) (10 ng, 100 ng, 500 ng, and 1,000 ng) were cotransfected with the *HESX1* promoter (Hesx1-PP) luciferase reporter. Gal4-SOX3 led to a dose-dependent activation of the *HESX1* promoter (a 6-fold activation at the highest concentration tested), whereas Gal4-SOX3($A_{(7)}$240∧241 ins) was associated with impaired activation (a 3-fold activation at the highest concentration tested). *b,* Impaired activation of Gal4-SOX3($A_{(7)}$240∧241 ins) (labeled "SOX3 (22 ala)") at the SV40 promoter. Increasing concentrations of Gal4-SOX3 (labeled "SOX3 (15 ala)") and Gal4-SOX3($A_{(7)}$240∧241 ins) (10 ng, 100 ng, 500 ng, and 1,000 ng) were cotransfected with the SV40 promoter reporter construct. Gal4-SOX3 led to a dose-dependent activation of the SV40 promoter (a 3.3-fold activation at the highest concentration tested), whereas Gal4-SOX3($A_{(7)}$240∧241 ins) was associated with impaired activation (a 2-fold activation at the highest concentration tested). *a* and *b,* One asterisk (*) indicates $P < .05$, two asterisks (**) indicate $P < .001$, and three asterisks (***) indicate $P < .0001$. The results represent the means of three independent experiments, each performed in triplicate. *c,* Gal4-SOX3($A_{(7)}$240∧241 ins) (labeled "SOX3 (22 ala)") binds to SOX binding sites in a manner that is similar to that of wild-type SOX3 (labeled "SOX3 (15 ala)"). Identical amounts of in vitro translated wild-type SOX3 or SOX3($A_{(7)}$240∧241 ins) (10 μl) were added to the consensus SOX DNA-binding site (*lanes* 2 and 4). Duplicate experiments—but with the addition of 15 pmol of cold probe, showing specific loss of DNA binding—are shown in lanes 3 and 5. Lane 1 shows the effect of free probe in the absence of protein. Western blot analysis showed equivalent expression levels of the constructs (data not shown). *d,* Impaired nuclear localization in Gal4-SOX3($A_{(7)}$240∧241) (labeled "SOX3 (22 ala)"). CHO cells were transfected with 50 ng of the respective plasmid construct, as indicated. Nuclei in the cells were counterstained with DAPI. *Panels i–vi,* wild-type SOX3 (labeled "SOX3 (15 ala)"), using either α-GAL4 (*panels i–iii*) or α-cSOX3 (*panels iv–vi*) antibodies; *panels vii–xii,* Gal4-SOX3($A_{(7)}$240∧241) (labeled "SOX3 (22 ala)"), using either α-GAL4 (*panels vii–ix*) or α-cSOX3 (*panels x–xii*) antibodies.

studies is that the gene dosage of *SOX3* appears to be critical for the normal development of the diencephalon and the infundibulum in humans, since both overdosage and underdosage of *SOX3* are associated with somewhat similar phenotypes. The phenotype is predominantly that of infundibular hypoplasia with variable effects on the corpus callosum. As *SOX3* is not expressed in Rathke's pouch or in the developing anterior pituitary (Collignon et al. 1996; Solomon et al. 2004), the resulting APH is probably secondary, confirming the importance of inductive mechanisms from the hypothalamus and infundibulum on normal anterior pituitary development. An ectopic/undescended posterior pituitary may well directly reflect the effects of infundibular hypoplasia. A similar phenotype has previously been observed in connection with mutations within *HESX1* and *LHX4,* both of which are associated with APH and an ectopic/undescended posterior pituitary (Machinis et al. 2001; Thomas et al. 2001).

These data are consistent with observations in mice, in which *Sox3* is expressed throughout the CNS but particularly in the ventral diencephalon and infundibulum (Rizzoti et al. 2004; Solomon et al. 2004). Mice with *Sox3* deletions are affected with variable reductions in growth rate and in pituitary concentrations of GH, TSH, LH, and FSH, in mice that survived to adulthood. Also, as observed in some of the human patients with the longer PA expansion, 50% of the mutant mice displayed craniofacial defects (Rizzoti et al. 2004). *Sox3* was shown to be required at different levels for the development and function of the hypothalamopituitary axis; indeed, *Sox3* is first necessary in the infundibulum, for correct morphogenesis of Rathke's pouch, and it is also necessary, later, in the hypothalamus, for normal hypothalamopituitary function (Rizzoti et al. 2004). More precisely, in heterozygous female embryos in which one copy of *Sox3* had been deleted and replaced with green fluorescent protein, which was expressed under the control of the *Sox3* promoter, *Sox3* null cells, in which the wild-type copy has been X inactivated, were shown to be clustered in the infundibulum/hypothalamic region. Within this cluster, cell proliferation was reduced, showing a specific requirement for Sox3 in this region. Moreover, the infundibulum was less evaginated, and expression of secreted factors within this territory was expanded, probably explaining the bifurcations that were observed in the pouch and that persist in the adult gland as extra clefts. However, since heterozygous female mice displayed dysmorphic glands but were not affected with hypopituitarism, it is very likely that the hypothalamus, where *Sox3* expression is maintained, is also affected in the *Sox3* null animals. The null mutants also showed dysgenesis of the corpus callosum and failure of the dorsal hippocampal commissure to cross the midline. A similarly variable phenotype was reported in connection with an independent *Sox3*-targeted mutation in mice (Weiss et al. 2003).

The similarity between the null mutant mice and the pedigrees with the PA expansion and duplication described in the present study encourage us in the notion that the PA expansion reflects a loss of function. Given the similarity in phenotype, we cannot rule out the possibility that the duplication could also represent a loss of functional SOX3. It will be interesting to know whether overexpression of *Sox3* in mice generates a phenotype that is similar to that of *Sox3* null mice.

None of the patients in the present study manifested craniofacial defects or any evidence of MR, in contrast to findings in previous reports (Laumonnier et al. 2002). Given that the PA expansion observed in our patients may represent only a partial loss of function and that the duplication reported in the present study is the smallest reported to date, there may indeed be some correlation between the genotype and phenotype, but further studies are required to explore this possibility. Similar dosage dependence has also been suggested in patients with mutations and duplications encompassing *PAX6* (MIM 607108), *SOX9* (MIM 608160), *WNT4* (MIM 603490), and *DAX1* (MIM 300473) (Huang et al. 1999; Jordan et al. 2001; Hanson 2003; Meeks et al. 2003; Vincent et al. 2003). Indeed, normal development of the pituitary gland itself appears to be critically dependent on the timing of expression and dosage of *Hesx1* and *Prop1* in the mouse (Dasen et al. 2001). The underlying mechanism whereby both under- and overdosage of *SOX3* can lead to an abnormal phenotype remains unknown. Although our data are consistent with those of previous studies that have suggested that Sox3 is a transcriptional activator (Uchikawa et al. 1999), recent data have suggested that, in *Xenopus laevis,* Sox3 can repress expression of *Xnr5,* a nodal-related gene that is expressed early in embryonic development (Zhang et al. 2003). This phenomenon—whereby a transcription factor can act as both an activator and a repressor, in a context-dependent manner—has been described elsewhere (Scully and Rosenfeld 2002). In this context, target genes could be critically sensitive to dosage of *SOX3.* It is interesting that our preliminary data suggest that the prevalence of *SOX3* duplications (1/18) and mutations (1/74) in unselected patients with hypopituitarism is comparable to the prevalence of mutations in other transcription factors, such as *HESX1,* but is lower than the prevalence of mutations in the pituitary-specific genes *POU1F1* and *PROP1* (J.T. and M.T.D., unpublished data), although the prevalence increases if the cohort is carefully selected for familial CPHD.

In conclusion, we have shown that the dosage of *SOX3* is critical for the normal development of the infundibulum and, hence, the anterior pituitary in humans. We report the smallest duplication interval containing

SOX3, which suggests that this candidate is the gene most likely to be responsible for the hypopituitarism observed in individuals with duplications of Xq26-27. We also describe patients with a seven-alanine expansion in a PA tract within SOX3 that is associated with impaired transcriptional activity possibly consequent to incorrect cellular localization of the protein. Two of the patients in the present study had abnormalities of the corpus callosum in addition to hypopituitarism, but, in contrast to previous studies, none of our patients showed evidence of learning difficulties or MR. This marked phenotypic variation should be borne in mind when considering potential X-linked GH deficiency and/or MR.

Acknowledgments

We thank all the pediatricians and patients who participated in the study. This study was supported by grants from the Medical Research Council U.K. (to M.T.D., K.S.W., J.T., A.M., and M.C.), the Wellcome Trust (to K.J.W.), Novo Nordisk (to A.M.), and the Child Growth Foundation (to A.M.). Research at the Institute of Child Health and the Great Ormond Street Hospital for Children NHS Trust benefits from research-and-development funding received from the NHS Executive.

Electronic-Database Information

The accession number and URLs for data presented herein are as follows:

Ensembl Genome Browser, http://www.ensembl.org (for *ENST00000343662*, *ENSG00000329997*, and *ENSMUSG 00000036258*)

GenBank, http://www.ncbi.nlm.nih.gov/Genbank/ (for reference sequence [accession number X71135])

Online Mendelian Inheritance in Man (OMIM), http://www.ncbi.nlm.nih.gov/Omim/ (for *POU1F1, PROP1, HESX1, LHX3, LHX4,* mental retardation, X-linked, with isolated growth hormone deficiency, *SOX3, SOX2, FOXL2, HOXA13, HOXD13, PABPN1, RUNX2, ZIC2, ARX, PHOX2, PAX6, SOX9, WNT4,* and *DAX1*)

References

Albrecht AN, Kornak U, Boddrich A, Suring K, Robinson PN, Stiege AC, Lurz R, Stricker S, Wanker EE, Mundlos S (2004) A molecular pathogenesis for transcription factor associated poly-alanine tract expansions. Hum Mol Genet 13:2351–2359

Allen RC, Zoghbi HY, Moseley AB, Rosenblatt HM, Belmont JW (1992) Methylation of HpaII and HhaI sites near the polymorphic CAG repeat in the human androgen-receptor gene correlates with X chromosome inactivation. Am J Hum Genet 51:1229–1239

Bienvenu T, Poirier K, Friocourt G, Bahi N, Beaumont D, Fauchereau F, Ben Jeema L, Zemni R, Vinet MC, Francis F, Couvert P, Gomot M, Moraine C, Van Bokhoven H, Kalscheuer V, Frints S, Gecz J, Ohzaki K, Chaabouni H, Fryns JP, Desportes V, Beldjord C, Chelly J (2002) *ARX,* a novel Prd-class-homeobox gene highly expressed in the telencephalon, is mutated in X-linked mental retardation. Hum Mol Genet 11:981–991

Brais B, Bouchard JP, Xie YG, Rochefort DL, Chretien N, Tome FM, Lafreniere RG, Rommens JM, Uyama E, Nohira O, Blumen S, Korczyn AD, Heutink P, Mathieu J, Duranceau A, Codere F, Fardeau M, Rouleau GA, Korcyn AD (1998) Short GCG expansions in the *PABP2* gene cause oculopharyngeal muscular dystrophy. Nat Genet 18:164–167

Brickman JM, Adam M, Ptashne M (1999) Interactions between an HMG-1 protein and members of the Rel family. Proc Natl Acad Sci USA 96:10679–10683

Brickman JM, Clements M, Tyrell R, McNay D, Woods K, Warner J, Stewart A, Beddington RS, Dattani M (2001) Molecular effects of novel mutations in *Hesx1/HESX1* associated with human pituitary disorders. Development 128:5189–5199

Brickman JM, Jones CM, Clements M, Smith JC, Beddington RS (2000) Hex is a transcriptional repressor that contributes to anterior identity and suppresses Spemann organiser function. Development 127:2303–2315

Brown LY, Brown SA (2004) Alanine tracts: the expanding story of human illness and trinucleotide repeats. Trends Genet 20:51–58

Brown LY, Odent S, David V, Blayau M, Dubourg C, Apacik C, Delgado MA, Hall BD, Reynolds JF, Sommer A, Wieczorek D, Brown SA, Muenke M (2001) Holoprosencephaly due to mutations in *ZIC2:* alanine tract expansion mutations may be caused by parental somatic recombination. Hum Mol Genet 10:791–796

Cohen LE, Radovick S (2002) Molecular basis of combined pituitary hormone deficiencies. Endocr Rev 23:431–442

Collignon J, Sockanathan S, Hacker A, Cohen-Tannoudji M, Norris D, Rastan S, Stevanovic M, Goodfellow PN, Lovell-Badge R (1996) A comparison of the properties of *Sox-3* with Sry and two related genes, *Sox-1* and *Sox-2.* Development 122:509–520

Crisponi L, Deiana M, Loi A, Chiappe F, Uda M, Amati P, Bisceglia L, Zelante L, Nagaraja R, Porcu S, Ristaldi MS, Marzella R, Rocchi M, Nicolino M, Lienhardt-Roussie A, Nivelon A, Verloes A, Schlessinger D, Gasparini P, Bonneau D, Cao A, Pilia G (2001) The putative forkhead transcription factor FOXL2 is mutated in blepharophimosis/ptosis/epicanthus inversus syndrome. Nat Genet 27:159–166

Dasen JS, Barbera JP, Herman TS, Connell SO, Olson L, Ju B, Tollkuhn J, Baek SH, Rose DW, Rosenfeld MG (2001) Temporal regulation of a paired-like homeodomain repressor/TLE corepressor complex and a related activator is required for pituitary organogenesis. Genes Dev 15:3193–3207

Dasen JS, Rosenfeld MG (2001) Signaling and transcriptional mechanisms in pituitary development. Annu Rev Neurosci 24:327–355

Dattani MT, Martinez Barbera JP, Thomas PQ, Brickman JM, Gupta R, Martensson IL, Toresson H, Fox M, Wales JK, Hindmarsh PC, Krauss S, Beddington RS, Robinson IC (1998) Mutations in the homeobox gene *HESX1/Hesx1* associated with septo-optic dysplasia in human and mouse. Nat Genet 19:125–133

Dattani MT, Robinson IC (2000) The molecular basis for developmental disorders of the pituitary gland in man. Clin Genet 57:337–346

Ericson J, Norlin S, Jessell TM, Edlund T (1998) Integrated FGF and BMP signaling controls the progression of progenitor cell differentiation and the emergence of pattern in the embryonic anterior pituitary. Development 125:1005–1015

Eroshkin F, Kazanskaya O, Martynova N, Zaraisky A (2002) Characterization of cis-regulatory elements of the homeobox gene *Xanf-1*. Gene 285:279–286

Goodman FR, Bacchelli C, Brady AF, Brueton LA, Fryns JP, Mortlock DP, Innis JW, Holmes LB, Donnenfeld AE, Feingold M, Beemer FA, Hennekam RC, Scambler PJ (2000) Novel *HOXA13* mutations and the phenotypic spectrum of hand-foot-genital syndrome. Am J Hum Genet 67:197–202

Hamel BC, Smits AP, Otten BJ, van den Helm B, Ropers HH, Mariman EC (1996) Familial X-linked mental retardation and isolated growth hormone deficiency: clinical and molecular findings. Am J Med Genet 64:35–41

Hanson IM (2003) *PAX6* and congenital eye malformations. Pediatr Res 54:791–796

Heath KE, Day IN, Humphries SE (2000) Universal primer quantitative fluorescent multiplex (UPQFM) PCR: a method to detect major and minor rearrangements of the low density lipoprotein receptor gene. J Med Genet 37:272–280

Hol FA, Schepens MT, van Beersum SE, Redolfi E, Affer M, Vezzoni P, Hamel BC, Karnes PS, Mariman EC, Zucchi I (2000) Identification and characterization of an Xq26-q27 duplication in a family with spina bifida and panhypopituitarism suggests the involvement of two distinct genes. Genomics 69:174–181

Huang B, Wang S, Ning Y, Lamb AN, Bartley J (1999) Autosomal XX sex reversal caused by duplication of *SOX9*. Am J Med Genet 87:349–353

Jordan BK, Mohammed M, Ching ST, Delot E, Chen XN, Dewing P, Swain A, Rao PN, Elejalde BR, Vilain E (2001) Up-regulation of WNT-4 signaling and dosage-sensitive sex reversal in humans. Am J Hum Genet 68:1102–1109

Koster RW, Kuhnlein RP, Wittbrodt J (2000) Ectopic Sox3 activity elicits sensory placode formation. Mech Dev 95: 175–187

Lagerstrom-Fermer M, Sundvall M, Johnsen E, Warne GL, Forrest SM, Zajac JD, Rickards A, Ravine D, Landegren U, Pettersson U (1997) X-linked recessive panhypopituitarism associated with a regional duplication in Xq25-q26. Am J Hum Genet 60:910–916

Laumonnier F, Ronce N, Hamel BC, Thomas P, Lespinasse J, Raynaud M, Paringaux C, Van Bokhoven H, Kalscheuer V, Fryns JP, Chelly J, Moraine C, Briault S (2002) Transcription factor SOX3 is involved in X-linked mental retardation with growth hormone deficiency. Am J Hum Genet 71:1450–1455

Lazzaro D, Price M, de Felice M, Di Lauro R (1991) The transcription factor TTF-1 is expressed at the onset of thyroid and lung morphogenesis and in restricted regions of the foetal brain. Development 113:1093–1104

Lieber MR, Ma Y, Pannicke U, Schwarz K (2003) Mechanism and regulation of human non-homologous DNA end-joining. Nat Rev Mol Cell Biol 4:712–720

Lim HN, Berkovitz GD, Hughes IA, Hawkins JR (2000) Mutation analysis of subjects with 46,XX sex reversal and 46,XY gonadal dysgenesis does not support the involvement of SOX3 in testis determination. Hum Genet 107:650–652

Machinis K, Pantel J, Netchine I, Leger J, Camand OJ, Sobrier ML, Dastot-Le Moal F, Duquesnoy P, Abitbol M, Czernichow P, Amselem S (2001) Syndromic short stature in patients with a germline mutation in the LIM homeobox *LHX4*. Am J Hum Genet 69:961–968

Meeks JJ, Weiss J, Jameson JL (2003) Dax1 is required for testis determination. Nat Genet 34:32–33

Muragaki Y, Mundlos S, Upton J, Olsen BR (1996) Altered growth and branching patterns in synpolydactyly caused by mutations in *HOXD13*. Science 272:548–551

Nakano M, Yamada K, Fain J, Sener EC, Selleck CJ, Awad AH, Zwaan J, Mullaney PB, Bosley TM, Engle EC (2001) Homozygous mutations in *ARIX* (*PHOX2A*) result in congenital fibrosis of the extraocular muscles type 2. Nat Genet 29:315–320

Netchine I, Sobrier ML, Krude H, Schnabel D, Maghnie M, Marcos E, Duriez B, Cacheux V, Moers A, Goossens M, Gruters A, Amselem S (2000) Mutations in *LHX3* result in a new syndrome revealed by combined pituitary hormone deficiency. Nat Genet 25:182–186

Otto F, Kanegane H, Mundlos S (2002) Mutations in the *RUNX2* gene in patients with cleidocranial dysplasia. Hum Mutat 19:209–216

Pfaffle RW, DiMattia GE, Parks JS, Brown MR, Wit JM, Jansen M, Van der Nat H, Van den Brande JL, Rosenfeld MG, Ingraham HA (1992) Mutation of the POU-specific domain of Pit-1 and hypopituitarism without pituitary hypoplasia. Science 257:1118–1121

Radovick S, Nations M, Du Y, Berg LA, Weintraub BD, Wondisford FE (1992) A mutation in the POU-homeodomain of Pit-1 responsible for combined pituitary hormone deficiency. Science 257:1115–1118

Raverot G, Lejeune H, Kotlar T, Pugeat M, Jameson JL (2004) X-linked sex-determining region Y box 3 (*SOX3*) gene mutations are uncommon in men with idiopathic oligoazoospermic infertility. J Clin Endocrinol Metab 89:4146–4148

Rizzoti K, Brunelli S, Carmignac D, Thomas PQ, Robinson IC, Lovell-Badge R (2004) SOX3 is required during the formation of the hypothalamo-pituitary axis. Nat Genet 36: 247–255

Scully KM, Rosenfeld MG (2002) Pituitary development: regulatory codes in mammalian organogenesis. Science 295: 2231–2235

Smith JM, Koopman PA (2004) The ins and outs of transcriptional control: nucleocytoplasmic shuttling in development and disease. Trends Genet 20:4–8

Solomon NM, Nouri S, Warne GL, Lagerstrom-Fermer M, Forrest SM, Thomas PQ (2002) Increased gene dosage at Xq26-q27 is associated with X-linked hypopituitarism. Genomics 79:553–559

Solomon NM, Ross SA, Morgan T, Belsky JL, Hol FA, Karnes PS, Hopwood NJ, Myers SE, Tan AS, Warne GL, Forrest SM, Thomas PQ (2004) Array comparative genomic hybridisation analysis of boys with X linked hypopituitarism identifies a 3.9 Mb duplicated critical region at Xq27 containing SOX3. J Med Genet 41:669–678

Stromme P, Mangelsdorf ME, Shaw MA, Lower KM, Lewis

SM, Bruyere H, Lutcherath V, Gedeon AK, Wallace RH, Scheffer IE, Turner G, Partington M, Frints SG, Fryns JP, Sutherland GR, Mulley JC, Gecz J (2002) Mutations in the human ortholog of Aristaless cause X-linked mental retardation and epilepsy. Nat Genet 30:441–445

Takuma N, Sheng HZ, Furuta Y, Ward JM, Sharma K, Hogan LM, Pfaff SL, Westphal H, Kimura S, Mahon KA (1998) Formation of Rathke's pouch requires dual induction from the diencephalon. Development 125:4835–4840

Thomas PQ, Dattani MT, Brickman JM, McNay D, Warne G, Zacharin M, Cameron F, Hurst J, Woods K, Dunger D, Stanhope R, Forrest S, Robinson IC, Beddington RS (2001) Heterozygous *HESX1* mutations associated with isolated congenital pituitary hypoplasia and septo-optic dysplasia. Hum Mol Genet 10:39–45

Uchikawa M, Kamachi Y, Kondoh H (1999) Two distinct subgroups of group B Sox genes for transcriptional activators and repressors: their expression during embryonic organogenesis of the chicken. Mech Dev 84:103–120

Vincent MC, Pujo AL, Olivier D, Calvas P (2003) Screening for *PAX6* gene mutations is consistent with haploinsufficiency as the main mechanism leading to various ocular defects. Eur J Hum Genet 11:163–169

Weiss J, Meeks JJ, Hurley L, Raverot G, Frassetto A, Jameson JL (2003) Sox3 is required for gonadal function, but not sex determination, in males and females. Mol Cell Biol 23: 8084–8091

Woodward K, Cundall M, Palmer R, Surtees R, Winter RM, Malcolm S (2003) Complex chromosomal rearrangement and associated counseling issues in a family with Pelizaeus-Merzbacher disease. Am J Med Genet A 118:15–24

Wu W, Cogan JD, Pfaffle RW, Dasen JS, Frisch H, O'Connell SM, Flynn SE, Brown MR, Mullis PE, Parks JS, Phillips JA, Rosenfeld MG (1998) Mutations in *PROP1* cause familial combined pituitary hormone deficiency. Nat Genet 18:147–149

Xiang F, Buervenich S, Nicolao P, Bailey ME, Zhang Z, Anvret M (2000) Mutation screening in Rett syndrome patients. J Med Genet 37:250–255

Zhang C, Basta T, Jensen ED, Klymkowsky MW (2003) The β-catenin/VegT-regulated early zygotic gene Xnr5 is a direct target of SOX3 regulation. Development 130:5609–5624

Am. J. Hum. Genet. 76:850–858, 2005

Report

Identifying Candidate Hirschsprung Disease–Associated *RET* Variants

Grzegorz M. Burzynski,[1] Ilja M. Nolte,[2] Agnes Bronda,[1] Krista K. Bos,[1] Jan Osinga,[1] Ivan Plaza Menacho,[1] Bas Twigt,[1] Saskia Maas,[4] Alice S. Brooks,[5] Joke B. G. M. Verheij,[3] Charles H. C. M. Buys,[1,3] and Robert M. W. Hofstra[1]

Departments of [1]Medical Genetics and [2]Medical Biology, University of Groningen, and [3]Department of Clinical Genetics, Academic Hospital Groningen, Groningen, The Netherlands; [4]Department of Clinical Genetics, Academic Medical Center, Amsterdam; and [5]Department of Clinical Genetics, Erasmus Medical Center, Rotterdam

Patients with sporadic Hirschsprung disease (HSCR) show increased allele sharing at markers in the 5′ region of the *RET* locus, indicating the presence of a common ancestral *RET* mutation. In a previous study, we found a haplotype of six SNPs that was transmitted to 55.6% of our patients, whereas it was present in only 16.2% of the controls we used. Among the patients with that haplotype, 90.8% had it on both chromosomes, which led to a much higher risk of developing HSCR than when the haplotype occurred heterozygously. To more precisely define the HSCR-associated region and to identify candidate disease-associated variant(s), we sequenced the shared common haplotype region from 10 kb upstream of the *RET* gene through intron 1 and exon 2 (in total, 33 kb) in a patient homozygous for the common risk haplotype and in a control individual homozygous for the most common nonrisk haplotype. A comparison of these sequences revealed 86 sequence differences. Of these 86 variations, 8 proved to be in regions highly conserved among different vertebrates and within putative transcription factor binding sites. We therefore considered these as candidate disease-associated variants. Subsequent genotyping of these eight variants revealed a strong disease association for six of the eight markers. These six markers also showed the largest distortions in allele transmission. Interspecies comparison showed that only one of the six variations was located in a region also conserved in a nonmammalian species, making it the most likely candidate HSCR-associated variant.

Hirschsprung disease (HSCR [MIM 142623]) is caused by the absence of intrinsic ganglion cells in the myenteric and submucosal plexuses of the gastrointestinal tract, resulting in severe intestinal obstructions. HSCR is a heterogenic disorder: a number of genes have been shown to play a role in the disease etiology (Holschneider 1982; Badner et al. 1990; Amiel and Lyonnet 2001). The *RET* gene (MIM 164761) is a main factor in HSCR development. *RET* encodes a transmembrane tyrosine kinase receptor, a protein responsible for triggering a number of downstream signaling pathways involved in crucial processes, such as neural crest cell differentiation, migration, and proliferation (Manie et al. 2001). Mutations in *RET* have been found in up to 50% of familial cases of HSCR.

Received December 20, 2004; accepted for publication February 9, 2005; electronically published March 9, 2005.

Address for correspondence and reprints: Dr. R. M. W. Hofstra, Department of Medical Genetics, Antonius Deusinglaan 4, 9713 AW Groningen, The Netherlands. E-mail: r.m.w.hofstra@medgen.azg.nl

0002-9297/2005/7605-0012$15.00

For the more common sporadic form of HSCR, *RET* coding mutations have been found in not more than 20% of patients (Hofstra et al. 2000; Amiel and Lyonnet 2001). Several studies have shown, however, that the *RET* locus is linked to the disease in almost all familial cases, regardless of their mutation status (Bolk et al. 2000; Gabriel et al. 2002), and is also associated with HSCR in a large proportion of the patients with sporadic HSCR who do not have *RET* coding mutations. Furthermore, recently published articles revealed that similar haplotypes are found in the 5′ region of the *RET* locus in patients from several European populations with HSCR (Borrego et al. 2003; Fitze et al. 2003; Sancandi et al. 2003; Burzynski et al. 2004), indicating the segregation of the same ancestral mutation(s) in the whole European population of patients with HSCR. The identified region of association comprises intron 1 of the *RET* gene and, depending on the markers genotyped by the different groups, different lengths of upstream genomic sequence (Borrego et al. 2003; Fitze et al. 2003; Sancandi et al. 2003; Burzynski et al. 2004). In a previous study, we found that a hap-

Table 1

Sequence Variations in the Common Risk Haplotype, as Compared with the Most Common Nonrisk Haplotype

Position and Type of Variant	NCBI dbSNP Accession No.
−9557G→C	...
−9341C→T	rs3026719
−9256C→G	rs2505989
−7359A→C	rs2505990
−6347G→A	rs2505991
−6093T→C	...
−5669G→C	rs2505992
−4636G→C	rs732610
−4361C→G[a,b]	rs741763
−4201G→A	rs2082107
−4146C→G	...
−3820C→T	rs2505994
−3054G→A	rs2505995
−2897T→C	rs2505996
−2352T→C	rs2505997
−1782G→A	rs2505998
−1260T→C	rs2505999
−719C→T	rs2435366
−200G→A (SNP-5)[a,c]	rs10900296
−196A→C (SNP-1)[a,c]	rs10900297
IVS1+620C→A	rs3123712
IVS1+779T→C	rs2506010
IVS1+1813C→T	rs2435365
IVS1+2157C→T	rs2506011
IVS1+2820T→C	rs1864411
IVS1+2846G→T	rs1864410
IVS1+3104C→T	rs1864408
IVS1+3442A→G	rs2506013
IVS1+3460C→T	rs2435364
IVS1+3470G→A	...
IVS1+3788C→G	rs2506014
IVS1+3991del12	...
IVS1+4247C→G	rs2506015
IVS1+5094T→A	rs2506016
IVS1+5274insCT	...
IVS1+6000C→A[a,b]	rs2435362
IVS1+6136G→T	rs2506019
IVS1+6174G→A	rs2435361
IVS1+6294T→C	rs2506020
IVS1+6383G→C	...
IVS1+6384G→C	...
IVS1+6411G→A	...
IVS1+6751T→C	rs1897001
IVS1+6757A→G	rs1897000
IVS1+6813C→T	rs1896999
IVS1+7236G→A	rs2435359
IVS1+7436A→G	rs2435358
IVS1+7445A→C	rs2506008
IVS1+7994C→G	rs2506007
IVS1+9494C→A	rs2506004
IVS1+10371G→A	rs2435356
IVS1+10813A→G	...
IVS1+11369T→C	rs2506021
IVS1+11476C→T	rs2435342
IVS1−11490T→C	rs2506022
IVS1−11084insG	...
IVS1−10285G→T	rs2435343
IVS1−10032C→T	rs2435344
IVS1−10017C→T	rs2435345
IVS1−9651T→G	...
IVS1−8047C→T	rs2506023
IVS1−7593G→A	rs752975
IVS1−7525C→T	rs752977
IVS1−7477T→A	rs752978
IVS1−7298G→A	...
IVS1−6988G→A	rs2506024
IVS1−6567C→G	...
IVS1−6566G→C	...
IVS1−6393A→G	...
IVS1−6257G→C	rs3128726
IVS1−5791C→T	rs2505541
IVS1−5666C→T	rs2505540
IVS1−5127C→G	...
IVS1−5107T→C	...
IVS1−5038C→T	rs2505539
IVS1−5005A→G	rs2435346
IVS1−4925G→A	...
IVS1−4503G→A	rs2505538
IVS1−4073C→A	...
IVS1−3748C→T	rs2505537
IVS1−3702T→A	rs2505536
IVS1−2863G→A	rs2505535
IVS1−891A→T	...
IVS1−888G→C[a]	...
IVS1−881C→T	...
c135G→A (exon 2)[d]	rs1800858

(*continued*)

Table 1 (continued)

NOTE.—Positions of variations localized upstream the gene refer to *RET* ATG.

[a] SNPs from our previously characterized six-locus ancestral haplotype.

[b] Previously reported in Burzynski et al. 2004.

[c] Previously reported in Sancandi et al. 2003.

[d] Previously reported in Ceccherini et al. 1994.

lotype consisting of six SNPs, spanning 27 kb (from 4 kb upstream of the gene through the whole intron 1), was transmitted from the parents in 55.6% of our patients with sporadic HSCR and was not transmitted in only 16.2% (Burzynski et al. 2004). Moreover, for individuals homozygous for the risk haplotype, the odds ratio to develop HSCR was 21.9, whereas, for the heterozygotes, it was 2.2, suggesting dose dependence of the unknown variants (Burzynski et al. 2004). Three groups tried to correlate specific haplotypes of two SNPs (which were also part of our risk haplotype) located in the basal *RET* promoter (−5 bp and −1 bp from the transcription start site) with reduced *RET* expression by performing functional assays in human cell lines (Fitze et al. 2003; Garcia-Barcelo et al. 2005; Griseri et al. 2005). However, results were not consistent, so these SNPs cannot unambiguously be considered as being pathogenic.

In this study, we attempt to further investigate the region of interest by sequencing 33 kb—from 10 kb upstream of the gene through 23 kb of intron 1 and exon 2—in a patient homozygous for the common risk haplotype and in a healthy control individual homozygous for the most common nonrisk haplotype. To sequence this 33-kb region (NCBI genomic position: 42846516 bp–42880012 bp [chromosome 10]), 49 primer sets were designed. The average size of the amplification product was 750 bp, and, between amplicons, there was an overlap of ∼50 bp. Primer sequences can be found on the Hirschsprung Disease Web site of the University of Groningen Department of Genetics. Samples were sequenced by BaseClear. By restricting the comparison (for economic reasons) to a single patient and a single control individual, one runs the risk of missing SNPs in the comparison. However, since the haplotypes are quite common, one might expect that a SNP responsible for the difference will have a very high probability to be found.

Sequence comparison between the two sequences (the sequence of the common HSCR haplotype and that of the most common control haplotype) revealed 86 different sequence variants (table 1). In intron 1, a deletion of 12 bp was found (IVS+3991), as were two insertions (IVS1+5274insCT and IVS1−11084insG) and two 2-base substitutions (IVS1+6383−84GG→CC and IVS1−6567CG→GC). The remaining 81 variations are all SNPs. All the variations were found in a homozygous state in the patient's DNA as well as in the control's DNA. Table 1 includes, as indicated, five of the six SNPs that form our previously identified haplotype. The sixth marker, IVS1−126G→T, is not included, since the patient's DNA and the control's DNA had the same allele at this locus. Twenty variants were located in the region upstream of the gene, 65 are located in intron 1, and 1 is located in exon 2 (table 1). The sequence-variation frequency in the upstream region is 1/536 bp, and, for the intronic region, it is 1/353 bp. This might indicate a tighter selection mechanism on the upstream sequence, as a consequence of the possible presence of more-important regulatory regions. On the other hand, the common risk haplotype observed in our patients also spans the whole of intron 1, supporting the hypothesis that this intronic region might also be involved in the regulation of *RET* expression.

Since our aim was to delimit the HSCR-associated region by further genotyping, we selected from these 86 sequence variations the most likely candidate disease-associated variants. Variants were first selected on the basis of their location in regions that are conserved among vertebrate species. To identify evolutionarily conserved domains within this 33-kb region, we compared the human genomic sequence with the genomic DNA sequences of chimpanzee (*Pan troglodytes*), rat (*Rattus norvegicus*), mouse (*Mus musculus*), and chicken (*Gallus gallus*) (downloaded from the UCSC Genome Browser database). Sequence comparisons between these species were performed using the freely available tool MULAN (MUltiple sequence Local AligNment and conservation visualization tool) and the software package Clone Manager Professional Suite (Needleman-Wunsch method). Figure 1 shows the level of evolutionary conservation between the chimpanzee, mouse, rat, and chicken, with the human sequence as a reference. Rat and mouse genomes show a comparable level of conservation with the human sequence. There are 11 regions with a similarity >70%. The distal part of the human intron 1 shows no homology with the mouse and rat counterparts, except for the short region just downstream of exon 2 and exon 2 itself. Furthermore, it has to be noticed that the rodents' intron 1 is only 12 kb long—roughly half as long as the human intron 1. Moreover, in the mouse genome, homology to the human intron 1 is found in a region 30 kb upstream of the gene and also in intron 18 of the mouse *Ret* gene (data not shown). This could mean that this region has been translocated either in rodents or in primates, since the chimpanzee's intron 1 is highly similar to that of humans.

A region that is almost identical between rodents and primates (99.5%) is located between the positions −5.7 kb and −5.2 kb, with reference to *RET* ATG (fig. 1). Between the human and chicken sequences, there is hardly any significant similarity. This might imply that conserved transcriptional regulation of *RET* is restricted to mammals. However, similarity was found in the region between positions +9.3 kb and +9.7 kb (corresponding to the human sequence), where strong homology with chimpanzee, rat, and mouse sequences is observed as well (fig. 1). This is the only region conserved among all of the species studied. The second region of moderate conservation in chicken is located in the distal part of the sequence at the beginning of exon 2.

The sequence of the chimpanzee is almost identical to the human sequence, except for a number of repeats, point mutations, and small deletions/insertions. A puzzling observation is that exon 1 is missing from the chimpanzee genome database. Instead, there is a repeated sequence in this position. This is probably a sequencing error, since the chimpanzee genome database is still not assembled well enough, and many gaps exist between contigs.

The occurrence of sequence homology between different species in noncoding regions (including promoter and intron regions) might suggest that these conserved regions contain binding sites for relevant transcription factors. We therefore checked the sequenced genomic region for the presence of specific consensus binding elements for mammalian transcription factors, and we determined whether the identified DNA variants were present in these putative transcription factor consensus binding elements. For this, we used the UCSC Genome Browser and the program GENEQUEST from the DNASTAR software package. We

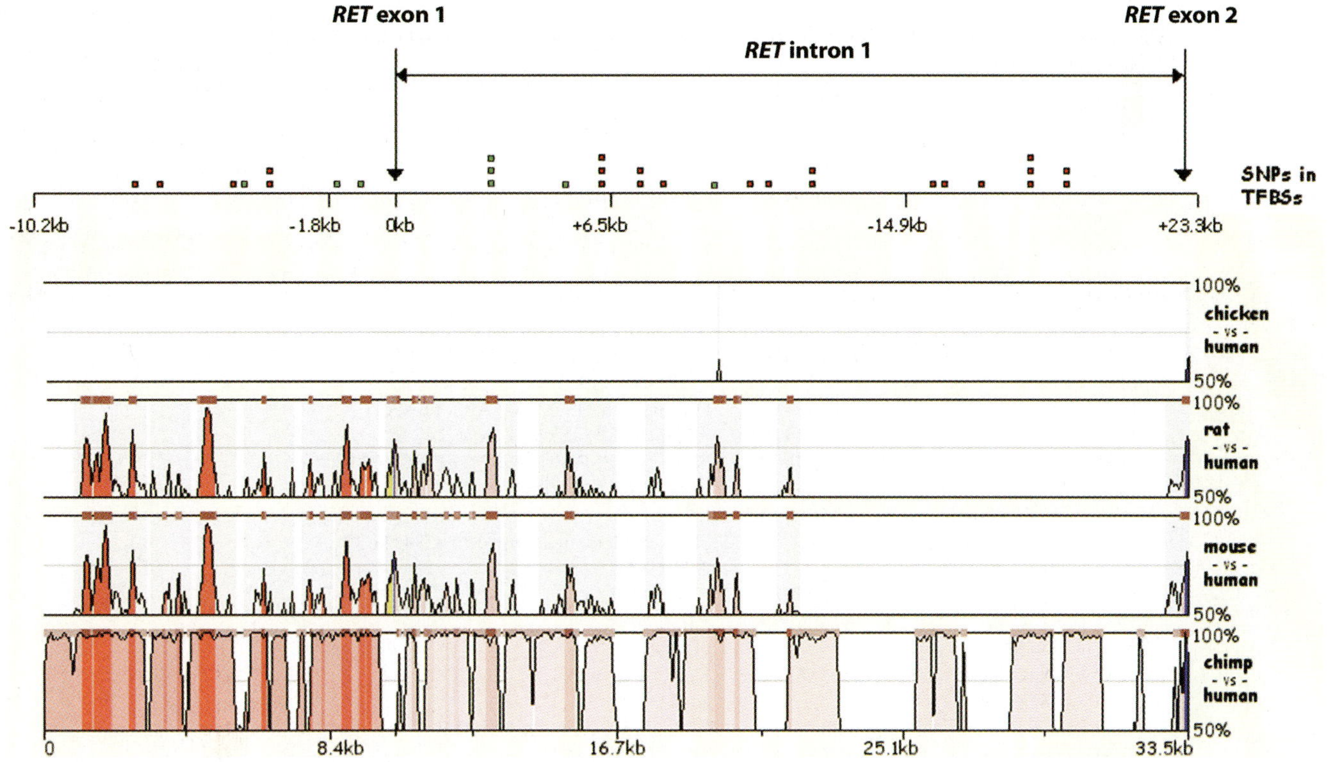

Figure 1 MULAN plots displaying the percentages of similarity of the 5′ region of the *RET* locus in the chicken, rat, mouse, and chimpanzee genomic sequences, compared with the human sequence as a reference. The horizontal gray line indicates 70% identity. The top panel of the figure depicts the positions of the 31 SNPs that are located within putative transcription factor binding sites. Those indicated in green fall in one of the evolutionarily conserved regions. The upper scale refers to *RET* ATG (0 kb). The lower scale represents the length of the whole region. TFBSs = transcription factor binding sites.

aimed to find DNA elements that were lost in the patient's DNA that might result in diminished expression and might thereby explain the HSCR phenotype. We detected 31 base changes that led to the loss of such a binding site (table 2). Among the binding sites that were found, many were recognized by ubiquitous transcription factors such as SP1, AP2, or NF. We also found, however, consensus binding elements for more specifically acting factors, such as Msx1, that play a role in neural tube development (table 2). At the top of figure 1, the approximate positions are given of those SNPs that cause loss of the putative transcription factor binding sites. Eight of them fall in the previously mentioned evolutionarily conserved regions (−4201G→A, −1260T→C, −719C→T, IVS1+2820T→C, IVS1+2846G→T, IVS1+3104C→T, IVS1+5094T→A, and IVS1+9494C→A) (fig. 1; table 2).

Previously, we reported 23 different haplotypes (Burzynski et al. 2004), of which 4 were homozygously present in our patients or controls (2 risk haplotypes and 2 nonrisk haplotypes). We typed individuals homozygous for these four haplotypes by direct sequencing (used for seven SNPs) and by digestion (HpyCH4IV) of amplified PCR products (used for one SNP, IVS1+9494C→A). For four of the eight markers, including the two most proximal SNPs, −4201G→A and −1260T→C, the same alleles were identified on both the risk and nonrisk haplotypes (fig. 2). Four SNPs (−719C→T, IVS1+2846, IVS1+3104, and IVS1+9494) showed perfect segregation with the disease, meaning that one allele was present on a risk haplotype and the other was on a nonrisk haplotype. Therefore, the candidate region for the causal mutation in HSCR is likely bordered by SNP−1260C→A and SNP IVS1−126G→T. As SNPs, −4201G→A and −1260T→C are not part of the candidate region; only SNPs −719C→T, IVS1+2820T→C, IVS1+2846G→T, IVS1+3104C→T, IVS1+5094T→A, and IVS1+9494C→A were subsequently genotyped in all of our families with HSCR. DNA samples used for genotyping were obtained after the receipt of written informed consent from patients with sporadic HSCR and from their parents (only those who resided in the Netherlands); the DNA samples were subsequently referred to clinical genetics centers. Almost all of the families in our study (113 of 117) consist of two parents and an affected child (trios). In three cases, only one parent was available for the study, and one patient participated with his child and spouse. Sixty-four

Table 2

Sequence Variations in the Common Risk Haplotype with Loss of a Hypothetical Consensus Binding Element

Position and Type of Variant	NCBI dbSNP Accession No.	Transcription Factor
−7359A→C	rs2505990	CSS(2)
−6347G→A	rs2505991	AP2/SP1, SP1erk
−4201G→A	rs2082107	SP1-YB1, ApoE-B1
−3820C→T	rs2505994	USF-APP, IgHC.4, NF-mu-E1-CS, GT-2B-RS
−3054G→A	rs2505995	HC5
−2897T→C	rs2505996	NF-E1, NF-E1.6
−1260T→C	rs2505999	MEF3_B
−719C→T	rs2435366	SP1erk, AP2/SP1, SP1-TPI(4), SP1-hsp70, hsp70.2, SP1-IE-3.3,4.5
IVS1+2820T→C	rs1864411	Uteroglobin HS-2.4-C, AP2-TBXAS1
IVS1+2846G→T	rs1864410	AP2/SP1, SP1-erk1(1), JCV
IVS1+3104C→T	rs1864408	NFI-CS3, ELP/SF1/FT2F1, SF1-CYP21
IVS1+5094T→A	rs2506016	BPV-E2.CS2, E2-RS1
IVS1+6294T→C	rs2506020	ETS-1
IVS1+6383−84GG→CC	...	SP1 complement factor, SP1-CS4, HC3
IVS1+6411G→A	...	AP2 CS4
IVS1+6751T→C	rs1897001	PEA3, IE1.2
IVS1+6813C→T	rs1896999	Site-I(2)
IVS1+7445A→C	rs2506008	HNF-5
IVS1+9494C→A	rs2506004	E1AF
IVS1+10813A→G	...	Msx1
IVS1−10032C→T	rs2435344	E2A-CAMLG, E2A, USFAPP
IVS1−10017C→T	rs2435345	SP1-TPI(4), AP-2-β
IVS1−7593G→A	rs752975	GR-MT-IIA
IVS1−7298G→A	...	AP2-CS5
IVS1−5791C→T	rs2505541	AP2-CS5
IVS1−5127C→G	...	TFIID-EIIa
IVS1−5038C→T	rs2505539	Uteroglobin HS-2.4-C, T antigen
IVS1−5005A→G	rs2435346	SP1YB1, MyoD-MCK right site, site F (4,5), AP2-APP
IVS1−3748C→T	rs2505537	AP2-β
IVS1−3702T→A	rs2505536	GR-uteroglobin(1,2), GR/Prconnexin43

patients were screened by means of denaturing gradient gel electrophoresis and sequence analysis (Hofstra et al. 2000) and were found to be negative for *RET* mutations. These 64 were selected from an initial group of 72 patients with sporadic HSCR, of whom 8 appeared to carry a *RET* mutation. Fifty-three of the patients included in the study have not been screened for a *RET* mutation, which therefore may be present in a few of them. As controls for the transmitted haplotypes, the nontransmitted haplotypes of unaffected parents were used, as is also the case in the haplotype-relative-risk method (Falk and Rubinstein 1987; Terwilliger and Ott 1992). The two nontransmitted haplotypes within each trio form pseudocontrol genotypes. Under the hypothesis of random mating in our study population, these pseudocontrol genotypes are expected to be similar to genotypes of population controls and can be used to provide estimates of the number of heterozygotes and homozygotes in the population, as well as estimates of the odds ratios of their risk of developing HSCR. The results of the transmission/disequilibrium tests (TDTs) and the association tests for the six newly selected SNPs and the six SNPs from our previous study are shown in figure 3. All SNPs were strongly associated. For six of them (−200G→A [SNP-5], IVS1+2820T→C, IVS1+2846G→T, IVS1+3104C→T, IVS1+5094T→A, and IVS1+9494C→A), the association was stronger than for the other six. Corresponding allele frequencies were all in the range of 66.7%−68.6% among patients and 21.8%−25.4% among pseudocontrols. Haplotype analysis showed that these six risk alleles are present on the same risk haplotype, CTACCTTAAATA (table 3). Its frequency is estimated to be 53.3% among patients and 15.9% among controls (table 3). Another haplotype, CCACCTTAAATA, which only differs from the risk haplotype at the second SNP (which also contains the risk alleles of our previous six-locus risk haplotype), was present in 6.01% of patients and in 1.5% of controls. Since this haplotype also confers an increased risk, it does not contribute to further restriction of our candidate region.

The question remains: which of the identified variants is contributing to the disease development? Several candidates have already been put forward. SNPs −200G→A

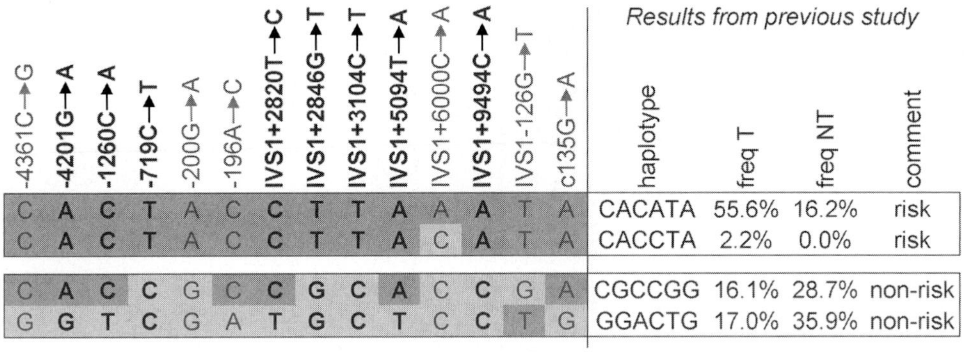

Figure 2 Haplotypes consisting of 14 SNPs—6 from our previous risk haplotype and 8 newly selected ones—of four homozygous individuals. Individuals homozygous for one of the haplotypes identified in our previous study (the corresponding SNPs are indicated in *plain typeface*) were typed for eight new SNPs (indicated in **bold typeface**). They were also homozygous for all eight new SNPs. Risk alleles are in dark gray boxes; nonrisk alleles are in light gray boxes. freq T = frequency of transmitted haplotype; freq NT = frequency of nontransmitted haplotype.

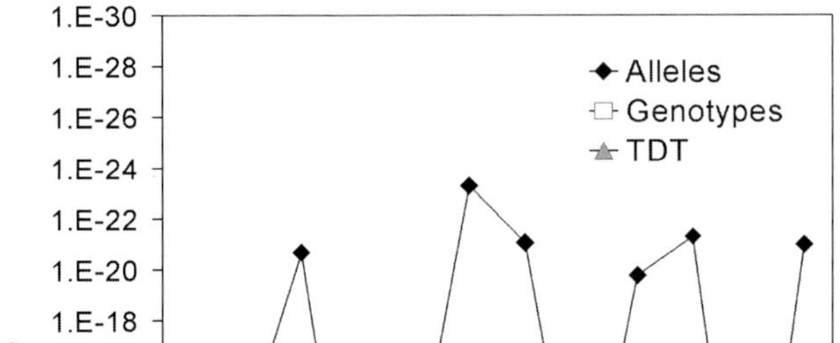

Figure 3 Results of allelic and genotypic association tests and TDT for the 5′ *RET* locus SNPs. Results presented regard markers characterized in the previous study (Burzynski et al. 2004) as well as six new loci. For the single-locus allelic and genotypic association analyses, the frequencies of the alleles and the genotypes, respectively, were compared between patients and pseudocontrols by use of a χ^2 test. Transmission distortion of each allele versus all other alleles together was tested and combined in a multiallelic TDT (Spielman and Ewens 1996). All *P* values and CIs were corrected for multiple testing for independent tests by use of a Bonferroni correction.

(SNP-5) and −196A→C (SNP-1), which were subjects of functional studies (Fitze et al. 2003; Garcia-Barcelo et al. 2005; Griseri et al. 2005) and are part of the risk haplotype identified in our previous study (Burzynski et al. 2004), were not present among the eight variants we selected. These two candidate variations did not fulfill our current criteria, which are based on interspecies sequence conservation and changes in transcription factor binding sites. Nevertheless, Fitze et al. (2003) claimed that SNP −200G→A, in particular, caused reduced *RET* promoter activity. Griseri et al. (2005) found rather contradictory results, as they observed strong cell line dependency and no consistent results in promoter activity assays. These two SNPs are localized in close proximity to a transcription start site. They are part of the *RET* basal promoter, which is conserved in human, mouse, and rat. Because of these contradictory results and because of our findings presented here, it is likely that they are in linkage disequilibrium with mutation(s) lying nearby. The closest polymorphism that we found upstream of SNP-5 is SNP −719C→T, one of our eight selected polymorphisms. It causes the loss of several putative sites recognized by the *SP1* and *AP2* transcription factors. It is likely that this SNP is still a part of the basal promoter and, thus, is a good candidate for future promoter activity studies. Three other SNPs (IVS1+2820T→C, IVS1+2846G→T, and IVS1+3104C→T) lie close together and are located in the proximal part of intron 1, in a region of strong sequence conservation between species (fig. 1, peak from −5.7 kb to −5.2 kb). The most distal SNP of the eight, IVS1+9494C→A, lies in an interesting region, since all species, including chicken, show homology with the human genome at this position (fig. 1, peak from +9.3 kb to +9.7 kb). The occurrence of evolutionarily conserved regions

Table 3

Haplotype Frequencies over 12 SNPs

Allele at Marker												% of Patients	% of Controls
−4361C→G	***−719C→T***	SNP-5	SNP-1	***IVS1+2820T→C***	***IVS1+2846G→T***	***IVS1+3104C→T***	***IVS1+5094T→A***	IVS1+6000C→A	***IVS1+9494C→A***	IVS1−126G→T	c135G→A	(n = 230)	(n = 290)
C	***C***	G	C	***C***	***G***	***C***	***A***	C	***C***	G	G	11.04	20.88
C	***C***	G	C	***C***	***G***	***C***	***A***	C	***C***	G	G	.00	3.43
G	***C***	G	A	***T***	***G***	***C***	***T***	C	***C***	T	G	11.05	24.41
G	***T***	G	A	***T***	***G***	***C***	***T***	C	***C***	T	G	.91	4.64
C	***C***	A	C	***C***	***T***	***T***	***A***	A	***A***	T	A	6.05	1.46
C	***T***	A	C	***C***	***T***	***T***	***A***	A	***A***	T	A	53.31	15.94

NOTE.—Frequencies were estimated by means of an expectation-maximization algorithm implemented in our own software. Newly selected SNPs are in bold italics.

located in an intronic sequence supports the idea that intron 1 is involved in transcriptional regulation. Downstream of the last SNP, IVS1+9494C→A, there is only one more short region of moderate homology in the human and rodent sequences (fig. 1, peak from +11.5 kb to +11.6 kb). Intron 1 in the mouse and rat genomes is only 12 kb long, whereas, in humans, it is 23 kb. This likely results either from a translocation or deletion of this sequence in rodent genomes or from an insertion in primate genomes, since, in the mouse, we found regions of partial homology to the missing sequence 30 kb upstream of *Ret* and also in intron 18 (data not shown).

On the basis of the statistical analyses, no single SNP could be identified as being the causal one (fig. 3). Since the region around SNP IVS1+9494 is the best-conserved region—not only in mammals but also in chicken—this DNA variation is a good candidate for disease susceptibility, although we cannot fully exclude the possibility that a nearby DNA variation(s) that we might have missed could actually be responsible for HSCR or could act in combination with the candidate proposed here. Marker IVS1+9494C→A causes the loss of a binding site of the *ETV4* enhancer (ETS variant gene 4 *E1A* enhancer binding protein, E1AF [DNA-binding sequence TGGACGT]). *ETV4* is a member of the ETS transcription factor family and is a downstream nuclear target of RAS-MAP kinase signaling. Its disturbed functioning was implicated in malignant tumors, such as ovarian carcinoma and breast cancer (Davidson et al. 2004). Transcription factors with an evolutionarily conserved ETS domain play (in general) important roles in cell development, cell differentiation, cell proliferation, apoptosis, and tissue remodeling (Oikawa 2004), which suggests that *ETV4* can influence the HSCR phenotype. Functional studies of *ETV4* and its interaction with *RET* regulatory sequences should follow, to determine the importance of this enhancer in *RET* transcription.

Acknowledgments

This study was supported by the Nederlandse organisatie voor Wetenschappelijk Onderzoek (grants 901-04-210 and 901-04-225).

Electronic-Database Information

The URLs for data presented herein are as follows:

Hirschsprung Disease, University of Groningen Department of Medical Genetics, http://www.rug.nl/med/faculteit/disciplinegroepen/medischegenetica/hereditarydiseases/hirschprungDisease (for additional information about HSCR)
MULAN, http://mulan.dcode.org/
NCBI Home Page, http://www.ncbi.nlm.nih.gov/
Online Mendelian Inheritance in Man (OMIM), http://www.ncbi.nlm.nih.gov/Omim/ (for HSCR and *RET*)
UCSC Genome Browser, http://genome.ucsc.edu/

References

Amiel J, Lyonnet S (2001) Hirschsprung disease, associated syndromes, and genetics: a review. J Med Genet 38:729–739

Badner J, Sieber W, Garver K, Chakravarti A (1990) A genetic study of Hirschsprung disease. Am J Hum Genet 46:568–580

Bolk S, Pelet A, Hofstra RMW, Angrist M, Salomon R, Croaker D, Buys CHCM, Lyonnet S, Chakravarti A (2000) A human model for multigenic inheritance: phenotypic expression in Hirschsprung disease requires both the *RET* gene and a new 9q31 locus. Proc Natl Acad Sci USA 97:268–273

Borrego S, Wright F, Fernandez R, Williams N, Lopez-Alonso M, Davuluri R, Antinolo G, Eng C (2003) A founding locus within the *RET* proto-oncogene may account for a large proportion of apparently sporadic Hirschsprung disease and a subset of cases of sporadic medullary thyroid carcinoma. Am J Hum Genet 72:88–100

Burzynski GM, Nolte IM, Osinga J, Ceccherini I, Twigt B, Maas S, Brooks A, Verheij J, Plaza Menacho I, Buys CHCM, Hofstra RMW (2004) Localizing a putative mutation as the major contributor to the development of sporadic Hirschsprung disease to the RET genomic sequence between the promoter region and exon 2. Eur J Hum Genet 12:604–612

Ceccherini I, Hofstra RM, Luo Y, Stulp RP, Barone V, Stelwagen T, Bocciardi R, Nijveen H, Bolino A, Seri M (1994) DNA polymorphisms and conditions for SSCP analysis of the 20 exons of the ret proto-oncogene. Oncogene 9:3025–3029

Davidson B, Goldberg I, Tell L, Vigdorchik S, Baekelandt M, Berner A, Kristensen GB, Reich R, Kopolovic J (2004) The clinical role of the PEA3 transcription factor in ovarian and breast carcinoma in effusions. Clin Exp Metastasis 21:191–199

Falk CT, Rubinstein P (1987) Haplotype relative risks: an easy reliable way to construct a proper control sample for risk calculations. Ann Hum Genet 51:227–233

Fitze G, Appelt H, Konig I, Gorgens H, Stein U, Walther W, Gossen M, Schreiber M, Ziegler A, Roesner D, Schackert HK (2003) Functional haplotypes of the RET proto-oncogene promoter are associated with Hirschsprung disease (HSCR). Hum Mol Genet 12:3207–3214

Gabriel SB, Salomon R, Pelet A, Angrist M, Amiel J, Fornage M, Attie-Bitach T, Olson JM, Hofstra R, Buys C, Steffann J, Munnich A, Lyonnet S, Chakravarti A (2002) Segregation at three loci explains familial and population risk in Hirschsprung disease. Nat Genet 31:89–93

Garcia-Barcelo M, Ganster RW, Lui VC, Leon TY, So MT, Lau AM, Fu M, Sham MH, Knight J, Zannini MS, Sham PC, Tam PK (2005) TTF-1 and RET promoter SNPs: regulation of RET transcription in Hirschsprung's disease. Hum Mol Genet 14:191–204

Griseri P, Bachetti T, Puppo F, Lantieri F, Ravazzolo R, Devoto M, Ceccherini I (2005) A common haplotype at the 5′ end of the *RET* proto-oncogene underlies genetic susceptibility to

HSCR development through reduced gene expression. Hum Mutat 25:189–195

Hofstra RM, Wu Y, Stulp RP, Elfferich P, Osinga J, Maas SM, Siderius L, Brooks AS, vd Ende JJ, Heydendael VM, Severijnen RS, Bax KM, Meijers C, Buys CH (2000) RET and GDNF gene scanning in Hirschsprung patients using two dual denaturing gel systems. Hum Mutat 15:418–429

Holschneider A (1982) Hirschsprung's congenital megacolon: the concept of physiopathology and therapy. Med Welt 33: 210–213

Manie S, Santoro M, Fusco A, Billaud M (2001) The RET receptor: function in development and dysfunction in congenital malformation. Trends Genet 17:580–589

Oikawa T (2004) ETS transcription factors: possible targets for cancer therapy. Cancer Sci 95:626–633

Sancandi M, Griseri P, Pesce B, Patrone G, Puppo F, Lerone M, Martucciello G, Romeo G, Ravazzolo R, Devoto M, Ceccherini I (2003) Single nucleotide polymorphic alleles in the 5′ region of the *RET* proto-oncogene define a risk haplotype in Hirschsprung disease. J Med Genet 40:714–718

Spielman RS, Ewens WJ (1996) The TDT and other family-based tests for linkage disequilibrium and association. Am J Hum Genet 59:983–989

Terwilliger JD, Ott J (1992) A haplotype-based "haplotype relative risk" approach to detect allelic associations. Hum Hered 42:337–346

Report

Single- and Multilocus Allelic Variants within the $GABA_B$ Receptor Subunit 2 (*GABAB2*) Gene Are Significantly Associated with Nicotine Dependence

Joke Beuten,[1] Jennie Z. Ma,[1] Thomas J. Payne,[2] Randolph T. Dupont,[3] Karen M. Crews,[2] Grant Somes,[4] Nancy J. Williams,[4] Robert C. Elston,[5] and Ming D. Li[1]

[1]Department of Psychiatry, University of Texas Health Science Center at San Antonio, San Antonio; [2]A Comprehensive Tobacco Center, University of Mississippi Medical Center, Jackson, MS; [3]Department of Criminology and Criminal Justice, University of Memphis, and [4]Departments of Preventive Medicine and Dental Hygiene, University of Tennessee Health Science Center, Memphis; and [5]Department of Epidemiology and Biostatistics, Case Western Reserve University, Cleveland

Twelve single-nucleotide polymorphisms (SNPs) in the human γ-aminobutyric acid type B ($GABA_B$) receptor subunit 2 gene (*GABAB2*) were tested for association with nicotine dependence (ND) in an extensively phenotyped cohort of 1,276 smokers and nonsmokers, representing ~404 nuclear families of African American (AA) or European American (EA) origin. The *GABAB2* gene encodes a subunit of the $GABA_B$ receptor for GABA, an inhibitory neurotransmitter involved in the regulation of many physiological and psychological processes in the brain. The gene is located within a region of chromosome 9q22 that showed a "suggestive" linkage to ND. Individual SNP analysis performed using the PBAT-GEE program indicated that two SNPs in the AAs and four SNPs in the EAs were significantly associated with ND. Haplotype analysis using the Family-Based Association Test revealed that, even after Bonferroni correction, the haplotype C-C-G of *rs2491397-rs2184026-rs3750344* had a significant positive association with ND in both the pooled and the AA samples. In the EAs, we identified two haplotypes, C-A-C-A and T-A-T-A, formed by SNPs *rs1435252-rs378042-rs2779562-rs3750344*, that showed a highly significant negative and positive association with ND, respectively. In summary, our findings provide evidence of a significant association of *GABAB2* variants with ND, implying that this gene plays an important role in the etiology of this drug addiction.

Tobacco use is a major worldwide health problem, and nearly one-third of the global adult population smokes tobacco products (United States Department of Health and Human Services [USDHHS] 2000). Nicotine is the primary reward component in tobacco that maintains continued use and results in addiction (USDHHS 2000). Nicotine dependence (ND [MIM 188890]), like many other substance dependencies, is a complex trait determined by strong genetic and environmental factors (Sullivan and Kendler 1999; Li et al. 2003*a*). Our previous meta-analysis of the genetic parameter for ND, which was based on 17 reported twin studies, indicated an average weighted mean polygenic heritability of 0.56 for adult smokers (Li et al. 2003*a*). On the basis of the results from genomewide linkage analyses for smoking behavior, several chromosomal regions appear to harbor susceptibility loci for ND (for recent reviews, see the studies by Uhl et al. [2002] and Li et al. [2004]). However, no susceptibility genes for ND have yet been identified within these positive regions. In addition, although numerous population-based association studies have been conducted to examine the effects of functional candidate genes on ND, only a limited number of variants have been confirmed in multiple cross-sectional studies (Li et al. 2004).

We previously identified an ~13-cM interval on chromosome 9q22 that showed "suggestive" linkage with ND (measured as the number of cigarettes smoked per day, called "smoking quantity") in the Framingham Heart Study (FHS) samples (Li et al. 2003*b*). Furthermore, three additional independent studies reported linkage—at a nominally significant level—of smoking to a region on chromosome 9 overlapping with our linked region (Ber-

Received September 15, 2004; accepted for publication February 21, 2005; electronically published March 9, 2005.

Address for correspondence and reprints: Dr. Ming D. Li, MSC 7792, 7703 Floyd Curl Drive, San Antonio, TX 78229. E-mail: lim2@uthscsa.edu

0002-9297/2005/7605-0013$15.00

Table 1

Clinical Characteristics of the AA, EA, and Pooled Sample Groups

Characteristic	AA	EA	Pooled
No. of families	253	151	404
Average no. of members/family (mean ± SD)	3.1 ± .8	3.2 ± .7	3.2 ± .8
No. of subjects	793	483	1,276
% Female	64.6	68.7	66.1
Age (years) (mean ± SD)	40.0 ± 14.5	41.1 ± 15.2	40.4 ± 14.8
No. of smokers	622	468	990
Age at smoking onset (years) (mean ± SD)	17.2 ± 4.7	15.5 ± 4.4	16.6 ± 4.7
Years smoked (mean ± SD)	21.0 ± 12.7	24.1 ± 12.8	22.1 ± 12.8
SQ/day (mean ± SD)	17.9 ± 12.5	18.0 ± 13.7	18.0 ± 12.9
HSI score (mean ± SD)	3.7 ± 1.4	3.9 ± 1.4	3.8 ± 1.4
FTND score (mean ± SD)	6.3 ± 2.1	6.2 ± 2.2	6.2 ± 2.2

gen et al. 1999; Bierut et al. 2004; Gelernter et al. 2004). The gene encoding the human γ-aminobutyric acid (GABA) type B receptor subunit 2 (*GABAB2*, also called "G-protein–coupled receptor 51" [MIM 607340]) has been mapped to the 9q22.1 region, spans ~420,000,000 bp, and consists of a 3.1-kb coding region that is distributed over 19 exons (Martin et al. 2001). GABA is a major neurotransmitter in the mammalian brain and controls neuronal excitability. The $GABA_B$ receptor inhibits neuronal activity through G-protein–coupled second-messenger systems, which regulate the release of neurotransmitters and the activity of ion channels and adenylyl cyclase (Kaupmann et al. 1998). Two types of $GABA_B$ receptors ($GABA_{B1}$ and $GABA_{B2}$) have been identified (Jones et al. 1998; Kaupmann et al. 1998). Although no unique pharmacological or physiological roles have been determined for either subtype of the $GABA_B$ receptor to date (Schuler et al. 2001), studies in both humans and animals have implicated GABAergic mechanisms in drug dependence, including ND (Dewey et al. 1999; Corrigall et al. 2000). Moreover, baclofen, a widely used $GABA_B$ agonist, is able to antagonize nicotine-rewarding effects in mice and rats (Fattore et al. 2002). Although there are lines of evidence suggesting biological links between *GABAB2* and smoking behavior (Cousins et al. 2001; Fattore et al. 2002), few genetic studies have examined the role of *GABAB2* in the etiology of ND, and no polymorphism in the *GABAB2* gene has been reported to be associated with any addictive behavior. On the other hand, association of the $\alpha 2$ subunit of the $GABA_A$ receptor with alcohol dependence has been reported (Edenberg et al. 2004). The linkage results in the chromosomal 9q22 region, together with a likely biological function of *GABAB2* in drug addiction, make this gene a plausible candidate for association with ND.

The subjects used in this study were of either African American (AA) or European American (EA) origin and were recruited primarily from the mid-South states in the United States from 1999 to 2004. The symptoms of ND of probands and other smoker participants were assessed with the Fagerstrom Test for Nicotine Dependence (FTND) scale (Heatherton et al. 1991). Once a proband was recruited, additional siblings and parents were recruited whenever possible, regardless of smoking status. Extensive clinical data were collected on all participants, including demographics (e.g., sex, age, race, biological relationships, weight, height, years of education, and marital status), medical history, smoking history, smoking experience, ND, and personality characteristics, as assessed by various questionnaires (National Institute on Drug Abuse, Center for Genetic Studies). Of the families recruited, 75.7% (EAs: 74.2%; AAs: 76.7%) had at least two siblings whose FTND score was 5 or above. All subjects agreed to participate in this study and signed the consent form, which was approved by each institutional review board.

In the present study, the ND of each smoker was ascertained by the three most commonly used measures in the literature: smoking quantity (SQ) (also used in our previous linkage study for ND in the FHS samples [Li et al. 2003*b*]); the heaviness of smoking index (HSI [0–6 scale]), which includes SQ and smoking urgency (i.e., how soon after waking up does the subject smoke the first cigarette?); and the FTND score (0–10 scale). Given the presence of overlap in the contents of the three ND measures, there exist fairly robust correlations among them ($r = 0.88$–0.94). The primary reason for running similar analyses for each of the three ND measures was for comparison with previous findings. Demographic and clinical characteristics are presented in table 1. DNA from the participants was obtained using a blood extraction kit from Qiagen. Selection of the SNPs for association analysis was based on (1) a preference for SNPs located in coding or regulatory regions of the gene, (2) high heterozygosity (minor-allele frequency ≥ 0.15), and (3) a uniform coverage of the gene. The 12 SNPs used were selected from the dbSNP, JSNP, and Celera Genomics databases. SNPs *rs3750344* and *rs2304389* are synonymous variants located in exons 2 and 15, respectively, of *GABAB2* (*rs3750344* has an A/G transition at the third

Table 2

***P* Values of PBAT-GEE Statistic for Significant Association (*P* < .05) for Individual *GABAB2* SNPs with Three ND Measures**

SNP ID	Pooled SQ	Pooled HSI	Pooled FTND	AA SQ	AA HSI	AA FTND	EA SQ	EA HSI	EA FTND
rs2304389	***.01***[a,b]	***.01***[a,b]	***.03***[a,b]	.53	.74	.81	.07	.06	.14
rs1435252	***.03***[a,b]	.10	.13	.07	.09	.09	***.003***[a,b]	***.009***[a,b]	***.004***[a], ***.005***[b]
rs3780422	.35	.28	.21	.43	.56	.49	.09	.08	***.04***[a,b]
rs1537959	.09	***.03***[a,b]	.07	***.02***[a,b]	***.007***[a,b]	***.02***[a,b]	.49	.40	.38
rs2491397	***.03***[a,b]	***.03***[a,b]	.07	***.02***[a,b]	***.04***[a,b]	.11	.17	.19	.12
rs2779562	.40	.29	.38	.78	.71	.44	.06	***.01***[a,b,c]	***.008***[c]
rs3750344	.14	.30	.35	.33	.56	.74	***.004***[c], ***.003***[a,b]	***.03***[c], ***.02***[a,b]	***.01***[c], ***.007***[a], ***.006***[b]

NOTE.—Significant *P* values are shown in bold italics. The adjusted *P* value after correction for multiple testing at the .05 significance level is .0043. For the pooled samples, the three ND measures were adjusted for age, sex, and ethnicity; for each ethnic-specific sample group, only age and sex were used as covariates for the ND measures.

[a] Dominant model.

[b] Recessive model

[c] Additive model.

position of the 120th codon for alanine; *rs2304389* has a G/A transition at the third position of the 684th codon for proline). The remaining 10 SNPs are located within intronic regions of *GABAB2*. Data for these SNPs, including their locations within the gene, chromosomal position, allele frequency, and primer/probe sequences, are provided in table A1 (online only). SNPs were genotyped using the TaqMan assay in a 384-well microplate format (Applied Biosystems). Briefly, 15 ng of DNA was amplified in a total volume of 7 μl containing a minor groove binder (MGB) probe and 2.5 μl of TaqMan Universal PCR Master Mix. Amplification conditions were 2 min at 50°C and 10 min at 95°C, followed by 40 cycles of 95°C for 25 s and 60°C for 1 min. Allelic discrimination analysis was performed on the ABI Prism 9700 Sequence Detection System. We applied the PedCheck program (O'Connell and Weeks 1998) to identify any inconsistent Mendelian inheritance, nonpaternity, or other typing errors. To avoid bias, 135 inconsistencies (88 in the AA samples and 47 in the EA samples) among ~18,000 reactions for 12 SNPs were excluded from further statistical analyses.

The pairwise $|D'|$ values for the 12 selected SNPs within *GABAB2* were calculated using the GOLD program (Abecasis and Cookson 2000) and showed a $|D'|$ value of >0.72 for pairwise combinations of *rs1547272*, *rs1930139*, and *rs509747* in the AA, EA, and pooled sample groups (see fig. A1 [online only]). In the AA samples, an additional SNP pair (*rs1537959* and *rs3780422*) showed a $|D'|$ value of >0.72. These findings suggest that the SNPs *rs1547272-rs1930139-rs509747* and SNPs *rs1537959-rs3780422* are part of a single haplotype block. We noticed differences for several SNPs, compared with the allele frequencies presented on various SNP Web sites, when we calculated the allele frequency by directly counting the numbers of each allele from the progenitors of our samples, especially in the AA samples (see table A2 [online only]), suggesting an ethnicity-specific allele distribution.

Association between a single SNP and three ND measures was determined by the Pedigree-Based Association Test (PBAT) program with the use of generalized estimating equations (Lange et al. 2003). Association between each ND measure and a haplotype was examined using the Family-Based Association Test (FBAT) program, with the option of computing *P* values of the *Z* statistic with the use of Monte Carlo sampling under the null distribution of no linkage and no association (Horvath et al. 2004). Three genetic models (additive, dominant, and recessive) were tested, with correction for sex and age in the AA or EA samples and for sex, age, and ethnicity in the pooled samples.

Analysis of individual SNPs indicated a significant association for 4 of the 12 SNPs with at least one age-, sex-, or ethnicity-adjusted ND measure in the pooled samples (table 2). Given the potential genetic differences in ND between ethnic groups, we analyzed all 12 SNPs in the two ethnic groups separately. Two SNPs in the AA samples and four SNPs in the EA samples showed significant or highly significant association with at least one ND measure under different genetic models. The association of SNPs *rs1435252* and *rs3750344* in the EA samples remained significant with the adjusted SQ and FTND after correction for multiple testing, on the basis of the SNP spectral decomposition approach (Nyholt 2004).

Haplotype analysis of SNPs *rs2491397*, *rs2184026*, and *rs3750344*, which cover ~135 kb of *GABAB2*, revealed four major haplotypes (⩾5%) in the AA samples and five major haplotypes in the pooled and EA samples.

Table 3

Z Values and Permutation P Values for Highly Significant Association ($P < .01$) of Major Haplotypes Formed by a Three- or Four-SNP Combination within *GABAB2* with Three ND Measures

No. of SNPs and Haplotype	Pooled %	Pooled SQ	Pooled HSI	Pooled FTND	AA %	AA SQ	AA HSI	AA FTND	EA %	EA SQ	EA HSI	EA FTND
Three:[a]												
C-C-G	6.2	***3.65 (.0002)***[b], ***3.73 (.0002)***[c]	***3.69 (.0002)***[b], ***3.74 (.0002)***[c]	***3.98 (.0001)***[b], ***4.02 (.0001)***[c]	7.6	***3.03 (.002)***[b], ***3.12 (.002)***[c]	***3.20 (.001)***[b], ***3.26 (.001)***[c]	***3.50 (.0003)***[b], ***3.55 (.0004)***[c]	3.9	1.98 (.05)	1.59 (.12)	1.73 (.10)
Four:[d]												
C-A-C-A	7.7	−1.05 (.33)	−1.19 (.24)	−1.07 (.29)	4.6	2.22 (.028)[b], 2.24 (.02)[c]	2.21 (.03)[b], 2.2 (.02)[c]	2.10 (.03)[b], 2.07 (.04)[c]	12.8	***−3.05 (.001)***[b], ***−3.28 (.0006)***[c]	***−3.22 (.0009)***[b], ***−3.40 (.0003)***[c]	***−3.03 (.001)***[b], ***−3.16 (.0008)***[c]
T-A-T-A	3.8	1.61 (.11)	1.30 (.18)	1.69 (.09)	2.6	−.11 (.90)	−.47 (.64)	−.24 (.81)	6.6	2.41 (.015)[b], 2.28 (.024)[c]	2.43 (.014)[b], 2.42 (.017)[c]	***2.73 (.006)***[b], ***2.69 (.007)***[c]

Note.—Significant P values are shown in bold italics. The adjusted P value at the .01 significance level after Bonferroni correction for five major haplotypes formed by the three SNPs in the pooled samples is .002, and, for the four major haplotypes in the AA samples, the adjusted P value is .0025. The adjusted P values for six major haplotypes formed by the four SNPs in the EA samples are .0083 and .0016 for the .05 and .01 significance levels, respectively. The ND measures used in the analysis were corrected for age, sex, and ethnicity in the pooled samples and for age and sex in each ethnic-specific sample group.

[a] *rs2491397-rs2184026-rs3750344.*

[b] Additive model.

[c] Dominant model.

[d] *rs1435252-rs3780422-rs2779562-rs3750344.*

In both the pooled and the AA samples, the C-C-G haplotype of the three SNPs, with a frequency of 6.2% and 7.6%, respectively, showed a highly significant positive association with the three adjusted ND measures (max $Z = 4.02$ and permutation $P = .00001$ for association with FTND in the pooled samples and max $Z = 3.55$ and permutation $P = .0004$ for association with FTND in the AA samples, with 76 and 58 families contributing to the associations, respectively) (see table 3). These results remained highly significant after Bonferroni correction for testing of the major haplotypes in each sample group. In the EA samples, we did not find a haplotype for these three SNPs that remained significantly associated with ND after Bonferroni correction.

Haplotype analysis of the *rs1435252-rs3780422-rs2779562-rs3750344* combination, which covers a region extending from exon 2 to intron 13 of *GABAB2* (~237 kb), revealed eight major haplotypes in the pooled and AA samples and six major haplotypes in the EA samples. In the EA samples, the haplotype consisting of alleles C-A-C-A at a frequency of 12.8% showed a highly significant inverse association, even after Bonferroni correction, with all three adjusted ND measures (max $Z = -3.40$ and permutation $P = .0003$ for HSI, with 33 families contributing to the analysis) (see table 3). Additionally, in this EA sample group, we found another haplotype (T-A-T-A) that was formed by the same four SNPs at a frequency of 6.6% and that showed a significant association with the three adjusted ND measures; however, this haplotype only remained significant for FTND after Bonferroni correction (table 3). These findings indicate haplotype specificities in the two ethnic groups and further suggest different effects of haplotypes within *GABAB2* on ND in AAs and EAs.

Our study has several advantages. We chose to use the single-marker PBAT program because it allows correction for covariates such as age, sex, and/or ethnicity. This represents an important feature for our analysis, as age, sex, and ethnic differences have been documented for ND (Heath et al. 1999; Madden et al. 1999; Li et al. 2003*a*; Tyndale 2003). We used a family-based approach for association analysis, which has an advantage over unconditional analyses (e.g., case-control analysis), in that it minimizes the potential for the confounding effects of population stratification. Furthermore, large samples of smokers and nonsmokers from two ethnic groups were analyzed, which allowed analysis of interethnic differences. Extensive phenotypic data on the individuals were collected, which can be used to investigate different aspects of ND in future studies. The three ND measures analyzed herein are commonly employed in the genetic research and clinical settings of tobacco smoking and thus would be readily available for cross-study replication. To our knowledge, this cohort represents one of the largest family-based genetic samples designed specifically for studies of tobacco smoking.

We here provide the first evidence of an association between the allelic variants of *GABAB2* and ND. We are aware that none of the *GABAB2* SNPs included in the current study represents an obvious causative variant. Only one significantly associated SNP (*rs3750344*) is located within a coding region of *GABAB2,* but the polymorphism does not result in an amino acid change. Thus, no coding differences are present in any of the *GABAB2* SNPs from the higher-risk or protective haplotypes. Because the associated SNPs are not necessarily exclusive to *GABAB2,* a functional allelic variant(s) close to or in strong linkage disequilibrium (LD) with these SNPs may be responsible for ND vulnerability. We therefore plan to analyze more SNPs within *GABAB2,* as well as adjacent genes in this 13-cM region on chromosome 9, not only because 9 of the 12 SNPs do not show significant LD but also because of the data of the haplotype analyses: the higher-risk haplotypes C-C-G and T-A-T-A were found in 7.6% of the AA smokers and in 6.6% of the EA smokers, respectively, and the protective haplotype C-A-C-A was found in 12.8% of the EA smokers. This suggests that these haplotypes play an important role in a relatively small proportion of smokers.

In summary, our association results provide evidence of a significant impact of *GABAB2* on ND—both for individual SNPs and for multilocus haplotypes. We also demonstrate that ethnic differences exist in the association between *GABAB2* and vulnerability to ND. This study not only confirms molecular and pharmacological data about the importance of the family of GABA receptor genes in addictive/behavioral traits but it also provides new information on the genetics of ND, showing the importance of the *GABAB2* gene as a biological candidate in future studies of ND.

Acknowledgments

We acknowledge the invaluable contributions of personal information and blood samples by all participants in the study, as well as the dedicated work of many research staff at different clinical sites. This project was funded by National Institutes of Health grants DA12844 (to M.D.L.) and RR03655 and GM28356 (to R.C.E.).

Electronic-Database Information

The URLs for data presented herein are as follows:

Celera Genomics, http://www.celera.com/
dbSNP Home Page, http://www.ncbi.nlm.nih.gov/SNP/
JSNP, http://snp.ims.u-tokyo.ac.jp/
National Institute on Drug Abuse, Center for Genetic Studies, http://zork.wustl.edu/nida/ (for questionnaires used in the study)

Online Mendelian Inheritance in Man (OMIM), http://www.ncbi.nlm.nih.gov/Omim/ (for ND and *GABRB2*)

References

Abecasis GR, Cookson WO (2000) GOLD—graphical overview of linkage disequilibrium. Bioinformatics 16:182–183

Bergen AW, Korczak JF, Weissbecker KA, Goldstein AM (1999) A genome-wide search for loci contributing to smoking and alcoholism. Genet Epidemiol Suppl 17:S55–S60

Bierut LJ, Rice JP, Goate A, Hinrichs AL, Saccone NL, Foroud T, Edenberg HJ, Cloninger CR, Begleiter H, Conneally PM, Crowe RR, Hesselbrock V, Li TK, Nurnberger JI Jr, Porjesz B, Schuckit MA, Reich T (2004) A genomic scan for habitual smoking in families of alcoholics: common and specific genetic factors in substance dependence. Am J Med Genet 124A:19–27

Corrigall WA, Coen KM, Adamson KL, Chow BL, Zhang J (2000) Response of nicotine self-administration in the rat to manipulations of mu-opioid and γ-aminobutyric acid receptors in the ventral tegmental area. Psychopharmacology (Berl) 149:107–114

Cousins MS, Stamat HM, de Wit H (2001) Effects of a single dose of baclofen on self-reported subjective effects and tobacco smoking. Nicotine Tob Res 3:123–129

Dewey SL, Brodie JD, Gerasimov M, Horan B, Gardner EL, Ashby CR Jr (1999) A pharmacologic strategy for the treatment of nicotine addiction. Synapse 31:76–86

Edenberg HJ, Dick DM, Xuei X, Tian H, Almasy L, Bauer LO, Crowe RR, Goate A, Hesselbrock V, Jones K, Kwon J, Li TK, Nurnberger JI Jr, O'Connor SJ, Reich T, Rice J, Schuckit MA, Porjesz B, Foroud T, Begleiter H (2004) Variations in GABRA2, encoding the $\alpha 2$ subunit of the GABA(A) receptor, are associated with alcohol dependence and with brain oscillations. Am J Hum Genet 74:705–714

Fattore L, Cossu G, Martellotta MC, Fratta W (2002) Baclofen antagonizes intravenous self-administration of nicotine in mice and rats. Alcohol Alcohol 37:495–498

Gelernter J, Liu X, Hesselbrock V, Page GP, Goddard A, Zhang H (2004) Results of a genomewide linkage scan: support for chromosomes 9 and 11 loci increasing risk for cigarette smoking. Am J Med Genet B Neuropsychiatr Genet 128B: 94–101

Heath AC, Kirk KM, Meyer JM, Martin NG (1999) Genetic and social determinants of initiation and age at onset of smoking in Australian twins. Behav Genet 29:395–407

Heatherton TF, Kozlowski LT, Frecker RC, Fagerstrom KO (1991) The Fagerstrom Test for Nicotine Dependence: a revision of the Fagerstrom Tolerance Questionnaire. Br J Addict 86:1119–1127

Horvath S, Xu X, Lake SL, Silverman EK, Weiss ST, Laird NM (2004) Family-based tests for associating haplotypes with general phenotype data: application to asthma genetics. Genet Epidemiol 26:61–69

Jones KA, Borowsky B, Tamm JA, Craig DA, Durkin MM, Dai M, Yao WJ, Johnson M, Gunwaldsen C, Huang LY, Tang C, Shen Q, Salon JA, Morse K, Laz T, Smith KE, Nagarathnam D, Noble SA, Branchek TA, Gerald C (1998) GABA(B) receptors function as a heteromeric assembly of the subunits GABA(B)R1 and GABA(B)R2. Nature 396:674–679

Kaupmann K, Malitschek B, Schuler V, Heid J, Froestl W, Beck P, Mosbacher J, Bischoff S, Kulik A, Shigemoto R, Karschin A, Bettler B (1998) GABA(B)-receptor subtypes assemble into functional heteromeric complexes. Nature 396:683–687

Lange C, Silverman EK, Xu X, Weiss ST, Laird NM (2003) A multivariate family-based association test using generalized estimating equations: FBAT-GEE. Biostatistics 4:195–206

Li MD, Cheng R, Ma JZ, Swan GE (2003*a*) A meta-analysis of estimated genetic and environmental effects on smoking behavior in male and female adult twins. Addiction 98:23–31

Li MD, Ma JZ, Beuten J (2004) Progress in searching for susceptibility loci and genes for smoking-related behaviour. Clin Genet 66:382–392

Li MD, Ma JZ, Cheng R, Dupont R, Williams KC, Payne TJ, Elston RC (2003*b*) A genome-wide scan to identify loci for smoking quantity in the Framingham Heart Study populations. BMC Genetics Suppl 4:S103

Madden PA, Heath AC, Pedersen NL, Kaprio J, Koskenvuo MJ, Martin NG (1999) The genetics of smoking persistence in men and women: a multicultural study. Behav Genet 29: 423–431

Martin SC, Russek SJ, Farb DH (2001) Human GABA(B)R genomic structure: evidence for splice variants in GABA(B)R1 but not GABA(B)R2. Gene 278:63–79

Nyholt DR (2004) A simple correction for multiple testing for single-nucleotide polymorphisms in linkage disequilibrium with each other. Am J Hum Genet 74:765–769

O'Connell JR, Weeks DE (1998) PedCheck: a program for identification of genotype incompatibilities in linkage analysis. Am J Hum Genet 63:259–266

Schuler V, Luscher C, Blanchet C, Klix N, Sansig G, Klebs K, Schmutz M, Heid J, Gentry C, Urban L, Fox A, Spooren W, Jaton AL, Vigouret J, Pozza M, Kelly PH, Mosbacher J, Froestl W, Kaslin E, Korn R, Bischoff S, Kaupmann K, van der Putten H, Bettler B (2001) Epilepsy, hyperalgesia, impaired memory, and loss of pre- and postsynaptic GABA(B) responses in mice lacking GABA(B(1)). Neuron 31:47–58

Sullivan PF, Kendler KS (1999) The genetic epidemiology of smoking. Nicotine Tob Res Suppl 1:S51–S57, S69–S70

Tyndale RF (2003) Genetics of alcohol and tobacco use in humans. Ann Med 35:94–121

Uhl GR, Liu QR, Naiman D (2002) Substance abuse vulnerability loci: converging genome scanning data. Trends Genet 18:420–425

United States Department of Health and Human Services (USDHHS) (2000) Reducing tobacco use: a report of the Surgeon General. United States Department of Health and Human Services, Center for Disease Control and Prevention, National Center for Chronic Disease Prevention and Health Promotion, Atlanta, GA

Am. J. Hum. Genet. 76:865–876, 2005

Report

Microduplication and Triplication of 22q11.2: A Highly Variable Syndrome

Twila M. Yobb,[1] Martin J. Somerville,[2] Lionel Willatt,[3] Helen V. Firth,[4] Karen Harrison,[5] Jennifer MacKenzie,[6] Natasha Gallo,[5] Bernice E. Morrow,[7] Lisa G. Shaffer,[8] Melanie Babcock,[7] Judy Chernos,[9] Francois Bernier,[9] Kathy Sprysak,[2] Jesse Christiansen,[2] Shelagh Haase,[2] Basil Elyas,[2] Margaret Lilley,[2] Steven Bamforth,[2] and Heather E. McDermid[1]

Departments of [1]Biological Sciences and [2]Medical Genetics, University of Alberta, Edmonton; [3]Addenbrooke's National Health Service Trust and [4]Department of Medical Genetics, University of Cambridge, Cambridge, United Kingdom; [5]Departments of Pathology and [6]Pediatrics Queen's University, Kingston, Ontario; [7]Department of Molecular Genetics, Albert Einstein College of Medicine, Bronx, NY; [8]School of Molecular Biosciences, Health Research and Education Center, Washington State University, Spokane; and [9]Department of Medical Genetics, Alberta Children's Hospital, Calgary

22q11.2 microduplications of a 3-Mb region surrounded by low-copy repeats should be, theoretically, as frequent as the deletions of this region; however, few microduplications have been reported. We show that the phenotype of these patients with microduplications is extremely diverse, ranging from normal to behavioral abnormalities to multiple defects, only some of which are reminiscent of the 22q11.2 deletion syndrome. This diversity will make ascertainment difficult and will necessitate a rapid-screening method. We demonstrate the utility of four different screening methods. Although all the screening techniques give unique information, the efficiency of real-time polymerase chain reaction allowed the discovery of two 22q11.2 microduplications in a series of 275 females who tested negative for fragile X syndrome, thus widening the phenotypic diversity. Ascertainment of the fragile X–negative cohort was twice that of the cohort screened for the 22q11.2 deletion. We also report the first patient with a 22q11.2 triplication and show that this patient's mother carries a 22q11.2 microduplication. We strongly recommend that other family members of patients with 22q11.2 microduplications also be tested, since we found several phenotypically normal parents who were carriers of the chromosomal abnormality.

Chromosomal rearrangements of 22q11.2 result in several genomic disorders, including the 22q11.2 deletion syndrome (also known as "DiGeorge syndrome" [MIM 188400] and "velocardiofacial syndrome" [MIM 192430]), and partially overlapping duplications result in cat eye syndrome (CES [MIM 115470]) and der(22) syndrome (reviewed by McDermid and Morrow [2002]) (fig. 1). These rearrangements are thought to be the result of nonallelic homologous recombination between low-copy repeats found in the region (LCR22s) (Edelmann et al. 1999*b*; Stankiewicz and Lupski 2002). In particular, the 22q11.2 deletion syndrome represents the most commonly ascertained deletion syndrome in humans, with a frequency estimated at 1/4,000–6,000 live births (Shaffer and Lupski 2000; Botto et al. 2003). Features of the 22q11.2 deletion syndrome include cleft palate, velopharyngeal insufficiency, hypernasal speech, characteristic facial features, heart defects, learning disabilities, and behavioral disorders (Shprintzen et al. 1978; Swillen et al. 1999). More-severely affected patients may have a reduced or absent thymus, as well as hypocalcemia (DiGeorge 1965). Since this microdeletion results from unequal crossing over—usually between the LCR22s separated by 3 Mb and usually on different chromosome 22 homologues (Saitta et al. 2004)—one would expect the reciprocal 3-Mb microduplication of the region to be present with a frequency equal to that of the 22q11.2 deletion. However, there are few reports of microduplications of this region of 22q11.2 (Edelmann et al. 1999*b*; Papenhausen et al. 2002; Ensenauer et al. 2003; Hassed et al. 2004). A small number of patients with larger duplications that include the critical regions for both CES and 22q11.2 deletion syndrome have also been reported (Reiss et al. 1985; Knoll et al. 1995; Lindsay et al. 1995), but these patients have fea-

Received November 30, 2004; accepted for publication February 21, 2005; electronically published March 30, 2005.

Address for correspondence and reprints: Dr. Heather McDermid, Department of Biological Sciences, University of Alberta, Edmonton, AB T6G 2E9, Canada. E-mail: hmcdermi@ualberta.ca

0002-9297/2005/7605-0014$15.00

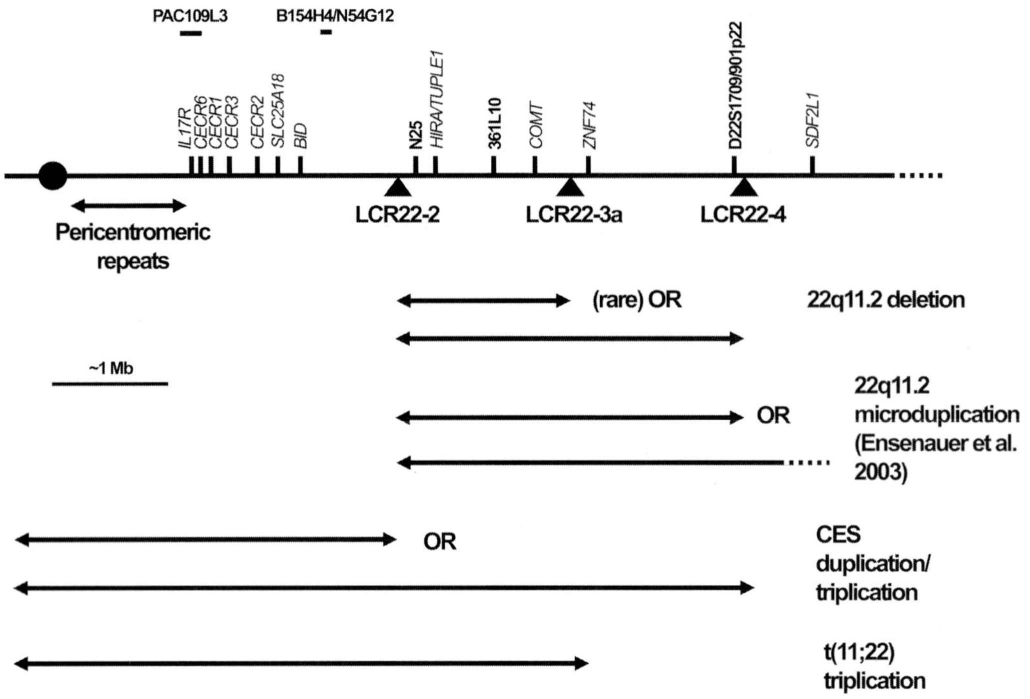

Figure 1 Duplications and deletions on chromosome 22q11.2. Arrows indicate the size of the various deletions and duplications. Triangles below the line representing the chromosome show the location of the LCR22s. Probes located above the line were used in the various FISH and dosage techniques.

tures typical of CES. These duplications also overlap with critical regions in patients with der(22) syndrome, who have partial trisomy for the 22pter-q11 regions, including half of the region typically deleted in 22q11.2 deletion syndrome (Funke et al. 1999; Kurahashi et al. 2000) (fig. 1). Similarly, Smith-Magenis syndrome (SMS) is a microdeletion syndrome associated with 17p11.2 (Smith et al. 1986) and is characterized by mental retardation, neurobehavioral abnormalities, sleep disorders, speech and motor delays, midface hypoplasia, short stature, and brachydactyly. The reciprocal microduplication of 17p11.2 has only recently been identified. It has a phenotype that is milder than that of the deletion (Potocki et al. 2000), including behavioral problems, mild-to-borderline mental retardation, short stature, dental anomalies, normal facies, and a lack of major-organ malformations.

Microduplications of 22q11.2 may be largely undetected, as a result of a less-distinct, unpredictable, and/or milder phenotype, which leads not only to problems with ascertainment and choosing the patient cohort to search but also to technical difficulties involved in identifying microduplications. A recent report described the clinical, cytogenetic, and molecular findings of 10 independent patients with 22q11.2 microduplications. Seven of the microduplications include only the 22q11.2 deletion syndrome region (Ensenauer et al. 2003). These individuals were ascertained from 653 patients tested for the 22q11.2 deletion; the latter syndrome was diagnosed in 40 of 653 patients. The patients with 22q11.2 microduplications had a variable phenotype, including heart defects, velopharyngeal insufficiency with and without cleft palate, hearing loss, growth delay, cognitive deficits, motor delay, learning disabilities, behavioral problems, and mild dysmorphic features. Whereas the phenotype of some individuals with a 22q11.2 microduplication may overlap with that of individuals with the 22q11.2 deletion syndrome, this overlap may (as a result of ascertainment bias) represent only one part of this syndrome's phenotypic spectrum. If these reciprocal chromosomal rearrangements are of equal frequency, then the difference in frequency between patients with 22q11.2 deletion syndrome (6.1%) and those with 22q11.2 microduplications (1.5%) in the test group used by Ensenauer et al. (2003) indicates that the majority of patients with microduplications do not fall within this test group.

In this report, we present seven unrelated patients/families (one reported elsewhere [Edelmann et al. 1999*b*]) with increased copy number in the 22q11.2 deletion syndrome region. Table 1 compares the clinical features of these patients with the features of patients published elsewhere. Figure 2 illustrates features of two patients. The microduplications in patients 1–5 were originally

Table 1

Clinical Characterization of Eight Patients with Increased Dosage of 22q11.2

Feature	Finding for Patient 1	2	3	4	4M	5	6	7	Results (No. Affected/No. Tested) of Ensenauer et al. (2003)
22q11.2 copy number	3	3	3	4	3	3	3	3	
Age at last evaluation	8 years	4 years	1 mo	8 years		4 mo	3 years	34 years	
Sex	M	F	M	F	F	F	F	F	
Heart defect	−	−	+[a]	−		+[b]	−	−	2[c,d]/6
Velopharyngeal insufficiency	−	+		−			−	−	5/5
Palatal defect	A		−	−		−	−		4/7
Hearing impairment	+[e]	−	−	+[e]		+	+[f]	−	4/6
Failure to thrive	−	+	−	−		+	+	−	
Sleep apnea		+		−			−		
Absent thymus/asplenia	−		−	−		−	−	−	1/6
Urogenital abnormality	−		−	−		−	−	−	2/5
Hypotonia	−	+	−	−		+	+	−	1/5
Gastrointestinal abnormality	−		−	−		−	+	−	
Cognitive deficits	+[g,h]	+[g,h]		+[g,i]			+[h]	+[i]	5/5
Behavioral problems	+[j]			+[k]			−	+[l]	3/3
Seizures	+	+		−		+			1/6
Dysmorphic features:									6/6
Broad nasal bridge			+	+		+	+		
Hand/foot abnormality	+[m]		+[n]	+[o]	+[o]	−	−	−	4[p,q]/5
Hypertelorism	+					+	+		
Epicanthal folds	+			+					2/5
Micrognathia	+			−		+	+		3/5
Microcephaly				−		+	+		1/6
Additional features	+[r]	+[s]	+[t]	+[u]		+[v]	+[w]		6/6
Other	+[x]	+[y]	+[z]	+[aa]			+[bb]		

NOTE.—"+" = feature present; "−" = feature absent; blank cells indicate unknown or patient too young to determine; A = arched.

[a] Hypoplastic left heart.
[b] Tetrology of Fallot and right-sided aortic arch.
[c] Tetrology of Fallot.
[d] Hypoplastic left heart and interrupted aortic arch.
[e] Impairment secondary to recurrent otitis media.
[f] Mild conductive deafness.
[g] Speech delay.
[h] Developmental delay.
[i] Learning difficulties.
[j] Impulsivity and aggression.
[k] Short concentration span and social immaturity.
[l] Childhood aggression and childhood ADD.
[m] Clinodactyly of the fifth fingers.
[n] Hypoplastic fifth fingernail and toenails smaller than normal.
[o] Broad hands, with square tipped fingers and prominent fetal finger pads.
[p] Abnormal palmar creases.
[q] Long fingers and/or toes.
[r] High forehead, round face, flat supraorbital ridge, short nose, thin upper lip, and long, smooth philtrum.
[s] Narrow face and downslanting palpebral fissures.
[t] Prominent eyes, medial deficiency of the eyebrows, and prominent chin and lower lip.
[u] Eversion of the lateral eye lids and bulbous nasal tip.
[v] Facial asymmetry.
[w] Mild synophrys, tented peak in the middle of each eyebrow, facial asymmetry, and small, downslanting mouth.
[x] Maternal half brother (aged 16 years) with developmental delay, paternal cousin (aged 9 years) with behavioral problems, and another paternal cousin with cleft lip and palate.
[y] Gross motor delay and poor fine-motor skills.
[z] Nystagmus and myopia; prominent metopic suture, with an anterior fontanel of a width of three fingers; sagittal sutures widely separated; and open posterior fontanel.
[aa] Left ear pit.
[bb] Chorioretinal coloboma, visual impairment, and preauricular skin tags.

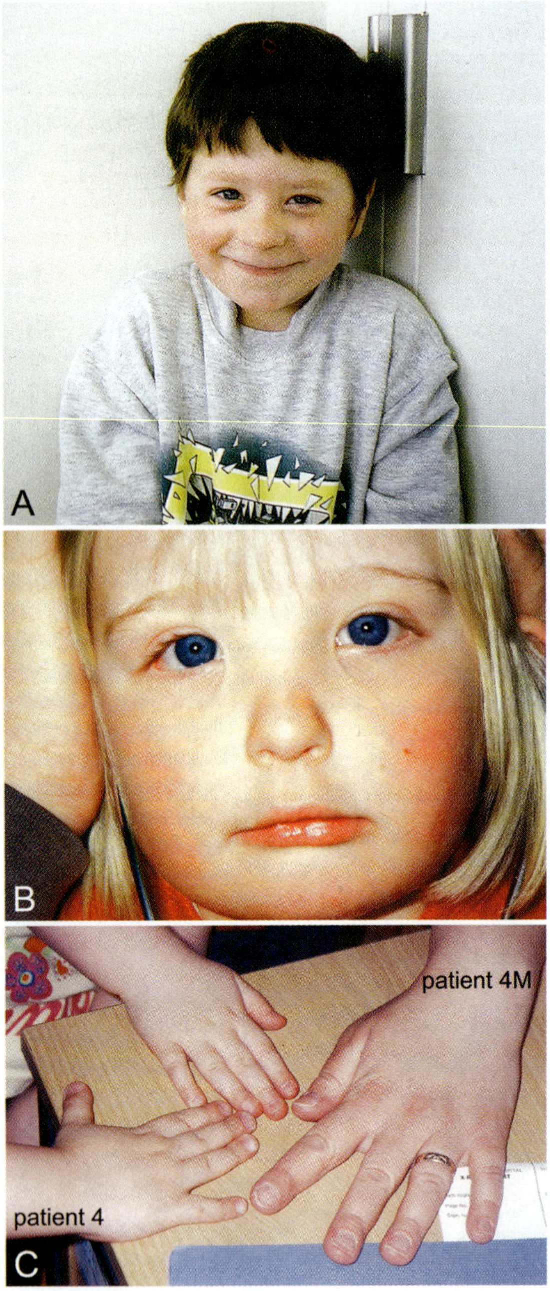

Figure 2 Photographs of patients with increased dosage of 22q11.2. *A*, Patient 1. *B*, Patient 4. *C*, Hands of patient 4 and her mother (patient 4M). The unlabeled hand is an unaffected sister of patient 4.

identified during tests for the 22q11.2 deletion syndrome at five different centers. Patients 6 and 7 were ascertained by screening 275 female patients referred for diagnostic fragile X syndrome testing. The seven patients show a remarkable variation in phenotype, with some showing little-to-no resemblance to the phenotype of 22q11.2 deletion syndrome.

Most patients in this study were analyzed by several different methods to confirm an increased copy number within 22q11.2. Patients 1–5 were originally identified by FISH. Analysis of interphase nuclei of patients 1 and 3 showed a microduplication of the Vysis *TUPLE1* probe (fig. 3*A* [patient 1]). To narrow the extent of microduplication, cells from patient 1 were further tested using a number of BAC clones (obtained from the Wellcome Trust Sanger Institute and M. Rocchi) within and surrounding the 22q11.2 deletion syndrome region. Probes proximal (109L3, N54G12, and BK154H4) and distal (BA24N11, BCR, and BA297B9) to the 22q11.2 deletion syndrome region were not duplicated. Only probes D22S75/N25 and *TUPLE1,* located within the 22q11.2 deletion syndrome region, were duplicated. Duplications of the 22q11.2 deletion syndrome region were shown in patient 2 by use of Oncor probe N25 (Edelmann et al. 1999*b*). Interphase FISH analysis was performed on patient 4 with the use of two BAC probes located within the 22q11.2 deletion syndrome region. Probe 361L10 (*green*) was clearly triplicated and showed four hybridization spots (fig. 3*B*), whereas 901P22 (*red*) gave ambiguous results (three copies in most cells, but four copies in some cells [see fig. 3*B*]). Analysis could not be repeated, as a result of a lack of sample. The consistent clustering of three of the four copies of 361L10 indicates the presence of three copies on one chromosome 22 and one copy on the other homologue. FISH on interphase nuclei of patient 5 showed three *TUPLE1* (*red*) signals, compared with two *ARSA* (*green*) signals (fig. 3*C*). On review of signals for metaphase chromosomes, a *TUPLE1* signal on one chromosome 22 was subjectively larger (fig. 3*D*), supporting a tandem duplication of this region, rather than a cryptic translocation. FISH studies of the parents of patient 5 revealed the same microduplication in the infant's father, who was healthy but had a history of significant learning difficulties, unilateral hearing loss, and poor vision in one eye. No FISH analysis was done for patients 6 and 7.

The triplication in patient 4 was analyzed using the microsatellite marker *D22S1709,* which is located in the distal portion of the 22q11.2 deletion syndrome region (fig. 1). Four different alleles are present at this locus, confirming four copies of the region (fig. 4). This probe is located within BAC 901P22, which gave ambiguous FISH results of three or four copies. The microsatellite analysis confirms the involvement of four different chromosome 22 homologues in the production of this triplication. Microsatellite analyses were also done on patients 3, 5, 6, and 7. Several loci within the 22q11.2 deletion syndrome region were informative for the presence of three distinct alleles in all four patients (results not shown).

Since it is cumbersome, expensive, and labor-intensive to screen for 22q11.2 interstitial microduplications by

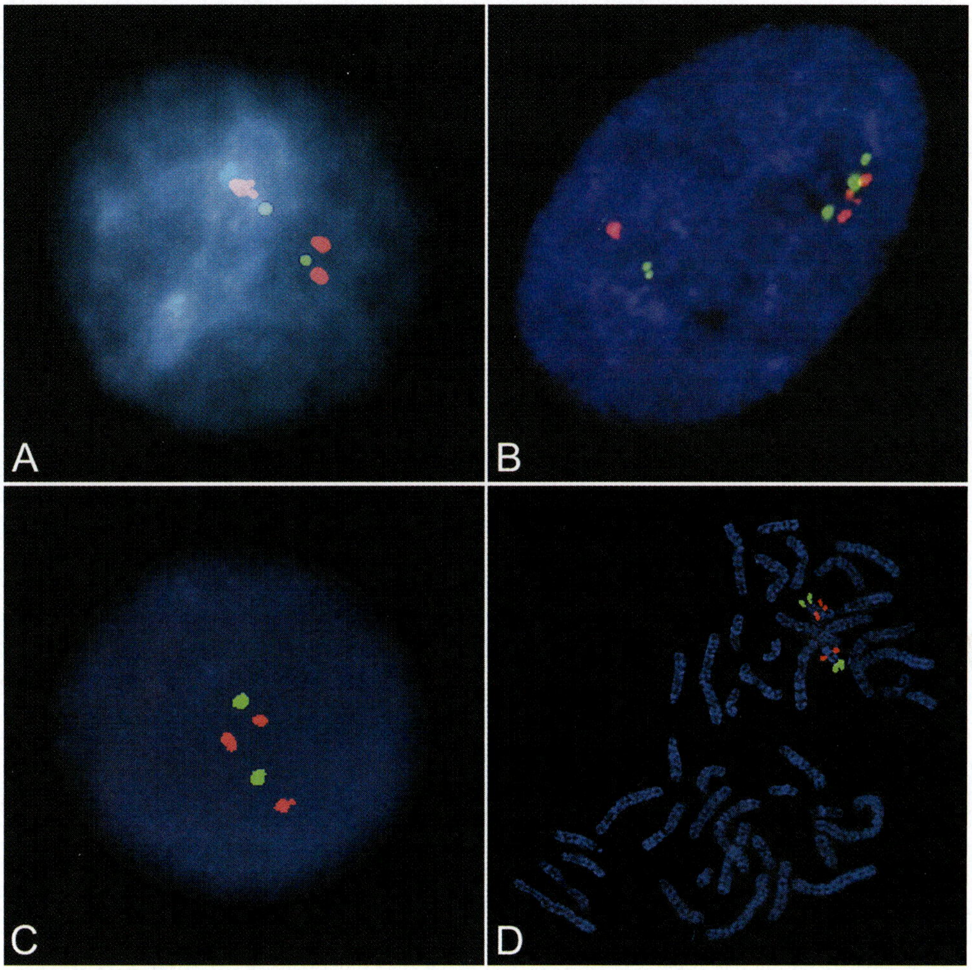

Figure 3 FISH analyses. *A*, Patient 1 test probe *TUPLE1* (*red*) shows three copies for an interphase cell; control probe *ARSA* (*green*) shows two copies. *B*, Patient 4 test probes 361L10 and 901P22 (*green* and *red*, respectively) show four copies for this cell. *C*, Patient 5 test probe *TUPLE1* (*red*) shows three copies; control probe *ARSA* (*green*) shows two copies. *D*, Metaphase spread from patient 5 shows the duplication of the *TUPLE1* probe.

use of interphase FISH, we sought a more efficient screening method. Real-time PCR analysis of two genes in the proximal 1.5 portion (fig. 1) of the 22q11.2 deletion syndrome region (*HIRA* and *COMT*) was performed on all patients (fig. 5) with the use of a multiplexed array of two quantitative reactions (Thiel et al. 2003). A *Taq*Man *GJA5* gene Pre-Developed Assay Reagent (PDAR [Applied Biosystems]) was multiplexed as a two-copy control in both reactions. Reactions from patients with 22q11.2 deletion syndrome, from wild-type DNA, and from "no template" controls were included in each analysis. All real-time PCR amplifications were performed on an ABI Prism 7900 HT Sequence Detection System (Applied Biosystems) with the use of a 384-well plate. *HIRA* and *COMT* were assayed in separate reactions, and each assay was performed in triplicate. Sequence Detection Software (SDS, version 2.0 [Applied Biosystems]) was used to process raw fluorescence data and to produce a threshold cycle number (Ct) for each sample. The Ct value was the cycle number at which the fluorescence emission of the reporter dye passed a fixed threshold on the amplification plot. The default setting for the threshold was 10 SDs above the mean baseline emission. All Ct settings were manually checked and adjusted within the logarithmic curve between background and plateau levels. The ABI 7900 HT data were exported to a Microsoft Excel macro in which all Ct values were normalized to the multiplexed PDAR and were compared with the wild-type and positive-control values.

Patients 1, 2, 3, and 5 have three copies of *HIRA* and *COMT*, indicating a microduplication of the 22q11.2 deletion syndrome region of 22q11.2. Patient 4 was found to have four copies of *HIRA* and *COMT*, con-

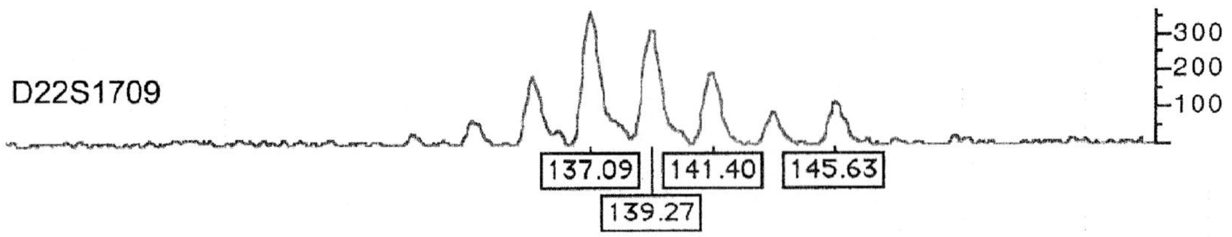

Figure 4 Microsatellite analysis of probe D22S1709, showing four different alleles in patient 4, with sizes (in bp) marked below the peaks. Unmarked peaks are due to stutter bands, an artifact of PCR. The method has been described elsewhere (Edelmann et al. 1999*a*).

firming a triplication of the 22q11.2 deletion syndrome region. Interestingly, the mother of patient 4 (patient 4M) was found to have only three copies of 22q11.2, indicating an expansion of the 22q11.2 deletion syndrome region from three to four copies between mother and child. This was confirmed cytogenetically. In addition to FISH analysis, patients 3 and 5 were independently ascertained by real-time PCR among 671 22q11.2 deletion syndrome referrals (0.3%). In this same cohort, 26 cases of 22q11.2 deletion were detected (3.9%).

The efficiency of the real-time PCR analysis allowed us to quickly screen for microduplications in a set of 275 unrelated females who were negative for fragile X syndrome; the individuals in this set were collected from multiple referrals, with little or no clinical data available. However, since common features of patients with the 22q11.2 microduplication are behavioral and cognitive problems, the fragile X–negative cohort would be a reasonable group to screen. Only females were screened, to minimize the contribution of X-linked conditions to the analysis. Our screen resulted in the discovery of two patients (0.7%) with duplications in the 22q11.2 deletion syndrome region (fig. 5 [patients 6 and 7]). Permission from the Health Research Ethics Board of the University of Alberta Health Sciences Faculties allowed us to access the clinical data for these two patients (table 1). As controls, 520 unrelated individuals referred for hemochromatosis testing were also screened for microduplication of 22q11.2. None of the control individuals had a microduplication of 22q11.2 ($P < .00003$), indicating that this chromosomal abnormality is not a polymorphism. Interestingly, one patient (0.4%) in the fragile X–negative female group had a deletion of 22q11.2.

Although real-time PCR allowed the rapid analysis of a large number of individuals, it did not allow us to define the size of the microduplication, since only two probes in the 22q11.2 deletion syndrome region were examined. Sizing of microduplications requires the examination of multiple sites along 22q11.2, which is expensive to set up for real-time PCR and is time-consuming to test by FISH and microsatellites. We therefore analyzed the patients by use of our CES/22q11.2 deletion syndrome multiplex amplifiable probe hybridization (MAPH) probe set that covered regions both distal and proximal to the 22q11.2 deletion syndrome region (table 2). Seven probes were located within the CES region, one probe was within the 3-Mb 22q11.2 deletion syndrome region (*ZNF74* [position 19073420 bp in the UCSC Genome Browser May 2004 Assembly Map]), and one probe was ~600 kb distal to the 22q11.2 deletion syndrome region (*SDF2L1* [position 20321160 bp in the UCSC Genome Browser May 2004 Assembly Map]) (fig. 1). Control probes, supplied by J. Armour (University of Nottingham), were located on other chromosomes (5, 15, 16, and 17). In addition to patient DNA samples, three control samples were used: the two-copy control was a normal lymphoblast cell line GM03657 (Coriell Institute for Medical Research); the three-copy control was a lymphoblastoid cell line from a patient with a duplication including the CES region and the 22q11.2 deletion syndrome region (Reiss et al. 1985; McDermid et al. 1986; H.E.M., unpublished results); and the four-copy control was patient CM01, who has CES and is known to have four copies of both the CES region and the 22q11.2 deletion syndrome region (McTaggart et al. 1998). Genescan software was used to calculate the peak area for each probe. Peak ratios were calculated by dividing the peak area of a test probe by the sum of the peak areas of the two closest control probes. Each experiment contained four to eight replicates of the two-copy control, the three-copy control, and a patient. Each peak-ratio replicate for all samples was normalized to the mean peak ratio of the two-copy control. The mean and SD of the normalized peak ratios for each probe were calculated for the two-copy control, the three-copy control, and the patient. One experiment also contained a four-copy control.

A graph of the normalized mean peak ratio (± 1 SD) for each probe, compared with a two-copy and three-copy control, was plotted for patients 1–4 (fig. 6), as well as for patient 6 and the mother of patient 4 (data for the latter two not shown). DNA was not available for MAPH analysis of patients 5 and 7. A four-copy control was included for patient 4. In all cases, a ratio of ~1:1 with the two-copy control was calculated for all the probes within the CES region and distal to the 22q11.2 deletion syndrome region, indicating no duplication of these probes. Thus, in each patient tested, the

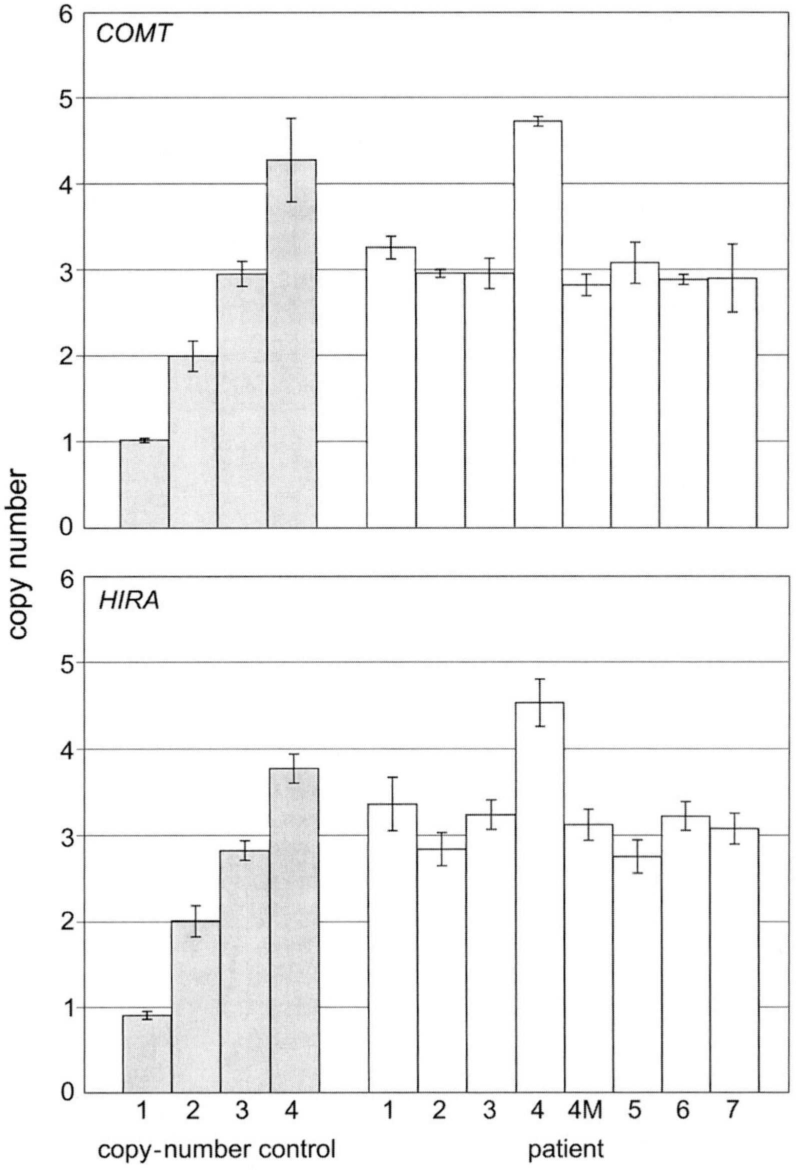

Figure 5 Real-time PCR analysis of probes *COMT* and *HIRA* (also known as "*TUPLE1*"). Copy number was calculated by multiplying the ΔΔCt ratio by 2. A two-copy control was run for each set of experiments, but only the most variable two-copy control is shown in each graph. Error bars represent 1 SD above and below the mean. Each reaction mixture consisted of 200 nmol/L of each primer, 50 nmol/L of *Taq*Man probe, 40 ng of genomic DNA, 0.3 μl of PDAR (Applied Biosystems), and 7.5 μl of 2 × *Taq*Man mix (Applied Biosystems), in a total volume of 15 μl. Thermal cycling conditions included a presoak for 2 min at 50°C and for 10 min at 95°C. Samples were amplified for 40 cycles at 95°C for 15 s and at 60°C for 1 min.

region of increased dosage was confined to the 22q11.2 deletion syndrome region, and no cases extended proximally, as in the study by Ensenauer et al. (2003). The size of the duplication could not be determined for patients 5 and 7. In all cases, the previous results showing microduplications and triplications were confirmed. On the basis of the ratios calculated for the *ZNF74* probe (~1.5:1 with the two-copy control), patients 1, 2, 3, and 6 have a microduplication of the 22q11.2 deletion syndrome region. In each experiment, the three-copy control showed a ratio of ~1.5:1 with the two-copy control. In patient 4 and the four-copy control, a ratio of ~2:1 with the two-copy control was calculated for *ZNF74*, confirming that patient 4 has a triplication of the 22q11.2 deletion syndrome region. The mother of patient 4 (patient 4M) was confirmed to have three copies of *ZNF74* (data not shown).

In summary, we report seven unrelated patients/families with duplication or triplication of the 3-Mb 22q11.2 deletion syndrome region. Ensenauer et al. (2003) de-

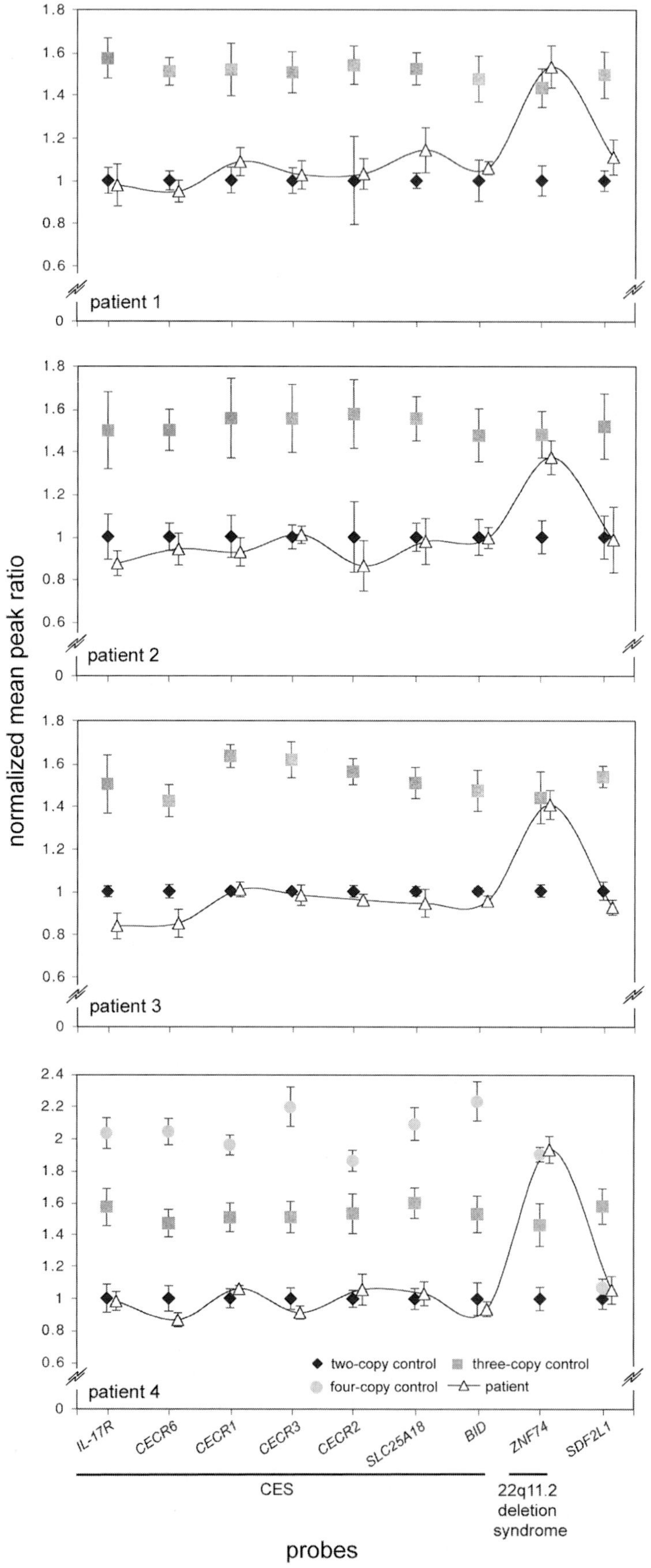

normalized mean peak ratio
patient 1
patient 2
patient 3
patient 4
two-copy control
three-copy control
four-copy control
patient
IL-17R
CECR6
CECR1
CECR3
CECR2
SLC25A18
BID
ZNF74
SDF2L1
CES
22q11.2 deletion syndrome
probes

scribed seven unrelated patients with just the 22q11.2 deletion syndrome region duplicated, as well as an additional three independent patients with duplications that included the 22q11.2 deletion syndrome region and extended distally. All were ascertained from 653 patients referred for 22q11.2 deletion testing. Although distinct dysmorphic features for the microduplication were suggested, the other features of the seven patients have a strong bias toward 22q11.2 deletion syndrome features, including conotruncal heart defects (2/6), velopharyngeal insufficiency (5/5), cleft palate (4/7), cognitive defects (5/5), and absent thymus with T-cell deficiency (1/6). This is not surprising, considering the method of ascertainment. However, although our patients 1–5 were also identified through 22q11.2 deletion testing, they show a less distinct phenotype, with fewer instances of velopharyngeal insufficiency (1/4) and no cases of cleft palate or abnormal thymus. Developmental/speech delay, behavioral problems, and mild dysmorphic features are the major phenotypes observed in our patients 1–5 (table 1). Aggressive behavior and attention deficit disorder (ADD) were seen in patients from both studies.

The true spectrum of 22q11.2 microduplication syndrome will not be apparent until patients are ascertained independently of the 22q11.2 deletion syndrome symptoms. We have initiated this by screening 275 females who were referred for diagnostic fragile X syndrome testing but with no *FMR1* expansion detected. We identified two patients with 22q11.2 microduplications in this group and no microduplications in 520 controls ($P < .00003$). Patient 6 showed an eye defect, as well as dysmorphic features and developmental delay, but her phenotype did not particularly resemble that of 22q11.2 deletion syndrome. In fact, the presence of a coloboma and preauricular tags in this patient suggested an association with the CES duplication, yet the CES critical region was not duplicated. Patient 7 showed only behavioral symptoms, with no similarity to the 22q11.2 deletion syndrome. The analysis of these patients suggests that a large number of individuals with 22q11.2 microduplications do not show similarity to 22q11.2 deletion syndrome and, therefore, are currently undiagnosed, which would explain the imbalance between reported deletions and duplications of this region. The lack of similarity of our patients to each other underscores the remarkable variability in the phenotype of this syndrome, which will make ascertainment of the majority of cases extremely difficult.

A significant number of 22q11.2 microduplications may also be associated with a normal phenotype. The mother and grandmother of patient 2 both carry the microduplication and are normal (Edelmann et al. 1999*b*). The mother of patient 4 shows a normal phenotype, except for her hands, but has a 22q11.2 microduplication. The father of patient 5 has the microduplication and showed learning difficulties and hearing loss. This suggests that parents of children with 22q11.2 duplications should also be tested for the same microduplication, since it could be responsible for other mild abnormalities within the pedigree and is a potential risk to future children of the parents and of other relatives.

The normal or near-normal phenotype associated with a significant proportion of patients with 22q11.2 microduplications could also explain why there appears to be no correlation between patients with CES with increased dosage of the 22q11.2 deletion syndrome region and those without increased dosage, in addition to triplication of the CES region (McTaggart et al. 1998). Since the sample size of patients with CES was small (10 individuals) and the phenotype of CES is highly variable, small additions to the phenotype from microduplication or triplication of the 22q11.2 deletion syndrome region may not be detectable unless a very large number of patients are analyzed. Interstitial duplications including both the CES and the 22q11.2 deletion syndrome regions have also shown predominantly CES-like fea-

Table 2

MAPH Probes, Primer Sequences, and Sizes

The table is available in its entirety in the online edition of *The American Journal of Human Genetics.*

Figure 6 MAPH analysis of the 22q11.2 region for patients 1, 2, 3, and 4. Probes are shown below the four graphs and are listed in order along the chromosome (centromere at left), with the CES region and the 22q11.2 deletion syndrome region indicated. Normalized mean peak ratios (error bars represent 1 SD above and below the mean) are graphed for all probes for each patient (*unblackened triangles* connected by a line) and control (two-copy control sample represented by *blackened diamonds;* three-copy control sample represented by *squares*). The four-copy control sample (*circles*) has four copies of the CES region and the 22q11.2 deletion syndrome region; however, distal to the 22q11.2 deletion syndrome region, the copy number is 2. Probes and probe mixes, membrane preparation, and hybridization were performed in accordance with the study by Armour et al. (2000) and the Multiplex Amplifiable Probe Hybridization (MAPH) Web site, with the following changes. Genomic DNA was blotted onto a Hybond N membrane (Amersham Biosciences). After hybridization, the membranes were washed six times for 10 min each at 65°C in 1 × SSC/1% SDS solution and six times for 10 min each at 65°C in 0.1 × SSC/0.1% SDS solution. Membranes were each placed in a 0.2-ml PCR tube with 50 μl of 1 × AB gene buffer IV and were heated to 95°C to release the probes; 3.75 μl of this solution was used as a template for a fluorescent PCR containing 1 × AB gene buffer IV, 2 mM $MgCl_2$, 0.4 mM dNTPs, 2 μM PZA-FAM, 1 μM PZB, and 2.5 U *Taq* polymerase (Invitrogen). Finally, 1 μl of the PCR was mixed with 1 μl of formamide loading dye, and 1.2 μl of the mixture was run on a polyacrylamide gel for 3.5 h by use of the ABI Prism 377 DNA sequencer.

tures (Reiss et al. 1985; Knoll et al. 1995; Lindsay et al. 1995).

Patient 4 has a triplication of the 22q11.2 deletion syndrome region, which has been confirmed by four independent methods (figs. 3, 4, 5, and 6). To our knowledge, this is the first reported triplication of the 22q11.2 deletion syndrome region. Microsatellite analysis of patient 4 showed the presence of four different alleles of locus *D22S1709,* located in the distal portion of the 22q11.2 deletion syndrome region. This implies that four different chromosome 22 homologues were involved in the creation of the triplication. FISH analysis showed that the two extra copies are on the same chromosome. This could be explained by an interchromosomal exchange in a maternal heterozygous grandparent—which would have created the microduplication in the mother—followed by a second interchromosomal exchange involving the same chromosome in the heterozygous mother, leading to the tandem triplication in the child. It is unknown whether the presence of the first microduplication predisposed to the second rearrangement. Interestingly, the phenotype of this patient is very mild. The patient's mother has a microduplication of the 22q11.2 deletion syndrome region and a normal phenotype, except for dysmorphic hands, suggesting that modifier loci in this family are ameliorating the effect of the chromosomal defect.

To ascertain a significant proportion of 22q11.2 microduplications, a very large number of individuals would need to be screened. However, microduplications have generally been more difficult to detect than deletions. Microduplications of 22q11.2 have previously been diagnosed primarily using interphase FISH (Edelmann et al. 1999*b*; Ensenauer et al. 2003). Although this method is effective, it is time-consuming and is not suited for quickly screening large numbers of patients. However, this technique does give unique information about the position and arrangement of the duplicated segments. In our study, FISH analysis of patient 4 revealed that the two additional copies of the 22q11.2 deletion syndrome region are both located on the same homologue, indicating a tandem triplication (fig. 3). Duplications of 22q11.2 have also previously been seen by use of chromosome banding; however, a resolution greater than what is routinely used was necessary (Ensenauer et al. 2003).

Microsatellite analysis has also been used to detect 22q11.2 microduplications and to define breakpoints (Edelmann et al. 1999*a*; Ensenauer et al. 2003). However, because dosage analysis with microsatellites is, at best, only semiquantitative, unambiguous results are obtained only when the number of different allele sizes is equal to the copy number of the region. Preferential amplification of the smaller alleles leads to inaccuracies, as do stuttering effects, which produce smaller peaks preceding the major-allele peak (Armour et al. 2002). However, in the case of patient 4, microsatellite analysis gave unique information about possible mechanisms of the formation of the triplication.

Real-time PCR (Thiel et al. 2003) and MAPH (Armour et al. 2000) are two methods used to study changes in dosage that generally give unambiguous results and only require a small amount of DNA from the patient. Real-time PCR is a quick, straightforward, and reproducible test that uses minute amounts of DNA. As many as 185 patients can be analyzed in a single run for the dosage (deletion or duplication) of one probe. The disadvantage of this technique is the cost of both the initial equipment and the individual probes. Alternatively, MAPH was specifically designed to analyze a large number of probes at once and, therefore, is suited to more-complex detection projects, such as breakpoint comparisons. In this study, we scanned for microduplications over seven genes in the CES region, as well as single genes within and distal to the 22q11.2 deletion syndrome region.

All four methods were used in our study, although not all methods were used on each patient. All patients were examined with more than one method, and, in each case, the results concurred. Each technique has advantages and disadvantages. However, for screening large numbers of individuals, real-time PCR is the method of choice; microarray-based comparative genomic hybridization (array CGH) has also been used to detect abnormalities of 22q11.2 (Mantripragada et al. 2004). Large screens of different patient cohorts would aid in defining the full phenotypic spectrum of the 22q11.2 microduplication syndrome. The finding of 22q11.2 microduplications in 2 of 275 females who tested negative for fragile X syndrome implies that these microduplications are not uncommon and that they may be associated more with neurological and behavioral features in many patients. The remaining challenge is to identify these patients, and this syndrome is likely to remain underdiagnosed until this is done. Large-scale real-time PCR screens of neurologically impaired individuals (those with developmental delay, mild dysmorphology, minor behavioral problems, and learning disabilities with mild dysmorphology), such as diagnostic fragile X referrals, followed by family studies to detect relatives with 22q11.2 microduplications, would be a reasonable place to start. Indeed, our success rate for detecting 22q11.2 microduplications among fragile X referrals (0.7%) approaches half of the success rate for detecting fragile X itself in this cohort (2%) and is twice the number of 22q11.2 microduplications found in the 22q11.2 deletion syndrome referrals. By widening the scope of the patients tested, we will gain a better understanding of the phenotype associated with 22q11.2 microduplications.

Acknowledgments

We thank John Armour for providing control MAPH probes and invaluable advice. We also thank John Gaspar, for performing the microsatellite analysis of patient 4; Catherine Kashork (Baylor College of Medicine, Houston, TX), for performing the FISH analysis of patient 4; Lucy Osborne, for helpful discussions; and Jack Scott, for help with the figures. H.E.M. was supported by a grant from the Canadian Institutes of Health Research (MOP11639). This work was also supported by the March of Dimes (1-FY00-768 [to B.E.M.]) and the National Institutes of Health (1 P01 HD39420-01 [to B.E.M. and L.G.S.] and 5 P01 HD34980-05 [to B.E.M.]). This study was approved by the Health Research Ethics Board of the University of Alberta Health Sciences Faculties.

Electronic-Database Information

The URLs for data presented herein are as follows:

Multiplex Amplifiable Probe Hybridization (MAPH) Web site, http://www.nott.ac.uk/~pdzjala/maph/maph.html
Online Mendelian Inheritance in Man (OMIM), http://www.ncbi.nlm.nih.gov/Omim/ (for DiGeorge syndrome, velocardiofacial syndrome, and CES)
Wellcome Trust Sanger Institute, http://www.sanger.ac.uk/ (for clones)

References

Armour JA, Barton DE, Cockburn DJ, Taylor GR (2002) The detection of large deletions or duplications in genomic DNA. Hum Mutat 20:325–337
Armour JA, Sismani C, Patsalis PC, Cross G (2000) Measurement of locus copy number by hybridisation with amplifiable probes. Nucleic Acids Res 28:605–609
Botto LD, May K, Fernhoff PM, Correa A, Coleman K, Rasmussen SA, Merritt RK, O'Leary LA, Wong LY, Elixson EM, Mahle WT, Campbell RM (2003) A population-based study of the 22q11.2 deletion: phenotype, incidence, and contribution to major birth defects in the population. Pediatrics 112:101–107
DiGeorge A (1965) A new concept of the cellular basis of immunity. J Pediatr 67:907
Edelmann L, Pandita RK, Morrow BE (1999*a*) Low-copy repeats mediate the common 3-Mb deletion in patients with velo-cardio-facial syndrome. Am J Hum Genet 64:1076–1086
Edelmann L, Pandita RK, Spiteri E, Funke B, Goldberg R, Palanisamy N, Chaganti RS, Magenis E, Shprintzen RJ, Morrow BE (1999*b*) A common molecular basis for rearrangement disorders on chromosome 22q11. Hum Mol Genet 8:1157–1167
Ensenauer RE, Adeyinka A, Flynn HC, Michels VV, Lindor NM, Dawson DB, Thorland EC, Lorentz CP, Goldstein JL, McDonald MT, Smith WE, Simon-Fayard E, Alexander AA, Kulharya AS, Ketterling RP, Clark RD, Jalal SM (2003) Microduplication 22q11.2, an emerging syndrome: clinical, cytogenetic, and molecular analysis of thirteen patients. Am J Hum Genet 73:1027–1040
Funke B, Edelmann L, McCain N, Pandita RK, Ferreira J, Merscher S, Zohouri M, Cannizzaro L, Shanske A, Morrow BE (1999) Der(22) syndrome and velo-cardio-facial syndrome/DiGeorge syndrome share a 1.5-Mb region of overlap on chromosome 22q11. Am J Hum Genet 64:747–758
Hassed SJ, Hopcus-Niccum D, Zhang L, Li S, Mulvihill JJ (2004) A new genomic duplication syndrome complementary to the velocardiofacial (22q11 deletion) syndrome. Clin Genet 65:400–404
Knoll JH, Asamoah A, Pletcher BA, Wagstaff J (1995) Interstitial duplication of proximal 22q: phenotypic overlap with cat eye syndrome. Am J Med Genet 55:221–224
Kurahashi H, Shaikh TH, Hu P, Roe BA, Emanuel BS, Budarf ML (2000) Regions of genomic instability on 22q11 and 11q23 as the etiology for the recurrent constitutional t(11;22). Hum Mol Genet 9:1665–1670
Lindsay EA, Shaffer LG, Carrozzo R, Greenberg F, Baldini A (1995) De novo tandem duplication of chromosome segment 22q11-q12: clinical, cytogenetic, and molecular characterization. Am J Med Genet 56:296–299
Mantripragada KK, Tapia-Paez I, Blennow E, Nilsson P, Wedell A, Dumanski JP (2004) DNA copy-number analysis of the 22q11 deletion-syndrome region using array-CGH with genomic and PCR-based targets. Int J Mol Med 13:273–279
McDermid HE, Duncan AM, Brasch KR, Holden JJ, Magenis E, Sheehy R, Burn J, Kardon N, Noel B, Schinzel A, Teshima I, White BN (1986) Characterization of the supernumerary chromosome in cat eye syndrome. Science 232:646–648
McDermid HE, Morrow BE (2002) Genomic disorders on 22q11. Am J Hum Genet 70:1077–1088
McTaggart KE, Budarf ML, Driscoll DA, Emanuel BS, Ferreira P, McDermid HE (1998) Cat eye syndrome chromosome breakpoint clustering: identification of two intervals also associated with 22q11 deletion syndrome breakpoints. Cytogenet Cell Genet 81:222–228
Papenhausen P, Singh-Kahlon P, Griffin S, Stone P, Rogers KK, Rosini JE, Gadi IK, Tepperberg JH, Mowery PM (2002) Two cases of interstitial duplications detected only by interphase FISH. Am J Hum Genet Suppl 71:302
Potocki L, Chen KS, Park SS, Osterholm DE, Withers MA, Kimonis V, Summers AM, Meschino WS, Anyane-Yeboa K, Kashork CD, Shaffer LG, Lupski JR (2000) Molecular mechanism for duplication 17p11.2—the homologous recombination reciprocal of the Smith-Magenis microdeletion. Nat Genet 24:84–87
Reiss JA, Weleber RG, Brown MG, Bangs CD, Lovrien EW, Magenis RE (1985) Tandem duplication of proximal 22q: a cause of cat-eye syndrome. Am J Med Genet 20:165–171
Saitta SC, Harris SE, Gaeth AP, Driscoll DA, McDonald-McGinn DM, Maisenbacher MK, Yersak JM, Chakraborty PK, Hacker AM, Zackai EH, Ashley T, Emanuel BS (2004) Aberrant interchromosomal exchanges are the predominant cause of the 22q11.2 deletion. Hum Mol Genet 13:417–428
Shaffer LG, Lupski JR (2000) Molecular mechanisms for constitutional chromosomal rearrangements in humans. Annu Rev Genet 34:297–329
Shprintzen RJ, Goldberg RB, Lewin ML, Sidoti EJ, Berkman MD, Argamaso RV, Young D (1978) A new syndrome involving cleft palate, cardiac anomalies, typical facies, and

learning disabilities: velo-cardio-facial syndrome. Cleft Palate J 15:56–62
Smith AC, McGavran L, Robinson J, Waldstein G, Macfarlane J, Zonona J, Reiss J, Lahr M, Allen L, Magenis E (1986) Interstitial deletion of (17)(p11.2p11.2) in nine patients. Am J Med Genet 24:393–414
Stankiewicz P, Lupski JR (2002) Molecular-evolutionary mechanisms for genomic disorders. Curr Opin Genet Dev 12: 312–319
Swillen A, Devriendt K, Legius E, Prinzie P, Vogels A, Ghesquiere P, Fryns JP (1999) The behavioural phenotype in velo-cardio-facial syndrome (VCFS): from infancy to adolescence. Genet Couns 10:79–88
Thiel CT, Kraus C, Rauch A, Ekici AB, Rautenstrauss B, Reis A (2003) A new quantitative PCR multiplex assay for rapid analysis of chromosome 17p11.2–12 duplications and deletions leading to HMSN/HNPP. Eur J Hum Genet 11:170–178

Report

Congenital Diaphragmatic Hernia and Chromosome 15q26: Determination of a Candidate Region by Use of Fluorescent In Situ Hybridization and Array-Based Comparative Genomic Hybridization

M. Klaassens,[1,2,*] M. van Dooren,[2,*] H. J. Eussen,[2] H. Douben,[2] A. T. den Dekker,[2] C. Lee,[4] P. K. Donahoe,[5] R. J. Galjaard,[2] N. Goemaere,[3] R. R. de Krijger,[3] C. Wouters,[2] J. Wauters,[6] B. A. Oostra,[2] D. Tibboel,[1] and A. de Klein[2]

Departments of [1]Paediatric Surgery and [2]Clinical Genetics, Erasmus Medical Centre, and [3]Department of Pathology, Josephine Nefkens Institute, Erasmus Medical Centre, Rotterdam, The Netherlands; [4]Department of Pathology, Brigham and Women's Hospital and Harvard Medical School, and [5]Department of Surgery and Pediatric Surgical Research Laboratories, Massachusetts General Hospital and Harvard Medical School, Boston; and [6]Department of Cytogenetics, University Hospital Antwerpen, Antwerpen, Belgium

Congenital diaphragmatic hernia (CDH) has an incidence of 1 in 3,000 births and a high mortality rate (33%–58%). Multifactorial inheritance, teratogenic agents, and genetic abnormalities have all been suggested as possible etiologic factors. To define candidate regions for CDH, we analyzed cytogenetic data collected on 200 CDH cases, of which 7% and 5% showed numerical and structural abnormalities, respectively. This study focused on the most frequent structural anomaly found: a deletion on chromosome 15q. We analyzed material from three of our patients and from four previously published patients with CDH and a 15q deletion. By using array-based comparative genomic hybridization and fluorescent in situ hybridization to determine the boundaries of the deletions and by including data from two individuals with terminal 15q deletions but without CDH, we were able to exclude a substantial portion of the telomeric region from the genetic etiology of this disorder. Moreover, one patient with CDH harbored a small interstitial deletion. Together, these findings allowed us to define a minimal deletion region of ~5 Mb at chromosome 15q26.1-26.2. The region contains four known genes, of which two—*NR2F2* and *CHD2*—are particularly intriguing gene candidates for CDH.

Congenital diaphragmatic hernia (CDH [MIM 142340]), a severe, life-threatening, congenital anomaly characterized by variable defect in the diaphragm, pulmonary hypoplasia, and postnatal pulmonary hypertension, is a relatively common anomaly (Torfs et al. 1992; Beresford and Shaw 2000). CDH can occur as an isolated defect, in combination with multiple congenital anomalies, or as part of a defined syndrome (Fryns et al. 1979; Enns et al. 1998). Little is known about the etiology of CDH. However, there is increasing evidence for a genetic cause of CDH. Various chromosomal anomalies have been described in CDH, with numerical abnormalities (such as trisomies 13, 18, and 21) as the most common type. Structural chromosomal anomalies, involving almost every chromosome, have been reported (Lurie 2003). Since 1988, clinical data from all Erasmus Medical Centre patients with CDH have been stored in a database. Cytogenetic data from 200 patients with CDH were available, and 24 patients (12%) showed an abnormality. Fourteen patients (7%) showed a numerical abnormality (trisomy 18 or 21). The remaining 10 patients (5%) had a structural anomaly, and 3 of those patients (1.5%) were shown to have a deletion of part of chromosome 15q. The present study focuses on this subset of patients with CDH and chromosome 15q deletions. Data from four previously published patients with CDH and small chromosome 15q deletions were generously made available to us (table 1) (de Jong et al. 1989; Rosenberg et al. 1992; Chen et al. 1998; Schlembach et al. 2001). Clinical evaluation of the seven patients revealed a left-sided diaphragmatic hernia of the Bochdalek type, in-

Received December 9, 2004; accepted for publication February 21, 2005; electronically published March 4, 2005.

Address for correspondence and reprints: Dr. A. de Klein, Department of Clinical Genetics, Erasmus MC, Postbus 1738, 3000 DR Rotterdam, The Netherlands. E-mail: a.deklein@erasmusmc.nl

* These authors contributed equally to this article.

0002-9297/2005/7605-0015$15.00

Table 1

Summary of Clinical and Cytogenetic Data for Patients with Deletions Involving Chromosome 15

Patient	Karyotype	CDH[a]	Other Abnormalities[b]	Deletion Size (Mb)
1	46,XY,t(1;14),inv(6),del(15)(q26)	Yes	Genital anomalies; IUGR	6.3
2	46,XY,r(15)(p11q26)	Yes	Dysmorphic features; cardiac, renal, genital, and limb abnormalities; IUGR	19.9
3	46,XY,r(15)(p11q26)	Yes	Dysmorphic features; cardiac abnormalities; IUGR	23.3
4	46,XX,der(15)t(3;15)(q29;q26.1)	Yes	Dysmorphic features; cardiac and limb abnormalities; two-vessel umbilical cord; IUGR	22.8
5	46,XY,r(15)(p11q26.1)	Yes	Dysmorphic features; genital and limb abnormalities; IUGR	23
6	46,XX,der(15)t(8;15)(q24.1;q26.1)	Yes	Hydrocephaly; dysmorphic features; cardiac, renal, limb, and spine abnormalities; IUGR	16.8
7	46,XX,del(15)(q25q26.3)	Yes	Dysmorphic features; renal and limb abnormalities; IUGR	22.3
8	46,XX,r(15)(p11.1q26.3)	No	Mental retardation; mild dysmorphic features; IUGR	16.3
9	46,XY,del(15)(q26)	No	Mental retardation	15.6

NOTE.—Sources for patients 1–3 and 8, Erasmus Medical Centre, Rotterdam, The Netherlands; patient 4, Rosenberg et al. 1992 (case 2); patient 5, de Jong et al. 1989; patient 6, Chen et al. 1998; patient 7, Schlembach et al. 2001; patient 9, J. Wauters, University Hospital Antwerpen, Antwerpen, Belgium.

[a] Left-sided, Bochdalek-type CDH (if present).

[b] IUGR = intrauterine growth retardation (birth weight <3rd percentile).

trauterine growth retardation (all patients had birth weights <3rd percentile), and multiple other congenital anomalies, such as cardiac and renal abnormalities. In addition to the seven patients with CDH, we analyzed data from two patients with mental retardation and 15q deletions but without CDH manifestation. Genomic DNA was extracted from cultured cells (from patients 1, 2, 3, 4, and 9) or paraffin-embedded tissue (from patients 5 and 6).

To delineate the possible candidate region, array-based comparative genomic hybridization (array CGH) was performed using the 1-Mb Human BAC Array (Spectral Genomics) in accordance with the manufacturer's instructions. A dye-swap experimental strategy was used as an additional internal control. Fluorescent signals on the arrays were visualized using the ScanArray Express HT scanner. Images were analyzed with Spectral Ware 2 (Spectral Genomics). Results for patients 1, 3, 4, 7, and 8 are shown in figure 1.

To further delineate the deleted region and to deter-

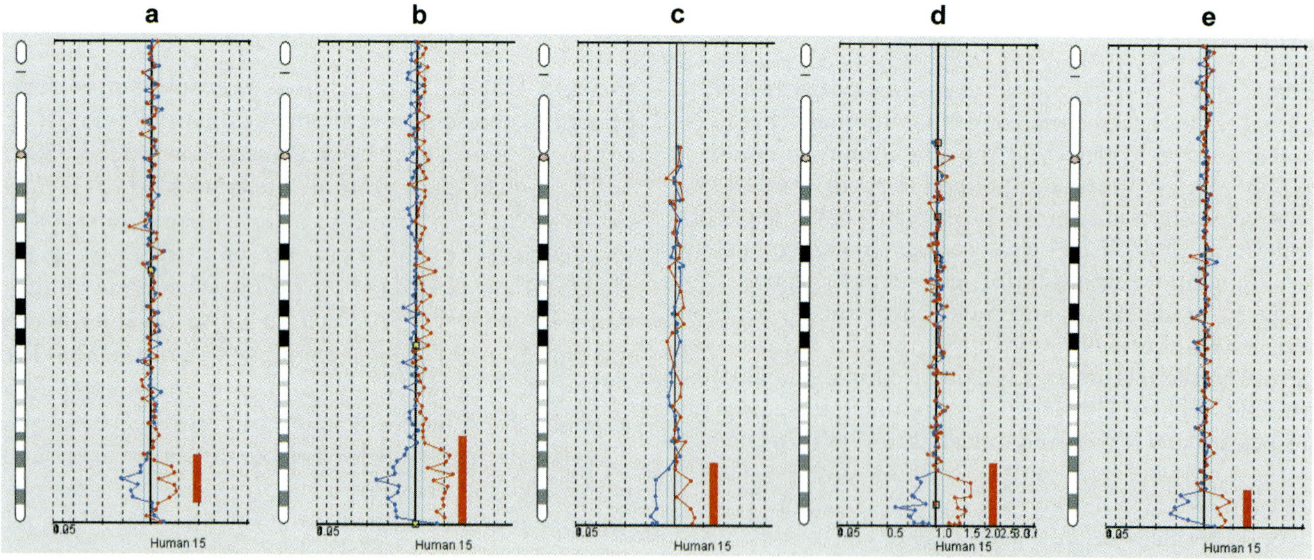

Figure 1 Array CGH results. *a,* Patient 1, with CDH and del(15) interstitial deletion. *b,* Patient 3, with CDH and r(15)(p11q26). *c,* Patient 4, with CDH and der(15)t(3;15)(q29;q26.1). *d,* Patient 7, with CDH and del(15)(q25q26.3). *e,* Patient 8, without CDH and with r(15)(p11.1q26.3).

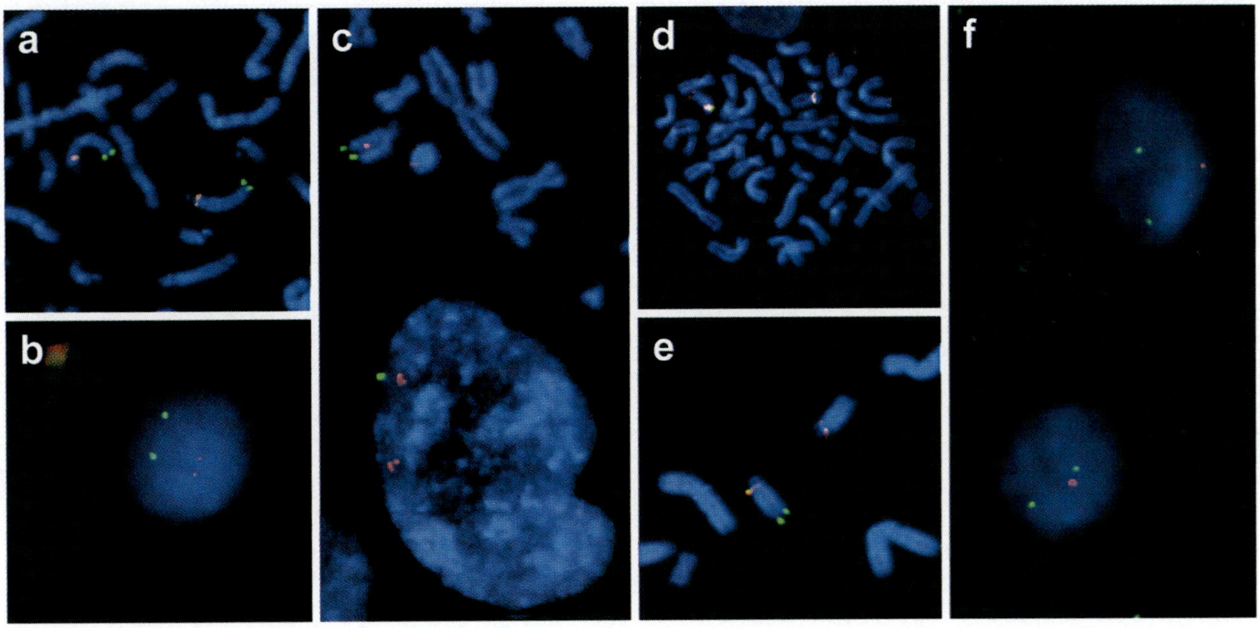

Figure 2 FISH results. *a*, Patient 1: partial metaphase, probe D15Z4 (*red signal*) at chromosome 15 centromeric locus and probe RP11-114I24 (*green signal*) at 15q26.3. *b*, Patient 2: interphase, probe RP11-369K8 (*red signal*) and RP11-253B9 (*green signal*) near the chromosome 5 centromeric region at 5p13.2. *c*, Patient 3: partial metaphase and interphase, deletion probe RP11-143C19 (*green signal*) and normal probe RP11-64K10 (*red signal*) at 15q23. *d*, Patient 4: metaphase spread, gain of chromosome 3q29; probe RP1-196F4 (*red signal*) (3qtel) present on der(15) and normal signal probe *D15Z4* (*yellow/red signal*) at the centromeric region of chromosome 15. The der(15) contains both signals. *e*, Patient 4: partial metaphase, deletion probe RP11-183E24 (*green signal*) at 15q26.2 and normal probe *D15Z4* (*yellow/red signal*). *f*, Patient 6: interphase, deletion probe RP11–57P19 (*red signal*) and normal probe *D15Z4* (*green signal*). Patients 1–6 all have CDH.

mine the deletions in patients 4, 5, and 9, ∼110 BAC clones were selected from the University of California Santa Cruz (UCSC) and Ensembl genome browsers to cover the distal part of chromosome 15. Using the appropriate BAC clones, we performed FISH on metaphase chromosomes from patients 1, 3, and 4 (fig. 2*a* and 2*c*–2*e*). Interphase FISH was performed on nuclei extracted from paraffin-embedded tissues from patients 2, 5, and 6 (fig. 2*b* and 2*f*; data for patient 5 not shown). Only genomic DNA was available from patients 7 and 8, so the size of the deletion in these patients was determined using only array CGH. FISH slides were analyzed using the Axioplan 2 Imaging microscope (Zeiss), and images were collected using the Isis Software System (Metasystems). Combining FISH and array CGH data, we were able to approximately determine the breakpoints in all patients (fig. 3). In patient 1, the interstitial deletion found by array CGH was confirmed and was narrowed to a 6-Mb deletion between BAC clones RP11-79A7 and RP11-616M17. In patient 2, the deletion extended from a region distal to RP11-79A7; in patient 3, it extended from a region distal to RP11-300G22. The proximal breakpoint in patient 4 lies within BAC clone RP11-617F23. In patient 5, the break occurs distal to RP11-300G22. In patient 6, the most distal probe tested that was present on the deleted chromosome 15 was RP11-79A7. The terminal deletion in patient 7 occurs distal to RP11-360F18. The proximal breakpoints of the deletion interval in the two patients without CDH were similarly determined (fig. 3). In the first patient without CDH, who had a ring chromosome 15, the most distal BAC clone tested that was present on the ring chromosome was RP11-120N1. In the second patient without CDH, the most distal BAC clone present was RP11-262P8. Combining all data, we determined the smallest common deletion interval in patients with CDH to be at 15q26.1-26.2 (which we have termed the "CDH region"). This region is ∼5 Mb in size and is bordered by BAC clones RP11-79A7 and RP11-80F4.

CDH is unlike many genetic disorders, for which candidate genes can be determined by using linkage analyses of familial cases, because the vast majority of CDH cases occur de novo. For this type of disorder, the best way to determine which genes are involved is by analyzing a large number of patients for common aberrations by use of different high-resolution genetic methodologies, such as FISH or array CGH. This strategy has already been used successfully to identify genes involved in CHARGE syndrome (MIM 214800) (Vissers et al. 2004) and Cornelia de Lange syndrome (CdLS [MIM 122470]) (Krantz et al. 2004; Tonkin et al. 2004).

Isolated reports of distal chromosome 15 deletions

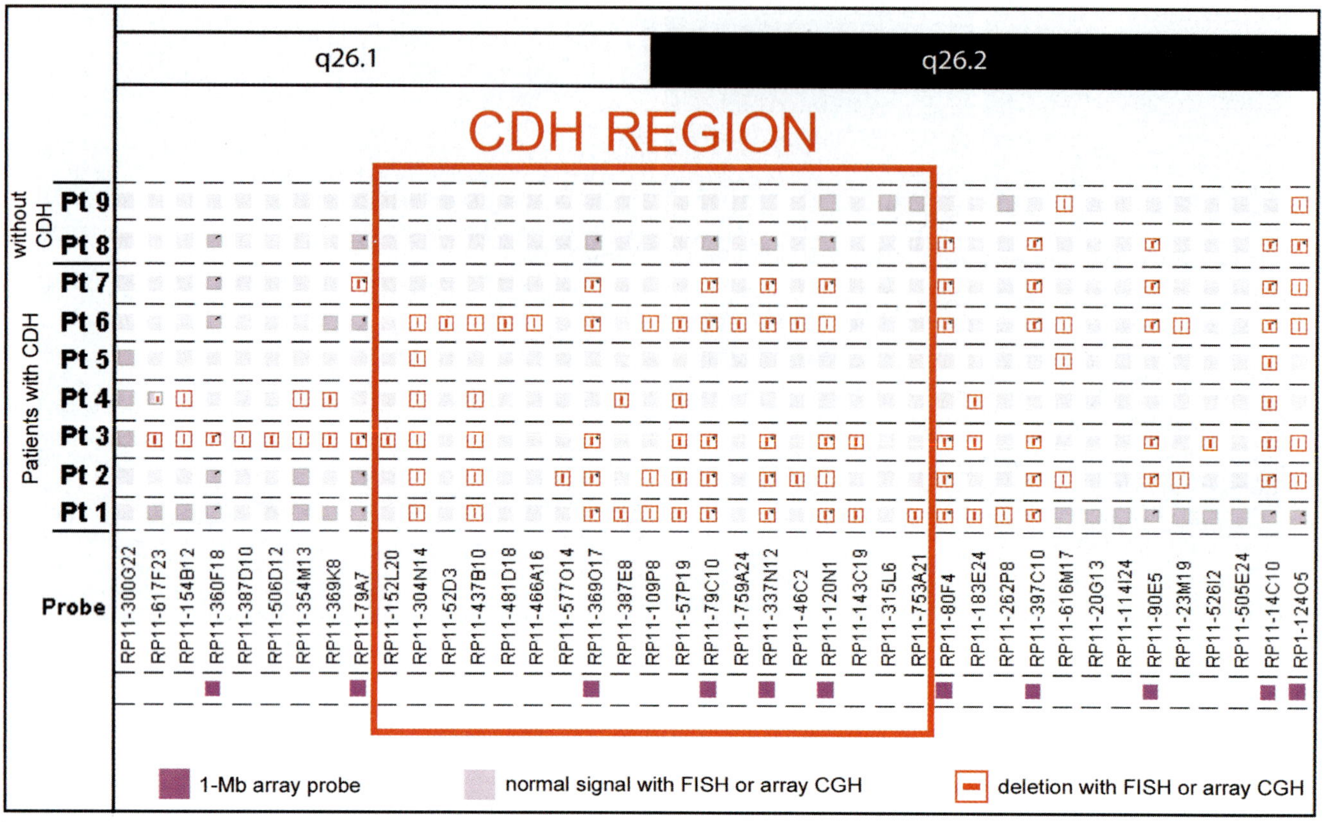

Figure 3 Schematic representation of the critical CDH region, with partial ideogram of chromosome 15q. Patients (Pt) 1–7 have CDH; patients 8 and 9 do not have CDH. BAC clones that were tested by array CGH and FISH are listed. The black dots inside boxes indicate that probes have been tested only on the array and not by FISH. The smallest common overlapping deletion interval involved in CDH is denoted by the large red square.

in patients with CDH have been described elsewhere (reviewed by Hengstschlager et al. [2004] and Schlembach et al. [2001]), suggesting involvement of this region in the pathogenesis of CDH. In the past year, three new cases of CDH have been reported (Biggio et al. 2004; Hengstschlager et al. 2004; Tonks et al. 2004). However, detailed molecular cytogenetic analyses of these cases are currently unavailable. To find other possible cases to study, we performed systematic FISH analysis on data from 25 patients with CDH, with the use of BAC clones spanning the CDH region. We identified no additional 15q deletions.

With array CGH and systematic FISH analysis performed on the seven patients with CDH and 15q deletions and the two patients without CDH but with 15q deletions, our study is the first to analyze data from multiple patients with CDH in detail and to refine the chromosome 15q critical CDH region to an ~5-Mb area within 15q26.1-26.2. In all patients, clinical abnormalities resembled the features described for other patients with a 15q deletion or with related syndromes, such as Fryns syndrome (MIM 229850) (Fryns et al. 1979). As can be expected, the r(15) patients, with or without CDH, had phenotypes similar to those seen with ring chromosome 15 syndrome (Butler et al. 1988; Rogan et al. 1996). To our knowledge, CDH has not yet been described as a main feature in ring chromosome 15 syndrome.

In our study, there appears to be a relationship between the number of abnormalities present and the size of the deletion. For example, the first patient, who had the smallest deletion, has few additional congenital defects. All other patients have deletions that are similar in size and have a similar spectrum of anatomical anomalies. In the two patients with an unbalanced translocation, the variation in phenotype could also be due, in part, to the presence of extra material from another chromosome.

The region of the smallest common deletion contains four known genes, none of which have been previously shown to be involved in diaphragm development or diaphragmatic hernia. On the basis of their structure and function, two of these genes are very interesting with respect to a potential relationship with CDH. The first gene, *NR2F2* (MIM 107773; also known as "*COUP-*

TFII"), is a member of the steroid/thyroid hormone receptor subfamily and is involved in retinoic acid metabolism (Kimura et al. 2002). A knockout mouse model of *NR2F2* showed that $Nr2f2^{-/-}$ mice are not viable and die at E9 in utero because of arrest of cardiac development (Pereira et al. 1999). Heterozygous knockout mice have poor viability in the neonatal period and are smaller than wild-type mice. However, the exact cause of death in these mice is not clear. The second interesting gene is the chromodomain helicase 2 gene (*CHD2* [MIM 602119]), a member of the SNF2/RAD54 helicase gene family. Recently, mutations in another member of this family (*CHD7*) have been found to cause CHARGE syndrome (Vissers et al. 2004). The third gene in the CDH region is the repulsive guidance molecule gene, *RGMA* (MIM 607362), which is involved in the guidance of growth cones in developing neurons (Brinks et al. 2004). This gene is not known to play a role in diaphragm development, nor has it been described in muscle or lung development. The fourth gene located in the smallest region of overlap is the sialyltransferase 8B gene (*SIAT8B* [MIM 602546]), which plays a role in the adhesive properties of neural cell adhesion molecules (Angata et al. 1997).

Haploinsufficiency due to the loss of a copy of one of these genes may be enough to result in a diaphragmatic defect. At the present time, the precise mechanism by which a deletion of or within one of these genes or a related gene mutation causes this developmental defect can only be speculated.

Elsewhere, other genes on chromosome 15q have been suggested as being involved in the pathogenesis of diaphragmatic defects. Biggio et al. (2004) suggested that the myocyte enhancer factor 2A gene, *MEF2A* (MIM 600660), could be involved in the pathogenesis of diaphragmatic defects. *MEF2A* maps to 15q26.3 and is involved in the differentiation of muscle cells from their precursors. Some genes involved in vitamin A metabolism—for example, *RALDH2* (MIM 603687), which maps to 15q21—have also been implicated in the pathogenesis of CDH (Greer et al. 2003). Both *MEF2A* and *RALDH2* are located outside our candidate critical CDH region, which limits their possible role in CDH in our subgroup of patients.

In conclusion, we have mapped a potential critical CDH region to 5 Mb at chromosome 15q26.1-26.2, a region that contains four genes, of which two are especially intriguing candidates in the etiology of diaphragmatic defects. Further research is needed to confirm their exact role in CDH and to determine the pathogenic mechanism. As a first step, we are performing FISH and mutation analyses of a large group of patients with CDH who have normal karyotypes. In the future, prenatal screening for 15q abnormalities when a diaphragmatic hernia is detected could give better clues for predicting the outcome and could provide more information for genetic counseling.

Acknowledgments

We thank C. P. Chen, G. de Jong, D. Schlembach, G. Stetten, and B. Ceulemans, for kindly providing us with data from patients with chromosome 15 deletions; T. de Vries Lentsch, for assistance with manuscript preparation; B. Pober, for critical reading of the manuscript; and M. Listewnik, for array CGH technical assistance. This research was funded in part by the Sophia Foundation for Scientific Research, Rotterdam, The Netherlands (SSWO project 441), and National Institute of Health program project grant HD39942 (to P.K.D. and C.L.).

Electronic-Database Information

The URLs for data presented herein are as follows:

Ensembl Genome Browser, http://www.ensembl.org/Homo_Sapiens/

Online Mendelian Inheritance in Man (OMIM), http://www.ncbi.nlm.nih.gov/Omim/ (for CDH, CHARGE syndrome, CdLS, Fryns syndrome, *NR2F2, CHD2, RGMA, SIAT8B, MEF2A,* and *RALDH2*)

UCSC Genome Browser, http://genome.cse.ucsc.edu/

References

Angata K, Nakayama J, Fredette B, Chong K, Ranscht B, Fukuda M (1997) Human STX polysialyltransferase forms the embryonic form of the neural cell adhesion molecule: tissue-specific expression, neurite outgrowth, and chromosomal localization in comparison with another polysialyltransferase, PST. J Biol Chem 272:7182–7190

Beresford MW, Shaw NJ (2000) Outcome of congenital diaphragmatic hernia. Pediatr Pulmonol 30:249–256

Biggio JR Jr, Descartes MD, Carroll AJ, Holt RL (2004) Congenital diaphragmatic hernia: is 15q26.1-26.2 a candidate locus? Am J Med Genet A 126:183–185

Brinks H, Conrad S, Vogt J, Oldekamp J, Sierra A, Deitinghoff L, Bechmann I, Alvarez-Bolado G, Heimrich B, Monnier PP, Mueller BK, Skutella T (2004) The repulsive guidance molecule RGMa is involved in the formation of afferent connections in the dentate gyrus. J Neurosci 24:3862–3869

Butler MG, Fogo AB, Fuchs DA, Collins FS, Dev VG, Phillips JA III (1988) Two patients with ring chromosome 15 syndrome. Am J Med Genet 29:149–154

Chen CP, Lee CC, Pan CW, Kir TY, Chen BF (1998) Partial trisomy 8q and partial monosomy 15q associated with congenital hydrocephalus, diaphragmatic hernia, urinary tract anomalies, congenital heart defect and kyphoscoliosis. Prenat Diagn 18:1289–1293

de Jong G, Rossouw RA, Retief AE (1989) Ring chromosome 15 in a patient with features of Fryns' syndrome. J Med Genet 26:469–470

Enns GM, Cox VA, Goldstein RB, Gibbs DL, Harrison MR, Golabi M (1998) Congenital diaphragmatic defects and associated syndromes, malformations, and chromosome anomalies: a retrospective study of 60 patients and literature review. Am J Med Genet 79:215–225

Fryns JP, Moerman F, Goddeeris P, Bossuyt C, Van den Berghe H (1979) A new lethal syndrome with cloudy corneae, diaphragmatic defects and distal limb deformities. Hum Genet 50:65–70

Greer JJ, Babiuk RP, Thebaud B (2003) Etiology of congenital diaphragmatic hernia: the retinoid hypothesis. Pediatr Res 53:726–730

Hengstschlager M, Mittermayer C, Repa C, Drahonsky R, Deutinger J, Bernaschek G (2004) Association of deletions of the chromosomal region 15q24-ter and diaphragmatic hernia: a new case and discussion of the literature. Fetal Diagn Ther 19:510–512

Kimura Y, Suzuki T, Kaneko C, Darnel AD, Moriya T, Suzuki S, Handa M, Ebina M, Nukiwa T, Sasano H (2002) Retinoid receptors in the developing human lung. Clin Sci (Lond) 103: 613–621

Krantz ID, McCallum J, DeScipio C, Kaur M, Gillis LA, Yaeger D, Jukofsky L, Wasserman N, Bottani A, Morris CA, Nowaczyk MJ, Toriello H, Bamshad MJ, Carey JC, Rappaport E, Kawauchi S, Lander AD, Calof AL, Li HH, Devoto M, Jackson LG (2004) Cornelia de Lange syndrome is caused by mutations in *NIPBL*, the human homolog of *Drosophila melanogaster Nipped-B*. Nat Genet 36:631–635

Lurie IW (2003) Where to look for the genes related to diaphragmatic hernia? Genet Couns 14:75–93

Pereira FA, Qiu Y, Zhou G, Tsai MJ, Tsai SY (1999) The orphan nuclear receptor COUP-TFII is required for angiogenesis and heart development. Genes Dev 13:1037–1049

Rogan PK, Seip JR, Driscoll DJ, Papenhausen PR, Johnson VP, Raskin S, Woodward AL, Butler MG (1996) Distinct 15q genotypes in Russell-Silver and ring 15 syndromes. Am J Med Genet 62:10–15

Rosenberg C, Blakemore KJ, Kearns WG, Giraldez RA, Escallon CS, Pearson PL, Stetten G (1992) Analysis of reciprocal translocations by chromosome painting: applications and limitations of the technique. Am J Hum Genet 50:700–705

Schlembach D, Zenker M, Trautmann U, Ulmer R, Beinder E (2001) Deletion 15q24-26 in prenatally detected diaphragmatic hernia: increasing evidence of a candidate region for diaphragmatic development. Prenat Diagn 21:289–292

Tonkin ET, Wang TJ, Lisgo S, Bamshad MJ, Strachan T (2004) *NIPBL*, encoding a homolog of fungal Scc2-type sister chromatid cohesion proteins and fly Nipped-B, is mutated in Cornelia de Lange syndrome. Nat Genet 36:636–641

Tonks A, Wyldes M, Somerset DA, Dent K, Abhyankar A, Bagchi I, Lander A, Roberts E, Kilby MD (2004) Congenital malformations of the diaphragm: findings of the West Midlands Congenital Anomaly Register 1995 to 2000. Prenat Diagn 24:596–604

Torfs CP, Curry CJ, Bateson TF, Honore LH (1992) A population-based study of congenital diaphragmatic hernia. Teratology 46:555–565

Vissers LE, Van Ravenswaaij CM, Admiraal R, Hurst JA, De Vries BB, Janssen IM, Van Der Vliet WA, Huys EH, De Jong PJ, Hamel BC, Schoenmakers EF, Brunner HG, Veltman JA, Van Kessel AG (2004) Mutations in a new member of the chromodomain gene family cause CHARGE syndrome. Nat Genet 36:955–957

Report

Saami and Berbers—An Unexpected Mitochondrial DNA Link

Alessandro Achilli,[1] Chiara Rengo,[1] Vincenza Battaglia,[1] Maria Pala,[1] Anna Olivieri,[1] Simona Fornarino,[1] Chiara Magri,[1] Rosaria Scozzari,[2] Nora Babudri,[3] A. Silvana Santachiara-Benerecetti,[1] Hans-Jürgen Bandelt,[4] Ornella Semino,[1] and Antonio Torroni[1]

[1]Dipartimento di Genetica e Microbiologia, Università di Pavia, Pavia, Italy; [2]Dipartimento di Genetica e Biologia Molecolare, Università "La Sapienza," Rome; [3]Dipartimento di Biologia Cellulare e Ambientale, Università di Perugia, Perugia, Italy; and [4]Fachbereich Mathematik, Universität Hamburg, Hamburg

The sequencing of entire human mitochondrial DNAs belonging to haplogroup U reveals that this clade arose shortly after the "out of Africa" exit and rapidly radiated into numerous regionally distinct subclades. Intriguingly, the Saami of Scandinavia and the Berbers of North Africa were found to share an extremely young branch, aged merely ~9,000 years. This unexpected finding not only confirms that the Franco-Cantabrian refuge area of southwestern Europe was the source of late-glacial expansions of hunter-gatherers that repopulated northern Europe after the Last Glacial Maximum but also reveals a direct maternal link between those European hunter-gatherer populations and the Berbers.

Because of maternal transmission and lack of recombination, the sequence differentiation of human mtDNA has been generated by only the sequential accumulation of new mutations along radiating maternal lineages. Over the course of time, this process of molecular divergence has given rise to monophyletic units that are called "haplogroups." Because this process of molecular differentiation occurred mainly during and after the process of human colonization of and diffusion into the different continents and regions, haplogroups and subhaplogroups tend to be restricted to specific geographic areas and population groups (Wallace 1995; Achilli et al. 2004).

Only the founders of the sister superhaplogroups M and N (which includes haplogroup R) (Quintana-Murci et al. 1999) participated in the "out of Africa" exit (Cann et al. 1987; Stringer and Andrews 1988; Cavalli-Sforza et al. 1994; Underhill et al. 2000; Forster et al. 2001) and were successful in colonizing the rest of the Old World. Superhaplogroup N is globally distributed outside Africa, encompassing virtually all of the western Eurasian mtDNA variation, and embraces haplogroup U, nested in haplogroup R. Haplogroup U has an extremely broad geographic distribution that ranges from Europe and North Africa to India and Central Asia and has a very high overall frequency (15%–30%) (Richards et al. 2000; Kivisild et al. 2003; Quintana-Murci et al. 2004)

To assess the nature and extent of haplogroup U variation, we initially sequenced 28 entire U mtDNAs (see authors' Web site and GenBank) from a wide range of populations. These were selected through a preliminary sequence analysis of the mtDNA control region to include the widest possible range of haplogroup U internal variation. A tree of the mtDNA sequences (fig. 1) reveals that haplogroup U first splits into two major subsets, distinguished by the mutation at nt 1811, and that there is a very large number of independent basal branches. Among these, representatives of all known subhaplogroups (U1–U9) were included. However, subhaplogroup U5 provided a rather intriguing result. A Yakut from northeastern Siberia (27 in fig. 1) and a Fulbe from Senegal (29 in fig. 1) harbored mtDNAs that differed at only two coding-region nucleotide positions.

To investigate this striking similarity, the portion of the tree encompassing these two mtDNAs was enriched by sequencing 11 additional mtDNA sequences (22–26,

Received January 21, 2005; accepted for publication March 3, 2005; electronically published March 24, 2005.

Address for correspondence and reprints: Dr. Antonio Torroni, Dipartimento di Genetica e Microbiologia, Università di Pavia, Via Ferrata 1, 27100 Pavia, Italy. E-mail: torroni@ipvgen.unipv.it

0002-9297/2005/7605-0016$15.00

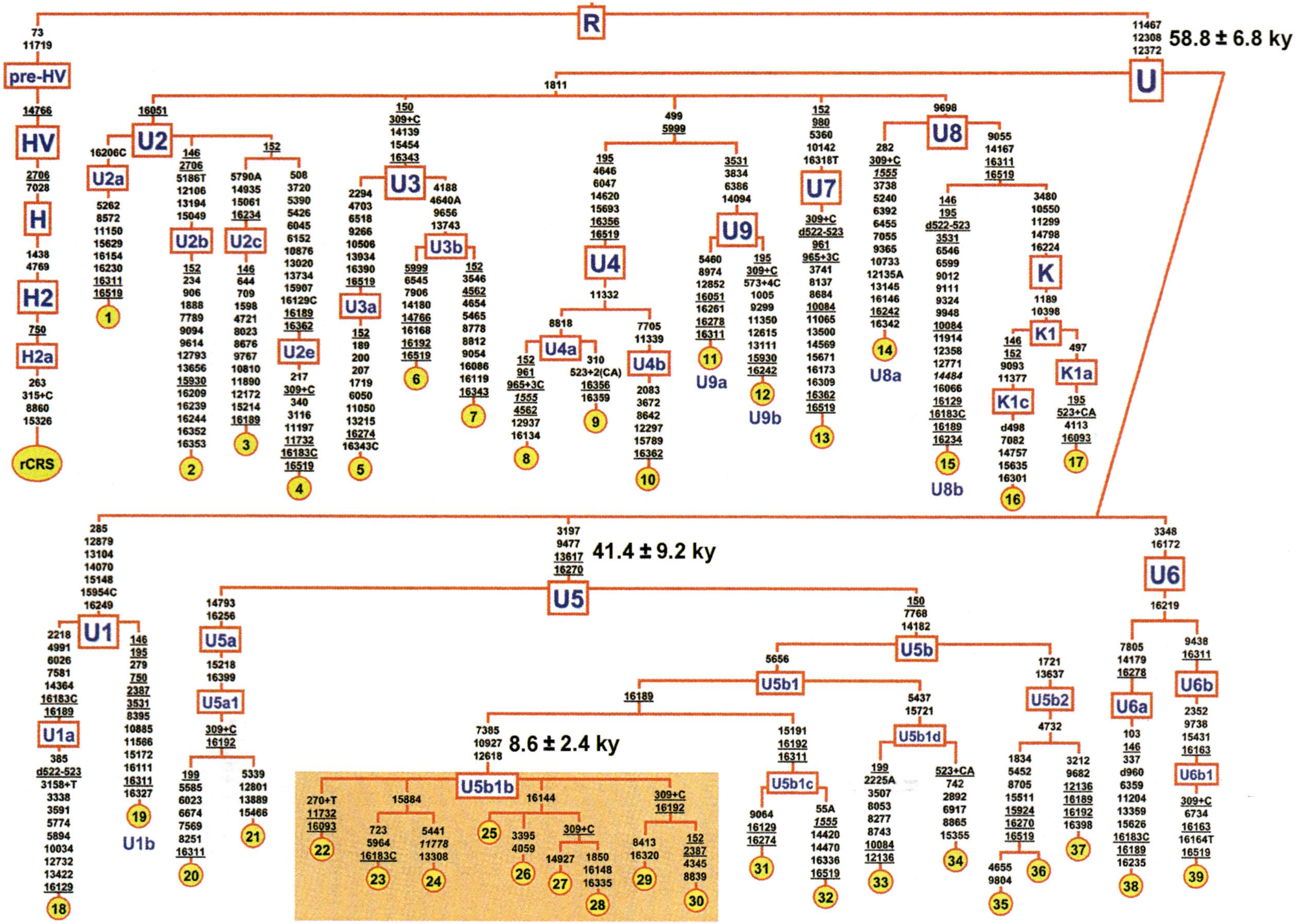
R
pre-HV
HV
H
H2
H2a
rCRS
U
58.8 ± 6.8 ky
U2
U2a
U2b
U2c
U2e
U3
U3a
U3b
U4
U4a
U4b
U9
U9a
U9b
U7
U8
U8a
U8b
K
K1
K1a
K1c
U5
41.4 ± 9.2 ky
U1
U1a
U1b
U5a
U5a1
U5b
U5b1
U5b1b
8.6 ± 2.4 ky
U5b1c
U5b1d
U5b2
U6
U6a
U6b
U6b1

28, 30, 32, 34, 36, and 37 in fig. 1) bearing the control-region motif 16270-150, a motif found generally at low frequencies (<2%) in Berber populations and in other African groups (such as the Fulbe) known to have intermingled with Berbers (Rosa et al. 2004). The motif also shows similarly low frequencies in virtually all European populations, except the Saami of northern Scandinavia, in which it reaches ~48% (Tambets et al 2004). Because virtually all Saami mtDNAs with 16270-150 harbor the transitions at nts 16189 and 16144 seen in the Yakut mtDNA, three Saami mtDNAs were included among the additional samples.

Seven of the new sequences (one Berber from Algeria, two Italian, one Spanish, and three Saami) clustered into U5b1b, the subclade encompassing the Yakut and Fulbe mtDNAs. The Saami and the Yakut mtDNAs formed a minor branch distinguished only by the transition at nt 16144, the Berber and the Fulbe mtDNAs clustered in a second minor branch also characterized only by control-region mutations, and the Italian and Spanish mtDNAs formed other minor branches.

The average sequence divergence ($\pm$ SE, computed as per Saillard et al. [2000]) of the 39 coding-region sequences from the root of haplogroup U was 11.4 ± 1.3 substitutions (disregarding indels and pathological mutations), a value which corresponds—according to the mutation-rate estimate of Mishmar et al. (2003)—to a coalescence time estimate of 58.8 ± 6.8 thousand years (ky) for the entire haplogroup U. This value agrees well with the corresponding estimate of 61.6 ± 12.5 ky, based on the hypervariable segment I (HVS-I) mutation rate (Forster et al. 1996), for these 39 mtDNAs. An age of ~60 ky indicates that haplogroup U arose very soon after the "out of Africa" exit. As for U5, its sequence divergence was 8.1 ± 1.8 substitutions, corresponding to 41.4 ± 9.2 ky, a time estimate in full agreement with its proposed proto-European origin (Richards et al. 2000). It is striking that the sequence divergence of U5b1b, the subclade encompassing mtDNAs from the Saami, Yakut, Berbers, and Fulbe, was 1.7 ± 0.5 substitutions, thus corresponding to only 8.6 ± 2.4 ky.

Such a recent common ancestry of maternal lineages found in populations living as far as 9,000 miles apart and whose anthropological affinities are not at all obvious is, to say the least, unexpected. Can we provide a reasonable explanation? The recent molecular dissection of other mtDNA haplogroups reveals some clues. H1 and H3, two frequent subhaplogroups of H, display frequency peaks centered in Iberia and surrounding populations, including the Berbers of Morocco, and coalescence ages of ~11 ky (Achilli et al. 2004). Furthermore, their frequency patterns and ages resemble those reported for haplogroup V (Torroni et al. 2001*a*)—which, similar to U5b1b, is extremely common only in the Saami (together, U5b1b and V encompass almost 90% of the Saami mtDNAs) (Torroni et al. 1996; Tambets et al. 2004). Thus, although these previous studies have highlighted the role of the Franco-Cantabrian refuge area as a major source of the hunter-gatherer populations that gradually repopulated much of central and northern Europe when climatic conditions began to improve ~15 ky ago, the identification of U5b1b now unequivocally links the maternal gene pool of the ancestral Berbers to the same refuge area and indicates that European hunter-gatherers also moved toward the south and, by crossing the Strait of Gibraltar, contributed their U5b1b, H1, H3, and V mtDNAs to modern North Africans.

In conclusion, this study is a paradigmatic example of the power of genetic inference in human-origin and evolutionary studies. It shows that mtDNA data—in this case, at the highest possible level of molecular resolution—can be used not only to evaluate models proposed by other disciplines and based on the direct survey of ancient material but also to identify previously unknown links between populations and geographic areas. Thus, the study of human genetics directly fosters the development of new research avenues in paleontology, archaeology, linguistics, and history.

Acknowledgments

This research was supported by CNR-MIUR Genomica Funzionale-Legge 449/97, Fondo Investimenti Ricerca di Base 2001, the Istituto Pasteur Fondazione Cenci Bolognetti, and Progetti Ricerca Interesse Nazionale 2003.

Figure 1 Tree of 39 mtDNA sequences belonging to haplogroup U. The tree, rooted using the reference sequence (rCRS) (Andrews et al. 1999) as an outgroup, illustrates subhaplogroup affiliations. The sequencing procedure and phylogeny construction were performed as described elsewhere (Torroni et al. 2001*b*; Achilli et al. 2004). For phylogeny construction, the highly variable site 16519 and the length variation in the poly-C stretch at nts 309–315 were not used, and half the weight was assigned to the control-region mutations, relative to that assigned to coding-region mutations. Mutations are shown on the branches; they are transitions unless a base change is explicitly indicated. Insertions are suffixed with a plus sign (+) and the inserted nucleotide(s), and deletions have a "d" prefix. Recurrent mutations are underlined; pathological mutations are in italics. The ethnic/geographic origins of mtDNAs are as follows: Pakistan (1–3, 12, and 13), Spain (4, 8, 14, 23, 36, and 39), Yemen (5 and 7), Adygei (6, 10, 18, and 20), Italy (9, 15–17, 19, 21, 22, 24, 31–33, 35, and 37), Ethiopia (11 and 38), Berber (30 and 34), Saami (25, 26, and 28), Yakut (27), and Fulbe from Senegal (29).

Electronic-Database Information

Accession numbers and URLs for data presented herein are as follows:

Author's Web site, http://ipvgen.unipv.it/docs/projects/torroni_data/torroni_sequences.html (for the complete mtDNA sequences)

GenBank, http://www.ncbi.nlm.nih.gov/Genbank/ (for the complete mtDNA sequences [accession numbers AY882379–AY882417])

References

Achilli A, Rengo C, Magri C, Battaglia V, Olivieri A, Scozzari R, Cruciani F, Zeviani M, Briem E, Carelli V, Moral P, Dugoujon JM, Roostalu U, Loogväli EL, Kivisild T, Bandelt HJ, Richards M, Villems R, Santachiara-Benerecetti AS, Semino O, Torroni A (2004) The molecular dissection of mtDNA haplogroup H confirms that the Franco-Cantabrian glacial refuge was a major source for the European gene pool. Am J Hum Genet 75:910–918

Andrews RM, Kubacka I, Chinnery PF, Lightowlers RN, Turnbull DM, Howell N (1999) Reanalysis and revision of the Cambridge reference sequence for human mitochondrial DNA. Nat Genet 23:147

Cann RL, Stoneking M, Wilson AC (1987) Mitochondrial DNA and human evolution. Nature 325:31–36

Cavalli-Sforza LL, Menozzi P, Piazza A (1994) The history and geography of human genes. Princeton University Press, Princeton, NJ

Forster P, Harding R, Torroni A, Bandelt H-J (1996) Origin and evolution of Native American mtDNA variation: a reappraisal. Am J Hum Genet 59:935–945

Forster P, Torroni A, Renfrew C, Rohl A (2001) Phylogenetic star contraction applied to Asian and Papuan mtDNA evolution. Mol Biol Evol 18:1864–1881

Kivisild T, Rootsi S, Metspalu M, Mastana S, Kaldma K, Parik J, Metspalu E, Adojaan M, Tolk HV, Stepanov V, Golge M, Usanga E, Papiha SS, Cinnioglu C, King R, Cavalli-Sforza L, Underhill PA, Villems R (2003) The genetic heritage of the earliest settlers persists both in Indian tribal and caste populations. Am J Hum Genet 72:313–332

Mishmar D, Ruiz-Pesini E, Golik P, Macaulay V, Clark AG, Hosseini S, Brandon M, Easley K, Chen E, Brown MD, Sukernik RI, Olckers A, Wallace DC (2003) Natural selection shaped regional mtDNA variation in humans. Proc Natl Acad Sci USA 100:171–176

Quintana-Murci L, Chaix R, Wells RS, Behar DM, Sayar H, Scozzari R, Rengo C, Al-Zahery N, Semino O, Santachiara-Benerecetti AS, Coppa A, Ayub Q, Mohyuddin A, Tyler-Smith C, Qasim Mehdi S, Torroni A, McElreavey K (2004) Where west meets east: the complex mtDNA landscape of the southwest and Central Asian corridor. Am J Hum Genet 74:827–845

Quintana-Murci L, Semino O, Bandelt HJ, Passarino G, McElreavey K, Santachiara-Benerecetti AS (1999) Genetic evidence of an early exit of *Homo sapiens sapiens* from Africa through eastern Africa. Nat Genet 23:437–441

Richards M, Macaulay V, Hickey E, Vega E, Sykes B, Guida V, Rengo C, et al (2000) Tracing European founder lineages in the Near Eastern mtDNA pool. Am J Hum Genet 67:1251–1276

Rosa A, Brehm A, Kivisild T, Metspalu E, Villems R (2004) MtDNA profile of West Africa Guineans: towards a better understanding of the Senegambia region. Ann Hum Genet 68:340–352 (erratum 68:658)

Saillard J, Forster P, Lynnerup N, Bandelt H-J, Nørby S (2000) mtDNA variation among Greenland Eskimos: the edge of the Beringian expansion. Am J Hum Genet 67:718–726

Stringer CB, Andrews P (1988) Genetic and fossil evidence for the origin of modern humans. Science 239:1263–1268

Tambets K, Rootsi S, Kivisild T, Help H, Serk P, Loogväli EL, Tolk HV, et al (2004) The western and eastern roots of the Saami—the story of genetic "outliers" told by mitochondrial DNA and Y chromosomes. Am J Hum Genet 74: 661–682

Torroni A, Bandelt H-J, Macaulay V, Richards M, Cruciani F, Rengo C, Martinez-Cabrera V, et al (2001*a*) A signal, from human mtDNA, of postglacial recolonization in Europe. Am J Hum Genet 69:844–852

Torroni A, Huoponen K, Francalacci P, Petrozzi M, Morelli L, Scozzari R, Obinu D, Savontaus ML, Wallace DC (1996) Classification of European mtDNAs from an analysis of three European populations. Genetics 144:1835–1850

Torroni A, Rengo C, Guida V, Cruciani F, Sellitto D, Coppa A, Calderon FL, Simionati B, Valle G, Richards M, Macaulay V, Scozzari R (2001*b*) Do the four clades of the mtDNA haplogroup L2 evolve at different rates? Am J Hum Genet 69:1348–1356

Underhill PA, Shen P, Lin AA, Jin L, Passarino G, Yang WH, Kauffman E, Bonne-Tamir B, Bertranpetit J, Francalacci P, Ibrahim M, Jenkins T, Kidd JR, Mehdi SQ, Seielstad MT, Wells RS, Piazza A, Davis RW, Feldman MW, Cavalli-Sforza LL, Oefner PJ (2000) Y chromosome sequence variation and the history of human populations. Nat Genet 26:358–361

Wallace DC (1995) Mitochondrial DNA variation in human evolution, degenerative disease and aging. Am J Hum Genet 57:201–223

Report

A Note on Exact Tests of Hardy-Weinberg Equilibrium

Janis E. Wigginton,[1] David J. Cutler,[2] and Gonçalo R. Abecasis[1]

[1]Center for Statistical Genetics, Department of Biostatistics, University of Michigan, Ann Arbor; and [2]Institute of Genetic Medicine, Johns Hopkins University School of Medicine, Baltimore

Deviations from Hardy-Weinberg equilibrium (HWE) can indicate inbreeding, population stratification, and even problems in genotyping. In samples of affected individuals, these deviations can also provide evidence for association. Tests of HWE are commonly performed using a simple χ^2 goodness-of-fit test. We show that this χ^2 test can have inflated type I error rates, even in relatively large samples (e.g., samples of 1,000 individuals that include ~100 copies of the minor allele). On the basis of previous work, we describe exact tests of HWE together with efficient computational methods for their implementation. Our methods adequately control type I error in large and small samples and are computationally efficient. They have been implemented in freely available code that will be useful for quality assessment of genotype data and for the detection of genetic association or population stratification in very large data sets.

In the absence of migration, mutation, natural selection, and assortative mating, genotype frequencies at any locus are a simple function of allele frequencies. This phenomenon, now termed "Hardy-Weinberg equilibrium" (HWE), was first described in the early part of the twentieth century (Hardy 1908; Weinberg 1908). The original descriptions of HWE are an important landmark in the history of population genetics (Crow 1988), and it is now common practice to check whether observed genotypes conform to Hardy-Weinberg expectations. These expectations appear to hold for most human populations, and deviations from HWE at particular markers may suggest problems with genotyping or population structure or, in samples of affected individuals, an association between the marker and disease susceptibility.

Here, we describe efficient implementations of exact tests for HWE, which are suitable for use in large-scale studies of SNP data, even when hundreds of thousands of markers are examined. The availability of data on patterns of linkage disequilibrium across the genome (International HapMap Consortium 2003), interest in identifying susceptibility alleles for complex diseases (Cardon and Abecasis 2003), and advances in genotyping technology (Kwok 2001; Weber and Broman 2001) suggest that such large studies will be increasingly common. The principles and procedures used for testing HWE are well established (Levene 1949; Haldane 1954; Hernandez and Weir 1989; Wellek 2004), but the lack of a publicly available, efficient, and reliable implementation for exact tests has led many scientists to rely on asymptotic tests that can perform poorly with realistic sample sizes.

Consider a sample of SNP genotypes for N unrelated diploid individuals measured at an autosomal locus. The sample includes $2N$ alleles, including n_A copies of the rarer allele and n_B copies of the common allele. Let the number of heterozygous AB genotypes be n_{AB}, and note that the numbers of AA and BB homozygous genotypes are $n_{AA} = (n_A - n_{AB})/2$ and $n_{BB} = (n_B - n_{AB})/2$. Note that there are $(2N)!/n_A!n_B!$ possible arrangements for the alleles in the sample and that $2^{n_{AB}}N!/(n_{AA}!n_{AB}!n_{BB}!)$ of these arrangements correspond to exactly n_{AB} heterozygotes. Thus, under the assumption of HWE, the probability of observing exactly n_{AB} heterozygotes in a sample of N individuals with n_A minor alleles is

$$P(N_{AB} = n_{AB}|N, n_A) = \frac{2^{n_{AB}}N!}{n_{AA}!n_{AB}!n_{BB}!} \times \frac{n_A!n_B!}{(2N)!} \quad . \quad (1)$$

This equation holds for each possible number of heterozygotes, n_{AB}. When n_A is odd, possible numbers of

Received November 18, 2004; accepted for publication February 22, 2005; electronically published March 23, 2005.

Address for correspondence and reprints: Dr. Janis E. Wigginton, Department of Biostatistics, School of Public Health, University of Michigan, Ann Arbor, MI 48109. E-mail: goncalo@umich.edu

0002-9297/2005/7605-0017$15.00

heterozygotes are 1, 3, 5,...,n_A. When n_A is even, possible numbers of heterozygotes are 0, 2, 4,...,n_A. The expression for $P(n_{AB}|N,n_A)$ given in equation (1) leads to natural tests for HWE. For example, one could define one-sided tests that focus on detection of a deficit of heterozygotes, by calculating the statistic $P_{low} = P(N_{AB} \leqslant n_{AB}|N,n_A)$, or detection of an excess of heterozygotes, by calculating the statistic $P_{high} = P(N_{AB} \geqslant n_{AB}|N,n_A)$. In each case, the statistic can be calculated by simply summing over equation (1), to include all possible values of N_{AB} that are lower (for P_{low}) or higher (for P_{high}) than those observed in the actual data. A test for a deficit of heterozygotes in relation to Hardy-Weinberg expectations is appropriate when deviations from HWE due to inbreeding or population stratification are suspected, since both of these increase the proportion of homozygotes in the population. A test for an excess of heterozygotes is appropriate when one suspects problems in genotyping due to the existence of highly homologous regions in the genome, since these low-copy repeats often lead to an increase in the proportion of apparent heterozygotes in the sample. In other settings, it might be appropriate to use both tests. For example, many technologies score genotypes by clustering signals, and misspecified clusters can result in either vast excesses or vast deficits of heterozygotes.

When neither an increase nor a decrease in the proportion of heterozygotes is specifically expected, one could perform two separate one-sided tests or, instead, use a two-sided test statistic (Weir 1996). A natural two-sided test statistic could be defined as $P_{2\alpha} = \min(1.0, 2P_{high}, 2P_{low})$. This two-sided statistic is appealing because it leads to rejection of HWE at significance level 2α in instances in which the one-sided tests lead to the rejection of HWE at significance level α. However, because of the asymmetric nature of the distribution of heterozygote counts in a sample, the statistic is quite conservative in practice, and we do not recommend its use. Instead, an appealing approach, analogous to Fisher's exact test for contingency tables (Fisher 1934), is to calculate the probability of observing a sample configuration that is even less likely than the one being evaluated, conditional on the observed allele counts. This can be achieved using a statistic similar to the Monte Carlo statistic proposed by Guo and Thompson (1992) for multiallelic markers:

$$P_{HWE} = \sum_{n^*_{AB}} I\big[P(N_{AB} = n_{AB}|N,n_A) \geqslant P(N_{AB} = n^*_{AB}|N,n_A)\big] \times P(N_{AB} = n^*_{AB}|N,n_A) \ .$$

In this definition, $I[x]$ is an indicator function that is equal to 1 when the comparison is true and equal to 0 otherwise. The sum should be performed over all heterozygote counts n^*_{AB} that are compatible with the observed number of minor alleles, n_A.

Most of the computational effort required for performing exact tests of linkage disequilibrium is spent evaluating the factorials in equation (1) for each possible value of n_{AB}. By use of a naive approach, evaluating equation (1) requires $5N$–$6N$ multiplications and one division for each possible value of n_{AB}. We simplify calculations by using the recurrence relationships previously recognized by Guo and Thompson (1992) in the implementation of their Markov chain–Monte Carlo sampler:

$$P(N_{AB} = n_{AB} + 2|N, n_A) = P(N_{AB} = n_{AB}|N, n_A)\frac{4n_{AA}n_{BB}}{(n_{AB}+2)(n_{AB}+1)} \ , \text{ and}$$

$$P(N_{AB} = n_{AB} - 2|N, n_A) = P(N_{AB} = n_{AB}|N, n_A)\frac{n_{AB}(n_{AB}-1)}{4(n_{AA}+1)(n_{BB}+1)} \ . \quad (2)$$

In this way, evaluating the probability for each possible number of heterozygotes takes only four multiplications and one division, whatever the sample size N. To avoid underflow, it is best to first calculate the probability of observing the expected number of heterozygotes (in this case, the most likely outcome) and then use the recurrence relationships to calculate probabilities for all other outcomes. A further reduction of computational effort is possible by noting that one need only calculate relative probabilities for each outcome and then scale these to ensure that their sum is 1.0. This means that the probability of observing the expected number of heterozygotes can be replaced with an arbitrary constant when using the recurrence relations in equation (2), provided that the final result is scaled.

Table 1 illustrates the performance of the statistics for a sample of 100 individuals in which 21 copies of the minor allele are present. The observed number of heterozygotes will vary from 1 to 21 and must be odd. Note that only a small number of distinct sample configurations are possible, and each of these is associated with a specific probability for the exact tests. If the desired significance level α does not correspond exactly to one of these discrete outcomes, then the exact test statistics will be conservative (Hernandez and Weir 1989). For example, at the significance level $\alpha = 0.05$, the P_{HWE} and P_{low} statistics both reject the hypothesis of HWE if $\leqslant 13$ heterozygotes are observed in this setting. Since the probability of observing $\leqslant 13$ heterozygotes is 0.010, the tests are conservative. In contrast, the asymptotic χ^2 test statistic results in rejection of HWE when $\leqslant 15$ heterozy-

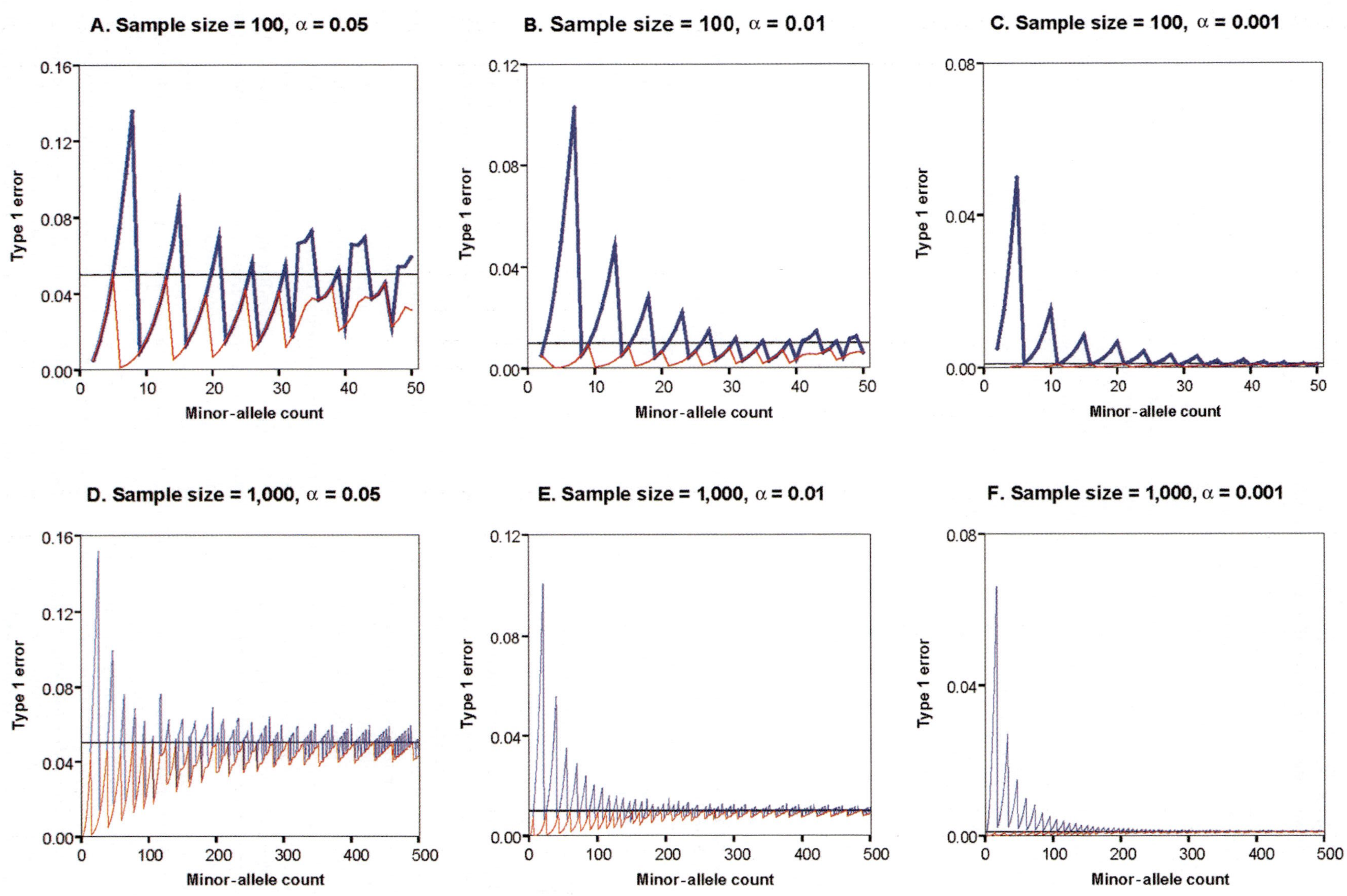

Figure 1 Type I error rates as a function of minor-allele counts for rare alleles, for samples of either 100 or 1,000 chromosomes and corresponding to a significance threshold of $\alpha = 0.05$, 0.01, or 0.001. Results are plotted as a function of the number of minor alleles in the sample for the exact P_{HWE} statistic (*red*) and for the asymptotic χ^2 test statistic (*blue*). A gray line denotes the nominal error rate. Note that the *Y*-axes in figures 1 and 2 differ.

Table 1

Possible Sample Configurations and Their Probabilities for a Sample of 100 Individuals and 21 Minor-Allele Copies Are Tabulated

No. of Heterozygotes (n_{AB})	Probability[a]	χ^2 Test P	Exact Test P Values		
			P_{HWE}	P_{high}	P_{low}
5	<.000001	<.000001[b]	<.000001[b]	1.000000	<.000001[b]
7	.000001	<.000001[b]	.000001[b]	1.000000	.000001[b]
9	.000047	<.000001[b]	.000048[b]	.999999	.000048[b]
11	.000870	.000039[b]	.000919[b]	.999952	.000919[b]
13	.009375	.002228[b]	.010293[b]	.999081	.010293[b]
15	.059283	.045180[b]	.069576	.989707	.069576
17	.214465	.342972	.284042	.930424	.284042
19	.406355	.906529	1.000000	.715958	.690396
21	.309604	.244336	.593645	.309604	1.000000

NOTE.—The probability of observing each possible outcome is given, together with the corresponding P values for tests of HWE based on the χ^2 statistic and on the exact test statistics P_{HWE}, P_{low}, and P_{high} (described in the main text).

[a] $P(n_{AB}|N = 100, n_A = 21)$.

[b] Configurations that would be rejected at the significance level $\alpha = 0.05$.

gotes are observed (for $\leqslant$15 heterozygotes, the χ^2 test statistic corresponds to an asymptotic $P \leqslant .045$). This results in an inflated type I error rate of 0.070 and therefore is inappropriate. In this sample, it is not possible to reject HWE because of an excess of heterozygous individuals—the probability of observing the maximum of 21 heterozygotes is 0.31, and none of the test statistics gives a P value <.05 for this extreme configuration. Additional examples of the performance of exact test statistics for HWE can be found in the work by Vithayasai (1973).

In general, the exact test statistics are conservative when a small number of minor-allele copies are present in the sample, but they approximate nominal significance levels as the sample size (and number of minor-allele copies) increases. In contrast, the commonly used χ^2 statistic can produce excessively small or large P values for specific outcomes (Hernandez and Weir 1989). To comprehensively evaluate the performance of the χ^2 and exact test statistics, we calculated their type I error rates for specified significance levels of $\alpha = 0.05$, 0.01, or 0.001, for sample sizes of $N = 100$ or $N = 1,000$ individuals and varying minor-allele counts. The results are summarized in figure 1 (for samples in which <25% of chromosomes carry the minor allele) and figure 2 (for samples in which >10% of chromosomes carry the minor allele), and it is clear that the statistics exhibit some periodicity in their type I error rates. As expected, both the exact P_{HWE} statistic and the χ^2 statistic perform better as the sample size and minor-allele counts increase. Nevertheless, one important difference is that the χ^2 statistic can sometimes be extremely anticonservative (e.g., in a sample of 1,000 individuals, when nominal $\alpha = 0.001$, the true type I error rate can exceed 0.06 and is often >0.01 for minor-allele counts <100), whereas the exact statistic never exceeds the nominal significance level. In practical settings, the χ^2 statistic could lead to many false rejections of HWE that depend on only the particular count of minor alleles in the sample.

To understand the periodicity of the statistics, it is important to consider the discrete nature of the data. For example, for a sample of $N = 100$ individuals including 2–5 copies of the minor allele, we reject HWE at the $\alpha = 0.05$ significance level (fig. 1*A*) when there is at least one homozygote for the minor allele. The probability of observing more than one homozygote for the minor allele increases gradually from 0.0050 when there are two copies of the allele in the sample up to 0.0499 when there are five copies of the minor allele in the sample. When there are 6–14 copies of the minor allele in the sample, we reject HWE at the $\alpha = 0.05$ significance level (fig. 1*A*) when at least two homozygotes for the rare allele are observed. Again, the probability of a more extreme event is quite low for small numbers of the rare allele ($P = .0011$ with six copies of the minor allele in the sample) but gradually increases if there are additional copies of the minor allele in the sample ($P = .0482$ with 13 copies of the minor allele).

In table 2, the overall type I error rates for each statistic are summarized for sample sizes of 100 or 1,000 individuals and various ranges of minor-allele counts. It is clear that, on average, the χ^2 test approximates nominal significance levels as the number of minor alleles in the sample increases. Nevertheless, as illustrated in figure 1, this is achieved at the cost of inflated error rates for samples with specific numbers of minor alleles. Even in a sample of 1,000 individuals, the type I error rate at $\alpha = 0.001$ for the χ^2 test is inflated when there are <200 copies of the minor allele (corresponding to an allele frequency of ~10%). The exact tests approximate nom-

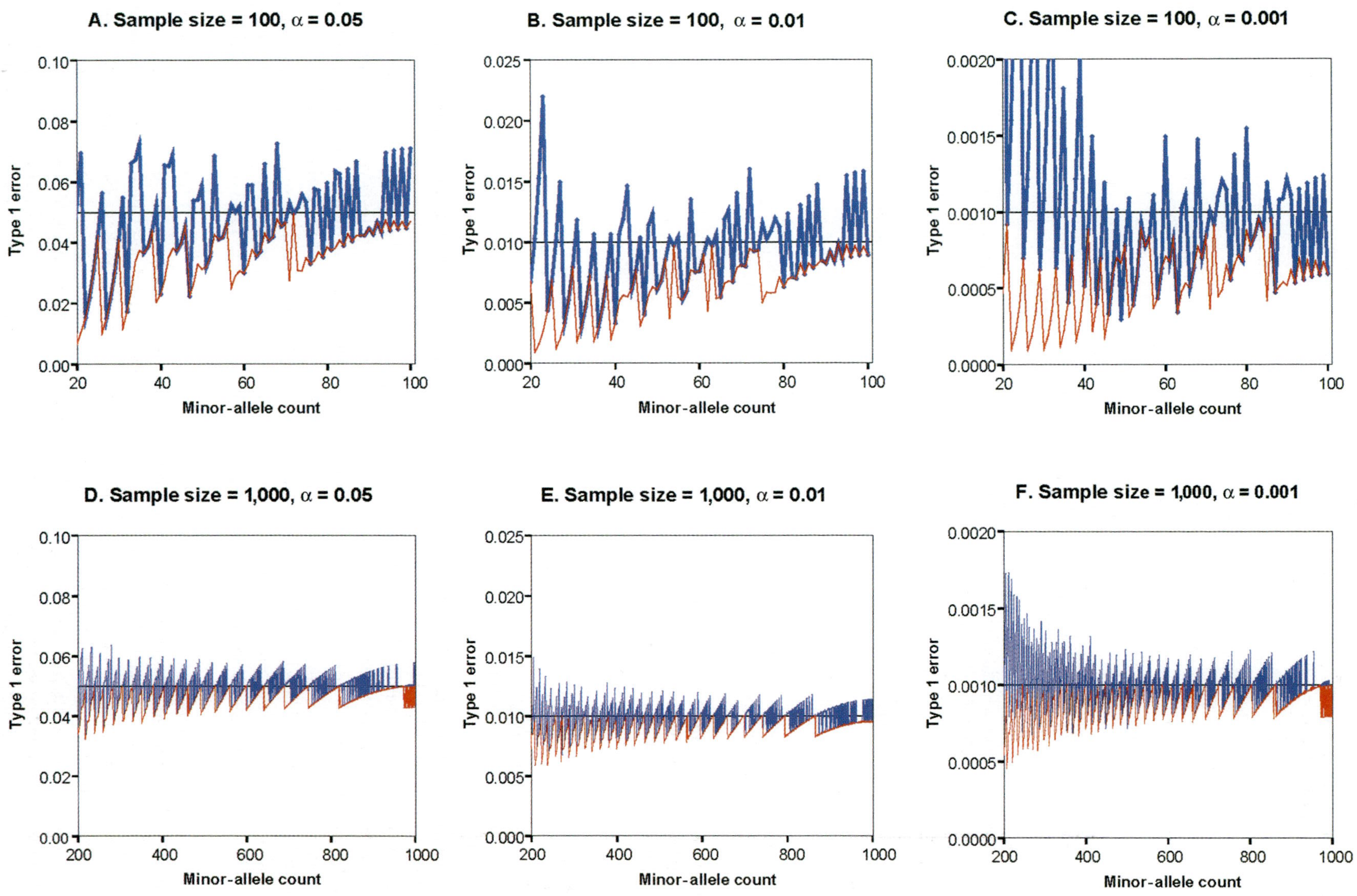

Figure 2 Type I error rates as a function of minor-allele counts for common alleles, for samples of either 100 or 1,000 chromosomes and corresponding to a significance threshold of $\alpha = 0.05$, 0.01, or 0.001. Results are plotted as a function of the number of minor alleles in the sample for the exact P_{HWE} statistic (*red*) and for the asymptotic χ^2 test statistic (*blue*). A gray line denotes the nominal error rate. Note that the *Y*-axes in figures 1 and 2 differ.

Table 2

Actual Error Rates for the χ^2 Test Statistic and the P_{HWE} Test Statistic for Nominal Significance Level α = 0.01 or 0.001

Sample and Minor-Allele Count	$\alpha = 0.01$[a]		$\alpha = 0.001$[a]	
	χ^2	P_{HWE}	χ^2	P_{HWE}
N = 1,000				
1–100	.0208[b] (.0208)[b]	.0039 (.0039)	.0088[b] (.0088)[b]	.0004 (.0004)
101–200	.0100 (.0154)[b]	.0065 (.0052)	.0017[b] (.0053)[b]	.0006 (.0005)
201–400	.0097 (.0126)[b]	.0083 (.0067)	.0010 (.0032)[b]	.0008 (.0006)
401–1,000	.0100 (.0110)[b]	.0090 (.0081)	.0010 (.0018)[b]	.0009 (.0008)
N = 100				
1–10	.0292[b] (.0292)[b]	.0024 (.0024)	.0114[b] (.0114)[b]	.0001 (.0001)
11–20	.0191[b] (.0242)[b]	.0035 (.0030)	.0035[b] (.0074)[b]	.0003 (.0002)
21–40	.0083 (.0162)[b]	.0037 (.0033)	.0016[b] (.0045)[b]	.0004 (.0003)
41–100	.0099 (.0124)[b]	.0072 (.0057)	.0009 (.0023)[b]	.0006 (.0005)

NOTE.—Results are tabulated for samples of 100 and 1,000 individuals and represent simple averages for each range of minor-allele counts.

[a] The error rate for each bin is tabulated, followed by the cumulative error rate in parenthesis. The cumulative error rate is calculated by including each bin and all previous bins. For example, for a sample of size 1,000, when α = 0.001, the type I error rate for the standard χ^2 test in a sample with 101–200 copies of the minor allele is 0.0017 and the cumulative error rate, corresponding to samples with 1–200 copies of the minor allele, is 0.0053.

[b] Exceeds nominal significance level.

inal significance levels with increasing sample size but remain conservative because of the discrete nature of the data.

As a final evaluation of our approach, we applied our method to a subset of the genotypes collected by the International HapMap Consortium (2003). We focused on a set of 18,460 SNP markers genotyped independently by two different centers with no discrepancies between the two sets of experimental results. For each of these markers, we evaluated evidence against HWE by using both the exact P_{HWE} statistic and the asymptotic χ^2 statistic. Results were broadly similar for 14,889 markers with minor-allele frequencies ≥20%. However, we observed noticeable differences for 3,571 markers with minor-allele frequencies <20%. For example, the χ^2 test rejected HWE for 71 of these markers at α = 0.01 (twice as many as the 35 markers expected to fail this test by chance), whereas the exact test rejected HWE for only 33 markers. At the more stringent α = 0.001 significance level, the χ^2 test rejected HWE for 28 markers (rejection for 3 markers is expected by chance), whereas the exact P_{HWE} statistic rejected HWE for only 5 markers.

Although we focus on testing the agreement of observed genotypes with HWE proportions, computationally efficient exact tests can be constructed for any desired genotype proportions. In brief, let the expected proportion of heterozygotes be p_{AB} and the two homozygote proportions be p_{AA} and p_{BB}. For example, in a population with inbreeding coefficient f, we might expect the proportion of heterozygotes to be $2(1-f)p_A p_B$. Define the quantity $\theta = p_{AB}^2/p_{AA}p_{BB}$ so that $\theta = 4$ when HWE holds. Then, the probability of observing n_{AB} heterozygotes is

$$P(N_{AB} = n_{AB}|N,n_A) = \frac{\theta^{n_{AB}/2}N!}{n_{AA}!n_{AB}!n_{BB}!} \times \frac{1}{C} ,$$

where

$$C = \sum_{n^*_{AB}} \frac{\theta^{n^*_{AB}/2}N!}{n^*_{AA}!n^*_{AB}!n^*_{BB}!}$$

(Wellek 2004). It is simple to verify that the recurrence relationships given in equation (2) can be extended to this setting by replacing the number 4 with the quantity θ in each expression.

The exact test statistics for HWE described here are accurate for a variety of allele frequencies and can be computed in an inexpensive manner. We recommend that they be used instead of the standard χ^2 test statistic in all situations. For large data sets, rather than fixing an arbitrary threshold for rejecting HWE, we suggest that methods based on the false-discovery rate (Benjamini and Hochberg 1995) be used to identify a subset of markers whose genotypes do not conform to the expected equilibrium distribution.

The P_{HWE} test statistic described here is implemented in the Pedstats software package (see Pedstats Web site), which generates summaries and checks the integrity of genetic data. In addition, code for calculating P_{low}, P_{high}, and P_{HWE} in C/C++, R, and Fortran is available from the authors' Web site. With appropriate citation, our code is freely available for use and can be incorporated into other programs. The HapMap Project genotype data are freely available at the HapMap Web site.

Acknowledgments

We gratefully acknowledge grant support from the National Human Genome Research Institute and the National Eye Institute. The manuscript was improved by helpful comments from reviewers.

Electronic-Database Information

The URLs for data presented herein are as follows:

Authors' Web site, http://www.sph.umich.edu/csg/abecasis/
HapMap, http://www.hapmap.org/
Pedstats, http://www.sph.umich.edu/csg/abecasis/Pedstats/

References

Benjamini Y, Hochberg Y (1995) Controlling the false discovery rate: a practical and powerful approach to multiple testing. J R Stat Soc Ser B 57:289–300

Cardon LR, Abecasis GR (2003) Using haplotype blocks to map human complex trait loci. Trends Genet 19:135–140

Crow JF (1988) Eighty years ago: the beginnings of population genetics. Genetics 119:473–476

Fisher RA (1934) Statistical methods for research workers. Oliver and Boyd, Edinburgh

Guo SW, Thompson EA (1992) Performing the exact test of Hardy-Weinberg proportion for multiple alleles. Biometrics 48:361–372

Haldane JBS (1954) An exact test for randomness of mating. J Genet 52:631–635

Hardy HG (1908) Mendelian proportions in a mixed population. Science 28:49–50

Hernandez JL, Weir BS (1989) A disequilibrium coefficient approach to Hardy-Weinberg equilibrium testing. Biometrics 45:53–70

International HapMap Consortium (2003) The International HapMap Project. Nature 426:789–796

Kwok PY (2001) Methods for genotyping single nucleotide polymorphisms. Annu Rev Genomics Hum Genet 2:235–258

Levene H (1949) On a matching problem arising in genetics. Ann Math Stat 21:91–94

Vithayasai C (1973) Exact critical values of the Hardy-Weinberg test statistic for two alleles. Communic Stat 1:229–242

Weber JL, Broman KW (2001) Genotyping for human whole-genome scans: past, present, and future. Adv Genet 42:77–96

Weinberg W (1908) On the demonstration of heredity in man. In: Boyer SH, trans (1963) Papers on human genetics. Prentice Hall, Englewood Cliffs, NJ

Weir BS (1996) Genetic data analysis II. Sinauer Associates, Sunderland, MA

Wellek S (2004) Tests for establishing compatibility of an observed genotype distribution with Hardy-Weinberg equilibrium in the case of a biallelic locus. Biometrics 60:694–703

Am. J. Hum. Genet. 76:894–901, 2005

Report

The Dual Origin of the Malagasy in Island Southeast Asia and East Africa: Evidence from Maternal and Paternal Lineages

Matthew E. Hurles,[1,2] Bryan C. Sykes,[3] Mark A. Jobling,[4] and Peter Forster[2]

[1]Wellcome Trust Sanger Institute, Wellcome Trust Genome Campus, Hinxton, United Kingdom; [2]McDonald Institute for Archaeological Research, University of Cambridge, Cambridge, United Kingdom; [3]Weatherall Institute for Molecular Medicine, University of Oxford, Oxford, United Kingdom; and [4]Department of Genetics, University of Leicester, Leicester, United Kingdom

Linguistic and archaeological evidence about the origins of the Malagasy, the indigenous peoples of Madagascar, points to mixed African and Indonesian ancestry. By contrast, genetic evidence about the origins of the Malagasy has hitherto remained partial and imprecise. We defined 26 Y-chromosomal lineages by typing 44 Y-chromosomal polymorphisms in 362 males from four different ethnic groups from Madagascar and 10 potential ancestral populations in Island Southeast Asia and the Pacific. We also compared mitochondrial sequence diversity in the Malagasy with a manually curated database of 19,371 hypervariable segment I sequences, incorporating both published and unpublished data. We could attribute every maternal and paternal lineage found in the Malagasy to a likely geographic origin. Here, we demonstrate approximately equal African and Indonesian contributions to both paternal and maternal Malagasy lineages. The most likely origin of the Asia-derived paternal lineages found in the Malagasy is Borneo. This agrees strikingly with the linguistic evidence that the languages spoken around the Barito River in southern Borneo are the closest extant relatives of Malagasy languages. As a result of their equally balanced admixed ancestry, the Malagasy may represent an ideal population in which to identify loci underlying complex traits of both anthropological and medical interest.

The island of Madagascar lies in the Indian Ocean, ~250 miles from the African coast and ~4,000 miles from Indonesia. Paleoecological and archaeological evidence suggest that, by 1,500–2,000 years ago, Madagascar had become the last great island landmass to be settled (Dewar and Wright 1993; Burney et al. 2004). The Malagasy language shares 90% of its basic vocabulary with Maanyan, a language spoken in the Barito River region of southern Borneo, which indicates that the predominant ancestry of the Malagasy language most likely derives from Borneo (Dahl 1951; Adelaar 1995). Malagasy also contains linguistic borrowings from the Bantu languages spoken in East Africa (Dahl 1988). Furthermore, substantial components of Malagasy material culture (e.g., cattle pastoralism) could be derived only from African sources.

At the time of the first Madagascan settlement, the entire Indian Ocean was a vast trading network connecting China with the Mediterranean and all societies in between (Vérin and Wright 1999). There is substantial evidence of Islamic influence and limited evidence of Indian influence on the Malagasy, in both language and culture.

In contrast to these cultural and linguistic traces of Malagasy ancestry, the genetic origins of the Malagasy are relatively poorly understood, and conflicting signals of African, Asian, and Pacific origin have appeared from studies of different loci (Migot et al. 1995; Soodyall et al. 1995; Hewitt et al. 1996). These contradictions result, in part, from being able to identify the likely origins of only a subset of lineages present at any single locus.

In the present study, we employed the detailed phylogenetic and geographic resolution of paternally inherited Y-chromosomal lineages and maternally inherited mtDNA lineages to apportion Malagasy lineages to ancestral populations. In this way, the contributions of the different ancestral populations to the modern Mala-

Received January 4, 2005; accepted for publication March 1, 2005; electronically published March 25, 2005.

Address for correspondence and reprints: Dr. Matthew E. Hurles, Wellcome Trust Sanger Institute, Wellcome Trust Genome Campus, Hinxton, Cambridge, CB10 1SA, United Kingdom. E-mail: meh@sanger.ac.uk

0002-9297/2005/7605-0018$15.00

gasy gene pool can be estimated directly, and likely geographic origins can be pinpointed with precision.

We assayed mtDNA and Y-chromosomal diversity in a Malagasy population sample comprising four different ethnic populations: Bezanozano ($n = 6$), Betsileo ($n = 18$), Merina ($n = 10$), and Sihanaka ($n = 3$). Ten potential ancestral populations ($n = 327$) representing major population groups within Island Southeast Asia and Oceania were also analyzed with Y-chromosomal markers. To type all these samples for the required number of Y-chromosomal and mitochondrial (mt) markers, it was necessary to perform whole-genome amplification. Degenerate oligonucleotide-primed PCR (Nrich [Genetix]) (Telenius et al. 1992) performed better than multiple displacement amplification (Molecular Staging) (Dean et al. 2002) in early trials and, consequently, was used throughout.

We selected 44 binary markers in the present Y-haplogroup phylogeny (Y Chromosome Consortium [YCC] 2002; Jobling and Tyler-Smith 2003) that were predicted to be particularly informative in this study. These markers were typed using a combination of single-plex PCRs described elsewhere (Hurles et al. 2002; YCC 2002) and nine novel PCR multiplexes, each analyzing between three and seven SNPs. These multiplexes were designed to facilitate hierarchical typing, which minimizes the amount of genomic DNA required to define lineages at high resolution. These multiplexes use locus-specific primers tagged with universal primers to enable a two-step amplification protocol that equalizes the simultaneous amplification of multiple loci (Belgrader et al. 1996; Paracchini et al. 2002). SNPs lying within these PCR products were subsequently genotyped by single-base extension (SNaPshot [Applied Biosystems]) and capillary electrophoresis. Primer extension reactions were performed in half the recommended reaction volume but were otherwise processed in accordance with the manufacturer's instructions. The amplification and extension primers used in the present study are detailed in table 1.

Together, these markers define 41 Y-chromosomal lineages, of which 10 are found in the Malagasy, 16 are found within Island Southeast Asia and Oceania, and 8 are found in East African populations (Luis et al. 2004). The Y-chromosomal lineages in East Africa are nonoverlapping with those found in Island Southeast Asia and Oceania (see fig. 1). As a consequence of this population differentiation, it is simple to apportion lineages found in the Malagasy to either an African or an Asian origin. All but two Malagasy lineages can be found in either East African or Southeast Asian populations. The two unaccounted-for lineages are single chromosomes belonging to haplogroups L* and R1b. Haplogroup L* is found at appreciable frequencies only in populations bordering the northern Indian Ocean, and haplogroup R1b reaches highest frequencies in northwestern Europe

Table 1

Primers for Y Binary and mt Variant Marker Multiplexes

The table is available in its entirety in the online edition of *The American Journal of Human Genetics.*

(Jobling and Tyler-Smith 2003). We believe these two lineages most likely reflect recent admixture events as a result of Indian Ocean trading links (Duplantier et al. 2002) and European colonization, respectively.

To identify which Island Southeast Asian or Oceanic population represents the most likely source population for the Asian lineages found in the Malagasy, we computed pairwise F_{ST} distances, using the Arlequin software, to determine the closest populations, in terms of genetic distance to the Malagasy. This analysis indicates that, among the populations we sampled, the two populations from Borneo are the best candidates for the likely source of these lineages (table 2). This genetic proximity between the Malagasy and Borneo populations reflects the presence of appreciable frequencies of lineages O1b and O2a* in both populations, as well as a relative lack of chromosomes belonging to O3 lineages. The closest single Island Southeast Asian or Oceanic population to the Malagasy is that from Banjarmasin.

To explore the statistical significance of these observations, we devised a permutation test to assess whether the genetic distance between the Malagasy (A) and one population (B) is significantly smaller than that between the Malagasy and another population (C). In this test, the individual haplotypes observed in populations B and C are pooled and are randomly reassigned 10,000 times into two simulated populations (B′ and C′) with the same sample sizes as B and C. The P value of the difference in genetic distance—$F_{ST}(A:B) - F_{ST}(A:C)$—is then calculated as the fraction of simulated population pairs in which the difference in genetic distance between each of the populations and the Malagasy is greater than that observed in the real data—$(F_{ST}[A:B'] - F_{ST}[A:C']) > (F_{ST}[A:B] - F_{ST}[A:C])$. By use of this test, it was observed that there is no significant difference between the two Borneo populations ($P = .8374$) but that the resultant pooled Borneo population is significantly closer to the Malagasy than any other Island Southeast Asian population ($P < .001$).

The phylogeny of mtDNA variation present in modern humans can be crudely characterized as comprising L lineages, present almost exclusively in Africa, and M and N lineages, present almost exclusively outside of Africa. Thus, classifying mt genomes into these major clades has significant power for discriminating between African and Asian origins. We devised a novel multiplex using the single base–extension method described above to type seven coding-region base substitutions (transitions at po-

A

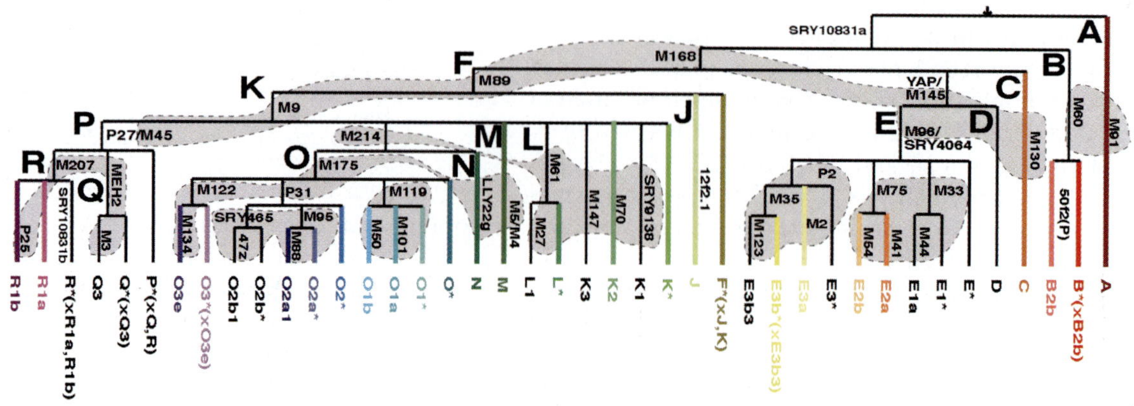

	R1b	R1a	O3e	O3*(xO3e)	O2a1	O2a*	O2*	O1b	O1a	O1*	O*	N	M	L*	K2	K*	J	F*(xJ,K)	E3b*(xE3b3)	E3a	E2b	E2a	C	B2b	B*(xB2b)	A	Total
Banjarmasin		1		1	1	7		2		3						1	1						5				**22**
Cook Islands				4																			16				**20**
Kapingamarangi						1										14							6				**21**
Kota Kinabalu		3	3	11	2	14		6	1	12		1					1	1					10				**65**
Majuro								2								7	1	1									**11**
Philippines			3	14				1		9						1											**28**
Papua New Guinea				4									28			9		1					2				**44**
Taiwan			2	5	2		1	13		15	1																**39**
Vanuatu				4				1					7			30	1						9				**52**
Western Samoa				7		1				1						1							15				**25**
S.E. Asian + Oceanic		***4***	***8***	***50***	***5***	***23***	***1***	***25***	***1***	***40***	***1***	***1***	***35***			***63***	***4***	***3***					***63***				**327**
Wiarak (Tanzania)															2				16	18		1		2	1	3	**43**
Bantu (Kenya)																			4	15	4	1			1	4	**29**
E. Africa															***2***				***20***	***33***	***4***	***2***		***2***	***2***	***7***	**72**
Malagasy	**1**	**1**				**6**		**6**						**1**			**2**			**12**	**3**			**1**	**2**		**35**
All	***1***	***5***	***8***	***5***	***5***	***29***	***1***	***31***	***1***	***40***	***1***	***1***	***35***	***1***	***2***	***63***	***6***	***3***	***20***	***45***	***7***	***2***	***63***	***3***	***4***	***7***	***434***

B

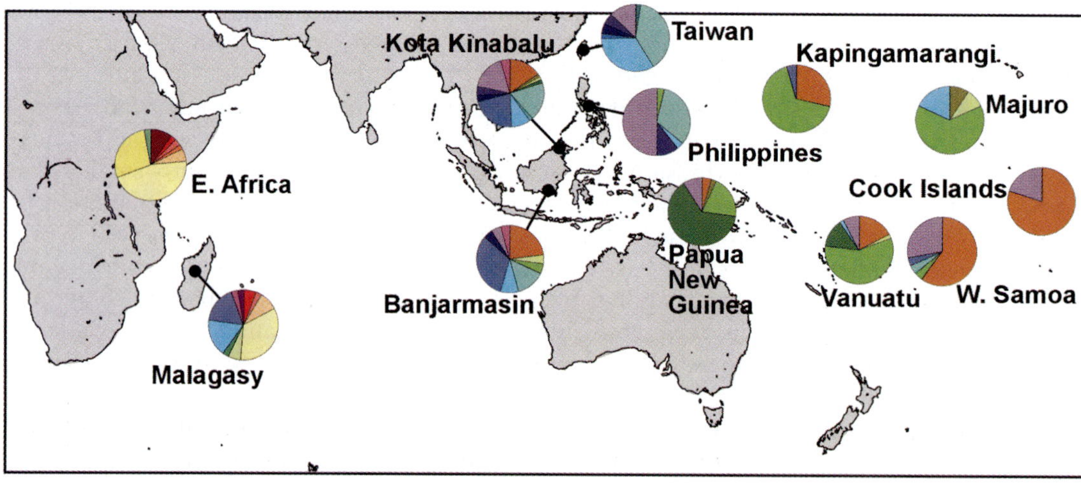

Figure 1 *A,* Y-chromosomal haplogroup frequencies in the Malagasy and in potential ancestral populations. The maximum parsimony phylogeny relating the 41 Y-chromosomal haplogroups defined in the present study is shown above the absolute frequencies of those lineages in the different populations. The phylogeny is labeled with single-letter clades, and branches are labeled with the markers that define them. The lineage nomenclature is the updated version of that proposed by the YCC (YCC 2002; Jobling and Tyler-Smith 2003). The gray shading on the phylogeny indicates the nine sets of markers typed together in multiplexes. *B,* Pie charts illustrating the relative frequencies of the different haplogroups (colored to agree with the coloring of the phylogeny) shown on a map of the Indian Ocean. The Taiwanese population sample represents individuals pooled from four different aboriginal groups. Samples in these Island Southeast Asian and Pacific populations that were identified elsewhere as representing recent paternal European admixture in published lower-resolution Y-chromosomal marker typing of the same populations (Hurles et al. 2002) were not typed in the present study. East African data come from Luis et al. (2004).

sitions 15043, 10400, 10398, 15301, 6455, 9824, and 10310) that define the M and N lineages, as well as the R9 sublineage within haplogroup N and the M7 sublineage within haplogroup M (Kivisild et al. 2002), both of which are known to be present in Island Southeast Asian populations (primers used in this multiplex assay are detailed in table 1). Among 37 Malagasy mt genomes, we found 23 that belong to M and N lineages and 14 that belong to L lineages (fig. 2 and table 3).

To further localize the geographical origins of Asian

Table 2

Pairwise Genetic Distances (F_{ST}) to the Malagasy on the Basis of Y-Haplogroup Frequencies

Population Location	Distance (F_{ST})
East Africa[a]	.083
Banjarmasin	.094
Kota Kinabalu	.102
Taiwan	.170
Majuro	.237
Philippines	.249
Vanuatu	.276
Western Samoa	.283
Papua New Guinea	.313
Kapingamarangi	.316
Cook Islands	.386

[a] From the publication by Luis et al. (2004).

mtDNA lineages found in the Malagasy, we studied the hypervariable segment I (HVSI) sequence of the mt genome, for which a large volume of comparative data is available, we amplified and sequenced HVSI, using primers TTAACTCCACCATTAGCACC and GAGGATGG-TGGTCAAGGGAC (Forster et al. 2002*a*) (between positions 16093 and 16362) in mtDNA from these 37 Malagasy individuals, and, by combining these data with the coding SNP haplotypes described above, we defined 14 distinct maternal lineages in the Malagasy (fig. 2).

A recently developed method for identifying the likely ancestry of a set of mt sequences is to perform a "center of gravity" (CoG) analysis of individual sequence types observed within a population (Röhl et al. 2001; Forster et al. 2002*b*). In our CoG analysis, the best matches to an HVSI sequence type were identified within a manually curated database of HVSI sequences associated with a precise geographical location. A CoG was then calculated by weighted interpolation of all best-match locations (see fig. 2). The relative lack of published Island Southeast Asian HVSI data could hamper a CoG analysis. To counteract this sampling bias, we added 82 HVSI sequences from Banjarmasin ($n = 21$), Kota Kinabalu ($n = 36$), and the Philippines ($n = 25$) to the analysis. These sequence types are given in table 3. Exact matches within our database of 19,371 HVSI sequences can be found for all six maternal lineages in the Malagasy that appear to be Africa derived. By contrast, exact matches can be found for only three of eight Asia-derived maternal lineages.

The CoGs observed in the Malagasy fall within either Island Southeast Asia or sub-Saharan Africa. These CoGs accord exactly with the lineage classifications: all sequence types that belong to L haplogroups are found in Africa, and all sequence types that belong to M and N haplogroups are found in Island Southeast Asia. The relatively broad distribution of the Asian CoGs suggests that the present level of geographical resolution afforded by a CoG analysis is not sufficient to enable us to identify a single likely source population in Island Southeast Asia. It does, however, allow us to exclude the possibility that a Pacific Island population was the sole source of these mt lineages.

We calculated Nei's gene diversity (using the Arlequin software) in HVSI sequences from the Malagasy and compared it with diversity apparent in the three Island Southeast Asian populations described above, as well as in published data on Mozambique (Pereira et al. 2001) and Oceanic populations (Hurles et al. 2003*b*). The Malagasy appear to have diversity that is significantly lower than that seen in Island Southeast Asia and Mozambique populations (Pereira et al. 2001) but that is higher than that seen in Pacific islands colonized within the past 3,500 years (table 4).

The amount of genetic diversity observed in a population is heavily influenced by demography and thus gives insights into settlement patterns. We might expect that the presence of HVSI sequences from two diverse ancestral populations would inflate HVSI sequence diversity; however, the lower genetic diversity in the Malagasy compared with both ancestral populations suggests either that early migrations were relatively restricted in numbers, duration, and origin or that subsequent population bottlenecks resulted in a postsettlement reduction of diversity. Recently colonized islands often exhibit reduced genetic diversity as a result of a combination of founder events and elevated genetic drift due to lower population sizes. However, this impact does not appear to be as severe in the Malagasy as it is for Pacific Island populations with a similarly recent settlement (reviewed by Hurles et al. [2003*a*]). This observation holds true even when only Asia-derived lineages are considered. This suggests that the sequential founder events and bottlenecks that were a feature of Pacific Island settlement were not paralleled in the colonization of Madagascar from the East and provides support for a direct rather than multistep process of migration from Indonesia. Alternatively, successive waves of migration from Asia may have brought different sets of lineages to Madagascar.

If we calculate gene diversity separately for Asia-derived and Africa-derived maternal lineages in the Malagasy, we find that the Asian lineages are significantly more diverse. These observations are largely explained by the predominance of a single African HVSI sequence type (found in 9 of 14 Africa-derived mt lineages). This sequence type is found in all four Malagasy ethnic populations sampled in the present study, so its predominance does not result from genetic drift in a single Malagasy subpopulation. Intuitively, one might expect fewer founders and therefore lower genetic diversity from the more geographically distant ancestral population. However, this does not appear to be the case in this situation. Given

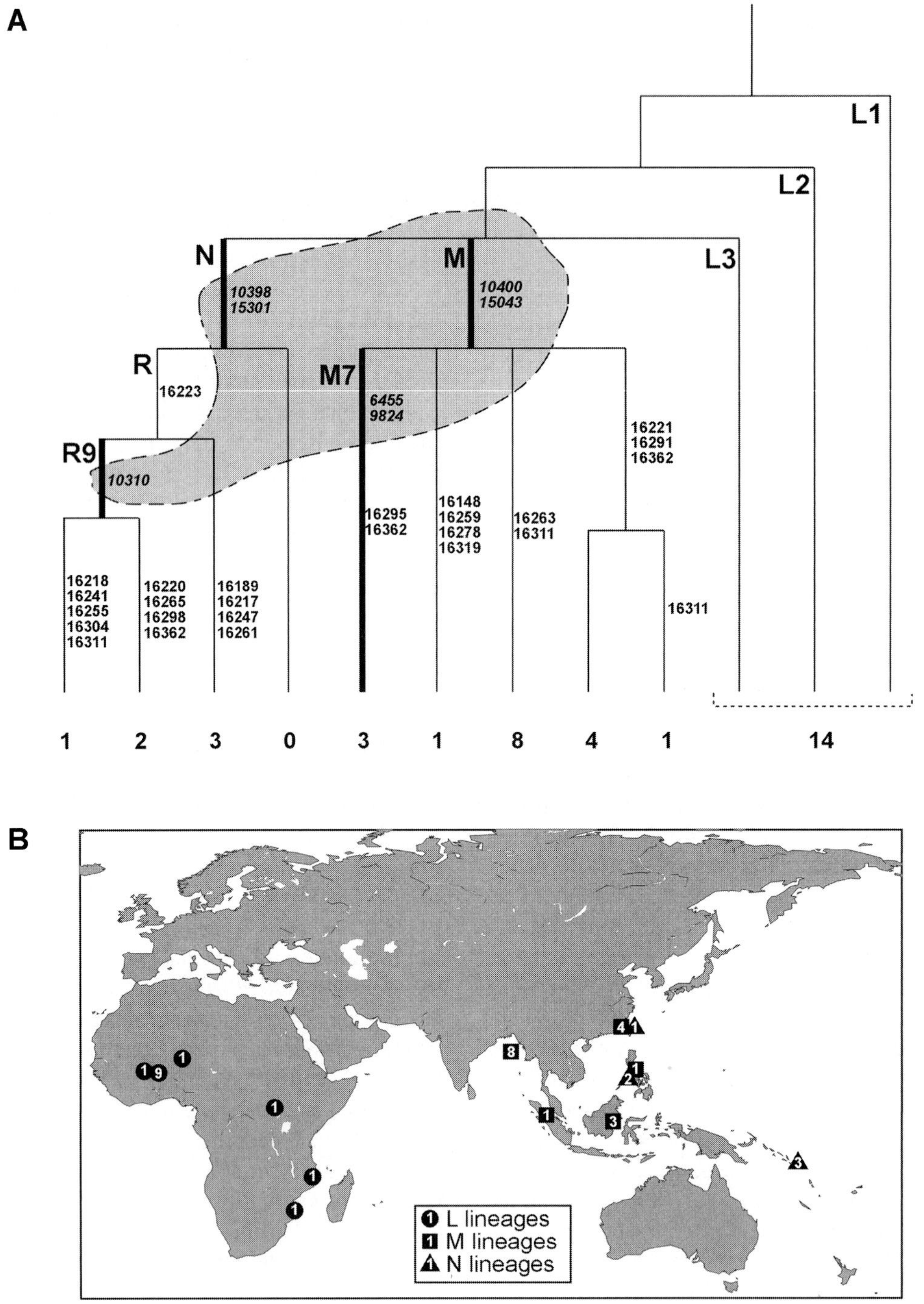

Figure 2 *A*, Phylogeny of mt sequence types found in the Malagasy and their CoGs. The maximum parsimony phylogeny of the 14 maternal lineages defined in the present study builds on the phylogeny constructed by Kivisild et al. (2002). The tips of the phylogeny are labeled with the number of Malagasy mt genomes found in each lineage. The phylogeny is also labeled with the major clades and the variable sites that define individual branches. The gray shading on the phylogeny indicates the seven coding variants that are typed together in a single multiplex. *B*, A map of the Old World, showing the positions of the CoGs of the 14 different mt sequence types (blackened circles, triangles, and squares) and the lineage group to which that sequence type belongs. Strictly speaking, mtDNA type "L" encompasses mtDNA types "M" and "N," which are Eurasian subgroups of "L"; however, for simplicity, "L" here denotes "L" lineages excluding "M" and "N" types. The number within each shape indicates the frequency of that lineage within the data set. For most mt types, it was sufficient to enter only their HVSI sequences. However, to obtain monophyletic hits in the geographic database for two Malagasy HVSI sequence types found in paraphyletic mt lineages, it was also necessary to consider their coding SNP haplotypes, to eliminate spurious matches in geographical regions in which these haplotypes are known to be absent. Full HVSI sequence types are given in table 3.

Table 3

mt Haplotypes Found in Study Populations

The table is available in its entirety in the online edition of *The American Journal of Human Genetics.*

that the diversity apparent within the two ancestral populations is comparable, this implies that migrations from Africa may have been more limited than those from Indonesia.

In principle, it would be interesting to test whether these differences in Africa-derived and Asia-derived lineage diversity are replicated in the paternal lineages of the Malagasy. However, it is well documented that estimates of diversity that are based on genotyping known SNPs are biased by the markers selected for genotyping and the geographic distribution of the initial screening set used to identify these markers (Jobling and Tyler-Smith 2003). As a consequence, it is not appropriate to compare apparent SNP diversity between African and Asian Y-chromosomal lineages.

The above analyses demonstrate that we can consider the Malagasy to be an admixed population derived from two ancestral populations, one African and the other Indonesian; we can now estimate the admixture proportions of these populations. The mutual exclusivity of Y-chromosomal and mtDNA lineages between these two ancestral populations means that we can obtain a point estimate of admixture proportions simply by counting lineages. Of Malagasy mtDNA lineages, 38% (14/37) can be traced to Africa, whereas 51% (18/35) of Y-chromosomal lineages have an African origin. This increases to 55% (18/33) when the two putative recently admixed Y chromosomes are removed.

When estimating admixture proportions, we are estimating the cumulative contributions made by different ancestral populations to a hybrid population (Chakraborty 1986). We do not know the true frequencies of the different lineages in these three populations at the time that admixture occurred, and we can only infer these frequencies from sampling the contemporary populations that best approximate these ancient populations. Various factors influence the accuracy and precision of estimates of admixture proportions from contemporary populations, including sampling errors, genetic drift in all populations, the degree of population differentiation between the ancestral populations, and mutations. Various statistical methods that take into account some of these factors are available for estimating admixture proportions (reviewed by Jobling et al. [2004]). Using the software LEADMIX (Wang 2003), we employed three different statistical methods to estimate the proportion of African ancestry in Malagasy paternal lineages; in order of increasing complexity, these estimators are RH62 (Roberts and Hiorns 1962), L91 (Long 1991), and W03 (Wang 2003), the last of which is a recently derived likelihood estimator that estimates rates of genetic drift simultaneously in the ancestral and hybrid populations. These three methods all gave very similar estimates of African admixture proportions, which do not differ greatly from the estimate obtained from lineage counting: 58% for RH62, 56% for L91, and 56% for W03. There are broad confidence limits (19%–82%) for the latter likelihood estimate of paternal African admixture, which encompasses the point estimate of the proportion (38%) of African ancestry from maternal lineages. Consequently, the paternal and maternal estimates of the proportion of African ancestry in the Malagasy are statistically indistinguishable; there is no evidence of ancient sex-biased admixture. Further microgeographic sampling within Madagascar will be required to explore how admixture proportions vary among different Malagasy ethnic populations.

Characterization of genetic ancestry in the Malagasy has hitherto remained partial and imprecise. By contrast, in this study, because we generated comparative data from a wide range of potential ancestral populations, we have been able to identify the likely origins of all paternal and maternal lineages found in four different Malagasy ethnic populations.

We have confirmed the presence of the mt "Polynesian motif" among maternal Malagasy lineages, as was reported elsewhere (Soodyall et al. 1995). However, direct migration from Polynesia can be discounted, since the predominant Y-chromosomal haplogroups found in Polynesians, O3 and C, are not found at all among Malagasy paternal lineages.

Among the 10 potential ancestral populations in Island Southeast Asia and Oceania that we sampled, the Borneo populations had Y-chromosomal haplogroup distributions that were the most similar to those observed

Table 4

Diversity of mt HVSI Sequences in Different Populations

HVSI Sequence Source	Nei's Gene Diversity ± SE
Malagasy	.884 ± .031
Malagasy Asian lineages[a]	.838 ± .053
Malagasy African lineages[a]	.582 ± .150
Mozambique[b]	.960 ± .008
Kota Kinabalu	.989 ± .010
Banjarmasin	.986 ± .019
Philippines	.973 ± .018
Samoa[c]	.805 ± .053
New Zealand Maori[c]	.239 ± .096

[a] "Malagasy Asian" and "Malagasy African" refer, respectively, to the HVSI gene diversity among the Asia-derived and Africa-derived mt lineages in the Malagasy.

[b] Mozambique mtDNA data are from the publication by Pereira et al. (2001).

[c] Samoan and New Zealand Maori gene-diversity values are from the publication by Hurles et al. (2003*b*).

among the Malagasy. This observation is in striking agreement with the linguistic evidence that the Malagasy language is most closely related to the Maanyan language from the Barito River Valley in southern Borneo. Now that we have identified the region of origin for this Asian migration to Madagascar, further microgeographic sampling within Indonesian islands may pinpoint more precisely the origins of the Malagasy. Populations that possess both the paternal (e.g., O1b and O2a*) and maternal lineages (e.g., Polynesian motif) that are common in the Malagasy would be of particular interest. It is intriguing that the majority of Asia-derived mtDNA types present in the Malagasy do not have exact matches in an extensive database of HVSI sequences, and identification of these specific mtDNA sequence motifs within potential ancestral populations in Indonesia should be a priority. However, it must be remembered that genetic diversity in contemporary populations is an imperfect proxy for variation within ancient populations. The ongoing processes of population fission and fusion as well as genetic drift may prohibit the identification of a precise contemporary population that exactly represents the ancient population from which migrants departed. In addition, the possibility remains that migration either occurred from several genetically distinct sources within Indonesia or was kin structured (Fix 1999), such that no ancient population ever had the same lineage distribution as that of the migrants to Madagascar.

Admixture between two highly differentiated populations generates long-range allelic associations that decay over time (Chakraborty and Weiss 1988). The amount of linkage disequilibrium (LD) exhibited by an admixed population depends on a number of factors, including proportions of admixture, differentiation between ancestral populations, time since admixture, and demography (Pfaff et al. 2001). It has been proposed that it will be possible to efficiently map genes underlying complex traits by focusing on association studies in admixed populations, and a range of potentially informative populations has been identified (Halder and Shriver 2003). Although the time since admixture in the Malagasy is comparatively long, the high degree of differentiation between the two ancestral populations and the even balance of their contributions suggest that excess LD might still exist. Admixture mapping of genes underlying complex traits is predicated on the observation that the trait itself is differentially manifested among the ancestral populations. Therefore, although most attention has focused on European and African admixture in African Americans (Halder and Shriver 2003), it would be of interest to identify a range of admixed populations that are derived from various different ancestral combinations. The admixture of Indonesian and African lineages present in the Malagasy may be uniquely informative. Further characterization of LD in the Malagasy will be necessary for determining whether the Malagasy can be added to the list of admixed populations suitable for the identification of genes underlying complex traits that are of interest to anthropologists and medical geneticists alike.

Acknowledgments

The authors thank John Clegg, for his generosity in donating samples for this project, and Jinliang Wang, for his assistance with the LEADMIX software. We are grateful to Robert Dewar, for his comments on an earlier manuscript, and to Sue Adams, for support with genotyping. This work was funded by the Royal Society Research grant "Prehistory in Oceanic Populations," the Wellcome Trust, and the McDonald Institute for Archaeological Research. M.A.J. was supported by a Wellcome Trust Senior Fellowship in Basic Biomedical Science (grant 057559).

References

Adelaar A (1995) Asian roots of the Malagasy: a linguistic perspective. Bijdragen tot de Taal-Land en Volkenkunde 151: 325–356

Belgrader P, Marino MM, Lubin M, Barany F (1996) A multiplex PCR-ligase detection reaction assay for human identity testing. Genome Sci Technol 1:77–87

Burney DA, Burney LP, Godfrey LR, Jungers WL, Goodman SM, Wright HT, Jull AJ (2004) A chronology for late prehistoric Madagascar. J Hum Evol 47:25–63

Chakraborty R (1986) Gene admixture in human populations: models and predictions. Yearb Phys Anthropol 29:1–43

Chakraborty R, Weiss KM (1988) Admixture as a tool for finding linked genes and detecting that difference from allelic association between loci. Proc Natl Acad Sci USA 85:9119–9123

Dahl OC (1951) Malgache et Maanyan: une comparison linguistique. Egede Intitutett, Oslo

——— (1988) Bantu substratum in Malagasy. Études Océan Indien 9:91–132

Dean FB, Hosono S, Fang L, Wu X, Faruqi AF, Bray-Ward P, Sun Z, Zong Q, Du Y, Du J, Driscoll M, Song W, Kingsmore SF, Egholm M, Lasken RS (2002) Comprehensive human genome amplification using multiple displacement amplification. Proc Natl Acad Sci USA 99:5261–5266

Dewar RE, Wright HT (1993) The culture history of Madagascar. J World Prehistory 7:417–466

Duplantier JM, Orth A, Catalan J, Bonhomme F (2002) Evidence for a mitochondrial lineage originating from the Arabian peninsula in the Madagascar house mouse (*Mus musculus*). Heredity 89:154–158

Fix AG (1999) Migration and colonisation in human microevolution. Cambridge University Press, Cambridge, United Kingdom

Forster L, Forster P, Lutz-Bonengel S, Willkomm H, Brinkmann B (2002*a*) Natural radioactivity and human mitochondrial DNA mutations. Proc Natl Acad Sci USA 99:13950–13954

Forster P, Cali F, Röhl A, Metspalu E, D'Anna R, Mirisola M, De Leo G, Flugy A, Salerno A, Ayala G, Kouvatsi A, Villems

R, Romano V (2002*b*) Continental and subcontinental distributions of mtDNA control region types. Int J Legal Med 116:99–108

Halder I, Shriver MD (2003) Measuring and using admixture to study the genetics of complex diseases. Hum Genomics 1:52–62

Hewitt R, Krause A, Goldman A, Campbell G, Jenkins T (1996) β-globin haplotype analysis suggests that a major source of Malagasy ancestry is derived from Bantu-speaking Negroids. Am J Hum Genet 58:1303–1308

Hurles ME, Matisoo-Smith E, Gray RD, Penny D (2003*a*) Untangling Oceanic settlement: the edge of the knowable. Trends Ecol Evol 18:531–540

Hurles ME, Maund E, Nicholson J, Bosch E, Renfrew C, Sykes BC, Jobling MA (2003*b*) Native American Y chromosomes in Polynesia: the genetic impact of the Polynesian slave trade. Am J Hum Genet 72:1282–1287

Hurles ME, Nicholson J, Bosch E, Renfrew C, Sykes BC, Jobling MA (2002) Y chromosomal evidence for the origins of Oceanic-speaking peoples. Genetics 160:289–303

Jobling MA, Hurles ME, Tyler-Smith C (2004) Human evolutionary genetics: origins, peoples and disease. Garland Science, New York

Jobling MA, Tyler-Smith C (2003) The human Y chromosome: an evolutionary marker comes of age. Nat Rev Genet 4:598–612

Kivisild T, Tolk HV, Parik J, Wang Y, Papiha SS, Bandelt HJ, Villems R (2002) The emerging limbs and twigs of the East Asian mtDNA tree. Mol Biol Evol 19:1737–1751

Long JC (1991) The genetic structure of admixed populations. Genetics 127:417–428

Luis JR, Rowold DJ, Regueiro M, Caeiro B, Cinnioğlu C, Roseman C, Underhill PA, Cavalli-Sforza LL, Herrera RJ (2004) The Levant versus the Horn of Africa: evidence for bidirectional corridors of human migrations. Am J Hum Genet 74: 532–544

Migot F, Perichon B, Danze PM, Raharimalala L, Lepers JP, Deloron P, Krishnamoorthy R (1995) HLA class II haplotype studies bring molecular evidence for population affinity between Madagascans and Javanese. Tissue Antigens 46:131–135

Paracchini S, Arredi B, Chalk R, Tyler-Smith C (2002) Hierarchical high-throughput SNP genotyping of the human Y chromosome using MALDI-TOF mass spectrometry. Nucleic Acids Res 30:e27

Pereira L, Macaulay V, Torroni A, Scozzari R, Prata MJ, Amorim A (2001) Prehistoric and historic traces in the mtDNA of Mozambique: insights into the Bantu expansions and the slave trade. Ann Hum Genet 65:439–458

Pfaff CL, Parra EJ, Bonilla C, Hiester K, McKeigue PM, Kamboh MI, Hutchinson RG, Ferrell RE, Boerwinkle E, Shriver MD (2001) Population structure in admixed populations: effect of admixture dynamics on the pattern of linkage disequilibrium. Am J Hum Genet 68:198–207

Roberts DF, Hiorns RW (1962) The dynamics of racial admixture. Am J Hum Genet 14:261–277

Röhl A, Brinkmann B, Forster L, Forster P (2001) An annotated mtDNA database. Int J Legal Med 115:29–39

Soodyall H, Jenkins T, Stoneking M (1995) "Polynesian" mtDNA in the Malagasy. Nat Genet 10:377–378

Telenius H, Carter NP, Bebb CE, Nordenskjold M, Ponder BA, Tunnacliffe A (1992) Degenerate oligonucleotide-primed PCR: general amplification of target DNA by a single degenerate primer. Genomics 13:718–725

Vérin P, Wright H (1999) Madagascar and Indonesia: new evidence from archaeology and linguistics. Indo Pac Prehist Assoc Bull 18:35–42

Wang J (2003) Maximum-likelihood estimation of admixture proportions from genetic data. Genetics 164:747–765

Y Chromosome Consortium (YCC) (2002) A nomenclature system for the tree of human Y-chromosomal binary haplogroups. Genome Res 12:339–348

Report

The *Epsin 4* Gene on Chromosome 5q, Which Encodes the Clathrin-Associated Protein Enthoprotin, Is Involved in the Genetic Susceptibility to Schizophrenia

Jonathan Pimm,[1,2] Andrew McQuillin,[1] Srinivasa Thirumalai,[5] Jacob Lawrence,[1] Digby Quested,[3,6] Nicholas Bass,[1] Graham Lamb,[2] Helen Moorey,[2] Susmita R. Datta,[1] Gursharan Kalsi,[1] Allison Badacsonyi,[4] Katie Kelly,[7] Jenny Morgan,[5] Bhaskar Punukollu,[3] David Curtis,[4] and Hugh Gurling[1]

[1]Molecular Psychiatry Laboratory, Department of Mental Health Sciences, University College London Medical School, Windeyer Institute of Medical Sciences, [2]Camden and Islington Mental Health and Social Care Trust, St. Pancras Hospital, [3]West London Mental Health Trust, Hammersmith and Fulham Mental Health Unit and St. Bernard's Hospital, and [4]Queen Mary College, University of London and East London and City Mental Health Trust, Royal London Hospital, London; [5]West Berkshire National Health Service (NHS) Trust, Reading, United Kingdom; [6]Department of Psychiatry, University of Oxford, Warneford Hospital, Oxford, United Kingdom; and [7]Gloucestershire Partnership NHS Trust, Gloucester, United Kingdom

Chromosome 5q33 is a region that has previously shown good evidence of linkage to schizophrenia, with four LOD scores >3.00 in independent linkage studies. We studied 450 unrelated white English, Irish, Welsh, and Scottish research subjects with schizophrenia and 450 ancestrally matched supernormal controls. Four adjacent markers at the 5′ end of the *Epsin 4* gene showed significant evidence of linkage disequilibrium with schizophrenia. These included two microsatellite markers, *D5S1403* ($P = .01$) and *AAAT11* ($P = .009$), and two single-nucleotide–polymorphism markers within the *Epsin 4* gene, *rs10046055* ($P = .007$) and *rs254664* ($P = .01$). A series of different two- and three-marker haplotypes were also significantly associated with schizophrenia, as confirmed with a permutation test (HapA, $P = .004$; HapB, $P = .0005$; HapC, $P = .007$; and HapD, $P = .01$). The *Epsin 4* gene encodes the clathrin-associated protein enthoprotin, which has a role in transport and stability of neurotransmitter vesicles at the synapses and within neurons. A genetically determined abnormality in the structure, function, or expression of enthoprotin is likely to be responsible for genetic susceptibility to a subtype of schizophrenia on chromosome 5q33.3.

Important genetic effects in the susceptibility to schizophrenia have now been established by twin, adoption, genetic-linkage, and allelic-association studies. Linkage studies have proven that there is heterogeneity of linkage or locus heterogeneity for different genetic subtypes of schizophrenia. We originally obtained LOD scores >3.00 showing linkage to the first schizophrenia locus (*SCZD1* [MIM 181150]) on chromosome 5 in a sample of 23 highly selected large multiplex families, by use of a limited set of RFLP markers that were not well localized but were thought to be within the cytogenetic region 5q11-12 (Sherrington et al. 1988; Kalsi et al. 1999). Later, we completed a genome linkage scan in a subsample of these families (Gurling et al. 2001) but found two positive regions of linkage to schizophrenia that were adjacent on either side of the original 5q11-12 region. In this later genome scan, we used better localized markers that were evenly spread along the whole chromosome 5. Some of the families that produced positive LOD scores at 5q11-12 in the original study (Sherrington et al. 1988) then showed linkage near the centromere on chromosome 5, with a LOD score of 2.5, and other families showed linkage to markers on the long arm in the 5q22-33 region (Gurling et al. 2001).

The more distal of the two regions we implicated was

Received December 15, 2004; accepted for publication March 4, 2005; electronically published March 25, 2005.

Address for correspondence and reprints: Dr. Hugh Gurling, Molecular Psychiatry Laboratory, Department of Mental Health Sciences, University College London Medical School, Windeyer Institute of Medical Sciences, 46 Cleveland Street, London W1T 4JF, United Kingdom. E-mail: rejuhxg@ucl.ac.uk

0002-9297/2005/7605-0019$15.00

at 5q22-34, where we obtained a LOD score of 3.6 (nominal $P = .0001$). The chromosome 5q22-34 region had also been found to be linked to schizophrenia in a sample of Irish families (Straub et al. 1997), with a heterogeneity LOD score of 3.35 near locus *D5S804* ($P = .0002$).

Subsequently, analysis of a single large kindred from Palau, Micronesia, resulted in a LOD score of 3.4 and showed linkage to schizophrenia with markers in the 5q22-31 region (Devlin et al. 2002). Later, a study of Finnish families also found linkage to schizophrenia, with a LOD score of 3.56, at 5q22-31 (Paunio et al. 2001). A collaborative study of the 5q22-31 region (Levinson 1999) found that four of eight independent linkage samples of families with schizophrenia resulted in LOD scores >1.00. For example, analysis of a sample of German families resulted in a LOD score of 1.8 at 5q22-31, at marker *D5S399* (Schwab et al. 1997).

These studies suggest that there must be at least two—and possibly three or more—different regions of chromosome 5 that harbor susceptibility loci for schizophrenia. The evidence implicating the more distal region of chromosome 5 at 5q33 is derived from four independent linkage studies that report LOD scores >3.00. We attempted to identify exactly which gene might be involved, by the detection of linkage disequilibrium (LD) in a case-control genetic-association study, using markers we had previously found to show maximal evidence of linkage to schizophrenia.

We recruited a sample of 450 volunteers with schizophrenia and 450 controls from London and southern England. All subjects were included only if both parents were of English, Irish, Welsh, or Scottish descent and if three of four grandparents were of the same descent. One grandparent was allowed to be of other white European origin but not of Jewish or non–European Union (EU) ancestry (on the basis of the EU countries before the recent enlargement). U.K. National Health Service (NHS) multicenter and local research ethics committee approval was obtained, and all subjects signed an approved consent form after reading an information sheet. All 450 schizophrenic research subjects had been diagnosed and assessed by NHS psychiatrists as part of routine clinical diagnosis and treatment. Research subjects with short-term drug-induced psychoses, learning disabilities, head injuries, and other symptomatic psychoses were excluded from the present study. Research subjects were selected on the basis of having an International Classification of Diseases version 10 diagnosis of schizophrenia recorded in the NHS medical case notes. That information together with personal, medical, and psychiatric histories and all other available information were taken into consideration to complete data collection and interviewing with the Schizophrenia and Affective Disorders Schedule–Lifetime Schedule (SADS-L) interview (Spitzer and Endicott 1977). The SADS-L protocol expects data items to be recorded accurately from previous medical records and does not rely on the accuracy of statements made during the interview by mentally ill research subjects. After the SADS-L interview was completed using all sources of information, the subject individuals received the diagnosis of schizophrenia in accordance with the probable level of the Research Diagnostic Criteria (RDC). The "supernormal" control subjects were also interviewed in accordance with SADS-L guidelines, by use of the initial clinical screening questions, and were selected on the basis of having no family history of schizophrenia, alcoholism, or bipolar disorder and having no past or present personal history of any RDC-defined mental disorder.

Genomic DNA was extracted from frozen whole-blood samples by use of a standard cell lysis, proteinase K digestion, and phenol/chloroform ethanol precipitation method. All DNA samples were quantified with pico green by laser fluorimetry. The first set of five markers genotyped was selected on the basis of having shown maximal linkage and minimal recombination fraction to a chromosome 5q33 schizophrenia-susceptibility locus, with the assumption of admixture, in our previous genome linkage scan in large kindreds with schizophrenia. Specific loci were not targeted by genotyping markers next to known genes. The microsatellite marker *AAAT11* was identified, formatted, and genotyped for the present study and was amplified with the primers (forward) CTAGTT-GGGAGGCTGAGGTG and (reverse) AAGAGGGAGC-CTCAATCTGG. Primer sequences for PCR amplification of the microsatellite marker *D5S1403* and the SNPs were obtained from ENSEMBL, the University of California–Santa Cruz (UCSC) Genome Bioinformatics Web site, or the National Center for Biotechnology Information SNP Database. PCR amplification of microsatellite markers was performed using an M13-tailed primer and a second nontailed oligonucleotide primer. A third universal M13 sequence primer labeled with infrared dye IRD 700 or IRD 800 was used to hybridize against the M13-tailed locus-specific primer. Microsatellite marker–fragment sizes were separated and visualized using dual argon laser LiCor 4200L sequencers. Genotyping was performed with the SAGA2 genotyping software and was checked by eye. Allele calling by SAGA2 was checked by a second independent person, blind to diagnosis. The genotype data were automatically stored in a database. Any genotypes that were discrepant between the two checkers were PCR amplified and were genotyped again.

SNPs were determined by the Amplifluor SNP genotyping method, as modified by K Biosciences. Of samples on each microtiter plate, 17% were duplicated to detect error and to confirm the reproducibility of genotypes. The data were then analyzed to confirm Hardy-Weinberg equilibrium (HWE). Markers with lack of HWE in the control group were rejected, and genotyping was

Table 1

Tests of Allelic Association with Schizophrenia at the *Epsin 4* Gene Locus

Marker and Sample	Location (in bp) on Chromosome 5	Distance (in bases) from Previous Marker	Observed Allele Frequencies at: Allele			Fragment Size																										χ^2	P[a]
			C	T	A	232	240	244	248	252	197	199	203	207	211	215	219	223	353	356	362	365	368	371	374	377	380	383	386	389		
rs254664:	157,246,580																														6.11	.01[a]
Control			638	242																												
Schizophrenic			522	258																												
5′ Start of *Epsin 4*	157,267,063																															
rs1186930:	157,272,308	2,984																													2.39	.12[a]
Control			483	363																												
Schizophrenic			470	302																												
rs10046055:	157,297,912	25,604																													9.83	.002[a]
Control				613	265																											
Schizophrenic				471	283																											
AAAT11:	157,301,697	3,785																													9.61	.007[b]
Control						0	50	3	471	236																						
Schizophrenic						1	63	1	392	265																						
D5S1403:	157,346,617	44,920																													11.28	.01[b]
Control											0	4	262	158	127	125	44	2														
Schizophrenic											2	3	201	162	148	140	34	0														
D5S1400:	157,439,237	92,620																													6.67	.06[c]
Control																			1	1	2	20	137	281	1	85	72	88	12	6		
Schizophrenic																			3	0	2	18	146	228	1	94	91	88	14	3		

[a] P from 2×2 χ^2, with 1 df.
[b] P from CLUMP Monte Carlo T4.
[c] P from CLUMP Monte Carlo T3.

Table 2

Results of Tests of Haplotypic Association with Schizophrenia at the *Epsin 4* Gene Locus

No. of Markers and Haplotype (Allele)	χ^2	P[a]
2 (440 controls; 396 cases):		
HapA: *rs254664* (T) and *rs10046055* (A)[b]	13.2	.004
HapB: *rs1186930* (T) and *rs10046055* (A)[b]	18.3	.0005
HapC: *rs10046055* (A) and *AAAT11* (252 bp)[b]	21.2	.007
3 (442 controls; 408 cases):		
HapD: *rs254664* (T), *rs10046055* (A), and *AAAT11* (252 bp)[b]	28.1	.01
HapE: *rs1145603* (T), *rs10046055* (A), and *AAAT11* (252 bp)[b]	28.3	.01

[a] Haplotype permutation test empirical *P*, on the basis of 99,999 permutations.
[b] Most likely to be specific alleles that show association in each haplotype.

repeated. Before association analysis, genotype data for each 96-well microtiter plate were analyzed for LD, by use of GENECOUNTING/LDPAIRS, to check that closely linked markers had consistent LD relationships on each plate.

Next, these data were analyzed for allelic association with schizophrenia by use of CLUMP, which employs an empirical Monte Carlo test of significance and which does not require correction for multiple alleles (Sham and Curtis 1995). Subtests of the CLUMP program are T1, Pearson's χ^2 statistic of the "raw" contingency table; T2, the χ^2 statistic of a table with rare alleles grouped together to prevent small expected cell counts; T3, the largest of the χ^2 statistics of 2×2 tables, each of which compares one allele with the rest grouped together; and T4, the largest of the χ^2 statistics of all possible 2×2 tables, comparing any combination of alleles with the rest. The genotypes were then analyzed for marker-to-marker LD and for haplotypic association with schizophrenia by use of GENECOUNTING/LDPAIRS, which computes D' and Cramer's V tests of LD and maximum-likelihood estimates of haplotype frequencies from phase-unknown case-control data (Zhao et al. 2000, 2002). The significance of any overall haplotype association with schizophrenia was computed using permutation testing. Fifteen genetic markers at chromosomal loci thought to be not involved in schizophrenia were genotyped in a subset of the sample (200 cases and 300 controls) and were analyzed to detect genetic heterogeneity between cases and controls, to confirm that the samples were genetically well matched. In addition, a statistical test (CHECKHET) for detecting subjects with atypical genetic background was employed (Curtis et al. 2002).

No evidence of genetic heterogeneity between cases and controls was found from using the reference markers. The CHECKHET test detected two subjects with schizophrenia with abnormal genotypes; these were excluded from further study before any chromosome 5 markers were genotyped. After five microsatellite markers—*D5S1480, D5S1507, D5S1499, D5S820,* and *D5S1403*—had been genotyped, a positive allelic association was found with *D5S1403,* as shown in table 1 (CLUMP T4, $P = .01$). Therefore, 11 additional markers close to *D5S1403* were selected and genotyped. One of these 11 markers was the microsatellite marker *AAAT11,* which was 40 kb from *D5S1403.* This marker also showed significant evidence of association with schizophrenia, with an empirical *P* value of .007. Two of four SNP markers within the *Epsin 4* gene (*rs10046055* [$P = .002$] and *rs254664* [$P = .02$]) were also found to be associated with schizophrenia. Flanking markers on each side of the *Epsin 4* gene did not show association.

The allele frequencies, positions on chromosome 5 for the *Epsin 4* gene, and markers showing significant evidence or a trend toward association with schizophrenia are shown in tables 1 and 2, in their order on chromosome 5q, in accordance with the June 2004 release of the UCSC Genome Browser. Two-marker haplotype

Table 3

Results of Pairwise LD Statistics between All Pairs of Associated Markers

	Absolute Value of D' and LD P Values[a]					
Marker	*rs254664*	*rs1186930*	*rs10046055*	*AAAT11*	*D5S1403*	*D5S1400*
rs254664		.992	.220	.395	.414	.044
rs1186930	<.00001		.242	.058	.383	.057
rs10046055	<.00001	<.00001		.883	.252	.339
AAAT11	<.00001	<.00001	<.00001		.238	.357
D5S1403	<.00001	<.00001	.006	.157		.220
D5S1400	<.00001	.856	<.00001	<.00001	<.00001	

[a] D' values shown above the diagonal; P values shown below diagonal.

HapA (see table 2), derived from combining the SNP markers *rs254664* and *rs10046055*, showed association with schizophrenia, on the basis of permutation testing ($P = .004$). Significant association verified through permutation testing ($P = .0005$) was also found with the SNP markers *rs1186930* and *rs10046055* when combined into haplotype HapB and with the markers *rs10046055* and *AAAT11* in HapC. Two three-marker haplotypes (HapD and HapE) that combined the microsatellite marker *ATTT11* with two of the three SNP markers *rs254664*, *rs10046055*, and *rs1145603* also showed significant association (permutation test $P =$ .001 and .007, respectively). Each of the markers that showed association with schizophrenia was in strong LD ($P < .00001$) with one or more of the other associated markers, as shown in table 3.

The five originally genotyped markers were selected as the closest markers to the chromosome 5q33 linkage peak obtained in our previously published genome analysis of large schizophrenic kindreds. One of these markers showed some evidence for association; hence, new markers nearby were genotyped. Individually, some of these markers produced more highly significant evidence for association. Because these markers are in LD with each other, it is not possible to state the overall significance of all the tests for association obtained from individual markers and from marker combinations, but, together, the results do indicate that a locus conferring susceptibility to schizophrenia is likely to be present in this narrowly defined region.

The schizophrenic subjects studied were routine cases from United Kingdom NHS facilities in London and southern England. They were not selected for having a positive family history of schizophrenia. An important implication of this finding is that genetic effects detected by linkage studies in large multiply affected pedigrees also apply to routinely treated patients in London and southern England NHS mental health facilities. The only gene in the chromosomal region that we implicated by LD was the *Epsin 4* gene. *Epsin 4* is a member of a class of proteins with an "epsin N-terminal homology (ENTH) domain." This protein sequence is evolutionarily conserved and is found in association with other proteins that participate in clathrin-mediated pit formation and endocytosis and in vesicle stability (Koshiba et al. 2002). Enthoprotin is highly enriched on clathrin-coated vesicles isolated from the rat brain and is probably involved in memory by its effects on reuptake and storage of neurotransmitters (Wasiak et al. 2002). Replication studies are needed to fully establish this new genetic association with schizophrenia. Etiological base-pair changes present in the coding and control regions of the *Epsin 4* gene can now be sought by resequencing or mutation screening of genomic DNA from subjects with schizophrenia who have inherited the alleles and haplotypes on chromosome 5q33.3 that are associated with schizophrenia.

Acknowledgments

This research was funded by the Neuroscience Research Charitable Trust and by a Priory Hospital research lectureship to J.L. The authors have no commercial conflicts of interest.

Electronic-Database Information

The URLs for data presented herein are as follows:

ENSEMBL, http://www.ensembl.org/ (for SNPs and microsatellites)

National Center for Biotechnology Information SNP Database, http://www.ncbi.nlm.nih.gov/projects/SNP/ (for SNPs)

Online Mendelian Inheritance in Man (OMIM), http://www.ncbi.nlm.nih.gov/Omim/ (for *SCZD1*)

University of California–Santa Cruz (UCSC) Genome Bioinformatics, http://www.genome.ucsc.edu/ (for SNPs and microsatellites)

References

Curtis D, North BV, Gurling HM, Blaveri E, Sham PC (2002) A quick and simple method for detecting subjects with abnormal genetic background in case-control samples. Ann Hum Genet 66:235–244

Devlin B, Bacanu SA, Roeder K, Reimherr F, Wender P, Galke B, Novasad D, Chu A, TCuenco K, Tiobek S, Otto C, Byerley W (2002) Genome-wide multipoint linkage analyses of multiplex schizophrenia pedigrees from the Oceanic nation of Palau. Mol Psychiatry 7:689–694

Gurling HM, Kalsi G, Brynjolfson J, Sigmundsson T, Sherrington R, Mankoo BS, Read T, Murphy P, Blaveri E, McQuillin A, Petursson H, Curtis D (2001) Genomewide genetic linkage analysis confirms the presence of susceptibility loci for schizophrenia, on chromosomes 1q32.2, 5q33.2, and 8p21-22 and provides support for linkage to schizophrenia, on chromosomes 11q23.3-24 and 20q12.1-11.23. Am J Hum Genet 68:661–673

Kalsi G, Mankoo B, Curtis D, Sherrington R, Melmer G, Brynjolfsson J, Sigmundsson T, Read T, Murphy P, Petursson H, Gurling H (1999) New DNA markers with increased informativeness show diminished support for a chromosome 5q11-13 schizophrenia susceptibility locus and exclude linkage in two new cohorts of British and Icelandic families. Ann Hum Genet 63:235–247

Koshiba S, Kigawa T, Kikuchi A, Yokoyama S (2002) Solution structure of the epsin N-terminal homology (ENTH) domain of human epsin. J Struct Funct Genomics 2:1–8

Levinson DF (1999) Multicenter linkage study of schizophrenia candidate regions on chromosomes 5q, 6q, 10p and 13q. Am J Hum Genet Suppl 65:A259

Paunio T, Ekelund J, Varilo T, Parker A, Hovatta I, Turunen JA, Rinard K, Foti A, Terwilliger JD, Juvonen H, Suvisaari J, Arajarvi R, Suokas J, Partonen T, Lonnqvist J, Meyer J, Peltonen L (2001) Genome-wide scan in a nationwide study sample of schizophrenia families in Finland reveals susceptibility loci on chromosomes 2q and 5q. Hum Mol Genet 10:3037–3048

Schwab SG, Eckstein GN, Hallmayer J, Lerer B, Albus M, Borrmann M, Lichtermann D, Ertl MA, Maier W, Wildenauer DB (1997) Evidence suggestive of a locus on chromosome 5q31 contributing to susceptibility for schizophrenia in German and Israeli families by multipoint affected sib-pair linkage analysis. Mol Psychiatry 2:156–160

Sham PC, Curtis D (1995) Monte Carlo tests for associations between disease and alleles at highly polymorphic loci. Ann Hum Genet 59:97–105

Sherrington R, Brynjolfsson J, Petursson H, Potter M, Dudleston K, Barraclough B, Wasmuth J, Dobbs M, Gurling H (1988) Localization of a susceptibility locus for schizophrenia on chromosome 5. Nature 336:164–167

Spitzer R, Endicott J (1977) The schedule for affective disorders and schizophrenia, lifetime version, 3rd ed. New York State Psychiatric Institute, New York

Straub RE, MacLean CJ, O'Neill FA, Walsh D, Kendler KS (1997) Support for a possible schizophrenia vulnerability locus in region 5q22-31 in Irish families. Mol Psychiatry 2: 148–155

Wasiak S, Legendre-Guillemin V, Puertollano R, Blondeau F, Girard M, de Heuvel E, Boismenu D, Bell AW, Bonifacino JS, McPherson PS (2002) Enthoprotin: a novel clathrin-associated protein identified through subcellular proteomics. J Cell Biol 158:855–862

Zhao JH, Curtis D, Sham PC (2000) Model-free analysis and permutation tests for allelic associations. Hum Hered 50: 133–139

Zhao JH, Lissarrague S, Essioux L, Sham PC (2002) GENECOUNTING: haplotype analysis with missing genotypes. Bioinformatics 18:1694–1695

Announcements[1]

EMPLOYMENT OPPORTUNITIES

Clinical Biochemical Genetics Fellowship.—The University of Utah Health Sciences Center invites applications for a 3-year fellowship position in clinical biochemical genetics starting July 1, 2005. The medical genetics program at the University of Utah was established in 1978 and currently offers training programs in clinical genetics, molecular genetics, cytogenetics, and biochemical genetics, all of which are accredited by the American Board of Medical Genetics (ABMG). Fellows in the program have the opportunity to work with a diverse group of clinicians (dysmorphologists, medical geneticists, biochemical geneticists, and neurologists), laboratory-based biochemical geneticists, pathologists, and molecular biologists. The biochemical genetics laboratory is part of ARUP Laboratories, a national reference laboratory owned by the University of Utah. It features a wide spectrum of analyses on biological specimens, performed by gas chromatography, ion-exchange chromatography, tandem mass spectrometry, high-performance liquid chromatography, enzymology, and various spectrophotometric methods. Services include pediatric and adult testing for aminoacidopathies, organic acidemias, fatty-acid oxidation disorders, and other inherited metabolic diseases, in addition to newborn screening. Research and development are directed toward both the development of new diagnostic tests for inborn errors of metabolism and the elucidation of the molecular bases/pathophysiology of inborn errors of metabolism. Prospective trainees in clinical biochemical genetics must have an M.D. or a Ph.D. in a relevant basic science (biochemistry, molecular biology, clinical chemistry, genetics, human genetics, etc.). Ph.D. candidates with at least 2 years of postdoctoral research experience are preferred. M.D. candidates will normally have at least 2 years of full-time training in a residency program that is accredited by the Accreditation Council for Graduate Medical Education. The training program satisfies the requirements for the ABMG examination in clinical biochemical genetics. All applicants should send a copy of their curriculum vitae, the names of three references, and a one-page letter with career goals to Nicola Longo, M.D., Ph.D., Medical Genetics/Pediatrics, University of Utah, 2C412 SOM, 50 North Medical Drive, Salt Lake City, UT 84132; telephone: (801) 585-2457; fax: (801) 585-7252; e-mail: Nicola.Longo@hsc.utah.edu

---

Director of Education.—The American Society of Human Genetics (ASHG) has established a new position of Director of Education to implement programs to address the vision of genetic literacy in the classroom as well as in the general public. The Director will work with the Executive Vice President, under the direction of the officers and the Board, to achieve the goals of ASHG, including making genetics-education programs and materials more accessible to all classrooms. ASHG, the primary professional organization for researchers and clinicians in the field, has a strong commitment to educational goals. The duties of the Director will include (1) providing staffing for the Information and Education Committee, (2) initiating and enhancing partnerships with organizations that focus on teaching science in grades K–12, (3) enhancing capabilities of the Mentor Network of volunteer members, (4) planning professional development programs, and (5) procuring funding to implement programs. The ideal candidate will have an M.S. or a Ph.D. in genetics or a related field and experience in developing educational programs and materials. Requirements include outstanding written and oral communication, grant-writing skills, and demonstrated ability to lead projects. Applicants should send a curriculum vitae, a letter of interest, and the names of three potential references to Joann Boughman either by e-mail, tojboughman@ashg.org, or by mail, to the following address: Joann Boughman, Ph.D., Executive Vice President, American Society of Human Genetics, 9650

1. Announcements are published free of charge for members of The American Society of Human Genetics (ASHG). Please e-mail announcements to ajhg@emory.edu. Submission must be received *at least 7 weeks* before the month of issue in which publication is requested. They must be double spaced with a $1\frac{1}{2}$-inch margin on all sides. The maximum length is *250 words,* excluding the address for correspondence. Please include a cover letter indicating the name of the sponsoring ASHG member.

Rockville Pike, Bethesda, MD 20814. Review of applications will begin in March 2005, and the position may start as early as June 1, 2005.

Program Associate.—The Cleft Lip and Palate Clinic and Craniofacial Anomalies Research Center seeks a program associate to identify and enroll patients in birth-defects research projects and to provide genetic evaluation in the Cleft Lip and Palate Clinic. The program associate will also conduct clinical, educational, administrative, and liaison activities as directed and will maintain a database of demographic, clinical, and genetic information on patients enrolled in genetic research studies. Basic qualifications include a master's degree in genetic counseling with board certification/board eligibility as a genetic counselor, a masters degree in nursing with an emphasis on genetics and a license to practice in Iowa, or an equivalent combination of education and experience. Desirable qualifications include reasonable experience in research, a background in research activities related to craniofacial or other birth defects, phlebotomy skills, computer experience with Microsoft Office, some grant-writing experience, excellent organizational skills, and demonstrated oral and written communication and interpersonal skills. Applicants should submit a resume to Cindy Fetters/#51184, 2625 JCP, University of Iowa, Department of Pediatrics, 200 Hawkins Drive, Iowa City, IA 52242-1083. The University of Iowa is an equal employment opportunity/affirmative action employer and strongly encourages women and minorities to apply.

Postdoctoral Research Fellows.—Positions for postdoctoral research fellows are available, to start between April 2005 and September 2005, in the Department of Dermatology at Columbia University. The laboratory is highly international, and its members have broad interests in skin and hair-follicle biology, as well as in translational research aimed at therapies for genetic skin diseases. The successful applicants will be involved in one of two main projects in the group. The first project is aimed at the genetic mapping of mouse and human disease genes for both Mendelian and complex disorders involving skin and/or hair phenotypes. The individual should have experience in statistical genetics for linkage analysis, molecular biology techniques, cytogenetics, FISH, genotyping, in situ hybridization, and RT-PCR and should have proficiency with genomic databases, etc. Good communication skills are also beneficial in dealing with genetic counselors and clinical colleagues. Another position is available in the area of stem-cell biology. Our laboratory's main focus is the study of epidermal and hair-follicle stem cells. Specific areas of knowledge that are a plus include cell, developmental, and molecular biology, as well as past work with in vitro and in vivo mouse models. Good written and oral communication skills are desirable. Interested candidates should send a curriculum vitae and two or three references to Dr. Angela M. Christiano, Departments of Dermatology and Genetics and Development, Columbia University, College of Physicians and Surgeons, 630 West 168th Street VC15-204, New York, NY 10032; telephone: (212) 305-9565; fax: (212) 305-7391; e-mail: amc65@columbia.edu

---

Assistant/Associate Professor.—The Division of Medical Genetics in the Department of Child Health at the University of Missouri–Columbia School of Medicine is seeking a full-time assistant/associate professor on either the clinical or tenure track. Candidates should have expertise in the clinical and laboratory diagnosis and treatment of children with metabolic disorders. Applicants must be board-certified/board-eligible in medical genetics and must also be board-certified in either pediatrics or internal medicine; applicants must have a record of medical and academic excellence. The successful applicant will join a busy Medical Genetics Division and will be responsible for (1) managing the metabolic genetics program, including clinics in Columbia and at outreach locations throughout rural Missouri; (2) directing the metabolic screening laboratory; and (3) participating in the Medical Genetics Clinic. The Childrens Hospital at University of Missouri Health Care has >100 inpatient beds, a wide variety of pediatric medical and surgical subspecialists, and comprehensive laboratory services. The department will begin screening applications immediately. Please direct all inquiries—as well as your letters of reference and curriculum vitae—to Bert Bachrach, M.D., Assistant Professor, Department of Child Health, Columbia, MO 65212; e-mail: bachrachb@missouri.edu. We also invite you to visit our Web site (http://www.genetics.missouri.edu/). Columbia, MO, has a lot to offer you! Visit the Chamber of Commerce Web site (http://chamber.columbia.mo.us/visitors.html) for additional information. The University of Missouri is an equal opportunity employer and complies with the guidelines of the Americans with Disabilities Act (ADA) of 1990. The department welcomes applications from underrepresented physician groups. For ADA accommodations, please contact our ADA coordinator; telephone: (573) 884-8278.

UCLA Intercampus Medical Genetics and Pediatric Genetics Training Programs.—The University of California, Los Angeles (UCLA) intercampus postdoctoral research and clinical training programs in medical genetics utilize the resources of the universitys affiliated campuses and teaching hospitals to offer academically oriented individuals a wide variety of clinical and/or research opportunities in molecular genetics, biochemical genetics, immunogenetics, cancer genetics, cytogenetics, somatic cell genetics, and population genetics. Five-year combined pediatric/medical genetics residencies are also available at each of the affiliated hospitals, and applications are accepted through the Electronic Residency Application Service. These programs meet all the requirements of the American Board of Medical Genetics and the Accreditation Council for Graduate Medical Education. Applicants must have an M.D., a Ph.D., a D.D.S., or an equivalent degree. Application forms are available from Patricia Kearney, Coordinator, Academic Affairs, Medical Genetics Institute, Cedars-Sinai Medical Center, 8700 Beverly Boulevard, West Tower 665, Los Angeles, CA 90048; application forms and additional information can also be found on our Web site (http://www.uclamedgeneticspostdoc.org).

Conference

Jefferson Matrix Biology Days 2005.—The 12th International Symposium on Basement Membranes will be held at Jefferson Medical College in Philadelphia, PA, on June 15–18, 2005. The conference is sponsored by the Lennox K. Black International Prize for Excellence in Medicine, in memory of Rupert Timpl. A special Matrix Biology Symposium will be held to honor Darwin J. Prockop. For further information on the programs, topics, abstract submissions/deadlines, and hotel accommodations and to register for this event, please visit our Web site (http://www.jeffersonhospital.org/matrixbiology2005) or contact Eileen O'Shaughnessy, Executive Secretary; telephone: (215) 503-5786; fax: (215) 503-5788; e-mail: eileen.oshaughnessy@jefferson.edu

Information for Contributors

Postal address: **Stephen T. Warren, Ph.D., Editor, The American Journal of Human Genetics, Department of Human Genetics, Emory University School of Medicine, 615 Michael Street, Room 301, Atlanta, GA 30322-3050.** Telephone: (404) 712-9980. Fax: (404) 712-9984. E-mail: ajhg@emory.edu. Web page: http://www.ajhg.org/.

The American Journal of Human Genetics is a record of research and review relating to heredity in humans; to the applications of genetic principles in medicine, psychology, anthropology, and social services; and to areas of molecular and cell biology relevant to human genetics. It is published monthly. The *Journal* is owned and controlled by The American Society of Human Genetics and is edited, in conjunction with the publisher, by a staff appointed by the Board of Directors of the Society.

Electronic Edition

The entire content of the *Journal* is published electronically on the World Wide Web, at http://www.ajhg.org/. The full text is available to subscribers, as is material supplemental to the print version, including video and archival databases. Articles will be posted as they are ready for publication. Approximately 2 weeks before publication of the hard copy, the table of contents for that issue will be posted with final pagination, along with editorials and other material.

Editorial Policy

The *Journal* welcomes submissions of articles and reports on timely subjects concerning all aspects of human genetics, including studies of model organisms that are of direct relevance to human genetics. Letters commenting on material previously published in the *Journal* are also welcome. Review articles, editorials, and book reviews usually are solicited by the editor. The *Journal* does not publish reports of either single mutations or mutational surveys of previously identified loci unless they have unusual significance and substantial insight. Descriptions of new linkage assignments will be considered only if they are of unusual interest and significance. Reports of negative data, without substantial insight and interest, will not normally be considered. Membership in The American Society of Human Genetics is not a prerequisite for publication in the *Journal.* Papers will be considered for publication on condition that they are not currently under consideration by any other publication and that no portion of them has been published elsewhere.

• *Review process.* Manuscripts will be considered for appropriateness to the *Journal* by the editor in conjunction with the editorial board. Those considered appropriate will be reviewed by two or more external reviewers or by members of the editorial board, and those not considered appropriate will be returned to the authors. Authors are requested to suggest appropriate referees. Manuscripts will be judged on their value as original contributions to the field and on their overall presentation. Authors whose manuscripts are returned without external review may appeal by writing the editor.

• *Return of figures.* For manuscripts that are reviewed but not accepted, all figures submitted as glossy prints will be returned whenever possible.

• *Editing.* Manuscripts will be edited to conform to *Journal* style, to correct spelling and grammar where necessary, and to improve conciseness, clarity, and precision of expression. Significant editorial changes will be identified on the page proofs.

• *Publication costs.* For papers published—except for invited contributions and Letters to the Editor—authors will be charged $50.00 per printed *Journal* page or portion thereof. Each *Journal* page contains ~800 words. If authors wish, they may instead pay a single publication fee of $5,000 for an article or $2,700 for a report, to make their work freely and immediately available to all readers at publication, rather than after the usual 6-month delay for nonsubscribers. All authors will also be charged for printing of color figures (see Illustrations, below).

• *Copyright agreement.* All authors of all manuscripts accepted for publication (except U.S. government employees) must sign an agreement transferring copyright to The American Society of Human Genetics. Corresponding authors must assume responsibility for obtaining the signatures of all coauthors. Material published in the *Journal* may not be reproduced or published elsewhere without written consent of the Society and the publisher. Requests for such permission should be addressed to the publisher: Copyright, University of Chicago Press, 1427 East 60th Street, Chicago, IL 60637. Fax: (773) 702-9756.

• *Research materials.* It is assumed that authors whose research is published in the *Journal* will make cell lines, antibodies, cloned DNA sequences, and similar materials available to other investigators in noncommercial institutions, so as to permit replication of the reported work.

• *Page proofs.* Page proofs will be sent to the corresponding author for correction of typographical errors only. Corresponding authors are responsible for the return of corrected page proofs to the publisher by the designated deadline.

• *Reprints.* The corresponding author will receive an order form for reprints, along with the page proofs.

Manuscript Submission

Manuscripts should now be submitted via the *AJHG* Web Peer Review System at http://mss.uchicago.edu/AJHG. Basic instructions for submission via the WPR system can be found at the Web site (http://mss.uchicago.edu/AJHG/auth_msprep_AJHG.epl), and detailed instructions are given below.

Manuscript Preparation

Manuscripts must be written in English. MS Word, Rich Text, or LaTeX formats are acceptable. All components of the text (including references and figure legends but not tables) must

be typed double spaced in 12-point type. Tables must be single spaced. *Manuscripts that are not double spaced throughout will not be sent out for review.* Use a 1-inch margin on all four sides of each page, and do not justify the right margin. Begin each manuscript component on a separate page, and arrange components in the following order: title page, Summary (abstract), text (articles separated into Introduction, Material and Methods, Results, and Discussion), Acknowledgments, appendices (if any), Electronic-Database Information, References, tables, and figure legends. Number all pages consecutively in the upper-right-hand corner, beginning with the title page.

Cover letter. Include a letter from the author who will be responsible for correspondence regarding the manuscript as well as for communications among authors in regard to revisions, publication agreements, and approval of proofs. This letter should indicate the category of manuscript being submitted (e.g., article, report, letter, review) and highlight the significance of the manuscript in a few sentences. It should also disclose the source of funding and any affiliations with or involvement in any companies, trade associations, unions, litigants, or other groups with a direct financial interest in the subject matter or materials discussed in the manuscript by any authors and/or their immediate family within the last 5 years. Also indicate whether the first author is a student or postdoctoral fellow and a member of The American Society of Human Genetics (to be eligible for the Cotterman awards, presented at the ASHG's annual meeting).

Please indicate the category of your manuscript in the cover letter:

Articles are full-length, original research articles.

Reports are short (approximately four *Journal* pages, 800 words per page) scientific correspondence with a brief abstract but without further subdivision of the manuscript. This category is designed for timely publication of original findings that may substantially impact their field.

Letters to the Editor are brief commentaries (less than one printed page) concerning articles published in the *Journal* within the past 2 months. They may also present new data. Also included in this section are short general news items of interest to the Society. Any letter concerning a previously published article will first be sent for external review, to determine whether it meets an appropriate level of significance for publication in the *Journal.* If the letter achieves this basic level of significance, it will then be sent to the corresponding author of the pertinent article, who will be given an opportunity to submit a response. This response will be provided to the corresponding author of the letter to the editor. After considering the response, the authors may choose to withdraw their letter or to proceed with publication without further revision.

Fast-track review. If circumstances so warrant, you may request in the cover letter a fast-track review of your paper. At the editor's discretion, a 24- to 48-hour fast-track review is available to expedite manuscripts that deserve rapid review and publication.

Related manuscripts. Please submit a copy of any related papers, by any of the authors, that have been submitted but not published elsewhere or that are in press. For citation of such manuscripts, see "*Work submitted to a publication but not yet accepted, personal communications, and unpublished data,*" below.

All papers should adhere to the guidelines that follow, with two exceptions:

1) *Reports* should contain a brief summary of five sentences or fewer, but the remainder of the text should not be divided into sections.

2) *Letters to the Editor* do not contain a summary, nor should the text be divided into sections.

Otherwise, please prepare all submissions according to the following directives:

Title page. This page should contain a concise title; a running title of no more than 40 characters (including spaces); the names and institutional affiliations of all authors at the time of the study (and present affiliations, if different); and the corresponding author's name, complete current mailing address, telephone number, fax number, and e-mail address. Each paper can be assigned only one corresponding author. Joint authorship is permitted only for the first author position, with a maximum of two individuals being given this designation.

Summary (abstract). The Summary should state the purpose of the study, the basic procedures and analytical methods, the findings, and the principal conclusions. The Summary must not exceed 275 words.

Text. The text should be as concise as possible and should be organized into the following sections: Introduction, Material and Methods (or Subjects and Methods), Results, and Discussion. Some manuscripts may require different formats appropriate to their content. Brief subheadings may be used where necessary.

The Introduction should summarize the rationale for the study, without reviewing the subject extensively. Using the past tense, describe the selection of subjects and identify the methods, apparatus, and procedures in detail. Provide references for established methods and brief descriptions of those that are not well known. Describe any new or modified methods used, including reasons for their use and evaluations of their limitations.

Present results in logical sequence in the text, tables, and illustrations. Do not repeat in the text all the data that appear in the tables and illustrations. Detailed results of statistical analyses may be presented as an appendix.

Electronic-Database Information. Please provide accession numbers along with the URL of any genome or locus-specific database in which information has been deposited. (This is required for establishing links in the electronic edition of the *Journal.*) Place this information in the text and in a separate section entitled "Electronic-Database Information," following the Acknowledgments. Please do not include URLs in the text or in the References.

MIM numbers should be listed in the text after the first mention of the relevant disorder or gene. Example: adrenal hypoplasia congenita (AHC [MIM 300200]). In the Electronic-Database Information section, only the URL for the OMIM database, and not the individual MIM numbers, should be noted. Example: Online Mendelian Inheritance in Man (OMIM), http://www.ncbi.nlm.nih.gov/Omim/.

Human subjects. If the manuscript reports results of studies of either human subjects or materials obtained from human subjects, state in the Material and Methods section that the study was approved by the appropriate institutional review board and/or that appropriate informed consent was obtained from human subjects. Copies of signed consent forms from identifiable persons appearing in any photographs submitted with the manuscript must be faxed to the *AJHG* office at the time of submission: (404) 712-9984. To avoid violation of HIPAA regulations, this consent form should state that the subject understands that his or her identity (but not his or her medical records) will be divulged to the *Journal* office by the transmission of the signed consent form. Alternatively, a letter from a member of your institutional review board (IRB) can be sent to us confirming that signed consent forms have been obtained from the individuals pictured in the manuscript without naming these individuals. Your manuscript cannot be processed until we receive these consent forms or a letter from your IRB.

Acknowledgments. Acknowledge those who have made substantive contributions to the study reported, as well as the institution(s) or grant sponsor(s) that supported the research.

Reference citations. Authors must assume responsibility for the accuracy of reference citations. Reference citations in the text, tables, or figure legends should be in parentheses and include author surname(s) and year of publication. When citing a work by two authors, provide both authors' names joined by "and." When citing a work by three or more authors, provide the first author's name followed by "et al." When the author name(s) and the year of publication are identical for two or more works, distinguish between the works by appending a lowercase italic letter to the year, to match the order in which the works appear in the References section. Examples: (Charlesworth 2001), (Peters and Sandkuijl 1992), (Devriendt et al. 1997), (Stack et al. 1995*a*). List two or more works in the same citation in chronological order, separated by semicolons. When two or more works in a citation were published in the same year, arrange them alphabetically by the first author's surname. When the same author name(s) are used for two or more works in the same citation, group those works together in chronological order, with the years separated by commas. If such a group occurs in a citation that includes other works, place the group chronologically within the citation according to the first year in the group, using semicolons between the group and the other works cited. Examples: (Erdmann 1994; Braverman et al. 1997; Purdue et al. 1997), (Hellsten 1995; Redding et al. 1996*a*, 1996*b*, 2000; Kessler et al. 1997).

References section. References should be arranged alphabetically by author surname(s). References by the same author(s) should be arranged chronologically. References by the same author(s) for which the year of publication is also the same should be arranged alphabetically by title. List the names of up to 25 authors; if more than 25, list the first 7 plus "et al." Use standard abbreviations for journal titles. Do not use excess punctuation.

References examples:

Journal: Devriendt K, Matthijs G, Legius E, Schollen E, Blockmans D, van Geet C, Degreef H, Cassiman J-J, Fryns J-P (1997) Skewed X-chromosome inactivation in female carriers of dyskeratosis congenita. Am J Hum Genet 60:581–587

Chapter: Peters DJM, Sandkuijl LA (1992) Genetic heterogeneity of polycystic kidney disease in Europe. In: Breuning MH, Devoto M, Romeo G (eds) Contributions to nephrology 97: polycystic kidney disease. Karger, Basel, pp 128–139

Entire volume: Dayhoff MV (ed) (1978) Atlas of protein sequence and structure. Vol 5, suppl 3. National Biomedical Research Foundation, Washington, DC

Meeting paper: Kessler S (1997) Transcripts of genetic counseling sessions: exercises in missed opportunities. Paper presented at Talking Human Genetics: Verbal Communication, Knowledge and Genetic Makeup. Hamburg, April 24–27

Thesis/dissertation: Hellsten E (1995) Positional cloning of the infantile ceroid lipofuscinosis gene. PhD thesis, National Public Health Institute, Helsinki

Computer software: SAS Institute (1997) SAS release 6.12, Cary, NC

Work "in press": Jones TM, Peterson RW. Ethical issues in screening for genetic diseases. Am J Hum Genet (in press)

Work submitted to a publication but not yet accepted, personal communications, and unpublished data: Do not list in References. Cite in the text as "personal communication" (if none of the individuals cited are authors of the manuscript being submitted) or "unpublished data" (if at least one of the individuals cited is also an author of the manuscript being submitted). List the names (including first initials) of all individuals responsible for the unpublished data or personal communication, and include letters of authorization from the individuals named.

Tables. Each table should appear on a separate page and should be single spaced. Whenever possible, construct exceptionally large tables and pedigree diagrams in sections. Number tables consecutively and give each a brief title. Give each column a short heading. Use footnotes to explain all abbreviations that are used in each table, and denote them by letter. Titles and footnotes should be included on the same page with the tables themselves. Use the table editor of a word-processing program to create tables. Do not use tabs or spaces, and omit vertical and horizontal lines from tables. Each row of data must be in a separate row of table cells. Do not submit tables as photographs. For more detailed instructions about tables, see "Special Instructions for Tables" at the *AJHG* homepage. For further guidelines, see *Scientific Style and Format: The CBE Manual for Authors, Editors, and Publishers* and *The Chicago Manual of Style* (cited in Style Guidelines, below).

Illustrations (figures). For complete instructions on preparing figures, please refer to http://www.ajhg.org/artguide.html. Design and prepare the figures carefully; they are the visual presentation of the scientific findings and will be carefully evaluated by the reviewers and editors. Figures should be saved as Encapsulated Postscript (EPS) files or Tagged Image File Format (TIF) files. Common Web formats, such as GIF or JPEG, are not acceptable; neither are proprietary application

formats, such as PowerPoint. Most figures will be set as single column (80 mm), some as double column (175 mm), and some broadside on a page (230 mm). Prepare the figures in publication size or larger (the lettering must be large enough so that the smallest letter will be at least 2.0 mm in height when the figure is reduced to publication size).

Use patterns, such as diagonal lines, rather than shading, which does not reproduce evenly. For pedigree construction, follow the guidelines described in Bennett et al.'s "Recommendations for Standardized Human Pedigree Nomenclature" (Am J Hum Genet 56:745–752, 1995). Include the key (explanation of symbols) within the figure. For micrographs, indicate magnification either by means of a micron bar or in the legend.

Use Helvetica lettering throughout the figure. Insert uppercase letters, in a larger font size, to designate panels.

For initial submission, we require that all figures and tables be included in the main text file. The figures may be converted to the file format of the main text file, since they are being used only for evaluation purposes. External reviewers are only permitted access to the main text file, so they will see only figures and tables included in that file. Thus, it is preferable that you include supplementary materials in the main text file as well. However, if including the supplementary materials makes the main text file too large to upload on our server, they may be uploaded separately.

In submission of revised manuscripts, the figure files should be uploaded as separate files in the appropriate format (EPS or TIFF) but should also be included in the main text file, as they were in the original submission, in case your paper is sent for further external review. Hard copies of figures are required for publication, but, if you wish, you may wait to send them until acceptance of the manuscript.

Color illustrations. Authors must sign an agreement to pay the costs of production of color figures when a manuscript with color figures is accepted. Each page containing a color figure will incur a charge of $450 for the first figure or separate part of a figure, plus $200 for each additional figure.

Figure legends. These should be double spaced, beginning on a separate page. The legend should begin with a brief phrase describing the figure content. The legend should describe the illustration so that it can be understood apart from the text and should explain any labels or symbols that are not included in a key.

Supplemental material. Authors may submit additional data, at the discretion of the editor, as a supplement to the *AJHG* electronic edition.

Supplemental clinical data. For manuscripts containing clinical information, it is important that as much clinical detail as possible be provided for others to verify the conclusions drawn. Photographs, radiographs, and imaging data as well as other laboratory, historical, and clinical data outside the immediate scope of the manuscript may be included as a supplement to the *AJHG* electronic edition.

Style Guidelines

For questions of grammar, punctuation, abbreviation, and scientific style, refer to *The Chicago Manual of Style* (15th ed., University of Chicago Press, Chicago) and *Scientific Style and Format: The CBE Manual for Authors, Editors, and Publishers* (6th ed., Cambridge University Press, Cambridge, UK). The preferred or first spelling of a word in *Merriam-Webster's Collegiate Dictionary* (11th ed., Merriam-Webster, Springfield, MA) is used by the *Journal.* Mathematical equations must be typed and spaced as they should appear in print. Use metric or other internationally accepted units for all quantitative measurements.

Genetic nomenclature and notation. For human genes, use genetic notation and symbols approved by the Human Gene Mapping Workshop. Approved gene symbols may be obtained, prior to submission, from Dr. Sue Povey of the HUGO Gene Nomenclature Committee (HGNC), Department of Biology, University College London, Wolfson House, 4 Stephenson Way, London NW1 2HE, United Kingdom (telephone: 44-20-7679-7410; fax: 44-20-7387-3496; e-mail: nome@galton.ucl.ac.uk). Nomenclature guidelines are available and the Gene Name Proposal form may be completed on the HGNC Web page: http://www.gene.ucl.ac.uk/nomenclature/. See Wain et al.'s "Guidelines for Human Gene Nomenclature" (Genomics 79:464470, 2002). Use ISCN nomenclature for cytogenetic notation (see Mitelman F [ed] ISCN 1995: an international system for human cytogenetic nomenclature. S. Karger, Basel). Human gene names and loci should be written in italicized capital letters and Arabic numerals. Protein product names are not italicized. For human-mutation nomenclature, see Antonarakis et al.'s "Recommendations for a Nomenclature System for Human Gene Mutations" (Hum Mutat 11:1-3, 1998) (http://www3.interscience.wiley.com/cgi-bin/fulltext/5001291/PDFSTART).

Approved mouse nomenclature may be obtained, prior to submission, from Lois Maltais, The Jackson Laboratory, Bar Harbor, ME 04609-0800; telephone: (207) 288-6429; fax: (207) 288-6132; e-mail: nomen@informatics.jax.org; Web page: http://www.informatics.jax.org/mgihome/nomen. For other organisms, consult the appropriate authorities.

Nucleotide sequence deposition. New nucleotide data must be submitted to and deposited in the DNA Data Bank of Japan (DDBJ)/European Molecular Biology Laboratory (EMBL)/GenBank databases, and accession number(s) must be obtained before the paper can be accepted for publication. Submission to any one of the three collaborating databases is sufficient to ensure data entry in all. The accession number(s) should be included in the manuscript's Electronic-Database Information section, and the following footnote should appear on the title page: "Nucleotide sequence data reported herein are available in the DDBJ/EMBL/GenBank databases; for details, see the Electronic-Database Information section of this article." The database will withhold release of data until publication, at authors' request. The most convenient method for submission of sequence data is by World Wide Web: DDBJ, via SAKURA (http://sakura.ddbj.nig.ac.jp/); EMBL, via WEBIN (http://www.ebi.ac.uk/embl/Submission/webin.html); or GenBank, via BankIt (http://www.ncbi.nlm.nih.gov/Sequin/).

Single-nucleotide polymorphisms. Newly described single-nucleotide polymorphisms (SNPs) should be submitted to an appropriate database such as dbSNP (http://www.ncbi.nlm

.nih.gov/SNP/) prior to submission of revised manuscripts. The identification numbers should be included in the "Electronic-Database Information" section of the manuscript.

Microarray data. All newly generated microarray data referred to in the text must be submitted for publication as a supplement to the *AJHG* electronic edition. Tables of quantitated raw data and processed data are acceptable, as outlined in guidelines proposed by the Microarray Gene Expression Data Society (for full details, see http://www.mged.org/Workgroups/MIAME/miame_checklist.html). For submission, please save the tables as tab-delimited ASCII text files and submit an electronic copy (no hard copies are necessary).

Computer programs. Authors of manuscripts that describe a novel computer program must make the relevant program publicly available by the time the manuscript is published.

Manuscript-Preparation Checklist

○ Cover letter

○ Copies of signed consent forms for all identifiable photographs of patients

○ Manuscript and figures

○ All pages of text and References *fully double spaced*

○ 1-inch margin on all four sides of each page

○ Title and running title

○ Order of manuscript elements: title page, Summary, text (Introduction, Material and Methods, Results, Discussion), Acknowledgments, appendixes, Electronic-Database Information, References, tables, figure legends

○ Summary: no more than 275 words

○ Acknowledgments: all sources of support and those who have made substantive contributions to the work reported

○ References: accurate, complete, and proper style in text and reference list; up to 25 authors' names included (if more than 25, list the first 7 plus "et al.")

○ Tables: *single spaced, no vertical lines, created with the table editor of a word-processing program, not with tabs;* title and footnotes included with table

○ Figures: all guidelines followed; figure legends on a separate page, double spaced

○ A copy of related manuscripts submitted or in press

Additional Components Required at Revision

○ Permission to reproduce previously published material

○ Letters of authorization from sources of personal communications and unpublished data

Submission via the Web Peer Review System

Formatting Electronic Files

Please follow the manuscript preparation requirements above to submit a new or revised manuscript via this system. The system relies on automated processing to create an Adobe Acrobat (PDF) file from your submission. If you do not follow these instructions, your submission cannot be processed automatically and will not be received by the journal office.

The following file formats are acceptable:

- Microsoft Word (.doc; any version that can be read by Word 2000 for Windows)
- Rich Text Format (.rtf)
- Adobe Acrobat (.pdf)
- LaTeX (see special instructions below)

File contents. For initial submission, manuscripts should be submitted as single files, in one of the formats listed above, with all figures, tables, and images embedded (inserted) directly into the document. We also request that supplementary materials be included in the same file, if possible. The figures may be converted to the file format of the main text file, since they are being used only for evaluation purposes. Only materials included in the main text file (and separate supplementary files, if necessary) will be examined by external reviewers.

If we request a revision, in addition to the main text file containing all figures and tables, each figure should be uploaded separately in EPS or TIFF format. Consult your word processing program's "Help" documentation for instructions on how to embed tables and figures. You must also submit in a second file, in one of the acceptable formats, a cover letter that includes your responses to reviewer comments.

Filename requirements. All filenames must be lowercase. (All file processing by the Web Peer Review system is done on Unix machines, where filenames are case-sensitive.)

File compression and archives. Although your manuscript itself must be provided in one file that includes the tables and figures, you will have at least two files to upload into our system (i.e. the cover letter, manuscript file, and any related manuscripts). Therefore, we strongly recommend that you combine these files into an archive so that you can upload a single file for submission. Applications for Mac OS (such as StuffIt) and Windows (such as WinZip) can create this archive.

The following archive formats may be used:

- Windows or Unix zip (e.g., "archiv.zip")
- Unix tar (e.g., "archive.tar" or compressed with gzip as "archive.tar.gz" or "archive.tgz")

If you cannot create archives in these formats, you may still compress individual files to shorten upload time:

- Unix compress (e.g., "ms.tex.Z")

Electronic File Specifications

Program	Main Text File	Cover Letter	Figures	Tables
Word	ms.doc	cover_letter.doc or cover_letter.txt	[embedded in main file]	[embedded in main file]
RTF	ms.rtf	cover_letter.rtf or cover_letter.txt	[embedded in main file]	[embedded in main file]
Acrobat	ms.pdf	cover_letter.pdf or cover_letter.txt	[embedded in main file]	[embedded in main file]
LaTeX	ms.tex	cover_letter.txt	f1.eps, f2.eps, etc.	tb1.tex, tb2.tex, etc.

- Unix gzip (e.g., "ms.tex.gz")

Revisions. If you are submitting a revised manuscript and have a response to the reviewers' comments, include your response as part of the cover letter file. When submitting a revised manuscript with figures, include all the figures even if they have not changed since the previous version.

Online Submission Instructions

Preparing the manuscript file. The preferred format for submitting manuscripts online is Microsoft Word (.doc files). If you are unable to submit a Microsoft Word file, the Web Peer Review system will also accept manuscripts in Acrobat (.pdf), Rich Text Format (.rtf) or LaTeX (.tex). We have provided a drop box in the "File format" area in which to indicate the document type.

As mentioned above, manuscripts should be submitted as single files with all figures, tables, and images embedded (inserted) directly into the document. Embedded figures must be in EPS or TIF format, as these formats result in the best overall outcome when manuscripts are converted to PDF. Please note that authors whose manuscripts are accepted for publication may be required by the publisher to submit high-resolution hard copies (e.g., glossy prints) after the review process is complete and press production is about to begin.

Special instructions for LaTeX. LaTeX files prepared with the AASTeX macro package are preferred. This package uses the "natbib" style for references. If you submit a LaTeX file, figures and tables may be kept in external files, as long as they are referenced within the main "ms.tex" file.

Submission Checklist

Please have the following items readily available before beginning the online submission process:

- Your manuscript as a MS Word, Acrobat (pdf), Rich Text, or LaTeX file including all tables, figures and images embedded in the document
- Cover letter
- Information from your title page for entry into the peer review database, including the title, running title, list of contributing authors and affiliations, word count, and contact information for the corresponding author
- A list of recommended reviewers and their e-mail addresses
- Related papers, by any of the authors, that have been submitted elsewhere or that are in press.
- Copies of signed consent forms for all identifiable photographs of patients (these should be faxed to the AJHG office at [404] 712-9984 at the time of submission).

Navigating the Peer Review Web Site

Step one: describing your manuscript. Go to the *AJHG* Peer Review Web site at http://mss.uchicago.edu/AJHG/. A username and password are required to enter the site. If you already have a username and password, click on "Login/See current tasks" to view the status of your account. If you are new to the site, click on "Create account" to register. After completing your login, click on the "Begin submission" button.

Once you have logged in, fill in the fields describing your manuscript. To move from one field to the next, press the "tab" key. When all the information is complete and you are sure it is correct, click "Ready to upload files" to proceed to step two.

Step two: uploading your file(s). Click the "Browse" button to locate a file on your local system. Once a file is specified in the field, click "Upload this file" to send the file to the Web Peer Review system. You must name your manuscript file "ms," using lowercase type. (All file processing by the Web Peer Review system is done on Unix machines, where filenames are case-sensitive.) The system will assign an ID number to your manuscript during the upload.

As previously mentioned, your manuscript file must contain all figures and tables as well as the text. Remember that if you have multiple files (such as if you are providing a manuscript "in press" for the reviewers), you can compress all of them into a single archive and upload just one file. We recommend that you make an archive of all the files for your submission and then upload the single archive file.

Check your results. Only files listed in the box labeled "Files uploaded so far" have been uploaded successfully. If you need to delete a file, click the file name in the box to select it, and then click the "Delete selected file" button.

When you have uploaded all the files for your submission, click "Process uploaded files" to proceed. The system will attempt to make a PDF version of your file. The conversion to PDF reduces the size of the file and makes it easier for editors and reviewers to read. PDF files can be viewed with Adobe Acrobat Reader version 3 or higher (available free at http://www.adobe.com) or with Ghostscript 5.1 or higher compiled with PDF support turned on (available free at http://www.cs.wisc.edu/~ghost). If successful, there will be a link to the PDF on the next Web page that appears.

If you want to delete all the uploaded files and make no submission, click "Cancel submission" instead.

Step three: submitting your information. After your file has been converted to a PDF file, view the file that was generated from your submission by clicking on "ms.pdf" (a link that will be provided on the next Web page that appears). Only the manuscript file, not the cover letter or related manuscript files, will be viewable at this time. After you finish viewing the manuscript PDF file, indicate how you would like to proceed.

If you select "Approve and submit now," you assert that you have viewed the PDF file via the link provided and that the file accurately shows your manuscript as reviewers should see it. If you select "Fix and resubmit later," the files you have already uploaded will be saved (for 30 days) so that you can return later and upload new or corrected files to make a new PDF file. If you wish to return later to upload other files, please make note of the file upload ID number.

Click "Finish" to complete the final process. Click "Cancel" if you wish to abort the submission.

If your manuscript has been successfully submitted to the *AJHG* Web Peer Review system, a confirmation screen, which includes your assigned manuscript number, will appear. Please carefully note this number and use it in all future correspondence with the *AJHG* editorial office. An e-mail message confirming your submission will be sent to you.

If you do not receive either a manuscript number or confirmation e-mail message, your manuscript was not success-

fully submitted to the journal and thus cannot be sent on to peer review. Please try again or contact ajhg-help@mss.uchicago.edu for assistance.

Announcements

Announcements are posted to the electronic edition of the *Journal* as soon as they are accepted, and they are published in the earliest possible print issue. They may also be viewed at http://www.journals.uchicago.edu/AJHG/journal/announce.html. Announcements are published free of charge for members of The American Society of Human Genetics. They should be submitted via e-mail (ajhg@emory.edu). For publication in print, announcements must be received at least 7 weeks before the month of issue in which publication is desired.

Who else needs paperless chain of custody?

Starfruit IdentiTrack®

Laboratory Information Management System(LIMS)
Software, database, computer hardware, and barcode/label supply for
Parentage Testing Laboratories
DNA Profiling Testing Laboratories
Forensic DNA Biology Laboratories

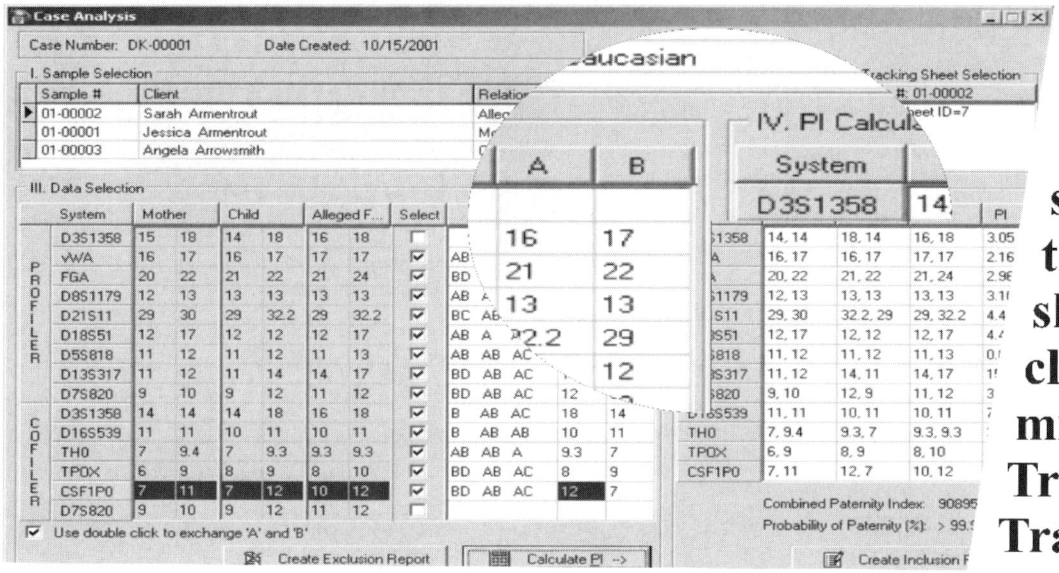

Track samples, Track derivative samples, Track sample consumption, Track sample ship-out, Track clients, Track submitting agencies, Track worksheets, Track worklists, Track plates, Track chain of custody, Create gel tracking data to export, Import allele data, Manage allele frequencies, Determination of sibship in any two persons, Assess paternity and likelihood ratio mathematically, Automate reporting inclusion or exclusion paternity test results and forensic matching, Population statistics, Reagent Management, Avoidance of expiration, Monitor inventory threshold, Inventory control, SOP, case archival, vendor management, electronic signature, Genetics labeling application, and more...

Your lab can be AABB/CAP/NFSTC/ASCLD compliant.

Data Unlimited International, Inc.
362A Christopher Ave.
Gaithersburg, MD 20879
Call (240) 631-7933
Fax (240) 631-7937
www.duii.com

Phone
USA 240-631-7933

Powered By
Starfruit® TECHNOLOGIES

Starfruit Resellers: Hong Kong www.bio-asia.com Japan: www.netwell.co.jp

Sf-1.9

2005 MEMBERSHIP APPLICATION • THE AMERICAN SOCIETY OF HUMAN GENETICS

9650 Rockville Pike • Bethesda, Maryland 20814-3998 • (301) 634-7300 • Fax: (301) 634-7079 • Toll free: (1-866) HUMGENE
E-mail: babbott@ashg.org • http://www.ashg.org/

Please keep information page for description of membership categories and discount subscriptions. Mail completed application, including profile form, and remittance to the above address. ***Type or print****. Use the URL above to apply online!*

Name ____ Degree(s) ____________________
Last First Middle

Department ____

Institution ____

Street address ____

City, state, zip, country ____

Telephone ( ) ____________________ Fax ( ) ____________________ E-mail Address ____________________
Area code Area code

Signature and membership start date: I, the undersigned, wish my membership in The American Society of Human Genetics to begin (check one): _________January 1, 2005 or_________January 1, 2006. Applications for 2006 will be accepted after September 1, 2005.
I will receive all applicable subscriptions beginning in January of the calendar year indicated above.

______________________________________ ____________________
Applicant's signature *Date*

We will acknowledge receipt of application and send it through the process established by the Board of Directors. Notification of the Board's action is usually sent in April or November. In the interim, you will be accorded all rights and privileges of a member in good standing, except that prior to Board approval you may not vote in ASHG elections.

DUES PAYMENT (Dues include 12 monthly issues of *The American Journal of Human Genetics* and are payable on a calendar year basis.)

1. Check one box and enter dues payment on line 1 .... $ ____________ 1
☐ $130 Regular ☐ $65 Trainee with Journal ☐ $70 Overseas Trainee
☐ $135 Overseas Affiliate ☐ $25 Trainee without Journal ☐ $190 Husband/Wife

2. Optional air mail postage for *AJHG* outside the United States .... $ ____________ 2
☐ $40 Canada, Mexico, Central America ☐ $70 all other areas
☐ Check here if you do not want to receive commercial mailings
☐ Check here if you do not wish to receive the printed Journal.

DISCOUNT SUBSCRIPTIONS

3. $650 North America, $850 elsewhere (print only) for ***American Journal of Medical Genetics*** .... $ ____________ 3
$530 North America, $690 elsewhere (print only) for ***AJMG*** *without* ***Neuropsychiatric Genetics***
4. $120 (print & online); $110 (online only) for ***BioEssays*** .... $ ____________ 4
5. $115 North America, $195 elsewhere (print & online); $104 (online only) for ***Birth Defects Research: Clinical and Molecular Teratology*** .... $ ____________ 5
6. $115 North America, $165 elsewhere (print & online); $104 (online only) for ***Birth Defects Research: Developmental and Reproductive Toxicology*** .... $ ____________ 6
7. $799 for ***Cancer Genetics and Cytogenetics*** .... $ ____________ 7
8. $159 Europe, $163 elsewhere for ***Clinical Dysmorphology*** .... $ ____________ 8
9. $258 US/elsewhere not otherwise specified (online only), $271 (print & online); $276 Canada (online only), $290 (print & online); $271 Europe (online only), $285 (print & online) for ***Clinical Genetics*** .... $ ____________ 9
10. $114 Europe, $117 elsewhere (print & online); $83 (online only) for ***Community Genetics*** .... $ ____________ 10
11. $125 US, $134 Canada, $186 elsewhere for ***Current Biology*** .... $ ____________ 11
12. $231 for ***Current Opinion in Cell Biology*** .... $ ____________ 12
13. $231 for ***Current Opinion in Genetics & Development*** .... $ ____________ 13
14. $623 Europe, $626 elsewhere (print & online); $557 (online only) for ***Cytogenetic and Genome Research*** .... $ ____________ 14
15. $165 for ***European Journal of Human Genetics*** (includes membership in ESHG) .... $ ____________ 15
$500 (print only); $550 (print & online) for ***European Journal of Human Genetics***
16. $330 North America, $390 elsewhere (print & online); $300 North America (online only) for ***Genes, Chromosomes, and Cancer*** .... $ ____________ 16
17. $105 US, $189 Canada, Mexico; $225 elsewhere for ***Genes & Development*** .... $ ____________ 17
18. $160 North America, $200 elsewhere (print & online); $145 (online only) for ***Genetic Epidemiology*** .... $ ____________ 18
19. $316 for ***Genetics in Medicine*** .... $ ____________ 19
20. $179 US, $258 elsewhere (print only); $213 US, $292 elsewhere (print & online); $179 (online only) for ***Genetic Testing*** .... $ ____________ 20
21. $98 US, $154 Canada, Mexico; $178 elsewhere for ***Genome Research*** .... $ ____________ 21
22. $124 for ***Genomics*** .... $ ____________ 22
23. $336 US, $395 elsewhere (print only); $402 US, $462 elsewhere (print & online); $336 (online only) for ***Human Gene Therapy*** .... $ ____________ 23
24. $495 for ***Human Genetics*** .... $ ____________ 24
25. $394 Europe, $397 elsewhere (print & online), $356 (online only) for ***Human Heredity*** .... $ ____________ 25
26. $369 US/elsewhere (print & online); $307 (online only); $394 Canada (print & online); $328 (online only) for ***Human Molecular Genetics*** (not available Europe) .... $ ____________ 26
27. $280 North America, $340 elsewhere (print & online); $255 North America (online only) for ***Human Mutation*** .... $ ____________ 27
28. $459 (print only) for ***Journal of Human Genetics*** .... $ ____________ 28
29. $289 (print & online), $130 (online only) for ***Journal of Medical Genetics*** .... $ ____________ 29
30. $113 for ***Molecular Genetics and Metabolism*** .... $ ____________ 30
31. $169 US, Canada, Mexico; $215 elsewhere for ***Nature Genetics*** (not available: Japan, Korea, & China) .... $ ____________ 31
32. $169 US, Canada, Mexico; $215 elsewhere for ***Nature Medicine*** (not available: Japan, Korea, & China) .... $ ____________ 32
33. $169 US, Canada, Mexico; $215 elsewhere for ***Nature Reviews Genetics*** (not available: Japan, Korea, & China) .... $ ____________ 33
34. $247 Europe, $254 elsewhere for ***Pharmacogenetics and Genomics*** .... $ ____________ 34
35. $157 for ***Trends in Genetics*** .... $ ____________ 35
36. Identify ***Annual Reviews*** by title, volume, year and price: Member price $72 per year US, $77 per year elsewhere

____________________ ________ ____________ $ ____________
Title Vol. Year Price

California and Indiana residents add state sales tax for ***Annual Reviews***: $ ____________
Canadian residents add 7% GST for ***Annual Reviews***: $ ____________

Enter total payment for ***Annual Reviews*** .... $ ____________ 36
37. Optional contribution to ASHG general fund: $25 ____ $50 ____ $75 ____ $100 ____ other ____ .... $ ____________ 37
38. **TOTAL REMITTANCE ENCLOSED** .... $ ____________ 38

PLEASE RETURN THIS NOTICE WITH YOUR REMITTANCE (U.S. currency only). See reverse for credit card information.

METHOD OF PAYMENT - 2005 ASHG MEMBER DUES

Payment may be made via money order; a check drawn on a U.S. bank, in U.S. currency only, and made payable to The American Society of Human Genetics; MasterCard, Visa, American Express (AMEX) or Discover credit card. Checks drawn on foreign banks cannot be accepted. Persons in countries with currency restrictions may apply to the Administrative Office for assistance.

For credit card remittance, please supply the following information:

Signature ______________________________

Cardholder name ______________________________
(please print)

Circle type of card: MasterCard VISA AMEX Discover
(no other cards accepted).

Credit card number ______________________________ ☐

VISA only: Supply final 3 digits on reverse of card

Expiration date ______________________________

Please note: ASHG is qualified as a 501(C) (3) organization. Dues and contributions are deductible as allowed by law. Dues payment includes $60 for a calendar year subscription to *The American Journal of Human Genetics*.

Member Profile Form

Name: ______________________________
Please type or print.

PRIMARY AFFILIATION *Check one:*

MEDICAL SCHOOL DEPTS.

A. ___ Genetics
B. ___ Pediatrics
C. ___ Pathology
D. ___ Psychiatry/Psychology
E. ___ Medicine
F. ___ Ob/Gyn
G. ___ Repro. Med.
H. ___ Neurology
I. ___ Family Medicine
J. ___ Internal Medicine

OTHER

K. ___ Hospitals and Clinics
L. ___ HMO
M. ___ Dental Schools
N. ___ Pub Hlth & Grad School
O. ___ College or University
P. ___ Nursing School
Q. ___ Veterinary School
R. ___ Priv Practice/Consultant
S. ___ Commercial Company
T. ___ Institutes/Foundations
U. ___ Federal Government
V. ___ State/Local Government
W. ___ Retired
X. ___ Other
Y. ___ Consultant

See box at right for codes:

Earned Degrees ☐☐☐☐ **Academic Rank** ☐ **Position** ☐☐

MAJOR TYPE OF WORK *Check one that accounts for more than 50% of your time:*
A. ___ Research B. ___ Teaching C. ___ Administration D. ___ Clinical E. ___ Counseling

SECONDARY TYPE OF WORK *Check one if it represents a significant portion of time and is different from your major type of work:*
A. ___ Research B. ___ Teaching C. ___ Administration D. ___ Clinical E. ___ Counseling

LABORATORY SETTING *If you are primarily in a laboratory setting, indicate focus:*
A. ___ private diagnostic/reference lab
B. ___ univ affiliated diagnostic/reference lab
C. ___ gov't affiliated research lab
D. ___ private research lab
E. ___ univ affiliated research lab

SPECIAL INTEREST AREAS *Do not check more than two:*
A. ___ cancer genetics
B. ___ cytogenetics
C. ___ DNA forensics
D. ___ differentiation & development
E. ___ dysmorphology
F. ___ ethics/social/legal/policy issues
G. ___ gene structure & function
H. ___ inborn errors/biochemical genetics
I. ___ late onset/adult genetic disorders
J. ___ linkage mapping & polymorphisms
K. ___ molecular genetics
L. ___ pediatric genetics
M. ___ physical mapping
N. ___ population genetics/epidemiology
O. ___ prenatal/perinatal genetics
P. ___ genomics
Q. ___ model systems
R. ___ informatics
S. ___ neurogenetics/behavorial genetics
T. ___ public health genetics

CURRENT GRANT SUPPORT *Check all that apply (US and Canadian members only):*
A. ___ NSF (NSERC in Canada)
B. ___ NIH (CIHR) training grant
C. ___ private industry
D. ___ NIH (CIHR in Canada)
E. ___ postdoc fellowship
F. ___ private foundation or charity
G. ___ state
H. ___ province
I. ___ institutional
J. ___ other national agencies
K. ___ HHMI

DESIGNATIONS(S) FOR YOUR RESEARCH
You may check more than one:
A. ___ Applied clinical research
B. ___ Applied lab research
C. ___ Applied mathematical research
D. ___ Basic clinical research
E. ___ Basic lab research
F. ___ Basic mathematical research
G. ___ Other

Degree Code
A. MD
B. PhD
C. MSW
D. DVM
E. SCD
F. DDS/DMD
G. EDD
H. MS
I. MA
J. MSN
K. JD
L. MPH
M. RN
N. BSN
O. BS/BA
P. Other

Academic Rank Code
A. Professor
B. Associate Professor
C. Assistant Professor
D. Instructor
E. Nonfaculty

Position Code
A. Dean
B. Department Chair
C. Division Chief
D. Institute Center Director
E. Laboratory Director
F. Training Program Director
G. Research Program Director
H. Program Coordinator/Administrator
I. Senior Research Associate
J. Research Associate
K. Research Assistant
L. Genetic Counselor
M. Postdoctoral Research Fellow
N. Postdoctoral Clinical Fellow
O. Resident
P. Graduate Student
Q. Private Practice
R. Corporate Executive
S. Consultant
T. Other
U. Principal Investigator/Professor

OPTIONAL:
Year of Birth: _____
Gender: F ☐ M ☐

Check Box(es):
A. ☐ American Indian, Eskimo and Aleut
B. ☐ Asian, Pacific Islander
C. ☐ Black
D. ☐ White
E. ☐ Other
F. ☐ Mixed
Hispanic (Yes ☐ No ☐)

2005 ASHG MEMBERSHIP AND SUBSCRIPTIONS INFORMATION
Please keep this page for your reference.

Line 1. MEMBERSHIP CATEGORIES

Regular Membership is open to any resident of the Americas (U.S., Canada, Mexico, Caribbean, Central and South America) who is interested in research in human genetics or in issues pertaining to human genetics.

Overseas Affiliate Status is open to individuals residing outside the Americas (U.S., Canada, Mexico, Caribbean, Central and South America).

Husband/Wife Membership is open to couples who are both Regular members, but who receive only one Journal subscription. Please fill out one membership application for each person.

Trainee Membership is open to postdoctoral fellows and bona fide students enrolled in degree-granting programs at institutions in the Americas (U.S., Canada, Mexico, Caribbean, Central and South America).

Overseas Trainee Membership is open to postdoctoral fellows and bona fide students enrolled in degree-granting programs at institutions outside the Americas.

Please note: ASHG is qualified as a 501(C) (3) organization. Dues and contributions are deductible as allowed by law. Dues payment includes $60 for a calendar year subscription to *The American Journal of Human Genetics.*

Line 2. OPTIONAL AIR MAIL POSTAGE OUTSIDE THE U.S.

For those who would like to receive *The American Journal of Human Genetics* via airmail, note additional postage on line 2.

DISCOUNT SUBSCRIPTIONS

To obtain these discounts, orders must be placed through the ASHG Administrative Office. It is understood that these orders are intended for personal use only. Standing orders are not available through ASHG. Typically, the publisher will begin mailing issues one or two months after your order is received in the Administrative Office. *Annual Reviews* will be mailed at the book rate in the month of issue.

Line 3. ***American Journal of Medical Genetics,*** 40 issues, list price $685, **member price $650 North America,** list price $855, **$850 elsewhere** (print only)
AJMG without Neuropsychiatric Genetics, 32 issues, list price $565, **member price $530 North America,** list price $707, **$690 elsewhere** (print only)

Line 4. ***BioEssays, Volume 27,*** 12 issues, list price $170, **member price $120** (print & online); **$110** (online only)

Line 5. ***Birth Defects Research: Clinical & Molecular Teratology,*** 16 issues, **member price $115 North America, $195 elsewhere** (print & online); **$104** (online only)

Line 6. ***Birth Defects Research: Developmental & Reproductive Toxicology,*** 10 issues, **member price $115 North America, $165 elsewhere** (print & online); **$104** (online only)

Line 7. ***Cancer Genetics and Cytogenetics,*** 16 issues, list price $3,169 US, **member price $799**

Line 8. ***Clinical Dysmorphology,*** 4 issues, **member price $159 Europe, $163 elsewhere**

Line 9. ***Clinical Genetics,*** 12 issues, list price $371 US/elsewhere not otherwise specified, **member price $258** (online only), **$271** (print & online); **$276 Canada** (online only), **$290** (print & online); **$271 Europe** (online only), **$285** (print & online)

Line 10. ***Community Genetics,*** 4 issues, list price $147 US, **member price $114 Europe, $117 elsewhere** (print & online), **$83** (online only)

Line 11. ***Current Biology,*** 24 issues, list price $165, **member price $125 US, $134 Canada,** list price $249, **$186 elsewhere**

Line 12. ***Current Opinion in Cell Biology,*** 6 issues, list price $271, **member price $231**

Line 13. ***Current Opinion in Genetics & Development,*** 6 issues, list price $271, **member price $231**

Line 14. ***Cytogenetic and Genome Research,*** 16 issues, list price $1,841, **member price $623 Europe, $626 elsewhere** (print & online); **$557** (online only)

Line 15. ***European Journal of Human Genetics,*** 12 issues, $165 (includes membership in ESHG); **member price $500** (print only); **$550** (print & online)

Line 16. ***Genes, Chromosomes, and Cancer,*** 12 issues, list price $365, **member price $330 North America, $390 elsewhere** (print & online); **$300 North America** (online only)

Line 17. ***Genes & Development,*** 24 issues, list price $140, **member price $105 US;** list price $260, **$189 Canada, Mexico; $225 elsewhere**

Line 18. ***Genetic Epidemiology,*** 8 issues, **member price $160 North America, $200 elsewhere** (print & online); **$145** (online only)

Line 19. ***Genetics in Medicine,*** 9 issues, list price $366, **member price $316**

Line 20. ***Genetic Testing,*** 4 issues, **member price $179 US, $258 elsewhere** (print only); **$213 US, $292 elsewhere** (print & online); **$179** (online only)

Line 21. ***Genome Research,*** 12 issues, list price $123, **member price $98 US;** list price $179, **$154 Canada, Mexico,** list price $203, **$178 elsewhere**

Line 22. ***Genomics,*** 12 issues, list price $458, **member price $124**

Line 23. ***Human Gene Therapy,*** 18 issues, **member price $336 US, $395 elsewhere** (print only); **$402 US, $462 elsewhere** (print & online); **$336** (online only)

Line 24. ***Human Genetics,*** 12 issues, list price $3,799 Europe, **member price $495**

Line 25. ***Human Heredity,*** 8 issues, list price $746 US, **member price $394 Europe, $397 elsewhere** (print & online); **$356** (online only)

Line 26. ***Human Molecular Genetics,*** 26 issues, list price $391, **member price $369 US/elsewhere** (print & online); **$307 US/elsewhere** (online only); **$394 Canada** (print & online); **$328 Canada** (online only) **(not available Europe)**

Line 27. ***Human Mutation,*** 12 issues, **member price $280 North America, $340 elsewhere** (print & online); **$255 North America** (online only)

Line 28. ***Journal of Human Genetics,*** list price $544, **member price $459** (print only)

Line 29. ***Journal of Medical Genetics,*** 12 issues, list price $478, **member price $289** (print & online); **$130** (online only)

Line 30. ***Molecular Genetics and Metabolism,*** 12 issues, list price $430, **member price $113**

Line 31. ***Nature Genetics,*** 12 issues, list price $199 US, **member price $169 US, Canada, Mexico; $215 elsewhere (not available: Japan, Korea & China)**

Line 32. ***Nature Medicine,*** 12 issues, list price $199 US, **member price $169 US, Canada, Mexico; $215 elsewhere (not available: Japan, Korea & China)**

Line 33. ***Nature Reviews Genetics,*** 12 issues, list price $199 US, **member price $169 US, Canada, Mexico; $215 elsewhere (not available: Japan, Korea & China)**

Line 34. ***Pharmacogenetics and Genomics,*** 12 issues, **member price $247 Europe, $254 elsewhere**

Line 35. ***Trends in Genetics,*** 12 issues, list price $182, **member price $157**

Line 36. ***Annual Reviews,*** **member price $72* per year US, $77* per year elsewhere**

Annual Review of:	*Genetics*	*Microbiol*	*Cell & Dev Biol*	*Ecol & Sys*	*Immunology*	*Medicine*	*Public Hlth*	*Biochem*	*Genomics & HG*
2003 Volumes	Vol. 37	Vol. 57	Vol. 19	Vol. 34	Vol. 21	Vol. 54	Vol. 24	Vol. 72	Vol. 4
2004 Volumes	Vol. 38	Vol. 58	Vol. 20	Vol. 35	Vol. 22	Vol. 55	Vol. 25	Vol. 73	Vol. 5
2005 Volumes	Available late 2005, will be offered on 2006 dues notice				Vol. 23	Vol. 56	Vol. 26	Vol. 74	Vol. 6
Month of Publication	Dec.	Oct.	Nov.	Dec.	April	February	May	July	Sept.

***California and Indiana residents add applicable sales tax. Canadian residents add 7% GST on total.**

Line 37: OPTIONAL CONTRIBUTIONS Optional contributions to the general fund are welcome. Contributions received will support projects designed to attract more young people to the field of human genetics and are tax deductible to the extent permitted by law.

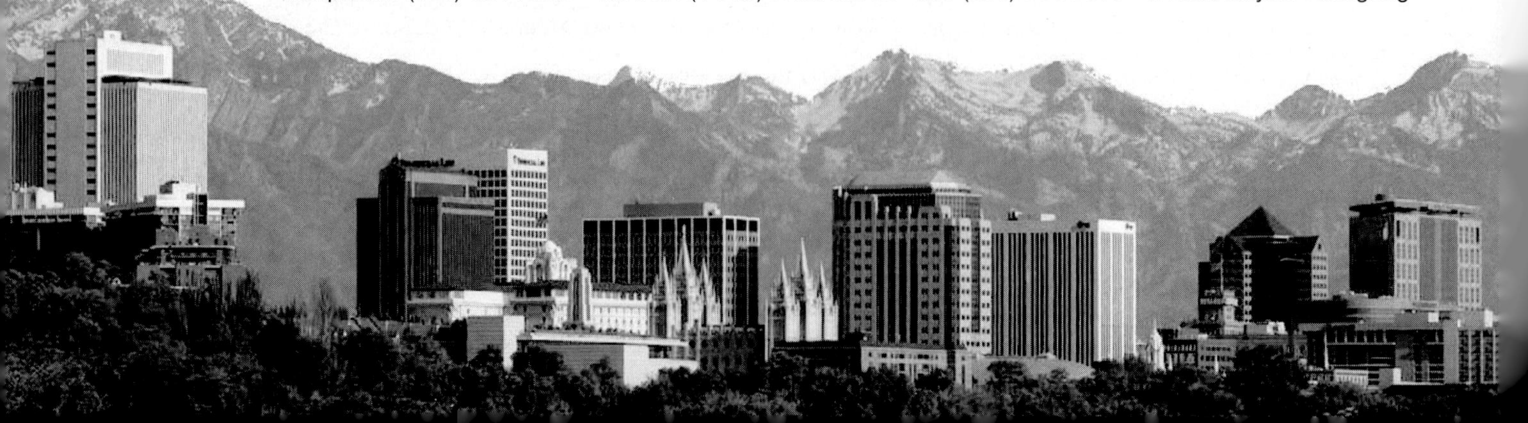

THE AMERICAN SOCIETY OF HUMAN GENETICS

was organized in 1948. Its purpose is to encourage and integrate research, scholarship and education in all areas of human genetics, to bring into close contact investigators in the many general fields of research that involve human genetics, and to encourage discourse on applications of human genetics to society at large.

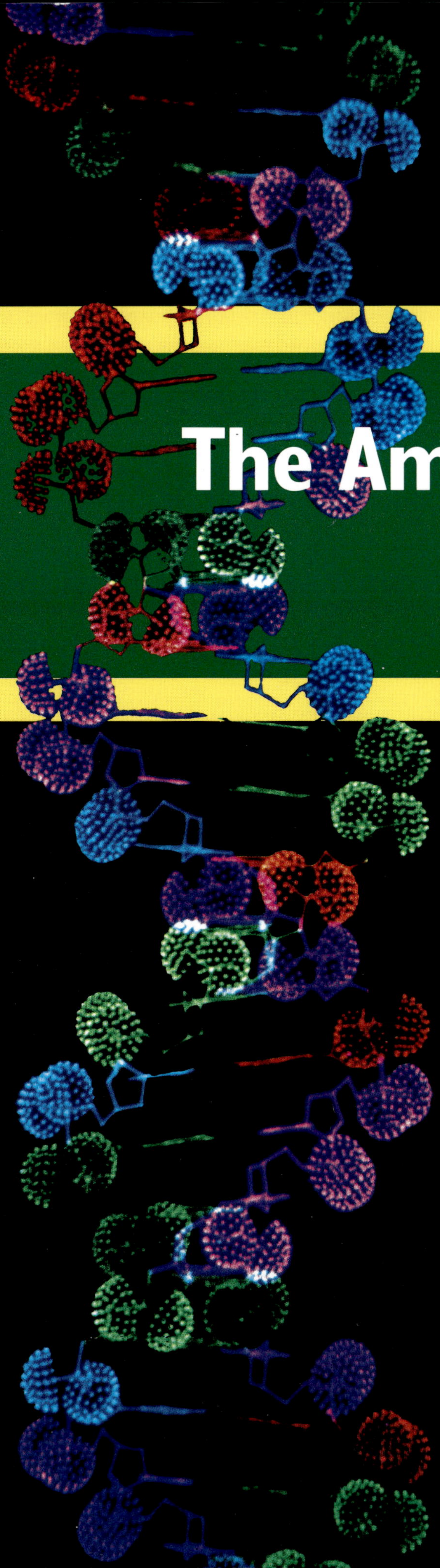

The American Journal of Human Genetics

VOLUME 76 NUMBER 6 JUNE 2005

THE AMERICAN SOCIETY OF HUMAN GENETICS

ASHG

Published for The American Society of Human Genetics
by The University of Chicago Press

DIRECT INQUIRIES AND SUBMISSIONS TO

The American Journal of Human Genetics
Department of Human Genetics
Emory University School of Medicine
615 Michael Street, Room 301
Atlanta, GA 30322-3050

Telephone: (404) 712-9980
Fax: (404) 712-9984
E-mail: ajhg@emory.edu
Web page: http://www.ajhg.org

PAST EDITORS

Subscription orders and correspondence should be addressed to the University of Chicago Press, P.O. Box 37005, Chicago, IL 60637. Checks should be made out to the University of Chicago Press. All orders must be in U.S. currency. Telephone: (8:00 A.M.–5:00 P.M. Central Standard Time, Monday–Friday) U.S. & Canada toll free, (877) 705-1878; Rest of World, (773) 753-3347. Fax: U.S. & Canada toll free, (877) 705-1879; Rest of World, (773) 753-0811. E-mail: subscriptions@press.uchicago.edu; Web site: http://www.journals.uchicago.edu. Remittance for nonmember subscription is payable to the publisher on a calendar-year basis. For domestic nonmember individuals and institutions, the single-copy rate is $88.00 and the calendar-year rate is $995.00; for foreign nonmember individuals and institutions, the single-copy rate is $88.00 (U.S. currency) and the calendar-year rate is $1050.00 (U.S. currency); the calendar-year rate for Canadian citizens, which includes GST, is $1088.65 (U.S. currency). All rates above include International Surface Airlift (ISAL) delivery to addresses outside the U.S. Subscription agent for Japan: Kinokuniya Company, Ltd. Individuals have the option to order directly from the University of Chicago Press.

Memberships.—A membership application and dues schedule appear at the back of each issue of the *Journal.*

The American Journal of Human Genetics (ISSN 0002-9297) is published monthly at 1427 East 60th Street, Chicago, IL 60637. Periodicals postage is paid at Chicago, IL, and at additional mailing offices by the American Society of Human Genetics. All rights reserved.

Postmaster: send address changes to *The American Journal of Human Genetics*, The University of Chicago Press, Journals Division, P.O. Box 37005, Chicago, IL 60637.

The American Journal of Human Genetics

Volume 76 Number 6 June 2005

i **This Month in the *Journal***
Kathryn Garber

Review Article

911 **Single-Gene Disorders: What Role Could Moonlighting Enzymes Play?**
Ganesh Sriram, Julian A. Martinez, Edward R. B. McCabe, James C. Liao, and Katrina M. Dipple

Articles

925 **A Genomewide Exploration Suggests a New Candidate Gene at Chromosome 11q23 as the Major Determinant of Plasma Homocysteine Levels: Results from the GAIT Project**
Juan Carlos Souto Francisco Blanco-Vaca, José Manuel Soria, Alfonso Buil, Laura Almasy, Jordi Ordoñez-Llanos, Jesús Mª Martín-Campos, Mark Lathrop, William Stone, John Blangero, and Jordi Fontcuberta

934 **Joint Modeling of Linkage and Association: Identifying SNPs Responsible for a Linkage Signal**
Mingyao Li, Michael Boehnke, and Gonçalo R. Abecasis

950 **Candidate-Gene Screening and Association Analysis at the Autism-Susceptibility Locus on Chromosome 16p: Evidence of Association at *GRIN2A* and *ABAT***
Gabrielle Barnby, Aaron Abbott, Nuala Sykes, Andrew Morris, Daniel E. Weeks, Richard Mott, Janine Lamb, Anthony J. Bailey, Anthony P. Monaco, and the International Molecular Genetics Study of Autism Consortium (IMGSAC)

967 **Rational Inferences about Departures from Hardy-Weinberg Equilibrium**
Jacqueline K. Wittke-Thompson, Anna Pluzhnikov, and Nancy J. Cox

987 **Alternative Splicing Suggests Extended Function of *PEX26* in Peroxisome Biogenesis**
Sabine Weller, Ivelisse Cajigas, James Morrell, Cassandra Obie, Gary Steel, Stephen J. Gould, and David Valle

1008 **Heterozygous Mutations of *OTX2* Cause Severe Ocular Malformations**
Nicola K. Ragge, Alison G. Brown, Charlotte M. Poloschek, Birgit Lorenz, R. Alex Henderson, Michael P. Clarke, Isabelle Russell-Eggitt, Alistair Fielder, Dianne Gerrelli, Juan Pedro Martinez-Barbera, Piers Ruddle, Jane Hurst, J. Richard O. Collin, Alison Salt, Simon T. Cooper, Pamela J. Thompson, Sanjay M. Sisodiya, Kathleen A. Williamson, David R. FitzPatrick, Veronica van Heyningen, and Isabel M. Hanson

1023 **Germline *BHD*-Mutation Spectrum and Phenotype Analysis of a Large Cohort of Families with Birt-Hogg-Dubé Syndrome**
Laura S. Schmidt, Michael L. Nickerson, Michelle B. Warren, Gladys M. Glenn, Jorge R. Toro, Maria J. Merino, Maria L. Turner, Peter L. Choyke, Nirmala Sharma, James Peterson, Patrick Morrison, Eamonn R. Maher, McClellan M. Walther Berton Zbar, and W. Marston Linehan

1034 **Fatal Congenital Heart Glycogenosis Caused by a Recurrent Activating R531Q Mutation in the γ2-Subunit of AMP-Activated Protein Kinase (*PRKAG2*), Not by Phosphorylase Kinase Deficiency**
Barbara Burwinkel, John W. Scott, Christoph Bührer, Frank K. H. van Landeghem, Gerald F. Cox, Callum J. Wilson, D. Grahame Hardie, and Manfred W. Kilimann

Reports

1050 **Replication of Autism Linkage: Fine-Mapping Peak at 17q21**
Rita M. Cantor, Naoko Kono, Jackie A. Duvall, Ana Alvarez-Retuerto, Jennifer L. Stone, Maricela Alarcón, Stanley F. Nelson, and Daniel H. Geschwind

1057 **A Novel Linkage to Generalized Vitiligo on 4q13-q21 Identified in a Genomewide Linkage Analysis of Chinese Families**
Jian-Jun Chen, Wei Huang, Jin-Ping Gui, Sen Yang, Fu-Sheng Zhou, Quan-Geng Xiong, Hong-Bo Wu, Yong Cui, Min Gao, Wei Li, Jin-Xian Li, Kai-Lin Yan, Wen-Tao Yuan, Shi-Jie Xu, Jian-Jun Liu, and Xue-Jun Zhang

1066 ***In Silico* Analysis of Disease-Association Mapping Strategies Using the Coalescent Process and Incorporating Ascertainment and Selection**
Ying Wang and Bruce Rannala

1074 **Identification of FOXP2 Truncation as a Novel Cause of Developmental Speech and Language Deficits**
Kay D. MacDermot, Elena Bonora, Nuala Sykes, Anne-Marie Coupe, Cecilia S. L. Lai, Sonja C. Vernes, Faraneh Vargha-Khadem, Fiona McKenzie, Robert L. Smith, Anthony P. Monaco, and Simon E. Fisher

1081 **Deficiency of the ADP-Forming Succinyl-CoA Synthase Activity Is Associated with Encephalomyopathy and Mitochondrial DNA Depletion**
Orly Elpeleg, Chaya Miller, Eli Hershkovitz, Maria Bitner-Glindzicz, Gili Bondi-Rubinstein, Shamima Rahman, Alistair Pagnamenta, Sharon Eshhar, and Ann Saada

Book Reviews

1087 **Human Evolutionary Genetics: Origins, Peoples, and Disease**
Written by M. A. Jobling, M. E. Hurles, and C. Tyler-Smith
Reviewed by Stephen L. Zegura

1088 **Facioscapulohumeral Muscular Dystrophy: Clinical Medicine and Molecular Cell Biology**
Edited by Meena Upadhyaya and David N. Cooper
Reviewed by Katherine D. Mathews

Erratum

1089 **Functional Analysis of Genetic Variation in Catechol-O-Methyltransferase (*COMT*): Effects on mRNA, Protein, and Enzyme Activity in Postmortem Human Brain**
Chen et al. (November 2004 [75:807-821])

Announcements

1090 **Employment Opportunities; Conferences; Symposium**

1094 **Contents of Volume 76**

Information for Contributors

This Month in the *Journal*

When we think of complex traits, we often think of the contribution of multiple genes and environmental factors to the phenotype. This month in the *Journal*, Sriram et al. discuss a factor that may contribute to the complexities of phenotypes associated with single-gene disorders: moonlighting activities. Moonlighting enzymes are metabolic enzymes with more than one unrelated function. One can imagine that, when researchers are blind to one or more functions of a moonlighting enzyme, there may be aspects of a phenotype that are not explained by the main function of the protein. The authors discuss known moonlighting activities as well as methods for identifying additional moonlighting activities. As new functions are identified for some proteins, it is likely that we will resolve some of the mysteries of complex phenotypes related to those proteins, leaving us better able to make genotype-phenotype correlations.

SNPs Responsible for a Linkage Signal, by Li et al. (p. 934)

Many research groups follow a similar procedure in their attempts to identify a genetic locus: start with a genome scan and follow that up with an association study in the regions that showed linkage with the trait. But it can be difficult to determine which associated markers are responsible for the linkage signal. To get around this problem, Li et al. developed a method that uses affected sib pairs and jointly models linkage and association. This allows them to determine whether a candidate SNP accounts for the linkage to a region. Further, they can estimate the amount of linkage disequilibrium between the candidate SNP and the actual disease alleles to get an idea of the degree to which a SNP accounts for the linkage signal. Simulations indicate that their method has good power to detect an association even when the sibling recurrence risk is low.

OTX2 *Mutations in Ocular Malformations,* by Ragge et al. (p. 1008)

Ragge et al. report the first *OTX2* mutations associated with ocular malformations. Their results stem from a candidate-gene approach that included *OTX2* because of reports that the murine version of the gene is a key regulator of photoreceptor-cell development and the finding that deletions of the region surrounding *OTX2* are sometimes observed in people with anophthalmia. Of the 333 individuals with ocular malformations who were screened for *OTX2* mutations, 8 had heterozygous sequence changes in the coding region, although the significance of two of these variants is not clear. Ocular phenotypes ranged from borderline microphthalmia to bilateral anophthalmia, and some individuals also had severe learning disabilities and seizures. Reduced penetrance, parental mosaicism, and phenotypic variability appear to be commonly associated with these mutations and may make genetic counseling of affected families less than straightforward. In contrast with the craniofacial malformations reported in heterozygous *Otx2* knockout mice, there was an absence of craniofacial abnormalities in the study individuals, although the authors point out that this could have been due to the sample ascertainment. In conjunction with expression studies, these mutations give greater insight into the role of *OTX2* in ocular development.

FOXP2 Truncation Impairs Speech and Language, by MacDermot et al. (p. 1074)

In 2001, Lai et al. (see references in MacDermot et al.) reported a family with a missense mutation in *FOXP2* and a proband with a translocation disrupting the same gene; both mutations were associated with a severe speech and language disorder. The report of Lai et al. generated a lot of interest in *FOXP2,* and subsequent studies were designed to look for mutations in individuals with such language-related phenotypes as autism, dyslexia, and speech-language impairment. Despite these efforts, the missense mutation in the original family is the only unequivocal *FOXP2* mutation that has been found. MacDermot et al. reasoned that their chances of finding additional *FOXP2* mutations would increase if they focused on individuals with a phenotype similar to the cases in the original report. The hallmark of this phenotype was verbal dyspraxia, which is a deficit in the coordination of the orofacial movements required for speech. They screened *FOXP2* in 49 probands with difficulties in speech articulation but no mental retardation, congenital abnormalities, or hearing problems, and they report a nonsense mutation that segregates with the phenotype and results in functional, if not actual, *FOXP2* haploinsufficiency. Two other coding changes in *FOXP2* were identified but were not present in affected siblings of the probands and are therefore of uncertain significance. A preliminary characterization of the phenotype in the family with the nonsense mutation suggests that the language defects are similar to those reported in the earlier *FOXP2*-associated family. Comparisons of these

0002-9297/2005/7606-0001$15.00

families may yield further insight into the role of FOXP2 in neurological and cognitive development.

SUCLA2 *Mutation in mtDNA Depletion,* *by Elpeleg et al.* (*p. 1081*)

While we're talking about moonlighting proteins (see the review article in this issue), it might be interesting to mention that Elpeleg et al. report a somewhat unexpected mutation associated with encephalomyopathy and mtDNA depletion. It was found in a family with severely retarded psychomotor development, muscle hypotonia, impaired hearing, and seizures. The activities of oxidative phosphorylation complexes containing mtDNA-encoded proteins were decreased in the affected individuals, which was consistent with the 50% reduction in the mtDNA-nuclear ratio in these kids. Homozygosity mapping localized the critical region to chromosome 13, and predictions for mitochondrial localization based on the ORFs in this region were used to prioritize the candidates therein. The affected individuals all had a rearrangement in *SUCLA2,* a gene encoding part of the ADP-forming succinyl-CoA synthetase (SCS-A), which plays a role in the tricarboxylic acid cycle. So what does this have to do with mtDNA levels? It turns out that SCS-A is tightly associated with a nucleoside diphosphate kinase (NDPK) that is critical for maintaining homeostasis of deoxyribonucleotides. Although the significance of this association is not clear, it appears that SCS-A disruption might alter NDPK function and lead to mtDNA depletion. Although a true moonlighting activity for SCS-A hasn't yet been demonstrated, these results point to a secondary and unexpected role for the protein.

KATHRYN GARBER
Deputy Editor

Am. J. Hum. Genet. 76:911–924, 2005

REVIEW ARTICLE
Single-Gene Disorders: What Role Could Moonlighting Enzymes Play?

Ganesh Sriram,[1,3] Julian A. Martinez,[2,4] Edward R. B. McCabe,[1,2,4] James C. Liao,[3] and Katrina M. Dipple[1,2,4]

[1]Department of Human Genetics and [2]Division of Medical Genetics, Department of Pediatrics, David Geffen School of Medicine, [3]Department of Chemical Engineering, Henry Samueli School of Engineering and Applied Science, and [4]Mattel Children's Hospital, University of California–Los Angeles, Los Angeles

Single-gene disorders with "simple" Mendelian inheritance do not always imply that there will be an easy prediction of the phenotype from the genotype, which has been shown for a number of metabolic disorders. We propose that moonlighting enzymes (i.e., metabolic enzymes with additional functional activities) could contribute to the complexity of such disorders. The lack of knowledge about the additional functional activities of proteins could result in a lack of correlation between genotype and phenotype. In this review, we highlight some notable and recent examples of moonlighting enzymes and their possible contributions to human disease. Because knowledge and cataloging of the moonlighting activities of proteins are essential for the study of cellular function and human physiology, we also review recently reported and recommended methods for the discovery of moonlighting activities.

Introduction

We now recognize that single-gene disorders, with deceptively simple Mendelian inheritance patterns, do not always show evidence of predictable relationships between genotypes and phenotypes (Scriver and Waters 1999; Dipple and McCabe 2000*a*, 2000*b*). This has been observed in the case of metabolic disorders such as glycerol kinase deficiency (GKD [MIM 307030]), phenylketonuria (MIM 261600), and Gaucher disease (MIM 230800), in which the mutations identified in the genomes of affected patients do not correlate clearly with their symptoms. This is a source of disappointment to clinical geneticists, since it presents a serious challenge to the concept that genotype can predict the clinical phenotype (Dipple and McCabe 2000*b*).

Previous reviews from our group have proposed three reasons for the absence of a clear genotype-phenotype relationship in such cases: the presence of indeterminate ranges in protein activities (Dipple and McCabe 2000*b*), the existence of modifier genes or loci that modulate the phenotype (Dipple and McCabe 2000*a*), and the role of systems dynamics (including flux through related metabolic pathways) in imparting a phenotype that is not easily deduced from the genotype (Dipple et al. 2001*a*, 2001*b*; Clipsham et al. 2002; Clipsham and McCabe 2003).

In this review, we point out an additional factor that could contribute to the complexity of metabolic disorders—the existence of moonlighting enzymes. "Moonlighting," a term coined by Jeffery (1999), refers to the phenomenon that many metabolic enzymes can exhibit unrelated functional activities within or outside the cell. The definition of moonlighting proteins excludes proteins that result from alternative mRNA splicing, posttranslational modifications, and gene fusions; proteins capable of utilizing multiple substrates (e.g., aldolase); and proteins catalyzing multiple steps in the same metabolic pathway (e.g., phosphofructokinase/fructose-2,6-bisphosphatase); nevertheless, there are a few dozen moonlighting proteins (Jeffery 2003*b*).

Examples of moonlighting activities include, but are not limited to, transcriptional regulation and apoptosis. If the gene of interest in a metabolic single-gene disorder encodes a metabolic enzyme whose moonlighting activities are as yet unknown, and if one or more of these moonlighting activities contribute to the phenotype of the disorder, then this could result in a phenotype that cannot be explained by the loss of the metabolic activity of the enzyme, thus causing an apparent uncorrelation between genotype and phenotype.

Here, we illustrate moonlighting proteins with specific examples and discuss their possible roles in disease. We also review methods of discovery of moonlighting activities and emphasize the need for reliable discovery methods.

Received February 24, 2005; accepted for publication April 5, 2005; electronically published April 22, 2005.

Address for correspondence and reprints: Dr. Katrina M. Dipple, David Geffen School of Medicine at UCLA, Departments of Human Genetics and Pediatrics, Gonda 5335B, 695 Charles E. Young Drive South, Los Angeles, CA 90095-7088. E-mail: kdipple@mednet.ucla.edu

0002-9297/2005/7606-0002$15.00

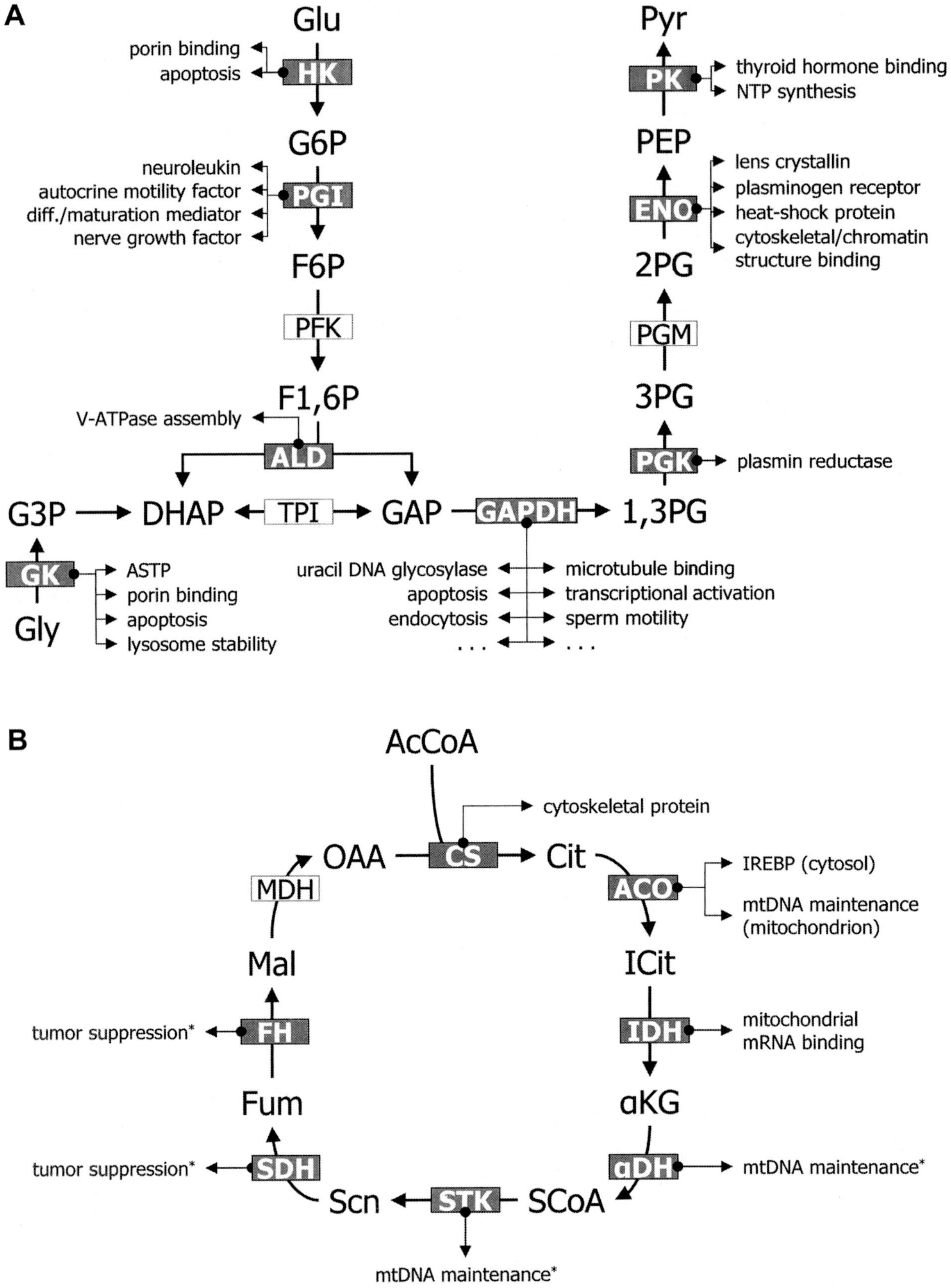

A
Glu
HK
porin binding
apoptosis
G6P
PGI
neuroleukin
autocrine motility factor
diff./maturation mediator
nerve growth factor
F6P
PFK
F1,6P
ALD
V-ATPase assembly
G3P
DHAP
TPI
GAP
GAPDH
1,3PG
GK
Gly
ASTP
porin binding
apoptosis
lysosome stability
uracil DNA glycosylase
apoptosis
endocytosis
...
microtubule binding
transcriptional activation
sperm motility
...
PGK
plasmin reductase
3PG
PGM
2PG
ENO
lens crystallin
plasminogen receptor
heat-shock protein
cytoskeletal/chromatin structure binding
PEP
PK
thyroid hormone binding
NTP synthesis
Pyr
B
AcCoA
cytoskeletal protein
OAA
CS
Cit
ACO
IREBP (cytosol)
mtDNA maintenance (mitochondrion)
ICit
IDH
mitochondrial mRNA binding
αKG
αDH
mtDNA maintenance*
SCoA
STK
mtDNA maintenance*
Scn
SDH
tumor suppression*
Fum
FH
tumor suppression*
Mal
MDH

Examples of Moonlighting Proteins

In this section, we highlight selected examples of metabolic enzymes that have demonstrated moonlighting activities. It should be noted that we present only a representative sample of the numerous metabolic enzymes that display additional functional activities. Previous reviews provide exhaustive lists (Ramasarma 1994; Jeffery 1999, 2003*a*, 2003*b*, 2004*b*), and we have chosen to draw attention only to moonlighting proteins that are not covered in those reviews (aldolase, enolase, glycerol kinase, and glycogen synthase kinase 3β), have additional moonlighting activities elucidated since those reviews were published (aconitase and glyceraldehyde-3-phosphate dehydrogenase), and/or are notable for the variety of moonlighting activities they exhibit (glyceraldehyde-3-phosphate dehydrogenase and phosphoglucose isomerase).

Figure 1 illustrates the high prevalence of moonlighting among familiar enzymes. A metabolic map of glycolysis (fig. 1*A*) reveals that 7 of the 10 glycolytic enzymes exhibit various moonlighting activities. In addition, other metabolic enzymes closely linked to glycolysis (e.g., glycerol kinase and fructose-1,6-bisphosphatase) also moonlight. Similarly, figure 1*B* shows that at least seven of the eight enzymes of the tricarboxylic acid (TCA) cycle have moonlighting or suspected-moonlighting activities.

The diversity of nonenzymatic additional functions exhibited by moonlighting enzymes is shown in figure 2. The moonlighting activities range from signal transduction events, such as transcriptional regulation and apoptosis; to growth and motility; to structural functions, such as those of lens crystallins.

Aconitase

Aconitase is an enzyme of the TCA cycle, and it catalyzes the reaction that converts isocitrate to α-ketoglutarate (fig. 1*B*). Cytosolic aconitase also plays a role in iron metabolism by functioning as an iron-responsive element-binding protein (IREBP), which regulates the mRNAs corresponding to ferritin, which is an iron-sequestration protein, and the transferrin receptor, a protein involved in iron uptake (Kennedy et al. 1992; Rouault et al. 1992). The aconitase and IREBP activities of this protein are mutually exclusive and are dictated by cytosolic iron levels. When iron levels in the cytosol are low, aconitase loses its enzymatic activity and functions as an IREBP (Kennedy et al. 1992). A recent study found an inverse correlation between the iron-responsive element-binding activity and the nonheme iron content in the livers of various mammals (Starzynski et al. 2004). The IREBP functions by binding to the iron-responsive element, which is located in the 5′ UTR of ferritin mRNA and in the 3′ UTR of transferrin receptor mRNA. This binding regulates the translation initiation of ferritin mRNA or the half-life of the transferrin receptor mRNA, thus exercising control of iron metabolism (Basilion et al. 1994; Jeffery 1999). Furthermore, it has been shown recently that, in yeast, mitochondrial aconitase is essential for mtDNA maintenance and that this activity is independent of catalytic activity or flux through aconitase (Chen et al. 2005).

Aldolase

Aldolase is a glycolytic enzyme that catalyzes the cleavage of fructose-1,6-bisphosphate into dihydroxyacetone phosphate and glyceraldehyde phosphate (fig. 1*A*). Lu et al. (2001, 2004) reported that aldolase binds to vacuolar H^+-ATPase (V-ATPase) in yeast, and adolase was found to be associated with intact V-ATPase in bovine kidney microsomes and in osteoclast-containing mouse marrow cultures. V-ATPases are essential for the acidification of intracellular compartments and for proton secretion from the plasma membrane in kidney epithelial cells and osteoclasts. Aldolase has been reported elsewhere to bind to actin (Arnold and Pette 1970).

Enolase

Enolase catalyzes the conversion of 2-phosphoglycerate to phosphoenolpyruvate in glycolysis (fig. 1*A*). It has

Figure 1 High prevalence of moonlighting enzymes. Most metabolic enzymes in familiar pathways—for example, glycolysis (and glycerol metabolism) (*A*) and the TCA cycle (*B*)—exhibit moonlighting activities. Moonlighting enzymes are shown in white font in gray boxes, and their known moonlighting activities are listed on the side. Suspected moonlighting activities are marked with an asterisk (*). Metabolite abbreviations are as follows: 1,3PG = 1,3-bisphosphoglycerate; 2PG = 2-phosphoglycerate; 3PG = 3-phosphoglycerate; AcCoA = acetyl coenzyme A; Cit = citrate; DHAP = dihydroxyacetone phosphate; F1,6P = fructose-1,6-phosphate; F6P = fructose-6-phosphate; Fum = fumarate; G3P = glycerol-3-phosphate; G6P = glucose-6-phosphate; GAP = glyceraldehyde-3-phosphate; Glu = glucose; Gly = glycerol; ICit = isocitrate; Mal = malate; OAA = oxaloacetate; PEP = phosphoenolpyruvate; Pyr = pyruvate; SCoA = succinyl coenzyme A; Scn = succinate; aKG = α-ketoglutarate. Enzyme abbreviations are as follows: ACO = aconitase; ALD = aldolase; CS = citrate synthase; ENO = enolase; FH = fumarate hydratase; HK = hexokinase; IDH = isocitrate dehydrogenase; MDH = malate dehydrogenase; PFK = phosphofructokinase; PGK = phosphoglycerate kinase; PGM = phosphoglycerate mutase; PK = pyruvate kinase; STK = succinate thiokinase; TPI = triose phosphate isomerase; aDH = α-ketoglutarate dehydrogenase. diff. = differentiation. Enzymes shown here but not discussed in the main text (and their corresponding references) are HK (Fiek et al. 1982; Linden et al. 1982; Ostlund et al. 1983), PGK (Lay et al. 2000, 2002), CS (Numata et al. 1991; Numata 1996), IDH (Elzinga et al. 1993; Chen et al. 2005), aDH (Chen et al. 2005), and STK (Chen et al. 2005).

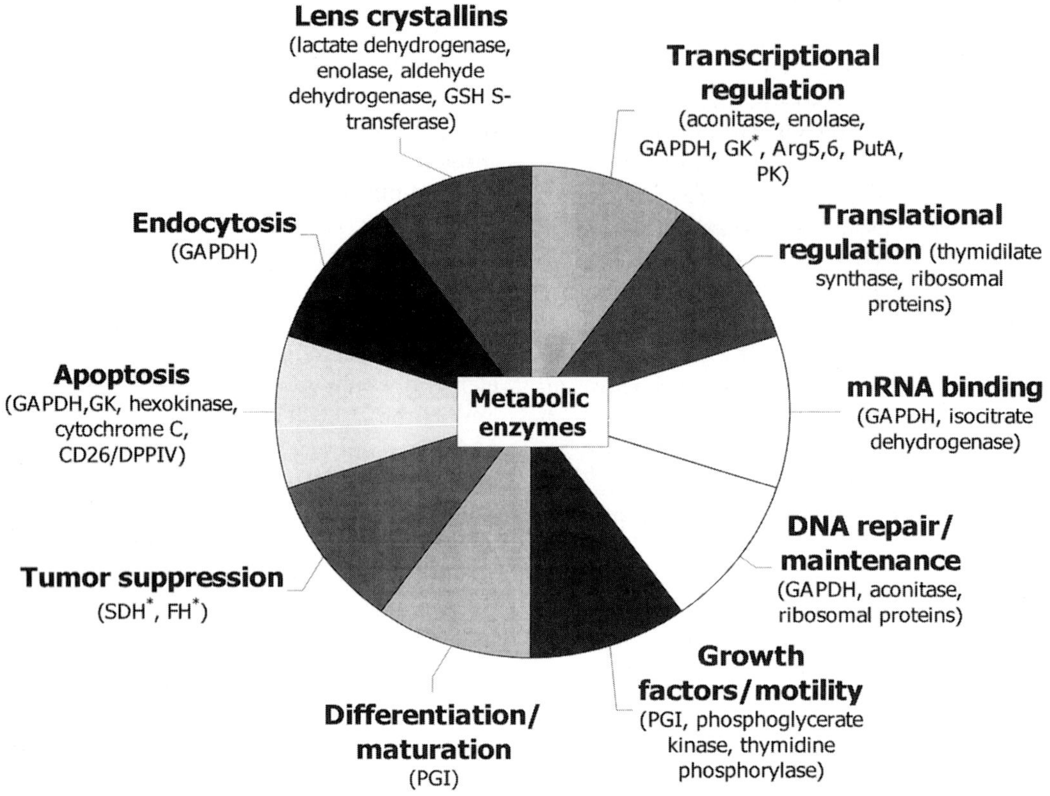

Figure 2 A representative sample of the wide variety of moonlighting activities of common metabolic enzymes. Suspected moonlighting activities are marked with an asterisk (*). FH = fumarate hydratase; PK = pyruvate kinase; GSH = glutathione. Moonlighting proteins shown here but not discussed in the main text (and their corresponding references) are CD26/dipeptidyl peptidase IV (CD26/DPPIV) (Boonacker and Van Noorden 2003) and cytochrome C, ribosomal proteins, thymidilate synthase, and thymidine phosphorylase (Jeffery 2003*b*).

been reported to function as a plasminogen receptor (Miles et al. 1991; Dudani et al. 1993; Nakajima et al. 1994) and a heat-shock protein and to bind to cytoskeletal and chromatin structures (Pancholi 2001). Enolase serves as a crystallin in the eye lens (Wistow et al. 1988). Recently, Wang et al. (2005) identified α-enolase as a nuclear DNA-binding protein in the zona fasciculata of the human adrenal cortex. The transfection of an α-enolase expression vector into human adenocortical cells enhanced the promoter activity of the type II 3β-hydroxysteroid dehydrogenase gene, which indicates that enolase may have a functional role in regulating the expression of this gene (Wang et al. 2005).

Glyceraldehyde-3-Phosphate Dehydrogenase

Glyceraldehyde-3-phosphate dehydrogenase (GAPDH) has been discovered to have several moonlighting activities (Sirover 1999)—it has at least 10 distinct, confirmed nonenzymatic activities apart from its enzymatic function of converting glyceraldehyde-3-phosphate to 1,3-diphosphoglycerate (fig. 1*A*). GAPDH is the same protein as uracil DNA glycosylase, which repairs DNA by excising uracil (Meyer-Siegler et al. 1991). It is also involved in endocytosis (Robbins et al. 1995), microtubule bundling (Kumagai and Sakai 1983), phosphate group transfer (Kawamoto and Caswell 1986; Duclos-Vallee et al. 1998; Engel et al. 1998), nuclear tRNA export (Singh and Green 1993), and vesicular transport (Tisdale 2001). GAPDH plays a structural role in the eye, where it acts as a lens crystallin (Jeffery 1999). It also binds to biomolecules, including RNA (Ryazanov 1985), RNA polymerase (Mitsuzawa et al. 2005), and diadenosine tetraphosphate ($A_{p4}A$) (Baxi and Vishwanatha 1995), one of whose functions is to decrease blood insulin levels (Rusing and Verspohl 2004). Recently, GAPDH has also been demonstrated to be important in sperm motility and, therefore, in male fertility (Miki et al. 2004).

Moreover, GAPDH plays a significant role in apoptosis. This is apparent from a mounting body of indirect and direct evidence (Berry and Boulton 2000; Tatton et al. 2000). For example, GAPDH binds to $A_{p4}A$, which is involved in apoptosis (Vartanian 2003; Wang et al. 2003). Low extracellular K^+ levels in cerebellar granule cell cultures that induced apoptosis also resulted in an increase in GAPDH mRNA and protein (Sunaga et al. 1995). Furthermore, treatment with GAPDH antisense oligonucleotides affected both GAPDH levels and apoptosis, establishing a direct link between the two (Sunaga et al. 1995; Ishitani et al. 1997). Although the lowering of extracellular K^+ levels can result in both apoptosis and necrosis (Berry and Boulton 2000), GAPDH antisense treatment affected apoptosis only and did not prevent necrosis (Ishitani et al. 1997).

The apoptotic activity of GAPDH involves the translocation of the protein into the nucleus (Sawa et al. 1997; Shashidharan et al. 1999) and is independent of both its glycolytic and uracil DNA glycosylase activities (Berry and Boulton 2000). Although the exact mechanism of nuclear translocation and subsequent initiation of apoptosis are not yet well understood (Chuang et al. 2005), some recent evidence has suggested a potential mode of action. This includes the binding of GAPDH to a nuclear localization signal–containing protein, Siah, to initiate nuclear translocation and an apparent change in the structure of GAPDH after its nuclear translocation (Chuang et al. 2005).

Also, GAPDH was recently shown to be involved in the formation of Lewy body–like inclusions in cultured cells and the concomitant apoptosis (Tsuchiya et al. 2005). Lewy bodies are intraneuronal proteinaceous cytoplasmic inclusions and are a pathological characteristic of Parkinson disease, which is linked to apoptosis of dopaminergic cells (Tsuchiya et al. 2005).

Glycerol Kinase

Glycerol kinase (GK) catalyzes the conversion of glycerol to glycerol-3-phosphate (fig. 1*A*) and is known to be an important enzyme in glycerol metabolism. Independently, Okamoto et al. (1993) cloned the gene responsible for the ATP-stimulated translocation protein (ASTP) from rat liver, and Huq et al. (1996) found that ASTP had 99% homology to the amino acid sequence of mouse GK. ASTP is an ATP-stimulated factor that enhances the nuclear binding of the activated glucocorticoid-receptor complex (Okamoto et al. 1984). Additionally, GK/ASTP has been shown to bind to histones (Okamoto et al. 1989), to interact with porin or the voltage-dependent anion channel on the outer surface of the outer mitochondrial membrane (McCabe 1983; Ostlund et al. 1983), and to be a lysosomal stabilization factor (Arai et al. 2002). Recently, our group has shown that GK may have a role in apoptosis (Martinez and McCabe 2004).

Glycogen Synthase Kinase 3β

Glycogen synthase kinase 3 (GSK3) was initially discovered as a kinase involved in the regulation of glucose metabolism, in which it phosphorylates glycogen synthase A to glycogen synthase B. In mammals, it occurs as two closely related isoforms, GSK3α and GSK3β. The GSK3β isoform is highly expressed in neural tissue. It has functions in various neuronal signal-transduction pathways and is emerging as a promising drug target for CNS therapies (Bhat et al. 2004). Most recently, GSK3β has been reported to play a critical role in the establishment and maintenance of neuronal polarity (Jiang et al. 2005; Yoshimura et al. 2005). In particular, it regulates collapsin-response mediator protein 2, which is crucial for axon outgrowth and for determining of the fate of the axon and dendrites and, therefore, in establishing and maintaining neuronal polarity (Yoshimura et al. 2005).

Lens Crystallins

Many crystallins present in the lens of the eye as refractive proteins have been identified as well-known metabolic enzymes, such as lactate dehydrogenase, arginosuccinate lyase, glutathione-S-transferase, enolase, and aldehyde dehydrogenase (Ramasarma 1994; Piatigorsky 1998*b*, 2003; Jeffery 1999). A recent study that analyzed the proteomes of human lens epithelial cells reported high abundances of the aforementioned enzymes among the proteins present, along with the glycolytic enzymes aldolase, phosphoglycerate kinase, and triose phosphate isomerase (Wang-Su et al. 2003). Lens crystallins are believed to have been recruited as structural proteins during the evolution of the eye (Piatigorsky 1998*a*, 1998*b*, 2003). Some crystallins may also serve additional functions. For instance, aldehyde dehydrogenase is postulated to function as a UV filter in the human lens, because of its binding to nicotinamide adenine dinucleotide (Bateman et al. 2003).

Phosphoglucose Isomerase

Phosphoglucose isomerase (PGI) catalyzes the second step in glycolysis, the conversion of glucose-6-phosphate to fructose-6-phosphate (fig. 1*A*). Mammalian PGI also functions as a neurotrophic factor, a neuroleukin (Chaput et al. 1988; Faik et al. 1988), an autocrine motility factor (Watanabe et al. 1996), and a nerve growth factor (Gurney et al. 1986), as well as a differentiation and maturation mediator (Xu et al. 1996). Interestingly, not all these activities are exhibited by PGI in other organisms. For example, bacterial or yeast PGI does not exhibit autocrine motility factor activity (Amraei and Nabi 2002).

Pyruvate Kinase

Pyruvate kinase mediates the final step of glycolysis—the conversion of phosphoenolpyruvate to pyruvate (fig. 1*A*). As a metabolic enzyme, it is a homotetramer in almost all organisms (Munoz and Ponce 2003). However, it can exist as a monomer, and its monomeric form in mammalian muscle is a thyroid hormone–binding protein that regulates the transcriptional responses of the thyroid-hormone receptor (Ashizawa et al. 1991, 1992). Additionally, it can synthesize nucleotide triphosphate

(NTP) under anaerobic conditions in bacteria (Saeki et al. 1974; Sundin et al. 1996).

Switching between Functions

One or more factors may be responsible for the function exhibited by a moonlighting protein. A partial list of such factors includes cellular sublocalization, expression in different cell types, presence inside or outside the cell, oligomeric state, substrate or ligand concentration, binding sites, and phosphorylation. Although a similar list was presented in an earlier publication by Jeffery (1999), it is revisited here with recently elucidated examples.

Cellular Sublocalization

GAPDH functions as an enzyme outside the nucleus but has an apoptotic function in the nucleus. Similarly, GK plays an enzymatic role outside the nucleus and an ASTP role within the nucleus. Aconitase functions as an enzyme in the mitochondrion and the cytosol; however, its compartmentation determines the nature of its moonlighting activity—it functions as an IREBP in the cytosol and has an mtDNA maintenance function in the mitochondrion.

Expression in Different Cell Types

Enolase functions as a glycolytic enzyme in most cell types but also as a structural crystallin in the eye lens. Furthermore, the DNA-binding function of enolase in the human adrenal cortex was observed only in the zona fasciculata and not in the zona reticularis (Wang et al. 2005).

Presence Inside or Outside the Cell

Ku70/Ku80 is a protein complex involved in DNA strand–break recognition and repair within the cell, but it participates in proteolytic processes outside the cell (Muller et al. 2005).

Oligomeric State

Pyruvate kinase exhibits metabolic activity as a tetramer and thyroid hormone–binding activity as a monomer.

Concentration of Ligand or Substrate

As mentioned above, iron levels determine whether aconitase functions as an enzyme or as an IREBP.

Binding Sites

Moonlighting proteins may employ different binding or catalytic sites for different functions. For example, ceruloplasmin, an oxidase that participates in copper metabolism, moonlights as a copper-independent glutathione peroxidase (Bielli and Calabrese 2002), and it employs distinct catalytic sites to bind to the substrates of either function. Similarly, mammalian $InsP_6$ kinase (an inositol phosphate kinase) binds to the guanine nucleotide exchange factor, and this binding does not require the catalytic site of the enzyme (Shears 2004).

Phosphorylation

It is likely that phosphorylation is sometimes responsible for switching between functions. There is recent evidence that phosphorylation of PGI at the residue Ser185 by protein kinase CK2 causes it to lose its enzymatic activity but does not affect its function as an autocrine motility factor (Yanagawa et al. 2005). However, there are instances in which phosphorylation is critical for both activities of a protein, as in the case of aconitase, in which loss of phosphorylation at Ser711 results in loss of both the aconitase and the IREBP activities (Fillebeen et al., in press).

Why Do Moonlighting Activities Exist?

There are two nonexclusive hypotheses about the existence of moonlighting activities: that these activities simply evolved and were not lost and that they offer definite advantages to the cell or organism (Jeffery 1999).

Evolution

Since many moonlighting proteins are familiar metabolic enzymes (fig. 1) and are present in a wide variety of organisms that have evolved over billions of years, it is likely that the additional activities of the proteins evolved, possibly to make use of unused sites on the protein surface. It is notable that active sites usually do not occupy a large fraction of the protein surface area, leaving considerable solvent-exposed surface that can be recruited for other functions (Jeffery 1999).

A recent study of lens crystallins (Piatigorsky 2003) provides interesting insights into the evolution of moonlighting activities. Ancestral enzymes may have been recruited as crystallins, following a gene duplication (with one gene encoding a protein with enzymatic activity and the other gene encoding a lens-specific crystallin) or a regulatory change (high expression of the ancestral protein in the lens), or both. Gene duplication is evidenced by the presence of two genes encoding α-crystallin/heat-shock protein (αA and αB), which are situated on separate chromosomes in mice and humans. The protein encoded by the αB-crystallin gene has remained a heat-shock protein, is expressed constitutively, and is inducible by stress. In contrast, αA-crystallin is expressed predominantly in the lens and is not stress inducible. However, certain other crystallins, such as ε-crystallin/lactate dehydrogenase and γ-crystallin/α-enolase, are encoded by single-copy genes, indicating that a transcriptional regulatory change conducive to high expression in the lens must have preceded the evolution of the refractory role for the protein. The fact that many crystallin genes are regulated by similar transcription factors (e.g., Pax-6, retinoic acid receptors, maf, Sox, AP-1, and cAMP response element B) reinforces the idea that the common feature of lens-specific expression may have played an important role in the recruitment of diverse enzymes as lens crystallins (Piatigorsky 2003).

Advantages to the Cell or Organism

Moonlighting activities can also be advantageous to the cell. One simple reason is that they reduce the number of proteins that the organism has to synthesize—thus, less energy is expended for DNA replication, and the genome is more compact (Jeffery 1999). The cell can benefit from the increased complexity with relatively fewer genes. Additionally, moonlighting can serve to coordinate related cellular activities or to switch between pathways (Jeffery 1999). For example, the interaction of aldolase with V-ATPase links two related pathways: the ATP-producing glycolytic pathway and the ATP-hydrolyzing proton pump (Lu et al. 2004; Sautin et al. 2005). The use of moonlighting activities to switch between proximate pathways is exemplified by mitochondrial aconitase (Chen et al. 2005) and rat liver mitochondrial Lon protease, an ATP-dependent protease that degrades certain mitochondrial proteins but that is also a mitochondrial chaperone (Jeffery 1999).

Moonlighting Proteins and Human Disease

As mentioned above, moonlighting proteins can add to the complexity of single-gene disorders. In a majority of cases, there is as yet no confirmed evidence that the nonmetabolic activity of a moonlighting enzyme encoded by a disease gene is responsible for the phenotype of a disorder. Nevertheless, there are strong indicators that this may be occurring, as discussed below.

GAPDH

We noted above that GAPDH plays a role in apoptosis. Excessive apoptosis is involved in many neurodegenerative diseases, such as Huntington disease (MIM 143100), Alzheimer disease (MIM 104300 and 104310), Parkinson disease (MIM 168601), and brain ischemia (Chuang et al. 2005), and recent findings support the role of GAPDH in these diseases. For example, nuclear-aggregated GAPDH was found in neurons of affected areas in postmortem brains of individuals who had Alzheimer disease (Tsuchiya et al. 2004). A proteomic analysis of neurofibrillary tangles in Alzheimer disease by mass spectroscopy identified GAPDH to be associated with neurofibrillary tangles (Wang et al., in press). A linkage analysis of patients with late-onset Alzheimer disease (MIM 104310) revealed an association with SNPs in the GAPDH gene, indicating that this gene is a risk factor for the disease (Li et al. 2004). Furthermore, potential drugs for treatment of Alzheimer disease, such as tetrahydroaminoacridine and ONO-1603, suppress GAPDH expression and its nuclear translocation in rat brain neurons undergoing apoptosis in cultures (Katsube et al. 1996, 1999).

These results suggest a role for GAPDH-induced apoptosis in Alzheimer disease. The role of GAPDH in Parkinson disease is indicated by its participation in the formation of Lewy body–like inclusions in cultured cells and subsequent apoptosis (Tsuchiya et al. 2005). For a full review that identifies the role of GAPDH in the aforementioned neurodegenerative diseases, see the article by Chuang et al. (2005).

Xanthine Oxidoreductase

Xanthine oxidoreductase (XOR) is the rate-limiting enzyme in purine catabolism. Vorbach et al. (2002) noted that XOR is expressed at very high levels in the lactating mammary epithelium and suggested that it may serve a structural role. They confirmed this hypothesis by studying XOR-deficient mice. XOR+/− females, although they appeared healthy, were unable to maintain lactation, and their pups died of starvation. Further investigations showed that the mammary epithelium collapsed in the knockout mice, and this resulted in premature involution of the mammary gland. XOR−/− mice, on the other hand, were runted and did not survive beyond 6 wk. Although this shows that XOR is necessary for survival, it does not indicate whether the protein's metabolic function (purine catabolism) or moonlighting function (structural role in mammary epithelium) is responsible for survival.

However, previous and recent reports provide strong indications that XOR plays a moonlighting structural role in the mammary gland. For example, XOR protein levels selectively increased in mammary tissue during pregnancy and lactation (McManaman et al. 1999, 2002), and XOR in human mammary epithelial cells had low specific activities despite high mRNA levels (Page et al. 1998; Harrison 2004), suggesting that XOR may be playing a nonenzymatic role.

Recent findings have also shown that XOR structurally interacts with milk-fat globule proteins, including butyrophilin and adipophilin (McManaman et al. 2004; Ogg et al. 2004). Ogg et al. (2004) have suggested that the butyrophilin-XOR interaction may contribute to the formation of a protein complex that stabilizes the milk droplet.

PGI

Deficiency of PGI is an autosomal recessive genetic disorder (MIM 172400), which manifests as hemolytic anemia but can also include neurological defects (Kugler et al. 1998). This is consistent with the enzyme's moonlighting role as a neuroleukin. A severe form of this disorder has been reported in which the mutations A59C (H20P) and T1016C (L339P) cause substitutions by prolines, with the consequent misfolding of the protein and the loss of both the enzymatic and neuroleukin activities. However, a less severe form of this disorder involved the mutations A1166G (H389R) and C1549G (L517V) located at the subunit surface, which affected the enzyme activity of PGI but not the neuroleukin activity. Not surprisingly, the latter mutations were not associated with neurological defects (Kugler et al. 1998). This example clearly illustrates that moonlighting activities of an enzyme can help to explain the apparent lack of genotype-phenotype correlation in a disease involving deficiency of the enzyme.

ERCC2

Mutations in the excision-repair, complementing defective, in Chinese hamster, 2 gene (*ERCC2* [MIM 126340], formerly known as the "xeroderma pigmentosum group D" gene), result in three disorders with markedly different clinical features (Lehmann 2001). Xeroderma pigmentosum (XP [MIM 278730]) is characterized by several skin abnormalities that range from excessive freckling to multiple skin cancers, with a high risk of skin cancer in affected individuals. Cockayne syndrome (MIM 216400) is characterized by severe cachectic dwarfism, mental retardation, microcephaly, and retinal and skeletal abnormalities. Trichothiodystrophy (TTD [MIM 601675]) is characterized by sulfur-deficient brittle hair, mental retardation, unusual facies, ichthyotic skin, and reduced stature, as well as sun sensitivity, but there are no reports of skin cancer. In addition, the XP-causing alleles of the gene were not observed in individuals with TTD, and vice versa (Petrini 2000).

The distinct phenotypes are now explained by the finding that *ERCC2* encodes a protein that has two distinct functions. It functions as a DNA helicase involved in the repair of DNA damaged by exposure to ultraviolet light, and it is also a subunit of TFIIH, a basal transcription factor (Lehmann 2001). XP is caused principally by defects in nucleotide-excision repair—that is, by the enzymatic (helicase) function of the gene product. In contrast, TTD and Cockayne syndrome are caused by defects in transcription (Lehmann 2003).

GK

GKD is a disorder that occurs because of mutations, deletions, or insertions in the GK gene (MIM 300474) on Xp21 (Dipple et al. 2001*b*). It can occur either as complex GKD, a contiguous-gene-deletion syndrome, or as isolated GKD. Isolated GKD can be symptomatic or asymptomatic (Sjarif et al. 2000; Dipple et al. 2001*b*). Thus far, there has been no satisfactory correlation between genotype and phenotype in patients with isolated GKD (Sargent et al. 2000; Dipple et al. 2001*b*). In fact, the exact same mutation has been observed in a symptomatic and an asymptomatic individual (Sargent et al. 2000), and this discrepancy has also been observed in two brothers with the identical mutation (Blomquist et al. 1996). The GK enzymatic activities in lymphoblastoid cell lines or fibroblasts were similar for the symptomatic and asymptomatic individuals. Also, mapping of the individuals' GK mutations to the *Escherichia coli* three-dimensional protein structure did not distinguish the symptomatic from the asymptomatic individuals (Dipple et al. 2001*b*).

As noted above, GK is a moonlighting enzyme, and it is likely that one of its additional functional activities, rather than its enzymatic activity, may help explain the GKD symptomatic phenotype. In particular, the role of GK in transcriptional regulation through nuclear translocation of the glucocorticoid receptor complex, or the role of GK in apoptosis, could provide clues to explain the complexity of GKD.

However, moonlighting might not by itself account for the perplexing fact that individuals or siblings with the same mutation exhibit different phenotypes. This could be a result of the action of modifier genes, as postulated elsewhere (Dipple and McCabe 2000*a*). Also, it is likely that the modifier genes interact with the moonlighting function of the protein, rather than the enzymatic function.

Succinate Dehydrogenase and Fumarate Hydratase

Succinate dehydrogenase (SDH [MIM 602690]) and fumarate hydratase (or fumarase [MIM 136850]) catalyze consecutive steps in the TCA cycle. Recently, it was discovered that a gene that predisposes to inherited multiple uterine leiomyomata (fibroids) (MIM 150800) and papillary renal cell cancer (MIM 650839) is the same as the gene encoding fumarate hydratase (Tomlinson et al. 2002). Along the same lines, germline SDH mutations were shown to be associated with paraganglioma (MIM 168000) and pheochromocytoma (MIM 171300) (Astuti et al. 2001). These findings suggest that these enzymes, directly or indirectly, play specific tumor-suppressing roles, which supports the potential existence of moonlighting activities for these metabolic enzymes, since the tumor suppression cannot be explained by the metabolic activity of the enzymes (Jeffery 2003*a*).

However, firm evidence is still lacking, and the investigation of the nature of the tumor-suppressing mechanism should shed more light on this interesting finding. A recent study showed that, at least in the case of SDH, metabolic activity may be indirectly responsible for tumor suppression; succinate, which accumulates as a result of SDH deficiency, inhibits hypoxia-inducible factor 1α (HIF-1α) prolyl hydroxylases, thereby stabilizing HIF-1α, which causes angiogenesis and tumor growth (Selak et al. 2005).

Aconitase

There is a myopathy (MIM 255125) that is associated with aconitase and SDH deficiency and in which the affected individual has an abnormal deposition of iron in the mitochondria (Haller et al. 1991; Hall et al. 1993). This affected individual experienced exertional muscle fatigue, dyspnea, and cardiac palpitations. Hall et al. (1993) have speculated that the dynamic Fe-S center of mitochondrial aconitase may respond to mitochondrial iron levels, as is seen with IREBP/aconitase. Although there is no evidence that the moonlighting function of aconitase is responsible for the myopathy, a recent article by Lipinski et al. (2005) shows that the IREBP function of this protein can have far-reaching effects, including DNA damage. Specifically, Lipinski et al. (2005) showed that increases in cellular iron (due to an increase in IR-EBP activity and a decrease in aconitase activity) may result in DNA damage induced by hydrogen peroxide through the Fenton reaction.

Elucidation of Moonlighting Activities

Serendipity

Serendipity has been a major contributor to the identification of moonlighting activities thus far. For example, the 10 moonlighting activities of GAPDH listed above were reported independently by 13 different research groups in five countries (see citations in the "Glyceraldehyde-3-Phosphate Dehydrogenase" section). Furthermore, 11 of those 13 research groups identified an unknown protein as GAPDH, so this enzyme was not even the initially intended subject of the study. A glimpse at articles that first reported moonlighting activities of many other proteins also reveals that many of the findings were unforeseen.

Nevertheless, the possible role of moonlighting proteins in metabolic disorders and the consequent urgency to identify them necessitates systematic methods of discovery. Below are some methods that have been reported and recommended.

Mass Spectrometry

Mass spectrometry (MS) is a powerful technique in proteomics. Jeffery (in press) has suggested the use of MS to identify potential moonlighting proteins. MS can provide two principal indicators of moonlighting activities. First, the presence of a protein in an unexpected location in the cell, in an unexpected cell type, or in an unexpected multiprotein complex could point to possible moonlighting activities. For example, large amounts of the glycolytic enzymes aldolase, phosphoglycerate kinase, and triose phosphate isomerase were detected in the proteomes of human lens epithelial cells by use of MS (Wang-Su et al. 2003), and this result indicates a possible role for these proteins in the lens. Second, if there are high protein expression levels that do not correlate with an enzyme's measured metabolic activity, that may indicate that the protein is performing a function distinct from its known metabolic activity (Jeffery, in press).

Since MS can be used in a high-throughput fashion, it holds promise for detection of possible moonlighting activities. However, it can provide only an indication, and further experimentation is essential to confirm whether the protein actually moonlights and to determine the nature of the moonlighting activity.

Proteome Arrays

A recent study reported that Arg5,6—a mitochondrial enzyme involved in arginine biosynthesis—binds to DNA and regulates transcription in yeast (Hall et al. 2004). That study employed a proteome array; a microarray containing 6,500 protein preparations of 5,800 yeast proteins was probed with genomic yeast double-stranded, fluorescently labeled DNA. Arg5,6 was identified among the positives found. Since transcriptional regulation by a moonlighting protein can play a potentially important role in disease, this technique of discovery is valuable, subject to the easy availability of proteome arrays for higher organisms.

Bioinformatic Approaches

Sequence-analysis algorithms, such as those used in BLAST, PROSITE, EMOTIF, PROTLOC, and many other programs, rely on sequence motifs to identify protein function (Jeffery 2004*b*). A recent study attempted to identify moonlighting activities of common moonlighting proteins by employing 11 different sequence-analysis algorithms (Gomez et al. 2003). It was observed that success rates were only moderate at best. For GAPDH, 7 of 11 algorithms identified the enzymatic function, and only 3 of 11 algorithms identified the uracil DNA glycosylase function. Among the algorithm-based programs, PSI-BLAST performed reasonably well in identifying moonlighting activities.

Network component analysis (NCA) is another bioinformatic approach that identifies possible new functions by recognizing novel connectivities between genes and transcription factors (Liao et al. 2003; Kao et al. 2004). NCA has been used with gene-expression microarray data from *E. coli* and yeast to uncover hidden regulatory signals and possible new network relationships when only partial knowledge of the underlying network topology exists. In *E. coli*, ~70% of randomly selected transcription-factor networks could be identified by NCA (Liao et al. 2003). NCA provides a powerful approach to mining microarray data and to gaining insight into new network connectivities and, therefore, novel putative functions.

Insights from the Structure-Function Relationships of Moonlighting Proteins

Many recent studies have focused on the elucidation of the structure-function relationships of moonlighting proteins. For example, a recent study of aconitase/IREBP (Fillebeen et al., in press) reported that, in HEK293 cells, phosphorylation of this protein at the residue Ser711 had devastating effects on both the enzymatic and IREBP activities, which indicates that Ser711 is a critical residue for the control of the activities of this protein. However, the exact mechanism by which phosphorylation controls the activities of this protein is yet to be elucidated.

The insights into multifunctionality obtained from three-dimensional crystal structures of moonlighting proteins (reviewed by Jeffery [2004*a*]) are of particular interest. For example, Lee et al. (2003) reported the crystal structure of PutA proline dehydrogenase, which moonlights as a transcriptional regulator of its own gene. Lee et al. (2003) noted that the structure contains a helical domain with three helices arranged in a helix-turn-helix pattern found in other DNA-binding domains, and they suggested that this could represent the DNA-binding domain responsible for transcriptional repression, although further experiments are needed to confirm this supposition (Jeffery 2004*a*).

Lee et al. (2004) investigated functional domains of the *Brevibacillus thermophilus* Lon protease (Bt-Lon), which is involved in the degradation of damaged and short-lived proteins, in ATPase and chaperone-like activities, and in DNA binding. This protein includes an N-terminal domain, a central sensor- and substrate-discrimination domain, and a C-terminal protease domain. Lee et al. (2004) prepared seven mutants of Bt-Lon, each of which lacked one or more domains. The truncation of the N-terminal domain led to the failure of oligomerization and the inactivation of proteolytic, ATPase, and chaperone-like activities, suggesting that oligomerization is essential for the catalytic and chaperone-like activities. Furthermore, gel-mobility shift assays indicated that the substrate-discrimination domain is involved in DNA binding.

Summary and Outlook

In this review, we highlighted some key and recently reported moonlighting enzymes that exhibit an astounding variety of additional functional activities. We also summarized mechanisms employed by moonlighting proteins to switch between functions, as well as hypotheses about the existence of moonlighting proteins.

The moonlighting activities of familiar metabolic enzymes include signal-transduction events such as transcriptional regulation and apoptosis, and it is likely that the moonlighting activities of these enzymes may contribute to the complex phenotype of a given disorder. It is very likely that the complex phenotypes observed in many single-gene disorders that cannot be explained solely by the loss of the enzymatic activity of the protein might be explained by a moonlighting activity of the protein.

The identification and cataloging of all activities of proteins in the proteome is therefore essential for understanding human genetic diseases. Thus, high-throughput methods of identification of moonlighting functions are required. Although most moonlighting activities reported to date were recognized by serendipity, the use of systematic methods is slowly gaining prominence, and we reviewed above some methodologies that hold promise in this area.

Acknowledgments

The research that led to the formulation of these models was supported in part by National Institute on Diabetes and Digestive and Kidney Diseases, National Institutes of Health (NIH), grant K08 DK60055 (to K.M.D.); National Institute of General Medical Science, NIH, grant R01 GM067929 (to K.M.D.); and National Institute of Child Health and Human Development, NIH, grant R01 HD22563 (to E.R.B.M.).

Electronic-Database Information

The URL for data presented herein is as follows:

Online Mendelian Inheritance in Man (OMIM), http://www.ncbi.nlm.nih.gov/Omim/

References

Amraei M, Nabi IR (2002) Species specificity of the cytokine function of phosphoglucose isomerase. FEBS Lett 525:151–155

Arai K, Yasuda N, Isohashi F, Okamoto K, Ohkuma S (2002) Inhibition of weak-base amine-induced lysis of lysosomes by cytosol. J Biochem (Tokyo) 132:529–534

Arnold H, Pette D (1970) Binding of aldolase and triosephosphate dehydrogenase to F-actin and modification of catalytic properties of aldolase. Eur J Biochem 15:360–366

Ashizawa K, Fukuda T, Cheng SY (1992) Transcriptional stimulation by thyroid hormone of a cytosolic thyroid hormone binding protein which is homologous to a subunit of pyruvate kinase M1. Biochemistry 31:2774–2778

Ashizawa K, McPhie P, Lin KH, Cheng SY (1991) An in vitro novel mechanism of regulating the activity of pyruvate kinase M2 by thyroid hormone and fructose 1,6-bisphosphate. Biochemistry 30:7105–7111

Astuti D, Latif F, Dallol A, Dahia PL, Douglas F, George E, Skoldberg F, Husebye ES, Eng C, Maher ER (2001) Gene mutations in the succinate dehydrogenase subunit SDHB cause susceptibility to familial pheochromocytoma and to familial paraganglioma. Am J Hum Genet 69:49–54

Basilion JP, Rouault TA, Massinople CM, Klausner RD, Burgess WH (1994) The iron-responsive element-binding protein: localization of the RNA-binding site to the aconitase active-site cleft. Proc Natl Acad Sci USA 91:574–578

Bateman OA, Purkiss AG, van Montfort R, Slingsby C, Graham C, Wistow G (2003) Crystal structure of η-crystallin: adaptation of a class 1 aldehyde dehydrogenase for a new role in the eye lens. Biochemistry 42:4349–4356

Baxi MD, Vishwanatha JK (1995) Uracil DNA-glycosylase/glyceraldehyde-3-phosphate dehydrogenase is an $A_{p4}A$ binding protein. Biochemistry 34:9700–9707

Berry MD, Boulton AA (2000) Glyceraldehyde-3-phosphate dehydrogenase and apoptosis. J Neurosci Res 60:150–154

Bhat RV, Budd Haeberlein SL, Avila J (2004) Glycogen synthase kinase 3: a drug target for CNS therapies. J Neurochem 89:1313–1317

Bielli P, Calabrese L (2002) Structure to function relationships in ceruloplasmin: a 'moonlighting' protein. Cell Mol Life Sci 59:1413–1427

Blomquist HK, Dahl N, Gustafsson L, Hellerud C, Holme E, Holmgren G, Matsson L, von Zweigbergk M (1996) Glycerol kinase deficiency in two brothers with and without clinical manifestations. Clin Genet 50:375–379

Boonacker E, Van Noorden CJ (2003) The multifunctional or moonlighting protein CD26/DPPIV. Eur J Cell Biol 82:53–73

Chaput M, Claes V, Portetelle D, Cludts I, Cravador A, Burny A, Gras H, Tartar A (1988) The neurotrophic factor neuroleukin is 90% homologous with phosphohexose isomerase. Nature 332:454–455

Chen XJ, Wang X, Kaufman BA, Butow RA (2005) Aconitase couples metabolic regulation to mitochondrial DNA maintenance. Science 307:714–717

Chuang DM, Hough C, Senatorov VV (2005) Glyceraldehyde-3-phosphate dehydrogenase, apoptosis, and neurodegenerative diseases. Annu Rev Pharmacol Toxicol 45:269–290

Clipsham R, McCabe ER (2003) DAX1 and its network partners: exploring complexity in development. Mol Genet Metab 80:81–120

Clipsham R, Zhang YH, Huang BL, McCabe ER (2002) Genetic network identification by high density, multiplexed reversed transcriptional (HD-MRT) analysis in steroidogenic axis model cell lines. Mol Genet Metab 77:159–178

Dipple KM, McCabe ER (2000*a*) Modifier genes convert "simple" Mendelian disorders to complex traits. Mol Genet Metab 71:43–50

——— (2000*b*) Phenotypes of patients with "simple" Mendelian disorders are complex traits: thresholds, modifiers, and systems dynamics. Am J Hum Genet 66:1729–1735

Dipple KM, Phelan JK, McCabe ER (2001*a*) Consequences of complexity within biological networks: robustness and health, or vulnerability and disease. Mol Genet Metab 74: 45–50

Dipple KM, Zhang YH, Huang BL, McCabe LL, Dallongeville J, Inokuchi T, Kimura M, Marx HJ, Roederer GO, Shih V, Yamaguchi S, Yoshida I, McCabe ER (2001*b*) Glycerol kinase deficiency: evidence for complexity in a single gene disorder. Hum Genet 109:55–62

Duclos-Vallee JC, Capel F, Mabit H, Petit MA (1998) Phosphorylation of the hepatitis B virus core protein by glyceraldehyde-3-phosphate dehydrogenase protein kinase activity. J Gen Virol 79:1665–1670

Dudani AK, Cummings C, Hashemi S, Ganz PR (1993) Isolation of a novel 45 kDa plasminogen receptor from human endothelial cells. Thromb Res 69:185–196

Elzinga SD, Bednarz AL, van Oosterum K, Dekker PJ, Grivell LA (1993) Yeast mitochondrial NAD^+-dependent isocitrate dehydrogenase is an RNA-binding protein. Nucleic Acids Res 21:5328–5331

Engel M, Seifert M, Theisinger B, Seyfert U, Welter C (1998) Glyceraldehyde-3-phosphate dehydrogenase and Nm23-H1/nucleoside diphosphate kinase A: two old enzymes combine for the novel Nm23 protein phosphotransferase function. J Biol Chem 273:20058–20065

Faik P, Walker JI, Redmill AA, Morgan MJ (1988) Mouse glucose-6-phosphate isomerase and neuroleukin have identical 3′ sequences. Nature 332:455–457

Fiek C, Benz R, Roos N, Brdiczka D (1982) Evidence for identity between the hexokinase-binding protein and the mitochondrial porin in the outer membrane of rat liver mitochondria. Biochim Biophys Acta 688:429–440

Fillebeen C, Caltagirone A, Martelli A, Moulis JM, Pantopoulos K. IRP1 Ser-711 is a phosphorylation site, critical for regulation of RNA-binding and aconitase activities. Biochem J (in press)

Gomez A, Domedel N, Cedano J, Pinol J, Querol E (2003) Do current sequence analysis algorithms disclose multifunctional (moonlighting) proteins? Bioinformatics 19:895–896

Gurney ME, Heinrich SP, Lee MR, Yin HS (1986) Molecular cloning and expression of neuroleukin, a neurotrophic factor for spinal and sensory neurons. Science 234:566–574

Hall DA, Zhu H, Zhu X, Royce T, Gerstein M, Snyder M (2004) Regulation of gene expression by a metabolic enzyme. Science 306:482–484

Hall RE, Henriksson KG, Lewis SF, Haller RG, Kennaway NG (1993) Mitochondrial myopathy with succinate dehydrogenase and aconitase deficiency: abnormalities of several iron-sulfur proteins. J Clin Invest 92:2660–2666

Haller RG, Henriksson KG, Jorfeldt L, Hultman E, Wibom R, Sahlin K, Areskog NH, et al (1991) Deficiency of skeletal muscle succinate dehydrogenase and aconitase: pathophysiology of exercise in a novel human muscle oxidative defect. J Clin Invest 88:1197–1206

Harrison R (2004) Physiological roles of xanthine oxidoreductase. Drug Metab Rev 36:363–375

Huq AH, Lovell RS, Sampson MJ, Decker WK, Dinulos MB, Disteche CM, Craigen WJ (1996) Isolation, mapping, and functional expression of the mouse X chromosome glycerol kinase gene. Genomics 36:530–534

Ishitani R, Sunaga K, Tanaka M, Aishita H, Chuang DM (1997) Overexpression of glyceraldehyde-3-phosphate dehydrogenase is involved in low K^+-induced apoptosis but not necrosis of cultured cerebellar granule cells. Mol Pharmacol 51:542–550

Jeffery CJ (1999) Moonlighting proteins. Trends Biochem Sci 24:8–11

——— (2003*a*) Moonlighting proteins: old proteins learning new tricks. Trends Genet 19:415–417

——— (2003*b*) Multifunctional proteins: examples of gene sharing. Ann Med 35:28–35

——— (2004*a*) Molecular mechanisms for multitasking: recent crystal structures of moonlighting proteins. Curr Opin Struct Biol 14:663–668

——— (2004*b*) Moonlighting proteins: complications and implications for proteomics research. Drug Discov Today Targets 3:71–78

——— Mass spectrometry and the search for moonlighting proteins. Mass Spectrom Rev (in press)

Jiang H, Guo W, Liang X, Rao Y (2005) Both the establishment and the maintenance of neuronal polarity require active mechanisms: critical roles of GSK-3β and its upstream regulators. Cell 120:123–135

Kao KC, Yang YL, Boscolo R, Sabatti C, Roychowdhury V, Liao JC (2004) Transcriptome-based determination of multiple transcription regulator activities in *Escherichia coli* by using network component analysis. Proc Natl Acad Sci USA 101:641–646

Katsube N, Sunaga K, Aishita H, Chuang DM, Ishitani R (1999) ONO-1603, a potential antidementia drug, delays age-induced apoptosis and suppresses overexpression of glyceraldehyde-3-phosphate dehydrogenase in cultured central nervous system neurons. J Pharmacol Exp Ther 288:6–13

Katsube N, Sunaga K, Chuang D-M, Ishitani R (1996) ONO-1603, a potential antidementia drug, shows neuroprotective effects and increases m3-muscarinic receptor mRNA levels in differentiating rat cerebellar granule neurons. Neurosci Lett 214:151–154

Kawamoto RM, Caswell AH (1986) Autophosphorylation of glyceraldehydephosphate dehydrogenase and phosphorylation of protein from skeletal muscle microsomes. Biochemistry 25:657–661

Kennedy MC, Mende-Mueller L, Blondin GA, Beinert H (1992) Purification and characterization of cytosolic aconitase from beef liver and its relationship to the iron-responsive element binding protein. Proc Natl Acad Sci USA 89:11730–11734

Kugler W, Breme K, Laspe P, Muirhead H, Davies C, Winkler H, Schroter W, Lakomek M (1998) Molecular basis of neurological dysfunction coupled with haemolytic anaemia in human glucose-6-phosphate isomerase (GPI) deficiency. Hum Genet 103:450–454

Kumagai H, Sakai H (1983) A porcine brain protein (35 K protein) which bundles microtubules and its identification as glyceraldehyde 3-phosphate dehydrogenase. J Biochem 93:1259–1269

Lay AJ, Jiang XM, Daly E, Sun L, Hogg PJ (2002) Plasmin reduction by phosphoglycerate kinase is a thiol-independent process. J Biol Chem 277:9062–9068

Lay AJ, Jiang XM, Kisker O, Flynn E, Underwood A, Condron R, Hogg PJ (2000) Phosphoglycerate kinase acts in tumour angiogenesis as a disulphide reductase. Nature 408:869–873

Lee AY, Hsu CH, Wu SH (2004) Functional domains of *Brevibacillus thermoruber* Lon protease for oligomerization and DNA binding: role of N-terminal and sensor and substrate discrimination domains. J Biol Chem 279:34903–34912

Lee Y-H, Nadaraia S, Gu D, Becker DF, Tanner JJ (2003) Structure of the proline dehydrogenase domain of the multifunctional PutA flavoprotein. Nat Struct Biol 10:109–114

Lehmann AR (2001) The xeroderma pigmentosum group D (XPD) gene: one gene, two functions, three diseases. Genes Dev 15:15–23

——— (2003) DNA repair-deficient diseases, xeroderma pigmentosum, Cockayne syndrome and trichothiodystrophy. Biochimie 85:1101–1111

Li Y, Nowotny P, Holmans P, Smemo S, Kauwe JSK, Hinrichs AL, Tacey K, et al (2004) Association of late-onset Alzheimer's disease with genetic variation in multiple members of the *GAPD* gene family. Proc Natl Acad Sci USA 101:15688–15693

Liao JC, Boscolo R, Yang YL, Tran LM, Sabatti C, Roychowdhury VP (2003) Network component analysis: reconstruction of regulatory signals in biological systems. Proc Natl Acad Sci USA 100:15522–15527

Linden M, Gellerfors P, Nelson BD (1982) Pore protein and the hexokinase-binding protein from the outer membrane of rat liver mitochondria are identical. FEBS Lett 141:189–192

Lipinski P, Starzynski RR, Drapier J-C, Bouton C, Bartlomiejczyk T, Sochanowicz B, Smuda E, Gajkowska A, Kruszewski M (2005) Induction of iron regulatory protein 1 RNA-binding activity by nitric oxide is associated with a concomitant increase in the labile iron pool: implications for DNA damage. Biochem Biophys Res Commun 327:349–355

Lu M, Holliday LS, Zhang L, Dunn WA Jr, Gluck SL (2001) Interaction between aldolase and vacuolar H^+-ATPase: evidence for direct coupling of glycolysis to the ATP-hydrolyzing proton pump. J Biol Chem 276:30407–30413

Lu M, Sautin YY, Holliday LS, Gluck SL (2004) The glycolytic enzyme aldolase mediates assembly, expression, and activity of vacuolar H^+-ATPase. J Biol Chem 279:8732–8739

Martinez JA, McCabe ERB (2004) Apoptosis in glycerol kinase deficiency: investigations in *Drosophila melangaster.* Paper presented at the American Society of Human Genetics Annual Meeting, Toronto, October 26–30

McCabe ER (1983) Human glycerol kinase deficiency: an inborn error of compartmental metabolism. Biochem Med 30: 215–230

McManaman JL, Neville MC, Wright RM (1999) Mouse mammary gland xanthine oxidoreductase: purification, characterization, and regulation. Arch Biochem Biophys 371:308–316

McManaman JL, Palmer CA, Anderson S, Schwertfeger K, Neville MC (2004) Regulation of milk lipid formation and secretion in the mouse mammary gland. Adv Exp Med Biol 554:263–279

McManaman JL, Palmer CA, Wright RM, Neville MC (2002) Functional regulation of xanthine oxidoreductase expression and localization in the mouse mammary gland: evidence of a role in lipid secretion. J Physiol 545:567–579

Meyer-Siegler K, Mauro DJ, Seal G, Wurzer J, deRiel JK, Sirover MA (1991) A human nuclear uracil DNA glycosylase is the 37-kDa subunit of glyceraldehyde-3-phosphate dehydrogenase. Proc Natl Acad Sci USA 88:8460–8464

Miki K, Qu W, Goulding EH, Willis WD, Bunch DO, Strader LF, Perreault SD, Eddy EM, O'Brien DA (2004) Glyceraldehyde 3-phosphate dehydrogenase-S, a sperm-specific glycolytic enzyme, is required for sperm motility and male fertility. Proc Natl Acad Sci USA 101:16501–16506

Miles LA, Dahlberg CM, Plescia J, Felez J, Kato K, Plow EF (1991) Role of cell-surface lysines in plasminogen binding to cells: identification of α-enolase as a candidate plasminogen receptor. Biochemistry 30:1682–1691

Mitsuzawa H, Kimura M, Kanda E, Ishihama A (2005) Glyceraldehyde-3-phosphate dehydrogenase and actin associate with RNA polymerase II and interact with its Rpb7 subunit. FEBS Lett 579:48–52

Muller C, Paupert J, Monferran S, Salles B (2005) The double life of the Ku protein: facing the DNA breaks and the extracellular environment. Cell Cycle 4:438–441

Munoz ME, Ponce E (2003) Pyruvate kinase: current status of regulatory and functional properties. Comp Biochem Physiol B Biochem Mol Biol 135:197–218

Nakajima K, Hamanoue M, Takemoto N, Hattori T, Kato K, Kohsaka S (1994) Plasminogen binds specifically to α-enolase on rat neuronal plasma membrane. J Neurochem 63: 2048–2057

Numata O (1996) Multifunctional proteins in Tetrahymena: 14-nm filament protein/citrate synthase and translation elongation factor-1α. Int Rev Cytol 164:1–35

Numata O, Takemasa T, Takagi I, Hirono M, Hirano H, Chiba J, Watanabe Y (1991) Tetrahymena 14-nm filament-forming protein has citrate synthase activity. Biochem Biophys Res Commun 174:1028–1034

Ogg SL, Weldon AK, Dobbie L, Smith AJH, Mather IH (2004) Expression of butyrophilin (Btn1a1) in lactating mammary gland is essential for the regulated secretion of milk-lipid droplets. Proc Natl Acad Sci USA 101:10084–10089

Okamoto K, Hirano H, Isohashi F (1993) Molecular cloning of rat liver glucocorticoid-receptor translocation promoter. Biochem Biophys Res Commun 193:848–854

Okamoto K, Isohashi F, Horiuchi M, Sakamoto Y (1984) An ATP-stimulated factor that enhances the nuclear binding of "activated" receptor-glucocorticoid complex. Biochem Biophys Res Commun 121:940–945

Okamoto K, Isohashi F, Ueda K, Sakamoto Y (1989) Properties of an adenosine triphosphate-stimulated factor that enhances the nuclear binding of activated glucocorticoid-receptor complex: binding to histone-agarose. Endocrinology 124:675–680

Ostlund AK, Gohring U, Krause J, Brdiczka D (1983) The binding of glycerol kinase to the outer membrane of rat liver mitochondria: its importance in metabolic regulation. Biochem Med 30:231–245

Page S, Powell D, Benboubetra M, Stevens CR, Blake DR, Selase F, Wolstenholme AJ, Harrison R (1998) Xanthine oxidoreductase in human mammary epithelial cells: activation in response to inflammatory cytokines. Biochim Biophys Acta 1381:191–202

Pancholi V (2001) Multifunctional α-enolase: its role in diseases. Cell Mol Life Sci 58:902–920

Petrini JH (2000) When more is better. Nat Genet 26:257–258

Piatigorsky J (1998*a*) Gene sharing in lens and cornea: facts and implications. Prog Retin Eye Res 17:145–174

——— (1998*b*) Multifunctional lens crystallins and corneal enzymes: more than meets the eye. Ann N Y Acad Sci 842: 7–15

——— (2003) Crystallin genes: specialization by changes in gene regulation may precede gene duplication. J Struct Funct Genomics 3:131–137

Ramasarma T (1994) One protein—many functions. Curr Sci 67:24–29

Robbins AR, Ward RD, Oliver C (1995) A mutation in glyceraldehyde 3-phosphate dehydrogenase alters endocytosis in CHO cells. J Cell Biol 130:1093–1104

Rouault TA, Haile DJ, Downey WE, Philpott CC, Tang C, Samaniego F, Chin J, Paul I, Orloff D, Harford JB, Klausner RD (1992) An iron-sulfur cluster plays a novel regulatory role in the iron-responsive element binding protein. Biometals 5:131–140

Rusing D, Verspohl EJ (2004) Influence of diadenosine tetraphosphate ($A_{p4}A$) on lipid metabolism. Cell Biochem Funct 22:333–338

Ryazanov AG (1985) Glyceraldehyde-3-phosphate dehydrogenase is one of the three major RNA-binding proteins of rabbit reticulocytes. FEBS Lett 192:131–134

Saeki T, Hori M, Umezawa H (1974) Pyruvate kinase of Escherichia coli: its role in supplying nucleoside triphosphates in cells under anaerobic conditions. J Biochem 76:631–637

Sargent CA, Kidd A, Moore S, Dean J, Besley GT, Affara NA (2000) Five cases of isolated glycerol kinase deficiency, including two families: failure to find genotype:phenotype correlation. J Med Genet 37:434–441

Sautin YY, Lu M, Gaugler A, Zhang L, Gluck SL (2005) Phosphatidylinositol 3-kinase-mediated effects of glucose on vacuolar H^+-ATPase assembly, translocation, and acidification of intracellular compartments in renal epithelial cells. Mol Cell Biol 25:575–589

Sawa A, Khan AA, Hester LD, Snyder SH (1997) Glyceraldehyde-3-phosphate dehydrogenase: nuclear translocation participates in neuronal and nonneuronal cell death. Proc Natl Acad Sci USA 94:11669–11674

Scriver CR, Waters PJ (1999) Monogenic traits are not simple: lessons from phenylketonuria. Trends Genet 15:267–272

Selak MA, Armour SM, Mackenzie ED, Boulahbel H, Watson DG, Mansfield KD, Pan Y, Simon MC, Thompson CB, Gottlieb E (2005) Succinate links TCA cycle dysfunction to oncogenesis by inhibiting HIF-α prolyl hydroxylase. Cancer Cell 7:77–85

Shashidharan P, Chalmers-Redman RM, Carlile GW, Rodic V, Gurvich N, Yuen T, Tatton WG, Sealfon SC (1999) Nuclear translocation of GAPDH-GFP fusion protein during apoptosis. Neuroreport 10:1149–1153

Shears SB (2004) How versatile are inositol phosphate kinases? Biochem J 377:265–280

Singh R, Green MR (1993) Sequence-specific binding of transfer RNA by glyceraldehyde-3-phosphate dehydrogenase. Science 259:365–368

Sirover MA (1999) New insights into an old protein: the functional diversity of mammalian glyceraldehyde-3-phosphate dehydrogenase. Biochim Biophys Acta 1432:159–184

Sjarif DR, Ploos van Amstel JK, Duran M, Beemer FA, Poll-The BT (2000) Isolated and contiguous glycerol kinase gene disorders: a review. J Inherit Metab Dis 23:529–547

Starzynski RR, Gralak MA, Smuda E, Lipinski P (2004) A characterization of the activities of iron regulatory protein 1 in various farm animal species. Cell Mol Biol Lett 9:651–664

Sunaga K, Takahashi H, Chuang DM, Ishitani R (1995) Glyceraldehyde-3-phosphate dehydrogenase is over-expressed during apoptotic death of neuronal cultures and is recognized by a monoclonal antibody against amyloid plaques from Alzheimer's brain. Neurosci Lett 200:133–136

Sundin GW, Shankar S, Chugani SA, Chopade BA, Kavanaugh-Black A, Chakrabarty AM (1996) Nucleoside diphosphate kinase from *Pseudomonas aeruginosa*: characterization of the gene and its role in cellular growth and exopolysaccharide alginate synthesis. Mol Microbiol 20:965–979

Tatton WG, Chalmers-Redman RM, Elstner M, Leesch W, Jagodzinski FB, Stupak DP, Sugrue MM, Tatton NA (2000) Glyceraldehyde-3-phosphate dehydrogenase in neurodegeneration and apoptosis signaling. J Neural Transm Suppl:77–100

Tisdale EJ (2001) Glyceraldehyde-3-phosphate dehydrogenase is required for vesicular transport in the early secretory pathway. J Biol Chem 276:2480–2486

Tomlinson IP, Alam NA, Rowan AJ, Barclay E, Jaeger EE, Kelsell D, Leigh I, et al (2002) Germline mutations in FH predispose to dominantly inherited uterine fibroids, skin leiomyomata and papillary renal cell cancer. Nat Genet 30:406–410

Tsuchiya K, Tajima H, Kuwae T, Takeshima T, Nakano T, Tanaka M, Sunaga K, Fukuhara Y, Nakashima K, Ohama E, Mochizuki H, Mizuno Y, Katsube N, Ishitani R (2005) Pro-apoptotic protein glyceraldehyde-3-phosphate dehydrogenase promotes the formation of Lewy body-like inclusions. Eur J Neurosci 21:317–326

Tsuchiya K, Tajima H, Yamada M, Takahashi H, Kuwae T, Sunaga K, Katsube N, Ishitani R (2004) Disclosure of a proapoptotic glyceraldehyde-3-phosphate dehydrogenase promoter: anti-dementia drugs depress its activation in apoptosis. Life Sciences 74:3245–3258

Vartanian AA (2003) Gelsolin and plasminogen activator inhibitor-1 are $A_{p3}A$-binding proteins. Ital J Biochem 52:9–16

Vorbach C, Scriven A, Capecchi MR (2002) The housekeeping gene xanthine oxidoreductase is necessary for milk fat droplet enveloping and secretion: gene sharing in the lactating mammary gland. Genes Dev 16:3223–3235

Wang Q, Woltjer RL, Cimino PJ, Pan C, Montine KS, Zhang J, Montine TJ. Proteomic analysis of neurofibrillary tangles in Alzheimer disease identifies GAPDH as a detergent-insoluble paired helical filament tau binding protein. FASEB J (in press)

Wang W, Wang L, Endoh A, Hummelke G, Hawks CL, Hornsby PJ (2005) Identification of α-enolase as a nuclear DNA-binding protein in the zona fasciculata but not the zona reticularis of the human adrenal cortex. J Endocrinol 184:85–94

Wang Y, Chang CF, Morales M, Chiang YH, Harvey BK, Su TP, Tsao LI, Chen S, Thiemermann C (2003) Diadenosine tetraphosphate protects against injuries induced by ischemia and 6-hydroxydopamine in rat brain. J Neurosci 23:7958–7965

Wang-Su ST, McCormack AL, Yang S, Hosler MR, Mixon A, Riviere MA, Wilmarth PA, Andley UP, Garland D, Li H, David LL, Wagner BJ (2003) Proteome analysis of lens epithelia, fibers, and the HLE B-3 cell line. Invest Ophthalmol Vis Sci 44:4829–4836

Watanabe H, Takehana K, Date M, Shinozaki T, Raz A (1996) Tumor cell autocrine motility factor is the neuroleukin/phosphohexose isomerase polypeptide. Cancer Res 56:2960–2963

Wistow GJ, Lietman T, Williams LA, Stapel SO, de Jong WW, Horwitz J, Piatigorsky J (1988) τ-Crystallin/α-enolase: one gene encodes both an enzyme and a lens structural protein. J Cell Biol 107:2729–2736

Xu W, Seiter K, Feldman E, Ahmed T, Chiao JW (1996) The differentiation and maturation mediator for human myeloid leukemia cells shares homology with neuroleukin or phosphoglucose isomerase. Blood 87:4502–4506

Yanagawa T, Funasaka T, Tsutsumi S, Raz T, Tanaka N, Raz A (2005) Differential regulation of phosphoglucose isomerase/autocrine motility factor activities by protein kinase CK2 phosphorylation. J Biol Chem 280:10419–10426

Yoshimura T, Kawano Y, Arimura N, Kawabata S, Kikuchi A, Kaibuchi K (2005) GSK-3β regulates phosphorylation of CRMP-2 and neuronal polarity. Cell 120:137–149

Am. J. Hum. Genet. 76:925–933, 2005

A Genomewide Exploration Suggests a New Candidate Gene at Chromosome 11q23 as the Major Determinant of Plasma Homocysteine Levels: Results from the GAIT Project

Juan Carlos Souto[1,*] Francisco Blanco-Vaca,[2,*] José Manuel Soria,[1] Alfonso Buil,[1] Laura Almasy,[3] Jordi Ordoñez-Llanos,[2] Jesús Mª Martín-Campos,[2] Mark Lathrop,[4] William Stone,[1,3] John Blangero,[3] and Jordi Fontcuberta[1]

[1]Unitat de Trombosi i Hemostàsia, Departament d' Hematologia, and [2]Servei de Bioquimica, Hospital de la Santa Creu i Sant Pau, Barcelona; [3]Department of Genetics, Southwest Foundation for Biomedical Research, San Antonio; and [4]Centre National de Genotypage, Evry, France

Homocysteine (Hcy) plasma level is an independent risk marker for venous thrombosis, myocardial infarction, stroke, congestive heart failure, osteoporotic fractures, and Alzheimer disease. Hcy levels are determined by the interaction of genetic and environmental factors. The genetic basis is still poorly understood, since only the *MTHFR* 677 C→T polymorphism has been consistently associated with plasma Hcy levels. We conducted a genomewide linkage scan for genes affecting variation in plasma Hcy levels in 398 subjects from 21 extended Spanish families. A variance-components linkage method was used to analyze the data. The strongest linkage signal (LOD score of 3.01; genomewide $P = .035$) was found on chromosome 11q23, near marker *D11S908,* where a candidate gene involved in the metabolism of Hcy (the nicotinamide N-methyltransferase gene [*NNMT*]) is mapped. Haplotype analyses of 10 single-nucleotide polymorphisms within this gene found one haplotype associated with plasma Hcy levels ($P = .0003$). Our results, to our knowledge, represent the first genomic scan for quantitative variation in Hcy plasma levels. They strongly suggest that the *NNMT* gene could be a major genetic determinant of plasma Hcy levels in Spanish families. Since this gene encodes an enzyme involved in Hcy synthesis, this finding would be consistent with known biochemical pathways. These data could be relevant in determining the relationships between Hcy level, cardiovascular disease, osteoporosis, and Alzheimer disease.

Introduction

Multiple case-control and prospective studies have established an association between moderate hyperhomocysteinemia and increased risk of ischemic heart disease and stroke (Welch and Loscalzo 1998; Cattaneo 1999; Homocysteine Studies Collaboration 2002; Wald et al. 2002), congestive heart failure (Vasan et al. 2003), and deep vein thrombosis (Cattaneo 1999). Furthermore, recent data from the Framingham Study indicate that plasma homocysteine (Hcy) level is also a dose-related risk marker for the development of dementia and Alzheimer disease (Seshadri et al. 2002). There have been additional reports on the association between hyperhomocysteinemia and Alzheimer disease (Morris 2003), mental deterioration (Morris et al. 2001), and vascular dementia (McIlroy et al. 2002). These associations seems to be independent of age, sex, apolipoprotein E gene (*APOE*) genotype, plasma vitamin levels, and other putative risk factors (Seshadri et al. 2002). Furthermore, elevated Hcy concentration has been associated with risk of osteoporotic fractures in elderly persons (McLean et al. 2004; van Meurs et al. 2004)

The plasma Hcy level is a quantitative phenotype that is influenced by genetic and environmental factors. The main environmental determinants are sex, age, renal function, and vitamin intake (Brattsström et al. 1994). However, the genetic component is still poorly understood. Currently, the most widely accepted polymorphism associated with Hcy variability is *MTHFR* 677 C→T (Frosst et al. 1995). Other common polymorphisms within genes for enzymes involved in Hcy metabolism have been described. These polymorphisms, along with *MTHFR* 677 C→T, account for <10% of the variance in plasma Hcy level (Kluijtmans et al. 2003). A recent family study, which involved a segregation analysis, suggested the existence of a major gene that regulates Hcy plasma level, even after adjusting for effects of *MTHFR* 677 C→T (Jee et al. 2002).

As part of our Genetic Analysis of Idiopathic Thrombophilia (GAIT) Project, we observed that the herita-

Received December 28, 2004; accepted for publication March 21, 2005; electronically published April 22, 2005.

Address for correspondence and reprints: Dr. Juan Carlos Souto, Unitat de Trombosi i Hemostàsia, Hospital de la Santa Creu i Sant Pau, Sant Antoni Mª Claret 167, 08025 Barcelona, Spain. E-mail: jsouto@hsp.santpau.es

* These authors contributed equally to this study.

0002-9297/2005/7606-0003$15.00

bility of Hcy plasma levels (± SD) was 0.25 ± 0.08, indicating that ~25% of the phenotypic variation in this trait is due to the additive effect of genes (Souto et al. 2000*b*). Additional results from the GAIT Project (Souto et al. 2000*a*) have demonstrated that Hcy levels are genetically correlated with thrombotic risk (ρ_G = 0.65). This implies that some genes influence simultaneously the plasma levels of Hcy and the risk of thromboembolic disease.

In an effort to localize the genes influencing variation in plasma Hcy levels, we conducted a genomewide linkage scan of DNA from individuals in the GAIT sample.

Material and Methods

Study Population

The GAIT Project includes 21 extended families, 12 of whom were ascertained through a proband with thrombophilia, and 9 of whom were obtained randomly from the general population. A total of 398 individuals were examined, with a mean of 19 individuals examined per family. The composition of the families and the collection of lifestyle, medical, and family history data have been detailed elsewhere (Souto et al. 2000*b*). The study was performed in accordance with the Declaration of Helsinki of 1975; all adult patients provided informed consent and parents of minors provided informed consent for their children. All procedures were approved by the institutional review board of the Hospital de la Santa Creu i Sant Pau, Barcelona, Spain.

Plasma Hcy Determination

EDTA blood samples were obtained by venipuncture after a 12-h fast. Measures to prevent the flow of Hcy from erythrocytes to plasma were strictly implemented. Total Hcy plasma concentration was measured by use of high-performance liquid chromatography (Millipore) and fluorescence detection (Kontron Instruments). The analytical characteristics of this method have been analyzed and compared to a widely used commercial immunoassay (Blanco-Vaca et al. 2000).

DNA Extraction and Genotype Analysis

DNA extraction was performed in accordance with a standard protocol (Souto et al. 2000*b*). Subjects were genotyped for an autosomal genomewide scan with 363 highly informative DNA markers. Microsatellites consisted primarily of the ABI Prism genotyping set MD-10 (Applied Biosystems). PCR products were analyzed on PE 310, PE 377, and PE 3700 automated sequencers and were genotyped using PE Genotyper software (Applied Biosystems). The average heterozygosity of the microsatellite markers was 0.79, and the average distance between markers was 9.5 cM. The 677 C→T polymorphism in the *MTHFR* gene was genotyped using PCR with primers described elsewhere (Frosst et al. 1995) and with minor modifications to the reaction conditions. Marker maps for multipoint analyses were obtained from ABI Prism and from the Marshfield Center for Medical Genetics.

Genetic Linkage Analysis

Levels of Hcy in the GAIT sample exhibited a kurtosis of 29.5. For this reason, we used a natural logarithm to transform the Hcy values to achieve a normal distribution, and the new logarithmically transformed Hcy (lnHcy) levels had a kurtosis of only 0.48. This level of kurtosis did not affect the distribution of LOD scores (Blangero et al. 2000). The standard nominal *P* values for LOD scores were appropriate for the lnHcy linkage tests. The calculations also incorporated a simultaneous correction for covariates like sex, age, and BMI. Estimation of heritability (h^2) and the covariate effects of lnHcy were done using methods described elsewhere (Souto et al. 2000*b*). All analyses included an ascertainment correction, achieved by conditioning the likelihood of these pedigrees on the likelihoods of their respective probands (Boehnke and Lange 1984)

Standard multipoint variance-components linkage methods were used for the genome scan (Almasy and Blangero 1998). These methods have been implemented in the program SOLAR (available at the Southwest Foundation for Biomedical Research Web site). The statistical analysis is based on specification of the expected genetic covariances between arbitrary relatives as a function of the identity-by-descent (IBD) relationships at a given marker locus. To estimate the IBD matrix in these complex pedigrees, we used a Markov chain–Monte Carlo method as implemented in SIMWALK2 (Sobel and Lange 1996), which estimates the IBD probabilities at each cM. Bivariate linkage analyses with the use of a mixed discrete-/continuous-trait multivariate model were conducted with a modified version of SOLAR (Williams et al. 1999)

SNP Identification and Haplotype Analysis

We sequenced the nicotinamide N-methyltransferase gene (*NNMT* [UniGene accession number Hs.364345]) in 42 unrelated individuals from the GAIT Project using standard sequencing methods on an ABI 3100 automated sequencer (Applied Biosystems). The use of this number of individuals provided a >99% probability of detecting any polymorphism that had a frequency ⩾0.05. To enrich the sequencing sample for functional variants, we chose 22 individuals from those in the higher tail of the Hcy distribution and 20 from those in the lower tail. We sequenced ~1.5 kb of the proximal promoter of *NNMT*, including exon 1, and we then con-

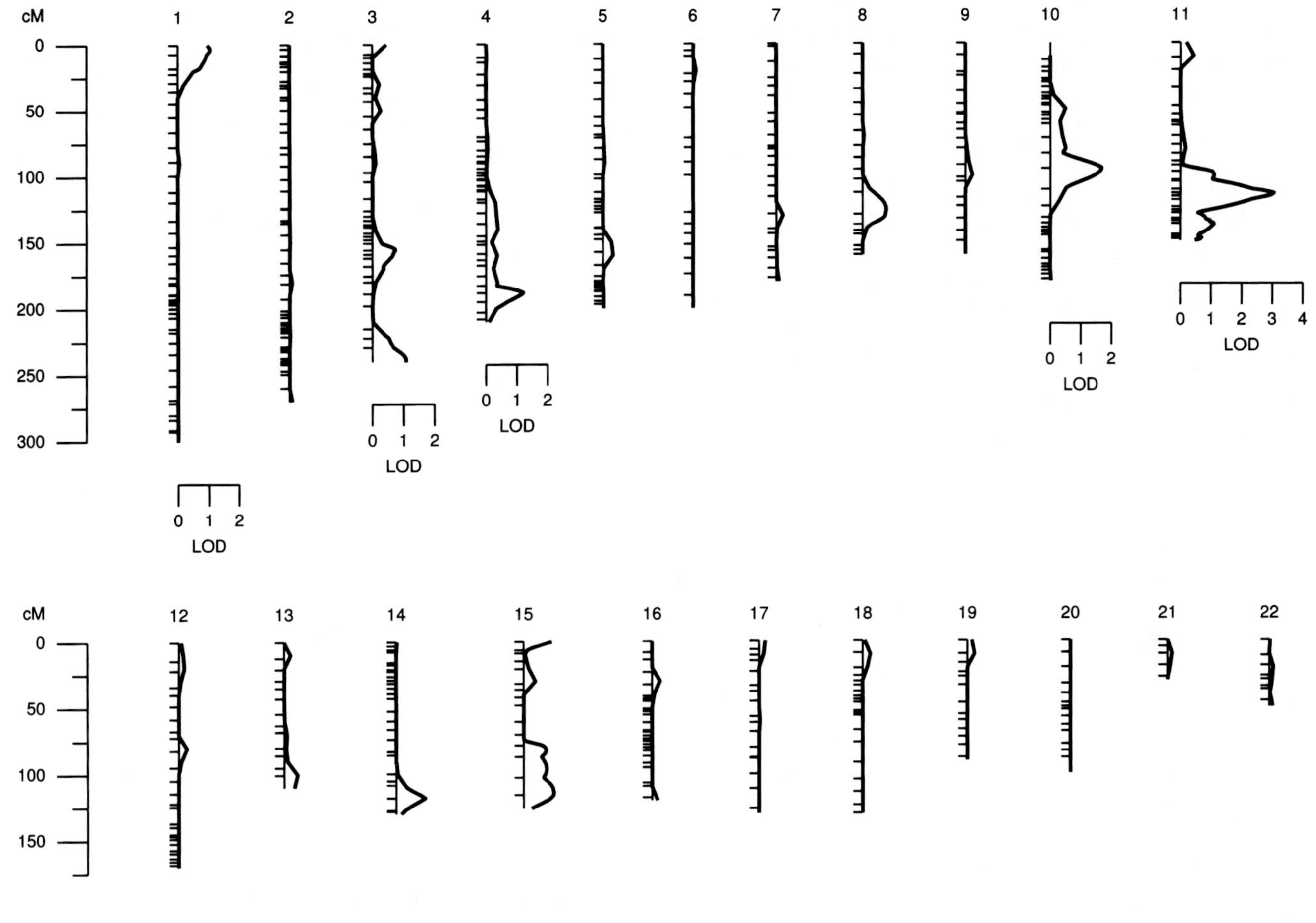

Figure 1 Linkage results from the autosomal multipoint genome scan. LOD score scales are shown for chromosomes 1, 3, 4, 10, and 11—the only chromosomes on which the maximum LOD score was >1. Hatch marks along the length of the chromosomes indicate the positions of the DNA markers.

tinued with the coding regions of exons 2, 3, 4, and 5. The latter included the 3′ UTR, with potential regulatory sequences.

Then, we genotyped the newly identified SNPs in our whole GAIT sample, as well as all previously reported *NNMT* SNPs (from the Celera database, available at the Applied Biosystems, myScience, Web site), by sequencing with the use of the SNP Genotyping Assays-on-Demand products from Applied Biosystems, in accordance with the recommendations of the manufacturer. The haplotypes with the SNPs detected in the *NNMT* gene were generated with the use of the "best" option in the MERLIN program (Abecasis et al. 2002). The association of each SNP or haplotype with Hcy plasma levels was tested by use of a quantitative-trait association analysis with the measured genotype approach, which involved testing for genotype-specific differences in the mean values of traits while allowing for the nonindependence among family members (Almasy and Blangero 2004). These analyses were performed using SOLAR.

Results

In the GAIT sample, the mean age-corrected Hcy plasma level (± SD) was 7.8 ± 3.1 μmol/liter. The range of Hcy values was 2.7–46.6 μmol/liter. After natural-logarithm transformation, lnHcy values showed a mean (± SD) of 2.05 ± 0.36. The significant regression coefficients for the covariates influencing lnHcy were 0.006 for age, −0.12 for female sex, and 0.004 for BMI. Together, they accounted for 18% of the variability of lnHcy levels. The heritability of the lnHcy phenotype (± SD) was 0.34 ± 0.08. This shows that genes play an important role in determining plasma levels (34% of phenotypic variability). This result is consistent with the previous estimate of $h^2 = 0.25 \pm 0.08$ for crude values of Hcy (Souto et al. 2000*b*).

Effects of the MTHFR *677 C→T Polymorphism*

The 677 C→T variant was present in 20 GAIT families. There were 174 heterozygotes and 59 homozygotes

Table 1

Genes Involved in Hcy Metabolism, with Their Chromosomal Locations and the Maximum LOD Score Obtained at Each Locus

Gene	Abbreviation	Location	LOD
Nicotinamide N-methyltransferase	*NNMT*	11q23	3.01
Methionine adenosyltransferase α I	*MATαI*	10q22	1.68
Methionine adenosyltransferase α II	*MATαII*	2p11	<1
Methionine adenosyltransferase β	*MATβ*	5q34	<1
5,10-Methylenetetrahydrofolate reductase	*MTHFR*	1p36	1.03
Other SAM-dependent methyltransferases[a]	...	...	<1
5-Methyltetrahydrofolate-homocysteine methyltransferase	*MTR*	1q43	<1
Methionine synthase reductase	*MTRR*	5p15	<1
Betaine-homocysteine methyltransferase	*BHMT*	5q14	<1
S-adenosylhomocysteine hydrolase	*AHCY*	20q11	<1
Cystathionine β-synthase	*CBS*	21q22	<1
Dihydrofolate reductase	*DHFR*	5q14	<1
Cystathionine γ-lyase	*CTH*	1p31	<1
Serine hydroxymethyltransferase 1	*SHMT1*	17p11	<1
Serine hydroxymethyltransferase 2	*SHMT2*	11q12	<1
Thymidylate synthase	*TS*	18p11	<1
Methylenetetrahydrofolate dehydrogenase 1	*MTHFD1*	14q23	<1
Methylenetetrahydrofolate dehydrogenase 2	*MTHFD2*	2p13	<1
S-adenosylmethionine decarboxylase	*AMD1*	6q21	<1
Choline dehydrogenase	*CHDH*	3p21	<1
Paraoxonase	*PON1*	7q21	<1
Folate receptor	*FOLR1*	11q13	<1
Folate carrier 19 member 1	*SLC19A1*	21q22	<1
Folate carrier 19 member 2	*SLC19A2*	1q24	<1
Folate carrier 19 member 3	*SLC19A3*	2q36	<1
Transcobalamin 1	*TCN1*	11q12	<1
Transcobalamin 2	*TCN2*	22q12	<1
Intrinsic factor	*GIF*	11q12	<1

[a] Apart from NNMT, there exist 38 other human SAM-dependent methyltransferases (Clarke and Banfield 2001); none of their respective gene loci showed a LOD score >1, and none is located on 11q23 or 10q22, where we obtained the highest LOD scores in our analysis.

for the T allele, and they exhibited higher mean Hcy levels than noncarriers (Hcy levels of 7.8 μmol/liter in CT heterozygotes, 9.5 μmol/liter in TT homozygotes, and 7.1 μmol/liter in CC noncarriers).

Nominal evidence of linkage was found between lnHcy levels and the *MTHFR* locus in a two-point linkage analysis (LOD score of 0.66; $P = .04$). Additionally, the 677 C→T polymorphism was strongly associated with lnHcy levels ($P < 1.6 \times 10^{-5}$).

Genomewide Linkage Analysis

Multipoint linkage analyses were performed across all 22 autosomes. The results of the genome scan for a QTL influencing lnHcy levels are shown in figure 1. One region, on chromosome 11q23, showed strong evidence of linkage (LOD score of 3.01; nominal $P = .0001$; genomewide $P = .035$). This peak was the highest LOD score found and occurred between markers *D11S908* and *D11S4142*. This suggests that there is a gene in this region that influences plasma levels of Hcy. The one-unit support interval surrounding this peak has a chromosomal location in the range of 112–118 cM from the p terminus. This region contains the gene *NNMT,* which is involved in Hcy metabolism and is thus a candidate gene to explain the linkage signal.

Another chromosomal region produced a LOD score of 1.68 (nominal $P = .003$), suggesting linkage. The region was on chromosome 10q22 (fig. 1 and table 1), corresponding to marker *D10S537*. Such a LOD score would be expected to occur by chance approximately once every genome scan and must be considered suggestive until supported by other evidence. Again, there is a gene within this region that is involved in Hcy metabolism and is a candidate to explain the observed linkage signal: the methionine adenosyltransferase α I gene (*MATαI*).

The maximum LOD score found in the region of the *MTHFR* gene on chromosome 1p36.3 was 1.03 (nominal $P = .015$) (fig. 1 and table 1). These multipoint results show only a marginal increase from the LOD score of 0.66 obtained in the two-point linkage analysis with only the 677 C→T polymorphism as a marker.

Because our previous studies have suggested that Hcy levels are genetically correlated ($\rho_G = 0.65$) with the sus-

Table 2

Genotyped SNPs within *NNMT* and Results from the Association Analysis with Hcy Plasma Levels

SNP	Celera ID[a]	dbSNP ID	Location	Position[b] (bp)	Allele Frequencies[c]	P^d
1	New[e]	*rs35077908*	Promoter	113,632,968	81/19	.38
2	c1058033	*rs505978*	Intron 1	113,634,267	76/24	.64
3	c1058034	*rs683271*	Intron 1	113,634,355	77/23	.65
4	***c2134722***	***rs694539***	Intron 1	113,638,629	85/15	***.017***
5	c2134725	*rs11214921*	Intron 2	113,642,022	19/81	.16
6	c2134727	*rs10891641*	Intron 2	113,644,291	21/79	.81
7	c10096025	*rs2852432*	Intron 2	113,669,214	27/73	.49
8	c10096016	*rs2852447*	Intron 4	113,684,911	75/25	.29
9	New[e]	*rs4646337*	3′ UTR	113,688,519	79/21	.98
10	c10096011	*rs11569688*	3′ UTR	113,688,653	18/81	.64

NOTE.—The SNP with a significant *P* value ($P < .05$) is shown in bold italics.

[a] Celera database available at the Applied Biosystems, myScience, Web site.

[b] The SNP position from the p terminus of chromosome 11.

[c] Estimated allele frequencies in the Spanish population, given as percentages (allele 1/allele 2), with family relationships taken into account.

[d] *P* value of association with Hcy levels. Values are not corrected for the number of markers tested.

[e] "New" indicates that the SNP was found in the present study and was not previously reported.

ceptibility to thrombosis (Souto et al. 2000*a*), we performed a bivariate linkage analysis. Bivariate analyses of related phenotypes have been shown to increase the power to detect linkage (Soria et al. 2002, 2003). In the combined analyses of lnHcy levels and thrombosis, the three LOD scores on chromosomes 11, 10, and 1 remained at their previous levels, with no significant QTL effects on susceptibility, providing no evidence that these QTLs influence thrombosis risk. Nevertheless, these results do not allow the possibility to be excluded.

Screening for SNPs in NNMT *and Haplotype Association Analysis*

We identified two novel SNPs. One (SNP 1 in table 2) is in the promoter region, and the other (SNP 9 in table 2) is in the 3′ UTR. These 2 identified SNPs, together with 10 SNPs previously reported in 2003 (Celera database), were genotyped for the whole GAIT sample. Of these 12 SNPs, 2 were excluded from the analysis because they correlated (i.e., showed perfect linkage disequilibrium) with other SNPs. The details of the 10 SNPs included in our analysis are given in table 2.

The measured-genotype association analysis revealed significant association between one of the SNPs (Celera accession number c2134722) and Hcy levels (table 2), supporting the presence of a QTL in the region of *NNMT.* In addition, in the GAIT sample, the 10 SNPs in the *NNMT* gene generated 31 haplotypes (table 3). In the measured-genotype association analysis, one of the haplotypes (Hap 18) was strongly associated with Hcy levels ($P = .00001$), even after correction for multiple testing (corrected $P = .00031$). Two other haplotypes (Hap 22 and Hap 31) showed an association with Hcy levels ($P = .01$ and .04, respectively), but the statistical significance was lost when the results were corrected for multiple testing. All carriers of Hap 18 ($n = 12$) were heterozygous and had a mean Hcy level ($\pm$ SD) of 13.2 $\pm$ 2.9 μmol/liter.

Discussion

A major challenge for medicine in the postgenomic era is to identify genetic variants that affect the risk of developing complex diseases such as cardiovascular or Alzheimer disease. It is usually extremely difficult to find these QTLs when the study focuses directly on disease status (i.e., disease or no disease). However, intermediate risk factors or risk markers can be analyzed by a genetic search. According to recent reports of epidemiological data, the Hcy plasma level is an independent intermediate risk marker for thromboembolic disease (both arterial and venous) (Welch and Loscalzo 1998; Cattaneo 1999; Homocysteine Studies Collaboration 2002; McIlroy et al. 2002; Wald et al. 2002), congestive heart failure (Vasan et al. 2003), Alzheimer disease (Morris et al. 2001; McIlroy et al. 2002; Seshadri et al. 2002; Morris 2003), and osteoporotic fractures (McLean et al. 2004; van Meurs et al. 2004).

In humans, the sole source of Hcy is the demethylation of methionine through the intervention of different methyltransferases. This pathway has several steps (fig. 2). First, methionine and ATP originate S-adeno-

Table 3

Haplotypes Observed within the *NNMT* Gene in the GAIT Sample, in Order of Frequency

Haplotype[a]	Hap ID	Frequency[b]	Hcy Level[c] (μmol/liter)	P[d]
1111222112	Hap 7	318	7.60	.69
2111222221	Hap 30	84	7.51	.99
1222111112	***Hap 22***	73	***6.94***	***.01***
2111222112	Hap 28	58	7.22	.87
1111221112	Hap 4	56	7.92	.89
1221222112	Hap 20	37	7.67	.59
1111222221	Hap 9	30	7.55	.69
1111221221	Hap 6	16	8.30	.09
1221211112	***Hap 18***	12	***13.18***	***.00001***
1222111212	Hap 24	9	7.97	.58
1111221212	Hap 5	8	8.55	.48
1221112112	Hap 16	8	7.64	.77
2111221212	Hap 27	8	9.80	.07
1112112112	Hap 13	7	6.66	.95
1111222212	Hap 8	5	6.42	.68
1112111221	Hap 12	5	8.00	.40
1111211222	Hap 3	4	6.22	.65
1112111212	Hap 11	3	7.10	.85
1221111112	Hap 14	3	10.76	.22
1221111222	Hap 15	3	7.37	.52
1221112221	Hap 17	3	7.00	.75
1221222221	Hap 21	3	6.00	.42
2111222211	Hap 29	3	8.20	.68
2112111112	***Hap 31***	3	***5.10***	***.04***
1111122112	Hap 2	2	10.00	.39
1111222222	Hap 10	2	9.85	.57
1221211222	Hap 19	2	5.90	.85
1222112112	Hap 26	2	5.50	.20
1111111221	Hap 1	1	7.70	.78
1222111122	Hap 23	1	3.90	.38
1222111221	Hap 25	1	8.20	.86

NOTE.—The haplotypes with significant *P* values ($P < .05$) are shown in bold italics.

[a] The composition of the haplotypes follows the same order of SNPs as in table 2.

[b] Frequency is given as the number of chromosomes containing the haplotype. There were only four haplotypes with homozygous carriers: Hap 7, Hap 20, Hap 22, and Hap 28. No statistically significant differences in Hcy levels between heterozygous and homozygous carriers were observed.

[c] Crude mean Hcy levels among haplotype carriers, without accounting for the nonindependence of family members.

[d] *P* value of association with Hcy levels. Values are not corrected for the number of haplotypes tested.

sylmethionine (SAM) by means of the enzyme methionine adenosyltransferase. Then, SAM is converted to S-adenosylhomocysteine (SAH) in a reaction catalyzed by SAM-dependent methyltransferases. This reaction originates a methyl group that is used for many different biochemical pathways through, in humans, at least 39 distinct methyltransferases (Clarke and Banfield 2001). SAH is subsequently broken down to form adenosine and Hcy that is remethylated to form methionine. Alternatively, Hcy can be converted to cysteine through the transsulfuration pathway.

The majority of potential candidate genes, which encode enzymes or proteins involved in Hcy metabolism (fig. 2 and table 1), did not produce a linkage signal for Hcy levels. The results of our genome scan suggest that the major QTL influencing variation in Hcy levels is located on chromosome 11q23 (fig. 1). Interestingly, this region has been linked to the risk of venous thrombosis in a genome scan performed with a single large pedigree with thrombosis and protein C deficiency (Hasstedt et al. 2004). This genetic protein C deficiency appeared insufficient to explain completely the venous thrombosis risk in the family. For this reason, Hasstedt et al. (2004) undertook a genomewide search of regions potentially harboring other genetic factors. In the search, a peak of significance was found at 113 cM from the p terminus of chromosome 11, just within our support interval (112–118 cM) for the Hcy QTL. We also investigated the possible pleiotropic effect of this QTL on the risk of thrombosis. The linkage signal in the bivariate linkage analysis was not significantly increased, and no significant QTL effect on susceptibility was observed. Thus, we can not directly replicate the observation by Hasstedt et al. (2004) of a thrombosis QTL on chromosome 11. However, lack of statistical power could be the reason for the failure to confirm this finding. A biologically plausible candidate gene, *NNMT,* is located within this region. NNMT is an enzyme involved in the synthesis of SAH, the precursor of Hcy, and it catabolizes nicotinamide and other pyridine compounds in a reaction that uses the methyl group generated during the conversion of SAM to SAH (Aksoy et al. 1994) (fig. 2). NNMT is widely synthesized in most tissues, especially in the liver (Yan et al. 1999). An important individual variability in the liver activity of this enzyme has been described, suggesting a trimodal distribution (Smith et al. 1998; Yan et al. 1999). In the absence of functional polymorphisms in the coding region of *NNMT,* this distribution has been shown to depend on variation at mRNA and protein levels (Smith et al. 1998; Yan et al. 1999).

To test whether *NNMT* variability accounts for the observed linkage signal for Hcy plasma levels, we studied 10 SNPs within this gene. One of them showed significant association with Hcy levels ($P = .017$), although this result was no longer significant when corrected for the testing of 10 markers. Moreover, a haplotype built with the 10 SNPs within *NNMT* was more strongly associated with higher Hcy levels than were the remaining haplotypes ($P = .00031$, corrected for multiple testing). Although we have not yet identified the functional variants that are responsible for the observed effects, the significant associations of the intragenic SNP and haplotype, in conjunction with the linkage signal in this QTL, strongly support the hypothesis that genetic variants in *NNMT* are the main determinants of plasma

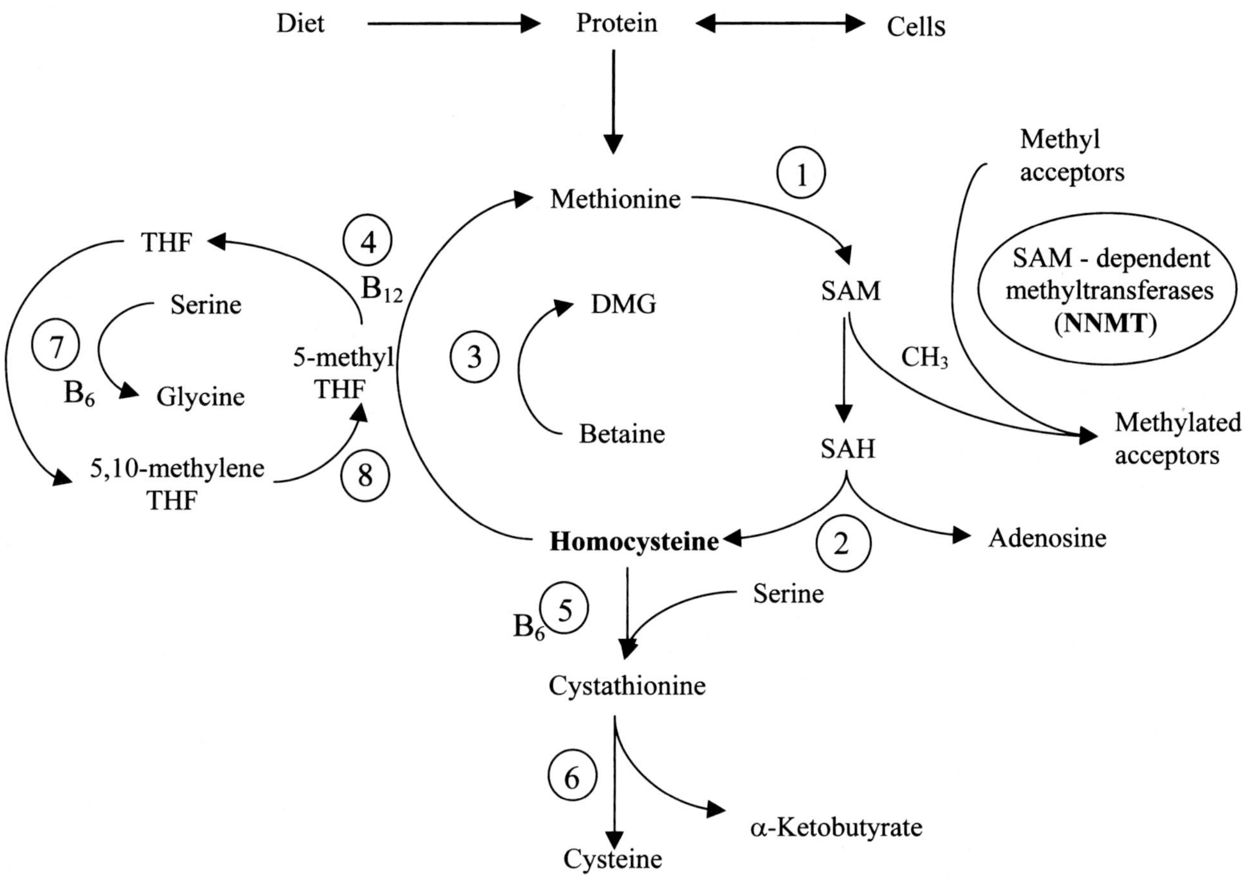

Figure 2 Metabolic pathways involved in Hcy regulation. Enzymes are numbered as follows: (1) methionine adenosyltransferase, (2) SAH hydrolase, (3) betaine-homocysteine methyltransferase, (4) 5-methyltetrahydrofolate-homocysteine methyltransferase, (5) cystathionine β-synthase, (6) cystathionine γ-lyase, (7) serine hydroxymethyltransferase, and (8) 5,10-methylenetetrahydrofolate reductase. B_6 = vitamin B_6; B_{12} = vitamin B_{12}; CH_3 = methyl group; DMG = dimethylglycine; THF = tetrahydrofolate. NNMT is one of at least 39 SAM-dependent methyltransferases described in mammals (Clarke and Banfield 2001). The gene encoding NNMT is located on chromosome 11q23, at the same QTL that has been linked to plasma Hcy levels.

Hcy variability in the GAIT sample. It is very probable that these variants will be located within noncoding regions, and they may influence the regulation of transcription. These regions were not included in our sequencing because of the huge size of the *NNMT* gene, which spans >50 kb. In support of the involvement of methyltransferases in plasma Hcy concentration, it is worth mentioning a recent report that demonstrated that mice deficient in another methyltransferase have a 50% decrease in plasma Hcy (Noga et al. 2003). Thus, we hypothesize a direct relationship between NNMT activity and plasma Hcy concentration.

The second-highest LOD score obtained in our genome scan is located on chromosome 10q22. This locus contains *MATαI,* a gene encoding another enzyme involved in Hcy formation (fig. 2). In the context of a genomewide exploration, a LOD score of 1.68 would be merely suggestive of linkage, but the presence of an obvious candidate gene reinforces the necessity of refining the search in this region. We genotyped three SNPs within *MATαI* that were reported in 2003 (Celera database), but none was significantly associated with Hcy levels (data not shown). Despite the attractiveness of *MATαI* as a candidate, the present study did not prove that it has an effect on Hcy levels. Nevertheless, an absence of association with some SNPs does not rule out implication of the gene in determining the phenotype. Other SNPs in the same gene that are not in linkage disequilibrium with those analyzed might be responsible for the linkage signal.

We have also examined the widely reported influence of the *MTHFR* 677 C→T genotype on Hcy levels. First, we used a two-point linkage analysis to assess the LOD score between this marker and the phenotype. We also explored this linkage in the genomewide scan. We confirmed previous findings of a direct effect of *MTHFR* on Hcy levels (Husemoen et al. 2003; Kluijtmans et al. 2003). However, our results indicate that the *MTHFR*

677 C→T polymorphism is not the major genetic determinant of the quantitative variation in Hcy plasma levels.

In conclusion, we found evidence that the *NNMT* gene, located in the region 11q23, influences plasma Hcy levels. It is probably the major genetic determinant of this phenotype in the Spanish population. It is possible that another gene on chromosome 10q22 also influences Hcy levels. Given the previous reports about the relevance of Hcy in certain diseases, further studies are warranted. These should include the exhaustive dissection (including exons, introns, and the 5′ and 3′ regulatory regions) of the *NNMT* gene. This task will require a high-throughput resequencing and genotyping effort, combined with advanced statistical genetic analyses, to determine the most likely functional variants.

Acknowledgments

This study was supported by National Institutes of Health (NIH) grant HL70751; Fondo de Investigación Sanitaria (FIS), Spanish Health Ministry, grants FIS PI020375 and FIS C03-08; grant SAF 2002-03449, partially supported by European Regional Development Funds (FEDER) (Spanish Ministry of Science and Technology); and grant RETICS C03/01 (Cardiovascular Network, FIS, Spanish Health Ministry). J.M.S. is supported by FIS 99/3048. A.B. is supported by FIS 01/A046. Statistical genetic analysis was supported by NIH grants MH59490 and HL70751. Fundació "La Caixa" and Fundació d'Investigació Sant Pau also contributed to the project. We are grateful to Rosa Arcelús, for homocysteine determinations, and Dr. Carlos Mª Díaz, for his help with *NNMT* sequencing. Finally, we are deeply grateful to all of the families who participated in the study.

Electronic-Database Information

The accession number and URLs for data presented herein are as follows:

Applied Biosystems, myScience, Web site, http://myscience.appliedbiosystems.com/ (for Celera database and *NNMT* SNPs)

dbSNP, http://www.ncbi.nlm.nih.gov/SNP/ (for *NNMT* SNPs)

Marshfield Center for Medical Genetics, http://research.marshfieldclinic.org/genetics/ (for the marker map used in multipoint linkage analysis)

Southwest Foundation for Biomedical Research, http://www.sfbr/org/ (for SOLAR program package)

UniGene, http://www.ncbi.nlm.nih.gov/UniGene/ (for *NNMT* [accession number Hs.364345] and other genes involved in Hcy metabolism)

References

Abecasis GR, Cherny SS, Cookson WO, Cardon LR (2002) Merlin-rapid analysis of dense genetic maps using sparse gene flow trees. Nat Genet 30:97–101

Aksoy S, Szumlanski CL, Weinshilboum RM (1994) Human liver nicotinamide N-methyltransferase: cDNA cloning, expression, and biochemical characterization. J Biol Chem 269:14835–14840

Almasy L, Blangero J (1998) Multipoint quantitative-trait linkage analysis in general pedigrees. Am J Hum Genet 62:1198–1211

——— (2004) Exploring positional candidate genes: linkage conditional on measured genotype. Behav Genet 34:173–177

Blanco-Vaca F, Arcelús R, González-Sastre F, Ordóñez-Llanos J, Queraltó-Compañó JM (2000) Comparison of the Abbott Imx and a high-performance liquid chromatography method for measuring total plasma homocysteine. Clin Chem Lab Med 38:327–329

Blangero J, Williams JT, Almasy L (2000) Robust LOD scores for variance component-based linkage analysis. Genet Epidemiol 19:S8–S14

Boehnke M, Lange K (1984) Ascertainment and goodness of fit of variance component models for pedigree data. Prog Clin Biol Res 147:173–192

Brattström L, Lindgren A, Israelsson B, Andersson A, Hultberg B (1994) Homocysteine and cysteine: determinants of plasma levels in middle-aged and elderly subjects. J Intern Med 236:633–641

Cattaneo M (1999) Hyperhomocysteinemia, atherosclerosis and thrombosis. Thromb Haemost 81:165–176

Clarke S, Banfield K (2001) S-adenosylmethionine-dependent methyltransferases. In: Carmel R, Jacobsen DW (eds) Homocysteine in health and disease. Cambridge University Press, Cambridge, United Kingdom, pp 63–78

Frosst P, Blom HJ, Milos R, Goyette P, Sheppard CA, Matthews RG, Boers GJH, den Heijer M, Kluijtmans LAJ, van den Heuvel LP, Rozen R (1995) A candidate genetic risk factor for vascular disease: a common mutation in methylenetetrahydrofolate reductase. Nat Genet 10:111–113

Hasstedt SJ, Scott BT, Callas PW, Vossen CY, Rosendaal FR, Long GL, Bovill EG (2004) Genome scan of venous thrombosis in a pedigree with protein C deficiency. J Thromb Haemost 2:868–873

Homocysteine Studies Collaboration (2002) Homocysteine and risk of ischemic heart disease and stroke: a meta-analysis. JAMA 288:2015–2022

Husemoen LLN, Thomsen TF, Fenger M, Jørgensen HL, Jørgensen T (2003) Contribution of thermolabile methylenetetrahydrofolate reductase variant to total plasma homocysteine levels in healthy men and women. Inter99 (2). Genet Epidemiol 24:322–330

Jee SH, Song KS, Shim WH, Kim HK, Suh I, Park JY, Won SY, Beaty TH (2002) Major gene evidence after MTHFR-segregation analysis of serum homocysteine in families of patients undergoing coronary arteriography. Hum Genet 111:128–135

Kluijtmans LA, Young IS, Boreham CA, Murray L, McMaster D, McNulty H, Strain JJ, McPartlin J, Scott JM, Whitehead AS (2003) Genetic and nutritional factors contributing to hyperhomocysteinemia in young adults. Blood 101:2483–2488

McIlroy SP, Dynan KB, Lawson JT, Patterson CC, Passmore AP (2002) Moderately elevated plasma homocysteine, methylenetetrahydrofolate reductase genotype, and risk for stroke, vascular dementia, and Alzheimer disease in Northern Ireland. Stroke 33:2351–2356

McLean RR, Jacques PF, Selhub J, Tucker KL, Samelson EJ, Broe KE, Hannan MT, Cupples LA, Kiel DP (2004) Homocysteine as a predictive factor for hip fracture in older persons. N Engl J Med 350:2042–2049

Morris MS (2003) Homocysteine and Alzheimer disease. Lancet Neurol 2:425–428

Morris MS, Jacques PF, Rosenberg IH, Selhub J (2001) National Health and Nutrition Examination Survey. Hyperhomocysteinemia associated with poor recall in the third National Health and Nutrition Examination Survey. Am J Clin Nutr 73:927–933

Noga AA, Stead LM, Zhao Y, Brosnan ME, Brosnan JT, Vance DE (2003) Plasma homocysteine is regulated by phospholipid methylation. J Biol Chem 278:5952–5955

Seshadri S, Beiser A, Selhub J, Jacques PF, Rosenberg IH, D'Agostina RB, Wilson PWF, Wolf PA (2002) Plasma homocysteine as a risk factor for dementia and Alzheimer disease. N Engl J Med 346:476–483

Smith ML, Burnett D, Bennet P, Waring RH, Brown HM, Williams AC, Ramsden DB (1998) A direct correlation between nicotinamide N-methyltransferase activity and protein levels in human liver cytosol. Biochim Biophys Acta 1442:238–244

Sobel E, Lange K (1996) Descent graphs in pedigree analysis: applications to haplotyping, location scores, and marker sharing statistics. Am J Hum Genet 58:1323–1337

Soria JM, Almasy L, Souto JC, Bacq D, Buil A, Faure A, Martínez-Marchán E, Mateo J, Borrell M, Stone W, Lathrop M, Fontcuberta J, Blangero J (2002) A quantitative-trait locus in the human factor XII gene influences both plasma factor XII levels and susceptibility to thrombotic disease. Am J Hum Genet 70:567–574

Soria JM, Almasy L, Souto JC, Buil A, Martínez-Marchán E, Mateo J, Borrell M, Stone WH, Lathrop M, Fontcuberta J, Blangero J (2003) A new locus on chromosome 18 that influences normal variation in activated protein C resistance phenotype and factor VIII activity and its relation to thrombosis susceptibility. Blood 101:163–167

Souto JC, Almasy L, Borrell M, Blanco-Vaca F, Mateo J, Soria JM, Coll I, Felices R, Stone W, Fontcuberta J, Blangero J (2000*a*) Genetic susceptibility to thrombosis and its relationship with physiological risk factors: the GAIT study. Am J Hum Genet 67:1452–1459

Souto JC, Almasy L, Borrell M, Garí M, Martínez E, Mateo J, Stone WH, Blangero J, Fontcuberta J (2000*b*) Genetic determinants of hemostasis phenotypes in Spanish families. Circulation 101:1546–1551

van Meurs JBJ, Dhonukshe-Rutten RAM, Pluijm SMF, van der Klift M, de Jonge R, Lindemans J, de Groot LC, Hofman A, Witteman JC, van Leeuwen JP, Breteler MM, Lips P, Pols HA, Uitterlinden AG (2004) Homocysteine levels and the risk of osteoporotic fracture. N Engl J Med 350:2033–2041

Vasan RS, Beiser A, D'Agostino RB, Levy D, Selhub J, Jacques PF, Rosenberg IH, Wilson PWF (2003) Plasma homocysteine and risk for congestive heart failure in adults without prior myocardial infarction. JAMA 289:1251–1257

Wald DS, Law M, Morris JK (2002) Homocysteine and cardiovascular disease: evidence on causality from a meta-analysis. BMJ 325:1202–1208

Welch GN, Loscalzo J (1998) Homocysteine and atherothrombosis. N Engl J Med 338:1042–1050

Williams JT, Van Eerdewegh P, Almasy L, Blangero J (1999) Joint multipoint linkage analysis of multivariate qualitative and quantitative traits. I. Likelihood formulation and simulation results. Am J Hum Genet 65:1134–1147

Yan L, Otterness DM, Weinshilboum RM (1999) Human nicotinamide N-methyltransferase pharmacogenetics: gene sequence analysis and promoter characterization. Pharmacogenetics 9:307–316

Am. J. Hum. Genet. 76:934–949, 2005

Joint Modeling of Linkage and Association: Identifying SNPs Responsible for a Linkage Signal

Mingyao Li, Michael Boehnke, and Gonçalo R. Abecasis

Department of Biostatistics, School of Public Health, and Center for Statistical Genetics, University of Michigan, Ann Arbor

Once genetic linkage has been identified for a complex disease, the next step is often association analysis, in which single-nucleotide polymorphisms (SNPs) within the linkage region are genotyped and tested for association with the disease. If a SNP shows evidence of association, it is useful to know whether the linkage result can be explained, in part or in full, by the candidate SNP. We propose a novel approach that quantifies the degree of linkage disequilibrium (LD) between the candidate SNP and the putative disease locus through joint modeling of linkage and association. We describe a simple likelihood of the marker data conditional on the trait data for a sample of affected sib pairs, with disease penetrances and disease-SNP haplotype frequencies as parameters. We estimate model parameters by maximum likelihood and propose two likelihood-ratio tests to characterize the relationship of the candidate SNP and the disease locus. The first test assesses whether the candidate SNP and the disease locus are in linkage equilibrium so that the SNP plays no causal role in the linkage signal. The second test assesses whether the candidate SNP and the disease locus are in complete LD so that the SNP or a marker in complete LD with it may account fully for the linkage signal. Our method also yields a genetic model that includes parameter estimates for disease-SNP haplotype frequencies and the degree of disease-SNP LD. Our method provides a new tool for detecting linkage and association and can be extended to study designs that include unaffected family members.

Introduction

Positional cloning is widely used for identification of genes involved in human diseases. To date, hundreds of disease genes have been identified solely on the basis of their chromosomal position (Botstein and Risch 2003); examples include hemochromatosis (Feder et al. 1996), inflammatory bowel disease (Hugot et al. 2001; Ogura et al. 2001), and lactose intolerance (Enattah et al. 2002). The first step in a traditional positional-cloning approach involves a genomewide linkage analysis performed on a collection of families with multiple affected individuals. Often, linkage analysis results in a candidate region of 10–20 Mb. To localize the susceptibility allele more precisely, disease-marker association analyses with additional genetic markers specific to the linked region can be performed. With recent progress on high-throughput SNP genotyping (Sachidanandam et al. 2001; Syvanen 2001; Oliphant et al. 2002; Olivier et al. 2002) and the HapMap project (International HapMap Consortium 2003), these follow-up association studies are becoming less expensive and now routinely include hundreds or thousands of markers.

Association analysis often compares marker-allele frequencies between unrelated case and control subjects. In this design, only a subset of the samples originally collected for linkage analysis can be reused. As an alternative, family-based association methods have been developed. Family-based association tests offer a compromise between traditional linkage studies and case-control association studies. The classic family-based transmission/disequilibrium test was proposed to test for association in the presence of linkage in family trios containing two parents and one affected offspring (Spielman et al. 1993). This approach has been extended to discordant sib pairs (Curtis 1997; Boehnke and Langefeld 1998), sibships with multiple affected and unaffected sibs (Spielman and Ewens 1998), general pedigrees (Martin et al. 2000), and quantitative traits (Allison 1997; Rabinowitz 1997; Abecasis et al. 2000*a*, 2000*b*).

A shortcoming of these family-based association methods is that, although they test for association, they cannot distinguish between potentially causal SNPs and other variants showing weaker association, except in the case of quantitative traits (Cardon and Abecasis 2000). Göring and Terwilliger (2000) proposed a unified theoretical model for linkage and linkage disequilibrium (LD) analysis through the use of a "pseudomarker" locus, but their approach cannot accommodate information contributed by flanking markers. Hori-

Received November 9, 2004; accepted for publication March 16, 2005; electronically published April 5, 2005.

Address for correspondence and reprints: Mingyao Li, Department of Biostatistics, School of Public Health, University of Michigan, 1420 Washington Heights, Ann Arbor, MI 48109-2029. E-mail: myli@umich.edu

0002-9297/2005/7606-0004$15.00

kawa et al. (2000) suggested a modified association approach by examining how the evidence of linkage was partitioned in accordance with the genotype at the associated SNP, but they did not explore the properties of this approach. Li et al. (2004) explored the relationship between family-specific weights based on the affected individuals' genotypes and family-specific nonparametric linkage (NPL) scores, but their method does not quantify the relationship between SNP alleles and the linkage signal. Sun et al. (2002) developed an approach that identifies SNPs whose genotypes can fully explain the observed linkage signal, but their test does not identify SNPs that play a partial role in explaining the linkage signal.

In this article, we describe a statistical framework that identifies candidate SNPs that can fully or partly explain the observed linkage signal, through joint modeling of linkage and association with the use of affected sib pairs (ASPs). Our method uses genotype information contributed by both the candidate SNP and the flanking markers. When a candidate SNP is identified as being able to account for linkage, our approach estimates the degree of LD between the candidate SNP and disease alleles. The estimate of disease-SNP LD quantifies the degree to which the linkage signal can be explained by the candidate SNP. We summarize the available information using a simple likelihood of the marker data conditional on the trait data, with disease penetrances and disease-SNP haplotype frequencies as parameters. We estimate model parameters by maximum likelihood and propose two likelihood-ratio tests to characterize the relationship between the candidate SNP and the putative disease locus. We calculate LD between disease and SNP alleles on the basis of haplotype-frequency estimates. Our method can identify both associated and potentially causal SNPs. Here, we focus on the ASP study design, but our method can be readily extended to accommodate unaffected individuals and other family structures, as well as unrelated individuals.

Methods

Assumptions and Definitions

We assume that there is a set of ASPs typed for a candidate SNP and $M \geqslant 0$ flanking markers that can help evaluate evidence for linkage. We wish to evaluate evidence for association at the candidate SNP and to estimate the degree of LD with the unobserved disease locus. If there are multiple SNPs, we consider them one at a time as the candidate SNP. We allow LD between the candidate SNP and the unobserved disease alleles, but we assume linkage equilibrium between the flanking markers and the candidate SNP. Our goal is to quantify the relationship between the candidate SNPs and the unobserved disease alleles. Our method assumes that a single diallelic polymorphism directly contributes to risk in each linked region. We address the implications of multiple disease variants in the "Discussion" section.

Consider a diallelic disease locus with disease-predisposing allele D (with frequency p_D) and wild-type allele d (with frequency $p_d = 1 - p_D$) and a nearby diallelic SNP with alleles A (with frequency p_A) and a (with frequency $p_a = 1 - p_A$). Denote the four disease-SNP haplotypes as DA, Da, dA, and da (with frequencies p_{DA}, p_{Da}, p_{dA}, and p_{da}, respectively). We assume Hardy-Weinberg equilibrium in the general population for all markers, including the superlocus formed by the combination of the disease and SNP loci. Let $f_g = P(\text{affected}|g)$ be the penetrance for a given genotype $g \in \{dd, Dd, DD\}$ at the disease locus. By definition, the population prevalence of the disease, K, is equal to $f_{dd}p_d^2 + 2f_{Dd}p_dp_D + f_{DD}p_D^2$, the attributable fraction equals $K - f_{dd}/K$, and the genotype relative risk (GRR) equals f_g/f_{dd}.

Let $X = (X_1, \ldots, X_k, X_{\text{SNP}}, X_{k+1}, \ldots, X_M)$ be the observed marker genotypes for the ASP, and let the probability of no change in identity-by-descent (IBD) status between consecutive markers be $\psi_m = \theta_m^2 + (1-\theta_m)^2$, where θ_m is the recombination fraction between markers m and $m+1$ $(1 \leqslant m \leqslant M-1)$. Let I_m, I_{SNP}, and I_D be the possibly unknown number of alleles shared IBD by an ASP at marker m, at the candidate SNP, and at the putative disease locus, respectively. For now, assume that there is no recombination between the candidate SNP and the disease locus, so that $I_{\text{SNP}} = I_D$. Denote disease locus IBD-sharing probabilities for an ASP by $z_i = P(I_D = i|\text{ASP})$, where $i = 0,1,2$, and $\mathbf{z} = (z_0, z_1, z_2)$. For ease of computation, we assume that there is no genetic interference, so that $\{I_m\}$ forms a hidden Markov chain.

Conditional Probability of Marker Data, Given an ASP

We wish to calculate $P(X|\text{ASP})$, the probability of the marker genotype data X for an ASP. By applying the forward and backward algorithms of Baum (1972), $P(X|\text{ASP})$ can be calculated as

$$\begin{aligned}
&\sum_{I_D} P(X|I_D;\text{ASP})P(I_D|\text{ASP}) \\
&= \sum_{I_D} P(X_1,\ldots,X_k|I_D)P(X_{k+1},\ldots,X_M|I_D) \\
&\quad \times P(X_{\text{SNP}},I_D|\text{ASP}) \\
&= \sum_{I_D} \left\{ \left(\sum_{I_k} P[I_k|I_D]L_k[I_k] \right) \right. \\
&\quad \left. \times \left(\sum_{I_{k+1}} P[I_{k+1}|I_D]R_{k+1}[I_{k+1}] \right) P(X_{\text{SNP}},I_D|\text{ASP}) \right\} , \qquad (1)
\end{aligned}$$

Table 1

Conditional Probabilities $P(X_m|I_m)$ for Ordered Sib-Pair Genotypes X_m

	$P(X_m\|I_m)$ FOR		
X_m	$I_m = 0$	$I_m = 1$	$I_m = 2$
(aa, aa)	p_a^4	p_a^3	p_a^2
(aa, ab)	$2p_a^3 p_b$	$p_a^2 p_b$	0
(aa, bb)	$p_a^2 p_b^2$	0	0
(aa, bc)	$2p_a^2 p_b p_c$	0	0
(ab, ab)	$4p_a^2 p_b^2$	$p_a p_b(p_a + p_b)$	$2p_a p_b$
(ab, ac)	$4p_a^2 p_b p_c$	$p_a p_b p_c$	0
(ab, cd)	$4p_a p_b p_c p_d$	0	0

NOTE.—a, b, c, and d are distinct alleles with frequencies p_a, p_b, p_c, and p_d, respectively.

where k and $k+1$ are the flanking markers on the left- and right-hand sides of the candidate SNP.

At an arbitrary marker m ($1 \leqslant m \leqslant M$),

$$L_m(I_m) = P(X_1,\ldots,X_m|I_m) = \sum_{I_{m-1}} L_{m-1}(I_{m-1})P(X_m|I_m)P(I_{m-1}|I_m)$$

and

$$R_m(I_m) = P(X_m,\ldots,X_M|I_m) = \sum_{I_{m+1}} R_{m+1}(I_{m+1})P(X_m|I_m)P(I_{m+1}|I_m) \ .$$

Special cases are $L_1(I_1) = P(X_1 \mid I_1)$ and $R_M(I_M) = P(X_M|I_M)$. The conditional probabilities of the genotype data, given the number of alleles shared IBD by the sib pair at marker m, $P(X_m|I_m)$, are given in table 1 (Thompson 1975). IBD transition probabilities, $P(I_{m+1}|I_m)$, are given in table 2 (Risch 1990). Recursive calculation of $L_m(I_m)$ and $R_m(I_m)$ allows the rapid evaluation of $P(X|\text{ASP})$ in a manner linear to the number of markers, M.

To calculate $P(X_{\text{SNP}},I_D|\text{ASP})$, let G_j denote the disease-SNP haplogenotype for sib $j = 1,2$. Summing over all ordered haplogenotypes that are consistent with the observed SNP genotypes, we get

$$P(X_{\text{SNP}},I_D|\text{ASP}) = \sum_{(G_1,G_2)\sim X_{\text{SNP}}} P(G_1,G_2,I_D|\text{ASP}) = \sum_{(G_1,G_2)\sim X_{\text{SNP}}} \frac{P(\text{ASP}|G_1,G_2)P(G_1,G_2|I_D)P(I_D)}{P(\text{ASP})} = \sum_{(G_1,G_2)\sim X_{\text{SNP}}} \frac{f_{G_1}f_{G_2}P(G_1,G_2|I_D)P(I_D)}{P(\text{ASP})} \ , \quad (2)$$

where $P(G_1,G_2|I_D)$ can be calculated from table 1 by regarding each haplogenotype as a genotype of the superlocus that has up to four alleles. For a sib pair, $P(I_D)$ takes the values (1/4, 1/2, 1/4). To illustrate how equation (2) is calculated, consider an ASP with SNP genotype A/A for the first sib and a/a for the second sib. The disease-SNP genotypes that are consistent with the observed SNP genotypes are $G_1 \in \{DA/DA, DA/dA, dA/dA\}$ and $G_2 \in \{Da/Da, Da/da, da/da\}$. If $I_D = 0$, then the numerator of equation (2) is

$$\sum_{(G_1,G_2)\sim X_{\text{SNP}}} f_{G_1}f_{G_2}P(G_1,G_2|I_D=0)P(I_D=0) = \frac{1}{4}\Big\{(f_{DD}p_{DA}^2 + 2f_{Dd}p_{DA}p_{dA} + f_{dd}p_{dA}^2) \times (f_{DD}p_{Da}^2 + 2f_{Dd}p_{Da}p_{da} + f_{dd}p_{da}^2)\Big\} \ .$$

Similarly, we can obtain the probability of an ASP, where

$$P(\text{ASP}) = \sum_{I_D}\sum_{(G_1,G_2)} f_{G_1}f_{G_2}P(G_1,G_2|I_D)P(I_D) \ . \quad (3)$$

In the calculation of equations (2) and (3), we assume that the disease-affection statuses of the ASP are conditionally independent, given their genotypes at the disease locus. This is a common assumption for parametric likelihood calculation. It is exactly true when there are no other genetic or environmental risk factors shared among siblings, and it is a reasonable approximation when there are multiple disease-causing variants or shared environmental risk factors.

Our calculation allows analysis with missing genotypes. For example, to accommodate ASPs in which only one sib is genotyped at the candidate SNP, we sum over all possible SNP genotypes for the sib with missing genotype. Our calculation can also be readily extended to sib-pair samples that include unaffected individuals, by replacing f_{G_j} in equations (2) and (3) with $1 - f_{G_j}$ for an unaffected individual.

Table 2

IBD Transition Probabilities $P(I_{m+1}|I_m)$ for a Sib Pair

	$P(I_{m+1}\|I_m)$ FOR		
I_m	$I_{m+1} = 0$	$I_{m+1} = 1$	$I_{m+1} = 2$
0	ψ_m^2	$2\psi_m(1-\psi_m)$	$(1-\psi_m)^2$
1	$\psi_m(1-\psi_m)$	$\psi_m^2 + (1-\psi_m)^2$	$\psi_m(1-\psi_m)$
2	$(1-\psi_m)^2$	$2\psi_m(1-\psi_m)$	ψ_m^2

NOTE.—$\psi_m = \theta_m^2 + (1-\theta_m)^2$, where θ_m is the recombination fraction between loci m and $m+1$.

Table 3

Relationship of Disease Locus and Candidate SNP

Likelihood	Linkage	Disease-SNP Relationship	r^2	Parameters[a]	Constraints[a]
L_{UL}	Unlinked	Linkage equilibrium	0	p_A	$0<p_A<1$
L_{LE}	Completely linked	Linkage equilibrium	0	z_0, z_1, p_A	$0 \leq z_1 \leq 0.5$; $0 \leq z_0 \leq 0.5z_1$; $0<p_A<1$
L_{LD}	Completely linked	Complete LD	1	$f_{dd}, f_{Dd}, f_{DD}, p=p_D=p_A$	$0 \leq f_{dd}, f_{Dd}, f_{DD} \leq 1$; $0<p<1$
L_{GM}	Completely linked	Any level of LD	[0, 1]	$f_{dd}, f_{Dd}, f_{DD}, p_{DA}, p_{Da}, p_{dA}$	$0 \leq f_{dd}, f_{Dd}, f_{DD} \leq 1$; $0 \leq p_{DA}, p_{Da}, p_{dA} \leq 1$; $0 \leq p_{DA}+p_{Da}+p_{dA} \leq 1$

[a] Disease penetrances f_{dd}, f_{Dd}, and f_{DD} are assumed to be not all equal.

The Relationship between Disease Locus and Candidate SNP

A useful measure of LD between two loci is the squared statistical correlation, defined as $r^2 = (p_{DA} - p_Dp_A)^2/[p_D(1-p_D)p_A(1-p_A)]$ in a sample of phased haplotypes. Multiplying r^2 by the sample size yields the χ^2 statistic for comparison of allele frequencies between cases and controls in a random population sample. r^2 measures the degree of LD between the candidate SNP and the putative disease locus, as represented by the observed linkage signal, and can quantify the degree to which the linkage signal is explained by the candidate SNP. The candidate SNP and the putative disease locus can be in linkage equilibrium ($r^2 = 0$), complete LD ($r^2 = 1$), or partial LD ($0<r^2<1$). Under linkage equilibrium, the candidate SNP is not associated with the putative disease locus and plays no causal role in the linkage signal. Under complete LD, the candidate SNP or a marker in complete LD with it can fully account for the linkage signal; we call this model "plausible causality." Under partial LD, the candidate SNP partially accounts for the linkage signal.

We parameterize our models by using three penetrances, f_{dd}, f_{Dd}, and f_{DD}, in addition to (1) allele frequencies p_D and p_A for the linkage equilibrium model, (2) single-allele frequency $p = p_D = p_A$ for the complete LD model, and (3) haplotype frequencies p_{DA}, p_{Da}, and p_{dA} for the general model. Given only ASPs, each of these models is identifiable, except the linkage equilibrium model, in which parameters (f_{dd}, f_{Dd}, f_{DD}, p_D, and p_A) are not all identifiable, because the data contain information for only p_A and $\mathbf{z} = (z_0,z_1,z_2)$, corresponding to a total of 3 df, since $z_0 + z_1 + z_2 = 1$. To achieve an identifiable model, note that, under linkage equilibrium, $P(X_{SNP}, I_D|ASP) = P(X_{SNP}|I_D)P(I_D|ASP)$ and that $P(X_{SNP}|I_D)$ depends on only p_A. Thus, the linkage equilibrium model can be reparameterized in terms of (z_0,z_1,p_A), resulting in a likelihood similar to the traditional maximum LOD score (MLS) linkage test (Risch 1990) but with an additional parameter, p_A. Here, we assume that the candidate SNP is completely linked to the putative disease locus. In theory, one could allow recombination between the candidate SNP and the putative disease locus as well. However, there is confounding between recombination and IBD sharing at the SNP (Risch 1990). A commonly used approach to avoid confounding in multipoint MLS calculation is to assume no recombination. IBD-sharing probabilities $\mathbf{z} = (z_0,z_1,z_2)$ should satisfy the triangle constraint $0 \leq z_1 \leq 0.5$ and $0 \leq z_0 \leq 0.5z_1$ (Holmans 1993).

The previous models assume that the candidate SNP is completely linked to the putative disease locus. If the

Table 4

Characteristics of Simulated Disease Models

	$\lambda_s = 1.1$						$\lambda_s = 1.3$					
MODEL	f_{dd}	f_{Dd}	f_{DD}	p_D	AF[a]	GRR	f_{dd}	f_{Dd}	f_{DD}	p_D	AF[a]	GRR
Dominant	.017	.047	.047	.05	.148	2.78	.015	.067	.067	.05	.256	4.53
	.014	.035	.035	.15	.283	2.42	.010	.046	.046	.15	.490	4.46
	.010	.029	.029	.30	.478	2.79	.003	.036	.036	.30	.828	10.41
Recessive	.019	.019	.261	.05	.030	13.48	.019	.019	.438	.05	.052	23.12
	.018	.018	.094	.15	.085	5.15	.017	.017	.149	.15	.148	8.72
	.017	.017	.053	.30	.165	3.19	.014	.014	.078	.30	.285	5.43
Additive	.017	.046	.075	.05	.145	2.70, 4.39	.015	.065	.115	.05	.251	4.36, 7.71
	.015	.032	.050	.15	.266	2.21, 3.41	.011	.041	.072	.15	.460	3.84, 6.68
	.012	.026	.039	.30	.414	2.18, 3.36	.006	.030	.053	.30	.717	5.23, 9.45

NOTE.—Population disease prevalence K was fixed at 2%.

[a] AF = attributable fraction.

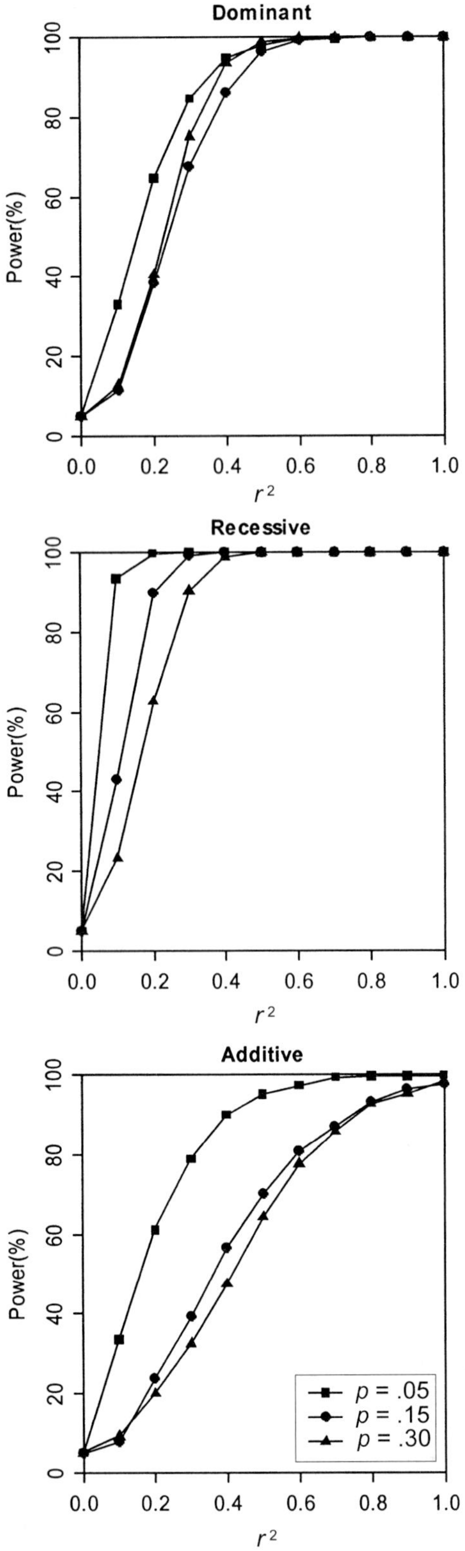

Figure 1 Power to reject linkage equilibrium ($r^2 = 0$). Results are based on 2,000 replicates of 500 ASPs. All models have population disease prevalence $K = 2\%$ and sibling recurrence-risk ratio $\lambda_s = 1.1$. Power was assessed at the 5% level.

candidate SNP is unlinked, then IBD-sharing probabilities at the SNP should be $\mathbf{z} = (1/4, 1/2, 1/4)$, and the only estimable parameter is p_A. As such, the relationship between the candidate SNP and the putative disease locus falls into one of four models (table 3).

For a sample of independent ASPs, the retrospective likelihood of the data is

$$L = \prod P(X|\mathrm{ASP}) \ , \qquad (4)$$

where the product is taken over all independent ASPs. Here, we chose to use a retrospective likelihood because the data are ascertained through the disease-affection statuses of the ASPs. The use of a retrospective likelihood can avoid the problem of ascertainment bias so that the parameter estimates are valid for the general population. To maximize equation (4), we use a simplex algorithm (Nelder and Mead 1965), an optimization method that does not require derivatives. Below, we represent the maximum of a particular likelihood subject to its parameter constraints by $\hat{L}$. In addition, we estimate r^2 from frequency estimates of disease-SNP haplotype frequencies. The estimate of r^2 is of particular interest in the case of partial disease-SNP LD; it reflects the degree to which a linkage result is explained by the candidate SNP.

Likelihood-Ratio Statistic

Given different relationships between the candidate SNP and the disease locus, we can test for linkage, association, and plausible causality. We evaluate evidence for linkage with $\mathrm{MLS} = \log_{10}(\hat{L}_{\mathrm{LE}}) - \log_{10}(\hat{L}_{\mathrm{UL}})$ (see table 3 for explanations of L_{LE}, L_{UL}, L_{GM}, and L_{LD}). We evaluate evidence for association by testing whether the candidate SNP is in linkage equilibrium with the disease locus by use of the likelihood-ratio statistic $T_{LE} = 2[\ln(\hat{L}_{\mathrm{GM}}) - \ln(\hat{L}_{\mathrm{LE}})]$. Rejection of linkage equilibrium between the disease and SNP loci suggests the candidate SNP is associated with the disease locus and can account (in part) for the observed linkage signal. We examine plausible causality by testing whether the candidate SNP is in complete LD with the disease locus by use of the likelihood-ratio statistic $T_{\mathrm{LD}} = 2[\ln(\hat{L}_{\mathrm{GM}}) - \ln(\hat{L}_{\mathrm{LD}})]$. Rejection of complete LD for an associated SNP suggests that the SNP cannot fully account for the observed linkage signal. If there is a single disease causal variant in the region, then it must be another SNP; otherwise, there might be other disease causal variants in the region.

Empirical Null Distributions for Tests of Linkage Equilibrium and Complete LD

The asymptotic distributions of T_{LE} and T_{LD} under the null hypotheses might, in principle, be approximated by

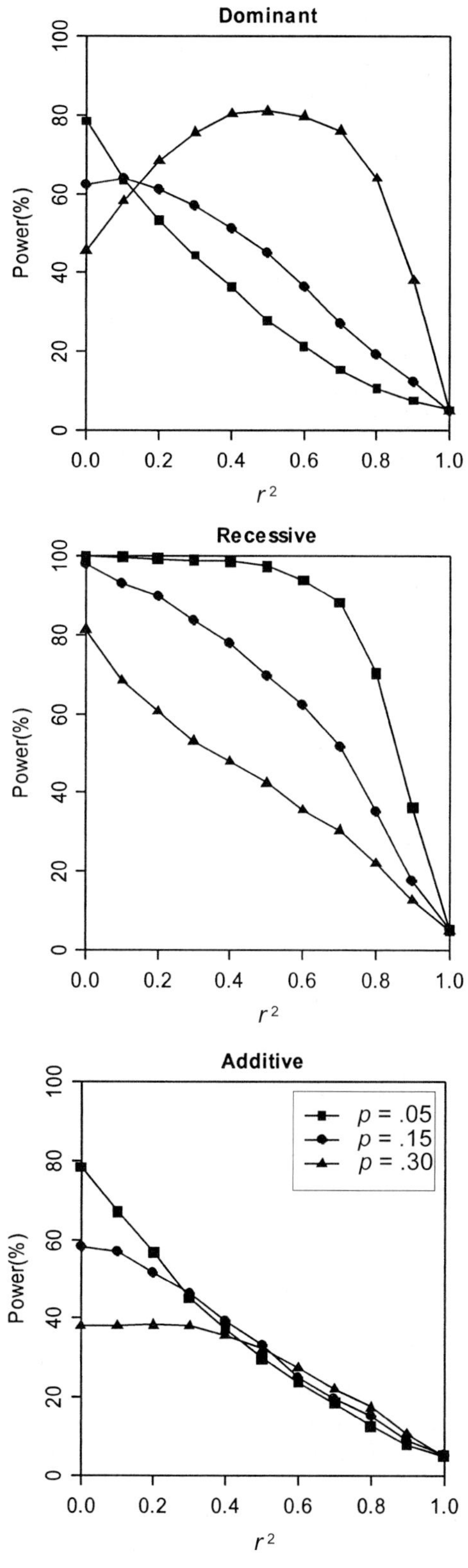

Figure 2 Power to reject complete LD ($r^2 = 1$). Results are based on 2,000 replicates of 500 ASPs. All models have population disease prevalence $K = 2\%$ and sibling recurrence-risk ratio $\lambda_s = 1.3$. Power was assessed at the 5% level.

a mixture of χ^2 distributions (Self and Liang 1987), but we have not derived the degrees of freedom and mixing parameters, because of the complexity of parameter constraints and boundaries. Alternatively, the significance of the tests can be assessed empirically by simulating marker genotypes under the null hypothesis and comparing the observed statistic with the simulated null distribution. One possibility would be to estimate disease-locus parameters and marker-allele frequencies under the null hypothesis and then to simulate genotypes for the candidate SNP and flanking markers conditional on the estimated parameters and observed phenotypes. In our preliminary investigations, this approach led to inflated type I error rates (data not shown), and we describe below, in detail, alternative strategies that may be theoretically less efficient but perform well in all the settings we examined.

For the T_{LE} statistic, employed when the null hypothesis assumes linkage equilibrium between trait and marker loci, we sample SNP genotypes conditional on flanking-marker genotypes and estimated model parameters. In contrast, for the T_{LD} statistic, employed when the null hypothesis assumes complete LD between the candidate SNP alleles and disease-susceptibility alleles, we sample flanking-marker genotypes conditional on the observed candidate SNP genotypes and estimated parameters.

For the linkage-equilibrium model, we use the observed data to obtain the SNP allele-frequency estimate $\hat{p}_A$ and the IBD-sharing probability estimates $\hat{\mathbf{z}} = (\hat{z}_0,\hat{z}_1,\hat{z}_2)$ at the candidate SNP. To obtain a simulated sample under linkage equilibrium, for each ASP, we retain flanking-marker data and simulate the IBD configuration at the candidate SNP in accordance with

$$P(I_D|X_1,\ldots,X_M,\mathrm{ASP}) \propto P(X_1,\ldots,X_k|I_D)P(X_{k+1},\ldots,X_M|I_D)\hat{z}_{I_D}\ ,$$

for $I_D = 0,1,2$ and where $P(X_1,\ldots,X_k|I_D)$ and $P(X_{k+1},\ldots,X_M|I_D)$ are the left- and right-chain probabilities calculated in equation (1). Given the IBD configuration at the candidate SNP, the ASP's candidate-SNP genotypes can then be sampled on the basis of the estimated candidate-SNP allele frequency, $\hat{p}_A$. Note that, when flanking-marker genotypes are not available, $P(X_1,\ldots,X_k|I_D) = P(X_{k+1},\ldots,X_M|I_D) = 1$, so that sampling is conditional on only the estimated parameter values and phenotypes. We obtain the null distribution of T_{LE} by simulating a large number of replicates and calculating the statistic for each simulated data set.

Our procedure for simulating the null distribution of T_{LD} is different. Note that, if the candidate SNP is in complete LD with the disease locus alleles (or it is the disease locus itself), then candidate SNP genotypes should be sufficient to explain IBD sharing in the region.

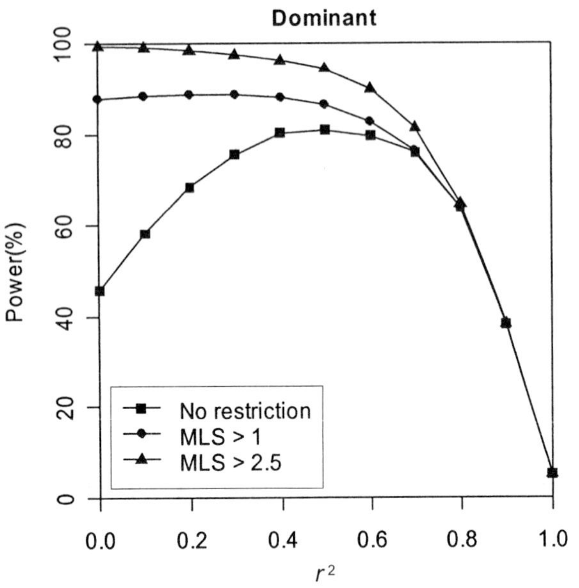

Figure 3 Impact of linkage evidence on test of complete LD. Results are based on 2,000 replicates of 500 ASPs under a dominant model with population disease prevalence $K = 2\%$, allele frequency $p_D = p_A = 0.30$, and sibling recurrence-risk ratio $\lambda_s = 1.3$. Power was assessed at the 5% level.

This observation has previously been used by Sun et al. (2002), who calibrated the significance of their test by sampling flanking-marker genotypes conditional on the observed SNP genotypes for each ASP. For each ASP, we leave the candidate SNP genotypes for the ASP unchanged from their observed values. Then, we sample an IBD configuration at the candidate SNP conditional on the observed SNP genotypes for the ASP and the estimated parameters $(\tilde{f}_{dd}, \tilde{f}_{Dd}, \tilde{f}_{DD})$ and $\tilde{p} = \tilde{p}_D = \tilde{p}_A$ obtained from the complete LD model in accordance with

$$P(I_D|X_{\mathrm{SNP}},\mathrm{ASP}) \propto P(X_{\mathrm{SNP}},I_D|\mathrm{ASP}) \ ,$$

which can be obtained from equation (2). Finally, we sample genotypes for flanking markers, conditional on the IBD configuration at the candidate SNP. Specifically, we sample genotypes at marker k in accordance with transition probabilities $P(I_k|I_D)$ and the allele frequencies of marker k. The genotypes of marker $k+1$ are sampled similarly but with transition probabilities $P(I_{k+1}|I_D)$. Moving left and right along the chromosome, we simulate flanking-marker genotypes on the basis of $P(I_{m-1}|I_m)$ and $P(I_{m+1}|I_m)$, respectively. We obtain the null distribution of T_{LD} by simulating a large number of replicates and calculating the statistic for each simulated data set. This procedure for generating the empirical distribution of T_{LD} has some limitations. In particular, when there are no flanking markers, our procedure leaves the original data unchanged, and so it is not possible to evaluate the significance of a particular value for T_{LD}. Nevertheless, and as shown in the "Results" section, flanking markers provide most of the information required to distinguish between markers in complete LD and those in partial LD with the disease locus; thus, the distribution of T_{LD} when there are no flanking markers is of little practical interest.

Simulations

We conducted a number of simulations to explore the properties of our proposed tests of no association and plausible causality and the resulting estimates of genetic model parameters. Table 4 describes the disease models we considered, which varied over a range of attributable fractions, disease-allele frequencies, GRRs, and sibling recurrence-risk ratio λ_s, defined as the recurrence risk for a sib of an affected individual divided by the population disease prevalence (Risch 1987). For all disease models, the population prevalence K of the disease was fixed at 2%.

In each model, we assumed the disease- and SNP-allele frequencies to be identical and, except where noted, used a map of 10 markers with eight equally frequent alleles (heterozygosity [H] of .875) evenly spaced at 11.16-cM intervals, corresponding to recombination fraction 0.10 under the no-interference map function of Haldane (1919). We centered the disease and SNP loci in the middle of the map and assumed zero recombination between them. We removed disease-locus genotypes prior to data analysis. For each of the disease models in table 4, we simulated 5,000 replicates of 500 ASPs under linkage equilibrium or complete LD to obtain null distributions and to determine critical values for each test. We simulated 2,000 replicates of 500 ASPs with various levels of disease-SNP LD to assess the empirical power of the corresponding tests. Here, we simulated the null distributions by using their generating values. In the "Discussion" section, we consider the impact of the use of null distributions estimated using our computationally intensive resampling procedures.

Results

Power to Reject Linkage Equilibrium (No Association)

Figure 1 displays the estimated power to reject the hypothesis of linkage equilibrium as a function of r^2 for the disease models in table 4. As expected, the power of T_{LE} increases as r^2 increases, for all disease models, and it is at its maximum when $r^2 = 1$. Figure 1 also shows that, for models with the same λ_s, it is relatively easier to detect association for a less-common disease allele than for a common one. More generally, we found that the power of the test is closely related to the GRR. We found that, for a fixed λ_s, lower disease-allele frequencies

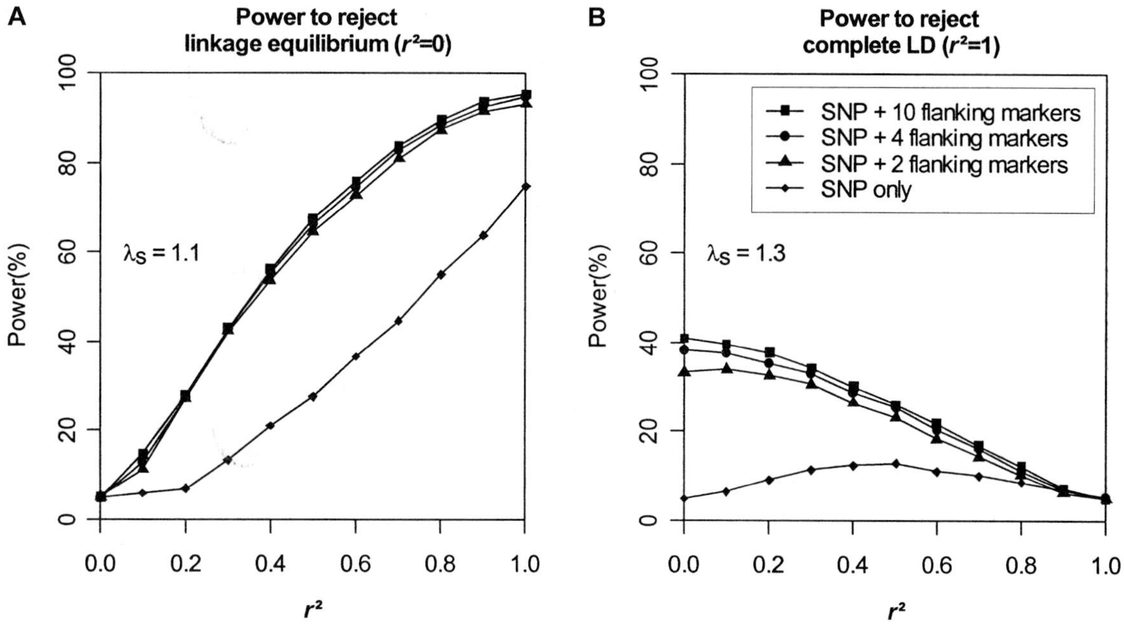

Figure 4 Impact of the number of flanking markers. Results are based on 2,000 replicates of 500 ASPs simulated under an additive model with population disease prevalence $K = 2\%$, allele frequency $p_D = p_A = 0.15$, and sibling recurrence-risk ratios $\lambda_s = 1.1$ (*A*) and 1.3 (*B*). Data were simulated using 10 flanking markers, each with two equally frequent alleles. Intermarker recombination fraction is 0.1. Power was assessed at the 5% level.

generally corresponded to a higher GRR for the disease models we considered.

These simulation results indicate that our method has good power to detect whether a candidate SNP is associated with the putative disease locus, even when the genetic effect is modest ($\lambda_s = 1.1$). In each set of simulations, we found that the power of the test of linkage equilibrium to detect disease-SNP association does not depend on the magnitude of the observed linkage signal. Our results show that, given the same genetic effect as measured by λ_s, the power of T_{LE} estimated using replicates with smaller MLS is nearly identical to the power of T_{LE} estimated using replicates with larger MLS. For complex diseases with modest genetic effects, increased sharing near a disease locus can be overwhelmed by sampling variation in IBD estimates. Even when the evidence for linkage is absent, our method still yields a valid and useful test of association.

Power to Reject Complete LD (Plausible Causality)

Intuitively, one would expect the power to reject the hypothesis of complete LD to increase as r^2 decreases from 1, with maximum power when $r^2 = 0$. Figure 2 shows that the simulation results agree well with this expectation for our recessive and additive models but not for our dominant models. In our simulations, we found that the magnitude of the T_{LD} statistic is highly correlated with the MLS when r^2 is low, and the dependence becomes less strong as r^2 increases. To illustrate this effect, we estimated power using those replicate data sets in which MLS is >1 or >2.5 for a dominant model with $p_D = p_A = 0.30$ and $\lambda_s = 1.3$. Figure 3 suggests that our ability to detect complete LD is dramatically enhanced as the MLS increases. For example, when $r^2 = 0$, the power is 46% given no minimum MLS requirement but increases to 88% when MLS >1 and increases to nearly 100% when MLS >2.5.

In general, determining that a SNP is not in complete LD with the disease allele is more difficult than detecting whether it is associated with the disease allele, and it generally requires a larger sample. Our simulation results suggest that, at the same level of genetic effect as measured by λ_s, it is easier to evaluate whether a SNP might be in complete LD with the disease allele if the disease is recessive. This might be because the ASPs are more likely to share two alleles IBD under a recessive model than under a dominant model, and such excess IBD sharing provides more information on linkage. Since the power of T_{LD} depends strongly on the magnitude of the observed linkage signal, this situation provides greater power to evaluate whether a candidate SNP is plausibly causal.

Parameter Estimates

Our method yields maximum-likelihood estimates of the disease-SNP haplotype frequencies directly, and,

Table 5

Results for Additive Model

$p_D = p_A$, r^2, and ASPs	MEAN (EMPIRICAL SD) VALUE							
	$\lambda_s = 1.1$				$\lambda_s = 1.3$			
	$\hat{P}_D$	$\hat{P}_A$	$\hat{\lambda}_S$	$\hat{r}^2$	$\hat{P}_D$	$\hat{P}_A$	$\hat{\lambda}_S$	$\hat{r}^2$
$p_D = p_A = .05$:								
$r^2 = .00$:								
500	.28 (.17)	.09 (.04)	1.08 (.07)	.28 (.36)	.23 (.13)	.08 (.06)	1.22 (.10)	.17 (.29)
2,000	.25 (.12)	.07 (.02)	1.08 (.04)	.16 (.23)	.20 (.08)	.07 (.03)	1.24 (.06)	.13 (.25)
$r^2 = .33$:								
500	.22 (.22)	.07 (.02)	1.11 (.06)	.31 (.33)	.11 (.15)	.07 (.02)	1.28 (.12)	.40 (.28)
2,000	.16 (.09)	.06 (.02)	1.10 (.04)	.35 (.29)	.05 (.06)	.06 (.02)	1.27 (.06)	.38 (.22)
$r^2 = .67$:								
500	.09 (.13)	.06 (.02)	1.13 (.07)	.55 (.37)	.05 (.03)	.06 (.02)	1.30 (.09)	.56 (.32)
2,000	.06 (.03)	.06 (.01)	1.11 (.03)	.65 (.30)	.04 (.02)	.06 (.01)	1.29 (.05)	.56 (.28)
$r^2 = 1.00$:								
500	.06 (.04)	.06 (.02)	1.15 (.07)	.64 (.33)	.05 (.02)	.06 (.02)	1.34 (.09)	.67 (.34)
2,000	.05 (.02)	.06 (.01)	1.12 (.03)	.69 (.31)	.04 (.01)	.06 (.01)	1.31 (.04)	.74 (.32)
$p_D = p_A = .30$:								
$r^2 = .00$:								
500	.48 (.22)	.34 (.08)	1.06 (.05)	.40 (.33)	.47 (.18)	.34 (.07)	1.17 (.11)	.20 (.24)
2,000	.45 (.12)	.34 (.03)	1.03 (.03)	.33 (.28)	.44 (.07)	.33 (.03)	1.16 (.05)	.08 (.11)
$r^2 = .33$:								
500	.33 (.15)	.33 (.06)	1.08 (.06)	.48 (.31)	.31 (.15)	.32 (.06)	1.21 (.10)	.44 (.27)
2,000	.31 (.10)	.32 (.03)	1.05 (.03)	.46 (.27)	.30 (.11)	.32 (.03)	1.20 (.05)	.38 (.18)
$r^2 = .67$:								
500	.28 (.12)	.33 (.06)	1.12 (.06)	.56 (.30)	.28 (.10)	.32 (.06)	1.27 (.10)	.65 (.27)
2,000	.27 (.08)	.32 (.03)	1.09 (.03)	.64 (.24)	.29 (.06)	.32 (.03)	1.26 (.05)	.68 (.18)
$r^2 = 1.00$:								
500	.27 (.10)	.32 (.06)	1.15 (.06)	.64 (.30)	.28 (.06)	.32 (.06)	1.34 (.11)	.82 (.23)
2,000	.27 (.06)	.31 (.03)	1.13 (.03)	.73 (.22)	.29 (.03)	.31 (.03)	1.32 (.05)	.90 (.13)

NOTE.—Results are based on 2,000 replicates of data sets simulated under an additive model with population disease prevalence $K = 2\%$.

from those, we can calculate estimates of LD measures, such as r^2. Mean parameter estimates and empirical SDs for the additive model, given 500 and 2,000 ASPs, are listed in table 5. The bias of parameter estimates is similar for dominant and recessive models (data not shown).

The bias of the maximum-likelihood allele-frequency estimates generally decreases as r^2 increases to values close to 1, corresponding to greater information about the disease locus. Maximum-likelihood estimates are asymptotically unbiased under appropriate regularity conditions, notably when no null hypothesis parameter value is on the boundary of the parameter space. In our case, $r^2 = 1$ results in two disease-SNP haplotypes with a frequency of 0, so our parameter estimates may be biased even in large samples. From table 5, we see that, when $r^2 = 1$, p_D can be underestimated and λ_s is slightly overestimated, with the bias decreasing as the sample size and magnitude of genetic effect increase.

Impact of Flanking Markers

To investigate the impact of flanking-marker data on our tests of disease-SNP LD, we simulated additional data sets using a map of 10 flanking markers, each with two equally frequent alleles ($H = .50$). We analyzed each of our data sets using 0, 2, 4, or all 10 flanking markers. Figure 4 suggests that having at least two flanking markers improves performance for both tests, but especially for the test of complete LD. Results based on 2, 4, or 10 flanking markers show only slight differences. Note that results are presented in figure 4*B* for the evaluation of the significance of T_{LD} when there are no flanking markers. Although this is possible for a simulation study such as this (in which the true population parameter values are known and were used to simulate the null distribution of the statistic), it is not practical for analysis of real data, since our procedure for evaluating the empirical distribution of T_{LD} requires information on flanking markers. In practice, this is not a serious limitation, because T_{LD} has very low power when there are no flanking markers, and we recommend that it should be used only when at least two flanking markers are available.

We next assessed the impact of flanking-marker heterozygosity on power estimation by conducting additional simulations using two flanking markers, each with two ($H = .50$), four ($H = .75$), or eight ($H =$

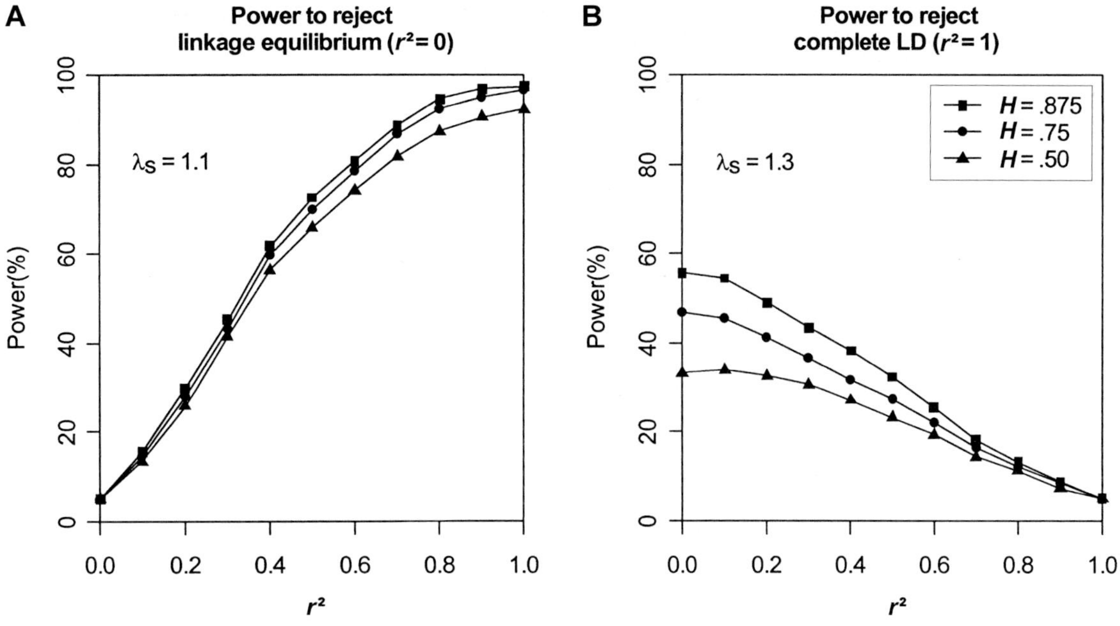

Figure 5 Impact of heterozygosity of flanking markers. Results are based on 2,000 replicates of 500 ASPs simulated under an additive model with population disease prevalence $K = 2\%$, allele frequency $p_D = p_A = 0.15$, and sibling recurrence-risk ratios $\lambda_s = 1.1$ (*A*) and 1.3 (*B*). Data were simulated using two flanking markers, each with two, four, or eight equally frequent alleles. Intermarker recombination fraction is 0.1. Power was assessed at the 5% level.

.875) equally frequent alleles. We found that, for the test of linkage equilibrium, the power for two and four equally frequent alleles is only slightly lower than for eight equally frequent alleles, but the difference in power is more pronounced for the test of complete LD (fig. 5). The differences between power for 2, 4, and 10 flanking markers when flanking-marker H was ≥ 0.75 were modest (data not shown), suggesting that even just two highly polymorphic flanking markers may provide substantial power to detect disease-SNP LD. The utility of even two flanking markers is especially helpful when linkage data are not available and additional genotyping is required.

We also evaluated the impact of flanking-marker densities on power (fig. 6) by simulating data sets using a map of 10 flanking markers, each with four equally frequent alleles ($H = .75$). Clearly, denser markers give greater power, but the increment of power is not substantial for the range of densities we considered. In practice, having flanking markers within ~10 cM should be enough for the initial evaluation of a candidate SNP.

Comparison of GIST and STEPC

Li et al. (2004) examined whether a SNP might account in part for an observed linkage signal by testing for a correlation between SNP genotypes and family-specific NPL scores. Their method is implemented in the software package GIST. Their simulations show that GIST is useful for identifying SNPs that are in LD with the disease locus and suggest that GIST could also identify associated SNPs in the absence of evidence for linkage. We compared our test of $r^2 = 0$ with GIST (table 6). We assessed the significance of T_{LE} at the 5% significance level by comparing the observed statistic with the empirical null distribution simulated in accordance with the resampling procedure described in the "Methods" section. Results are based on 500 replicates of 500 ASPs. For each replicate, the empirical null distribution of T_{LE} was obtained by resampling 1,000 times. The results indicate that our test has greater power than GIST for the models we considered. For example, our test has 89% power to reject linkage equilibrium when $r^2 = .67$ for an additive model with $p_D = p_A = 0.15$ and $\lambda_s = 1.1$ at the 5% significance level, whereas GIST has 76% power.

Sun et al. (2002) examined whether a SNP could fully explain the observed linkage signal and implemented their approach in the software package STEPC. The method of Sun et al. (2002) is based on the observation that if a SNP is the only variant in the region that influences the trait, then conditional on the affected relatives' SNP genotypes, there should be no increased IBD sharing in the region among affected individuals. We compared our test of $r^2 = 1$ with STEPC (table 6) by using 500 replicates of 500 ASPs. Again, the significance of T_{LD} was assessed empirically using the empirical null distribution simulation procedure for T_{LD} described in

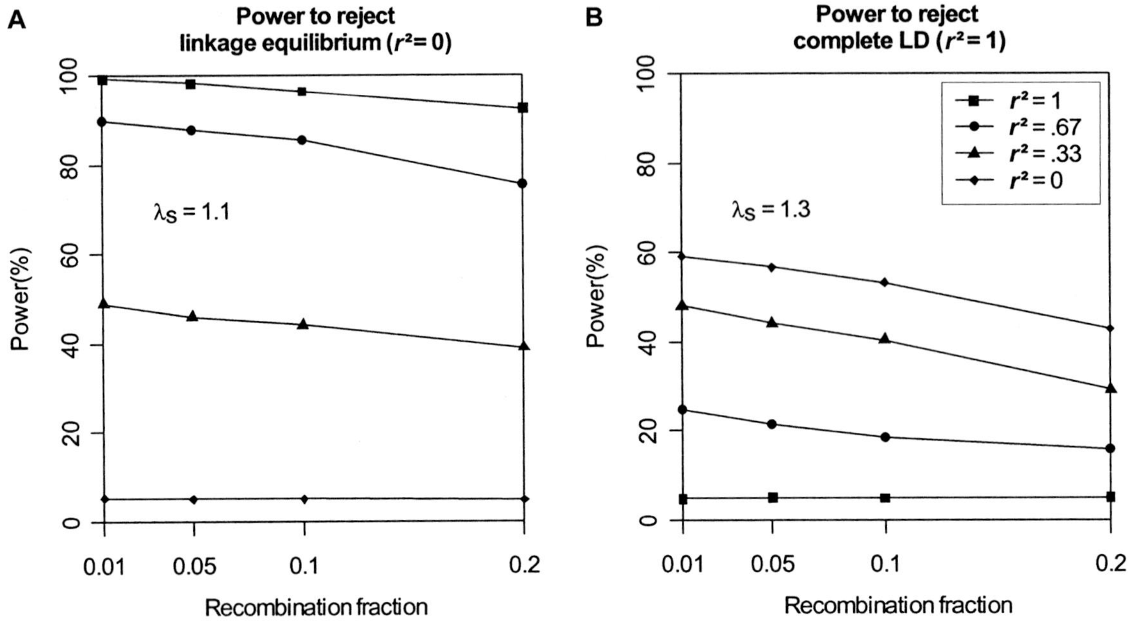

Figure 6 Impact of intermarker recombination of flanking markers. Results are based on 2,000 replicates of 500 ASPs simulated under an additive model with population disease prevalence $K = 2\%$, allele frequency $p_D = p_A = 0.15$, and sibling recurrence-risk ratios $\lambda_s = 1.1$ (*A*) and 1.3 (*B*). Data were simulated using 10 flanking markers, each with four equally frequent alleles. Power was assessed at the 5% level.

the "Methods" section. The two tests have nearly identical performance when $r^2 = 0$. However, the power of STEPC drops quickly as r^2 increases, so that, when SNPs are in moderate LD with the putative disease locus, our method has better resolving power and thus should identify a smaller set of potential explanatory SNPs.

Discussion

We have developed a statistical framework that quantifies the relationship between SNP alleles and unobserved trait alleles through joint modeling of linkage and association by use of ASP data. We described a parametric likelihood of the marker genotypes conditional on the trait data under the assumption that there is a single disease-causing variant in the region. Our unified likelihood framework naturally leads to two tests: (1) a test of whether a candidate SNP is in linkage equilibrium with the putative disease locus and (2) a test of whether the candidate SNP is in complete LD with the putative disease locus. In the first case, the rejection of linkage equilibrium suggests that the candidate SNP is associated with the putative disease locus and that the candidate SNP or one in LD with it accounts, at least in part, for the observed linkage signal. In the second case, the rejection of complete LD indicates that the candidate SNP cannot fully account for the linkage signal. Our method also yields estimates of interesting genetic parameters, including the disease-locus and SNP-allele frequencies, the locus-specific risk ratio λ_s, and the degree of disease-SNP LD. Our method uses ASPs and does not require parental genotypes. This feature is important for late-onset diseases, for which parents may not be available to study.

Simulation studies show that our method has good power to detect disease-SNP association, even when the sibling recurrence-risk ratio is as low as 1.1. We compared our test of linkage equilibrium with GIST (Li et al. 2004) and found our test to be more powerful in the models that we considered. The increase of power may come from the fact that our method is model-based, whereas GIST is nonparametric and is based on model-free NPL scores. Like GIST, the power of our test of linkage equilibrium does not depend on the overall strength of the linkage signal. Evidence of disease-SNP LD from our test also reveals underlying linkage, which might be overwhelmed by sampling variation in IBD estimates. This feature makes our method a useful tool for detecting linkage as well as association. We also compared our test of complete LD with STEPC (Sun et al. 2002) and found that the two tests have similar performance under linkage equilibrium, but our test has greater power to distinguish those SNPs that are in strong but incomplete LD with the putative disease locus.

In contrast to previous approaches (Sun et al. 2002; Li et al. 2004), our method yields disease-SNP haplotype-frequency estimates in the general population with-

Table 6

Comparisons with GIST and STEPC

	$r^2 = 0$				$r^2 = .33$				$r^2 = .67$				$r^2 = 1$			
λ_s, Test, and Model	T_{LE}	T_{LD}	GIST	STEPC	T_{LE}	T_{LD}	GIST	STEPC	T_{LE}	T_{LD}	GIST	STEPC	T_{LE}	T_{LD}	GIST	STEPC
1.1:																
Linkage equilibrium:																
Dominant	5	...	5	...	78	...	47	...	100	...	75	...	100	...	90	...
Recessive	6	...	5	...	100	...	95	...	100	...	100	...	100	...	100	...
Additive	5	...	5	...	54	...	46	...	89	...	76	...	98	...	87	...
1.3:																
Complete LD:																
Dominant	...	64	...	66	...	55	...	22	...	32	...	15	...	5	...	6
Recessive	...	97	...	98	...	82	...	62	...	57	...	27	...	5	...	5
Additive	...	56	...	58	...	44	...	26	...	24	...	12	...	6	...	5

NOTE.—Results are based on 500 replicates of 500 ASPs. All models have population disease prevalence $K = 2\%$ and allele frequency $p_D = p_A = 0.15$. Significance of T_{LE} and T_{LD} is assessed by comparing the observed statistics with the empirical null distributions generated in accordance with the resampling procedures described in the "Methods" section. Power is assessed at the 5% level.

out the requirement of a separate control sample. These quantities lead to the estimate of disease-SNP r^2, a measure that can be used to quantify the degree to which a linkage signal is explained by a candidate SNP. Our estimate of r^2 also provides information about the distance between the candidate SNP and the unobserved disease locus and helps refine the region in which further candidate SNPs should be examined. The disease-allele frequency estimate may be helpful to researchers in selecting additional nearby SNPs, by focusing on those with frequencies close to the predicted disease-allele frequency. This approach becomes increasingly useful as r^2 increases.

Our tests benefit from genotype information on flanking markers, which are available in many gene mapping studies. Our results show that even two highly polymorphic flanking markers can provide nearly as much information as many more markers for this purpose. Compared with other family-based association tests and a previous joint model of linkage and association (Göring and Terwilliger 2000), our model has the attractive feature of incorporating flanking-marker information when it is available. An alternative joint model of linkage and association was developed independently by Cantor et al. (2005). In contrast to our approach, theirs includes recombination as an additional parameter and fixes disease model parameters, including penetrances and the disease-allele frequency. Like the approach of Göring and Terwilliger (2000), the model of Cantor et al. (2005) does not readily incorporate genotype information contributed by flanking markers.

Since the test of linkage equilibrium does not depend strongly on the overall evidence of linkage, flanking-marker heterozygosity has less impact on power for this test than for the test of complete LD, which is highly dependent on the strength of linkage evidence. We assume linkage equilibrium between the flanking markers and the candidate SNP in our likelihood calculation. For flanking markers that are close together, they may show strong evidence of LD. For such data, we recommend selecting a small number of flanking markers in linkage equilibrium so that the linkage equilibrium assumption is satisfied.

The likelihood framework described in this article is applicable to dichotomous traits only. However, many disease-related traits—for instance, blood pressure and cholesterol level—are continuous in nature. Dichotomization can result in a loss of power of the corresponding tests. Fulker et al. (1999) developed a method that tests for linkage while simultaneously modeling allelic association by use of the variance-components framework. Their method was further extended to general pedigrees (Abecasis et al. 2000*a*; Cardon and Abecasis 2000). Attenuation of evidence for linkage when association to SNP alleles is modeled suggests that the candidate SNP accounts for linkage and provides information about unobserved trait alleles. Although these methods provide bounds on disease-allele frequencies and disease-marker LD (Cardon and Abecasis 2000), they provide no direct estimate of these quantities. To address the same question for quantitative traits, we plan to develop a statistical framework that summarizes the available information by a retrospective likelihood, with the putative trait locus and the SNP haplotype frequencies as parameters.

In most gene mapping studies, the ASPs are likely to be selected from a sample that was originally collected for linkage analysis and for which flanking-marker genotypes are available. Our likelihood calculation naturally allows for missing genotypes at the candidate SNP. Given fixed genotyping resources, researchers may initially type many SNPs in only one sib per ASP. This approach halves the genotyping costs, and additional

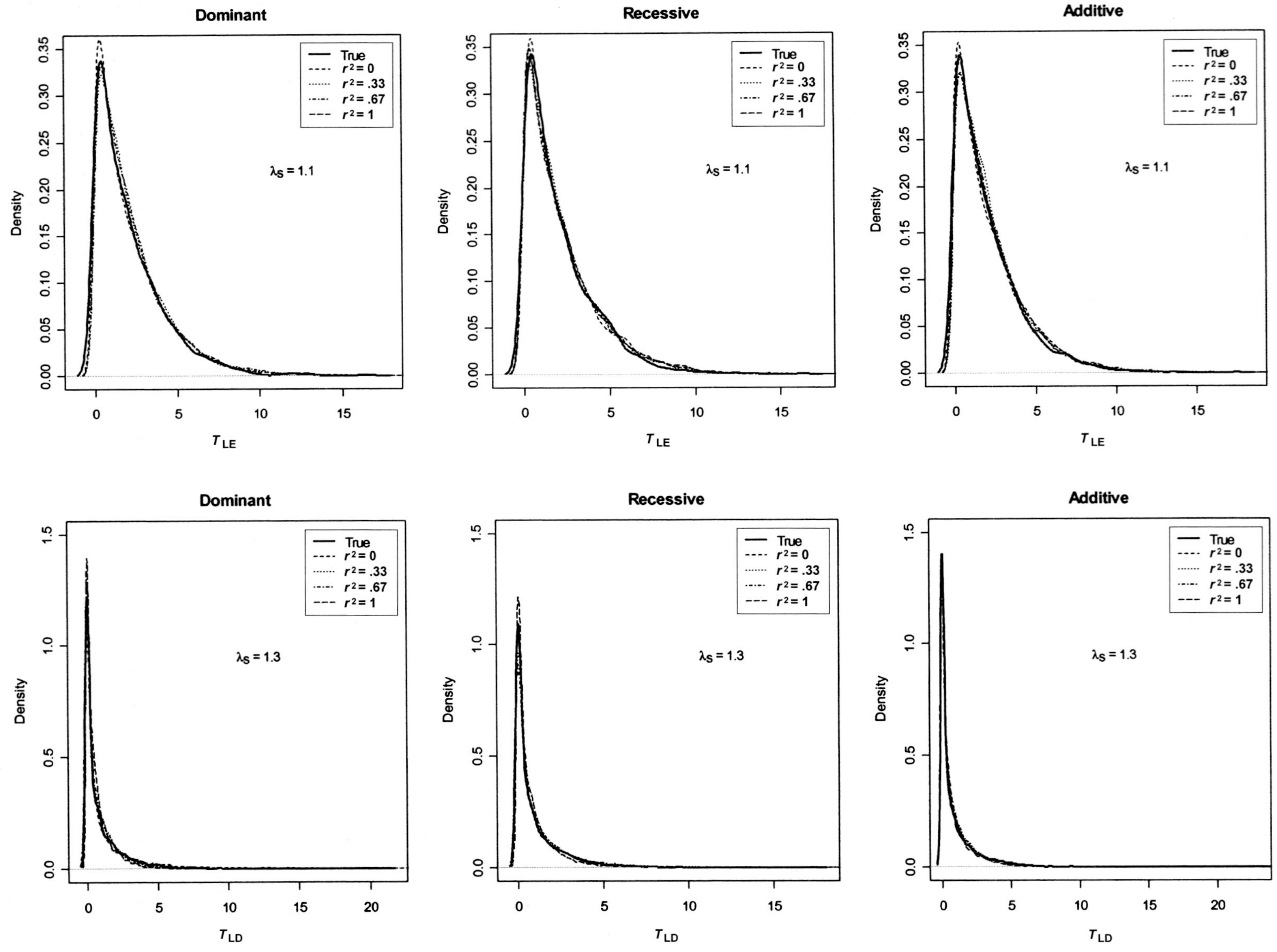
Dominant
Recessive
Additive
True
r² = 0
r² = .33
r² = .67
r² = 1
λS = 1.1
λS = 1.3
Density
T LE
T LD

simulations suggested that even one sib per ASP can provide meaningful information on whether a candidate SNP is associated with the disease locus. This suggests that, for an initial screen of SNPs, it may be cost effective to genotype only one sib per ASP, with genotyping of the other sibs done when a candidate SNP shows at least suggestive evidence of association.

In our simulations, we assessed the empirical power of T_{LE} and T_{LD} by simulating the null distributions generated using the true parameter values. For real data sets, these values are unknown, and the null distributions must be generated using the estimated parameter values. We described simulation procedures to obtain the empirical null distributions. For the test of linkage equilibrium, we simulate the SNP genotypes for each ASP, conditional on their flanking-marker genotypes, and leave the flanking-marker genotypes unchanged from their observed values. For the test of complete LD, we leave the SNP genotypes unchanged and simulate the flanking-marker genotypes, conditional on the observed SNP genotypes, to remove excess sharing explained by the flanking markers. The difference in these two simulation procedures is due to the inherent difference of the two tests. Under linkage equilibrium, the candidate SNP provides no information on the unobserved disease locus, and the SNP genotypes can be sampled by gene-dropping simulations. In contrast, under complete LD, the candidate SNP is statistically identical to the unobserved disease locus, and the SNP genotypes need to be preserved to retain complete information on the unobserved disease locus.

We examined the performance of our null distribution simulation procedures and found that the simulated null distributions for both tests agree well with those generated in accordance with their true parameter values at all levels of disease-SNP LD and that both simulation procedures give correct type I errors (fig. 7). Evaluation of the significance of our tests by use of their simulated null distributions can be computationally intensive in practice, especially when the sample size is large. For an initial screen of SNPs, one might choose to evaluate the significance of the linkage equilibrium test empirically only if $T_{LE} \geqslant 3.84$ (at the 5% significance level), since χ_1^2 approximates the lower bound for the asymptotic distribution of T_{LE}, and one may test whether a candidate SNP is potentially causal only if it shows significant evidence of association.

We described our likelihood framework in the context of ASPs, but our method can be readily extended to other study designs. We are extending our method to sibships of arbitrary size and disease-phenotype configuration and to include unrelated affected or unaffected individuals. Unaffected individuals are more representative of the general population and may help to infer the underlying genetic model parameters. We expect the power of our test of linkage equilibrium to increase when unrelated unaffected individuals are added to the study.

Despite its flexibility, our method has limitations. Like all statistical methods, ours is unable to distinguish the true disease causal variant from an allele that is in complete LD with it. We assume that there is a single disease causal variant in the candidate region. However, many complex diseases are influenced by multiple genetic variants and are possibly the result of gene-gene and gene-environment interactions. Individual variants may be neither necessary nor sufficient to explain the effect of a single locus on disease susceptibility—for example, three independent SNPs, a frameshift variant, and two missense variants of *NOD2* were identified as determining susceptibility to inflammatory bowel disease (Hugot et al. 2001). If only one causal variant is assumed, then we expect our model to indicate that each variant is associated with the underlying disease loci but none is causal (i.e., for all, $0 < r^2 < 1$). For complex diseases that are influenced by multiple genetic variants, fitting the data under the assumption of a single-locus disease model is equivalent to testing the marginal effect of a specific locus. If the marginal effect of that locus is modest, then we may have limited power to detect association. For those cases, it might be desirable to develop a method that allows the analysis of two-locus or even multilocus disease models.

In summary, we have developed a unified likelihood framework to estimate useful genetic parameters and to test for both linkage equilibrium and complete LD between a candidate SNP and the putative disease locus. Results from these two tests complement each other in answering the question of whether the candidate SNP can account in part or in full for the observed linkage signal. An estimate of the disease-SNP LD provides a measure to quantify the degree of contribution of the candidate SNP to linkage evidence. Together with the disease locus and the SNP-allele frequency estimates, our method will be valuable in helping researchers to evaluate the role of a candidate SNP in disease susceptibility and to fine-map disease genes. We have implemented our method in a C++ program, which can be

Figure 7 Comparison of empirical null distributions. Results are based on 2,000 replicates of 500 ASPs. All models have population disease prevalence $K = 2\%$ and allele frequency $p_D = p_A = 0.15$. The solid line in each plot is the density of the empirical null distribution simulated using true parameter values of the disease model. Dashed lines are density plots of the empirical null distributions generated using the resampling procedures described in the "Methods" section. The empirical null distribution was generated for each level of disease-SNP LD.

downloaded from the University of Michigan Center for Statistical Genetics Web site.

Acknowledgments

This research is supported by National Institutes of Health grants HG00376 (to M.B.) and HG02651 (to G.R.A.). M.L. is currently supported by a University of Michigan Rackham predoctoral fellowship. We gratefully thank two anonymous reviewers for their valuable comments.

Electronic-Database Information

The URL for data presented herein is as follows:

University of Michigan Center for Statistical Genetics, http://csg.sph.umich.edu/

References

Abecasis GR, Cardon LR, Cookson WO (2000*a*) A general test of association for quantitative traits in nuclear families. Am J Hum Genet 66:279–292

Abecasis GR, Cookson WO, Cardon LR (2000*b*) Pedigree tests of transmission disequilibrium. Eur J Hum Genet 8:545–551

Allison DB (1997) Transmission disequilibrium tests for quantitative traits. Am J Hum Genet 60:676–690

Baum LE (1972) An inequality and associated maximization technique in statistical estimation for probabilistic functions of Markov processes. Inequalities 3:1–8

Boehnke M, Langefeld CD (1998) Genetic association mapping based on discordant sib pairs: the discordant-alleles test. Am J Hum Genet 62:950–961

Botstein D, Risch N (2003) Discovering genotypes underlying human phenotypes: past successes for mendelian disease, future approaches for complex diseases. Nat Genet Suppl 33:228–237

Cantor RM, Chen GK, Pajukanta P, Lange K (2005) Association testing in a linked region using large pedigrees. Am J Hum Genet 76:538–542

Cardon LR, Abecasis GR (2000) Some properties of a variance components model for fine-mapping quantitative trait loci. Behav Genet 30:235–243

Curtis D (1997) Use of siblings as controls in case-control association studies. Ann Hum Genet 61:319–333

Enattah NS, Sahi T, Savilahti E, Terwilliger JD, Peltonen L, Jarvela I (2002) Identification of a variant associated with adult-type hypolactasia. Nat Genet 30:233–237

Feder JN, Gnirke A, Thomas W, Tsuchihashi Z, Ruddy DA, Basava A, Dormishian F, et al (1996) A novel MHC class I–like gene is mutated in patients with hereditary haemochromatosis. Nat Genet 13:399–408

Fulker DW, Cherny SS, Sham PC, Hewitt JK (1999) Combined linkage and association sib-pair analysis for quantitative traits. Am J Hum Genet 64:259–267

Göring HHH, Terwilliger JD (2000) Linkage analysis in the presence of errors IV: joint pseudomarker analysis of linkage and/or linkage disequilibrium on a mixture of pedigrees and singletons when the mode of inheritance cannot be accurately specified. Am J Hum Genet 66:1310–1327

Haldane JBS (1919) The combination of linkage values and the calculation of distances between the loci of linked factors. J Genet 8:299–309

Holmans P (1993) Asymptotic properties of affected-sib-pair linkage analysis. Am J Hum Genet 52:362–374

Horikawa Y, Oda N, Cox NJ, Li X, Orho-Melander M, Hara M, Hinokio Y, et al (2000) Genetic variation in the gene encoding calpain-10 is associated with type 2 diabetes mellitus. Nat Genet 26:163–175

Hugot JP, Chamaillard M, Zouali H, Lesage S, Cézard JP, Belaiche J, Almer S, Tysk C, O'Morain CA, Gassull M, Binder V, Finkel Y, Cortot A, Modigliani R, Laurent-Puig P, Gower-Rousseau C, Macry J, Colombel JF, Sahbatou M, Thomas G (2001) Association of NOD2 leucine-rich repeat variants with susceptibility to Crohn's disease. Nature 411: 599–603

International HapMap Consortium (2003) The International HapMap Project. Nature 426:789–796

Li C, Scott LJ, Boehnke M (2004) Assessing whether an allele can account in part for a linkage signal: the genotype-IBD sharing test (GIST). Am J Hum Genet 74:418–431

Martin ER, Monks SA, Warren LL, Kaplan NL (2000) A test for linkage and association in general pedigrees: the pedigree disequilibrium test. Am J Hum Genet 67:146–154

Nelder JA, Mead R (1965) A simplex method for function minimization. Comput J 7:308–313

Ogura Y, Bonen DK, Inohara N, Nicolae DN, Chen FF, Ramos R, Britton H, Moran T, Karaliuskas R, Duerr RH, Achkar JP, Brant SR, Bayless TM, Kirschner BS, Hanauer SB, Nunez G, Cho JH (2001) A frameshift mutation in *NOD2* associated with susceptibility to Crohn's disease. Nature 411: 603–606

Oliphant A, Barker DL, Stuelpnagel JR, Chee MS (2002) BeadArray technology: enabling an accurate, cost-effective approach to high-throughput genotyping. Biotechniques Suppl:56–58, 60–61

Olivier M, Chuang LM, Chang MS, Chen YT, Pei D, Ranade K, de Witte A, Allen J, Tran N, Curb D, Pratt R, Neefs H, de Arruda Indig M, Law S, Neri B, Wang L, Cox DR (2002) High-throughput genotyping of single nucleotide polymorphisms using new biplex invader technology. Nucleic Acids Res 30:e53

Rabinowitz D (1997) A transmission disequilibrium test for quantitative traits. Hum Hered 47:342–350

Risch N (1987) Assessing the role of HLA-linked and unlinked determinants of disease. Am J Hum Genet 40:1–14

——— (1990) Linkage strategies for genetically complex traits. II. The power of affected relative pairs. Am J Hum Genet 46:229–241

Sachidanandam R, Weissman D, Schmidt SC, Kakol JM, Stein LD, Marth G, Sherry S, Mullikin JC, et al (2001) A map of human genome sequence variation containing 1.42 million single nucleotide polymorphisms. Nature 409:928–933

Self SG, Liang KY (1987) Asymptotic properties of maximum likelihood estimators and likelihood ratio tests under nonstandard conditions. J Am Statist Assoc 82:605–610

Spielman RS, Ewens WJ (1998) A sibship test for linkage in

the presence of association: the sib transmission/disequilibrium test. Am J Hum Genet 62:450–458
Spielman RS, McGinnis RE, Ewens WJ (1993) Transmission test for linkage disequilibrium: the insulin gene region and insulin-dependent diabetes mellitus (IDDM). Am J Hum Genet 52:506–516
Sun L, Cox NJ, McPeak MS (2002) A statistical method for identification of polymorphisms that explain a linkage result. Am J Hum Genet 70:399–411
Syvanen AC (2001) Assessing genetic variation: genotyping single nucleotide polymorphisms. Nat Rev Genet 2:930–942
Thompson EA (1975) The estimation of pairwise relationships. Ann Hum Genet 39:173–188

Candidate-Gene Screening and Association Analysis at the Autism-Susceptibility Locus on Chromosome 16p: Evidence of Association at *GRIN2A* and *ABAT*

Gabrielle Barnby,[1] Aaron Abbott,[1] Nuala Sykes,[1] Andrew Morris,[1] Daniel E. Weeks,[3] Richard Mott,[1] Janine Lamb,[1] Anthony J. Bailey,[2] Anthony P. Monaco,[1] and the International Molecular Genetics Study of Autism Consortium (IMGSAC)*

[1]Wellcome Trust Centre for Human Genetics, University of Oxford, and [2]Section of Child and Adolescent Psychiatry, University Department of Psychiatry, Park Hospital for Children, Oxford, United Kingdom; and [3]Departments of Human Genetics and Biostatistics, Graduate School of Public Health, University of Pittsburgh, Pittsburgh

Autism is a highly heritable neurodevelopmental disorder whose underlying genetic causes have yet to be identified. To date, there have been eight genome screens for autism, two of which identified a putative susceptibility locus on chromosome 16p. In the present study, 10 positional candidate genes that map to 16p11-13 were examined for coding variants: *A2BP1, ABAT, BFAR, CREBBP, EMP2, GRIN2A, MRTF-B, SSTR5, TBX6,* and *UBN1*. Screening of all coding and regulatory regions by denaturing high-performance liquid chromatography identified seven non-synonymous changes. Five of these mutations were found to cosegregate with autism, but the mutations are not predicted to have deleterious effects on protein structure and are unlikely to represent significant etiological variants. Selected variants from candidate genes were genotyped in the entire International Molecular Genetics Study of Autism Consortium collection of 239 multiplex families and were tested for association with autism by use of the pedigree disequilibrium test. Additionally, genotype frequencies were compared between 239 unrelated affected individuals and 192 controls. Patterns of linkage disequilibrium were investigated, and the transmission of haplotypes across candidate genes was tested for association. Evidence of single-marker association was found for variants in *ABAT, CREBBP,* and *GRIN2A*. Within these genes, 12 single-nucleotide polymorphisms (SNPs) were subsequently genotyped in 91 autism trios (one affected individual and two unaffected parents), and the association was replicated within *GRIN2A* (Fisher's exact test, $P < .0001$). Logistic regression analysis of SNP data across *GRIN2A* and *ABAT* showed a trend toward haplotypic differences between cases and controls.

Introduction

Autism is a severe neurodevelopmental disorder that affects reciprocal communication and social interaction and is associated with repetitive and stereotyped behaviors. Recent epidemiological studies have revised the population prevalence of autism upward from 4 in 10,000 to 9–11 in 10,000 (Chakrabarti and Fombonne 2001; Fombonne 2003), and the overall rate of pervasive developmental disorders is ~60 in 10,000 (Fombonne 2002). Autism is highly heritable and shows strong familial clustering, with a λ (sibling relative risk) of 75–100, although the mode of inheritance is complex (Bailey et al. 1995; Pickles et al. 1995). Autism is found in three-to-four times as many males as females, which suggests a possible sex-linked effect, but multivariate analysis of the phenotype in relatives does not support X-linked inheritance (Pickles et al. 2000). Moderate evidence of linkage to the X chromosome has been observed in two genome screens (Liu et al. 2001; Shao et al. 2002). A single mutation in each of the X-linked neuroligin genes *NLGN3* and *NLGN4* has also been reported, but the low frequency of the mutations makes it unlikely that they contribute significantly to autism etiology (Jamain et al. 2003; Stone et al. 2003; Vincent et al. 2004). Autism is associated with phenotypes of known etiologies in ~6% of cases, including fragile-X syndrome, epilepsy, neurofibromatosis, and tuberous sclerosis (Fombonne 2002). The increased comorbidity of these disorders with autism may indicate a contribution to the autism phenotype by disruption of a common neurological—although not necessarily genetic—pathway.

Recently, the IMGSAC performed a whole-genome screen of 83 affected sib pairs (ASPs). Thirteen loci that displayed evidence of linkage were subsequently genotyped for 152 sib pairs (IMGSAC 2001). The three high-

Received November 1, 2004; accepted for publication March 23, 2005; electronically published April 13, 2005.

Address for correspondence and reprints: Dr. Anthony P. Monaco, Wellcome Trust Centre for Human Genetics, University of Oxford, Roosevelt Drive, Oxford, OX3 7BN, United Kingdom. E-mail: anthony.monaco@well.ox.ac.uk

* IMGSAC members are listed in the Acknowledgments.

0002-9297/2005/7606-0005$15.00

Table 1

Candidate Genes Screened for Autism-Susceptibility Variants

Gene Symbol	Gene Name	Position[a]	GenBank Accession Number	Genomic Region (kb)	mRNA Length (bp)	No. of Exons
A2BP1	Ataxin 2–binding protein	6009132–7700843	NM_018723	420.449	2,279	16
ABAT	4-Aminobutyrate aminotransferase	8675992–8782887	BC031413	106.895	1,705	14
BFAR	Bifunctional apoptosis regulator	14634296–14670193	NM_016561	35.898	2,531	8
CREBBP	CREB-binding protein	3716569–3870712	NM_004380	154.144	8,694	32
EMP2	Epithelial membrane protein 2	10533475–10582040	NM_001424	48.566	690	4
GRIN2A	Glutamate receptor, ionotropic, NMDA 2A	9762922–10184112	NM_000833	421.191	6,293	14
MRTF-B	Myocardin-related transcription factor B	14235623–14268130	NM_014048	32.508	7,815	8
SSTR5	Somatostatin receptor 5	1068869–1069964	NM_001053	1.096	1,095	1
TBX6	T-box 6	30004582–30010709	NM_004608	6.128	2,468	9
UBN1	Ubinuclein 1	4842216–4872364	NM_016936	30.149	5,747	18

[a] From the May 2004 release of the International Human Genome Sequencing Consortium.

est-scoring loci detected were on 2q21-33 at *D2S2118,* with a multipoint maximum LOD score (MLS) of 3.74; 7q22.2-31.3 at *D7S477,* with a multipoint MLS of 3.20; and 16p11-13 at *D16S3102,* with a multipoint MLS of 2.93. Detailed analysis of sex-specific and parent-of-origin effects at these loci has recently been reported (Lamb et al. 2005). The linkage to chromosome 16p was found in male-male ASPs (MLS of 2.48 for 145 male-male ASPs vs. MLS of 0 for 74 male-female or female-female ASPs) (Lamb et al. 2005). *D16S3102* at the peak of linkage was physically mapped at 12.46 Mb in the May 2004 release of the Human Genome Sequence. Linkage overlapping the region on chromosome 16p, between 10 cM and 23 cM, has been reported by Philippe et al. (1999), with a multipoint MLS of 0.74 at 10.6 cM ($n = 51$ multiplex families). Additionally, trisomy of 16p and duplications mapping to 16p11.2 and 16p12.2 have been reported for individuals with autism traits (Finelli et al. 2004).

To identify the autism-susceptibility gene at 16p11-13, positional functional candidate genes were selected, and their coding sequences were screened by denaturing high-performance liquid chromatography (DHPLC) for 48 individuals (from multiplex families) who contributed to linkage on 16p11-13. Variants detected by DHPLC were further characterized by sequencing, and missense variants were tested for cosegregation with autism. The candidate genes that were examined in the present study are described in table 1.

In total, 38 SNPs were selected for genotyping in 239 multiplex families and were tested for association by use of the pedigree disequilibrium test (PDT). These included three SNPs in *TSC2; TSC2* maps to 16p13 and encodes one of the genes that cause tuberous sclerosis, which has been reported to be associated with autism. Following the suggestion that there is a phenotypic overlap between attention-deficit/hyperactivity disorder (ADHD) and autism, four SNPs previously analyzed in a study of ADHD that found linkage to chromosome 16p were also genotyped (Smalley et al. 2002; Ogdie et al. 2003, 2004), as shown in table 2. All SNPs were also genotyped for 192 controls, and the allele and genotype frequencies were compared with those of 239 unrelated affected individuals. SNP data were analyzed for linkage disequilibrium (LD), association with autism, and haplotype

Table 2

SNPs Genotyped in *TSC2* and below ADHD Linkage Peak

Genomic Region anddbSNP Number	Position[a]	Allele Variant
TSC2[b]:		
rs2516740	2037111	G→T
rs2074968	2050572	G→C
rs1051771	2078585	G→C
ADHD linkage peak[c]:		
rs153783	15509867	G→A
rs1125972	15514488	G→A
rs1065838	15535539	T→C
rs1107143	15594082	T→C

[a] From the May 2004 release of the International Human Genome Sequencing Consortium.

[b] The distance between *rs2516740* and *rs2074968* is 13,461 bp; the distance between *rs2074968* and *rs1051771* is 28,013 bp.

[c] The distance between *rs153783* and *rs1125972* is 4,621 bp; the distance between *rs1125972* and *rs1065838* is 21,051 bp; the distance between *rs1065838* and *rs1107143* is 58,543 bp.

transmission disequilibrium. Twelve SNPs that showed evidence of association were subsequently genotyped for 91 autism trios (one affected individual and two unaffected parents). Logistic regression analysis was performed for haplotypes from genes containing SNPs that showed evidence of association.

Description of Candidate Genes

GRIN2A (MIM 138253) and *SSTR5* are cell-surface receptors. *GRIN2A* encodes one of four N-methyl-D-aspartate (NMDA) receptor 2 subunits that form an NMDA-receptor channel. NMDA receptors have been shown to be involved in long-term potentiation (LTP), an activity associated with learning and memory. Targeted disruption of the mouse homologue of *GRIN2A*, *GluRε*, reduces LTP and produces other behavioral deficits (Sakimura et al. 1995). Evidence of association between a *GRIN2A* exon 5 polymorphism and ADHD has also been reported recently (Turic et al. 2004). *SSTR5* (MIM 182455) encodes a G-protein–coupled receptor for the inhibitory hormonal regulator somatostatin. There is evidence that somatostatin and its receptors are transiently expressed in developing neurons; they are thought to control cell migration. Lauritsen et al. (2003) have performed analysis of 12 polymorphisms in *SSTR5* in 79 families with autism but found no evidence of association.

Three of the genes screened are involved in transcriptional regulation. *TBX6* (MIM 602427) is a member of the T-box family that encodes transcription factors involved in the regulation of developmental processes and is expressed in discrete embryonic domains (Papapetrou et al. 1999). *UBN1* encodes a ubiquitously expressed nuclear protein found to interact with EB1 and c-Jun, which, in turn, interact with cellular promoters and transcription factors. *CREBBP* (MIM 600140) encodes a large protein of 2,442 aa and binds specifically to the protein-kinase-A–phosphorylated form of the CREB protein (Chrivia et al. 1993). *CREBBP* can activate transcription through its C-terminus and acts to augment the ability of phosphorylated CREB to activate cAMP-responsive genes, interacting directly with transcription factor IIB. Mutations in *CREBBP* are responsible for Rubenstein-Taybi syndrome (RTS [MIM 180849]), which is characterized by mental retardation and broad thumbs and halluces. RTS has been associated with autism-like features in a minority of cases (Hellings et al. 2002).

EMP2 (MIM 602334) and *BFAR* are involved in cell-cycle control. *EMP2* has high sequence similarity with peripheral myelin protein 22, suggesting that it may have a similar function in cell proliferation and cell-cell interactions. *BFAR* encodes a protein that inhibits Bax-induced and Fas-induced apoptosis (Itoh et al. 1993; Wei et al. 2001).

The remaining three candidate genes were chosen because of their expression patterns and potential connection with neurological disease. *ABAT* (MIM 137150) is responsible for the catabolism of gamma-aminobutyric acid (GABA) into succinic semialdehyde (De Biase et al. 1995). GABA is an important inhibitory neurotransmitter in the brain and is estimated to be present in 20%–50% of human synapses. GABA is involved directly and indirectly in the pathogenesis of many neurological diseases, including convulsions, which may be relevant, given that approximately one-third of individuals with autism develop epilepsy (Fombonne 2002). *A2BP1* (MIM 605104) possesses a ribonucleoprotein motif, which is highly conserved among RNA-binding proteins. *A2BP1* binds to the C-terminus of ataxin-2 and may contribute to the pathology of spinocerebellar ataxia type 2 (SCA2 [MIM 183090]) (Shibata et al. 2000). *MRTF-B* was identified from cDNA libraries of size-fractioned adult and fetal human brain (Nagase et al. 1999). *MRTF-B* is highly expressed in the amygdala, caudate nucleus, hippocampus, and fetal brain and was recently found to be involved in muscle differentiation (Selvaraj and Prywes 2003).

Material and Methods

IMGSAC Family Collection

The IMGSAC has collected family data in successive stages, and details of assessment protocols are described elsewhere (IMGSAC 2001). To summarize, after an initial screen for medical disorders and a preliminary assessment, parents were administered the Autism Diagnostic Interview–Revised (ADI-R) and the Vineland Adaptive Behavior Scales (Sparrow et al. 1984; Le Couteur et al. 1989). Probands were administered the Autism Diagnostic Observation Schedule (ADOS) (Lord et al. 2000), and psychometric data were obtained. Affected individuals also underwent a thorough medical examination so that those with tuberous sclerosis and neurofibromatosis could be excluded, and any morphological abnormalities were recorded. All participating clinical sites followed the same assessment protocol, and ADI-R and ADOS consensus-coding meetings were held regularly by clinicians. DNA was extracted from blood, buccal swabs, or cell lines by use of the Nucleon kit and standard techniques. Samples from one affected individual per multiplex family were tested for fragile-X syndrome, and, when possible, all affected individuals underwent karyotypic analysis (Lamb et al. 2005). Relevant ethical committees have reviewed this study.

The IMGSAC has collected a further 67 sibling pairs since the publication of the completed genome screen, for a total of 219 sibling pairs from 207 families. In addition, 32 families containing extended relative pairs have been collected. The male:female ratio of affected individuals is 3.9 : 1. One affected individual was selected at random from each multiplex family, to create a group of 239 affected unrelated individuals for case-control analysis. A singleton sample consisting of 91 autism trios with a clinical diagnosis of autism has also been collected. The singleton sample consists of 22 trios from Denmark, 37 trios from the Netherlands, and 32 trios from the United Kingdom. Analysis of linkage data from the IMGSAC sample on chromosomes 2,7, and 16 does not indicate that country of origin significantly affects either the magnitude or location of the linkage signal or the evidence of association in the complete IMGSAC sample (authors' unpublished data) (Bonora et al. 2005).

Controls

Random controls from the European Collection of Cell Cultures (ECACC) ($n = 192$) were used for SNP typing. DNA was extracted at ECACC from lymphoblastoid cell lines derived from white randomly selected blood donors whose parents and grandparents were born in the United Kingdom or Ireland. The control samples were not characterized for autism phenotypes. Half of the controls were male and half female. Although the male : female ratio is different for cases and controls, only the presence of a very strong sex-specific allelic effect could reduce the ability to detect association. Linkage analysis based on the sex of APSs on chromosome 16 shows some evidence of a sex-specific effect, but it is unclear how this would affect the frequency of a disease-causing variant (Lamb et al. 2005).

Mutation Screening

Intron-exon boundaries were characterized *in silico* by use of National Center for Biotechnology Information LocusLink and University of California–Santa Cruz (UCSC) Golden Path (see UCSC Genome Browser Web site). The mRNA sequence was subjected to BLAST analysis, to determine or confirm genomic structure. Exon-specific primers were designed using Primer3. Large exons and promoter regions were covered by overlapping PCR products of ∼500 bp. PCRs were performed in a reaction mixture containing 40 ng of DNA and final concentrations of 2.5 mM KCl; 2.0, 2.5, or 3.0 mM $MgCl_2$; 0.2 mM primer; 0.2 mM dNTPs; 0.9 U Ampli*Taq* Gold polymerase; and 0.1 U *Pfu*Turbo (Stratagene). For GC-rich products of 2.5%–10%, DMSO was used with a mix of 0.2 mM dATP, dTTP, and dCTP; 0.1 mM dGTP; and 0.1 mM 7-deaz-2′-deoxyguanosine-5′-triphosphate (Amersham Pharmacia Biotech). The PCR consisted of touchdown protocols with a maximum annealing temperature of 50°C–67.5°C (T1) and a minimum annealing temperature of 42.5°C–60°C (T2) (15 min at 95°C, followed by 14 cycles of 30 s at 95°C, 30 s at T1−0.5°C per cycle, and 30 s at 72°C, followed by 29 cycles of 30 s at 95°C, 30 s at T2, and 30 s at 72°C). PCR products were denatured and reannealed using the following protocol: 4 min at 95°C, 30 s at 95°C, and 42 cycles of 30 s at −1.6°C per cycle.

The Transgenomic WAVE DNA Fragment Analysis System was used to detect heterozygous individuals by DHPLC. Gradients were designed using WAVEMAKER Software (version 4.1) and spanned a temperature range of 51.5°C–70°C. Crude PCR products were loaded onto the DNASep Column, and elution profiles were analyzed for heteroduplex formation. Melting curves for fragments containing c^7dGTP were experimentally determined.

Variant Identification

Common variants were identified by sequencing seven heteroduplex samples and a control sample with a homoduplex profile. Low-frequency variants were sequenced for all individuals showing the heteroduplex profile and for a control sample. Sequencing was performed with BigDye Terminator mix on ABI 377 machines, in accordance with standard protocols, and variants were analyzed with Sequence Analysis and Sequence Navigator.

SNP Typing

Mass-extension assay.—Primers and mass-extension assays were designed for Sequenom SNP typing with SpectroDESIGNER. PCRs were performed in 10-μl reactions with 8 ng of DNA template and final concentrations of 2.5 mM KCl and $MgCl_2$, 200 μM dNTPs, 1 U of HotStar*Taq* Polymerase (Qiagen), and primer concentration of 0.15 mM. Multiplex PCRs were performed using up to four primer pairs per reaction; 45 cycles of 20 s at 95°C, 30 s at 56°C, and 1 min at 72°C were performed. Nonincorporated dNTPs were removed with shrimp alkaline phosphatase for 20 min at 37°C and for 5 min at 85°C. The mass-extension reaction was performed using MassEXTEND enzymes—thermosequenase, hME termination mixes, and hME extension primers; 55 cycles were performed for 5 s at 94°C, for 5 s at 52°C, and for 5 s at 72°C. Unincorporated ddNTPs and dNTPs were removed with SpectroCLEAN resin, and products were transferred to a 384 SpectroCHIP by use of the SpectroPOINT robot. The chip was read using the Bruker Biflex III Mass Spectrometer system. Sequenom Genotype Analyzer was used to manually check failed genotypes and to assign alleles, when possible. Data either were exported from SpectroTYPER using Report Generator or were directly streamed into the Wellcome Trust Centre for Human Genetics Laboratory Information Management System Integrated Genotyping System (IGS).

Restriction digest.—PCR for *ABAT* exon 2 was performed in 10-μl reactions containing 24 ng of DNA and final concentrations of 2.5 mM KCl, 2.5 mM $MgCl_2$,

0.2 mM primer, 0.2 mM dNTPs, and 0.25 U Ampli*Taq* Gold polymerase. Touchdown PCR was performed with a maximum annealing temperature of 62.5°C. PCR product from each plate was tested on agarose and was incubated with 0.1 U of *Bso*B1 and 2 μl of buffer 2 (New England BioLabs), in a total volume of 20 μl at 37°C for 6 h. Digested products were visualized on a 3% agarose gel. Digests were genotyped blind to affection status and were entered into the IGS.

Statistical Analysis

Association analysis.—The PDT was used to test for transmission disequilibrium (Martin et al. 2000) for the multiplex and singleton samples. This test is more powerful than the transmission/disequilibrium test (TDT) for the multiplex sample and analyzes informative branches of extended families with all available data. The PDT retains the within-family nature of the TDT and provides a valid test for association, even in the presence of population substructure. A test for the transmission disequilibrium of genotypes—rather than alleles—was also performed using the geno-PDT, an extension of the PDT (Martin et al. 2003*a*). Case-control association analysis was performed using related cases from the multiplex families and controls, as proposed by Slager and Schaid (2001). This test accounts for the biological relationship between cases and compares genotype frequencies between cases and controls by comparing the trend in proportions as the dosage of the risk allele increases. Genotype-frequency differences between unrelated affected cases from the multiplex and singleton samples and controls were analyzed using Fisher's exact test for count data.

Haplotype analysis.—Haplotypes were determined using PHASE v2.0.2 for groups of SNPs within candidate genes. Any genotypes that were not assigned phase with >90% certainty were disregarded. Because PHASE v2.02 reconstructs haplotypes from population genotype data, two rounds of haplotype reconstruction were performed. First, multiplex case and control data were analyzed together, and, second, singleton case and control data were analyzed together, with the result of small differences in the numbers of haplotypes constructed for controls. PHASE v2.0.2 was selected instead of GENEHUNTER 2.0 for determination of haplotypes, because PHASE v2.0.2 does not assume linkage equilibrium over short distances and can be used to generate haplotypes for individuals without parental genotypes. Haplotype analysis was performed using TRANSMIT for both multiplex and singleton data (Clayton and Jones 1999). TRANSMIT implements a TDT that analyzes the transmission of multilocus haplotypes and has good power when parental genotypes are available, as is the case in this sample (~80%) (Martin et al. 2003*b*). For each haplotype, a χ^2 test with 1 df for excess transmission is produced. A global test for association is also produced with $H-1$ df (H = number of haplotypes for which information is available).

Logistic regression analysis.—Logistic regression analysis of haplotype data was performed with the program R (R Project for Statistical Computing), as described by Wallenstein et al. (1998). Unrelated affected individuals from the multiplex and singleton families, identical to those used in the case-control analyses, were used in the logistic regression analysis. They impose an assumption of additivity on the haplotype analysis, thus providing predictor variables that include the number of copies (0, 1, or 2) of each haplotype and that yield a logistic regression for which the outcome is either case or control. The model is constructed so that each coefficient gives the log odds ratio for disease for an individual with a single copy of the relevant haplotype and another copy of the baseline haplotype, compared with an individual with two copies of a baseline haplotype. Models were fitted in which each gene (*ABAT, CREBBP, GRIN2A,* and *TSC2*) was tested alone and jointly. Genotypes for an individual (i.e., the pairs of haplotypes) are denoted as $(x;y)$.

LD mapping.—Haplotype files were analyzed using HaploXT to generate an output file describing LD (Abecasis and Cookson 2000). Individual marker-by-marker contingency tables were produced and imported into the Graphical Overview of Linkage Disequilibrium (GOLD) program. Lewontin's standardized disequilibrium coefficient D' was used (Lewontin and Kojima 1960), because it accounts for allele frequency, although, like other measures of LD, it may be artificially inflated by rare haplotypes.

Error detection.—Mendelian consistency of SNP genotype data was checked using PedCheck (O'Connell and Weeks 1998), and any inconsistent genotypes were removed. Data were prepared for statistical analysis by use of Mega2 (Mukhopadhyay et al. 1999; see the University of Pittsburgh Department of Human Genetics Web site). Genotypes flanking double recombinants, detected after running GENEHUNTER 2.0, were checked and disregarded if ambiguous. SIBMED (sib-pair mutation error detection) was also used to remove possible genotyping errors (Douglas et al. 2000).

Permutation of affection status: Fisher's exact test.—An empirical experimentwise P value for association, to allow for multiple testing across all 28 SNPs, was obtained by random permutations of case and control status. For each permutation, the minimum P value from Fisher's exact test across all SNPs was recorded. An empirical estimate of the experimentwise P value was then given by the proportion of permutations for which the minimum P value exceeded that obtained for the original

Table 3

Missense Mutations in Candidate Genes Identified by DHPLC

Gene and Exon[a]	cDNA Nucleotide	Wild-Type/ Variant Allele	Amino Acid Substitution	No. of Heterozygotes in Screened Samples (n = 48)	Minor-Allele Frequency in: Multiplex Cases (n = 239)	Controls (n = 192)
ABAT:						
2	208	A/G	G56R	21	.457	.369
BFAR:						
3	563	G/T	M140R	6	.332	.388
6	1096	A/G	V315I	2	.018	.077
MRTF-B:						
5	1624	C/G	N543K	1	.024	.035
SSTR5:						
1	92	C/T	T333I	1	ND[b]	ND[b]
UBN1:						
3	422	A/C	A103N	1	.004	.000
9	1413	G/A	Y435C	2	.031	.027

[a] SNPs genotyped in the entire IMGSAC sample and controls for all but exon 1.
[b] ND = no data were available.

sample. The same procedure was repeated for the singleton cases and controls.

Permutation of affection status: logistic regression analysis.—To test the significance of the logistic haplotype regression analysis of the four genes, with consideration of multiple testing, PHASE v2.0.2 was used to generate "best pair" haplotypes for cases and controls; affection status was then permuted 10,000 times. An additive logistic regression model incorporating the joint haplotypic effects across *ABAT, CREBBP, GRIN2A,* and *TSC2* was fitted to the permuted data, and *P* values were recorded. The significance of the joint model was estimated as the proportion of permutations in which the regression *P* value was smaller than that observed in the joint analysis of the original sample data.

Bioinformatic Analysis

Variants found within 20 bp of intron-exon boundaries were analyzed for possible effects on splice-site signal by use of sequence analysis tools available at the Berkeley *Drosophila* Genome Project Web site (Brunak et al. 1991; Kulp et al. 1997). Variants within exons were analyzed for possible changes to exon-splice enhancers by use of the ESEfinder interface (Cartegni et al. 2003). The program Pfam was used to determine the location of coding variants within known protein domains (Bateman et al. 2004). Homology searches by use of PolyPhen were performed to determine the extent of conservation at the position of missense mutations in known sequences (Sunyaev et al. 2001). PolyPhen uses empirical rules and structural information to characterize the effect of an amino acid substitution.

Results

Failure Rates and Error Checking

Of the 38 SNPs initially selected for genotyping, 10 were disregarded because of failing multiplex PCR, failing extension reaction, poor success rate, or a weak extension assay. Additionally, the A/G SNP causing the G56R substitution in *ABAT* was genotyped by restriction enzyme digestion because of spurious heterozygotes in the mass-extension assay. Of a total of 47,646 SNP genotyping assays performed, 44,647 genotypes were generated, a 93.7% success rate. Analysis with PedCheck led to the removal of 35 genotypes from the IMGSAC data (0.08% error rate). Most of these were due to nonconservative SNP genotyping allele calls from the Sequenom Genotype Analyzer. Checking for double recombinants resulted in the removal of an additional 26 genotypes. All markers were analyzed for Hardy-Weinberg equilibrium and were not found to deviate from expected allele frequencies ($P < .01$); a small number of markers with low heterozygosity did deviate from expected allele frequencies ($P < .05$), but this is likely to be due to chance. Finally, SIBMED was run with all SNP data, and microsatellite data were generated from the completion of the IMGSAC genome screen; an additional 14 low-probability genotypes were removed.

Mutation Screening

Seven missense variants were detected during mutation screening of the coding sequence, as described in table 3. Additionally, 108 noncoding/silent variants were found, as shown in table 4. Several missense variants were found in a single family; the T333I change in *SSTR5*

Table 4

Nonmissense Variants in Candidate Genes Identified by DHPLC

Gene, Location, and cDNA Nucleotide	Major/Minor Allele	No. of Heterozygotes in Screened Samples (n = 48)	Minor-Allele Frequency[a] in Cases	Minor-Allele Frequency[a] in Controls
A2BP1:				
Intron 1:				
730−6	+/CTT del	2	...	...
Intron 2:				
804−47	A/C	24	...	...
804−48	A/T	24	...	...
Intron 3:				
852−20	+/T del	23	...	...
Exon 5:				
1067	C/G	2	...	...
1098	G/A	2	...	...
Intron 5:				
1182−25	A/C	4	...	...
Exon 6[b]:				
1271	A/G	1	.021	.003
Intron 7:				
1379+109	A/G	1	...	...
Intron 11:				
1673−17	−/CT ins	21	...	...
Intron 13:				
183−19	A/G	2	...	...
Intron 15[b]:				
1973+3	A/G	6	.004	0
3′ UTR:				
2102+141	G/T	23	...	...
ABAT:				
Intron 1[b]:				
102+49	T/C	15	.391	.2952
Intron 2:				
209+11	A/G	1	...	...
210−68	C/A	1	...	...
210−5	C/T	1	...	...
Exon 4[b]:				
350	C/T	10	...	...
Intron 8:				
582+14	−/CA ins	5	...	...
582+54	A/C	2	...	...
Exon 9:				
685	C/T	1	...	...
Exon 12:				
995	A/C	2	...	...
Intron 13:				
1313−120	−/G ins	10	...	...
Intron 14:				
1423+9	C/T	22	...	...
3′ UTR:				
1544+71	A/G	1	...	...
BFAR:				
Exon 1:				
50	T/C	1	...	...
Intron 1:				
89+105	G/A	4	...	...
Exon 2:				
178	T/A	1	...	...
Intron 6:				
937+84	−/GTG ins	1	...	...
3′ UTR:				
1507+794	A/G	1	...	...
1507+795	G/C	1	...	...

(*continued*)

Table 4 (continued)

Gene, Location, and cDNA Nucleotide	Major/Minor Allele	No. of Heterozygotes in Screened Samples (n = 48)	Minor-Allele Frequency[a] in Cases	Minor-Allele Frequency[a] in Controls
CREBBP:				
Exon 3:				
258	G/A	1	...	...
Exon 4:				
1037	T/C	3	...	...
Intron 3[b,c]:				
1995−8585	T/C	ND[d]	.005	0
Intron 4:				
1174−76	+/TTTG del	1	...	...
Intron 6:				
1530−31	G/T	3	...	...
Intron 7[b,c]:				
1730+215	G/A	ND[d]	.349	.363
1731−58	A/C	1	...	...
Exon 11:				
2152	T/C	1	...	...
Intron 11[b]:				
2311+78	C/T	3	.077	.007
Intron 13:				
2358+59	T/C	1	...	...
Intron 17[b]:				
3449+6163	C/T	23	.414	.522
Intron 20[b,c]:				
3898+3049	C/T	ND[d]	.033	.015
Intron 22[b]:				
4040−8	T/C	3	.014	.022
Exon 23:				
4097	A/C	1	...	...
Intron 26[b,c]:				
4480+42	G/A	11	.027	.015
Intron 29[b]:				
4937−19	C/G	3	.028	.019
Exon 31:				
5160	A/C	2	...	...
Exon 32:				
7411	G/A	3	...	...
3′ UTR:				
7525+26	−/C ins	2	...	...
EMP2:				
Exon 2:				
53	G/C	7	...	...
Exon 3:				
172	C/T	15	...	...
205	G/A	23	...	...
245	C/T	23	...	...
3′ UTR:				
Unidentified	Unidentified	13	...	...
GRIN2A:				
Intron 1:				
112−33	C/T	27	...	...
Intron 5:				
1318−15	G/C	1	...	...
Exon 6[b]:				
1576	T/C	21	.424	.597
Intron 7:				
1808−29	G/C	1	...	...
Intron 8:				
1964+31	−/GA ins	25	...	...
Intron 10[b]:				
2316−35	G/C	25	.447	.381
Intron 11:				
2316−21	−/GA ins	1	...	...

(*continued*)

Table 4 (continued)

Gene, Location, and cDNA Nucleotide	Major/Minor Allele	No. of Heterozygotes in Screened Samples (n = 48)	Minor-Allele Frequency[a] in	
			Cases	Controls
Exon 11:				
2396	G/A	2	...	...
Exon 14:				
3539	G/T	2	...	...
3′ UTR[b]:				
4705+39	C/A	2	.005	.014
4105+1213	A/G	26	.298	.510
MRTF-B:				
Exon 1:				
90	G/C	1	...	...
Exon 2:				
379	T/G	1	...	...
Intron 3:				
1475−12	G/T	2	...	...
Intron 4:				
1513+21	C/T	1	...	...
3′ UTR[b]:				
2487+67	T/C	1	...	...
2487+561	T/C	1	...	...
2487+1110	G/C	1	...	...
2487+1441	T/A	1	...	...
2487+1713	A/C	1	...	...
2487+1849	G/T	1	...	...
TBX6:				
5′ UTR:				
120+6	A/G	3	...	...
Intron 7:				
938−4	C/T	20	...	...
937+19	−/GAT ins	23	...	...
Exon 8:				
1252	A/G	1	...	...
Intron 8:				
1335+428	G/C	1	...	...
UBN1:				
5′ UTR:				
1−17	C/G	7	...	...
Intron 1:				
75−109	TA/AG	3	...	...
75−63	T/C	3	...	...
75−21	A/G	6	...	...
74+26	T/C	3	...	...
75+40	T/G	25	...	...
74+68	G/T	2	...	...
Exon 3:				
147	A/G	2	...	...
Intron 3:				
454+22	A/G	2	...	...
Intron 4:				
546+3	G/A	4	...	...
Exon 5:				
599+5	C/T	11	...	...
Intron 6:				
784+8	G/A	1	...	...
Intron 9:				
1296+11	−/G ins	1	...	...
1296+39	+/TT del	1	...	...
1425+62	C/T	3	...	...
Intron 14:				
1915+17	A/G	15	...	...
1915+53	A/G	2	...	...

(continued)

Table 4 (continued)

Gene, Location, and cDNA Nucleotide	Major/Minor Allele	No. of Heterozygotes in Screened Samples (n = 48)	Minor-Allele Frequency[a] in	
			Cases	Controls
Exon 15:				
2743	T/G	7	...	...
2994	T/G	6	...	...
Exon 18:				
3486	C/T	3	...	...
3519+1006	C/T	12	...	...
3′ UTR:				
3519+157	T/C	7	...	...
3519+1008	−/C ins	1	...	...
3519+1889	C/T	4	...	...
3519+2302	C/G	1	...	...
Exon 18:				
3519+2588	A/C	13	...	...
3519+2660	C/T	26	...	...

[a] No data were available unless values are shown. For cases, $n = 239$; for controls, $n = 192$.
[b] SNPs genotyped in the entire IMGSAC sample and controls.
[c] SNPs identified through dbSNP or Sequenom's RealSNP Array.
[d] ND = no data were available.

was found in an unaffected mother, and the N543K missense variant in *MRTF-B* was paternally transmitted to one of two affected sons. Bioinformatic analysis indicated that these variants do not occur in any known functional domain and that they were predicted to have a benign effect. However, there are few homologous sequences available for thorough conservation analysis of *MRTF-B*. Two missense variants were detected in *BFAR*. During screening, the first missense variant in exon 3, M140R, was found in six individuals and cosegregated with autism in these families, although three parents were found to be homozygous for arginine. The second missense variant in *BFAR*, V315I, was detected, during screening, in two individuals and cosegregated with autism in both families. Bioinformatic analysis of the missense variants in *BFAR* showed that they were likely to have only a benign effect on protein structure and that they do not occur at highly conserved residues. Two rare variants were found in *UBN1*. The A103N variant in exon 3 was detected in one family and was transmitted paternally to two affected offspring. This variant is in a region of low complexity without a strong domain identity. A variant in exon 9, Y435C, was detected in two individuals but cosegregated with autism in only one family. Although this variant was predicted to have a potentially harmful effect on protein function, no homologous sequences were available, and detailed comparative analysis was not possible.

One missense variant was found at a high frequency in *ABAT* exon 2. However, the G56R change is distant from the enzyme's catalytic site and is unlikely to hinder protein function. Sequence homology analysis also predicted that the variant is likely to be benign. All of the missense variants detected during screening, except that in *SSTR5*, were typed in the entire IMGSAC sample and 192 controls. No evidence of transmission disequilibrium was found, and no significant differences in case-control allele frequencies were observed for these missense variants, as shown in table 3. None of the variants detected by DHPLC within 20 bp of the intron/exon splice site were found to potentially affect splice signal.

Association Analysis and Logistic Regression Analysis for Candidate Genes

Twenty-eight SNPs were successfully genotyped in the IMGSAC families and controls, as shown in table 5. The family data were analyzed for allele and genotype transmission disequilibrium by use of the PDT. Fisher's exact test for count data was used to compare genotypes observed in cases and controls. Additionally, multiplex genotype data were compared with controls by use of a trend test that accounts for relatedness between affected individuals. No significant evidence of association was found with these tests either for SNPs in *A2BP1, BFAR, MRTF-B, TSC2,* and *UBN1* or for SNPs within the region of linkage with ADHD, as described in table 5. SNPs within *ABAT, GRIN2A, TSC2,* and *CREBBP* were analyzed for LD, to determine whether any haplotype blocks were present in the data. The SNPs within *ABAT* and *GRIN2A* were in strong LD with each other ($D' = 0.667$–1), whereas there was variability in LD between SNPs in *TSC2* and *CREBBP.* Because of the manner in which most of the SNPs were identified and the comparatively large inter-SNP distances, it is unlikely that any underlying haplotype-block structure is fully described by these analyses. But, given the evidence of LD between SNPs in candidate genes, haplotype transmission analysis was performed. No evidence of haplotype transmission disequilibrium was detected, using TRANSMIT, in the IMGSAC families, although an exhaustive analysis of all possible SNP combinations was not performed. There was evidence of association with SNPs genotyped in *ABAT, CREBBP,* and *GRIN2A,* and further logistic regression analysis was performed, as described below. The logistic regression analysis performed does not rely on any LD between SNPs and assesses only the risk of being affected, given a particular genotype. Haplotypes are described as sequential SNP alleles across the candidate genes, with alleles labeled as in table 5 (e.g., haplotype h12 for *ABAT* describes allele 1 at *rs1731017,* followed by allele 2 at the SNP within exon 2 of the gene).

ABAT.—Both SNPs within *ABAT* showed some evidence of association in the multiplex sample, with the trend-test and case-control analysis. The strongest evidence of association was from the SNP within *ABAT* intron 1, which, when analyzed using the trend test, indicated that allele 2 was responsible for increasing the risk of autism ($P < .001$). Fisher's exact test for count data gave a P value of .0089, which indicates a significant difference in genotype distribution between cases and controls, as shown in table 5. This result was supported by the analysis of the same SNP in the singleton sample with use of Fisher's exact test ($P = .0112$), as shown in table 5. Logistic regression of SNPs within *ABAT* did not indicate that a particular haplotype significantly increased the risk of autism, although there is an overall difference in haplotype distribution between cases, from the multiplex and singleton samples, and controls ($\chi^2 = 20.37$; $P = 1.422 \times 10^{-4}$ for multiplex cases; $\chi^2 = 6.18$; $P = .1031$ for singleton cases), as shown in table 6. An additional SNP was also genotyped in exon 4 of *ABAT* but was excluded from the final analysis, despite supporting the results described above, because of a low genotyping success rate (65.9% in the multiplex sample; 73.9% in the singleton sample).

CREBBP.—In the multiplex sample, association was found for *CREBBP* with two SNPs within introns 22 and 29, with use of the geno-PDT ($P = .0363$ and $P = .001$, respectively) and with use of the allelic PDT ($P = .0074$ and $P = .0024$, respectively). However, both these SNPs had a minor-allele frequency <6%, and the number of transmissions to affected individuals was small. There was some additional evidence of association from the trend test for the SNP in intron 17 ($P = .0103$), but these results were not replicated in the singleton sample. Conversely, SNPs within introns 7 and 20 showed evidence of association in the singleton sample ($P = .03078$ and $P = .0196$, respectively) but not in the multiplex sample. It should be noted that the minor-allele frequency was also low for the SNP in intron 20, and the P value was of marginal significance for the SNP in intron 7; it is likely these represent chance findings. These results are shown in table 5. There was no evidence from the logistic regression analysis to support the presence of a risk haplotype across *CREBBP,* as shown in table 6.

GRIN2A.—One SNP in *GRIN2A* intron 10 showed some evidence of transmission disequilibrium with the geno-PDT ($P = .013$) and the trend test ($P = .0337$). This was supported by SNPs within exon 6 and the 3′ UTR that also showed evidence of association with the trend test and case-control analysis, as shown in table 5. Although the singleton analysis does appear to support these results, closer inspection shows that the transmission of different genotypes is responsible for the significant result for the SNP within exon 6—genotype 1/1 in the singleton sample compared with genotype 1/2 in the multiplex sample, as shown in table 5. A significant difference in the distribution of haplotypes, between cases and controls, was found using logistic regression analysis

Table 5

Association Analysis of SNP Genotyping Data for Multiplex Families (n = 239) and Singleton Families (n = 91)

Genomic Region, Location, and dbSNP Number	Genotyping Success (%)	Percentage of Genotypes with Alleles									*P* for				Trend Test[a] Analysis				Fisher's Exact Test of Sample	
		1/1 in			1/2 in			2/2 in			Multiplex		Singleton		No. of Sibling Pairs/ Controls	*P* for High-Risk Allele(s)				
		Multiplex Cases	Singletons	Controls	Multiplex Cases	Singletons	Controls	Multiplex Cases	Singletons	Controls	Geno-PDT	Allelic PDT	Geno-PDT	Allelic PDT		1 and 2[b]	1[c]	2[c]	Multiplex	Singleton
A2BP1:																				
Exon 6	89.1	95.8	ND	99.4	4.2	ND	.6	0	ND	0			ND	ND	219/172				.0265	ND
Intron 15	54.3	0	ND	0	.8	ND	0	99.2	ND	100			ND	ND	103/113					ND
ABAT:																				
Intron 1:																				
rs1731017	76.8	37	47.3	49.7	42.5	33.8	40.8	20.4	18.9	9.5					142/147	.0061		.0113	.0089	.0112
Exon 2:	93.3	21	5.7	13.5	46.2	54	43.2	32.9	40.2	43.2					212/185		.0257		.0483	
BFAR:																				
Exon 3	91.6	44.5	ND	37.5	43.6	ND	47.8	11.8	ND	14.7			ND	ND	209/184					ND
Exon 6	84.5	0	ND	.6	3.6	ND	4.2	96.4	ND	95.2			ND	ND	186/167					ND
CREBBP:																				
Intron 3:																				
rs3025702	97	0	ND	0	.9	ND	0	99.1	ND	100			ND	ND	244/187					ND
Intron 7:																				
rs130021	94.5	42.5	39.3	40.6	45.3	40.4	50.3	12.3	20.2	9.1					210/187					.03078
Intron 11:																				
rs130002	55.3	.6	0	0	2.5	1.1	1.4	96.9	98.9	98.6					127/74					
Intron 17:																				
rs886528	89.2	17.1	14.6	27.2	45.5	48.3	41	37.4	37.1	31.8					166/173			.0103		
Intron 20:																				
rs130025	90.5	0	0	0	6.5	2.3	2.9	93.5	97.7	97.1			.0196	.0196	219/172					
Intron 22:																				
rs3025684	98.1	97.3	100	95.7	2.7	0	4.3	0	0	0	.036	.0074			225/186					
Intron 26:																				
rs129967	92.8	0	0	0	5.4	0	2.9	94.6	100	97.1					227/175					
Intron 29:																				
rs130008	94.9	0	1.1	0	5.6	4.5	3.7	94.4	94.3	96.3	.001	.0024			221/187					
GRIN2A:																				
Exon 6	93.7	18.1	47.7	35.6	75.8	43.2	58.8	6.2	9.1	5.6					239/177	.0013		<.0001	.0003	.0486
Intron 10	96.3	20	54.7	14.5	75.7	37.2	81.2	4.3	8.1	4.3	.013				242/186			.0337		2.32×10^{-12}
3′ UTR:	96.3	99.1	ND	97.3	.9	ND	2.7	0	ND	0			ND	ND	240/186					ND
rs1014531	75.5	8.9	19.7	26	78.5	49.3	50.4	12.6	31	23.6					218/127		.0214	<.0001	2.9×10^{-7}	.0439
MRTF-B:																				
Exon 5	75.9	0	ND	0	4.7	ND	6.8	95.3	ND	93.2			ND	ND	155/177					ND
TSC2:																				
5′ UTR:																				
rs2516740	93.5	62.6	ND	63.5	31.3	ND	30.7	6.1	ND	5.8			ND	ND	219/189					ND
Intron 10:																				
rs2074968	93.7	17.4	ND	15	48.2	ND	52.8	34.4	ND	32.2			ND	ND	231/180					ND
3′ UTR:																				
rs1051771	82.1	0	ND	0	2.1	ND	6.8	97.9	ND	93.2		.0143	ND	ND	169/162	.0023	.0022		.0346	ND
UBN1:																				
Exon 3	83.8	100	ND	0	0	ND	0	0	ND	0			ND	ND	183/161					ND
Exon 9	96.8	93.9	ND	94.7	5.7	ND	5.3	.4	ND	0			ND	ND	233/187					ND
ADHD linkage peak:																				
14–15 Mb[d]:																				
rs153783	92.1	54.6	ND	51.6	37.7	ND	37.4	7.7	ND	11.1			ND	ND	202/190					ND
rs1125972	96.8	88.7	ND	86.6	10.4	ND	12.9	.9	ND	.5			ND	ND	240/186					ND
rs1065838	93.7	8.4	ND	8.4	40.2	ND	41.6	51.4	ND	50			ND	ND	201/190					ND
rs1107143	96.1	38.2	ND	39.2	46.5	ND	46.2	15.4	ND	14.5			ND	ND	237/186					ND

NOTE.—Results shown only when $P < .05$. ND = no data were available.

[a] Trend test performed on multiplex sample.

[b] Additive allele effect.

[c] Dominant allele effect.

[d] Below linkage peak identified by Smalley et al. (2002).

Table 6

Haplotype Logistic Regression Analysis

Gene and Haplotype	No. of Multiplex Cases[a]	No. of Multiplex Controls[b]	Log Relative Risk	SE	P (>|z|)	χ^2	P	df
ABAT:						20.37	1.4226×10^{-4}	3
h11[c]	18	7		.8226	.1246			
h12	162	85	−.1536	.4397	.0727			
h21	225	219	−.726	.4209	.0845			
h22	15	3	.7212	.7466	.334			
CREBBP:						16.52	.0355	8
h12122222[c]	7	3		1.3986	.242			
h21121212	5	0	14.6899	649.2732	.982			
h21221212	4	5	−.9564	.9743	.326			
h22112222	4	2	−.1661	1.1172	.882			
h22121212	71	85	−.9602	.7079	.175			
h22121222	28	32	−.9925	.7698	.197			
h22122212	118	93	−.7084	.7217	.326			
h22122222	51	38	−.662	.732	.366			
Other[d]	10	2	.6144	1.0274	.558			
GRIN2A:						62.05	1.7232×10^{-11}	6
h1111[c]	34	42		.4716	.0103[e]			
h1112	5	3	1.4334	.8411	.0883			
h1122	168	73	.8251	.3143	.0086[f]			
h2111	217	85	1.5479	.306	4.21×10^{-7}[f]			
h2121	2	20	−2.5906	.791	.001[b]			
h2122	13	7	.4442	.5331	.4047			
Other[d]	5	2	1.3741	.9345	.1414			
TSC2:						1.63	.8033	4
h112[c]	135	103		.22961	.22			
h122	178	142	−.0364	.1733	.834			
h212	13	6	.4427	.5116	.387			
h222	45	33	.012	.2326	.959			
Other[d]	3	4	−.5625	.783	.472			

Gene and Haplotype	No. of Singleton Cases[a]	No. of Singleton Controls[b]	Log Relative Risk	SE	P (>|z|)	χ^2	P	df
ABAT:						6.18	.1031	3
h11[c]	2	7		1.6134	.2746			
h12	55	106	.4878	.8411	.562			
h21	120	244	.5369	.8129	.509			
h22	7	3	2.122	1.0626	.0458			
CREBBP:						9.77	.1346	6
h12122222[c]	4	2		1.5728	.422			
h21221212	0	5	−16.7436	1,072.0759	.988			
h22121212	35	86	−1.0608	.8039	.187			
h22121222	12	33	−1.2422	.8471	.143			
h22122212	49	96	−1.013	.8081	.21			
h22122222	30	40	−.6101	.8348	.465			
Other[d]	2	6	−1.4596	1.1374	.199			
GRIN2A:						37.05	5.8528×10^{-7}	5
h1111[c]	22	42		.5113	.138			
h1122	38	72	−.2564	.3701	.4885			
h2111	72	83	.7756	.3248	.0169[f]			
h2121	0	20	−17.5343	877.517	.9841			
h2122	4	7	−.4984	.6939	.4726			
Other[d]	0	4	−16.6823	1,972.8826	.9933			

[a] $n = 239$.
[b] $n = 192$.
[c] Referent haplotype.
[d] Haplotypes combined when <5.
[e] Haplotype has a protective effect $P < .05$.
[f] Haplotype has a deleterious effect $P < .05$.

for both the multiplex and singleton samples ($\chi^2 = 62.05$; $P = 1.7232 \times 10^{-11}$) compared with controls ($\chi^2 = 37.05$; $P = 5.8528 \times 10^{-7}$). Haplotype h2111—genotypes $x = (2,1,1,1)$, $y = (1,1,1,1)$—significantly increased the chances of being affected ($P = 4.21 \times 10^{-7}$), as did haplotype h1122—$x = (1,1,2,2)$, $y = (1,1,1,1)$—although not as strongly ($P = .0086$), as shown in table 6. The effect of the h2111 haplotype was replicated in the singleton sample but at a less significant level ($P = .0169$). Additionally, haplotype h2121—genotypes $x = (1,2,1,2)$, $y = (1,1,1,1)$—is found at a rate of 20/232 in controls, compared with 2/580 in multiplex cases, and appears to decrease the chances of being affected ($P = .001$).

Statistical significance of association and logistic regression analysis.—A simple Bonferroni correction, to reduce the chance of type 1 error to 0.05 across all tests, gives a significance threshold of .00714, if we consider that seven tests were performed: geno-PDT, allelic PDT, trend test for high-risk alleles 1 and 2, trend test for high-risk allele 1, and trend test for high-risk allele 2, Fisher's exact test, and logistic regression analysis. To reduce type 1 error to 0.001 across all tests, a Bonferroni significance threshold of .000142 is required. This represents a highly conservative correction, given that the PDTs and trend tests are correlated, although a number of the results in table 5 do exceed these significance levels.

Permutation tests, which provide more-accurate significance thresholds, were performed (see the "Material and Methods" section). For the single-point analysis with Fisher's exact test across 28 SNPs, the minimum P value of 2.9×10^{-7} for *rs1014531* in *GRIN2A* in the multiplex case-control analysis was smaller than any obtained in 10,000 permutations, for an empirical P value of $< 10^{-4}$. Similarly, for the joint logistic haplotype regression of all four genes, the observed χ^2 statistic of 102.9 with 34 df (nominal $P = 7.4 \times 10^{-9}$) was greater than for all 10,000 permutations; that is, an empirical P value of $< 10^{-4}$.

Separate haplotype logistic analysis of the four genes indicates that *GRIN2A* has by far the most significant contribution. A test comparing the fit of *GRIN2A* alone with that of all four genes gave a χ^2 value of 47.44 with 25 df ($P < .0043$), which suggests that, whereas the *GRIN2A* haplotypes are the principal contributors, there may be some effect associated with the *ABAT* haplotypes.

Discussion

Seven missense variants were detected during the screening of 10 positional candidate genes on chromosome 16p11-13 for autism. Although a number of these variants cosegregated with autism, both their presence at similar frequencies in controls and the lack of evidence of transmission disequilibrium suggest that they are unlikely to make a significant contribution to the etiology of autism.

A large number of noncoding and silent mutations were detected, but these are not predicted to alter splice-site recognition sequences. However, bioinformatic analysis alone may be insufficient to detect the effects of intronic and silent variants on splicing and transcriptional efficiency, as recently reported for *CFTR* and *SLC22A4* (Pagani et al. 2003; Tokuhiro et al. 2003), and it is possible that novel regulatory elements could be disrupted. A lack of missense mutations in coding sequence does not preclude the presence of harmful noncoding variants within a candidate gene. In fact, for a multigenic disorder such as autism, more subtle changes in gene regulation and expression are anticipated. This has been found for *PAD14,* a gene associated with rheumatoid arthritis (Suzuki et al. 2003). Suzuki et al. (2003) failed to detect any missense mutations in 48 affected individuals but found a functional SNP haplotype affecting mRNA stability.

The 28 SNPs genotyped in the IMGSAC families are unlikely to provide sufficient coverage of the genomic regions to conclusively exclude genes by association mapping. This was particularly true for genes such as *A2BP1,* which has a genomic region of 1,690 kb, from which only two SNPs with low heterozygosities were genotyped. Although a number of the SNPs genotyped in this study had low heterozygosities, it has been argued that they are useful for detecting association between disease variants with more-recent origins, despite reduced informativeness (Pritchard and Cox 2002). Additionally, even though most of the SNPs were successfully genotyped in 85% of individuals, the SNP-genotyping success rates had a range of 54.3%–98.1%. Although this failure rate could reduce confidence in the data used for analysis, Sequenom traces were manually inspected for markers with low success rates, and low-probability genotypes were removed when identified by software programs.

The association analysis performed in this study attempts to extract the maximum information from the data available and is, in some respects, exploratory. Family-based and case-control association analyses were performed for single-marker and multimarker haplotypes. Although this requires multiple testing of the data, it has been suggested that different approaches have varying power, depending on disease and marker-allele frequency. A family-based analysis benefits when parental genotypes are used as controls but may yield little informative data if marker heterozygosity is low and parental data is missing. Conversely, a case-control analysis may have more power at varying allele frequencies for the number of individuals genotyped but could provide an artifactual result because of population-specific differences between cases and controls (Risch and Teng 1998). It has also been suggested that the added information from haplotype analysis of SNPs has more power than single-marker analysis (Zaykin et al. 2002). A number of procedures have been suggested for correcting for multiple testing, including Bonferroni correction, but there is as yet little consensus as to an "ideal statistical framework" either for reporting *P* values or for analysis of SNP data (Roeder et al. 2005). We have presented raw *P* values uncorrected for multiple testing, but the significance of reported *P* values should be viewed with caution, given the number of statistical tests performed.

Empirical significance levels were determined by permutation of affection status for statistical tests involving cases and controls. These levels suggest that the results for the SNPs within *GRIN2A* for *rs1014531* ($P = 2.9 \times 10^{-7}$) in the multiplex case-control analysis and for intron 10 ($P = 2.32 \times 10^{-12}$) in the singleton case-control analysis are significant results. Additionally, the logistic regression analysis suggests *GRIN2A* haplotypes are significant contributors to genetic risk for autism. Determining empirical *P* values for the family-based tests for association, such as the PDT, requires correlations between transmitted alleles within pedigrees to be preserved, and "[i]t is not clear whether a simple permutation procedure can be developed for this purpose in general pedigrees" (Martin et al. 2000, p. 153). Additionally, simple permutation of affection status is inappropriate for the trend test, because the correlation between alleles in related cases must be preserved (Slager and Schaid 2001). Interpreting the results from these statistical tests is challenging, but, on balance, the strongest evidence of association with autism comes principally from *GRIN2A,* with *ABAT* accounting for the remaining association.

Both SNPs genotyped in *ABAT* have genotypes associated with autism in the case-control analysis of the multiplex sample, with use of Fisher's exact test for count data (Fisher's exact test provides more power than the PDT, given the sample sizes). The result for the intron 1 SNP was also replicated in the singleton sample. The result is further supported by the logistic regression analysis, which indicates a difference in haplotype distribution between cases and controls. *ABAT* is a good positional functional candidate for autism, especially given its involvement in the catabolism of GABA, which is known to be involved in neurological disease (Wong et al. 2003). Other genes involved in this pathway have been studied elsewhere, including the GABA receptor subunit $\beta 3$ (*GABRB3*) on 15q11-13, following reports of chromosomal abnormalities in autistic individuals. A number of studies have been published on the role of this pathway in autism (reviewed by Veenstra-VanderWeele and Cook [2004]).

Screening the coding sequence of *ABAT* revealed one high-frequency missense mutation, but this does not occur in a highly conserved position and was less strongly associated with autism, compared with the SNP within intron 1. It seems likely that any variants influencing the expression of *ABAT* in individuals with autism are located outside of the coding sequence within regulatory regions.

No missense variants were detected by DHPLC in *GRIN2A*. However, SNPs within *GRIN2A* gave strong evidence of association in the case-control analysis of the multiplex and singleton samples. There was also some evidence of transmission disequilibrium with the SNP in intron 10 in PDT results. Additionally, the logistic regression analysis found a significant difference in haplotype distribution between cases and controls. *GRIN2A* is an interesting candidate gene for autism, given its role in learning and memory and the evidence from mouse models of a complex behavioral phenotype (Bannerman et al. 2004). There is also evidence, from postmortem analysis, of expression differences in the glutamate system between cerebella of subjects with autism and of controls (Purcell et al. 2001). Variants within *GRIN2A* may also confer increased risk for ADHD, which indicates involvement in behavioral disorders (Turic et al. 2004).

The candidate-gene analysis presented here is substantial but not completely exhaustive. Candidate genes were screened for coding variants, and association analysis was performed, but additional SNPs with inter-SNP distances of 5–10 kb may be required to conclusively discount these genes having a role in autism susceptibility (Kruglyak 1999). Increasing the density of SNPs across candidate genes, on the basis of known patterns of LD, to capture the maximum information about haplotypic diversity is now increasingly feasible, as data become available from the International HapMap Project. Prior knowledge of the LD structure of a region will allow a more-intelligent and -efficient approach to association mapping in studies of candidate genes and perhaps will lead to less-tentative statistical analysis and more-definitive conclusions (Zondervan and Cardon 2004). A combination of strategies that include association mapping and complementary statistical and bioinformatic analysis will be needed to determine the significance of the results for *GRIN2A* and *ABAT,* as well as replication in independent samples. The design of subsequent studies should also include careful consideration of the control samples used for allele- and genotype-frequency comparisons, in terms of their ethnicity, sex, and independence. Chromosome 16p has been identified by a number of genome screens for autism and is likely to contain an autism-susceptibility variant. Although the 16p locus has been less consistently replicated than the chromosome 7 locus, it remains an important area for future research (Lamb et al. 2002). However, as with all multifactorial disorders, progressing from a broad linkage peak to identifiable functional genetic variants remains a significant challenge.

Acknowledgments

This work would not have been possible without the cooperation of the subjects, their families, and the many referring professionals. This work was funded by the U.K. Medical Research Council, The Wellcome Trust, BIOMED 2 grant CT-97-2759, European Community Fifth Framework grant QLG2-CT-1999-0094, Telethon-Italy grant GGP030227, Fondazione Cassa di Risparmio di Bologna, the Janus Korczak Foundation, Deutsche Forschungsgemeinschaft, Fondation France Télécom, Conseil Régional Midi-Pyrénées, Danish Medical Research Council, Sofiefonden, the Beatrice Surovell Haskells Fund for Child Mental Health Research of Copenhagen, Danish Natural Science Research Council grant 9802210, and National Institutes of Health (NIH) grants MO1 RR06022 GCRC NIH, NIH K05 MH01196, K02 MH01389, and U19 HD35482. A.J.B is the Cheryl and Reece Scott Professor of Psychiatry. A.P.M. is a Wellcome Trust Principal Research Fellow. Members of the IMGSAC follow and are grouped by institution. In the United Kingdom: Nicola Mathews, Jeremy Parr, Simon Wallace, and A.J.B. (Section of Child and Adolescent Psychiatry, University Department of Psychiatry, Park Hospital for Children, Oxford); G.B., Elena Bonora, J.L., Angela Marlow, N.S., and A.P.M. (Wellcome Trust Centre for Human Genetics, University of Oxford, Oxford); Patrick Bolton and Michael Rutter (Social, Genetic and Development Research Centre, Institute of Psychiatry, London); Gillian Baird (Newcomen Centre, Guy's Hospital, London); Stephen Abbs, Zoe Docherty, Caroline Ogilvie, and Pamela Warburton (South East Thames Regional Genetics Centre, Division of Medical and Molecular Genetics, Guy's Hospital, London); Tom Berney, Ann Le Couteur, and Helen McConachie (School of Clinical Medical Sciences, University of Newcastle, Newcastle); Petrus de Vries and Emma Weisblatt (Developmental Psychiatry Section, University of Cambridge Clinical School, Cambridge); Catherine Aldred, Julie-Anne Wilkinson, and Jonathan Green (Academic Department of Child Psychiatry, University of Manchester, Manchester); and Andrew Pickles (School of Epidemiology and Health Science, University of Manchester, Manchester); Philippa Bracegirdle, Ros Packer, and Bryan Bolton (ECACC Health Protection Agency, Porton Down). In Italy: Elena Bacchelli, Francesca Blasi, Simona Carone, and Elena Maestrini (Dipartimento di Biologia Evoluzionistica Sperimentale, University of Bologna, Bologna). In the Netherlands: Maretha De Jonge, Chantal Kemner, Margreet Scherpenisse, Karlijn Steggehuis, and Herman Van Engeland (Department of Child and Adolescent Psychiatry, Academisch Ziekenhuis Utrecht [AZU], Utrecht); and Ineke den Hartog (Department of Child Psychiatry, AZU, Utrecht). In Germany: Sabine M. Klauck, Bärbel Felder, Claudia Schuster, and Annemarie Poustka (Deutsches Krebsforschungszentrum, Molecular Genome Analysis, Heidelberg); and Sven Bölte, Sabine Feineis-Matthews, Nora Uhlig, Dorothea Rühl, Gabriele Schmötzer, and Fritz Poustka (Department of Child and Adolescent Psychiatry, J.W. Goethe-Universität, Frankfurt). In France: Eric Fombonne, Jeanne Fremolle-Kruck, Carine Mantoulan, and Kerstin Wittemeyer (Hôpital la Grave, Toulouse); and Bernadette Rogé (Centre d'Études et de Recherches en PsychoPathologie, Maison de la Recherche, Université de Toulouse le Mirail, Toulouse). In Denmark: Ester Ulsted Sorensen, Birgitte Viskum, Rodney Cotterill, Karen-Brondum-Nielsen, Gunna Eriksen, Demetrious Haracopos, Torben Isager, and Lennart Pedersen (Centre for Autisme, Bagsvaerd). In Greece: Katerina Papanikolaou and John Tsiantis (Agia Sophia Children's Hospital, Athens). In the United States: D.E.W. (Department of Human Genetics, University of Pittsburgh, Pittsburgh); Jeff Salt, Stephen Guter, Bennett Leventhal, and Edwin Cook (Department of Psychiatry, University of Chicago, Chicago); Stanley Nelson and Susan Smalley (Center for Neurobehavioral Genetics, University of California at Los Angeles [UCLA], Los Angeles); Jennifer Levitt (Child Psychiatry Division, UCLA Psychiatric Institute, Los Angeles); Christina Corsello and Catherine Lord (University of Michigan Autism and Communicative Disorders Center, Ann Arbor); and Joel Bregman, Ami Klin, Kathy Koenig, Rosalind Oti, and Fred Volkmar (Yale University, New Haven).

Electronic-Database Information

Accession numbers and URLs for data presented herein are as follows:

Berkeley *Drosophila* Genome Project, http:///www.fruitfly.org/seq_tools/splice.html (for SpliceSite analysis)
dbSNP Home Page, http://www.ncbi.nlm.nih.gov/SNP/index.html
ECACC, http://www.ecacc.org.uk/
ESEfinder, http://rulai.cshl.edu/tools/ESE/
GenBank, http://www.ncbi.nlm.nih.gov/Genbank/ (for *A2BP1* [accession number NM_018723], *ABAT* [accession number BC031413], *BFAR* [accession number NM_016561], *CREBBP* [accession number NM_004380], *EMP2* [accession number NM_001424], *GRIN2A* [accession number NM_000833], *MRTF-B* [accession number NM_014048], *SSTR5* [accession number NM_001053], *TBX6* [accession number NM_004608], and *UBN1* [accession number NM_016936])
IGS, http://bioinformatics.well.ox.ac.uk/project-lims.shtml
IMGSAC, http://www.ox.ac.uk/~maestrin/iat.html
International HapMap Project, http://www.hapmap.org/
LocusLink, http://www.ncbi.nih.gov/entrez/query.fcgi?db=gene
Online Mendelian Inheritance in Man (OMIM), http://www.ncbi.nlm.nih.gov/Omim/ (for *GRIN2A, SSTR5, TBX6, CREBBP,* RTS, *EMP2, ABAT, A2BP1,* and *SCA2*)
Pfam, http://www.sanger.ac.uk/Software/Pfam/
PolyPhen, http://tux.embl-heidelberg.de/ramensky
Primer3, http://www-genome.wi.mit.edu/cgi-bin/primer/primer3_www.cgi
R Project for Statistical Computing, http://www.r-project.org/
SIBMED program, http://www.sph.umich.edu/
UCSC Genome Browser, http://genome.ucsc.edu/
University of Pittsburgh Department of Human Genetics, http://watson.hgen.pitt.edu/ (for Mega2, version 2.5)

References

Abecasis GR, Cookson WO (2000) GOLD—graphical overview of linkage disequilibrium. Bioinformatics 16:182–183

Bailey A, Le Couteur A, Gottesman I, Bolton P, Simonoff E, Yuzda E, Rutter M (1995) Autism as a strongly genetic disorder: evidence from a British twin study. Psychol Med 25: 63–77

Bannerman DM, Deacon RM, Brady S, Bruce A, Sprengel R, Seeburg PH, Rawlins JN (2004) A comparison of GluR-A-deficient and wild-type mice on a test battery assessing sensorimotor, affective, and cognitive behaviors. Behav Neurosci 118:643–647

Bateman A, Coin L, Durbin R, Finn RD, Hollich V, Griffiths-Jones S, Khanna A, Marshall M, Moxon S, Sonnhammer EL, Studholme DJ, Yeats C, Eddy SR (2004) The Pfam protein families database. Nucleic Acids Res 32 D138–D141

Bonora E, Lamb JA, Barnby G, Sykes N, Moberly T, Beyer KS, Klauck SM, et al (2005) Mutation screening and association analysis of six candidate genes for autism on chromosome 7q. Eur J Hum Genet 13:198–207

Brunak S, Engelbrecht J, Knudsen S (1991) Prediction of human mRNA donor and acceptor sites from the DNA sequence. J Mol Biol 220:49–65

Cartegni L, Wang J, Zhu Z, Zhang MQ, Krainer AR (2003) ESEfinder: a Web resource to identify exonic splicing enhancers. Nucleic Acids Res 31:3568–3571

Chakrabarti S, Fombonne E (2001) Pervasive developmental disorders in preschool children. JAMA 285:3093–3099

Chrivia JC, Kwok RP, Lamb N, Hagiwara M, Montminy MR, Goodman RH (1993) Phosphorylated CREB binds specifically to the nuclear protein CBP. Nature 365:855–859

Clayton D, Jones H (1999) Transmission/disequilibrium tests for extended marker haplotypes. Am J Hum Genet 65:1161–1169

De Biase D, Barra D, Simmaco M, John RA, Bossa F (1995) Primary structure and tissue distribution of human 4-aminobutyrate aminotransferase. Eur J Biochem 227:476–480

Douglas JA, Boehnke M, Lange K (2000) A multipoint method for detecting genotyping errors and mutations in sibling-pair linkage data. Am J Hum Genet 66:1287–1297

Finelli P, Natacci F, Bonati MT, Gottardi G, Engelen JJ, de Die-Smulders CE, Sala M, Giardino D, Larizza L (2004) FISH characterisation of an identical (16)(p11.2p12.2) tandem duplication in two unrelated patients with autistic behaviour. J Med Genet 41:e90

Fombonne E (2002) Epidemiological trends in rates of autism. Mol Psychiatry (Suppl 2) 7:S4–S6

——— (2003) Epidemiological surveys of autism and other pervasive developmental disorders: an update. J Autism Dev Disord 33:365–382

Hellings JA, Hossain S, Martin JK, Baratang RR (2002) Psychopathology, GABA, and the Rubinstein-Taybi syndrome: a review and case study. Am J Med Genet 114:190–195

IMGSAC (2001) A genomewide screen for autism: strong evidence for linkage to chromosomes 2q, 7q, and 16p. Am J Hum Genet 69:570–581

Itoh N, Tsujimoto Y, Nagata S (1993) Effect of bcl-2 on Fas antigen-mediated cell death. J Immunol 151:621–627

Jamain S, Quach H, Betancur C, Rastam M, Colineaux C, Gillberg IC, Soderstrom H, Giros B, Leboyer M, Gillberg C, Bourgeron T, and the Paris Autism Research International Sibpair Study (2003) Mutations of the X-linked genes encoding neuroligins NLGN3 and NLGN4 are associated with autism. Nat Genet 34:27–29

Kruglyak L (1999) Prospects for whole-genome linkage disequilibrium mapping of common disease genes. Nat Genet 22:139–144

Kulp D, Haussler D, Reese MG, Eeckman FH (1997) Integrating database homology in a probabilistic gene structure model. Pac Symp Biocomput 232–244

Lamb JA, Barnby G, Bonora E, Sykes N, Bacchelli E, Blasi F, Maestrini E, Broxholme J, Tzenova J, Weeks D, Bailey AJ, Monaco AP (2005) Analysis of IMGSAC autism susceptibility loci: evidence for sex limited and parent of origin specific effects. J Med Genet 42:132–137

Lamb JA, Parr JR, Bailey AJ, Monaco AP (2002) Autism: in search of susceptibility genes. Neuromolecular Med 2:11–28

Lauritsen MB, Nyegaard M, Betancur C, Colineaux C, Josiassen TL, Kruse TA, Leboyer M, Ewald H (2003) Analysis of transmission of novel polymorphisms in the somatostatin receptor 5 (SSTR5) gene in patients with autism. Am J Med Genet B Neuropsychiatr Genet 121:100–104

Le Couteur A, Rutter M, Lord C, Rios P, Robertson S, Holdgrafer M, McLennan J (1989) Autism diagnostic interview: a standardized investigator-based instrument. J Autism Dev Disord 19:363–387

Lewontin R, Kojima K (1960) The evolutionary dynamics of complex polymorphisms. Evolution 14:458–472

Liu J, Nyholt DR, Magnussen P, Parano E, Pavone P, Geschwind D, Lord C, Iversen P, Hoh J, Autism Genetic Resource Exchange Consortium, Ott J, Gilliam TC (2001) A genomewide screen for autism susceptibility loci. Am J Hum Genet 69:327–340

Lord C, Risi S, Lambrecht L, Cook EH Jr, Leventhal BL, DiLavore PC, Pickles A, Rutter M (2000) The autism diagnostic observation schedule-generic: a standard measure of social and communication deficits associated with the spectrum of autism. J Autism Dev Disord 30:205–223

Martin ER, Bass MP, Gilbert JR, Pericak-Vance MA, Hauser ER (2003*a*) Genotype-based association test for general pedigrees: the genotype-PDT. Genet Epidemiol 25:203–213

Martin ER, Bass MP, Hauser ER, Kaplan NL (2003*b*) Accounting for linkage in family-based tests of association with missing parental genotypes. Am J Hum Genet 73:1016–1026

Martin ER, Monks SA, Warren LL, Kaplan NL (2000) A test for linkage and association in general pedigrees: the pedigree disequilibrium test. Am J Hum Genet 67:146–154

Mukhopadhyay N, Almasy L, Schroeder M, Mulvihill WP, Weeks DE (1999) Mega2, a data-handling program for facilitating genetic linkage and association analysis. Am J Hum Genet Suppl 65:A436

Nagase T, Ishikawa K, Kikuno R, Hirosawa M, Nomura N, Ohara O (1999) Prediction of the coding sequences of unidentified human genes. XV. The complete sequences of 100 new cDNA clones from brain which code for large proteins in vitro. DNA Res 6:337–345

O'Connell JR, Weeks DE (1998) PedCheck: a program for identification of genotype incompatibilities in linkage analysis. Am J Hum Genet 63:259–266

Ogdie MN, Fisher SE, Yang M, Ishii J, Francks C, Loo SK, Cantor RM, McCracken JT, McGough JJ, Smalley SL, Nelson SF (2004) Attention deficit hyperactivity disorder: fine mapping supports linkage to 5p13, 6q12, 16p13, and 17p11. Am J Hum Genet 75:661–668

Ogdie MN, Macphie IL, Minassian SL, Yang M, Fisher SE, Francks C, Cantor RM, McCracken JT, McGough JJ, Nelson SF, Monaco AP, Smalley SL (2003) A genomewide scan for attention-deficit/hyperactivity disorder in an extended sample: suggestive linkage on 17p11. Am J Hum Genet 72: 1268–1279

Pagani F, Stuani C, Tzetis M, Kanavakis E, Efthymiadou A, Doudounakis S, Casals T, Baralle FE (2003) New type of disease causing mutations: the example of the composite exonic regulatory elements of splicing in CFTR exon 12. Hum Mol Genet 12:1111–1120

Papapetrou C, Putt W, Fox M, Edwards YH (1999) The human TBX6 gene: cloning and assignment to chromosome 16p11.2. Genomics 55:238–241

Philippe A, Martinez M, Guilloud-Bataille M, Gillberg C, Rastam M, Sponheim E, Coleman M, Zappella M, Aschauer H, Van Maldergem L, Penet C, Feingold J, Brice A, Leboyer M, and the Paris Autism Research International Sibpair Study (1999) Genome-wide scan for autism susceptibility genes. Hum Mol Genet 8:805–812

Pickles A, Bolton P, Macdonald H, Bailey A, Le Couteur A, Sim CH, Rutter M (1995) Latent-class analysis of recurrence risks for complex phenotypes with selection and measurement error: a twin and family history study of autism. Am J Hum Genet 57:717–726

Pickles A, Starr E, Kazak S, Bolton P, Papanikolaou K, Bailey A, Goodman R, Rutter M (2000) Variable expression of the autism broader phenotype: findings from extended pedigrees. J Child Psychol Psychiatry 41:491–502

Pritchard JK, Cox NJ (2002) The allelic architecture of human disease genes: common disease-common variant…or not? Hum Mol Genet 11:2417–2423

Purcell AE, Jeon OH, Zimmerman AW, Blue ME, Pevsner J (2001) Postmortem brain abnormalities of the glutamate neurotransmitter system in autism. Neurology 57:1618–1628

Risch N, Teng J (1998) The relative power of family-based and case-control designs for linkage disequilibrium studies of complex human diseases I. DNA pooling. Genome Res 8:1273–1288

Roeder K, Bacanu SA, Sonpar V, Zhang X, Devlin B (2005) Analysis of single-locus tests to detect gene/disease associations. Genet Epidemiol 28:207–219

Sakimura K, Kutsuwada T, Ito I, Manabe T, Takayama C, Kushiya E, Yagi T, Aizawa S, Inoue Y, Sugiyama H, Mishina M (1995) Reduced hippocampal LTP and spatial learning in mice lacking NMDA receptor epsilon 1 subunit. Nature 373:151–155

Selvaraj A, Prywes R (2003) Megakaryoblastic leukemia-1/2, a transcriptional co-activator of serum response factor, is required for skeletal myogenic differentiation. J Biol Chem 278:41977–41987

Shao Y, Wolpert CM, Raiford KL, Menold MM, Donnelly SL, Ravan SA, Bass MP, McClain C, von Wendt L, Vance JM, Abramson RH, Wright HH, Ashley-Koch A, Gilbert JR, DeLong RG, Cuccaro ML, Pericak-Vance MA (2002) Genomic screen and follow-up analysis for autistic disorder. Am J Med Genet 114:99–105

Shibata H, Huynh DP, Pulst SM (2000) A novel protein with RNA-binding motifs interacts with ataxin-2. Hum Mol Genet 9:1303–1313

Slager SL, Schaid DJ (2001) Evaluation of candidate genes in case-control studies: a statistical method to account for related subjects. Am J Hum Genet 68:1457–1462

Smalley SL, Kustanovich V, Minassian SL, Stone JL, Ogdie MN, McGough JJ, McCracken JT, MacPhie IL, Francks C, Fisher SE, Cantor RM, Monaco AP, Nelson SF (2002) Genetic linkage of attention-deficit/hyperactivity disorder on chromosome 16p13, in a region implicated in autism. Am J Hum Genet 71:959–963

Sparrow S, Balla D, Cicchetti D (1984) Vineland Adaptive Behavior Scales. Circle Pines, MN

Stone JL, Tsai S, Merriman B, Cantor-Chui RM, Geschwind D, Nelson SF, Consortium A (2003) High density SNP based association study of 21 candidate genes in autism spectrum disorder. Paper presented at The American Society of Human Genetics, Los Angeles, November 4–8

Sunyaev S, Ramensky V, Koch I, Lathe W 3rd, Kondrashov AS, Bork P (2001) Prediction of deleterious human alleles. Hum Mol Genet 10:591–597

Suzuki A, Yamada R, Chang X, Tokuhiro S, Sawada T, Suzuki M, Nagasaki M, Nakayama-Hamada M, Kawaida R, Ono M, Ohtsuki M, Furukawa H, Yoshino S, Yukioka M, Tohma S, Matsubara T, Wakitani S, Teshima R, Nishioka Y, Sekine A, Iida A, Takahashi A, Tsunoda T, Nakamura Y, Yamamoto K (2003) Functional haplotypes of PADI4, encoding citrullinating enzyme peptidylarginine deiminase 4, are associated with rheumatoid arthritis. Nat Genet 34:395–402

Tokuhiro S, Yamada R, Chang X, Suzuki A, Kochi Y, Sawada T, Suzuki M, Nagasaki M, Ohtsuki M, Ono M, Furukawa H, Nagashima M, Yoshino S, Mabuchi A, Sekine A, Saito S, Takahashi A, Tsunoda T, Nakamura Y, Yamamoto K (2003) An intronic SNP in a RUNX1 binding site of SLC22A4, encoding an organic cation transporter, is associated with rheumatoid arthritis. Nat Genet 35:341–348

Turic D, Langley K, Mills S, Stephens M, Lawson D, Govan C, Williams N, Van Den Bree M, Craddock N, Kent L, Owen M, O'Donovan M, Thapar A (2004) Follow-up of genetic linkage findings on chromosome 16p13: evidence of association of N-methyl-D aspartate glutamate receptor 2A gene polymorphism with ADHD. Mol Psychiatry 9:169–173

Veenstra-VanderWeele J, Cook EH (2004) Molecular genetics of autism spectrum disorder. Mol Psychiatry 9:819–832

Vincent JB, Kolozsvari D, Roberts WS, Bolton PF, Gurling HM, Scherer SW (2004) Mutation screening of X-chromosomal neuroligin genes: no mutations in 196 autism probands. Am J Med Genet B Neuropsychiatr Genet 129B:82–84

Wallenstein S, Hodge SE, Weston A (1998) Logistic regression model for analyzing extended haplotype data. Genet Epidemiol 15:173–181

Wei MC, Zong WX, Cheng EH, Lindsten T, Panoutsakopoulou V, Ross AJ, Roth KA, MacGregor GR, Thompson CB, Korsmeyer SJ (2001) Proapoptotic BAX and BAK: a requisite gateway to mitochondrial dysfunction and death. Science 292:727–730

Wong CG, Bottiglieri T, Snead OC 3rd (2003) GABA, gamma-hydroxybutyric acid, and neurological disease. Ann Neurol (Suppl 6) 54:S3–S12

Zaykin DV, Westfall PH, Young SS, Karnoub MA, Wagner MJ, Ehm MG (2002) Testing association of statistically inferred haplotypes with discrete and continuous traits in samples of unrelated individuals. Hum Hered 53:79–91

Zondervan KT, Cardon LR (2004) The complex interplay among factors that influence allelic association. Nat Rev Genet 5:89–100

Rational Inferences about Departures from Hardy-Weinberg Equilibrium

Jacqueline K. Wittke-Thompson,[1] Anna Pluzhnikov,[1] and Nancy J. Cox[1,2]

Departments of [1]Human Genetics and [2]Medicine, The University of Chicago, Chicago

Previous studies have explored the use of departure from Hardy-Weinberg equilibrium (DHW) for fine mapping Mendelian disorders and for general fine mapping. Other studies have used Hardy-Weinberg tests for genotyping quality control. To enable investigators to make rational decisions about whether DHW is due to genotyping error or to underlying biology, we developed an analytic framework and software to determine the parameter values for which DHW might be expected for common diseases. We show analytically that, for a general disease model, the difference between population and Hardy-Weinberg–expected genotypic frequencies (Δ) at the susceptibility locus is a function of the susceptibility-allele frequency (q), heterozygote relative risk (β), and homozygote relative risk (γ). For unaffected control samples, Δ is a function of risk in nonsusceptible homozygotes (α), the population prevalence of disease (K_P), q, β, and γ. We used these analytic functions to calculate Δ and the number of cases or controls needed to detect DHW for a range of genetic models consistent with common diseases ($1.1 \leqslant \gamma \leqslant 10$ and $0.005 \leqslant K_P \leqslant 0.2$). Results suggest that significant DHW can be expected in relatively small samples of patients over a range of genetic models. We also propose a goodness-of-fit test to aid investigators in determining whether a DHW observed in the context of a case-control study is consistent with a genetic disease model. We illustrate how the analytic framework and software can be used to help investigators interpret DHW in the context of association studies of common diseases.

Introduction

Hardy-Weinberg equilibrium (HWE) has been used for more than a century to better understand genetic characteristics of populations. In 1902, William E. Castle noted that, if the selective removal from the general population of individuals who have a recessive genotype at a particular locus ceases, then the future generation will establish an equilibrium value of recessive alleles. His conclusions assume that one allele is dominant with respect to the other(s), that the alleles do not affect fertility, that there is no migration into or out of the population, and that the population is large and randomly mating (Castle 1903; Li 1967). Five years later, G. H. Hardy and W. Weinberg individually came to the same conclusion but noted that the population allele frequencies could be used to calculate the equilibrium-expected genotypic proportions (Hardy 1908; Weinberg 1908). If p is the frequency of one allele (A) and q is the frequency of the alternative allele (a) for a biallelic locus, then the HWE-expected frequency will be p^2 for the AA genotype, $2pq$ for the Aa genotype, and q^2 for the aa genotype. The three genotypic proportions should sum to 1, as should the allele frequencies (Hardy 1908; Weinberg 1908).

The most common way to assess HWE is through a goodness-of-fit χ^2 test (Weir 1996). The null hypothesis is that alleles are chosen randomly, and the genotypic proportions thus follow HWE-expected proportions (i.e., p^2, $2pq$, and q^2). Alternatively, the second allele is dependent on the first allele being selected, resulting in the genotypic proportions deviating from the HWE-expected proportions. The χ^2 test for HWE has $k(k-1)/2$ df, where k is the number of alleles at the locus being studied (Weir 1996). Or, more intuitively, the degrees of freedom can be calculated by $g - k$, where g is the number of possible genotypes and k is the number of alleles. For example, a SNP that has two alleles and three possible genotypes yields 1 df for the χ^2 test that assesses the significance of departure from HWE (DHW).

Testing for HWE is commonly used for quality control of large-scale genotyping and is one of the few ways to identify systematic genotyping errors in unrelated individuals (Gomes et al. 1999; Hosking et al. 2004). However, there is little consensus on the correct threshold for identifying DHW in the context of large-scale studies or on what to do with markers that fit all other quality-control criteria but show a significant DHW, given the study-specific threshold. Some association studies do not consider DHW in patients to indicate genotyping error but prefer to assume a biological explanation for DHW in a patient sample, while requiring

Received January 18, 2005; accepted for publication March 24, 2005; electronically published April 15, 2005.

Address for correspondence and reprints: Dr. Nancy J. Cox, Department of Human Genetics, 507H CLSC, 920 East 58th Street, Chicago, IL 60637. Email: ncox@genetics.bsd.uchicago.edu

0002-9297/2005/7606-0006$15.00

control or random samples to be in HWE (Oka et al. 1999; Levecque et al. 2003; Nejentsev et al. 2003). Others require that both the patient and the control samples be in HWE for the marker to be used in further analyses (Martin et al. 2000; Xu et al. 2001; Wang et al. 2003). Bonferroni correction is commonly used to correct for multiple testing when many markers are tested for HWE but is a conservative approach if the markers are correlated (e.g., are in linkage disequilibrium [LD]). Another widespread approach is to assign a significance level, such as 5% or 1%, and to test each marker without regard for whether markers are independent. Sometimes, markers showing DHW are removed from a data set because subsequent genetic analysis requires HWE to be assumed. However, since the design of association studies is to partition cases and controls in the general population on the basis of their phenotype and genetic composition, cases and controls at a disease locus may be expected to show DHW under certain conditions. There is little guidance on how to distinguish between markers whose DHW is due to chance, genotyping error, or failure of one of the requisite assumptions of HWE from markers whose DHW is due to their proximity to an allele affecting a phenotype on which the sample is ascertained (Xu et al. 2002).

Our focus is to understand DHW observed in the context of association studies. When an investigator observes a marker with a significant DHW, a key question is "Are deviations from HWE due to genotyping error, chance, failure of assumptions underlying Hardy-Weinberg expectations, or, instead, to the underlying genetic disease model?" To address this question, we developed an analytic framework for assessing the difference between population and HWE-expected genotypic proportions (Δ), as well as software tools for calculating expectations over a range of single-locus genetic disease models. We use a single-locus context in our examination of DHW because it enables us to represent the marginal effects of the particular susceptibility locus being examined. For general disease models, we show that Δ in patients at the disease locus is determined by the population susceptibility-allele frequency (q), the homozygote relative risk (γ), and the heterozygote relative risk (β). For "true" control samples (i.e., those ascertained by being unaffected with respect to disease status), the value of Δ depends on the risk to nonsusceptible homozygotes (α), q, γ, and β. Using these formulations, we have examined a wide range of parameter values for genetic models commonly believed to be consistent with observations for complex disorders. Our results provide support for the notion that systematic examination of HWE has been underutilized as a tool for fine mapping. To aid investigators in distinguishing a DHW that is generated by the biological model underlying disease transmission from one that is generated by genotyping errors, chance, or failure of the requisite assumptions of HWE, we propose a general goodness-of-fit test to determine whether the observed genotype counts are significantly different from the expected genotype counts in patients and controls for the genetic disease model that best fits the observed data. We provide software for both the investigation of DHW in a generalized single-locus context and the examination of specific observations of DHW.

Methods

Common Disease Models

The prevalence of disease in the general population is defined as $K_P = p^2\alpha + 2pq\alpha\beta + q^2\alpha\gamma$, where p is the population frequency of the wild-type allele (A), q is the frequency of the disease-susceptibility allele (a), and α is the baseline penetrance of disease in homozygotes without a risk allele at this locus. By modeling the population prevalence of disease in the general population in this manner, we explicitly assume that the susceptibility locus will be in HWE in the general population. Note that, although this parameterization is for a single-locus model, there may be many genetic and nongenetic risk factors, in addition to the particular region being studied, that will determine values of the parameters α, β, and γ. Thus, we use this approach to model the marginal effects of a particular model, with the full recognition that, in general, there will be nongenetic risk factors and many other loci with genetic variation that affect the phenotype.

We explored dominant, recessive, additive, and multiplicative genetic models with K_P and γ values that are characteristic of a variety of common diseases, for which K_P values range from 0.005 to 0.2 and γ is equal to 1.1, 1.3, 1.5, 2, 5, or 10. All dominant, recessive, and additive models examined correspond to sibling relative risk (λ_s) values <2.5, although most models have $\lambda_s \leq 1.1$. Multiplicative models generally have higher λ_s values than dominant, recessive, and additive models with identical parameters. The maximum λ_s for a multiplicative model is 4.20, which occurs at the lowest population prevalence ($K_P = 0.005$) and the highest homozygote relative risk ($\gamma = 10$), but most multiplicative models considered have λ_s values <1.2.

The Difference between Population and Expected Genotypic Frequencies (Δ)

Weir (1996) defined a variable, Δ, as the difference between population and HWE-expected genotypic frequencies. Δ is population specific (e.g., Δ_p for patients and Δ_c for unaffected controls), and it ranges from $\max[-(1-q)^2, -q^2]$ to $(q-q^2)$.

To better understand the magnitude and direction of

DHW for different genetic disease models, we defined Δ in terms of key parameters of the genetic model, specified separately in patients and controls, and characterized how parameters interact to affect directionality of DHW (i.e., if $\Delta < 0$, there is a deficiency of homozygotes and an excess of heterozygotes; if $\Delta > 0$, there is an excess of homozygotes and a deficiency of heterozygotes). For patients in a general disease model,

$$\Delta_p = \frac{q^2(1-q)^2(\gamma-\beta^2)}{[(1-q)^2+2q(1-q)\beta+q^2\gamma]^2} . \qquad (1)$$

A more thorough derivation of the above equation and the simplified equations for the classic dominant, recessive, and additive models are given in appendix A. For a multiplicative model, Δ_p is equal to 0 and there is no expected DHW. Figure 1 highlights the direction and magnitude of Δ_p as the susceptibility-allele frequency at the susceptibility locus varies from 0 to 1.

Similarly, for an unaffected control sample,

$$\Delta_c = \frac{\alpha q^2(1-q)^2(2\beta-1-\gamma-\alpha\beta^2+\alpha\gamma)}{(1-K_P)^2} , \qquad (2)$$

and equations for the classic recessive, classic dominant, additive, and multiplicative models are given in appendix B. Figure 2 shows the direction and magnitude of Δ_c for several dominant, recessive, additive, and multiplicative models.

Number of Individuals Needed to Detect DHW

The χ^2 test of HWE for patients can be simplified to the following:

$$\chi^2_p = \frac{N_p\hat{\Delta}^2_p}{\hat{q}^2_p(1-\hat{q}_p)^2} , \qquad (3)$$

where N_p is the number of patients and $\hat{q}_p$ is the susceptibility-allele frequency estimated in patients (Weir 1996). A χ^2 value can also be determined for controls by using the susceptibility-allele frequency in controls ($\hat{q}_c$), Δ_c, and the number of controls in the sample (N_c). The power of the χ^2 test can be accounted for by using a noncentral χ^2 distribution with noncentrality parameter

$$v = \frac{N\hat{\Delta}^2}{\hat{q}^2(1-\hat{q})^2}$$

(Weir 1996).

Given the above equations, it is straightforward to determine the number of individuals required to detect DHW for a specified level of significance and power, for patients and controls under any disease model. In figure 3, results for a variety of models are graphed in terms of N_p or N_c and the overall susceptibility-allele frequency for patients or controls. The results presented in figure 3*A* (patients) and 3*B* (controls) use a central χ^2 distribution corresponding to a significance level of 5% and 50% power, and the results presented in figure 3*C* (patients) and 3*D* (controls) use a noncentral χ^2 distribution corresponding to a significance level of 5% and 80% power.

For congruence with other studies reporting the results in terms of λ_s, the risk of disease in siblings of an affected individual relative to the risk in the general population, are summarized in appendix C with respect to common disease models. We also summarize results with respect to λ_s and Δ in figure 4.

Goodness-of-Fit Test

Given the analytic framework characterized above and a set of observations in patients and controls with DHW in one or both samples, we proceed to identify the genetic disease model with the best fit to the genotypic proportions observed in patients and controls (constrained by the known lifetime prevalence of disease). If that "best-fit" model is, nevertheless, a poor fit to the observed data, as assessed by a χ^2 test with 1 df for a general model and 2 df for a restrictive (dominant, recessive, additive, or multiplicative) model (see appendix D), then it is unlikely that the underlying genetic disease model has generated the observed DHW; thus, alternative explanations for the DHW, including chance, genotyping error, and/or violations of the requisite assumptions of HWE, must be considered.

Examples

We chose several examples from the literature that illustrate how our results and software can help investigators distinguish a DHW consistent with genetic models from one that is not. The first example involves a DHW in patients but not in controls, with data derived from an association study of Crohn disease and a rare frameshift polymorphism (Leu3020fsinsC) in *CARD15/NOD2* (Ogura et al. 2001; J. Cho, personal communication). The second example includes data from an association study that identified a highly significant association ($P = 3.3 \times 10^{-6}$) between *LTA* and myocardial infarction (MI) (Ozaki et al. 2002), attributable in part to the effect of significant DHW in both patients and controls in opposite directions. We also took advantage of several recent surveys of polymorphisms with DHW (Xu et al. 2002; Györffy et al. 2004; Kocsis et al. 2004*a*, 2004*b*; Osawa et al. 2004) to determine the proportion that are consistent with a genetic disease model (table 1).

A

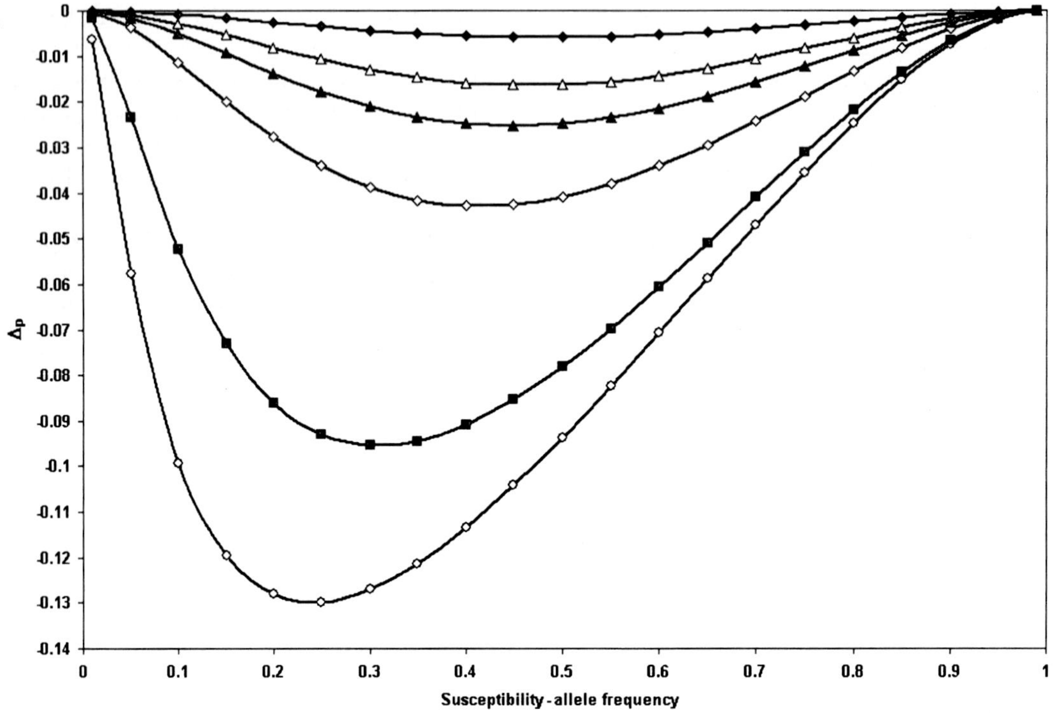

B

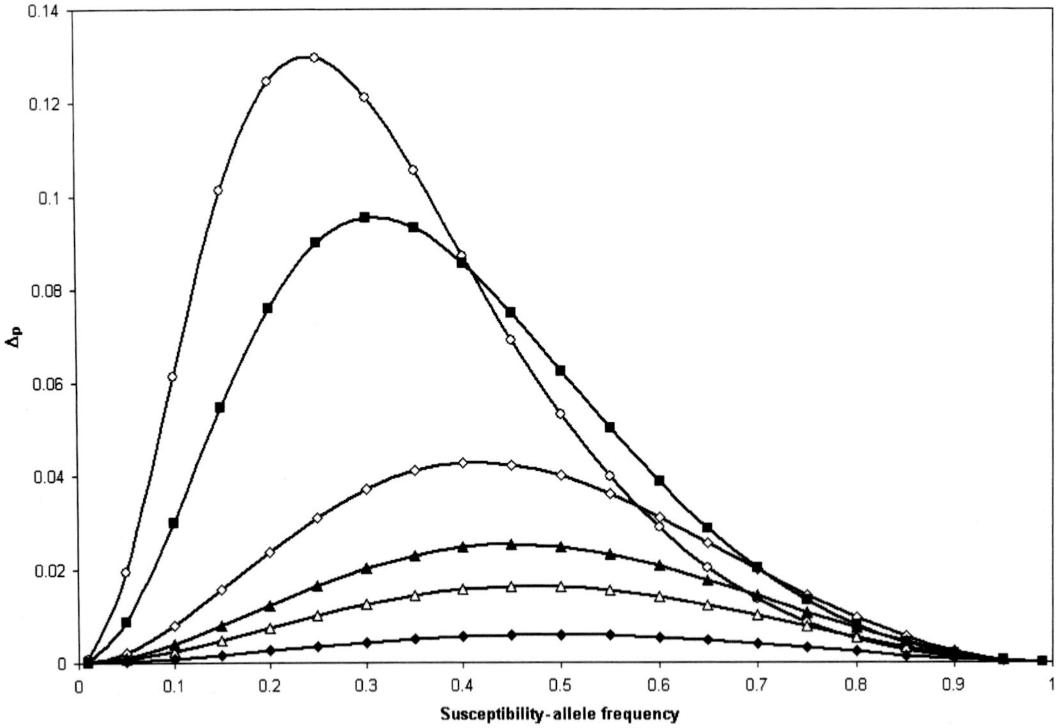

Figure 1 Δ_p plotted versus the susceptibility-allele frequency for patients. *A*, *B*, and *D*, Data points are as follows: $\gamma = 1.1$ (*blackened diamonds*), $\gamma = 1.3$ (*unblackened triangles*), $\gamma = 1.5$ (*blackened triangles*), $\gamma = 2$ (*unblackened diamonds*), $\gamma = 5$ (*blackened squares*), and $\gamma = 10$ (*unblackened circles*). *A*, Dominant model. *B*, Recessive model. *C*, Additive model. Since $\gamma < 2$ would not satisfy our definition of an additive model as $\gamma = 2\beta$ and $\beta > 1$, the data points in C are as follows: $\gamma = 2.2$ ($\beta = 1.1$) (*blackened diamonds*), $\gamma = 2.6$ ($\beta = 1.3$) (*unblackened triangles*), $\gamma = 3$ ($\beta = 1.5$) (*blackened triangles*), $\gamma = 5$ (*blackened squares*), $\gamma = 2$ (*unblackened diamonds*). *D*, Multiplicative model.

C

D

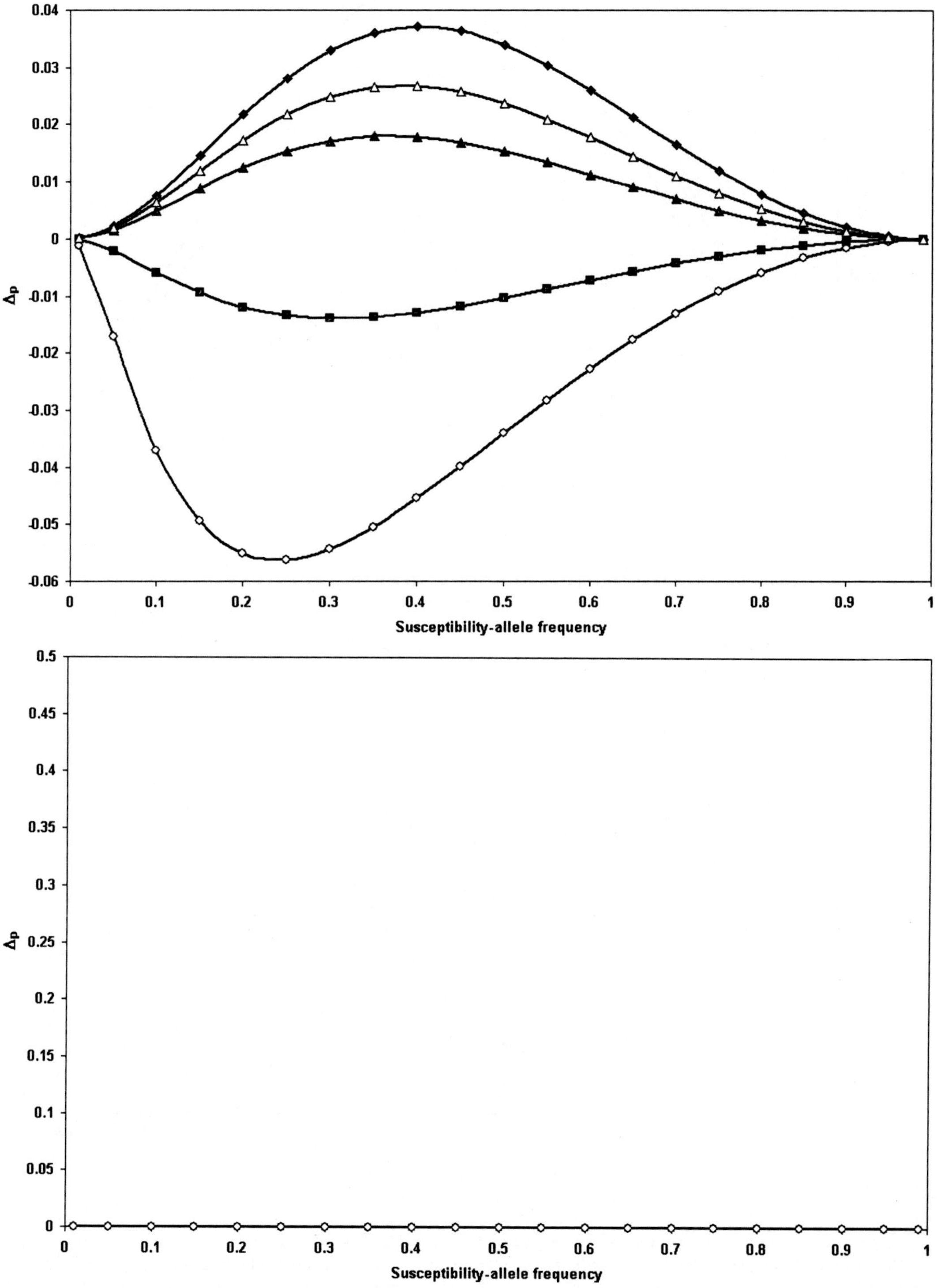
0.04
0.03
0.02
0.01
0
-0.01
-0.02
-0.03
-0.04
-0.05
-0.06
Δp
0
0.1
0.2
0.3
0.4
0.5
0.6
0.7
0.8
0.9
1
Susceptibility-allele frequency
0.5
0.45
0.4
0.35
0.3
0.25
0.2
0.15
0.1
0.05
0
Δp
Susceptibility-allele frequency

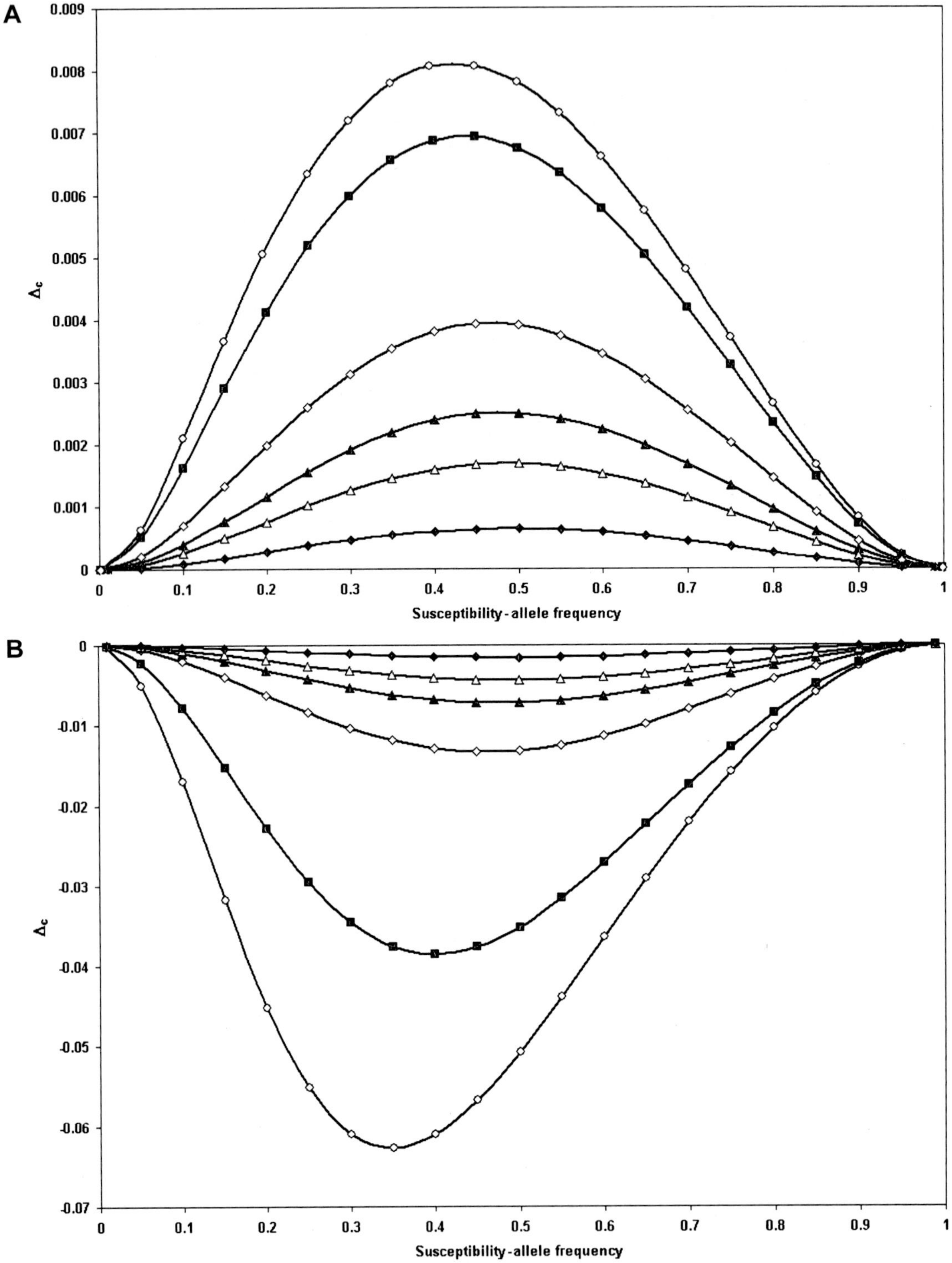

Figure 2 Δ_c plotted versus the susceptibility-allele frequency for controls. *A*, *B*, and *D*, Data points are as follows: $\gamma = 1.1$ (*blackened diamonds*), $\gamma = 1.3$ (*unblackened triangles*), $\gamma = 1.5$ (*blackened triangles*), $\gamma = 2$ (*unblackened diamonds*), $\gamma = 5$ (*blackened squares*), and $\gamma = 10$ (*unblackened circles*). *A*, Dominant model, $K_P = 0.1$. *B*, Recessive model, $K_P = 0.2$. *C*, Additive model, $K_P = 0.01$. As in figure 1, because of our definition of an additive model ($\gamma = 2\beta$ and $\beta > 1$), the data points in C are as follows: $\gamma = 4$ ($\beta = 2$) (*unblackened diamonds*), $\gamma = 2.2$ ($\beta = 1.1$) (*blackened diamonds*), $\gamma = 2.6$ ($\beta = 1.3$) (*unblackened triangles*), $\gamma = 3$ ($\beta = 1.5$) (*blackened triangles*), $\gamma = 2$ (*unblackened diamonds*), $\gamma = 5$ (*blackened squares*), and $\gamma = 10$ (*unblackened circles*). *D*, Multiplicative model, $K_P = 0.05$.

C

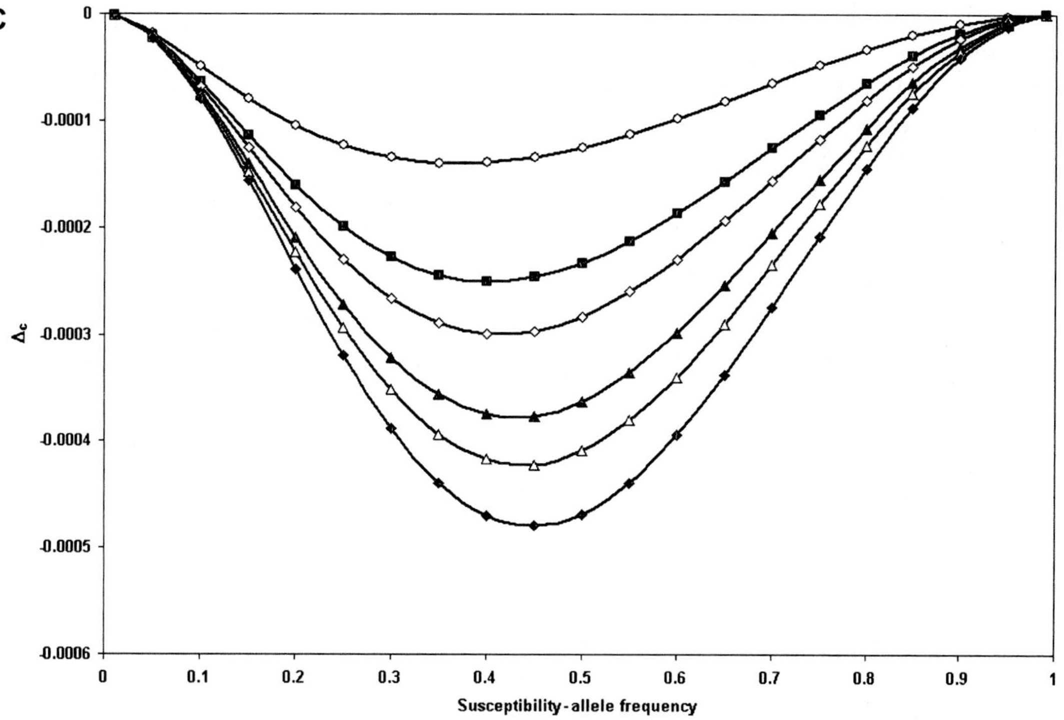

0
-0.0001
-0.0002
-0.0003
-0.0004
-0.0005
-0.0006
Δ_c
0
0.1
0.2
0.3
0.4
0.5
0.6
0.7
0.8
0.9
1
Susceptibility-allele frequency

D

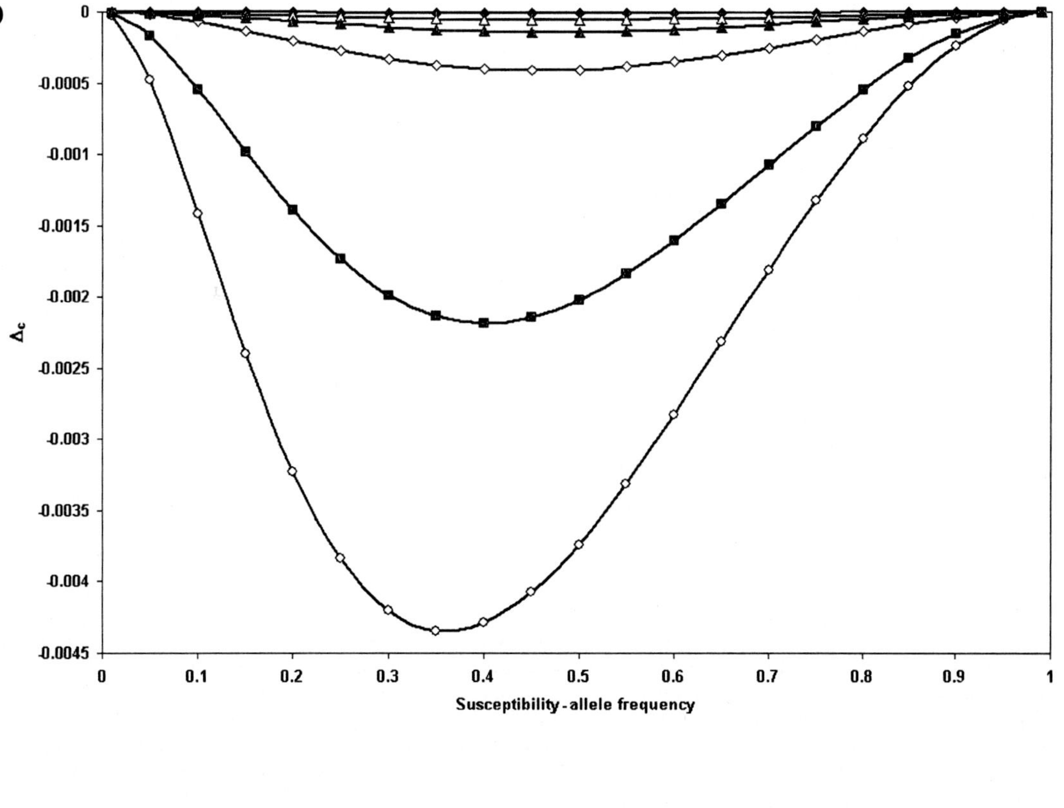

0
-0.0005
-0.001
-0.0015
-0.002
-0.0025
-0.003
-0.0035
-0.004
-0.0045
Δ_c
0
0.1
0.2
0.3
0.4
0.5
0.6
0.7
0.8
0.9
1
Susceptibility-allele frequency

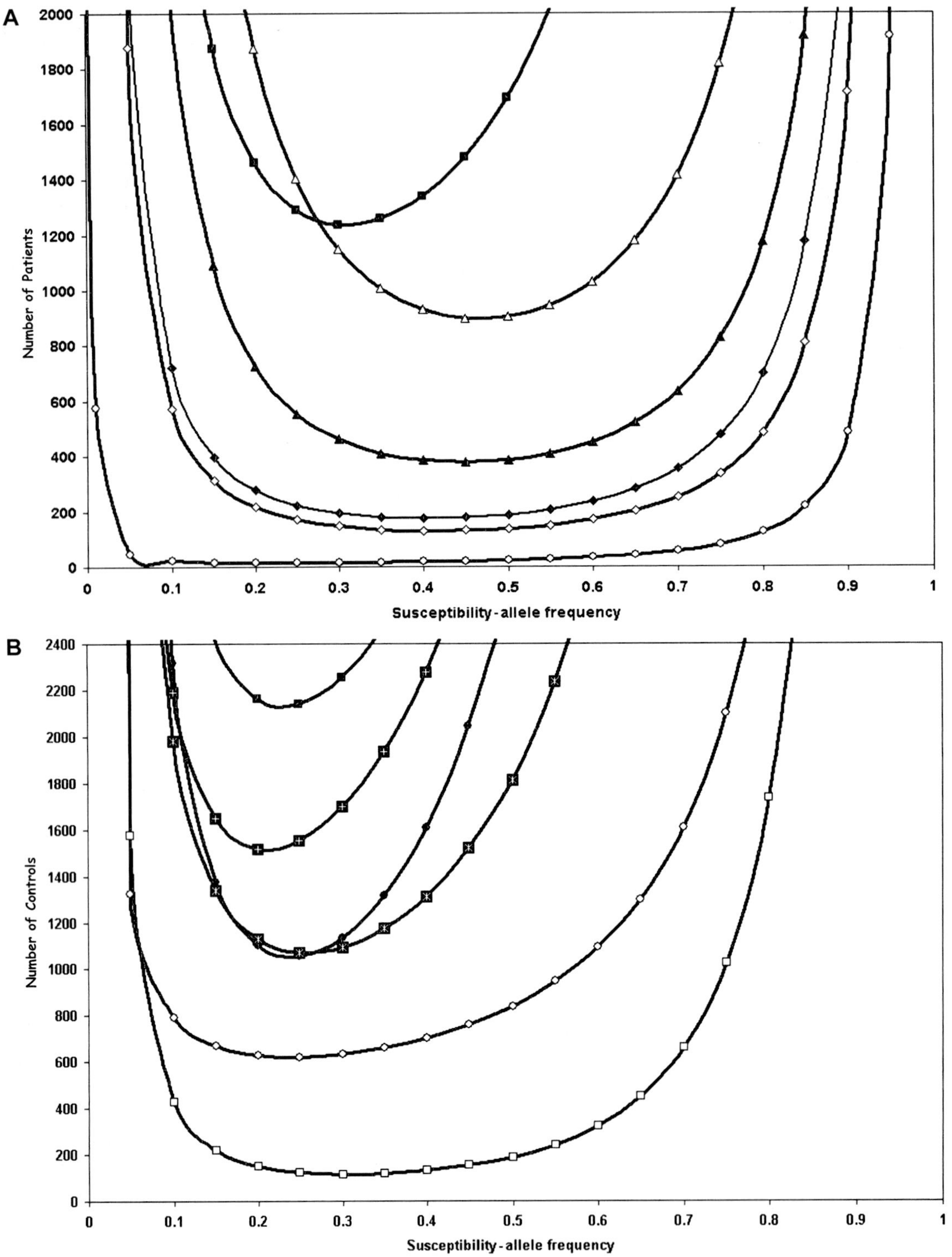

Figure 3 *A*, Number of patients needed to detect DHW as the susceptibility-allele frequency changes at a significance level of 5% and 50% power. Data points are as follows: dominant model with $\gamma = 1.3$ (*unblackened triangles*), dominant model with $\gamma = 10$ (*unblackened circles*), recessive model with $\gamma = 1.5$ (*blackened triangles*), recessive model with $\gamma = 2$ (*unblackened diamonds*), additive model with $\gamma = 2.2$ (*blackened diamonds*), and additive model with $\gamma = 5$ (*blackened squares*). *B*, Number of controls needed to detect DHW as the susceptibility-allele frequency changes at a significance level of 5% and 50% power. Data points are as follows: dominant model with $K_P = 0.2$ and $\gamma = 10$ (*blackened circles*), recessive model with $K_P = 0.05$ and $\gamma = 10$ (*blackened circles*), recessive model with $K_P = 0.2$ and $\gamma = 5$ (*unblackened squares*), additive model with $K_P = 0.2$ and $\gamma = 5$ (*blackened squares*), multiplicative model with $K_P = 0.1$ and $\gamma = 10$ (*blackened squares with white cross*), and multiplicative model with $K_P = 0.2$ and $\gamma = 5$ (*blackened squares with white star*). *C*, Same data points as *A* but assessed at 80% power. *D*, Same data points as *B* but assessed at 80% power.

C

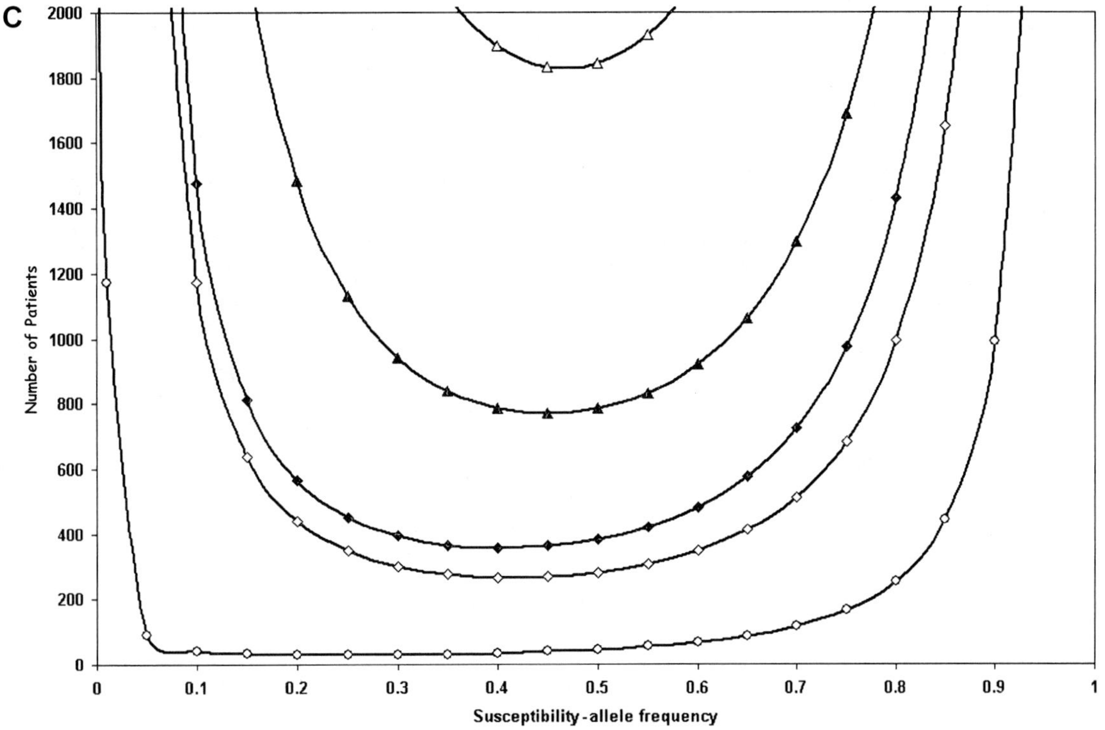
2000
1800
1600
1400
1200
1000
800
600
400
200
0
Number of Patients
0
0.1
0.2
0.3
0.4
0.5
0.6
0.7
0.8
0.9
1
Susceptibility-allele frequency

D

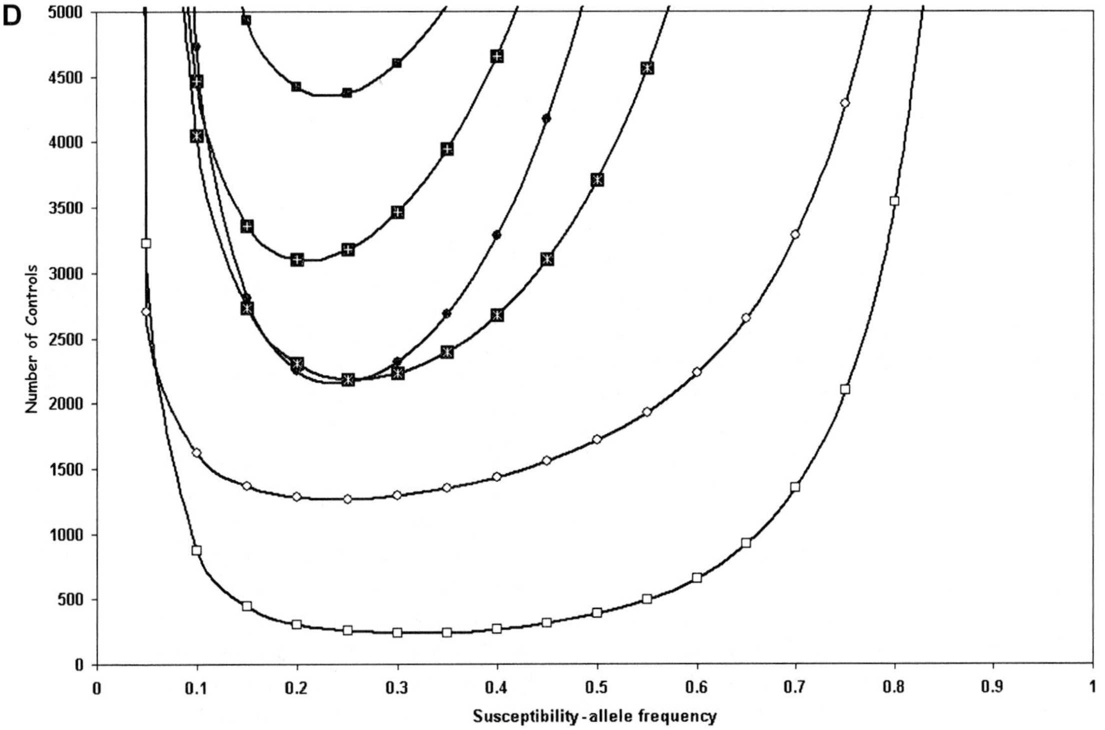
5000
4500
4000
3500
3000
2500
2000
1500
1000
500
0
Number of Controls
0
0.1
0.2
0.3
0.4
0.5
0.6
0.7
0.8
0.9
1
Susceptibility-allele frequency

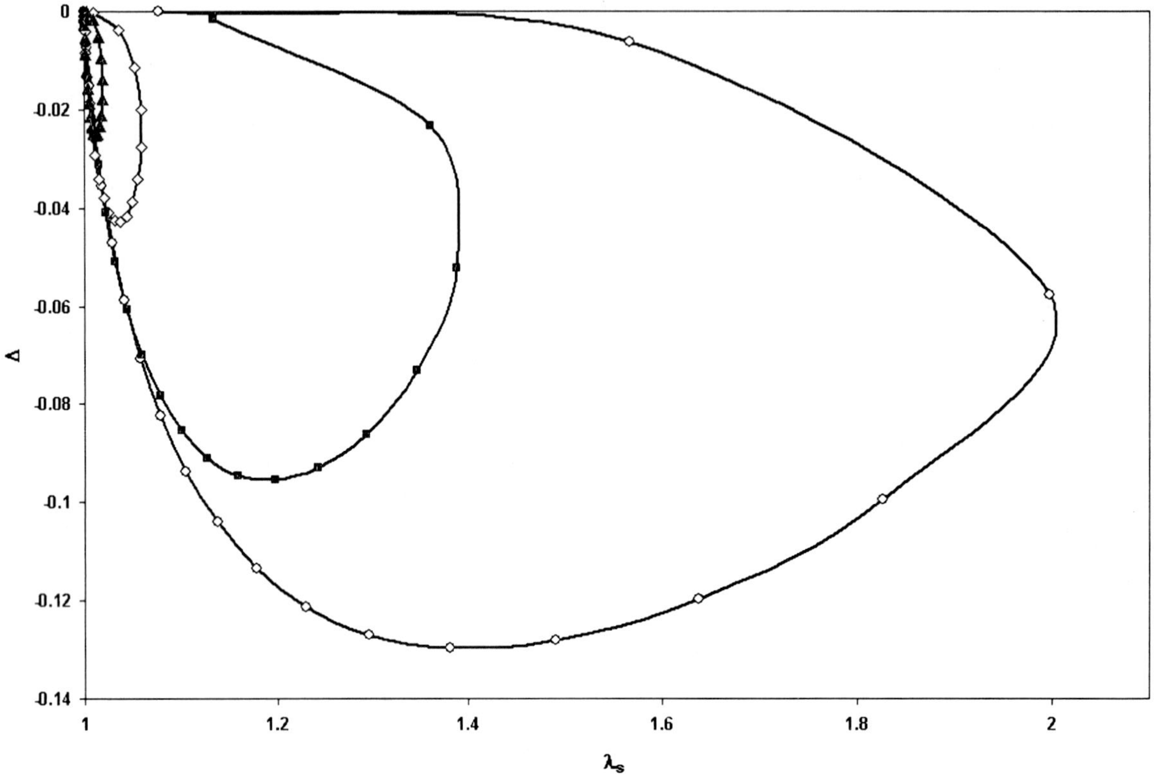

Figure 4 Sibling relative risk for dominant models with $K_P = 0.2$ and varied γ values: $\gamma = 10$ (*unblackened circles*), $\gamma = 5$ (*blackened squares*), $\gamma = 2$ (*unblackened diamonds*), and $\gamma = 1.5$ (*blackened triangles*).

Results

Magnitude of Δ

As noted elsewhere, the larger the value of Δ, the more the genotypic frequency departs from HWE expectations (Weir 1996). In patients, the magnitude of Δ_p is determined by q, γ, and β, as shown in equation (1) above. The maximum value for Δ_p, given a genetic disease model, occurs at the susceptibility-allele frequency that maximizes the HWE-expected proportion of heterozygotes affected with disease (g_{Aa}) and can be calculated by

$$\Delta_p = \frac{\gamma - \beta^2}{4\beta^2} g_{Aa}^2 .$$

For example, the maximum Δ_p for a dominant model with $\gamma = 1.5$ occurs when the allele frequency is 0.45, which corresponds to the highest proportion of HWE-expected heterozygotes among patients ($g_{Aa} = 0.5505$) under this model.

In controls, Δ_c is a function of K_P, α, β, γ, and q. Larger Δ_c values occur as the prevalence of disease in the general population increases, whereas, in patients, K_P has no direct effect on the size of Δ_p. For example, a dominant model with $\gamma = 1.5$ and $q = 0.33$ leads to a Δ_c of 0.00209 when $K_P = 0.1$ and a Δ_c of 0.000193 when $K_P = 0.01$. Larger Δ_c values also occur with higher γ values, as shown in figure 2. The susceptibility-allele frequency also affects the magnitude of Δ_c, with common allele frequencies ($0.1 \leq q \leq 0.8$) corresponding to larger Δ_c values and with allele frequencies at the tails of the frequency spectrum corresponding to smaller Δ_c values.

Direction of Δ

The direction of Δ is vital to understanding whether an observed DHW can be due to the underlying genetic model, and, for patients, the disease model specifies the direction of Δ_p (table 2). The additive model is different than the dominant, recessive, or multiplicative models, in that Δ_p can be positive, negative, or zero. Δ_p is positive when $2 < \gamma < 4$ and negative when $\gamma > 4$. However, when $\gamma = 4$, the additive model is equivalent to the multiplicative model ($\beta = 2$ and $\gamma = 4$), and Δ_p is equal to 0 (i.e., no DHW is expected). The general model is dependent on the value associated with β, where Δ_p is positive if $\gamma > \beta^2$ and negative if $\gamma < \beta^2$.

The direction of Δ in controls is also dependent on the underlying genetic disease model, and, for dominant and recessive models, Δ_c is in the direction opposite that observed in patients. Interestingly, Δ_c for controls under the additive model does not change with γ, as observed for patients, but always shows an excess of heterozygotes ($\Delta_c < 0$). However, there is an asymmetry in the homozygote classes when $\Delta \neq 0$ for both patients and controls, with patients showing an excess of disease-susceptible homozygotes and controls showing an excess of wild-type homozygotes. The multiplicative model generates Δ values for controls similar to those generated by the recessive and additive models, with $\Delta_c < 0$. The direction of DHW for a general disease model in controls is negative if $\gamma + 1 + \alpha\beta^2 > 2\beta + \alpha\gamma$ and positive if the inequality is reversed (i.e., $\gamma + 1 + \alpha\beta^2 < 2\beta + \alpha\gamma$).

Number of Individuals Needed to Detect DHW for a Specified Significance and Power

As might be expected, fewer patients are needed to detect DHW as the genotype relative risk increases. It is notable, however, that low γ values (e.g., 1.5) can produce DHW with relatively small samples of patients. For example, <500 patients are needed to detect DHW (at a significance level of 5% and 50% power) under a recessive model with $\gamma = 1.5$ and over a range of susceptibility-allele frequencies from 0.29 to 0.63. As γ increases to 2, the range of susceptibility-allele frequencies increases to 0.11–0.81, with a minimum sample size of ~130 patients when $q = 0.4$ with 50% power (fig. 3*A*) and 267 patients with 80% power (fig. 3*C*). An additive model, however, requires a minimum of ~750 patients at $q = 0.38$ to detect DHW with $\gamma = 3$, but the required sample size decreases to 176 patients with $\gamma = 2.2$. As shown above, Δ_p increases for additive models as γ increases or decreases from 4. Therefore, at a significance level of 5% and 50% power, an additive model can lead to detection of DHW in 176 patients when either $\gamma = 2.2$ or $\gamma = 7.56$. The difference between the two observations, however, is the direction of the DHW, in which the former ($\gamma = 2.2$) shows an excess of homozygotes and the latter ($\gamma = 7.56$) shows a deficiency of homozygotes.

The number of controls needed to detect DHW is generally much larger but is often still within the range of commonly collected sample sizes for a wide range of models. As with patients, the number of controls required to detect DHW decreases as γ increases. But, unlike in the calculations for patients, K_P also determines the number of controls needed to detect DHW. For dominant models, <1,000 unaffected individuals are needed to detect DHW when $K_P = 0.2$ and $\gamma \geq 5$ with 50% power (fig. 3*B*), and <2,000 controls with 80% power (fig. 3*D*). Because of the specifications of the additive model, the same effect is observed in controls as in patients, whereby a decrease in the number of controls needed to detect DHW occurs as γ increases or decreases from 4. Recessive models with $\gamma \geq 5$ can lead to detection of DHW in <200 controls with 50% power when $K_P = 0.2$. When K_P decreases to as low as 0.05, ~1,000 controls are needed to detect DHW for the recessive model with $\gamma \geq 10$ and $q = 0.23$ (fig. 3*B*). Multiplicative models show DHW in a sample of <2,000 controls when $K_P \geq 0.1$ and $\gamma \geq 10$ and in a sample of <1,200 controls when $K_P \geq 0.2$ and $\gamma \geq 5$ (at 50% power and a significance level of 5%). Generally, larger Δ_c values are associated with models specified by high K_P values (e.g., $K_P \geq 0.2$) and high γ values (e.g., $\gamma \geq 5$).

Sibling Relative Risk Values that Correspond to Expected DHW

We calculated λ_s for all models studied, to understand the results for these common disease models relative to those of previous studies that assessed power by using this parameter. As expected, λ_s increases as K_P decreases, and, overall, the resulting λ_s values (including those that are expected to give DHW in a small sample) are quite small. For dominant models or recessive models ($\gamma = 1.5$), in which DHW is expected for samples of <500 patients, λ_s is <1.03 (fig. 4). For additive models, in which <1,400 patients are needed to detect DHW, λ_s values do not exceed 1.18. Thus, DHW can be observed for strikingly low λ_s values in sample sizes currently being used for large-scale association studies.

Example 1: DHW in Patients Only

Ogura et al. (2001) conducted a case-control association study of Crohn disease to fine map *IBD1* in the pericentromeric region of chromosome 16. They identified a cytosine insertion (Leu3020fsinsC) in *CARD15/NOD2* that causes a truncated NOD2 protein and that results in deficient activation of NF-κB and the immune response. We calculated HWE for the Leu3020fsinsC (Cins) polymorphism in unrelated Jewish and European American patients with Crohn disease and in unrelated controls. Because of the low proportion of HWE-expected homozygotes, we used Fisher's exact test to determine DHW (Weir 1996). The distribution of genotypes in Jewish patients was 121 wild-type (wt)/wt homozygotes, 15 Cins/wt heterozygotes, and 4 Cins/Cins homozygotes, which yields $P = .0059$. The genotype distribution in European American patients was 314 wt/wt homozygotes, 41 Cins/wt heterozygotes, and 9 Cins/Cins homozygotes. Fisher's exact test generates $P = 1.28 \times 10^{-4}$, which is also highly significant. When all unrelated patients are tested for DHW (456 wt/wt homozygotes, 61 Cins/wt heterozygotes, and 13 Cins/Cins homozygotes), $P = 6.83 \times 10^{-6}$. All three populations of patients showed significant DHW, with an excess of homozygotes. The distribution of genotypes in all con-

Table 1

Survey of DHW

PubMed ID	Disease[a]	Gene	Genotype Distributions[b]		K_P	q	α	β	γ	χ^2	P^c
			Patients	Controls							
12221172	Alzheimer disease	*A2M*	61-48-23	98-77-9	.06	.264	.0513	1.085	2.966	1.016	NS
12105308	Alzheimer disease	*APOE*	4-18-94	6-53-74	.06	.758	.0269	1.000	3.137	1.013	NS
12105308	Alzheimer disease	*APOE*	31-49-29	67-102-19	.06	.381	.0449	1.251	2.509	4.221	.040
12105308	Alzheimer disease	*APOE*	57-118-100	58-97-48	.06	.482	.0462	1.118	2.027	.547	NS
12105308	Alzheimer disease	*APOE*	120-361-194	206-309-142	.06	.458	.0362	1.791	2.265	1.485	NS
11074789	Alzheimer disease	*CST3*	322-166-29	260-124-6	.05	.179	.0463	1.174	1.91	3.914	.048
11468325	Alzheimer disease	*CST3*	140-33-6	179-43-6	.06	.121	.059	1.000	2.114	4.064	NS
11468325	Alzheimer disease	*CST3*	137-34-8	180-40-8	.06	.13	.0587	1.000	2.343	9.671	.008
12034804	Alzheimer disease	*IL-1β*	5-40-39	15-107-95	.06	.679	.0365	1.718	1.718	4.812	NS
10869806	Alzheimer disease	*IL-6 promoter*	110-148-44	34-22-12	.05	.35	.043	1.257	1.377	5.111	.024
10815136	Alzheimer disease	*PS1*	3-45-45	3-24-18	.05	.66	.0141	3.803	3.94	1.929	NS
11124296	Macular degeneration	*mEPHX*	42-24-32	95-38-33	.01	.326	.00767	1.000	3.874	40.423	$\ll$.001
10843185	Autoimmune hypothyrodism	*IL-4*	2-7-68	3-23-75	.02	.847	.00917	1.000	2.645	2.909	NS
10781645	Acute myocardial infarction	*5-HT 2A receptor*	39-133-83	43-150-62	.05	.538	.0362	1.435	1.568	8.829	.003
11781417	Blepharospasm	*D1.1*	25-51-15	42-32-16	.001	.361	.000673	1.804	1.875	4.485	.034
11142420	Breast cancer	*CYP17*	39-63-10	112-132-33	.05	.352	.0412	1.367	1.367	3.161	NS
10698474	Breast cancer	*CYP1B1*	37-101-48	44-127-29	.05	.468	.0357	1.504	1.678	15.736	7.3×10^{-5}
10698474	Breast cancer	*CYP1B1*	26-68-27	26-78-17	.05	.464	.0379	1.446	1.446	11.11	.004
10698474	Breast cancer	*CYP1B1*	11-32-21	18-49-12	.05	.469	.0309	1.599	2.46	4.774	.029
11156391	Cancer toxicity (irinotecan)	*UGT1A1*	14-8-4	79-10-3	.01	.116	.00695	2.221	15.11	7.947	.005
12787424	Chronic allograft nephropathy	*TGF-β1*	0-22-8	23-83-67	.01	.613	0	11.76	11.76	4.204	NS
12787424	Chronic allograft nephropathy	*TNFα*	50-24-1	132-31-10	.01	.164	.00949	1.179	1.179	13.577	.001
10504487	Chronic renal failure	*VDR*	34-118-96	29-123-68	.005	.586	.00404	1.232	1.418	1.768	NS
10189842	Coeliac disease	*CTLA-4*	4-28-69	21-47-62	.01	.655	.00332	1.861	4.82	4.539	.033
10189842	Coeliac disease	*CTLA-4*	1-7-23	16-36-54	.01	.674	.003	1.731	5.43	5.198	.023
11889073	Colorectal cancer	*MTHFR*	28-35-12	204-229-34	.05	.324	.0415	1.231	1.995	7.478	.006
11889073	Colorectal cancer	*MTHFR*	28-64-94	114-560-533	.05	.669	.0455	1.000	1.223	10.133	.006
11889073	Colorectal cancer	*MTHFR*	14-66-73	39-116-148	.05	.678	.0431	1.161	1.195	4.313	.038
10794488	Colorectal polyps	*MTHFR*	98-72-26	297-258-71	.05	.315	.0484	1.000	1.338	4.323	NS
12631667	Crohn disease	*CYP1A1*	2-20-129	5-22-122	.05	.879	.0325	1.000	1.698	7.497	.024
12631667	Crohn disease	*EPXH*	20-60-71	59-58-32	.05	.428	.0201	2.046	6.307	6.759	.009

12631669	Crohn disease	*NOD2*	248-20-3	290-10-0	.05	.0206	.0478	1.929	20.71	.454	NS
11402126	Dementia	*ACE*	74-239-120	98-233-144	.1	.539	.0808	1.301	1.301	2.457	NS
12221164	Epilepsy	*OPRM1*	193-29-8	208-20-0	.01	.0451	.0092	1.592	18.719	.399	NS
9607207	Hypertension/nephroangiosclerosis	*ACE*	6-10-21	8-48-19	.05	.557	.0312	1.000	2.933	7.18	.028
10792336	IDDM	*VDR*	137-16-4	231-16-1	.05	.046	.0482	1.236	9.315	3.482	NS
11231353	IDDM nephropathy	*GLUT1*	3-29-10	21-60-23	.005	.495	.00139	4.482	4.482	3.604	NS
11097227	Lung cancer	*HRAS1*	17-86-209	21-134-276	.01	.789	.00882	1.000	1.214	3.239	NS
11097227	Lung cancer	*HRAS1*	8-19-49	8-38-54	.01	.71	.00742	1.000	1.692	3.583	NS
11097227	Lung cancer	*TP53*	9-16-26	57-192-197	.01	.652	.00883	1.000	1.311	4.33	NS
11045785	Lung cancer, squamous cell	*p53*	16-44-73	61-212-237	.01	.668	.00823	1.000	1.48	3.481	NS
9844142	Macroangiopathy	*PAI-1*	6-28-22	22-88-42	.05	.567	.0295	1.683	2.116	4.958	.026
11122322	Myocardial infarction	*ACE*	184-460-217	193-393-215	.1	.508	.0884	1.174	1.174	1.748	NS
10712418	Myocardial infarction	*TF-1208*	227-361-218	197-349-186	.1	.483	.0956	1.000	1.199	6.502	.039
10680782	Multiple sclerosis	*GSTM3*	276-97-14	221-64-15	.05	.161	.0496	1.000	1.336	11.722	.003
15338456[d]	NIDDM	*RETN*	48-85-16	63-83-12	.054	.336	.0396	1.649	1.649	6.384	.041
10231446	NIDDM nephropathy	*GLUT1*	43-78-10	77-41-6	.05	.219	.0269	3.199	3.199	.0884	NS
10231446	NIDDM nephropathy	*GLUT1*	12-48-4	77-41-6	.05	.219	.0153	6.818	6.818	1.099	NS
9844142	NIDDM nephropathy	*PAI-1*	64-116-28	66-80-31	.05	.388	.0409	1.357	1.357	2.616	NS
9844142	NIDDM nephropathy	*PAI-1*	28-58-12	66-80-31	.05	.392	.0383	1.484	1.484	2.745	NS
12675860	NIDDM nephropathy	*TGF-β1*	24-24-17	27-26-5	.3	.354	.258	1.000	2.29	.537	NS
10964048	Oral cancer	*CYP1A1*	96-36-13	104-54-6	.01	.186	.00943	1.000	2.732	1.638	NS
10964048	Oral cancer	*CYP1A1*	56-55-31	62-65-15	.01	.332	.0087	1.02	2.275	.0473	NS
11914402	Parkinson disease	*Nurr1*	162-48-15	174-45-2	.02	.112	.0183	1.172	5.822	.14	NS
11786085	Renal parenchymal scarring	*TGF-β1*	0-27-16	16-76-79	.01	.669	.001	11.11	11.11	3.973	NS
11786085	Renal parenchymal scarring	*TGF-β1*	13-27-3	73-72-26	.01	.303	.00551	4.001	3.95	.0627	NS
10430441	Stroke	*NOS3*	109-125-31	154-203-36	.15	.353	.15	1.000	1.004	7.466	.024
11027931	Venous thrombosis	*β-fibrogen*	2-6-82	0-22-163	.01	.926	.00892	1.000	1.141	9.55	.008
11027931	Venous thrombosis	*Factor 7*	67-19-5	148-33-4	.01	.115	.0094	1.096	4.351	1.758	NS
12753258	Vertebral fracture	*COLIA1*	10-2-5	75-35-6	.01	.2	.00754	1	9.125	2.24	NS

[a] IDDM = insulin-dependent diabetes mellitus; NIDDM = non–insulin-dependent diabetes mellitus.

[b] In the genotype distributions for patients and controls, the three numbers separated by hyphens represent the nonsusceptible homozygotes, the heterozygotes, and the susceptible homozygotes.

[c] NS = not significant.

[d] Osawa et al. (2004)

Table 2

Direction of DHW, Given a Genetic Disease Model and Parameter Values

	Direction of DHW in	
Model	Patients	Controls
Dominant	−	+
Recessive	+	−
Additive	If $\gamma < 2$, +; if $\gamma > 2$, −; if $\gamma = 2$, 0	−
Multiplicative	0	−
General	If $\gamma > \beta^2$, +; if $\gamma < \beta^2$, −	If $\gamma + 1 + \alpha\beta^2 > 2\beta + \alpha\gamma$, −; if $\gamma + 1 + \alpha\beta^2 < 2\beta + \alpha\gamma$, +

Note.—A plus sign (+) represents an excess of homozygotes, and a minus sign (−) represents a deficiency of homozogyotes.

trols was 311 wt/wt homozygotes, 25 Cins/wt heterozygotes, and 0 Cins/Cins homozygotes, which is consistent with HWE.

If the allele frequencies in both the patients (q_p = 0.082) and the controls (q_c = 0.037) are used to help delineate the general genetic disease model that best fits the observed genotypic distributions, we find that it can be characterized by $K_P = 0.002$, $q = 0.0379$, $\alpha = 0.00186$, $\beta = 1.696$, and $\gamma = 18.338$. If a χ^2 test is performed to determine the goodness-of-fit of the expected number of patients and controls, given the model that best fits the observed genotypic counts, $\chi^2 = 0.478$ ($P = .827$ with 1 df); thus, the best-fit model is a good fit to the observed data. Moreover, the model is consistent with what has been obtained elsewhere for other types of data (Hampe et al. 2001; Ogura et al. 2001).

Example 2: DHW in Opposite Directions in Patients and Controls

Ozaki et al. (2002) published a large-scale association study designed to identify genetic variation affecting risk of MI in a Japanese sample. The study involved an initial screen of >92,000 SNPs in a small sample and follow-up studies for those SNPs with evidence of association ($P < .01$ for a dominant or recessive model) performed in a larger sample (1,133 patients, 1,006 random controls, and 872 age-matched random controls). This led to more intensive studies of the *LTA* region (near *HLA* on 6p21), with 5 of 26 SNPs genotyped in the region showing highly significant association with MI (e.g., for *LTA* exon 1 polymorphism, $P = 3.3 \times 10^{-6}$).

Although Ozaki et al. (2002) reported that all 26 SNPs were in HWE, with $P > .01$, we note that each of the 5 SNPs for which genotype distributions are published show a significant DHW in opposite directions for patients and controls. The *LTA* exon 1 polymorphism is the most significantly associated with MI, with a genotype distribution among the 1,133 patients of 416 GG homozygotes, 504 GA heterozygtoes, and 213 AA homozygotes, which yields $\chi^2 = 7.40$ ($P = .0065$)—an excess of homozygotes relative to HWE-expected genotype proportions. The genotype distribution among the 1,006 random controls is 378 GG homozygotes, 512 GA heterozygotes, and 116 AA homozygotes. This sample of controls generates $\chi^2 = 8.51$ ($P = .0035$) but shows a deviation in the opposite direction of patients, with a deficiency of homozygotes. The age-matched random control group of 872 individuals has a genotype distribution of 344 GG homozygotes, 428 GA heterozygotes, and 100 AA homozygotes, corresponding to a nonsignificant $\chi^2 = 3.69$ ($P = .055$) but also showing a deficiency of homozygotes similar to that seen for the 1,006 random controls.

The first problem easily identified is that a significant DHW is observed in a sample that may be better characterized as a random sample than a control sample and thus would not be expected to show DHW, regardless of the underlying genetic disease model. If we assume that the control sample is a control sample, rather than a random sample, the best-fit model is $K_P = 0.01$, $q = 0.371$, $\alpha = 0.00932$, $\beta = 1.024$, and $\gamma = 1.469$. The goodness-of-fit to the observed data is significantly poor, with $\chi^2 = 5.024$ ($P = .025$ with 1 df). Given that the best-fit model is not a good fit to what is observed in the 1,133 patients and 1,006 controls, the underlying genetic disease model for a susceptibility locus in that region is therefore an unlikely explanation for the observed DHW.

Survey of DHW

We identified 41 association studies with 60 polymorphisms that depart from HWE, from several recent reviews (Xu et al. 2002; Györffy et al. 2004; Kocsis et al. 2004*a*, 2004*b*; Osawa et al. 2004) (table 1). All K_P values were either given by the association study or were identified on the World Health Organization Web site. There are 35 polymorphisms that depart from HWE in patients only, 21 that depart in controls only, 2 that depart in the same direction in patients and controls, and 1 that departs in the opposite direction in patients and controls. Of those that have a dominant or recessive model as the best-fit genetic model, 35.3% (12 of 34) did not have a genetic model that fit the observed genotype distributions. Of those for which the best-fit model was a general model, 53.8% (14 of 26) did not have a model that fit well the observed data. Therefore, 43.3% of the polymorphisms we identified from the reviews are inconsistent with a biological reason for the observed DHW. This highlights the importance not only of correctly assessing HWE for genotype data but also of understanding whether an observed DHW is consistent with a genetic model of disease susceptibility.

Discussion

Investigators have taken surprisingly inconsistent pathways in the interpretation and use of DHW. In some cases, investigators report significant association between variation at candidate genes and complex disorders that is quite dependent on the existence of DHW (i.e., the associations are genotypic rather than allelic, and the genotypic differences are driven by DHW). In at least some situations, the observed DHW is implausible from a biological perspective, which calls into question the association result. On the other hand, some investigators believe that any marker showing a DHW is likely to be erroneous and/or misleading; as a result, they may be throwing away information valuable for mapping and identifying causal polymorphisms. With the analytic framework and software we have developed, we provide a way for investigators to assess markers with DHW in a more logical and systematic way by distinguishing those that could be attributed to the underlying genetic model at the susceptibility locus from those due to genotyping errors, chance, and/or violations of the assumptions of HWE, thereby improving the quality of scientific inferences.

Given the increasing sample sizes contemplated for large-scale association studies, it would seem that DHW is a neglected and potentially fruitful avenue for further research to improve signal localization. Results of studies of the *CARD15/NOD2* region provide support for this notion. A common coding polymorphism (P268S) ($q = 0.35$ in patients with Crohn disease, and $q = 0.29$ in unaffected controls) shows significant DHW, with an excess of homozygotes in both Jewish patients ($P = .0277$) and in patients overall ($P = .00546$) (J. Cho, personal communication). The best-fit model for this polymorphism provides a good fit to the observed genotypic distributions ($\chi^2 = 1.501 \times 10^{-10}$; $P = 1.0$ with 1 df). Although this polymorphism is not thought to affect the risk of Crohn disease, three of the known susceptibility alleles (Leu3020fsinsC, Gly908Arg, and Arg702Trp) are in the same haplotype as the more rare allele at this site. If patients with any of those mutations are removed from the patient population and HWE is reassessed, the DHW is no longer significant ($P = .2115$ for Jewish patients, and $P = .632$ for patients overall). If none of the causative SNPs had been previously identified, the observation that the common polymorphism departed from HWE in a way that was consistent with a genetic model could have been used to support further investigation of the local region. This observation highlights the value of using DHW when fine mapping complex diseases, as originally hypothesized by Nielsen et al. (1998).

Given the relatively large sample sizes used in modern candidate-gene studies as well as in fine-mapping and positional cloning studies, and the fact that DHW should be expected for a wide range of genetic disease models (consistent with the modest genetic contributions likely to be relevant for complex disorders), it is perhaps surprising that we have not seen a larger number of markers reported to show DHW. Of 60 SNPs from association studies in which DHW has been identified in patients and/or controls and in which both patient and control genotype distributions are available, 34 (56.7%) have genotype distributions consistent with the expectations from a best-fit model (table 1). DHW in patients is never expected for a multiplicative model and is less likely to be detected as significant for a model with susceptibility-allele frequencies at the tails of the frequency spectrum. We have not examined the consequences for HWE in more-complex disease models with allelic or locus epistasis, profound sex effects, etc., and, if such models were standard for complex disorders, it is unclear what the consequences would be. Thus, the failure to more often observe DHW at polymorphisms hypothesized to affect susceptibility to complex disorders may reflect biological characteristics of the genetic disease model that make such DHW impossible or at least less likely.

It is also possible that investigators mistrust data with DHW and may sometimes ignore such polymorphisms with DHW in their studies. Systematic errors in genotyping or nonrandom patterns of missing data may generate a relatively consistent pattern of DHW (e.g., disproportionate missing data in heterozygotes may lead to a consistent pattern of DHW, with an excess of homozygotes). Other types of error may be more sporadic. An unrecognized polymorphism in primer sequences used in subsequent PCR may lead to DHW, with an excess of homozygotes, particularly when the primer polymorphism is in LD with one of the test alleles. Genomic duplications or deletions can also lead to DHW. Because even the systematic errors will not be universal, error and nonrandom patterns of missing data may be detectable in a single marker within a set that are in strong LD. In contrast, when markers have DHW due to violations of assumptions of HWE or to chance, markers in LD may show similar patterns of DHW. Independent samples will tend not to replicate chance DHW but may replicate DHW due to violations of HWE assumptions. Clearly, genomewide or large-scale studies offer additional information for interpretation of DHW, including, for example, the ability to examine potential population substructure. Many of the studies summarized in table 1, however, focus on one or a small number of candidate genes, and the approaches we propose offer a unique opportunity to improve the scientific inferences about observed DHW. It should also be noted that just because an observed DHW is consistent with genetic models does not mean that errors, missing data patterns, or violations of HWE assumptions did not generate or contribute to the observed DHW, and DHW can no doubt be attributable to a combination of factors. Finally, it should also be noted that investigators frequently underestimate the significance of observed DHW, probably because of a misunderstanding of the degrees of freedom associated with the test.

Acknowledgments

We acknowledge William Wen, for creating the DHW software, and Dr. Judy Cho, for giving us access to the association data on *NOD2/CARD15* and Crohn disease. We also acknowledge Drs. Mark Abney, Carole Ober, Dan Nicolae, Jonathan Pritchard, and Daniel Schaid, for their helpful discussions. This work was supported by grants DK-55889, DK-58026, and U01-GM61393. The DHW software is freely available and can be downloaded from the Web site given below.

Appendix A

Δ in Patients

Weir (1996) defines Δ as the difference between the population and HWE-expected genotypic frequencies. Therefore, we first define these genotypic frequencies in terms of q, the susceptibility-allele frequency in the general population; α, the baseline penetrance for wild-type homozgyotes; β, the relative risk to heterozygotes; γ, the relative risk to homozygotes for the susceptibility allele; and K_{P}, the population prevalence of disease. The expected genotypic proportions in patients, under the assumption of HWE in the general population, are as follows:

$$g_{AA}=\frac{(1-q)^2\alpha}{K_{\mathrm{P}}},\ g_{Aa}=\frac{2q(1-q)\alpha\beta}{K_{\mathrm{P}}},\ \text{and}\ g_{aa}=\frac{q^2\alpha\gamma}{K_{\mathrm{P}}}\ .$$

The expected susceptibility-allele frequency for patients is

$$q_{\mathrm{P}}=\frac{q^2\alpha\gamma+q(1-q)\alpha\beta}{K_{\mathrm{P}}}\ .$$

The frequency of the wild-type allele in patients is

$$p_{\mathrm{P}}=1-q_{\mathrm{P}}=\frac{(1-q)^2\alpha+q(1-q)\alpha\beta}{K_{\mathrm{P}}}\ .$$

Therefore,

$$\Delta_{\mathrm{P}}=g_{AA}-(1-q_{\mathrm{P}})^2=\frac{(1-q)^2\alpha}{K_{\mathrm{P}}}-\frac{[(1-q)^2\alpha+q(1-q)\alpha\beta]^2}{K_{\mathrm{P}}^2}\ ,$$

which then simplifies to equation (1).

For a classic recessive model, where $\beta=1$ and $\gamma>1$,

$$\Delta_{\mathrm{P}}=\frac{q^2(1-q)^2(\gamma-1)}{(1-q^2+q^2\gamma)^2}\ .$$

For a classic dominant model, where $\beta=\gamma$ and $\gamma>1$,

$$\Delta_{\mathrm{P}}=\frac{q^2(1-q)^2(\gamma-\gamma^2)}{[(1-q)^2+2q\gamma-q^2\gamma]^2}\ .$$

For an additive model, where $\gamma = 2\beta$ and $\beta > 1$,

$$\Delta_p = \frac{q^2(1-q)^2\left(\gamma - \frac{\gamma^2}{4}\right)}{[(1-q)^2 + q\gamma]^2} .$$

As explained in the "Methods" section, the multiplicative model for patients, where $\beta^2 = \gamma$ and $\beta > 1$, simplifies to $\Delta_p = 0$.

Appendix B

Δ in Controls

As defined for patients in appendix A, we define the genotypic proportions in controls for a general disease model as

$$g_{AA} = \frac{(1-q)^2(1-\alpha)}{1-K_P},\ g_{Aa} = \frac{2q(1-q)(1-\alpha\beta)}{1-K_P},\ g_{aa} = \frac{q^2(1-\alpha\gamma)}{1-K_P} .$$

The expected susceptibility-allele frequency in controls is

$$q_c = \frac{q^2(1-\alpha\gamma) + q(1-q)(1-\alpha\beta)}{1-K_P} .$$

The frequency of the wild-type allele in controls is

$$p_c = 1 - q_c = \frac{(1-q)^2(1-\alpha) + q(1-q)(1-\alpha\beta)}{1-K_P} .$$

Therefore,

$$\Delta_c = g_{AA} - (1-q_c)^2 = \frac{(1-q)^2(1-\alpha)}{1-K_P} - \frac{[(1-q)^2(1-\alpha) + q(1-q)(1-\alpha\beta)]^2}{(1-K_P)^2} ,$$

which simplifies to equation (2).

For a classic recessive model, where $\beta = 1$ and $\gamma > 1$,

$$\Delta_c = \frac{\alpha q^2(1-q)^2(1-\gamma)(1-\alpha)}{(1-K_P)^2} .$$

For a classic dominant model, where $\beta = \gamma$ and $\gamma > 1$,

$$\Delta_c = \frac{\alpha q^2(1-q)^2(1-\alpha\gamma)(\gamma-1)}{(1-K_P)^2} .$$

For an additive model, where $\gamma = 2\beta$ and $\beta > 1$,

$$\Delta_c = \frac{\alpha q^2(1-q)^2\left(\alpha\gamma - 1 - \frac{\alpha\gamma^2}{4}\right)}{(1-K_P)^2} .$$

Finally, for a multiplicative model, where $\gamma = \beta^2$ and $\beta > 1$,

$$\Delta_c = \frac{-\alpha q^2(1-q)^2(\sqrt{\gamma}-1)^2}{(1-K_P)^2} .$$

Appendix C

λ_s Values

Given that

$$\lambda_s = 1 + \left(\frac{1}{K_P^2}\right)\left(\frac{1}{2}V_A + \frac{1}{4}V_D\right)$$

(Risch 1990), where V_A is the additive variance that can be calculated by

$$V_A = 2pq[p(\alpha - \alpha\beta) + q(\alpha\beta - \alpha\gamma)]^2$$

and V_D is the dominance variance that can be calculated by

$$V_D = p^2q^2(\alpha\gamma + \alpha - 2\alpha\beta)^2 ,$$

λ_s under the classic dominant model can then be calculated as

$$\lambda_s = 1 + \frac{pq[p(\alpha - \alpha\gamma)]^2 + \frac{1}{4}[p^2q^2(\alpha - \alpha\gamma)^2]}{K_P^2} ,$$

λ_s under the classic recessive model can be calculated as

$$\lambda_s = 1 + \frac{pq[q(\alpha - \alpha\gamma)]^2 + \frac{1}{4}[p^2q^2(\alpha\gamma - \alpha)^2]}{K_P^2} ,$$

λ_s under the additive model can be calculated as

$$\lambda_s = 1 + \frac{pq\left(\alpha - \frac{\alpha\gamma}{2} - q\alpha\right)^2 + \frac{1}{4}p^2q^2(\alpha - \alpha\gamma)^2}{K_P^2} ,$$

and, finally, λ_s under the multiplicative model can be calculated as

$$\lambda_s = 1 + \frac{pq[p(\alpha - \alpha\sqrt{\gamma}) + q(\alpha\sqrt{\gamma} - \alpha\gamma)]^2 + \frac{1}{4}p^2q^2(\alpha\gamma + \alpha - 2\alpha\sqrt{\gamma})^2}{K_P^2} .$$

Appendix D

Goodness-of-Fit Test

The expected genotypic proportions for patients under a genetic disease model are $g_{AA\text{-p}}$, $g_{Aa-\text{p}}$, and $g_{aa\text{-p}}$, as found in appendix A. The expected genotypic proportions for controls under a genetic disease model are $g_{AA\text{-c}}$, $g_{Aa\text{-c}}$, and $g_{aa\text{-c}}$, as found in appendix B.

For a particular set of disease model parameter values (α, β, γ, and q), where the total number of patients is N_{p}, the total number of controls denoted is N_{c}, and the observed number of patients (or controls), given a specific genotype, is $N_{\text{genotype-p}}$ (or $N_{\text{genotype-c}}$), the goodness-of-fit test is as follows:

$$\chi^2 = \frac{(N_{\text{p}}g_{AA\text{-p}} - N_{AA\text{-p}})^2}{N_{\text{p}}g_{AA\text{-p}}} + \frac{(N_{\text{p}}g_{Aa\text{-p}} - N_{Aa\text{-p}})^2}{N_{\text{p}}g_{Aa\text{-p}}} + \frac{(N_{\text{p}}g_{aa\text{-p}} - N_{aa\text{-p}})^2}{N_{\text{p}}g_{aa\text{-p}}} + \frac{(N_{\text{c}}g_{AA\text{-c}} - N_{AA\text{-c}})^2}{N_{\text{c}}g_{AA\text{-c}}} + \frac{(N_{\text{c}}g_{Aa\text{-c}} - N_{Aa\text{-c}})^2}{N_{\text{c}}g_{Aa\text{-c}}} + \frac{(N_{\text{c}}g_{aa\text{-c}} - N_{aa\text{-c}})^2}{N_{\text{c}}g_{aa\text{-c}}} \ .$$

Minimizing the resulting test statistic over the entire parameter space, subject to appropriate constraints on α, β, γ, and q and where K_{P} is fixed, yields parameter estimates that are approximately maximum-likelihood estimates. The minimal value of the test statistic is approximately distributed as a χ^2 with 1 df for a general model and 2 df for restricted models (i.e., dominant, recessive, additive, and multiplicative models) (Cramer 1946). We verify through simulations that applying this test to data showing a DHW does not affect the resulting distribution of the test statistic. We generated 1,000 replicates of 1,000 patients and 1,000 controls under a dominant, recessive, or general disease model as specified by the penetrances, which offer an advantage in being bound between 0 and 1. We kept for further analysis only replicates that showed DHW in patients, in controls, or in both patients and controls. We used the goodness-of-fit test to find the best-fit genetic model for each simulation and compared the resulting χ^2 value to 1,000 simulated χ^2 values, given the specified degrees of freedom (fig. 5).

If the goodness-of-fit test, with 1 df for a general model or 2 df for a restrictive model, corresponds to a P value less than the specified threshold, the genetic disease model can be rejected as a poor fit to the observed data. Note that rare-allele frequencies, which may produce low genotype counts, may produce approximations from the goodness-of-fit test that do not perform as expected.

The figure is available in its entirety in the online edition of *The American Journal of Human Genetics.*

Figure 5 Simulations with the goodness-of-fit test. The legend is available in its entirety in the online edition of *The American Journal of Human Genetics.*

Electronic-Database Information

The URLs for data presented herein are as follows:

DHW software, http://hg-wen.uchicago.edu/dhw2.html
World Health Organization, http://www.who.int/en/

References

Castle WE (1903) The laws of heredity of Galton and Mendel, and some laws governing race improvement by selection. Proc Am Acad Arts Sci 39:223–242

Cramer H (1946) Mathematical methods of statistics. Princeton University Press, Princeton, NJ

Gomes I, Collins A, Lonjou C, Thomas NS, Wilkinson J, Watson M, Morton N (1999) Hardy-Weinberg quality control. Ann Hum Genet 63:535–538

Györffy B, Kocsis I, Vásárhelyi B (2004) Biallelic genotype distributions in papers published in *Gut* between 1998 and 2003: altered conclusions after recalculating the Hardy-Weinberg equilibrium. Gut 53:614–616

Hampe J, Cuthbert A, Croucher PJP, Mirza MM, Mascheretti S, Fischer S, Frenzel H, King K, Hasselmeyer A, MacPherson AJS, Bridger S, van Deventer S, Forbes A, Nikolaus S, Lennard-Jones JE, Foelsch UR, Krawczak M, Lewis C, Schreiber S, Mathew CG (2001) Association between insertion mutation in *NOD2* gene and Crohn's disease in German and British populations. Lancet 357:1925–1928

Hardy GH (1908) Mendelian proportions in a mixed population. Science 18:49–50

Hosking L, Lumsden S, Lewis K, Yeo A, McCarthy L, Bansal A, Riley J, Purvis I, Xu CF (2004) Detection of genotyping errors by Hardy-Weinberg equilibrium testing. Eur J Hum Genet 12:395–399

Kocsis I, Györffy B, Németh E, Vásárhelyi B (2004*a*) Examination of Hardy-Weinberg equilibrium in papers of *Kidney International*: an underused tool. Kidney Int 65:1956–1958

Kocsis I, Vásárhelyi B, Györffy A, Györffy B (2004*b*) Reanalysis of genotype distributions published in *Neurology* between 1999 and 2002. Neurology 63:357–358

Levecque C, Elbaz A, Clavel J, Richard F, Vidal J, Amouyel P, Tzourio C, Alpérovitch A, Chartier-Harlin M (2003) Association between Parkinson's disease and polymorphisms in the nNos and iNos genes in a community-based case-control study. Hum Mol Genet 12:79–86

Li CC (1967) Castle's early work on selection and equilibrium. Am J Hum Genet 19:70–74

Martin ER, Lai EH, Gilbert JR, Rogala AR, Afshari AJ, Riley J, Finch KL, Stevens JF, Livak KJ, Slotterbeck BD, Slifer SH, Warren LL, Conneally PM, Schmechel DE, Purvis I, Pericak-Vance MA, Roses AD, Vance JM (2000) SNPing away at complex diseases: analysis of single-nucleotide polymorphisms around *APOE* in Alzheimer disease. Am J Hum Genet 67:383–394

Nejentsev S, Laaksonen M, Tienari PJ, Fernandez O, Cordell H, Ruutiainen J, Wikström J, Pastinen T, Kuokkanen S, Hillert J, Ilonen J (2003) Intercellular adhesion molecule-1 K469E polymorphism: study of association with multiple sclerosis. Hum Immunol 64:345–349

Nielsen DM, Ehm MG, Weir BS (1998) Detecting marker-disease association by testing for Hardy-Weinberg disequilibrium at a marker locus. Am J Hum Genet 63:1531–1540

Ogura Y, Bonen DK, Inohara N, Nicolae DL, Chen FF, Ramos R, Britton H, Moran T, Karaliuskas R, Duerr RH, Achkar J-P, Brant SR, Bayless TM, Kirschner BS, Hanauer SB, Nuñez G, Cho JH (2001) A frameshift mutation in *NOD2* associated with susceptibility to Crohn's disease. Nature 411: 603–606

Oka A, Tamiya G, Tomizawa M, Ota M, Katsuyama Y, Makino S, Shiina T, Yoshitome M, Iizuka M, Sasao Y, Iwashita K, Kawakubo Y, Sugai J, Ozawa A, Ohkido M, Kimura M, Bahram S, Inoko H (1999) Association analysis using refined microsatellite markers localizes a susceptibility locus for psoriasis vulgaris within a 111 kb segment telomeric to the HLA-C gene. Hum Mol Genet 8:2165–2170

Osawa H, Yamada K, Onuma H, Murakami A, Ochi M, Kawata H, Nishimiya T, Niiya T, Shimizu I, Nishida W, Hashiramoto M, Kanatsuka A, Fujii Y, Ohashi J, Makino H (2004) The G/G genotype of a resistin single-nucleotide polymorphism at −420 increases type 2 diabetes mellitus susceptibility by inducing promoter activity through specific binding of Sp1/3. Am J Hum Genet 75:678–686

Ozaki K, Ohnishi Y, Iida A, Sekine A, Yamada R, Tsunoda T, Sato H, Sato H, Hori M, Nakamura Y, Tanaka T (2002) Function SNPs in the lymphotoxin-α gene that are associated with susceptibility to myocardial infarction. Nat Genet 32:650–654

Risch N (1990) Linkage strategies for genetically complex traits. I. Multilocus models. Am J Hum Genet 46:222–228

Wang L, Sato K, Tsuchiya N, Yu J, Ohyama C, Satoh S, Habuchi T, Ogawa O, Kato T (2003) Polymorphisms in prostate-specific antigen (*PSA*) gene, risk of prostate cancer, and serum PSA levels in Japanese population. Cancer Letters 202:53–59

Weinberg W (1908) On the demonstration of heredity in man. In: Boyer SH (ed) (1963) Papers on human genetics. Prentice-Hall, Englewood Cliffs, NJ

Weir BS (1996) Disequilibrium. In: Genetic data analysis II: methods for discrete population genetic data. Sinaur Associates, Sunderland, MA, pp 91–139

Xu J, Turner A, Little J, Bleecker ER, Meyers DA (2002) Positive results in association studies are associated with departure from Hardy-Weinberg equilibrium: hint for genotyping error? Hum Genet 111:573–574

Xu J, Zheng SL, Hawkins GA, Faith DA, Kelly B, Isaacs SD, Wiley KE, Chang B, Ewing CM, Bujnovszky P, Carpten JD, Bleecker ER, Walsh PC, Trent JM, Meyers DA, Isaacs WB (2001) Linkage and association studies of prostate cancer susceptibility: evidence for linkage at 8p22-23. Am J Hum Genet 69:341–350

Am. J. Hum. Genet. 76:987–1007, 2005

Alternative Splicing Suggests Extended Function of *PEX26* in Peroxisome Biogenesis

Sabine Weller,[1,*] Ivelisse Cajigas,[2] James Morrell,[3] Cassandra Obie,[1,4] Gary Steel,[1,4] Stephen J. Gould,[3] and David Valle[1,4]

[1]McKusick-Nathans Institute of Genetic Medicine, [2]Summer Internship Program, [3]Department of Biological Chemistry, and [4]Howard Hughes Medical Institute, Johns Hopkins University School of Medicine, Baltimore

Matsumoto and colleagues recently identified *PEX26* as the gene responsible for complementation group 8 of the peroxisome biogenesis disorders and showed that it encodes an integral peroxisomal membrane protein with a single C-terminal transmembrane domain and a cytosolic N-terminus that interacts with the PEX1/PEX6 heterodimer through direct binding to the latter. They proposed that PEX26 functions as the peroxisomal docking factor for the PEX1/PEX6 heterodimer. Here, we identify new *PEX26* disease alleles, localize the PEX6-binding domain to the N-terminal half of the protein (aa 29–174), and show that, at the cellular level, PEX26 deficiency impairs peroxisomal import of both PTS1- and PTS2-targeted matrix proteins. Also, we find that *PEX26* undergoes alternative splicing to produce several splice forms—including one, *PEX26-Δex5,* that maintains frame and encodes an isoform lacking the transmembrane domain of full-length PEX26 (PEX26-FL). Despite its cytosolic location, PEX26-Δex5 rescues peroxisome biogenesis in PEX26-deficient cells as efficiently as does PEX26-FL. To test our observation that a peroxisomal location is not required for PEX26 function, we made a chimeric protein (PEX26-Mito) with PEX26 as its N-terminus and the targeting segment of a mitochondrial outer membrane protein (OMP25) at its C-terminus. We found PEX26-Mito localized to the mitochondria and directed all detectable PEX6 and a fraction of PEX1 to this extraperoxisomal location; yet PEX26-Mito retains the full ability to rescue peroxisome biogenesis in PEX26-deficient cells. On the basis of these observations, we suggest that a peroxisomal localization of PEX26 and PEX6 is not required for their function and that the interaction of PEX6 with PEX1 is dynamic. This model predicts that, once activated in an extraperoxisomal location, PEX1 moves to the peroxisome and completes the function of the PEX1/6 heterodimer.

Introduction

Peroxisomes are ubiquitous, single-membrane–bound organelles that contain ⩾50 enzymes and participate in a variety of metabolic pathways. The importance of the peroxisome in development and metabolism is highlighted by inherited defects in peroxisome biogenesis in which most or all of peroxisomal metabolic functions are deficient (Wanders 2004*a,* 2004*b*). The clinical phenotype of the peroxisome-biogenesis disorders (PBDs) varies widely in severity and can be classified into two broad categories, the Zellweger spectrum and rhizomelic chondrodysplasia punctata (RCDP [MIM 215100]) (Gould et al. 2001). The Zellweger spectrum includes at least three overlapping phenotypes that represent segments of a phenotypic continuum, including Zellweger syndrome (ZS [MIM 214100]) at the severe end, neonatal adrenoleukodystrophy (NALD [MIM 202370]) as an intermediate form, and infantile Refsum disease (IRD [MIM 266510]) at the mild end of the spectrum. Dysmorphic features, neurological symptoms, hepatic disease, and skeletal abnormalities in varying degrees are common to all three (Gould et al. 2001). Reflecting the complexity of peroxisome assembly, somatic-cell-hybridization studies show that PBDs are genetically heterogeneous, with at least 13 human complementation groups (CGs) (Weller et al. 2003; Shimozawa et al. 2004).

At the cellular level, the PBDs can be divided into defects of peroxisomal membrane biogenesis and matrix protein import. Three CGs (9, 12, and 14) have blocks in peroxisome membrane biogenesis and lack identifiable peroxisomal structures entirely. The remaining 10 CGs (1, 2, 3, 4, 7, 8, 10, 11, 13, and K [Gifu]) display defects in peroxisome matrix protein import but retain the ability to form peroxisomal membranes (Sacksteder and Gould 2000; Shimozawa et al. 2004). Peroxisomal matrix proteins are synthesized on free cytosolic ribosomes and are targeted posttranslationally to the organ-

Received January 14, 2005; accepted for publication March 29, 2005; electronically published April 27, 2005.

Address for correspondence and reprints: Dr. David Valle, Johns Hopkins University School of Medicine, 519 Broadway Research Building, 733 North Broadway, Baltimore, MD 21205. E-mail: dvalle@jhmi.edu

* Present affiliation: Department of Pediatrics and Pediatric Neurology, Georg August University, Göttingen, Germany.

0002-9297/2005/7606-0007$15.00

elle by cytosolic receptors that bind to *cis*-acting sequences, the peroxisomal targeting signals (PTSs). The majority of matrix proteins are targeted by the PTS1, a C-terminal -SKL or conserved variant (Gould et al. 1988, 1989). A few matrix proteins are targeted by a different sequence, the PTS2, a degenerate sequence—(R/K)(L/V/I)X_5(H/Q)(L/A)—located near the N-terminus (Osumi et al. 1991; Swinkels et al. 1991). PTS1 and PTS2 sequences are recognized by the cytosolic receptors PEX5 and PEX7, respectively. The receptor/matrix protein complexes assemble in the cytosol and shuttle to the peroxisome, where they dock to PEX14, an integral peroxisomal-membrane protein. Unloading and translocation of the cargo proteins into the peroxisomal matrix involves interactions with several other membrane peroxins (PEX13, PEX10, and PEX12) (Weller et al. 2003). The receptors are recycled back to the cytosol to participate in another round of import (Dodt and Gould 1996). Decreased steady-state levels of PEX5 in cell lines from patients with primary deficiencies of PEX1 or PEX6 suggest a role for these peroxins in stabilization and/or recycling of the former (Yahraus et al. 1996; Reuber et al. 1997; Collins et al. 2000). PEX1 and PEX6 are AAA ATPases that, in yeast, form heterodimeric complexes in an ATP-dependent manner (Faber et al. 1998*a;* Birschmann et al. 2005). AAA ATPases are involved in a diverse set of cellular processes, many involving protein unfolding, refolding, or the disassembly of protein complexes (Vale 2000; Lupas and Martin 2002). Although the precise roles of PEX1 and PEX6 in the peroxisome membrane protein import process are unknown, epistasis analyses utilizing the decreased level of PEX5 in PEX1 and PEX6-deficient cells indicated that they may act in the disassembly of the multimeric PEX5-PTS protein complex (preimplex) prior to or during the import process (Collins et al. 2000; Gould and Collins 2002).

Using expression cloning in Chinese hamster ovary (CHO) cells defective for peroxisome biogenesis, Matsumoto and colleagues (2003*a*) recently identified *PEX26* as the gene responsible for CG8, the last unexplained human CG. In both human and mouse, PEX26 is a 305-aa protein with one transmembrane domain, located near the C-terminus of the protein (aa 252–269) and an N-terminal domain (NTD) exposed to the cytosol. Matsumoto and colleagues (2003*a*) showed that PEX26 binds PEX6 and proposed that it functions to recruit PEX1 and PEX6 to peroxisomal membranes. Interestingly, they also propose that PEX26 function is required for import of only catalase and PTS2-targeted proteins and is not required for import of classical PTS1-targeted proteins. To date, 12 pathologic *PEX26* alleles have been described in studies of 12 patients with CG8, all with phenotypes in the Zellweger spectrum (Matsumoto et al. 2003*a*, 2003*b*; Steinberg et al. 2004).

Here, we identify all mutant *PEX26* alleles in 10 CG8 probands, including five new *PEX26* mutations, and quantify the peroxisomal import phenotype in CG8 cells of known genotype, showing that both PTS1- and PTS2-mediated import is impaired. We also determine the effect of *PEX26* deficiency on PEX5 and PEX1 steady-state levels and map the PEX6-binding domain in PEX26. Additionally, we describe extensive alternative splicing of *PEX26* in fibroblasts and various human tissues that creates a cytoplasmic, but nevertheless functional, PEX26 isoform. Extending this observation, we show that PEX26 mislocalized to the outer mitochondrial membrane retains its function in peroxisome biogenesis. Our findings extend the consequences of *PEX26* deficiency to PTS1-mediated import and challenge the current model of PEX26 function as a docking factor for the PEX1-PEX6 protein complex at the peroxisomal membrane.

Material and Methods

PEX26 Amplification and Mutation Detection

We isolated genomic DNA and total RNA from transformed skin fibroblasts with the Puregene and Purescript kits (Gentra Systems), per the manufacturer's directions, and purchased additional human total cellular RNA from Ambion. We amplified *PEX26* exons 1–6 from genomic DNA (250 ng) and total RNA (0.5–2 μg), using *Taq* polymerase (Invitrogen) or the OneStep Cycle kit (Qiagen), per the manufacturer's directions. Oligonucleotide sequences are shown in table 1 (primers 26-1–26-24). PCR products were purified from agarose gel (QIAquick Gel Extraction kit [Qiagen]) and were sequenced directly by automated fluorescent sequencing. We confirmed each mutation in amplicons from both genomic DNA and RNA.

Allele-Specific Oligonucleotide Hybridization (ASO)

We performed ASO analysis to determine the frequency of missense mutations M1T, L44P, L45P, R98W, and P117L in exons 2 and 3, as described elsewhere (Gärtner et al. 1992; Braverman et al. 1997). Sequences of the wild-type and mutant-specific probes are listed in table 1 (probes 26-25–26-34).

Cell Lines, Transfections, and Immunofluorescence

We analyzed PBD skin fibroblast cell lines assigned to CG8 by somatic complementation analysis in the collec-

Table 1

Oligonucleotide Sequences

The table is available in its entirety in the online edition of *The American Journal of Human Genetics.*

tion of the Kennedy Krieger Institute, Baltimore. Cell lines are identified by a unique PBD number assigned to each proband and are used in all publications from our group. Cell lines PBD057, PBD111, PBD114, and PBD063 were also studied by Matsumoto and coworkers (2003*b*) (in which study they were designated GM11335, PDL35167, GM08771, and GM16865, respectively). Cell lines PBD059, PBD063, PBD057, and PBD114 from our study are also available from the Coriell cell repository (assigned numbers GM17398, GM16865, GM11335, and GM08771, respectively). Cell lines with null alleles for PEX1 (PBD009), PEX5 (PBD005), PEX6 (PBD106), and PEX3 (PBD400) have been reported elsewhere (Dodt et al. 1995; Yahraus et al. 1996; Reuber et al. 1997; South et al. 2000). All cell lines were transformed by transfection with a vector expressing SV40 large T-antigen, as described elsewhere (Dodt et al. 1995). Additionally, cell lines PBD009, PBD005, PBD106, and PBD400 were immortalized by stable transfection with a vector that constitutively expresses human telomerase (pBabePuro/hTER) (Hahn et al. 1999). We cultured the cells in Dulbecco's modified Eagle medium high-glucose supplemented with 10% fetal bovine serum and 100 U penicillin and 100 μg streptomycin/ml (Gibco). We transfected the cells by electroporation, as described elsewhere (Chang et al. 1997), and processed the cells for immunofluorescence 48 h later (Warren et al. 1998). We used monoclonal anti-HA, mono- and polyclonal anti-myc (BD Bioscience and Santa Cruz Biotechnology), polyclonal anti-PEX14 (South et al. 2000), and anti-PMP70 (Shani et al. 1997) as primary antibodies, and we obtained fluorescent secondary antibodies from Vector Laboratories. Mitochondria were visualized using MitoTracker (Molecular Probes). Microscopy was performed on a Zeiss LSM510 Meta confocal microscope with the Carl Zeiss LSM510 Imaging Software.

Plasmids

We constructed the recombinant plasmids to express full-length human PEX26 cDNA and its splice variants by cloning RT-PCR amplicons from human control fibroblast RNA spanning exons 1–6 (probes 26-15–26-16) (TOPO TA Cloning [Invitrogen]). After sequence analysis, we transferred the inserts representing full-length (-FL), exon 5–less (-Δex5) and exon 2–less (-Δex2) PEX26 cDNA into pcDNA3 (Invitrogen), using either the *Kpn*I and *Eco*RI restriction sites or the *Eco*RI restriction site only (PEX26-Δex2). To produce full-length PEX26 (PEX26-FL) and -Δex5 expression vectors with an N-terminal myc-tag, we modified the *Kpn*I–*Bsu36*I fragment, using PCR with a reverse primer incorporating the myc-sequence (primers 26-39–26-40). To obtain the myc-tagged PEX26 expression vector lacking exon 5 and exon 6 (mycPEX26-Δex5+6), we inserted a stop codon (c.667GGC→TGA; G223X) following the sequence encoded by exon 4 in the cDNA. We PCR amplified a fragment of mycPEX26-Δex5 with oligonucleotide primers 26-41 and 26-42, the latter containing the -TGA stop codon, and cloned the *Hin*dIII fragment from this PCR product into the *Hin*dIII sites of mycPEX26-Δex5.

To mislocalize the myc-tagged N-terminus of PEX26 to the outer mitochondrial membrane, we PCR-amplified the corresponding segment of mycPEX26-FL with primers that incorporated *Hin*dIII and *Eco*RI restriction sites (primers 26-51–26-52). Using RT-PCR of rat liver RNA, we isolated the segment of rat Omp25 cDNA that encodes the transmembrane segment of the protein flanked by *Eco*RI and *Not*I restriction sites (probes 26-53–26-54). We ligated these fragments into pcDNA3 (*Hin*dIII and *Not*I) to create a recombinant vector expressing a chimeric protein, mycPEX26 (aa 2–222)–OMP25 (aa 170–206) (PEX26-Mito). We used the QuickChange XL Site-Directed Mutagenesis Kit (Stratagene), per the manufacturer's directions, to introduce L44P (CTC→CCC) and L45P (CTG→CCG) into PEX26-FL cDNA expression vector and verified the mutations by sequencing (primers 26-35–26-38). For N-terminal myc-tagging of these clones, we used the PCR-modification strategy of the *Kpn* I-*Bsu*36 fragment that is described above (mycPEX26-L44P and -L45P). pcDNA3 with an N-terminal 3 × HA epitope tag was created by inserting a PCR product coding for MTSGRIFYPYDVPDYAG YPYDVPD YA GSYPY-DVPDYALQCGR, flanked by *Bgl*II and *Xho*I-*Not*I-*Xba*I restriction sites into *Bam*HI and *Xba*I sites of pcDNA3. To construct a plasmid with a 3 × HA-tag and a 3 × nuclear localization signal (HAnls) for N-terminal tagging of PEX26 fragments, we inserted a PCR amplicon containing the 3 × nls signal (Jones et al. 1999, 2001) flanked by *Sal*I and *Xho*I-*Not*I restriction sites, as a *Sal*I–*Not*I fragment into *Xho*I and *Not*I sites of the pcDNA3-3 × HA expression vector (probes 26-55–26-56). Using the new *Xho*I and the *Not*I restriction sites, we inserted PEX26 fragments obtained by PCR amplification with pcDNA3-PEX26-FL or PEX26-L44P/L45P as template for expression of PEX26 peptides corresponding to aa 2–222, aa 2-222-L44P, aa 2-222-L45P, aa 2–135, aa 2–163, aa 136–222, and aa 29–174 in frame with the HAnls signal at the N-terminus (probes 26-43–26-50). PCR-generated PEX26 fragments for expression of peptides corresponding to aa 2–174, aa 2–163, aa 29–174, and aa 69–174 were also inserted in frame with an N-terminal 3× myc-tag in pcDNA3 by use of *Xho*I and *Not*I restriction sites (Geisbrecht et al. 1998). pcDNA3-3 × HAPEX6 (JM721) and pcDNA3-3 × mycPEX6 (JM709) were constructed by inserting the *Sal*I-*Not*I fragment from pTY3 (Yahraus et al. 1996) that contained the PEX6 ORF in the *Xho*I-*Not*I sites of the pcDNA3-3 × HA (see above) and the pcDNA3-3 × myc expression vector (Geisbrecht et al.

1998), respectively. The expression vector for pcDNA3-PEX1 with a C-terminal 3 × HA-tag (pBER86) was made by inserting an *Apa*I-*Xho*I fragment that contained three repeats of the HA epitope tag (see above) between the *Apa*I-*Xho*I sites of pBER81 containing the *PEX1* ORF (Reuber et al. 1997), resulting in an in-frame C-terminal fusion.

Oligonucleotides used for cloning and mutagenesis are listed in table 1. We sequenced all recombinant constructs to verify absence of PCR-introduced mutations. As reporters for peroxisomal-protein import, we used the following plasmids: pcDNA3-PAHXmyc (Mihalik et al. 1997), pcDNA3-NmycPECI (Geisbrecht and Gould 1999), pcDNA3-NmycHAOX1 (Liu et al. 1999), pcDNA3-NmycCatalase (Liu et al. 1999), and GFP-SKL.

Characterization of the Cellular Phenotype and Relative Rescue

We processed cells grown on cover slips for immunofluorescence and counted the numbers of cells expressing the matrix-protein import markers with variations of the PTS consensus sequence (see above). We placed each expressing cell into one of the following categories on the basis of the distribution of the marker protein: no import for cytoplasmic-only staining, partial import for cells with cytoplasmic and peroxisomal staining, and complete import when the marker protein was exclusively peroxisomal. In a subset of these experiments, the observer was blind to the cell line and to the transfected constructs, with results indistinguishable from the nonblind quantification. Additionally, recounting the same experiment in a blind fashion gave values differing by no more than 10%. To calculate percentages of partial and complete import, we scored at least 500 expressing cells in each experiment. To determine the complementing activity of *PEX26* missense alleles L44P and L45P and PEX26 splice variants, we calculated the percentages of CG8 cells that displayed no import, partial import, and complete import of mycCAT or GFP-SKL after cotransfection with nonrecombinant pcDNA3, *PEX26*-FL, *PEX26*-L44P, *PEX26*-L45P, *PEX26*-$\Delta ex5$, *PEX26*-$\Delta ex2$, and *PEX26*-Mito expression vectors. Corrected rescue values were calculated by subtracting the percentage of import observed in cells transfected with nonrecombinant (empty) vector (typically with a range of 0%–10% for mycCAT/GFP-SKL in PBD059 cells) from the percentage of import observed in cells transfected with the *PEX26*-FL, *PEX26* mutant, *PEX26* splice variant, and *PEX26*-Mito expression vectors. Relative rescue values were obtained by dividing the corrected rescue values by the corrected rescue value determined for the cells transfected with the *PEX26*-FL expression vector.

Immunoblot Experiments

We used 15 μg of protein from whole-cell lysates from the indicated cells, electrophoresed in 7.5% or 10% Tris-HCl polyacrylamide gels (BioRad), and processed the gels for immunoblotting, following standard protocols. Mouse anti-PEX1 monoclonal antibody was purchased from BD Transduction Laboratories. Rabbit polyclonal anti-PEX5 antibody was described elsewhere (Dodt et al. 1995). Rabbit polyclonal anti-PEX13 antibody is directed against a C-terminal PEX13 peptide (South et al. 2000). We used anti-tubulin (Sigma) as a loading control. All results were obtained in duplicate in two experiments.

Antibodies directed against PEX26 were generated by immunization of rabbits with an N-terminal PEX26 peptide (NH_2-MKSDSSTSAAPLRGLC-COOH) conjugated to keyhole limpet hemocyanin as a carrier protein (Covance Research Products). In vitro transcription and translation of full-length PEX26 was performed with the TnT T7 Coupled Reticulocyte Lysate System (Promega), per the manufacturer's directions.

Results

PEX26 Full-Length Transcripts and Orthologs

PEX26 maps to 16.9 Mb at 22q11.21, just centromeric of the region typically deleted in DiGeorge/velocardiofacial syndrome (McDermid and Morrow 2002), and has seven predicted exons distributed over 13 kb, with the translation start site located in exon 2. In our RT-PCR experiments, we routinely use a primer (26-15) corresponding to the 5′ end of exon 1, as predicted by the *PEX26* cDNA with GenBank accession number NM_017929.

Using the human PEX26 amino acid sequence as a probe to screen public databases, we detected multiple vertebrate orthologs (*Mus musculus, Rattus norvegicus, Gallus gallus, Danio rerio, Fugu rubripes, Tetraodon nigriviridis*) but none in invertebrates. In *D. rerio* and *T. nigriviridis*, PEX26 orthologs show 30% and 32%, respectively, sequence identity with human PEX26 (fig. 1). *Saccharomyces cerevisiae* PEX15 resembles vertebrate PEX26 in topology (both are type II integral membrane proteins) and in binding of PEX6, but we found no detectable amino acid sequence similarity (12% overall identity between *S. cerevisiae* PEX15 and human PEX26, with no blocks of identical amino acids >2 residues).

PEX26 Mutation Analysis

Using RT-PCR of patient fibroblast RNA with confirmation by amplification of the indicated exons in genomic DNA, we found nine *PEX26* alleles that accounted for all 20 mutant *PEX26* genes in 10 CG8 probands (table

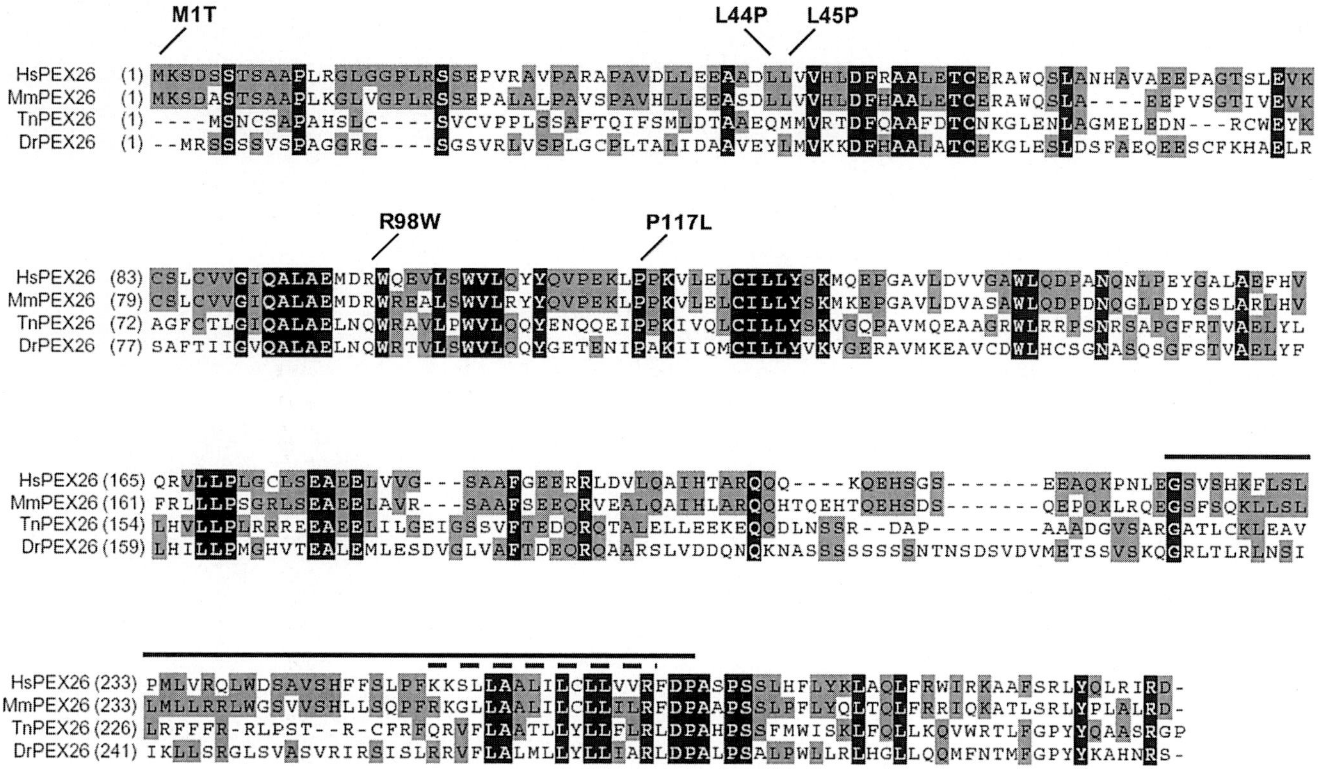

Figure 1 Sequence comparison of vertebrate PEX26 orthologs. Alignment of human (Hs), mouse (Mm), *T. nigroviridis* (Tn), and *D. rerio* (Dr) PEX26 amino acid sequence. HsPEX26 is 73%, 32%, and 31% identical to mouse, *T. nigriviridis,* and *D. rerio* PEX26, respectively. Amino acids identical across all four species are highlighted in black; those with a plurality are in gray. The positions of *PEX26* missense mutations identified in this study are indicated. The solid line marks the segment of human PEX26 encoded by the alternatively spliced exon 5; the dashed line indicates the predicted transmembrane domain.

2). Of these alleles, five are newly recognized (Matsumoto et al. 2003*a,* 2003*b;* Steinberg et al. 2004). One proband with a ZS phenotype (PBD059) is homozygous for a mutation in the splice-donor site of intron 2, c.230+1G→T, which leads to a frameshift at T77 and premature termination (T77fs139X) (see table 2). Four patients with an NALD or IRD phenotype (PBD111, PBD057, PBD161, and PBD065) are homozygous for a transition in exon 3, c.292C→T, which results in the previously reported missense mutation R98W. PBD063, with a ZS phenotype, is a compound heterozygote for R98W and an insertion of thymidine at position 254 in the cDNA (c.254insT; exon 3), which results in a frameshift and premature termination (C86fs114X). In PBD055, with an IRD phenotype, we detected three heterozygous mutations. In exon 3, a c.350C→T transition results in P117L; in exon 4, c.457C→G results in L153V; and, in exon 6, a single base-pair deletion (c.862delC) causes a frameshift at R288 with termination 79 aa downstream (R288fs366X). L153V is in *cis* with R288fs and is a known SNP (*rs12484657*). PBD110 is a compound heterozygote for L44P and R98W. PBD114 is a compound heterozygote for M1T and L45P. The first methionine downstream from M1 is M96, which is embedded in an acceptable Kozak consensus sequence (GCA**G**AA*AUG***G**, compared with the consensus GCC**Pu**CC*AUG***G**), which suggests that translation could initiate at this position (Kozak and Harper 2000). PBD109 is a compound heterozygote for R98W and a complicated allele with a 122-bp duplication separated by an inserted thymidine (c.426_548dup122bpinsT) that maintains frame and predicts a protein in which aa 134–182 are tandemly duplicated, with substitution of glycine by valine at position 183 (A134_V182dup+G183V).

Functional Consequence of PEX26 Missense Alleles L44P and L45P

Of these nine *PEX26* alleles, four (M1T, L45P, R98W, and c.254insT) were shown elsewhere to be functionally significant by expression in a *PEX26*-deficient CHO cell line (Matsumoto et al. 2003*b*). We assumed functional significance for three nonsense or frameshift mutations that disrupted a large segment of PEX26 (c.230+1G→T, L153V+R288fs, and A143_V182dup+G183C). To test the functional consequences of *PEX26*-L44P and -L45P,

Table 2

***PEX26* Mutations in CG8 Patients**

Patient, Clinical Phenotype, and *PEX26* Allele	*PEX26* Mutation in cDNA	Comment
PBD059:		
ZS:		
T77fs139X homozygote	c.230+1G→T	This donor splice-site mutation results in the insertion of 173, 236, or 650 bp of intron 2, with the result of addition of a nonspecific sequence of 61 or 82 aa. For clarity, we designate the allele by the shortest insert.
PBD111:		
NALD:		
R98W homozygote	c.292C→T[a]	Transition at CpG dinucleotide
PBD063:		
IRD:		
C86fs114X	c.254insT	Nonspecific sequence of 28 aa
R98W	c.292C→T	
PBD055:		
IRD:		
[L153V+R288fs366X]	[c.457C→G+c.862delC]	Nonspecific sequence of 78 aa; L153V and R288fs366C are in *cis*.
P117L	c.305C→T[a]	
PBD057:		
NALD:		
R98W homozygote	c.292C→T	
PBD110:		
NALD:		
L44P	c.131T→C[a]	
R98W	c.292C→T	
PBD114:		
IRD:		
M1T	c.2T→C[a]	Downstream initiation at M96 theoretically possible
L45P	c.134T→C[a]	
PBD109:		
IRD:		
R98W	c.292C→T	
A143_V182dup+G183V	c.426_548dup122bpinsT	Duplication within exon 4 maintains frame and predicts mutant PEX26p with duplication of aa 143–182 plus G183V
PBD161:		
IRD:		
R98W homozygote	c.292C→T	Clinical phenotype variant
PBD065:		
NALD:		
R98W homozygote	c.292C→T	

[a] Frequencies of cDNA changes have been determined by ASO in 106 control chromosomes (see text).

we expressed them in transformed fibroblasts from a CG8 patient (PBD059) who was homozygous for a *PEX26* null allele, and we compared their ability to restore matrix-protein import with wild-type *PEX26* (relative rescue). In two separate experiments, PEX26-L44P had 1% and 8% relative-rescue activity, whereas *PEX26*-L45P had 0% relative-rescue activity in both trials. Thus, both these mutants severely reduce the function of PEX26.

Frequency of Mutant Alleles

To estimate the frequency of the five missense alleles (M1T, L44P, L45P, R98W, and P117L) in the general population, we amplified *PEX26* exons 2 and 3 from genomic DNA of 53 individuals of mixed ethnicity, and we genotyped them by allele-specific oligonucleotide hybridization. We detected none of the mutations in these 106 control chromosomes and conclude all are relatively rare variants.

Cellular Phenotype of PEX26-Deficient Fibroblasts

A previous study concluded that PTS1 import is normal in PEX26-deficient cells, a result that is surprising, given that the clinical phenotype of the patients is in the Zellweger spectrum rather than RCDP (Matsumoto et al. 2003*b*). To determine the extent and severity of the import defect for peroxisomal matrix enzymes in *PEX26*-deficient fibroblasts from individuals with known genotype, we made use of the differing import efficiency associated with variation in the PTS1 (Liu et al. 1999). We determined the matrix-protein import of a series of PTS1-targeted proteins ranging from the canonical -SKL targeted peroxisomal Δ^3, Δ^2 enoyl-CoA isomerase (PECI) (Geisbrecht and Gould 1999); the near-consensus -SKI targeted human peroxisomal glycolate peroxidase (HAOX1) (Jones et al. 2000); and the most atypical PTS1, -KANL, found in catalase (CAT) (Lazarow et al. 1982; Bell et al. 1986; Purdue and Lazarow 1996). We also tested PTS2 import by analyzing the distribution of phytanoyl-CoA hydroxylase (PAHX) (Mihalik et al. 1997). We compared the peroxisomal matrix import of these reporters in transformed fibroblasts of patients PBD059, PBD111, PBD057, PBD110, and PBD114 to that in cells from *PEX1*-, *PEX5*-, and *PEX6*-deficient patients and a control individual. As predicted by the degree of conservation of the PTS1, import for these markers varied with PECI > HAOX1 > CAT (fig. 2). The cells of all *PEX26*-deficient patients had some residual import in this assay. PBD059, with a ZS phenotype (c.230+1G→T/c.230+1G→T), showed the most severe impairment, with residual import of mycPECI only. In contrast, cells from two R98W homozygotes (PBD111 and PBD057), both with an NALD phenotype, displayed the mildest import phenotype, with residual import for all marker proteins. Fibroblasts of PBD110 (L44P/R98W [NALD]) and PBD114 (M1T/L45P [IRD]) had minimal residual import for most marker proteins tested. Thus, there is a limited correlation between the cellular phenotype as measured in this assay and the clinical phenotype in these patients. Interestingly, cells from patients with null mutations in *PEX1, PEX6,* and *PEX5* all had a more severe import phenotype than we observed in any of the *PEX26*-deficient cells, including the presumed null, PBD059, which had some residual import of the reporter with the most conserved PTS1 signal (PECI; 24% residual import). Our results differ from those of Matsumoto and coworkers, who interpreted their immunofluorescence data with an antibody directed against the canonical PTS1 (-SKL) as showing normal import of PTS1-targeted matrix proteins (Matsumoto et al. 2003*a*, 2003*b*). Our results showing a generalized defect in PTS1-mediated import are consistent with the Zellweger spectrum clinical phenotype of the patients with CG8.

PEX26, PEX5, *and* PEX1 *Steady-State Levels in* PEX26*-Deficient Fibroblasts*

Immunoblot studies with anti-PEX26 antibody identified a protein of the size predicted for PEX26 (34 kD) in lysates of wild-type but not PBD059 cells. The antibody also detected a 34-kD protein produced in in vitro transcription and translation of a full-length *PEX26* cDNA. Preincubation of the antibody with the specific but not with a nonspecific peptide blocked binding to the 34-kD protein (fig. 3). We conclude that our antibody specifically detects PEX26. A larger, cross-reacting protein is present in the immunoblots of wild-type and CG8 samples and is detected with either preimmune or immune serum (fig. 3).

Immunoblots of lysates of all CG8 cell lines tested showed no detectable PEX26, which indicates that the *PEX26* mutations in these cell lines destabilize the protein product. Previous studies of monogenic defects in peroxisome biogenesis have shown that a primary defect in one component of the matrix-protein–import apparatus may result in a secondary deficiency of other components. For example, primary defects in PEX1 or PEX6 result in a marked secondary deficiency of PEX5 (Dodt and Gould 1996; Collins et al. 2000). Similarly, we found that, compared with wild type, PEX26 was reduced but detectable in lysates of reference *PEX1*-, *PEX5*-, and *PEX6*-deficient cell lines. In at least six CGs, including those caused by deficiency of *PEX1*, -5, and -6 (CG1, CG2, and CG4, respectively), peroxisomes are enlarged but show a 5-fold decrease in abundance (Chang et al. 1999). To exclude the possibility that the observed reduction in PEX26 level was secondary to a reduction of peroxisomal membrane, we examined the level of PEX13, an integral peroxisomal membrane protein, in this same

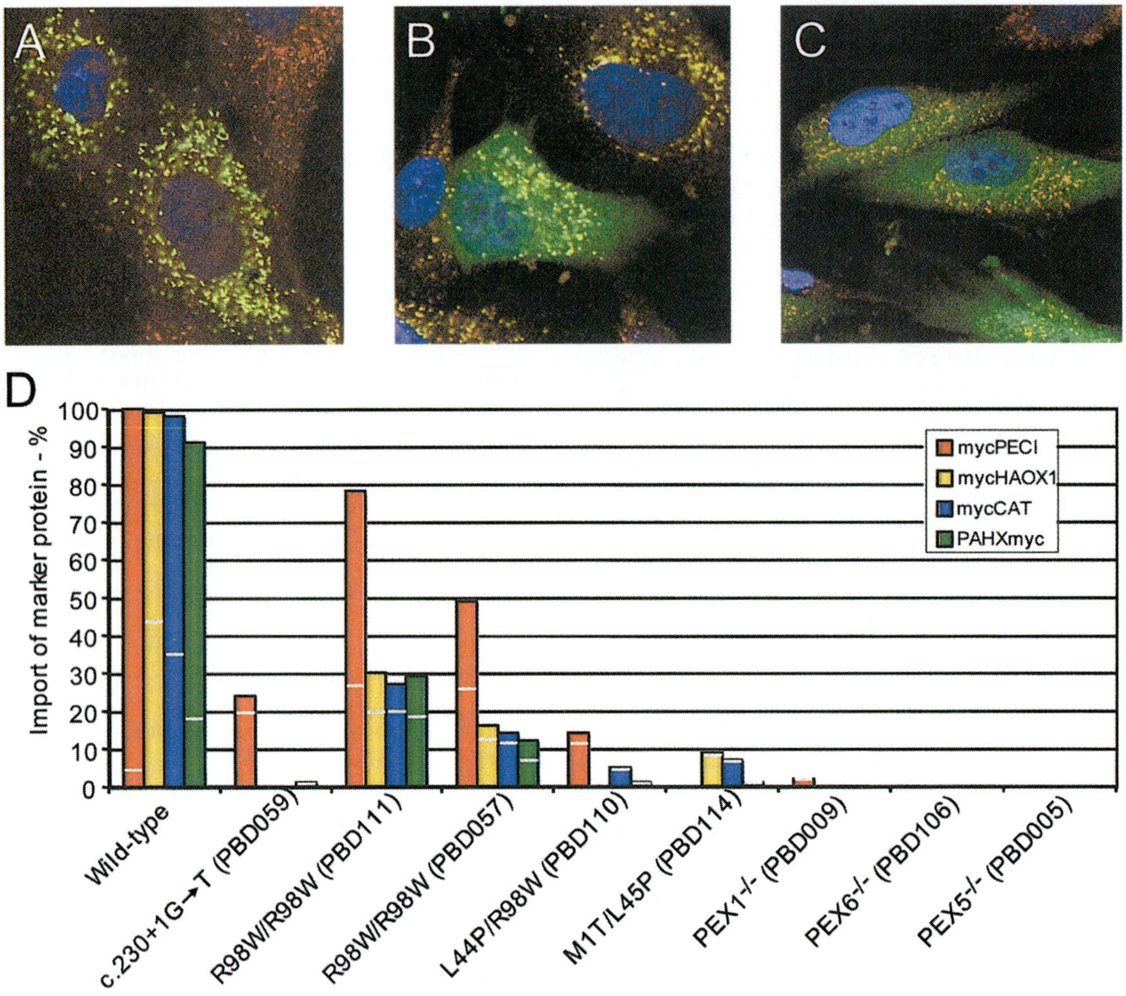

Figure 2 Cellular phenotype of cultured skin fibroblasts from *PEX26*-deficient patients. *A–C,* Example of merged images of transfected human fibroblasts showing complete (*A*), partial (*B*), or no (*C*) peroxisomal import of the indicated reporter. Indirect immunofluorescence staining of peroxisomal membranes was with anti-PEX14 antibody (Texas Red), and staining of a reporter peroxisomal matrix protein was with anti-myc antibody (FITC). Yellow indicates colocalization of the peroxisomal marker and the matrix-protein marker. *D,* Percentage of transfected cells displaying complete and partial import of the indicated matrix proteins. The vertical bars indicate the total percentage of cells showing import. The light horizontal line dividing each vertical bar indicates the fraction of cells scored as partial import (below the line) and complete import (above the line). The values represent the means of two experiments, except for (1) wild type, PBD059 and PBD111 transfected with mycPECI, and mycCAT (three experiments); and (2) PBD057 transfected with mycPECI, mycHAOX1, and PAHXmyc and PBD114 transfected with mycHAOX1, mycCAT, and PAHXmyc (one experiment); the value for PBD114 with mycPECI was not determined.

set of cell lines. The levels of PEX13 were essentially the same as in control cells (fig. 3). Thus, the decrease in PEX26 seems to be a specific consequence of deficiency of PEX1, PEX5, or PEX6.

To determine if *PEX26* deficiency affects the steady-state level of PEX5 or PEX1, we used total protein from whole-cell lysates from selected CG8-, CG1-, CG2-, and CG4-transformed fibroblasts for immunoblot experiments (fig. 3). As expected, we found no effect of *PEX26, PEX5,* or *PEX6* deficiency on PEX1 levels. Unfortunately, neither we nor others have been able to develop an antibody to assess PEX6 levels. PEX5 levels were equally reduced in all CG8 cell lines and in *PEX1*- and *PEX6*-deficient cells.

Alternative Splicing of PEX26

During the course of our RT-PCR experiments with fibroblast RNA, we detected three shorter amplified products in addition to the expected full-length product of 1,508 bp (*PEX26*-FL) (fig. 4). We cloned and sequenced these shorter cDNAs and found that they represented splice variants of *PEX26*. We found a similar pattern of these *PEX26* splice forms in RNA from sev-

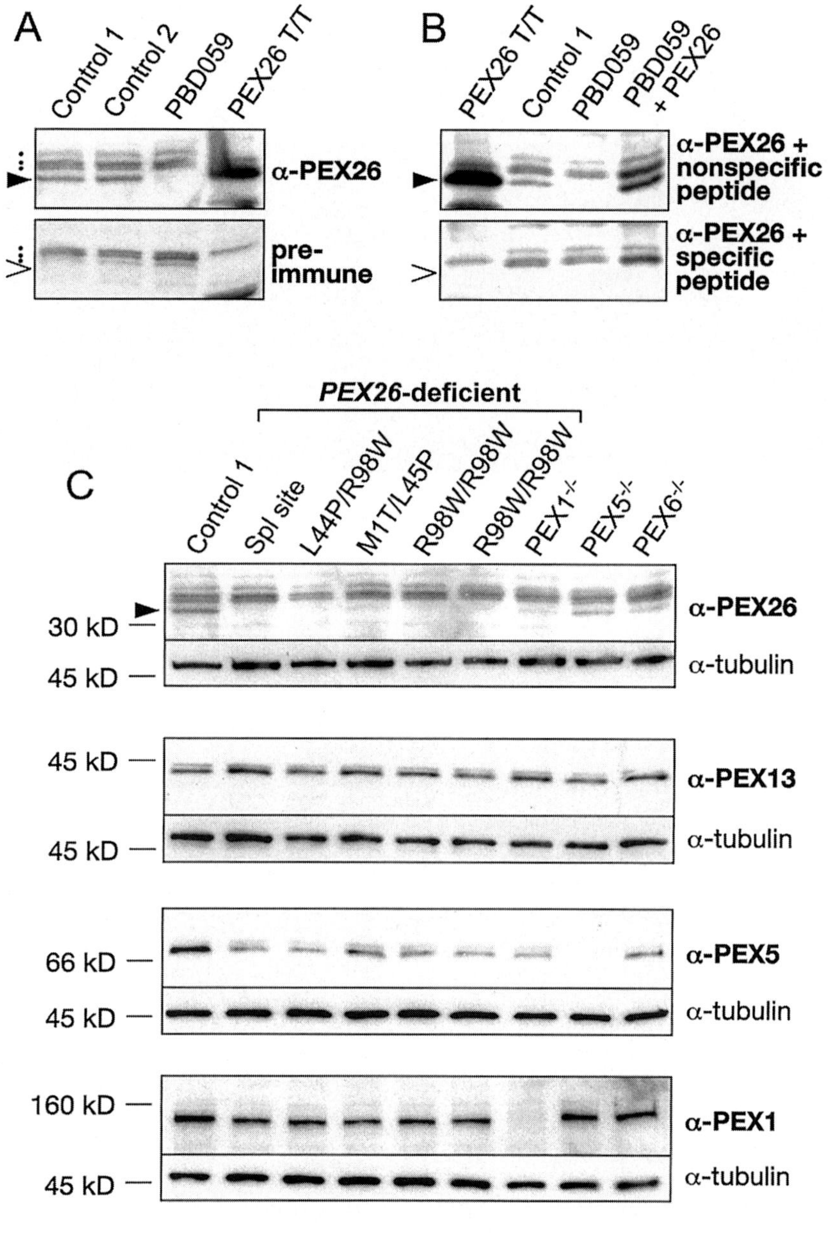

Figure 3 Immunoblot analysis of PEX26 and related peroxins in PBD fibroblasts. All panels show fibroblast lysates (15 μg/lane) or the products of in vitro transcribed and translated full-length PEX26 (PEX26T/T) electrophoresed in 7.5% or 10% polyacrylamide gels, under denaturing conditions, transferred to nylon filters, and detected with the indicated antibody or antiserum. Panels A and B show characterization of our anti-PEX26 N-terminal peptide (NH_2-MKSDSSTSAAPLRGLC-COOH) antibody. *A*, Blots of lysates from control fibroblasts, a *PEX26*-deficient cell (PBD059, c.230+1G→T/c.230+1G→T), and PEX26T/T detected either with anti-PEX26 (*top*) or preimmune serum (*bottom*). The filled wedge (►) indicates PEX26 (34 kDa), detected only in control fibroblasts and in the PEX26T/T products; the dots indicate nonspecific background bands present in fibroblast lysates; the unfilled wedge (>) indicates the expected location of PEX26 in the preimmune panel. *B*, Lysates from the indicated sources stained with anti-PEX26 antibody preincubated with either a nonspecific (unrelated) peptide (NH_2-QKQEHSGSEEAQKPNC-COOH) (*top*) or with the specific N-terminal PEX26 peptide used as immunogen (NH_2 -MKSDSSTSAAPLRGLC-COOH) (*bottom*). The lysate designated PBD059+PEX26 is from PEX26-null cells transfected with full-length *PEX26*. The filled wedge (►) indicates PEX26 (*top*); the unfilled wedge (>) indicates expected location of PEX26 (*bottom*). Note that preincubation with the specific immunizing peptide but not with the unrelated nonspecific peptide completely blocks detection of PEX26. *C*, Immunoblots of lysates from cells of the indicated genotype stained with anti-PEX26 antiserum and anti-tubulin as a loading control (*top panel*). The second panel shows the same lysates stained with anti-PEX13 as a measure of the amount of peroxisome membrane in each sample, also with anti-tubulin as a loading control. The third panel shows the same lysate stained with anti-PEX5 and the bottom panel with anti-PEX1. In all panels, the *PEX26* genotype is indicated above. The identity and genotypes of the cell lines with mutations in other PEX genes are as follows: $PEX1^{-/-}$, PBD009 (c.2097insT/IVS18+1G→A) (Reuber et al. 1997); $PEX5^{-/-}$, PBD005 (R390X/R390X) (Dodt et al. 1995); and $PEX6^{-/-}$, PBD106 (c.del2398−2417insT/c.1962−1G→A).

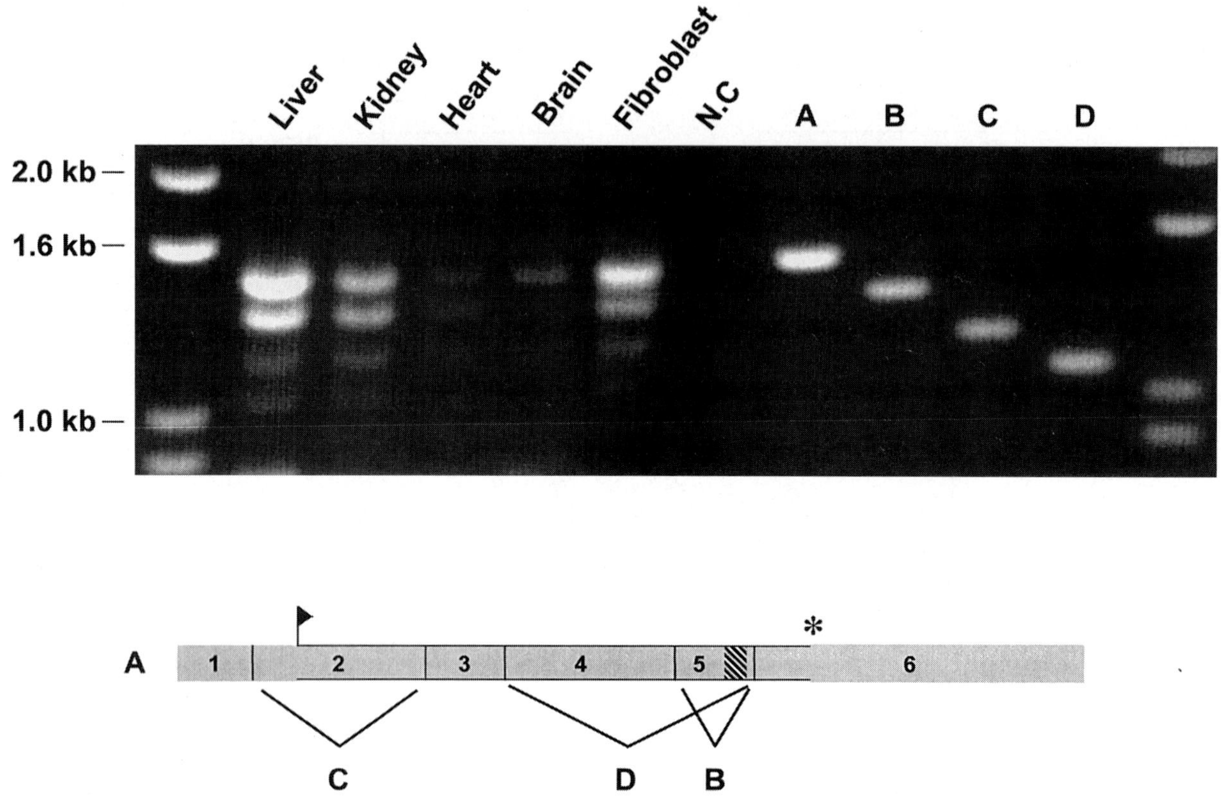

Figure 4 *PEX26*, alternatively spliced in fibroblasts and human tissues. *Top panel*, The products of RT-PCR amplification of *PEX26* transcripts. RT-PCR products with total RNA from human liver, kidney, heart, and brain, by use of primers complementary to the 5′ and 3′ ends of full-length *PEX26* transcript (probes 26-15 and 26-16, respectively), analyzed by agarose-gel electrophoresis and ethidium-bromide staining. The source of the RNA is indicated above the five lanes on the left. On the right, we cloned the RT-PCR products (1,508, 1,361, 1,197, and 1,065 bps) from fibroblast RNA, and the inserts representing full-length PEX26 cDNA (*A*), PEX26-Δex5 (*B*),PEX26-Δex2 (*C*), and PEX26-Δex4+5 (*D*) splice forms are shown as size references. *Lower panel*, Full-length PEX26 transcript, except for exon 7, which encodes 3′ untranslated sequence and is not included in the RT-PCR amplicons. The segments contributed by each exon are numbered and shown to scale. The flag shows the translation start site, the cross-hatched rectangle indicates the segment of exon 5 encoding the transmembrane domain, and the asterisk (*) indicates the translation stop site. The letters indicate the exon deleted from the similarly lettered splice form shown in the top panel.

eral tissues in relatively similar ratios (fig. 4). As compared with *PEX26*-FL, the next smaller product (1,361 bp) lacks exon 5 (*PEX26-Δex5*). The ORF of this splice form maintains frame and encodes a protein that is 49 aa shorter than full-length PEX26, lacking the 18-aa transmembrane domain of full-length PEX26 (fig. 4). The next shorter splice form (1,197 bp) results from skipping of exon 2 (*PEX26-Δex2*). Exon 2 encodes the N-terminus of PEX26, so this splice form would encode an N-terminal–truncated protein initiating at the next downstream methionine (M96). The next shorter splice form is 1,065 bp and lacks exons 4 and 5 (*PEX26-Δex4+5*). This splice form encodes a protein with the 124 N-terminal amino acids of PEX26, followed by a frameshift with an intact ORF, for 32 additional codons. In one RT-PCR experiment with heart mRNA, we also detected a faintly staining product that was 248 bp longer than *PEX26*-FL (data not shown). Cloning and sequencing revealed that intron 1 (248 bp) was retained in this product. Since the translation initiation site is located in exon 2, the complete ORF of *PEX26*-FL is intact in this splice form. A BLASTN search against the human EST database with use of *PEX26* exon 1 plus exon 2 as a probe identified 19 ESTs containing exon 1 and exon 2 sequences. Intron 1 was retained in nine. In BLASTN searches with *PEX26* cDNA exons 1–6, we found eight ESTs that contain or span the segment contributed by exon 5. Of these, two were the *PEX26-Δex5* splice variant. We did not find a *PEX26* EST corresponding to *PEX26-Δex2*.

Complementing Activity and Subcellular Localization of PEX26 *Isoforms*

To examine the functional significance of the two splice variants that retain frame (*PEX26-Δex5* and *PEX26-*

Δ*ex2*), we expressed them in control fibroblasts and in *PEX26*-deficient fibroblasts with various *PEX26* genotypes (PBD059, PBD111, PBD057, and PBD110). In control cells, neither *PEX26* splice form had an effect on matrix-protein import (data not shown), nor did *PEX26-*Δ*ex2* rescue-matrix–protein import in any of the PEX26-deficient cell lines. By contrast, the relative-rescue activity of *PEX26-*Δ*ex5* was the same as *PEX26*-FL (fig. 5). This result was surprising, given that *PEX26-*Δ*ex5* lacks the predicted transmembrane domain of PEX26, expected to be essential for its putative function as a docking protein for PEX1 and PEX6 (Matsumoto et al. 2003*b*).

To determine the subcellular localization of the complementing PEX26 isoforms, we added N-terminal myc-tags to *PEX26*-FL and *PEX26-*Δ*ex5*. We also produced a myc-tagged *PEX26* expression vector that lacked exon 5 and exon 6 (myc*PEX26-*Δ*ex5+6,* encoding PEX26 (aa 2–222). The relative-rescue activities for GFP-SKL import of myc*PEX26-*Δ*ex5* and myc*PEX26-*Δ*ex5+6*, as compared with myc*PEX26*-FL, were 84%/77% and 65%/34% for PBD059/PBD110 cell lines. Thus, addition of the N-terminal myc-tag did not have a deleterious effect on the function of the PEX26 isoforms and, consistent with our results with *PEX26-*Δ*ex5, PEX26-*Δ*ex5+6* encodes a partially functional protein. The subcellular localization of these various PEX26 isoforms is shown in figure 6. myc*PEX26*-FL is completely localized to peroxisomes, as indicated by a punctate staining pattern that colocalizes with PMP70. By contrast, the localization of mycPEX26-Δex5 and mycPEX26-Δex5+6 was similar and clearly different from that of mycPEX26-FL. Both show substantial localization to the cytosol, with some localization to the ER for mycPEX26-Δex5. These results suggest that a peroxisomal membrane location is not required for PEX26 function.

Mapping of PEX6 Binding in PEX26

Using Co-IP with epitope-tagged proteins and GST–pull down experiments, Matsumoto and colleagues (2003*b*) showed binding between full-length PEX26 and PEX6. We asked which part of PEX26 is essential for this interaction. To provide a discrete, easy-to-score subcellular location for these binding experiments, we mislocalized PEX26 fragments to the nucleus (HAnls-*PEX26*) (Sacksteder et al. 2000) in transformed fibroblasts from a PEX3-deficient patient (PBD400). These cells lack peroxisomes, as detected with antibodies to either peroxisome matrix or membrane proteins (South et al. 2000). We cotransfected PBD400 cells with myc-tagged *PEX6* and either pcDNA3 or recombinant pcDNA3 carrying HAnls-*PEX26* fragments (fig. 6). mycPEX6 was evenly distributed in the cytosol and was barely detectable in the nucleus when cotransfected with pcDNA3 vector alone. Cotransfection with HAnls-*PEX26* (aa 2–222), which includes ~90% of the cytoplasmic domain of PEX26, altered mycPEX6 localization to the nucleus. Using serial N- or C-terminal deletions of HAnls-*PEX26,* we identified aa 29–174 as a minimal fragment sufficient to localize mycPEX6 to the nucleus. HAnls-PEX26 (aa 2–163) had a variable effect on mycPEX6 localization, whereas two overlapping fragments, HAnls-PEX26 (aa 2–135) and HAnls-PEX26 (aa 136–222), showed no binding of mycPEX6. These results indicate that the segment of PEX26 required for interaction with PEX6 includes aa 29–163. Moreover, we found that HAnls-PEX26 (aa 2–222) with either the L44P or the L45P mutations produced a stable protein that did not direct mycPEX6 to the nucleus, which suggests that these mutations interfere with the binding of PEX6 to PEX26.

In line with these results, expression of full-length *PEX26*-L44P and *PEX26*-L45P does not result in the localization of mycPEX6 to peroxisomes that is observed with expression of wild-type *PEX26*-FL. We repeated this experiment with myc-tagged wild-type and mutant PEX26-FL (myc*PEX26*-FL, myc*PEX26*-L44P, and myc*PEX26*-L45P) and found that wild-type and mutant mycPEX26-FL are stable and localized on peroxisomal membranes, but only the wild-type protein directs HAPEX6 to peroxisomes (data not shown).

PEX26*-Deletion Mutants and the Minimal Complementing Fragment*

To determine whether the function of PEX26 necessary for peroxisome biogenesis can also be mapped to a smaller segment in the NTD, we constructed a series of deletion mutants with an N-terminal 3 × myc-tag. We verified the expression of the deletion mutants in the cytosol of PBD059 cells, with indirect immunofluorescence staining against the myc-tag. The smallest fragment able to complement PBD059 cells comprised aa 2–174 (53% and 56% relative rescue of GFP-SKL import over PEX26-FL in two trials). PEX26 fragments comprising aa 2–163 or less had no complementing activity. Using N-terminal deletions, we found that a peptide comprising aa 29–174 retained 36% relative-rescue activity, whereas fragments with aa 69–174 or smaller did not complement PBD059 cells (data not shown). Thus, the functional domain of PEX26 corresponds to aa 29–174—or nearly exactly to the PEX6-binding domain.

Expression of PEX26 *on the Outer Mitochondrial Membrane*

The results of our binding and splicing studies show that PEX26 does not require a peroxisomal location to rescue-matrix–protein import. To further test the function of extraperoxisomal PEX26, we elected to localize

A

	PEX26-Δex5	PEX26-Δex2
PBD059	101%	0%
PBD111	84%	0%
PBD057	106%	ND
PBD110	93%	0%

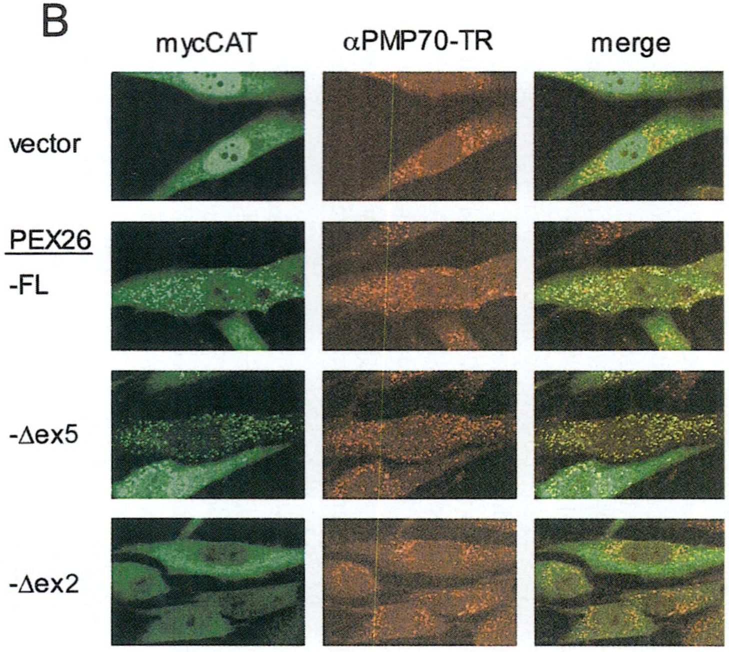

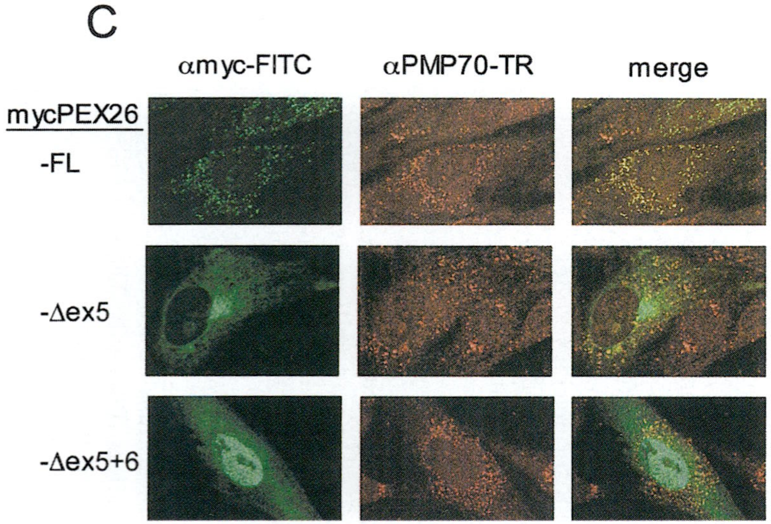

Figure 5 The PEX26-Δex5 splice form, which rescues *PEX26*-deficient cell lines without localizing to peroxisomal membranes. *A*, Relative-rescue activity of PEX26 isoforms for peroxisomal import of mycCAT. The numbers are the mean percent for import (partial plus complete) determined in three separate experiments for PBD059 (c.230+1G→T/c.230+1G→T), two trials for PBD111 (R98W/R98W) and PBD110 (L44P/R98W), and one trial for PBD057 (R98W/R98W). ND = not determined. *B*, Indirect immunofluorescence assays of the ability of *PEX26* splice forms to rescue matrix import. We cotransfected PBD059 cells with mycCAT as reporter for peroxisomal import and either nonrecombinant pcDNA3 vector alone or recombinant pcDNA3 expressing the indicated *PEX26* splice form. We localized peroxisomes, using a Texas Red–labeled αPMP70. *C*, Subcellular localization of the PEX26 isoforms. We transfected PBD059 cells with recombinant vectors expressing the indicated N-myc–tagged PEX26 isoform, and we localized the isoform (FITC) by indirect immunofluorescence and peroxisome membranes with anti-PM70 antibody (Texas Red ["TR"]). Images were made with a confocal laser scanning microscope (Zeiss). Colocalization is indicated by the yellow color in the merged images.

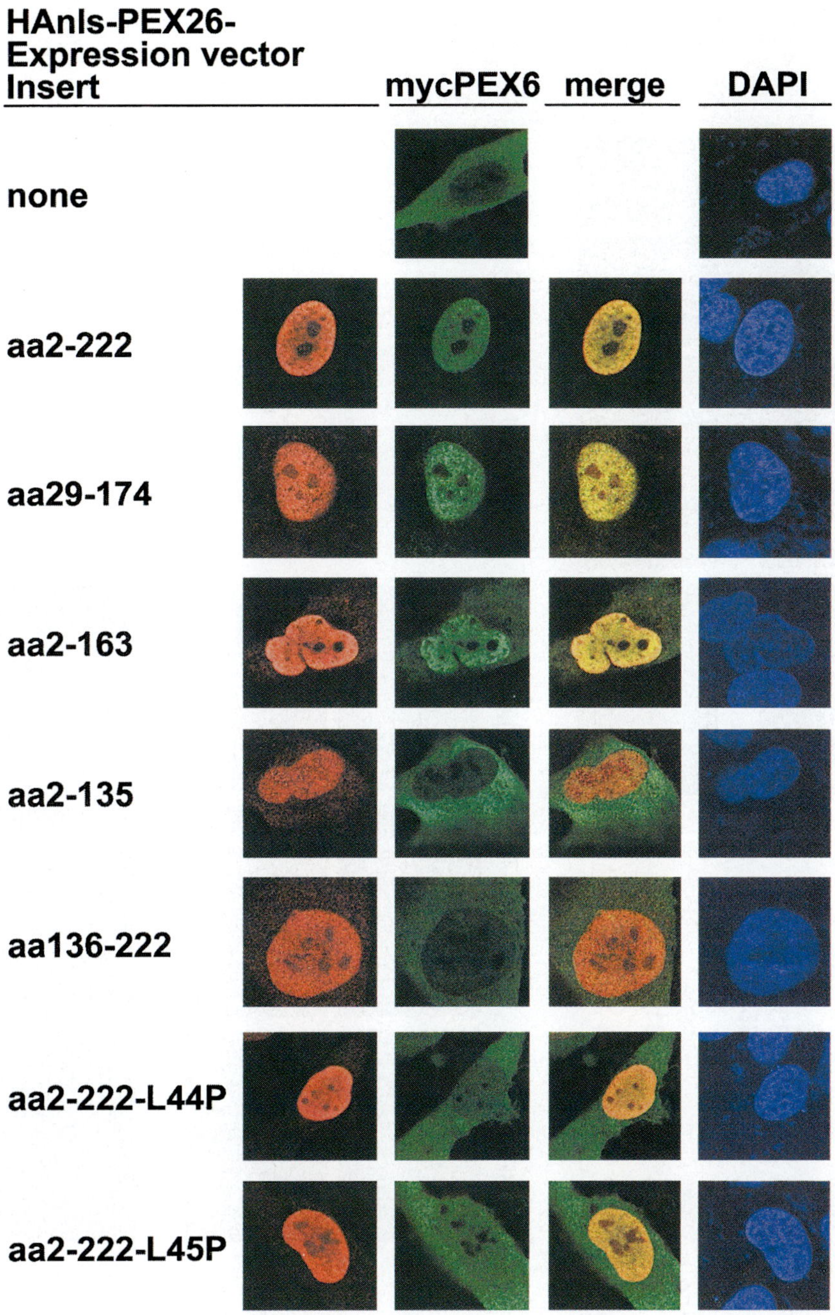

Figure 6 PEX26 segments aa 29–174 and 2–163, sufficient for PEX6 binding, as detected in a nuclear mislocalization assay. We transfected fibroblasts lacking peroxisomes due to an inherited deficiency of *PEX3* (PBD400) with pcDNA3–3 × myc*PEX6* and either nonrecombinant pcDNA3 vector alone or recombinant pcDNA3 expressing N-terminal HA-tagged, nls-PEX26 fragments comprising the indicated segments of PEX26, and we analyzed them by indirect immunofluorescence with anti-HA (Texas Red), anti-myc (FITC) antibodies, and DAPI counterstaining, to show nuclei. The bottom two rows show expression of PEX26 segments sufficient to bind PEX6 but with the indicated missense mutations.

it to a discrete and remote site, the outer mitochondrial membrane. To do this, we expressed a chimeric protein consisting of an N-terminus of Nmyc-tagged PEX26 (aa 2–222) and a C-terminus of rat OMP25 (aa 170–206) (PEX26-Mito) in PBD059 cells. Targeting to the mitochondrial outer membrane with an N_{out}-C_{in} orientation for N-terminal chimeric proteins, with use of this fragment of rat OMP25, has been described elsewhere (Horie et al. 2002). We found that PEX26-Mito is localized exclusively on mitochondria (fig. 7), which is consistent with these earlier studies. Surprisingly, despite this ectopic location, expression of PEX26-Mito in PBD059 cells resulted in complete restoration of peroxisome matrix-protein import. Relative-rescue activity of PEX26-

A

	Corrected rescue	Relative rescue (x/FL)
mycPEX26-FL	52% 58%	- -
mycPEX26(2-222)	33% 38%	63% 66%
mycPEX26(2-222)-Mito	50% 47%	96% 81%

B

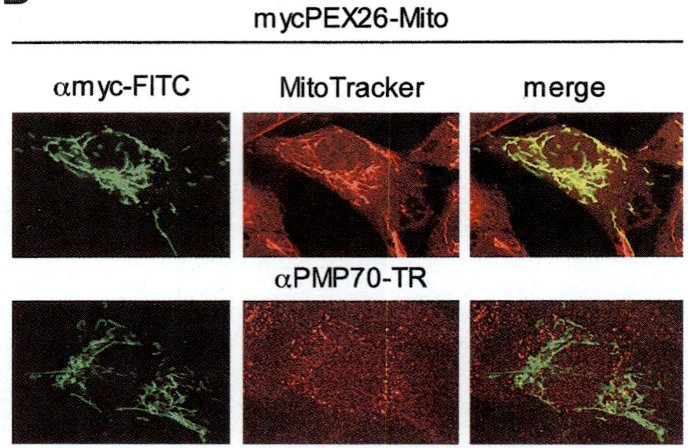

C

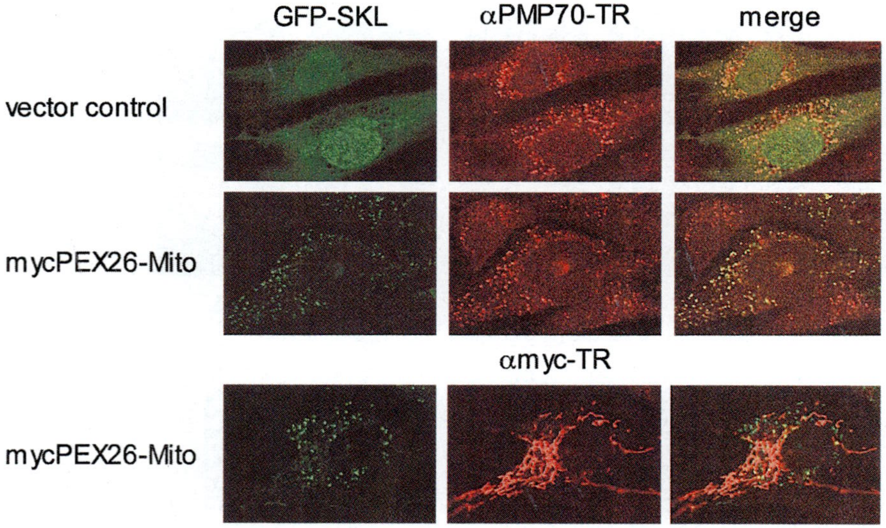

Figure 7 Expression of *PEX26*-Mito rescues the import defect of PBD059 cells. *A*, Relative rescue activity (partial plus complete) for a GFP-PTS1–tagged marker of mycPEX26 (aa 2–222) and *PEX26*-Mito (mycPEX26 [aa 2–222]–OMP25 [aa170–206]) in PBD059 cells. Values for two separate experiments are shown. Transfection of pcDNA3 vector alone as a control gave ~10% import of GFP-SKL. *B*, PBD059 cells transfected with *PEX26*-Mito and analyzed by indirect immunofluorescence by use of anti-myc antibodies (FITC), anti-PMP70 antibodies (Texas Red), and Mito-Tracker (*red*) to confirm the mitochondrial localization of PEX26-Mito. *C*, PBD059 cells transfected with GFP-SKL and nonrecombinant pcDNA3 vector alone or recombinant pcDNA3 expressing *PEX26*-Mito, analyzed by indirect immunofluorescence staining with anti-PMP70 antibodies (*red*) or anti-myc antibodies (*red*) to show that peroxisomal import of GFP-SKL is rescued by PEX26-Mito expression.

Mito compared with PEX26-FL was >80% and was even better than that of cytosolic mycPEX26-Δex5+6 (aa 2–222) in these experiments (63%–66%) (fig. 7).

Localization of PEX6 and PEX1 in PEX26-Deficient Cells Expressing Functional PEX26-Mito

Previous work showed that PEX26 binds PEX6 directly and PEX1 indirectly through the PEX6 interaction (Matsumoto et al. 2003*b*). Our data show that localization to peroxisomes is not essential for PEX26 function and that the minimal PEX26 fragment necessary to complement CG8 cells retains the ability to bind PEX6. To understand how PEX26 functions in an extraperoxisomal location, we determined the localization of PEX6 and PEX1 in PBD059 cells complemented with PEX26-Mito (fig. 8). Colocalization of these AAA ATPases with PEX26-Mito would support the hypothesis that PEX26-PEX6-PEX1 interaction is essential for peroxisome matrix-protein import but would be surprising, because current models predict that the PEX1-PEX6 hetero-oligomer acts at the peroxisomal membrane; for example, in the disassembly of PEX5-PTS1 and PEX7-PTS2 complexes just prior to translocation of PTS1 and PTS2 proteins into the organelle (Gould and Collins 2002). In PBD059 cells cotransfected with empty vector and 3 × HA-tagged PEX6 (JM721), we found that PEX6 localizes to the cytosol and does not accumulate on the membranes of either peroxisomes or mitochondria (fig. 8, *A* and *B*). Addition of PEX26-Mito results in a dramatic change, with complete colocalization of PEX6 with PEX26-Mito on the mitochondria (fig. 8, *C* and *D*). Under these conditions, we detected no colocalization of PEX6 with PMP70 on peroxisomal membranes (fig. 8, *E*).

Interestingly, PBD059 cells transfected with *PEX1*-3 × HA (pBER86)—untagged *PEX6* and empty vector—show a bimodal distribution of PEX1, with most in the cytosol but some on peroxisomal membranes, as marked by PMP70 (fig. 8, *F*). This result suggests that a fraction of PEX1 localizes to the peroxisome membrane despite the lack of detectable PEX26 and PEX6 in this location. Addition of PEX26-Mito dramatically alters the localization of PEX1, with most now colocalizing with PEX26-Mito on the mitochondrial outer membrane (fig. 8, *H* and *I*). Interestingly, in contrast to PEX6, a fraction of PEX1 retains a residual peroxisomal localization in cells cotransfected with PEX26-Mito (fig. 8, *J*).

We tested 3 × HA-PEX6 and PEX1-3 × HA for their ability to complement *PEX6*- and *PEX1*-deficient cell lines, respectively. In two independent experiments, they maintained 52%–62% and 61%–77% relative-rescue activity, respectively, compared with the untagged proteins for import of GFP-SKL (data not shown). The localization of 3 × HA-PEX6 and PEX1-3 × HA with and without cotransfection of *PEX26*-Mito was confirmed in at least three independent experiments. Although the amount varied, we found some PEX1 on peroxisomes in all cotransfection experiments with *PEX26*-Mito, untagged *PEX6,* and tagged *PEX1.* Panel J of figure 8 shows a cell with a typical ratio of peroxisomal to mitochondrial location of PEX1.

These results suggest that peroxisomal localization of neither PEX26 nor PEX6 is essential for peroxisome matrix-protein import. By contrast, we detected some PEX1 on peroxisomal membranes in cotransfection experiments with *PEX26*-Mito and *PEX6*. Thus, a peroxisomal location of some fraction of PEX1 may be required for matrix-protein import. The observations raise the question of how the interaction of PEX26-PEX6—and possibly of PEX1—at an extraperoxisomal localization participates in peroxisome matrix-protein import.

Discussion

The recent identification of *PEX26* by Matsumoto and colleagues completed the search for the genes responsible for the 12 recognized CGs for the Zellweger spectrum subgroup of the PBDs (Matsumoto et al. 2003*a,* 2003*b*) These investigators showed that *PEX26* encodes a 305-aa, 34-kD integral peroxisomal membrane protein with a single C-terminal transmembrane domain near the C-terminus, a short (~36 aa) intraperoxisomal C-terminal tail, and long (250 aa) N-terminus exposed to the cytosol. They also showed that PEX26 binds PEX6 directly and PEX1 indirectly, through the interaction with PEX6. The latter are AAA ATPases that have been proposed to act late in the peroxisomal matrix-protein import cycle (Collins et al. 2000; Vale 2000). Together, mutations in *PEX1, PEX6,* and *PEX26* account for a large fraction (~70%) of all patients with PBD (Gould and Valle 2000). In this work, we have identified 5 new *PEX26* mutant alleles, which brings the total to 17. Of these, six are missense mutations in the N-terminal, cytosolic 60% of the protein, a segment with greater sequence identity across the recognized PEX26 vertebrate orthologs, as compared with the remaining C-terminal segment (e.g., human compared with *Danio* has 38% identity vs. 24% identity, respectively) (fig. 1). We find that none of these missense mutations are common in the general population, although R98W accounts for 14 (39%) of the mutant *PEX26* genes in the total collection of 18 genotyped probands with CG8 (10 patients in our study and 7 in that of Matsumoto et al., with four overlaps, and 5 in that of Steinberg et al.). The high frequency of R98W may represent a founder effect, as has been described for certain alleles in other PBD CGs (Braverman et al. 1997), or recurrent mutations at a CpG dinucleotide in codon 98 (CGG→TGG). Haplotype studies will be necessary to distinguish between these possibilities.

In patient fibroblasts expressing endogenous *PEX26,*

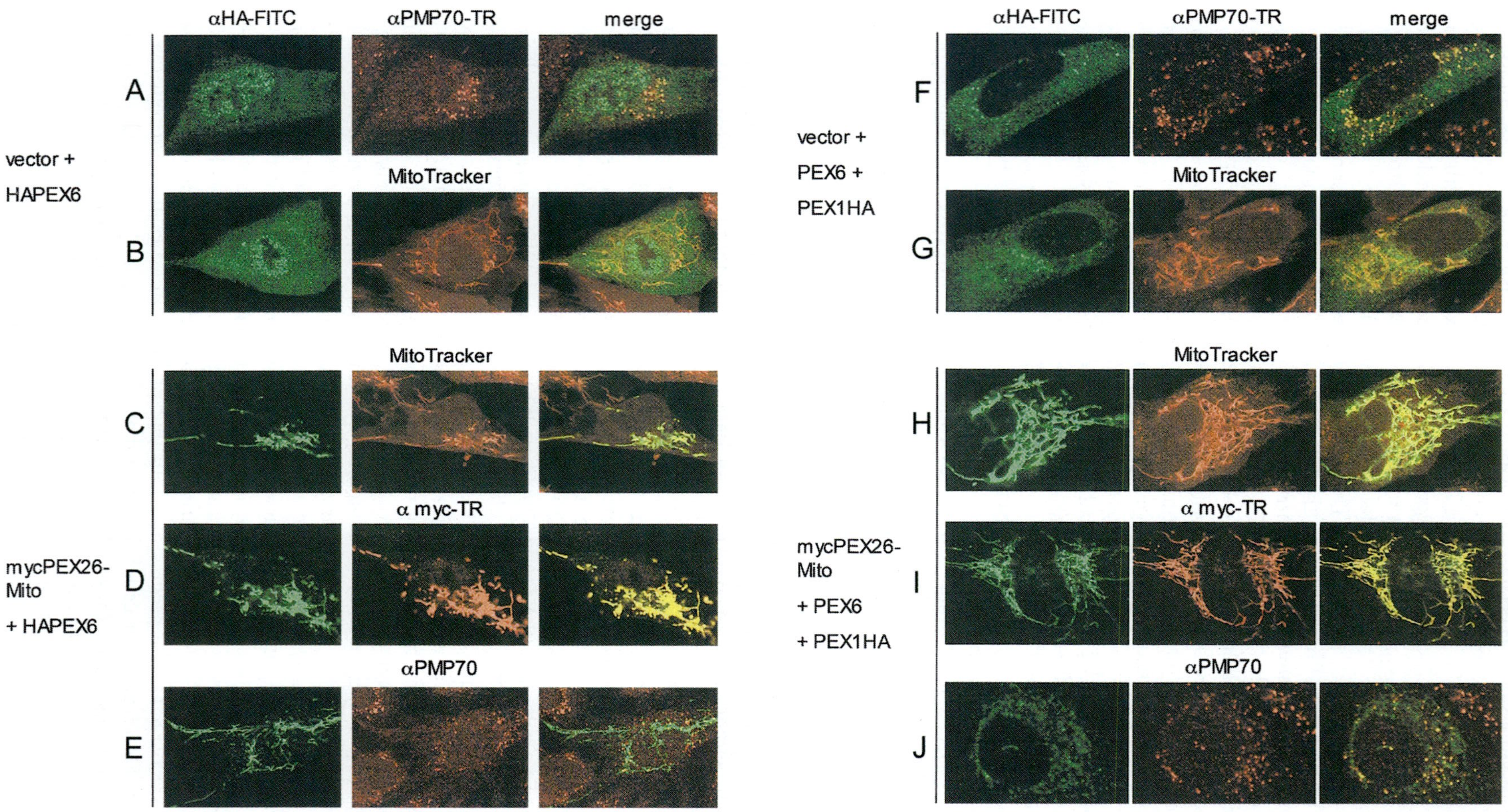

Figure 8 Expression of functional PEX26-Mito completely mislocalizes PEX6 and partially mislocalizes PEX1 to mitochondrial membranes. We analyzed PBD059 cells (c.230+1G→T/c.230+1G→T) by indirect immunofluorescence with anti-HA-FITC and anti-myc-Texas Red, as indicated. To mark peroxisomal or mitochondrial membranes, we used anti-PMP70 (Texas Red) or Mito-Tracker labeling (*red*), respectively. Yellow color in the merged column indicates colocalization. *A–E,* PBD059 cells were transfected with pcDNA3-HAPEX6 and either nonrecombinant pcDNA3 vector or recombinant pcDNA3 expressing myc*PEX26*-Mito (mycPEX26 [aa 2–222])–OMP25 [aa 170–206]). Panels A and B show a lack of colocalization of HAPEX6 with peroxisomes (*A*) or mitochondria (*B*) in cells cotransfected with pcDNA3 vector plus a recombinant vector expressing HAPEX6. By contrast, coexpression of mycPEX26-Mito redirects HAPEX6 to mitochondrial membranes (C), where it colocalizes with PEX26-Mito (*D*) but not with peroxisomes (*E*). In panels F–J, PBD059 cells were transfected with pcDNA3-PEX6 and pcDNA3-PEX1HA plus either nonrecombinant pcDNA3 (*F* and *G*) or recombinant pcDNA3 expressing mycPEX26-Mito (*H–J*). Panels F and G show a bimodal distribution of PEX1HA in the cytoplasm and on peroxisomes but no colocalization with mitochondria (*G*). Coexpression of myc*PEX26*-Mito redirects PEX1HA to mitochondrial membranes to a varying degree (*H–J*), with a fraction of PEX1 retaining a residual peroxisomal location (*J*). In multiple experiments, the amount of PEX1 on peroxisomes varied; in panel J, we show a typical ratio of peroxisomal to mitochondrial location of PEX1 from observations in three independent cotransfection experiments.

our immunoblot studies indicate that all of the missense mutations we tested are associated with a substantial reduction in steady-state levels of PEX26 (fig. 3). Thus, the major pathological consequence of these mutations in vivo appears to be destabilization of PEX26, a result that is similar to the consequences of disease-associated missense mutations at other loci (Brody et al. 1992). Additionally, our immunoblot studies suggest that cells with null mutations in *PEX1* or *PEX6* also appear to have some reduction in PEX26 that is not simply explained by alterations in the amount of peroxisomal membrane, as indicated by the similar levels of the integral peroxisome membrane protein PEX13 in all samples (fig. 3). The explanation for this observation is uncertain, but the finding is consistent with a model in which PEX26, PEX1, and PEX6 interact in a functional unit (see below).

As an additional aspect of the cellular phenotype, we also examined the steady-state levels of the PTS1 receptor PEX5 in the PEX26-deficient cells (fig. 3). Reduced abundance of PEX5 is characteristic of *PEX1*- and *PEX6*-deficient cell lines and has been reported elsewhere in a *PEX26*-deficient cell line (Dodt and Gould 1996) but is not observed in human cells with primary defects in *PEX2, PEX7, PEX10, PEX12,* or *PEX16* (Dodt and Gould 1996; Yahraus et al. 1996; Sacksteder and Gould 2000). Reduced PEX5 steady-state levels are also found in yeast cells with primary defects in *Pex1* and *Pex6* (Collins et al. 2000). In our studies, we found a severe reduction in PEX5 in five different *PEX26*-deficient cell lines, independent of their genotype and similar in extent to that we observed in *PEX1*- and *PEX6*-deficient cells (fig. 3). This result also is consistent with a model in which PEX26, -1, and -6 work together as a functional unit whose activity influences the levels of PEX5. The levels of PEX1, by contrast, in the same set of cell lines, are normal or nearly so, and we are unable to measure PEX6 levels because of lack of an appropriate antibody.

Curiously, Matsumoto et al.—using indirect immunofluorescence staining for endogenous PTS1-targeted matrix proteins (detected with an anti-peptide antibody directly against the consensus PTS1, -SKL), catalase (targeted by an atypical PTS1, -KANL), and peroxisomal thiolase (a PTS2-targeted protein)—concluded that the cellular phenotype of *PEX26*-deficient cells was characterized by impaired peroxisomal import of catalase and PTS2-targeted proteins with normal import of classical PTS1-targeted proteins. Given that the clinical phenotype of primary deficiency of catalase involves either adult-onset oral ulcers or no symptoms at all (Wanders et al. 2001), this conclusion suggests that the clinical phenotype of *PEX26*-deficient patients would mainly reflect deficiency of PTS2-targeted proteins and, therefore, should resemble RCDP (caused by deficiency of the PTS2 receptor, *PEX7*) rather than the Zellweger spectrum, as described for patients with CG8 (see table 2). To address this discrepancy, we performed quantitative studies of the peroxisomal import of a set of four matrix proteins targeted by consensus (-SKL, PECI), near consensus (-SKI, HAOX1), or atypical (-KANL, catalase) PTS1-targeting signals plus a consensus PTS2-targeted protein, PAHX, in four CG8 cell lines with a variety of *PEX26* genotypes. Although there is some residual import, our results show a clear and substantial defect in all three PTS1-targeted reporters, most severe for catalase but substantial for PECI and HAOX1 (14%–77% of control and 0%–30% of control, respectively, depending on cell line) (fig. 2). These results are consistent with the Zellweger spectrum clinical phenotype of *PEX26*-deficient patients and with a model of PEX26 function that involves interaction with PEX6 and PEX1, both of which are known to be necessary for the import of PTS1-targeted proteins. The reason(s) for the discrepancy between our results and those of Matsumoto et al. is unclear. It is possible that by using an antibody expected to detect any matrix protein with a classic (-SKL) PTS1-targeting signal, some or all of which may have a low level of residual import in *PEX26*-deficient cell lines, Matsumoto et al. may have underestimated the effect of *PEX26* mutations on PTS-1–mediated import. Our studies also show a rough correlation of *PEX26* genotype with cellular phenotype. The predicted null PBD059 (c.230+1G→T/c.230+1 G→T genotype) cells show the most severe defect in matrix-protein import and two cell lines homozygous for R98W showing the mildest defect, with some residual import for all four reporters. Moreover, there is a suggestion of correlation of genotype with clinical phenotype. PBD059 had ZS, the most severe clinical phenotype, whereas seven probands either homozygous or heterozygous for R98W had milder phenotypes, ranging from NALD to IRD (table 2).

At the mRNA level, we observed extensive alternative splicing of *PEX26* transcripts in RNA isolated from fibroblasts and in multiple human tissues (fig. 4). The most informative of these alternatively spliced transcripts skips exon 5 and encodes a PEX26 isoform of 256 aa that lacks the transmembrane domain of the full-length protein (fig. 1). If, as previously suggested, the function of PEX26 is to recruit the PEX1/PEX6 heterodimer to peroxisomes, this splice form seemed likely to encode a functionally inactive form of PEX26. Surprisingly, our expression studies showed this isoform is functionally active despite being located in the cytosol (fig. 5). This result shows that a peroxisomal location is not required for PEX26 function and that the essential function(s) of PEX26 in peroxisome biogenesis involves more than recruitment of PEX6 to the organelle (see below).

Although we find no sequence similarity between vertebrate PEX26 and *S. cerevisiae* Pex15 (see above), they share a type II membrane protein topology, and both have been described as a PEX1/PEX6 anchoring site at the peroxisomal membrane (Birschmann et al. 2003; Matsumoto et al. 2003*a*). In an attempt to establish additional functional similarities between human PEX26 and *S. cerevisiae* Pex15, we asked if a cytosolic form of Pex15 is functional in peroxisome biogenesis. We tested two TMD-less constructs of PEX15 (aa 2–330 and aa 2–260). In contrast to our results with PEX26 in human cells and with full-length PEX15 (aa 2–283) in *S. cerevisiae,* we found that the transmembrane domain–less, cytosolic form of Pex15 did not rescue peroxisome matrix-protein import in a Δ*pex15* yeast strain (I.C., S.W., S.J.G, and D.V., unpublished results).

Estimating from our RT-PCR results, the ratio of *PEX26-Δex5* transcript to full length is ~1:2 and seemed similar in all the tissues we examined, with the possible exception of a lower amount in brain (fig. 4). In immunoblot experiments, however, we did not detect the shorter PEX26 isoform (predicted molecular weight of 28 vs. 34 kD for full-length PEX26). This suggests that either the shorter transcript is not translated with the same efficiency as for the full-length transcript or the shorter isoform of PEX26 is less stable. Additional studies determining the relative ratio of these transcripts and the amount of the short PEX26 isoform in various cells and tissues in response to metabolic and/or developmental perturbations will be required to determine potential physiologic consequences of this alternative splicing.

The other alternatively spliced *PEX26* transcript we tested, *PEX26-Δex2,* lacks the normal translation start site and did not encode a functional PEX26 isoform. This result indicates that translation initiation at the most N-terminal internal methionine (Met96) either does not occur or produces an N-terminal–truncated protein that is unstable and/or nonfunctional. We favor the latter possibility. Met96 has an apparently acceptable Kozak consensus and might reasonably be expected to initiate translation. However, our functional studies (see below) and the N-terminal clustering of conserved sequence blocks and disease-producing missense mutations indicate that the N-terminus of PEX26 is essential for its function. These observations and conclusions contrast with those of Matsumoto et al., who report some residual activity for the PEX26-M1T allele expressed in PEX26-deficient CHO cells (ZP167) (Matsumoto et al. 2003*b*). The explanation for this difference is not clear, except possibly that the M1T transcript and/or its protein product behave differently in the CHO cell environment, as compared with our experiments in patient fibroblasts.

What do these results say about PEX26 function? First, our C- and N-terminal truncation studies of PEX26, mislocalized to the nucleus, delimit the PEX6-binding domain of PEX26 to the N-terminal half of the protein (residues 29–163). This result is consistent with the higher degree of sequence conservation among the vertebrate PEX26 orthologs in this segment of the protein and with the clustering of the disease-producing missense mutation to the same region. Moreover, our functional studies show that the minimal segment of PEX26 required to rescue peroxisome biogenesis in CG8 cells (residues 2–174) corresponds almost precisely to the minimal segment required for PEX6 binding. Additionally, we find that *PEX26* undergoes alternative splicing, and, surprisingly, a splice form lacking the transmembrane (*PEX26-Δex5*) is fully functional, despite a cytosolic rather than peroxisomal location. The conclusion that PEX26 does not require peroxisomal location to restore biogenesis is substantiated by our studies with a chimeric protein (PEX26-Mito) comprising the N-terminal half of PEX26 and a C-terminal segment from a rat mitochondrial outer membrane protein that is exclusively (within the limits of detection by indirect immunofluorescence methods) localized to mitochondria. In this extraperoxisomal location, PEX26-Mito sequesters PEX6 and a substantial fraction of PEX1 (fig. 8). Despite the mislocalization of these peroxins, we find that peroxisome matrix-protein import is restored by the expression of PEX26-Mito in PEX26-deficient cells (fig. 7). Although the interaction of PEX26 with PEX6 is essential for matrix-protein import, our results indicate that neither protein requires a peroxisomal location to perform its function in peroxisome biogenesis.

Ultimately, understanding the role of PEX26 in peroxisome biogenesis will require better understanding of the functions of PEX1 and PEX6. Observations in yeast and humans suggest that these two, closely related, type II AAA ATPases (Vale 2000; Frickey and Lupas 2004) form a dynamic hetero-oligomeric complex whose subunit interactions depend on ATP binding and whose function depends on ATP hydrolysis (Faber et al. 1998*b;* Tamura et al. 1998; Kiel et al. 1999). For example, in the yeast *Pichia pastoris,* PEX1 and PEX6 coimmunoprecipitate only in the presence of ATP or ATPγS. In this regard, PEX1 and PEX6 appear to resemble a few AAA ATPases (e.g., VPS4 and katanin) that cycle between monomeric and oligomeric forms and contrast to other AAA ATPases (e.g., NSF, p97) that form stable two-tiered hexameric rings (Vale 2000). Consistent with the hypothesis that the interaction between PEX1 and PEX6 is dynamic, their subcellular localizations appear to be overlapping but not identical. Using epitope-tagged constructs with expression driven by a strong promoter in wild-type cells, we found that PEX6 appears to be exclusively cytosolic, whereas PEX1 is mainly cytosolic but with detectable signal also colocalizing with peroxisomes. Similar overlapping but nonidentical subcellular localizations were described for *Pichia pastoris* PEX1 and PEX6 (Faber et al. 1998*b*). Moreover, our results with PEX26-Mito showing full restoration of peroxisome matrix-protein import in PEX26-deficient cells despite mislocalization of PEX26, PEX6, and a fraction of PEX1 to the mitochondrial outer membrane predict that some protein is able to move from the PEX26-PEX6 complex on the mitochondrial outer membrane to the peroxisome. PEX1 is the most obvious candidate, given that its interaction with PEX6 appears to be dynamic and that we find PEX1 at both mitochondrial and peroxisomal locations. We also speculate that, in these mislocalization experiments, PEX1 cycles between a location on the peroxisomal membrane and the complex with PEX6 tethered to the mitochondrial outer membrane by PEX26-Mito. We also speculate that the interaction with PEX6 serves to "activate" PEX1, perhaps through some conformational change in a manner that allows it to complete its function for matrix-protein import after it relocates to the peroxisome membrane. This function could involve disassembly of the matrix-protein–receptor complex or release of the N-terminus of PEX5 from the peroxisome membrane (Costa-Rodrigues et al. 2004) or some other, as yet unappreciated, function. Consistent with this model, Shiozawa et al. (2004) have recently examined the structure of the NTD of PEX1 (aa 1–180). Using bioinformatics analyses, they noted that the NTD of PEX1 but not that of PEX6 resembles that of two other AAA ATPases, NSF and p97. Using crystallographic studies at a 2.05-Å resolution, they showed that the NTD of PEX1 folds independently as a globular domain, with striking similarities to the structure of the NTDs of NSF and p97. On the basis of similarity to the NTDs of NSF and p97, Shiozama et al. predict that the PEX1 NTD functions in substrate binding and/or as a site for the binding of a hypothetical adaptor protein. Our hypothesized "activation" of PEX1 might involve a conformation change in the NTD similar to those involved in the function of NSF or p97 (Brunger and DeLaBarre 2003; Shimozawa et al. 2004; Whiteheart and Matveeva 2004). A corollary of our model is that activated PEX1 has some mechanism for localizing to the peroxisome membrane independent of the PEX26-PEX6 complex, possibly by docking to a site on one of the integral peroxisomal membrane proteins or to a site on PEX5, which appears to insert into the peroxisomal membrane as it delivers peroxisomal matrix proteins to the organelle but leaves its N-terminus exposed (Gouveia et al. 2003; Oliveira et al. 2003; Costa-Rodrigues et al. 2004). Given that the release of unloaded PEX5 from the organelle requires ATP hydrolysis (Dodt and Gould 1996; Oliveira et al. 2003), some interaction with PEX1 at this stage seems likely.

Acknowledgments:

We acknowledge helpful discussions and the long-term interest in PBDs of Ann and Hugo Moser. S.W. was funded by German Bundesministerium fur Bildung und Forschung grant BMBF-LPD 9901/8-51. David Valle is an Investigator in the Howard Hughes Medical Institute. We thank Sandy Muscelli for assistance in manuscript preparation.

Electronic-Database Information

The accession number and URLs for data presented herein are as follows:

GenBank, http://www.ncbi.nlm.nih.gov/Genbank/ (for PEX26 cDNA [accession number NM_017929])

Online Mendelian Inheritance in Man (OMIM), http://www.ncbi.nlm.nih.gov/Omim/ (for RCDP, ZS, NALD, and IRD)

References

Bell GI, Najarian RC, Mullenbach GT, Hallewell RA (1986) cDNA sequence coding for human kidney catalase. Nucl Acids Res 14:5561–5562

Birschmann I, Rosenkranz K, Erdmann R, Kunau WH (2005) Structural and functional analysis of the interaction of the AAA-peroxins Pex1p and Pex6p. FEBS J 272:47–58

Birschmann I, Stroobants AK, van den Berg M, Schafer AI, Rosenkranz AR, Kunau WH, Tabak HF (2003) Pex15p of *Saccharomyes cerevisiae* provides a molecular basis for recruitment of the AAA peroxin Pex6 to peroxisomal membranes. Mol Biol Cell 14:2226–2236

Braverman N, Steel G, Obie C, Moser A, Moser H, Gould SJ, Valle D (1997) Human *PEX7* encodes the peroxisomal PTS2 receptor and is responsible for rhizomelic chondrodysplasia punctata. Nat Genet 15:369–376

Brody LC, Mitchell GA, Obie C, Michaud J, Steel G, Fontaine G, Robert M-F, Kaiser-Kupfer MI, Valle D (1992) Ornithine-δ-aminotransferase mutations causing gyrate atrophy: allelic heterogeneity and functional consequences. J Biol Chem 267: 3302–3307

Brunger AT, DeLaBarre B (2003) NSF and p97/VCP: similar at first, different at last. FEBS Lett 555:126–133

Chang C-C, Lee W-H, Moser H, Valle D, Gould SJ (1997) Isolation of the human *PEX12* gene, mutated in group 3 of the peroxisome biogenesis disorders. Nat Genet 15:385–388

Chang C-C, South S, Warren D, Jones J, Moser AB, Moser HW, Gould SJ (1999) Metabolic control of peroxisome abundance. J Cell Sci 112:1579–1590

Collins CS, Kalish JE, Morrell JC, Gould SJ (2000) The peroxisome biogenesis factors Pex4p, Pex22p, Pex1p, and Pex6p act in the terminal steps of peroxisomal matrix protein import. Mol Cell Biol 20:7516–7526

Costa-Rodrigues J, Carvalho AF, Gouveia AM, Fransen M, Sa-Miranda C, Azevedo JE (2004) The N terminus of the peroxisomal cycling receptor, Pex5p, is required for redirecting the peroxisome-associated peroxin back to the cytosol. J Biol Chem 279:46573–46579

Dodt G, Braverman N, Wong C, Moser A, Moser HW, Watkins P, Valle D, Gould SJ (1995) Mutations in the PTS1 receptor gene, PXR1, define complementation group 2 of the peroxisome biogenesis disorders. Nat Genet 9:115–124

Dodt G, Gould SJ (1996) Multiple PEX genes are required for proper subcellular distribution and stability of Pex5p, the PTS1 receptor: evidence that PTS1 protein import is mediated by a cycling receptor. J Cell Biol 135:1763–1774

Faber KN, Elgersma Y, Heyman JA, Koller A, Luers GH, Nuttley WM, Terlecky SR, Wenzel TJ, Subramani S (1998*a*) Use of *Pichia pastoris* as a model eukaryotic system: peroxisome biogenesis. Methods Mol Biol 103:121–147

Faber KN, Heyman JA, Subramani S (1998*b*) Two AAA family peroxins, PpPex1p and PpPex6p, interact with each other in an ATP-dependent manner and are associated with different subcellular membranous structures distinct from peroxisomes. Mol Cell Biol 18:936–943

Frickey T, Lupas AN (2004) Phylogenetic analysis of AAA proteins. J Struct Biol 146:2–10

Gärtner J, Moser H, Valle D (1992) Mutations in the 70K peroxisomal membrane protein gene in Zellweger syndrome. Nat Genet 1:16–23

Geisbrecht BV, Collins CS, Reuber BE, Gould SJ (1998) Disruption of a *PEX1-PEX6* interaction is the most common cause of the neurologic disorders Zellweger syndrome, neonatal adrenoleukodystrophy, and infantile Refsum disease. Proc Natl Acad Sci USA 95:8630–8635

Geisbrecht BV, Gould SJ (1999) The human *PICD* gene encodes a cytoplasmic and peroxisomal $NADP^+$-dependent isocitrate dehydrogenase. J Biol Chem 274:30527–30533

Gould SJ, Collins CS (2002) Peroxisomal-protein import: is it really that complex? Nat Rev Mol Cell Biol 3:382–389

Gould SJ, Keller G-A, Hosken N, Wilkinson J, Subramani S (1989) A conserved tripeptide sorts proteins to peroxisomes. J Cell Biol 108:1657–1664

Gould SJ, Keller G-A, Subramani S (1988) Identification of peroxisomal targeting signals at the carboxy-terminus of four peroxisomal proteins. J Cell Biol 107:897–905

Gould SJ, Raymond GV, Valle D (2001) The peroxisome biogenesis disorders. In: Scriver CR, Beaudet AL, Sly WS, Valle D (eds) The metabolic and molecular bases of inherited disease. McGraw-Hill, New York, pp 3181–3217

Gould SJ, Valle D (2000) Peroxisome biogenesis disorders: genetics and cell biology. Trends Genet 16:340–344

Gouveia AM, Guimarães CP, Oliveira ME, Reguenga C, Sá-Miranda C, Azevedo JE (2003) Characterization of the peroxisomal cycling receptor, Pex5p, using a cell-free *in vitro* import system. J Biol Chem 278:226–232

Hahn SH, Lee EH, Jung JW, Hong CH, Yoon HR, Rinaldo P, Sims H, Gibson B, Strauss AW (1999) Very long chain acyl coenzyme A dehydrogenase deficiency in a 5 month old Korean boy: identification of a novel mutation. J Pediatr 135: 250–253

Horie C, Suzuki H, Sakaguchi M, Mihara K (2002) Characterization of signal that directs C-tail-anchored proteins to mammalian mitochondrial outer membrane. Mol Biol Cell 13:1615–1625

Jones JM, Morrell JC, Gould SJ (2000) Identification and characterization of HAOX1, HAOX2, and HAOX3, three human peroxisomal 2-hydroxy acid oxidases. J Biol Chem 275: 12590–12597

——— (2001) Multiple distinct targeting signals in integral peroxisomal membrane proteins. J Cell Biol 153:1141–1149

Jones JM, Nau K, Geraghty MT, Erdmann R, Gould SJ (1999) Identification of peroxisomal acyl-CoA thioesterases in yeast and humans. J Biol Chem 274:9216–9223

Kiel JA, Hilbrands RE, van der Klei IJ, Rasmussen SW, Salomons FA, van der Heide M, Faber KN, Cregg JM, Veenhuis M (1999) Hansenula polymorpha Pex1p and Pex6p are peroxisome-associated AAA proteins that functionally and physically interact. Yeast 15:1059–1078

Kozak LP, Harper M-E (2000) Mitochondrial uncoupling proteins in energy expenditure. Annu Rev Nutr 20:339–363

Lazarow PB, Robbi M, Fujiki Y, Wong L (1982) Biogenesis of peroxisomal proteins in vivo and in vitro. Ann NY Acad Sci 386:285–300

Liu Y, Björkman J, Urquhart A, Wanders RJA, Crane DI, Gould SJ (1999) *PEX13* is mutated in complementation group 13 of peroxisome-biogenesis disorders. Am J Hum Genet 65: 621–634

Lupas AN, Martin J (2002) AAA proteins. Curr Opin Struct Biol 12:746–753

Matsumoto N, Tamura S, Fujiki Y (2003*a*) The pathogenic peroxin Pex26p recruits the Pex1p-Pex6p AAA ATPase complexes to peroxisomes. Nat Cell Biol 5:454–460

Matsumoto N, Tamura S, Furuki S, Miyata N, Moser A, Shimozawa N, Moser HW, Suzuki Y, Kondo N, Fujiki Y (2003*b*) Mutations in novel peroxin gene *PEX26* that cause peroxisome-biogenesis disorders of complementation group 8 provide a genotype-phenotype correlation. Am J Hum Genet 73:233–246

McDermid HE, Morrow BE (2002) Genomic disorders on 22q11. Am J Hum Genet 70:1077–1088

Mihalik SJ, Morrell JC, Kim D, Sacksteder K, Watkins PA, Gould SJ (1997) Identification of *PAHX*, a Refsum-disease gene. Nat Genet 17:185–189

Oliveira ME, Gouveia AM, Pinto RA, Sa-Miranda C, Azevedo JE (2003) The energetics of Pex5p-mediated peroxisomal protein import. J Biol Chem 278:39483–39488

Osumi T, Tsukamoto T, Hata S, Yokota S, Miura S, Fujiki Y, Hijikata M, Miyazawa S, Hashimoto T (1991) Amino-terminal presequence of the precursor of peroxisomal 3-ketoacyl-CoA thiolase is a cleavable signal peptide for peroxisomal targeting. Biochem Biophys Res Comm 181:947–954

Purdue PE, Lazarow PB (1996) Targeting of human catalase to peroxisomes is dependent upon a novel COOH-terminal peroxisomal targeting sequence. J Cell Biol 134:849–862

Reuber BE, Collins CS, Germain-Lee E, Morrell JC, Ameritunga R, Moser HW, Valle D, Gould SJ (1997) Mutations in *PEX1* are the most common cause of Zellweger syndrome, neonatal adrenoleukodystrophy and infantile Refsum disease. Nat Genet 17:445–448

Sacksteder KA, Gould SJ (2000) The genetics of peroxisome biogenesis. Annu Rev Genet 34:623–652

Sacksteder KA, Jones JM, South ST, Li X, Liu Y, Gould SJ (2000) *PEX19* binds multiple peroxisomal membrane proteins, is predominantly cytoplasmic, and is required for peroxisome membrane synthesis. J Cell Biol 148:931–944

Shani N, Jimenez-Sanchez G, Steel G, Dean M, Valle D (1997) Identification of a fourth half ABC transporter in the human peroxisomal membrane. Hum Mol Genet 6:1925–1931

Shimozawa N, Tsukamoto T, Nagase T, Takemoto Y, Koyama N, Suzuki Y, Komori M, Osumi T, Gootjes J, Wanders RJ, Kondo N (2004) Identification of a new complementation

group of the peroxisome biogenesis disorders and *PEX14* as a mutated gene. Hum Mutat 23:552–558
Shiozawa K, Maita N, Tomii K, Seto A, Goda N, Akiyama Y, Shimizu T, Shirakawa M, Hiroaki H (2004) Structure of the N-terminal domain of PEX1 AAA-ATPase. J Biol Chem 279: 50060–50068
South ST, Sacksteder KA, Li X, Liu Y, Santos M, Gould SJ (2000) Inhibitors of COPI and COPII do not block *PEX3*-mediated peroxisome synthesis. J Cell Biol 149:1345–1360
Steinberg S, Chen L, Wei L, Moser A, Moser H, Cutting G, Braverman N (2004) The PEX gene screen: molecular diagnosis of peroxisome biogenesis disorders in the Zellweger syndrome spectrum. Mol Genet Metab 83:252–263
Swinkels BW, Gould SJ, Bodnar AG, Rachubinski RA, Subramani S (1991) A novel, cleavable peroxisomal targeting signal at the amino-terminus of the rat 3-ketoacyl-CoA thiolase. EMBO J 10:3255–3262
Tamura S, Shimozawa N, Suzuki Y, Tsukamoto T, Osumi T, Fujiki Y (1998) A cytoplasmic AAA family peroxin, Pex1p, interacts with Pex6p. Biochem Biophys Res Commun 245: 883–886
Vale RD (2000) AAA proteins: lords of the ring. J Cell Biol 150:F13–F19
Wanders RJ (2004*a*) Metabolic and molecular basis of peroxisomal disorders: a review. Am J Med Genet A 126:355–375
——— (2004*b*) Peroxisomes, lipid metabolism and peroxisomal disorders. Mol Genet Metab 83:16–27
Wanders RJ, Barth PG, Heymans HSA (2001) Single peroxisomal enzyme deficiencies. In: Scriver CR, Beaudet AL, Sly WS, Valle D (eds) The metabolic and molecular bases of inherited disease. McGraw-Hill, New York, pp 3219–3256
Warren DS, Morrell JC, Moser HW, Valle D, Gould SJ (1998) Identification of *PEX10,* the gene defective in complementation group 7 of the peroxisome-biogenesis disorders. Am J Hum Genet 63:347–359
Weller S, Gould SJ, Valle D (2003) Peroxisome biogenesis disorders. Annu Rev Genomics Hum Genet 4:165–211
Whiteheart SW, Matveeva EA (2004) Multiple binding proteins suggest diverse functions for the *N*-ethylmaleimide sensitive factor. J Struct Biol 146:32–43
Yahraus T, Braverman N, Dodt G, Kalish JE, Morrell JC, Moser HW, Valle D, Gould SJ (1996) The peroxisome biogenesis disorder group 4 gene, *PXAAA1,* encodes a cytoplasmic ATPase required for stability of the PTS1 receptor. EMBO J 15:2914–2923

Heterozygous Mutations of *OTX2* Cause Severe Ocular Malformations

Nicola K. Ragge,[1,6,8,*] Alison G. Brown,[9,*] Charlotte M. Poloschek,[11] Birgit Lorenz,[11] R. Alex Henderson,[12] Michael P. Clarke,[13] Isabelle Russell-Eggitt,[2] Alistair Fielder,[3] Dianne Gerrelli,[4] Juan Pedro Martinez-Barbera,[4] Piers Ruddle,[4] Jane Hurst,[7] J. Richard O. Collin,[6] Alison Salt,[2,6] Simon T. Cooper,[9] Pamela J. Thompson,[5] Sanjay M. Sisodiya,[5] Kathleen A. Williamson,[10] David R. FitzPatrick,[10] Veronica van Heyningen,[10] and Isabel M. Hanson[9]

[1]Department of Adnexal Surgery, Moorfields Eye Hospital, [2]Great Ormond Street Hospital for Children, [3]Department of Optometry and Visual Science, City University, [4]Neural Development Unit, Institute of Child Health, and [5]Department of Clinical and Experimental Epilepsy, Institute of Neurology, University College London, London; [6]Department of Human Anatomy and Genetics, University of Oxford, and [7]Clinical Genetics Department, Oxford Radcliffe Hospitals NHS Trust, Oxford, United Kingdom; [8]Birmingham Children's Hospital NHS Trust, Diana Princess of Wales Children's Hospital, Birmingham, United Kingdom; [9]University of Edinburgh, School of Molecular and Clinical Medicine, and [10]Medical Research Council Human Genetics Unit, Edinburgh; [11]University of Regensburg, Department of Pediatric Ophthalmology and Ophthalmogenetics, Regensburg, Germany; and [12]Institute of Human Genetics and [13]Claremont Wing Eye Department, Royal Victoria Infirmary, Newcastle upon Tyne, United Kingdom

Major malformations of the human eye, including microphthalmia and anophthalmia, are examples of phenotypes that recur in families yet often show no clear Mendelian inheritance pattern. Defining loci by mapping is therefore rarely feasible. Using a candidate-gene approach, we have identified heterozygous coding-region changes in the homeobox gene *OTX2* in eight families with ocular malformations. The expression pattern of *OTX2* in human embryos is consistent with the eye phenotypes observed in the patients, which range from bilateral anophthalmia to retinal defects resembling Leber congenital amaurosis and pigmentary retinopathy. Magnetic resonance imaging scans revealed defects of the optic nerve, optic chiasm, and, in some cases, brain. In two families, the mutations appear to have occurred de novo in severely affected offspring, and, in two other families, the mutations have been inherited from a gonosomal mosaic parent. Data from these four families support a simple model in which *OTX2* heterozygous loss-of-function mutations cause ocular malformations. Four additional families display complex inheritance patterns, suggesting that *OTX2* mutations alone may not lead to consistent phenotypes. The high incidence of mosaicism and the reduced penetrance have implications for genetic counseling.

Introduction

Abnormalities in the ocular development program can lead to a variety of major structural defects of the eye that present at birth (Graw 2003). At the severe end of the spectrum are anophthalmia (absence of the eye [MIM 206900]) and extreme microphthalmia (small eye [MIM 309700]), which are likely to result from a variety of developmental pathologies (Morrison et al. 2002). Other common malformations include sclerocornea (MIM 181700); anterior chamber malformations, including aniridia (MIM 106210), colobomata (MIM 120200), and congenital cataracts (MIM 116700); and disorders of early retinal differentiation. Diagnostically useful subclasses within these groups include optic-fissure closure defects (colobomata affecting iris, optic nerve, retina, and choroid) (Morrison et al. 2002), disorders of early retinal differentiation (Leber congenital amaurosis [LCA {MIM 204000}] and Walker-Warburg syndrome [MIM 236670]) (Dobyns et al. 1989), and disorders of lens induction or differentiation (congenital cataract/aphakia [MIM 177075]) (Jamieson et al. 2002). Each of these can be isolated or associated with microphthalmia and/or anophthalmia.

Ocular malformations display a broad range of inheritance patterns. Classic aniridia is almost always caused by *PAX6* (MIM 607108) haploinsufficiency and is transmitted with high penetrance and expressivity (Hanson 2003). In contrast, anophthalmia and severe microphthalmia show some evidence of familial recurrence but usually no clear Mendelian transmission pattern (Morrison et al. 2002). This is likely to be a reflection of several potentially interactive factors: oligogenic causation, gene-environment interactions, and stochastic variation in development. There is increasing recognition that, although non-Mendelian inheritance

Received February 2, 2005; accepted for publication April 1, 2005; electronically published April 21, 2005.

Address for correspondence and reprints: Dr. Veronica van Heyningen, Medical Research Council Human Genetics Unit, Western General Hospital, Edinburgh, EH4 2XU, United Kingdom. E-mail: v.vanheyningen@hgu.mrc.ac.uk

* These two authors contributed equally to this work.

0002-9297/2005/7606-0008$15.00

patterns make gene identification more difficult, they are ultimately very revealing about the complex molecular networks that contribute to normal development (Ming and Muenke 2002; van Heyningen and Yeyati 2004).

Several genes for anophthalmia, microphthalmia, and coloboma (*RAX* [MIM 601881], *CHX10* [MIM 142993], *PAX6*, *MAF* [MIM 177075], and *SOX2* [MIM 184429]) have been identified by different methods, ranging from the candidate-gene approach to positional identification, often using informative chromosomal rearrangements (Azuma et al. 1999; Ferda-Percin et al. 2000; Jamieson et al. 2002; Fantes et al. 2003; Graw 2003; Voronina et al. 2004). Apart from *SOX2*, which appears to account for ~10% of severe anophthalmias (Fantes et al. 2003; Ragge et al. 2005), none of these can be considered a major causative gene, because each examined cohort revealed mutations in a very small proportion of affected individuals. We decided to search for additional causative mutations, using a candidate-gene approach.

OTX2 (MIM 600037), a bicoid-type homeodomain gene, is a vertebrate ortholog of the *Drosophila* gene *orthodenticle* (*Otd*), which is required for anterior brain, eye, and antenna formation (Finkelstein and Boncinelli 1994) and for regulating the development of photoreceptors and the expression of rhodopsin (Tahayato et al. 2003). Mammals have three *Otx* genes: *Otx1*, *Otx2*, and the more diverged *Crx*, which is known as "*Otx5*" in lower vertebrates (Germot et al. 2001). All three genes are expressed in the developing eye—*Crx* almost exclusively so. Human *CRX* (MIM 602225) mutations have been reported in retinal degenerations, including cone-rod dystrophy (MIM 120970), late-onset pigmentary retinopathy, and LCA (Freund et al. 1997; Sohocki et al. 1998; Rivolta et al. 2001). Mouse *Otx1* and *Otx2* are expressed in developing neural and sensory structures, including the brain, ear, nose, and eye (Simeone et al. 1993; Martinez-Morales et al. 2001). The spatiotemporally complex expression pattern is reflected in the large flanking region that is occupied by enhancers required for the regulation of *Otx2* expression (Kurokawa et al. 2004*a*, 2004*b*). Ectopic expression studies in *Xenopus* suggest that *Otx2* operates early, interacting with a network of eye-field transcription factors, including *Rx1*, *Pax6*, and *Six3* (Zuber et al. 2003). During eye morphogenesis, initial expression in the entire optic vesicle becomes restricted to the presumptive retinal pigment epithelium (RPE) (Simeone et al. 1993; Bovolenta et al. 1997; Martinez-Morales et al. 2001), where OTX2 protein interacts with the transcription factor MITF (MIM 156845), leading to the activation of target genes, including tyrosinase (Martinez-Morales et al. 2003). Later, OTX2 is increasingly expressed in neural retinal cells, including postmitotic neuroblasts (Bovolenta et al. 1997; Nishida et al. 2003). Conditional ablation of *Otx2* in neural retina leads to loss of *Crx* expression and failure of photoreceptor development (Nishida et al. 2003).

Homozygous *Otx2*-knockout embryos have gastrulation defects and die at midgestation with severe brain anomalies (Acampora et al. 1995; Ang et al. 1996). Heterozygotes show highly variable phenotypes—ranging from acephaly; through micrognathia, anophthalmia, and microphthalmia; to normal—depending on genetic background (Acampora et al. 1995; Matsuo et al. 1995; Ang et al. 1996). Recurrent interstitial deletions of human chromosome 14q22-q23 have been consistently associated with anophthalmia (Brewer et al. 1998). No definitive analysis of *OTX2* has been reported in these cases, but the gene maps to the 14q22 genomic region and is a strong candidate for mutation studies in anophthalmia and related eye anomalies.

We therefore undertook mutation analysis of the *OTX2* gene. The common 289-aa isoform is transcribed from a 5-kb genomic region encompassing three exons. The protein has a homeodomain and a 192-aa proline-, serine-, and threonine-rich C-terminal region, which contains a highly conserved SIWSPA peptide sequence and a tandemly duplicated OTX tail, all motifs shared with OTX1 (MIM 600036) and CRX (Germot et al. 2001). Unrelated patients ($n = 333$) with a spectrum of ocular malformations were assessed by direct sequencing. Brain magnetic resonance imaging (MRI) data were obtained for two affected individuals and for an unaffected mutation carrier, and older diagnostic images from other patients were reassessed. The *OTX2* expression pattern was studied in early human embryos for comparison with the known mouse pattern.

Material and Methods

Patients and Controls

Patients with ocular malformation spectrum defects ($n = 333$) were recruited, with informed consent and with appropriate ethics review committee approvals. Detailed case histories of individuals with *OTX2* coding-region sequence changes are available in appendix A (online only). Control DNAs ($n = 164$) from apparently healthy adults were anonymized; they matched the patients in ethnicity (apart from patient 7, who was of African origin [see the "Results" section]). We sequenced 94 DNAs in full, and a further 70 partially, over the region of the proline missense mutations.

DNA Preparation

Genomic DNA was prepared from peripheral blood by use of a Nucleon DNA extraction kit (Tepnel Life Sciences). Buccal cell lysates were prepared from mouthwash samples by resuspending the cell pellet in 100 μl of 0.05 M NaOH, heating in a boiling water bath for 20 min, and then neutralizing with 12.5 μl of 1 M Tris (pH 7.6).

PCR and Sequencing

The human *OTX2* cDNA (GenBank accession number NM_172337) is encoded by three exons that are located in BAC AL161757 (GenBank) at positions 59950–60217 (exon 1), 61214–6138 (exon 2), and 6322–64868 (exon 3). The cDNA numbering is derived from the human *OTX2* cDNA (GenBank accession number NM_172337). We designed four genomic amplicons to cover the *OTX2* coding region and some flanking intronic sequences in each case: amplicon 1 contained exon 1, amplicon 2 contained exon 2, and overlapping amplicons 3a and 3b covered the coding part of exon 3. PCR primers are shown in table 1. PCRs were performed in 96-well plates. For amplicons 1 and 2, 50 ng genomic DNA was amplified in a volume of 50 μl containing 1 × Qiagen HotStar*Taq* PCR buffer, 1.5 mM $MgSO_4$, 5 μl PCR enhancer buffer (Invitrogen), 0.2 mM dNTPs, 250 nM forward primer, 250 nM reverse primer, and 2 U of HotStar*Taq* polymerase. For amplicons 3a and 3b, the PCR enhancer buffer was omitted and was replaced with 10 μl of Q solution (Qiagen). Thermal cycling was performed using an MJ PTC225 machine. PCR conditions were 1 cycle of 95°C for 15 min; 35 cycles of 94°C for 30 s, 55°C for 30 s, and 72°C for 1 min; and 1 cycle of 72°C for 5 min.

PCR products were run on a 2% agarose gel to ensure adequate yield and to check for the absence of nonspecific products. Unincorporated primers and dNTPs were removed by incubating 5 μl of PCR product with 1 μl of ExoSapIT (exonuclease I and shrimp alkaline phosphatase enzyme mix [USB]) for 45 min at 37°C, followed by 20 min at 80°C to inactivate the enzyme.

Direct Sequencing

Sequencing of PCR products was performed in a 96-well plate format, as described elsewhere (Aijaz et al. 2004), with the use of forward and reverse primers as shown in table 1. Individual sequence traces were inspected using Chromas software (Technelysium). Multiple sequence traces were aligned and compared using the phredPhrap program from the Consed package (see the Laboratory of Phil Green Web site). All changes were verified by performing a second PCR and sequencing reaction on the patient's DNA. Family members were analyzed if samples were available.

RNA In Situ Hybridization

The expression pattern of *OTX2* was investigated by nonradioactive RNA in situ hybridization in human embryos from Carnegie stages (CS) 14–22, which correspond approximately to mouse Theiler stages 18–23 (E11.25–E15.25). Human embryos were obtained from the Medical Research Council/Wellcome Trust Human Developmental Biology Resource, with full ethical approval. Preparation of embryo sections and nonradioactive RNA in situ hybridization was performed as described elsewhere (Lai et al. 2003).

Table 1

PCR Primers for Amplification of the *OTX2* Coding Region

The table is available in its entirety in the online edition of *The American Journal of Human Genetics.*

The template for the *OTX2* probe was a 1.1-kb fragment that was PCR amplified from exon 3 with the use of primers hOTX2A (5′-GCG GAT CCA GTG CTC CTG TGT CTA TCT GGA G-3′) and hOTX2D (5′-GCG AAT TCC AGA GGT GGA GTT CAA GGT TGC-3′) and that was cloned into pGEM-3Z. The construct was linearized with *Bam*HI and was transcribed with T7 RNA polymerase to synthesize the digoxygenin-labeled antisense riboprobe.

MRI Analysis

MRI scanning was approved by the local institutional ethics committees. All patients scanned for the present study provided written informed consent. Patient 5 and his unaffected mother underwent MRI scanning. MRI acquisition parameters were TE = 4.2, TI = 450, TR = 15, NEX = 1, flip angle = 20°, acquisition matrix 256 × 128, and field of view 24 cm; 124 contiguous slices were produced, with voxel dimension 0.9375 mm × 0.9375 mm × 1.5 mm. An equivalent sequence was used for patient 4B. These data were reformatted in multiple planes to allow careful examination of regions of interest. Additionally, signal changes were inspected on T2 and FastFLAIR sequences (T2 and PD sequence: TE1 = 30, TE2 = 120, TR = 2000, NEX = 1, acquisition matrix 256 × 128, field of view 24 cm × 18 cm, and slice thickness 5 mm contiguous; FastFLAIR sequence: TE1 = 152, TE2 = 2200, TR = 10002, NEX = 1, acquisition matrix 256 × 128, field of view 24 cm, and slice thickness 5 mm contiguous). Patient 4B underwent similar high-resolution T1-weighted MRI scanning. For patients 1, 2, and 6, existing MRI data were reviewed. For patient 3A, CT scan data were reviewed.

Psychometric Testing

Patient 5 and his mother underwent standard neuropsychometric testing, omitting any tests requiring visual function. This component of the study was also approved by the local institutional ethics committee and was undertaken after written informed consent was obtained.

Results

OTX2 *Mutation Analysis*

Of the 333 patients analyzed, 8 showed sequence variation in the *OTX2* coding region. The changes are distributed throughout the ORF (fig. 1). Additional family members were analyzed, if samples were available, for a total of 11 affected individuals in eight families (fig. 1). Detailed case histories of affected individuals are presented in appendix A (online only), and the phenotypes are summarized in table 2. In the course of the study, we uncovered evidence of mosaicism; therefore, when possible, we also analyzed oral epithelial DNA (obtained by mouthwash or buccal scrape).

Patient 1, with bilateral anophthalmia, has a de novo frameshifting insertion (c.635insGC) at codon 155 in exon 3, the A in the SIWSPA motif (figs. 1 and 2 and table 2). Subsequent out-of-frame translation of 22 amino acids is predicted to terminate at a TGA codon, beginning at c.701. Neither the parents nor the unaffected brother carry the mutation (fig. 1). Identical results were obtained with buccal cell DNA from all four individuals.

Patient 2, with bilateral optic-nerve aplasia (MIM 165550) and microphthalmia (fig. 3 and table 2), has a de novo transversion, c.436C→G, in exon 3 (fig. 1). This is predicted to produce an arginine-to-glycine (R89G) change at position 52 of the homeodomain. Neither parent carries the change in lymphocyte DNA (fig. 1).

Patient 3A, with severe bilateral microphthalmia, has an N-terminal domain frameshifting mutation, c.252delC, in codon 27 of exon 1 (figs. 1 and 2 and table 2). Out-of-frame translation is predicted until the first base of a termination codon is encountered at c.320 in exon 2. A fetus (patient 3B [fig. 1]), terminated after ultrasound diagnosis of affected status, also carried the same mutation. The phenotypically normal mother of patients 3A and 3B was found to have the mutation at low levels in blood and buccal DNA before the existence of the affected fetus was revealed. The unaffected father and maternal grandparents do not have the mutation in blood DNA (fig. 1). These data indicate that the mother is a gonosomal (gonadal and somatic) mosaic carrier of the mutation (Edwards 1989).

Siblings 4A and 4B—diagnosed with microphthalmia and severe developmental delay and with LCA, respectively (figs. 2 and 4 and table 2)—carry a transversion, c.708T→A, in exon 3 (fig. 1). The tyrosine-to-termination (TAT→TAA) change at codon 179 is in the C-terminal domain. Their mother (patient 4C) is a gonosomal mosaic for the Y179X mutation (fig. 1). She has a later-onset phenotype resembling pigmentary retinopathy (fig. 4).

Patient 5, with bilateral anophthalmia, has a frameshifting deletion, c.288delCC, in codons 39–40 in exon 2, at the start of the homeodomain (figs. 1 and 2 and table 2). This mutation is predicted to generate a 46-aa nonsense peptide before reaching a TAA termination codon, beginning at c.429 in exon 3. The phenotypically normal mother of this patient has full representation of the same mutation in both lymphocyte and buccal DNA, indicating that she is probably a nonmosaic mutation carrier. The unaffected father, brother, and sister do not carry the mutation (fig. 1).

Patient 6, with bilateral anophthalmia, has the transition c.466C→T in exon 3 (figs. 1 and 2 and table 2). Glutamine (CAA) is substituted by a termination codon (TAA) at the second amino acid of the C-terminal domain (Q99X). The phenotypically normal father shows full expression of the same mutation in his blood DNA, suggesting that he is a constitutive mutation carrier. The unaffected mother does not have the mutation (fig. 1).

Patient 7, with bilateral microphthalmia and left sclerocornea, has the transversion c.568C→A in exon 3 (figs. 1 and 2 and table 2). This results in replacement of proline (CCC) with threonine (ACC) at position 133 (P133T). The patient's phenotypically normal mother and brother have the same change, but the patient's unaffected father and sister do not (fig. 1). Identical results were obtained with DNA from blood and oral epithelium from all five family members. P133 occurs at the end of a highly conserved hexapeptide motif, SGQFTP, in the C-terminal domain of vertebrate Otx2, Otx1, and Crx proteins (Germot et al. 2001).

Patient 8, with unilateral anophthalmia, has the transversion c.571C→G in exon 3 (figs. 1 and 2 and table 2). This replaces proline (CCC) with alanine (GCC) at amino acid position 134 (P134A). The patient's similarly affected mother does not have this variant in blood or oral epithelium. The father was not available for analysis. The patient's unaffected maternal grandmother and maternal great-grandmother do not have the change, nor does a maternal half brother (fig. 1).

Ninety-four control individuals (188 chromosomes) were examined by direct sequencing for the presence of all the coding-region variants. An additional 70 individuals were sequenced for the region containing prolines 133 and 134. None of the changes was observed in the controls. Ethnic matching was not feasible for family 7, who are of African origin, and therefore no conclusion can be drawn about the frequency of this change in the population from which patient 7 comes.

We detected three SNPs during the course of the present study. All were located in noncoding regions: two newly reported sites (submitted to NCBI dbSNP) in the first intron, 268+12 C/T (dbSNP accession number

Table 2

Summary of Clinical Features

Feature	Patient 1	Patient 2	Patient 3A	Patient 4A	Patient 4B	Patient 5	Patient 6	Patient 7	Patient 8
Sex	Male	Male	Female	Female	Male	Male	Male	Female	Male
DNA mutation	c.635insGC	c.436C→G	c.252delC	c.708T→A	c.708T→A	c.288delCC	c.466C→T	c.568C→A	c.571C→G
Protein mutation	FS	R89G	FS	Y179X	Y179X	FS	Q99X	P133T	P134A
Exon with mutation	3	3	1	3	3	2	3	3	3
De novo mutation	Y	Y	N	N	N	N	N	N	Y?
Maternal age at patient's birth (years)	21		23	18	26	31	22	23	22
Paternal age at patient's birth (years)	22		24			39	25	29	21
Maternal genotype	WT	WT	mos c.252delC	(Patient 4C[a]) mos c.708T→A (Y179X)	(Patient 4C[a]) mos c.708T→A (Y179X)	c.288delCC	WT	c.568C→A	WT
Paternal genotype	WT	WT	WT			WT	c.466C→T	WT	
Maternal phenotype	Hypopigmented macula/fundus	Normal	Normal	(Patient 4C[a]) pigmentary retinopathy	(Patient 4C[a]) pigmentary retinopathy	Normal	Normal	Normal	Left anophthalmia
Paternal phenotype	No reported visual difficulties	Normal	Normal	Normal	Normal	Normal	Normal	Normal	Normal
Birth weight (g)	2,884	2,837	2,700	3,108		4,256		5,000	3,402
Birth OFC[b] (cm)		33		42	41	3rd–10th percentile			39
Gestation (wk)	38	38	40	40	39	42	38	42	42
Age at most recent assessment	4 years	6.3 years	12 years, 11 mo	33 years	25 years	24 years	11 years, 1 mo	4 years	9 years
Height (age)	25th–50th percentile (2.5 years)	10th–25th percentile, 113 cm (6.3 years)		149 cm	160 cm (25 years)	3rd percentile (24 years)		75th percentile, 113.5 cm	10th percentile, 78 cm (1 year)
Weight (age)	<3rd percentile (2.5 years)	25th–50th percentile, 21.4 kg (6.3 years)		65 kg	83.5 kg (25 years)	73.4 kg		97th percentile, 25.5 kg	25th percentile, 10.5 kg (1 year)
Head OFC[b] (age)	<.4th percentile, 48 cm (4 years)	46.2 cm (1 year, 1 mo)		53 cm (33 years)	54.3 cm (25 years)	3rd–10th percentile		97th percentile, 53.4 cm	44.6 cm (1 year)
Vision	None	None	None	None	6/60	None	None	None	R: 6/9.5
Clinical anophthalmia	Right	No	No	No	No	Bilateral	Bilateral	No	Left
Orbital cystic remnants	R: no; L: NA	No	No	NA	NA	None	Bilateral	NA	No
Microphthalmia	Left	Bilateral	Bilateral, severe	Bilateral	Bilateral, mild	NA	NA	Bilateral	NA
Axial length (mm)	L: 12				L: 20; R: 20	R: 4.4; L: 4.9		L: 12–14	R: 20; L: 14
Corneal diameter (mm)	R: NA; L: 8	R: 6.5; L: 7.5	NA	R: 4; L: 4	R: 11; L: 11	NA	NA	R: 3	L: NA; R: ?
Coloboma	Left chorioretinal	No	NA	Bilateral? (report at 1 year, 7 mo)	No	NA	NA	No	No
Anterior segment dysgenesis	No		NA	Corectopia with bilateral iris colobomata	Bilateral anterior synechiae	NA	NA	Left sclerocornea	No

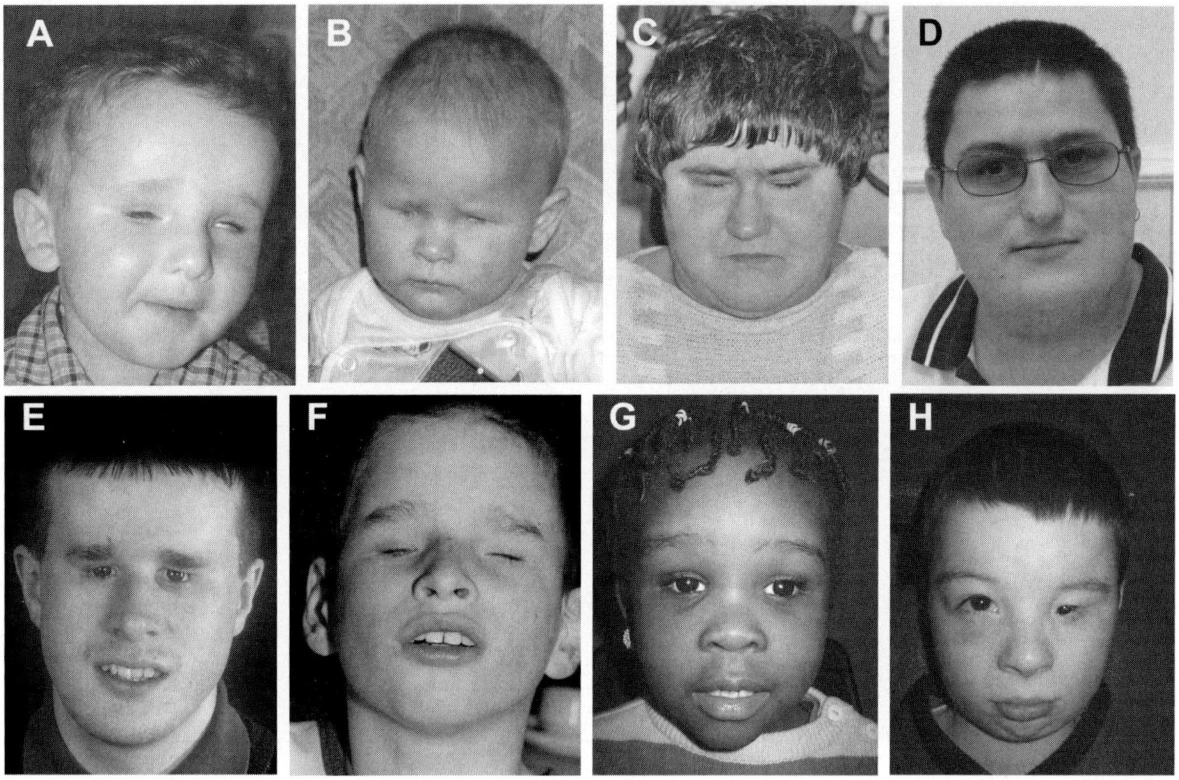

Figure 2 Facial views of eight patients with *OTX2* coding-region sequence changes: patient 1 (*A*), patient 3A (*B*), patient 4A (*C*), patient 4B (*D*), patient 5 (*E*), patient 6 (*F*), patient 7 (*G*), and patient 8 (*H*). Patients 5 and 7 are wearing prostheses in both eyes. Patient 8 is wearing a prosthesis in the left eye.

side and is hypoplastic on the microphthalmic side; the chiasm is thin.

Patients 3A and 5 both had slightly enlarged lateral ventricles. A striking cerebral anomaly is evident in patient 6, who has bilateral abnormal hippocampal morphology (fig. 5). A similar hippocampal malformation was seen, on review, in patient 1.

Patient 5 functions intellectually just within the average ability range (Wechsler Adult Intelligence Scale–Revised [WAIS-R]: verbal IQ [VIQ] 91). His verbal memory was good and was in keeping with his intellectual level (verbal learning and recall 25th–50th percentile). His performance on tests of executive skills was average. His 55-year-old mutation-carrying mother has no eye phenotype and functions intellectually at a level comparable to that found for her son (VIQ 96). Her memory was not as good as that of her son: after correcting for age, her scores were in the 10th–25th percentile. Executive skills were average.

Patient 2 was described as having cognitive and language skills at least age-appropriate for a blind child when a neurodisability assessment was performed at age 4.5 years.

RNA In Situ Hybridization

The developing human eye at CS16–CS19, like that of the mouse at a corresponding age, shows strong *OTX2* expression in the RPE layer and weaker *OTX2* expression in the neural retina (fig. 6*F*, 6*G*, and 6*H* and data not shown). Mice have low-level expression in the E11 neural retina, which becomes restricted to the neuroblastic layer by E17.5 and which remains present in the inner nuclear layer into the postnatal period (Martinez-Morales et al. 2001; Nishida et al. 2003).

OTX2 is widely expressed throughout the telencephalon and mesencephalon at CS14, with a sharp cutoff at the midbrain-hindbrain boundary (fig. 6*A*). *OTX2* expression was observed in the lamina terminalis and the floor of the telencephalon at CS16 (fig. 6*B* and 6*C*), sites that have also been reported in mouse (Simeone et al. 1993; Mallamaci et al. 1996; Simeone 2000). At CS22, *OTX2* was expressed in the choroid plexus, the dorsal thalamus, and the roof of the mesencephalon (fig. 6*E*). In the developing nasal structures, *OTX2* is seen in the olfactory epithelium of the nasal pits at CS18 (fig. 6*D*), again mirroring the mouse patterns.

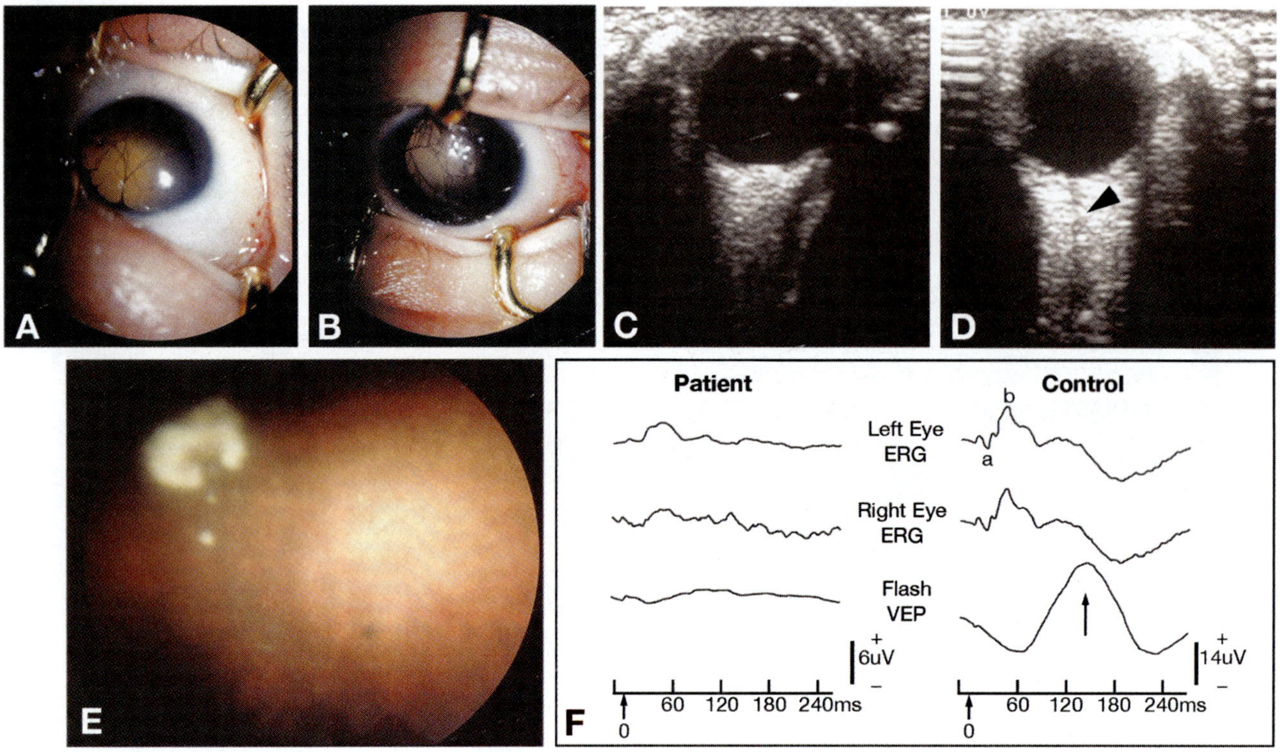

Figure 3 Ocular findings for patient 2 at age 6 wk. The right eye (*A*) and left eye (*B*) are shown, both with persistent pupillary membrane and tunica vasculosa lentis and a clear lens. Ultrasound scans of the right (*C*) and left (*D*) orbits show small eyes. In panel C, no optic nerve is visible. In panel D, the thin cord extending posteriorly from the globe (*arrowhead*) may be the optic-nerve sheath. The left fundus (*E*) has a white elevated area with a pigmented surrounding area and grayish tissue extending a short distance into the posterior segment. This may be a hyaloid remnant. No retinal vessels are visible. The fundus is hypopigmented, with a granular appearance and a few choroidal vessels. *F,* In electrophysiological tests, patient 2 (*left*) gave a small (<2 mV) but consistent response to flash "a" and "b" waves (control >10 mV). Visual evoked potential ("VEP") showed no consistent response to flash. Results from an age-matched control are shown (*right*).

Discussion

Using a candidate-gene approach, we found a wide spectrum of human phenotypes to be associated with *OTX2* coding-region sequence changes. The phenotypes were, however, significantly different from those in the mouse knockouts (Acampora et al. 1995; Matsuo et al. 1995; Ang et al. 1996). The inheritance patterns in the families are diverse.

Spectrum of OTX2 *Mutations and Genetic Mechanisms*

We found eight different heterozygous *OTX2* exonic changes in the patient cohort. Five of the eight changes are predicted to cause premature protein truncation either through direct creation of a stop codon or through a frameshift (fig. 1 and table 2). The only mutation predicted to lead to haploinsufficiency through nonsense-mediated decay (reviewed by Holbrook et al. [2004]) is in family 3, in which a stop codon is predicted in exon 2. In the other four families (1, 4, 5, and 6), termination is predicted in the last exon—making it likely that the truncated protein is expressed and that it may function in a dominant negative manner (Nussbaum et al. 2001).

The R89G de novo missense change found in patient 2 causes substitution of an invariant homeodomain arginine that is normally in contact with DNA phosphate residues. Missense mutations of the homologous residue have been identified in seven different homeodomain proteins, three of them (PITX2 [MIM 601542], SIX3 [MIM 603714], and CRX) associated with eye disease (Swaroop et al. 1999; D'Elia et al. 2001; Laflamme et al. 2004).

The mutations found in patient 1 (635insGC) and patient 2 (R89G) arose de novo. In siblings 3A and 3B (252delC) and siblings 4A and 4B (Y179X), the sequence changes were inherited from mothers who were found to carry, at a low level in blood DNA, the same mutation as their offspring. In both cases, the mother transmitted the mutation to two affected children, providing strong evidence that these mothers are gonosomal mosaics with a high frequency of mutant cells in their

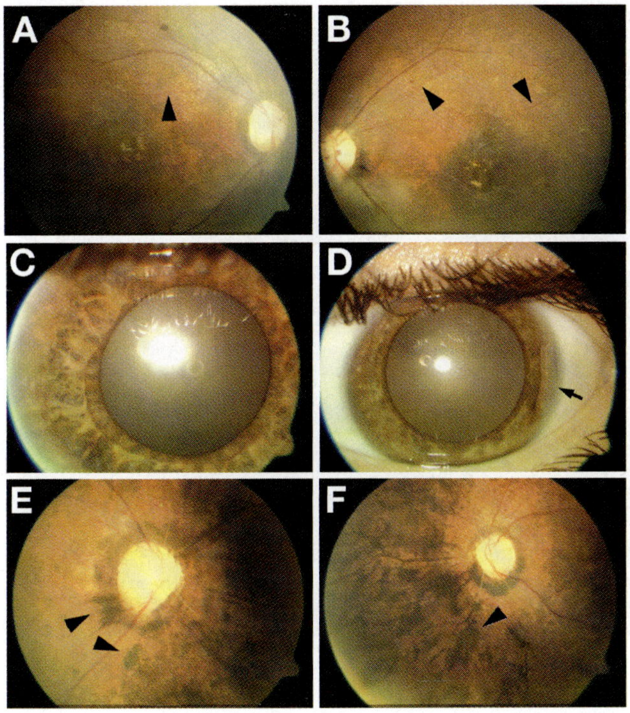

Figure 4 Ocular findings in family 4. Patient 4B at age 28 years: right fundus (*A*) and left fundus (*B*), both with pale optic disks, atrophic maculae, and thin retinal vessels (*arrowheads*); right iris (*C*) and left iris (*D*). The left iris has peripheral anterior synechiae (*arrow*). Patient 4C (mosaic mother of patients 4A and 4B) at age 51 years: right fundus (*E*) and left fundus (*F*), showing retinopathy with accumulated pigment clumps (*arrowheads*).

germ lines (Edwards 1989). The parents of the mosaic individual should not have the mutation, as observed in family 3 (fig. 1). Gonosomal mosaic individuals may or may not express clinical features themselves, depending on the proportion and distribution of mutant cells in their body. The mosaic mother in family 3 has undergone a full eye examination, including high-resolution multifocal electroretinogram (ERG), and is ophthalmologically normal. The mosaic mother in family 4 (patient 4C) has progressive retinal dystrophy (fig. 4*E* and 4*F*), with a self-reported history of undefined visual problems from an early age. Typically, an affected mosaic individual has a milder phenotype than his or her constitutive offspring (Zlotogora 1998). This seems to be true for patient 4C, since she has retinal pathology without the structural eye defects observed in her children.

Families 1–4 fit a model in which *OTX2* haploinsufficiency (loss of function in one allele) alone causes structural eye malformations. However, families 5 and 6 provide evidence of incomplete penetrance, since predicted protein-truncating mutations identified in bilateral anophthalmic children are also found in an unaffected mother and father, respectively (fig. 1 and table 2).

Results from families 7 and 8 are difficult to interpret. Both have missense substitutions at adjacent highly conserved proline residues, but the functional consequences of these sequence changes are unknown. Both families show discordance of phenotype and genotype. For family 7, no ethnically matched controls were available, so the frequency of the P133T change in the population of origin of family 7 is unknown. In family 8, the affected son has the P134A change, but his very similarly affected mother does not, making it highly unlikely that this sequence variant is a major contributor to the phenotype. We shall now focus on the loss-of-function mutations.

Two different models, based on recent insights from other human genetic diseases, may explain incomplete penetrance. First, if *OTX2* is the only locus involved, the level of gene expression may be affected by stochastic and/or genetic factors. This model assumes that an abnormal phenotype will be manifest if *OTX2* expression falls below a certain critical threshold level and if loss of function of one copy reduces gene expression levels close to this threshold. Stochastic fluctuations in transcription levels, possibly influenced by environmental factors but independent of genetic background, may reduce expression levels below the threshold. Evidence of this comes from the observation that genetically identical *Otx2*-knockout mice have highly variable phenotypes (Matsuo et al. 1995). Genetic factors at the mutant locus—specifically, regulatory polymorphisms of the normal allele—can also determine penetrance by controlling transcription levels (Gouya et al. 2002; Vithana et al. 2003). If the mutant allele is in *trans* to a strongly expressing normal allele, transcription is maintained above the threshold, which explains the clinically unaffected status of constitutive mutation carriers, but a weakly expressing normal allele leads to expression below the threshold required for normal development, and the abnormal phenotype is revealed (Gouya et al. 2002). The human *OTX2* locus spans >500 kb and has numerous distant enhancers that could be targets for regulatory polymorphisms (Kurokawa et al. 2004*b*).

Second, digenic or oligogenic inheritance may manifest as incomplete penetrance (Ming and Muenke 2002; van Heyningen and Yeyati 2004). An example of digenic inheritance is provided by a form of retinitis pigmentosa in which affected individuals have heterozygous mutations in both the *ROM1* (MIM 180721) and *RDS* (MIM 179605) genes, which encode related components of an oligomeric photoreceptor protein. Mutations at only one locus do not lead to an abnormal phenotype; penetrance is dependent on cosegregation of both mutations (Kajiwara et al. 1994). Perhaps more relevant to the developmental complexity of the eye and brain is holoprosencephaly (HPE [MIM 142945 and MIM 157170]), a disease that frequently shows non-Mendelian segregation patterns (Ming and Muenke 2002). The complex

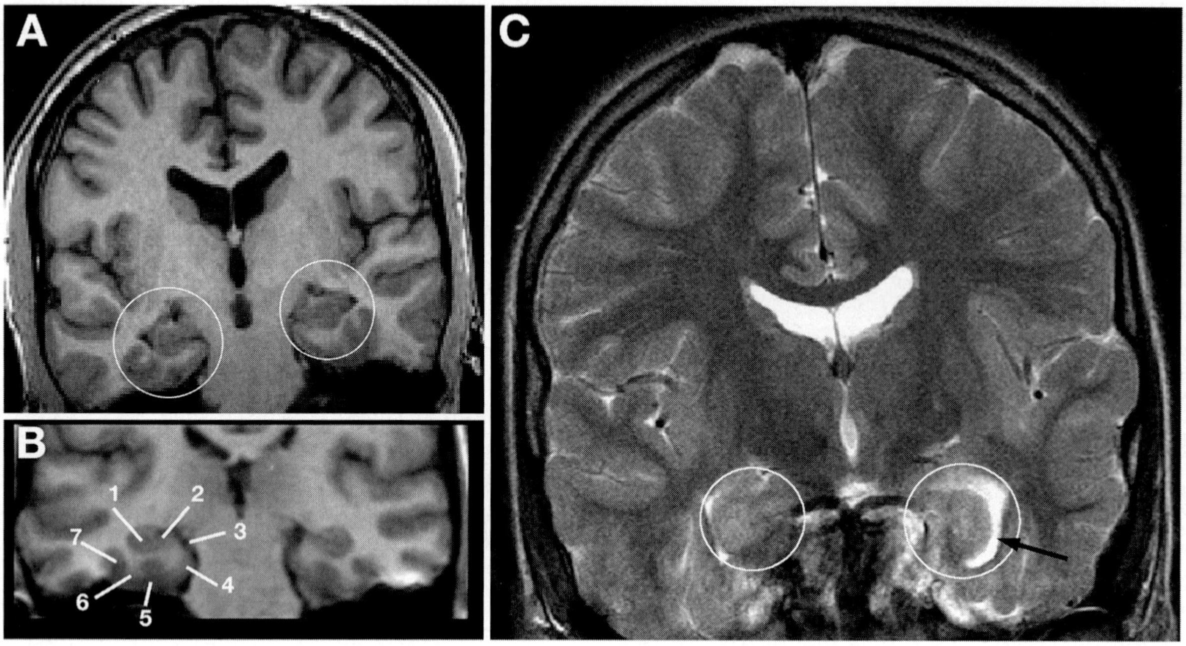

Figure 5 Coronal MRIs from patient 5 (T1-weighted image [*A*]), a normal control (T1-weighted image [*B*]), and patient 6 (T2-weighted image [*C*]). The left side of each image is the right side of the patient. In panels A and C, the hippocampi are circled. Panel B is labeled to show the normal hippocampal and parahippocampal structures: 1 = body of the hippocampus; 2 = subiculum; 3 = ambient cistern; 4 = parahippocampal gyrus; 5 = collateral sulcus; 6 = fusiform gyrus; 7 = lateral occipitotemporal sulcus. The hippocampi and parahippocampal structures are normal in panel A but are abnormal in panel C. Despite the different image parameters (T2 vs. T1 control), in panel C the hippocampi are more vertically aligned and are more globular than ovoid. Instead of being tucked laterally into the temporal horns of the lateral ventricles, the medial displacement and incomplete rotation of the hippocampi generate a cerebrospinal fluid–filled extension of the temporal horns of the lateral ventricle (*arrow*).

inheritance patterns and range of phenotypes we observe for *OTX2* are similar to those reported for *SHH* (MIM 600725) and *SIX3*, the major contributors toward HPE types 3 and 2, respectively (Nanni et al. 1999; Wallis et al. 1999). Whereas some HPE-associated *SHH* and *SIX3* mutations have arisen de novo, others have been inherited from completely unaffected carrier parents (Nanni et al. 1999; Wallis et al. 1999). The possibility that interaction with modifier gene variants at other loci may be required for full penetrance is supported by the observation that, in three reported cases, affected individuals carry mutations in two HPE genes (*SHH* with *TGIF* [MIM 602630] or *ZIC2* [MIM 603073]) (Nanni et al. 1999; Ming and Muenke 2002). Most HPE genes are involved in developmental signaling, and it is possible that reduction in the dosage of one protein can be buffered but two cannot, so that expression of an abnormal phenotype may depend on mutations in more than one gene (Ming and Muenke 2002).

Of six families with loss-of-function mutations, four have mutation-carrier parents (families 3, 4, 5, and 6 [fig. 1]), three of whom are unaffected. Two parents are probably constitutive mutation carriers, and two are gonosomal mosaics. This presents challenges for genetic counseling of families with *OTX2* mutations. Estimating the risk of having an affected child is extremely difficult. The relationship between levels of somatic and germline mosaicism is unpredictable. Little is known about either the precise stage at which the germ line is determined in humans or the number of precursor cells recruited. However, the number of cells ancestral to the germ line in mammals is thought to be small, so an individual who is gonosomal mosaic is likely to have a significant proportion of germ cells carrying the mutation (Zlotogora 1998; Leuer et al. 2001). Consequently, a relatively high recurrence risk is predicted for the offspring of gonosomal mosaic individuals, even if the proportion of mutant alleles in blood DNA is low. This has been observed in practice by others (Zlotogora 1998; Leuer et al. 2001) and in the present study, with both gonosomal mosaic mothers passing the mutation to two affected offspring. Constitutive-mutation-carrier parents are expected to be at 50% risk of having an affected child; however, recurrence was observed only in families with a mosaic parent. The lack of penetrance of *OTX2* mutations must also be taken into account; the recurrence risk will presumably be lower if, as we suggest, other factors are required for manifestation of an abnormal phenotype.

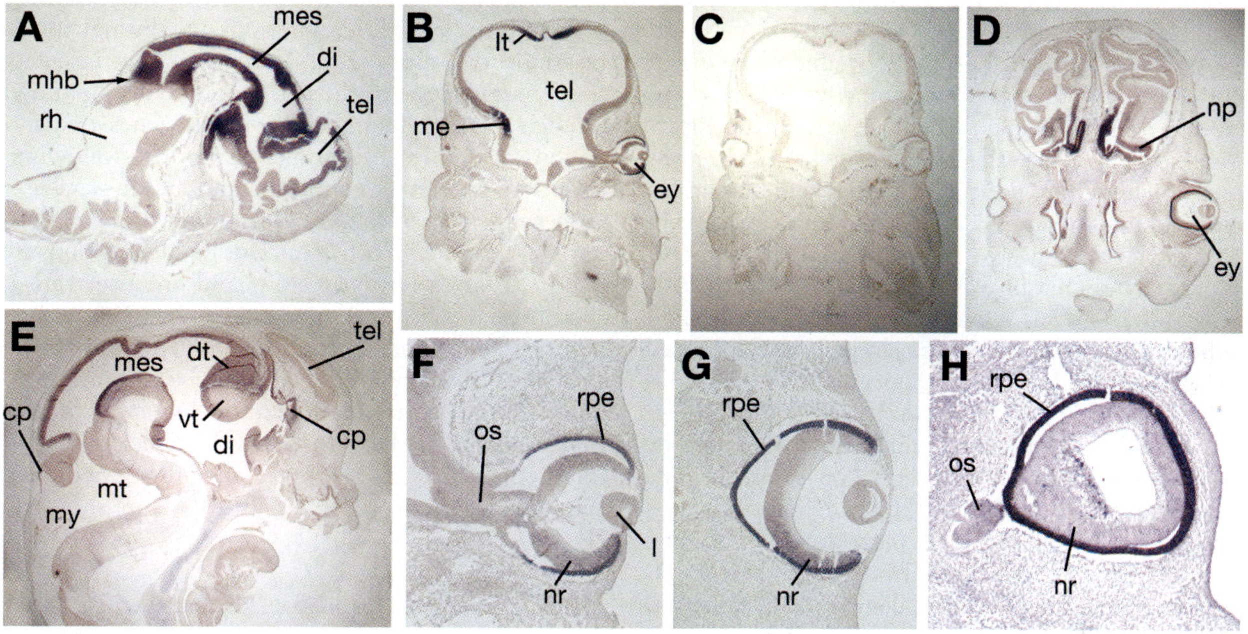

Figure 6 Expression pattern of the human *OTX2* gene in the developing head (*A–E*) and eye (*F–H*). Panels show representative results of nonradioactive in situ hybridization with a human *OTX2* probe. All panels (apart from panel C, which shows a sense control) show antisense hybridization: CS14 sagittal (*A*); CS16 coronal (*B* and *C*); CS18 (*D*); CS22 sagittal (*E*); CS16 5 × magnification of panel B (*F*); CS17 coronal (*G*); CS19 transverse (*H*). Strong expression is seen in the RPE (*panels B, D, F, G,* and *H*), and weaker expression is seen in the neural retina. Pigment formation has not yet begun at this stage; cp = choroid plexus; di = diencephalic vesicle; dt = dorsal thalamus; ey = eye; l = lens; lt = lamina terminalis; me = medial eminence; mes = mesencephalic vesicle; mhb = midbrain/hindbrain boundary; mt = metencephalic vesicle; my = myelencephalic vesicle; np = nasal pit; nr = neural retina; os = optic stalk; rh = rhombencephalic vesicle; rpe = retinal pigment epithelium; tel = telencephalic vesicle; vt = ventral thalamus.

The relevant factors are, however, already present in families with one or more affected offspring.

Unaffected parents may be constitutive or mosaic mutation carriers; therefore, it is essential to test them for any *OTX2* mutation identified in affected probands. However, accurate estimates of the recurrence risk await a molecular definition of the factors that determine penetrance of these mutations.

Phenotypic Variability

OTX2 loss-of-function mutations are associated with a broad spectrum of ocular phenotypes, ranging from bilateral anophthalmia to mild microphthalmia with retinal abnormalities. Asymmetry between the two sides, also noted in other genetic ocular malformations (Fantes et al. 2003; Ragge et al. 2005), is frequently seen. The spectrum of neurological phenotypes is broad, ranging from severe developmental delay to normal cognitive development. Variable expressivity is illustrated by the different phenotypes of siblings 4A and 4B.

The *OTX2* transcription pattern in human embryos is very similar to that described for mouse at the stages examined. This is not always the case (Fougerousse et al. 2000). The highly conserved expression pattern indicates conserved transcriptional control mechanisms. Analysis of the *Otx2* loci in human, mouse, *Xenopus*, zebrafish, and *Fugu* demonstrated that many of the distant enhancers that control *Otx2* expression are functionally conserved (Kurokawa et al. 2004*a*, 2004*b*). These elements, spread over hundreds of kilobases of genomic DNA, are possible targets for mutations/variations that might influence phenotypic severity and penetrance.

The ocular expression pattern of *OTX2* correlates well with the range of eye phenotypes observed in patients with loss-of-function mutations. *Otx2* interacts with *Mitf* to specify the RPE, which is essential for normal eye development (Martinez-Morales et al. 2003). Early RPE defects cause gross structural abnormalities of the eye (Raymond and Jackson 1995; Graw 2003). The anophthalmia and severe microphthalmia phenotypes in our cohort may result directly from loss of *OTX2* function in the developing RPE.

In the developing neural retina, OTX2 regulates *CRX*, and *CRX* mutations cause LCA and retinal degeneration (Sohocki et al. 1998; Rivolta et al. 2001; Nishida et al. 2003). The retinal phenotypes in patients 4B (with an original diagnosis of LCA) and 4C (resembling pigmentary retinopathy) may be due to disturbed OTX2 regulation of CRX function.

The optic nerve and chiasm were reduced or absent in four of the six patients for whom MRI, CT, or ultrasound data were available (patients 1, 2, 5 and 6 [fig. 3 and table 2]). Optic-nerve aplasia, which is very rare, was observed bilaterally in patients 2 and 6, with absence of the chiasm, and unilaterally on the anophthalmic side in patient 1, who also shows a thin chiasm. Hypoplasia of optic nerves and chiasm was observed in patient 5. Although *OTX2*/*Otx2* is expressed in the optic stalk and subsequently in the optic-nerve sheath, it is not expressed in the optic nerve itself (fig. 6) (Simeone et al. 1993; Bovolenta et al. 1997; Martinez-Morales et al. 2001). Hypoplasia of the optic nerve and chiasm may therefore be a secondary effect of abnormal retinal development. The optic nerve is formed when retinal ganglion-cell axons exit the globe. The majority of axons, encased in the optic sheath, project to the contralateral side of the brain, forming the optic chiasm in the ventral diencephalon (Rasband et al. 2003). *Otx2* is expressed in retinal ganglion cells (Bovolenta et al. 1997), so *OTX2* mutations may compromise the development of the optic nerve and the formation of the chiasm.

Pronounced hippocampal malformation was observed (fig. 5*C*) in patient 6, with bilateral anophthalmia, severe developmental delay, and seizures beginning in infancy. The hippocampus is derived from the alar plate, which develops from an OTX2-expressing domain of the neural plate (Fernandez-Garre et al. 2002). Patient 4A was the other individual in the cohort with severe developmental delay and seizures with teenage onset (table 2). Unfortunately, no MRI information is available for this patient. However, a hippocampal abnormality similar to that in patient 6 was observed in patient 1, a young child with severe developmental and speech delay, like patient 4B, but currently without seizures. The association of hippocampal malformation with seizures remains to be confirmed as additional patients are identified.

It is interesting to note that the ocular defects reported in heterozygous *Otx2*-knockout mice were usually accompanied by severe craniofacial malformations (Matsuo et al. 1995). Our data show that heterozygous *OTX2* mutations in humans are associated with structural eye malformations in the absence of gross craniofacial abnormalities. However, the phenotypic composition of our study cohort leads to biased ascertainment of *OTX2* mutations in ocular malformation cases. A broader human mutation study might reveal *OTX2* mutations associated with craniofacial malformation syndromes or seizure-associated brain defects in the absence of eye anomalies.

We have presented evidence that heterozygous loss-of-function mutations in the *OTX2* gene make a major contribution to the genetic basis of anophthalmia and microphthalmia in a small but significant proportion of patients. Two notable findings of our study are the lack of penetrance of *OTX2* mutations and the high incidence of gonosomal mosaicism. The factors that influence de novo mutagenesis in the early embryo are unknown; it is unclear at present whether some genes or genomic regions are more susceptible than others following fertilization or whether gonosomal mosaicism is more common than previously recognized and has simply been underascertained. Of five nucleotide substitutions in our cohort, four are transversions and one is a transition: this unusual bias (Nachman and Crowell 2000) may hint at novel mutational mechanisms. Elucidation of the factors that influence *OTX2* penetrance is a high priority and will assist with genetic counseling; in addition, further studies will help to unravel the complex genetic interactions that are responsible for the development of the human eye.

Acknowledgments

We gratefully acknowledge the cooperation of the patients and their families. We thank Marie Restori of Moorfields Eye Hospital, for performing ocular ultrasound; Alison Condie of the Wellcome Trust Clinical Research Facility, Edinburgh, for technical assistance; John Stevens, for expert neuroradiology; and the Medical Research Council/Wellcome Trust–funded Human Developmental Biology Resource. N.K.R. is a Senior Surgical Scientist and is supported by the Academy of Medical Sciences/The Health Foundation and the Medical Research Fund, Oxford. I.M.H. is supported by a Career Development Award from the U.K. Medical Research Council.

Electronic-Database Information

Accession numbers and URLs for data presented herein are as follows:

dbSNP, http://www.ncbi.nlm.nih.gov/SNP/ (for 268+12 C/T [accession number ss35522250], 269–70 C/A [accession number ss35522251], and c.1050 G/A [accession number rs171978])

GenBank, http://www.ncbi.nlm.nih.gov/Genbank/ (for human *OTX2* cDNA [accession number NM_172337] and BAC AL161757)

Laboratory of Phil Green, http://www.phrap.org/index.html

Online Mendelian Inheritance in Man (OMIM), http://www.ncbi.nlm.nih.gov/Omim/ (for anophthalmia, extreme microphthalmia, sclerocornea, aniridia, colobomata, congenital cataracts, LCA, Walker-Warburg syndrome, congenital cataract/aphakia, *PAX6*, *RAX*, *CHX10*, *MAF*, *SOX2*, *OTX2*, *CRX*, cone-rod dystrophy, MITF, OTX1, optic-nerve aplasia, PITX2, SIX3, *ROM1*, *RDS*, HPE, *SHH*, *TGIF*, and *ZIC2*)

References

Acampora D, Mazan S, Lallemand Y, Avantaggiato V, Maury M, Simeone A, Brulet P (1995) Forebrain and midbrain regions are deleted in Otx2$^{-/-}$ mutants due to a defective anterior neuroectoderm specification during gastrulation. Development 121:3279–3290

Aijaz S, Clark BJ, Williamson K, van Heyningen V, Morrison D, Fitzpatrick D, Collin R, Ragge N, Christoforou A, Brown A, Hanson I (2004) Absence of SIX6 mutations in microphthalmia, anophthalmia, and coloboma. Invest Ophthalmol Vis Sci 45:3871–3876

Ang SL, Jin O, Rhinn M, Daigle N, Stevenson L, Rossant J (1996) A targeted mouse Otx2 mutation leads to severe defects in gastrulation and formation of axial mesoderm and to deletion of rostral brain. Development 122:243–252

Azuma N, Yamaguchi Y, Handa H, Hayakawa M, Kanai A, Yamada M (1999) Missense mutation in the alternative splice region of the PAX6 gene in eye anomalies. Am J Hum Genet 65:656–663

Bovolenta P, Mallamaci A, Briata P, Corte G, Boncinelli E (1997) Implication of OTX2 in pigment epithelium determination and neural retina differentiation. J Neurosci 17: 4243–4252

Brewer C, Holloway S, Zawalnyski P, Schinzel A, FitzPatrick D (1998) A chromosomal deletion map of human malformations. Am J Hum Genet 63:1153–1159

D'Elia AV, Tell G, Paron I, Pellizzari L, Lonigro R, Damante G (2001) Missense mutations of human homeoboxes: a review. Hum Mutat 18:361–374

Dobyns WB, Pagon RA, Armstrong D, Curry CJ, Greenberg F, Grix A, Holmes LB, Laxova R, Michels VV, Robinow M, Zimmerman RL (1989) Diagnostic criteria for Walker-Warburg syndrome. Am J Med Genet 32:195–210

Edwards JH (1989) Familiarity, recessivity and germline mosaicism. Ann Hum Genet 53:33–47

Fantes J, Ragge NK, Lynch SA, McGill NI, Collin JR, Howard-Peebles PN, Hayward C, Vivian AJ, Williamson K, van Heyningen V, FitzPatrick DR (2003) Mutations in SOX2 cause anophthalmia. Nat Genet 33:461–463

Ferda-Percin E, Ploder LA, Yu JJ, Arici K, Horsford DJ, Rutherford A, Bapat B, Cox DW, Duncan AMV, Kalnins VI, Kocak-Altintas A, Sowden JC, Trabousli E, Sarfarazi M, McInnes RR (2000) Human microphthalmia associated with mutations in the retinal homeobox gene CHX10. Nat Genet 25:397–401

Fernandez-Garre P, Rodriguez-Gallardo L, Gallego-Diaz V, Alvarez IS, Puelles L (2002) Fate map of the chicken neural plate at stage 4. Development 129:2807–2822

Finkelstein R, Boncinelli E (1994) From fly head to mammalian forebrain: the story of otd and Otx. Trends Genet 10:310–315

Fledelius HC, Christensen AC (1996) Reappraisal of the human ocular growth curve in fetal life, infancy, and early childhood. Br J Ophthalmol 80:918–921

Fougerousse F, Bullen P, Herasse M, Lindsay S, Richard I, Wilson D, Suel L, Durand M, Robson S, Abitbol M, Beckmann JS, Strachan T (2000) Human-mouse differences in the embryonic expression patterns of developmental control genes and disease genes. Hum Mol Genet 9:165–173

Freund CL, Gregory-Evans CY, Furukawa T, Papaioannou M, Looser J, Ploder L, Bellingham J, Ng D, Herbrick JA, Duncan A, Scherer SW, Tsui LC, Loutradis-Anagnostou A, Jacobson SG, Cepko CL, Bhattacharya SS, McInnes RR (1997) Cone-rod dystrophy due to mutations in a novel photoreceptor-specific homeobox gene (CRX) essential for maintenance of the photoreceptor. Cell 91:543–553

Germot A, Lecointre G, Plouhinec JL, Le Mentec C, Girardot F, Mazan S (2001) Structural evolution of Otx genes in craniates. Mol Biol Evol 18:1668–1678

Gouya L, Puy H, Robreau AM, Bourgeois M, Lamoril J, Da Silva V, Grandchamp B, Deybach JC (2002) The penetrance of dominant erythropoietic protoporphyria is modulated by expression of wildtype FECH. Nat Genet 30:27–28

Graw J (2003) The genetic and molecular basis of congenital eye defects. Nat Rev Genet 4:876–888

Hanson I (2003) PAX6 and congenital eye malformations. Pediatr Res 54:791–796

Holbrook JA, Neu-Yilik G, Hentze MW, Kulozik AE (2004) Nonsense-mediated decay approaches the clinic. Nat Genet 36:801–808

Jamieson RV, Perveen R, Kerr B, Carette M, Yardley J, Heon E, Wirth MG, van Heyningen V, Donnai D, Munier F, Black GC (2002) Domain disruption and mutation of the bZIP transcription factor, MAF, associated with cataract, ocular anterior segment dysgenesis and coloboma. Hum Mol Genet 11:33–42

Kajiwara K, Berson EL, Dryja TP (1994) Digenic retinitis pigmentosa due to mutations at the unlinked peripherin/RDS and ROM1 loci. Science 264:1604–1608

Kurokawa D, Kiyonari H, Nakayama R, Kimura-Yoshida C, Matsuo I, Aizawa S (2004*a*) Regulation of Otx2 expression and its functions in mouse forebrain and midbrain. Development 131:3319–3331

Kurokawa D, Takasaki N, Kiyonari H, Nakayama R, Kimura-Yoshida C, Matsuo I, Aizawa S (2004*b*) Regulation of Otx2 expression and its functions in mouse epiblast and anterior neuroectoderm. Development 131:3307–3317

Laflamme C, Filion C, Labelle Y (2004) Functional characterization of SIX3 homeodomain mutations in holoprosencephaly: interaction with the nuclear receptor NR4A3/ NOR1. Hum Mutat 24:502–508

Lai CSL, Gerrelli D, Monaco AP, Fisher SE, Copp AJ (2003) FOXP2 expression during brain development coincides with adult sites of pathology in a severe speech and language disorder. Brain 126:2455–2462

Leuer M, Oldenburg J, Lavergne JM, Ludwig M, Fregin A, Eigel A, Ljung R, Goodeve A, Peake I, Olek K (2001) Somatic mosaicism in hemophilia A: a fairly common event. Am J Hum Genet 69:75–87

Mallamaci A, Di Blas E, Briata P, Boncinelli E, Corte G (1996) OTX2 homeoprotein in the developing central nervous system and migratory cells of the olfactory area. Mech Dev 58: 165–178

Martinez-Morales JR, Dolez V, Rodrigo I, Zaccarini R, Leconte L, Bovolenta P, Saule S (2003) OTX2 activates the molecular network underlying retina pigment epithelium differentiation. J Biol Chem 278:21721–21731

Martinez-Morales JR, Signore M, Acampora D, Simeone A, Bovolenta P (2001) Otx genes are required for tissue specification in the developing eye. Development 128:2019–2030

Matsuo I, Kuratani S, Kimura C, Takeda N, Aizawa S (1995) Mouse Otx2 functions in the formation and patterning of the rostral head. Genes Dev 9:2646–2658

Ming JE, Muenke M (2002) Multiple hits during early embryonic development: digenic diseases and holoprosencephaly. Am J Hum Genet 71:1017–1032

Morrison D, FitzPatrick D, Hanson I, Williamson K, van Heyningen V, Fleck B, Jones I, Chalmers J, Campbell H (2002) National study of microphthalmia, anophthalmia, and coloboma (MAC) in Scotland: investigation of genetic aetiology. J Med Genet 39:16–22

Nachman MW, Crowell SL (2000) Estimate of the mutation rate per nucleotide in humans. Genetics 156:297–304

Nanni L, Ming JE, Bocian M, Steinhaus K, Bianchi DW, Die-Smulders C, Giannotti A, Imaizumi K, Jones KL, Campo MD, Martin RA, Meinecke P, Pierpont ME, Robin NH, Young ID, Roessler E, Muenke M (1999) The mutational spectrum of the sonic hedgehog gene in holoprosencephaly: SHH mutations cause a significant proportion of autosomal dominant holoprosencephaly. Hum Mol Genet 8:2479–2488

Nishida A, Furukawa A, Koike C, Tano Y, Aizawa S, Matsuo I, Furukawa T (2003) Otx2 homeobox gene controls retinal photoreceptor cell fate and pineal gland development. Nat Neurosci 6:1255–1263

Nussbaum RL, McInnes RR, Willard HF (2001) Genetics in medicine, 6th ed. W.B. Saunders, Philadelphia, p 54

Ragge NK, Lorenz B, Schneider A, Bushby K, de Sanctis L, de Sanctis U, Salt A, Collin JRO, Vivian AJ, Free SL, Thompson P, Williamson K, Sisodiya SM, van Heyningen V, FitzPatrick DR (2005) SOX2 anophthalmia syndrome. Am J Med Genet. http://www3.interscience.wiley.com/cgi-bin/fulltext/110437025/HTMLSTART/ (electronically published April 5, 2005; accessed April 20, 2005)

Rasband K, Hardy M, Chien C-B (2003) Generating X: formation of the optic chiasm. Neuron 39:885–888

Raymond SM, Jackson IJ (1995) The retinal pigmented epithelium is required for development and maintenance of the mouse neural retina. Curr Biol 5:1286–1295

Rivolta C, Berson EL, Dryja TP (2001) Dominant Leber congenital amaurosis, cone-rod degeneration, and retinitis pigmentosa caused by mutant versions of the transcription factor CRX. Hum Mutat 18:488–498

Simeone A (2000) Positioning the isthmic organizer where Otx2 and Gbx2 meet. Trends Genet 16:237–240

Simeone A, Acampora D, Mallamaci A, Stornaiuolo A, D'Apice MR, Nigro V, Boncinelli E (1993) A vertebrate gene related to orthodenticle contains a homeodomain of the bicoid class and demarcates anterior neuroectoderm in the gastrulating mouse embryo. EMBO J 12:2735–2747

Sisodiya SM, Free SL, Williamson KA, Mitchell TN, Willis C, Stevens JM, Kendall BE, Shorvon SD, Hanson IM, Moore AT, van Heyningen V (2001) PAX6 haploinsufficiency causes cerebral malformation and olfactory dysfunction in humans. Nat Genet 28:214–216

Sohocki MM, Sullivan LS, Mintz-Hittner HA, Birch D, Heckenlively JR, Freund CL, McInnes RR, Daiger SP (1998) A range of clinical phenotypes associated with mutations in *CRX*, a photoreceptor transcription-factor gene. Am J Hum Genet 63:1307–1315

Swaroop A, Wang QL, Wu W, Cook J, Coats C, Xu S, Chen S, Zack DJ, Sieving P (1999) Leber congenital amaurosis caused by a homozygous mutation (R90W) in the homeodomain of the retinal transcription factor CRX: direct evidence for the involvement of CRX in the development of photoreceptor function. Hum Mol Genet 8:299–305

Tahayato A, Sonneville R, Pichaud F, Wernet MF, Papatsenko D, Beaufils P, Cook T, Desplan C (2003) Otd/Crx, a dual regulator for the specification of ommatidia subtypes in the *Drosophila* retina. Dev Cell 5:391–402

van Heyningen V, Yeyati PL (2004) Mechanisms of non-Mendelian inheritance in genetic disease. Hum Mol Genet 13 Spec No 2:R225–R233

Vithana EN, Abu-Safieh L, Pelosini L, Winchester E, Hornan D, Bird AC, Hunt DM, Bustin SA, Bhattacharya SS (2003) Expression of PRPF31 mRNA in patients with autosomal dominant retinitis pigmentosa: a molecular clue for incomplete penetrance? Invest Ophthalmol Vis Sci 44:4204–4209

Voronina VA, Kozhemyakina EA, O'Kernick CM, Kahn ND, Wenger SL, Linberg JV, Schneider AS, Mathers PH (2004) Mutation in the human RAX homeobox gene in a patient with anophthalmia and sclerocornea. Hum Mol Genet 13: 315–322

Wallis DE, Roessler E, Hehr U, Nanni L, Wiltshire T, Richieri-Costa A, Gillessen-Kaesbach G, Zackai EH, Rommens J, Muenke M (1999) Mutations in the homeodomain of the human SIX3 gene cause holoprosencephaly. Nat Genet 22: 196–198

Zlotogora J (1998) Germ line mosaicism. Hum Genet 102: 381–386

Zuber ME, Gestri G, Viczian AS, Barsacchi G, Harris WA (2003) Specification of the vertebrate eye by a network of eye field transcription factors. Development 130:5155–5167

Am. J. Hum. Genet. 76:1023–1033, 2005

Germline *BHD*-Mutation Spectrum and Phenotype Analysis of a Large Cohort of Families with Birt-Hogg-Dubé Syndrome

Laura S. Schmidt,[1] Michael L. Nickerson,[2,*] Michelle B. Warren,[2] Gladys M. Glenn,[3] Jorge R. Toro,[3] Maria J. Merino,[4] Maria L. Turner,[5] Peter L. Choyke,[6] Nirmala Sharma,[2] James Peterson,[7] Patrick Morrison,[8] Eamonn R. Maher,[9] McClellan M. Walther[7] Berton Zbar,[2] and W. Marston Linehan[7]

[1]Basic Research Program, Science Applications International Corporation–Frederick Inc., and [2]Laboratory of Immunobiology, Center for Cancer Research, National Cancer Institute (NCI)–Frederick, Frederick, MD; [3]Genetic Epidemiology Branch, Division of Cancer Epidemiology and Genetics, NCI, Rockville, MD; [4]Laboratory of Pathology, [5]Dermatology Branch, [6]Diagnostic Radiology, and [7]Urologic Oncology Branch, Center for Cancer Research, NCI, National Institutes of Health, Bethesda; [8]Clinical Genetics, Belfast City Hospital Trust, Belfast; and [9]Section of Medical and Molecular Genetics, Institute of Biomedical Research, University of Birmingham, Birmingham, United Kingdom

Birt-Hogg-Dubé syndrome (BHD), a genodermatosis characterized by multiple hamartomas of the hair follicle (fibrofolliculoma), predisposes individuals to an increased risk of developing renal neoplasms and spontaneous pneumothorax. Previously, we localized the *BHD* locus (also known as *FLCN*) to chromosome 17p11.2 by linkage analysis and subsequently identified germline mutations in a novel gene in probands from eight of the nine families with BHD in our screening panel. Affected members of five of the families inherited an insertion/deletion of a cytosine in a C_8 tract in exon 11. This mutation was also identified by exon 11 screening in probands from 22 of 52 additional families with BHD and therefore represents a hypermutable "hotspot" for mutation in *BHD*. Here, we screened the remaining 30 families from this large BHD cohort by direct sequence analysis and identified germline *BHD* mutations in 84% (51/61) of all families with BHD recruited to our study. Mutations were located along the entire length of the coding region, including 16 insertion/deletion, 3 nonsense, and 3 splice-site mutations. The majority of *BHD* mutations were predicted to truncate the BHD protein, folliculin. Among patients with a mutation in the exon 11 hotspot, significantly fewer renal tumors were observed in patients with the C-deletion than those with the C-insertion mutation. Coding-sequence mutations were not found, however, in probands from two large families with BHD whose affected members shared their family's BHD-affected haplotype. Of the 53 families with BHD whose members inherited either a germline mutation or the affected haplotype, 24 (45%) had at least one member with renal neoplasms. Three families classified with familial renal oncocytoma were identified with *BHD* mutations, which represents the first disease gene associated with this rare form of renal neoplasm. This study expands the *BHD*-mutation spectrum and evaluates genotype-phenotype correlations among families with BHD.

Introduction

Birt-Hogg-Dubé syndrome (BHD [MIM 135150]) was first described in 1977 by three Canadian physicians who studied a large family whose members were affected with multiple, small papules on the face, neck, and upper torso that developed after age 25 years (Birt et al. 1977). These lesions, called "fibrofolliculomas" (FFs), were characterized as benign hamartomas of the hair follicle. Histologically, FFs are characterized by strands of proliferating epithelial cells extending out from the infundibulum of the hair follicle, surrounded by a thick mantle of connective tissue and mucin-rich stroma (Birt et al. 1977). FFs are part of the triad of BHD skin lesions that also includes trichodiscomas and acrochordons. BHD is inherited in an autosomal dominant manner and has been reported to be associated with renal tumors (Roth et al. 1993; Toro et al. 1999), spontaneous pneumothorax (Binet et al. 1986; Toro et al. 1999), colon polyps, and colon carcinomas (Hornstein and Knickenberg 1975; Hornstein 1976; Rongioletti et al. 1989; Le Guyadec et al. 1998). A recent risk-assessment study of BHD-affected patients concluded that a diagnosis of BHD conferred a 7-fold increased risk of developing renal neoplasia and a 50-fold increased risk of spontaneous pneumothorax but no increased risk of colon polyps or colon cancer (Zbar et al. 2002). Renal tumors with a variety

Received March 2, 2005; accepted for publication April 7, 2005; electronically published April 25, 2005.

Address for correspondence and reprints: Dr. Laura S. Schmidt, Laboratory of Immunobiology, NCI-Frederick, Building 560, Room 12-69, Frederick, MD 21702. E-mail: schmidtl@ncifcrf.gov

* Present affiliation: Translational and Clinical Research, Transgenomic Inc., Gaithersburg, MD.

0002-9297/2005/7606-0009$15.00

of histologies are associated with BHD, including chromophobe renal cell carcinoma (RCC), benign renal oncocytoma, clear-cell RCC, and papillary type I RCC (Pavlovich et al. 2002, 2005). The most common form of renal tumor seen in patients with BHD is an oncocytic hybrid tumor with areas reminiscent of both chromophobe RCC and oncocytoma (Tickoo et al. 1999).

The BHD disease locus was mapped to chromosome 17p11.2 by genetic linkage analysis (Khoo et al. 2001; Schmidt et al. 2001); we subsequently identified germline mutations in a novel gene (*BHD* [GenBank accession number AF517523], or *FLCN* [MIM 607273]) in a panel of nine kindreds with BHD. These were insertions, deletions, and nonsense mutations that were predicted to truncate the BHD protein, folliculin (Nickerson et al. 2002). A majority of kindreds with BHD were found to harbor an insertion or deletion of a cytosine in a C_8 tract within exon 11, suggesting a hypermutable "hotspot" for mutation in *BHD* (Khoo et al. 2002; Nickerson et al. 2002).

Folliculin, is a 579-aa protein with no known functional domains, for which mouse, fly, worm, yeast, dog, and rat orthologs have been identified (Nickerson et al. 2002; Lingaas et al. 2003; Okimoto et al. 2004). *BHD* mRNA expression, measured by fluorescent in situ hybridization, is widespread in a variety of tissues, including skin and its appendages, the distal nephron of the kidney, and stromal cells and type I pneumocytes of the lung (Warren et al. 2004). Strong *BHD* mRNA expression was found in secretory cells, such as acinar cells of the parotid gland and pancreas, and ductal cells of the breast. Reduced *BHD* expression was seen in renal tumors from patients with BHD, regardless of histologic type.

Sixty-one families affected with BHD were recruited to the NCI for study over a 3-year period. Previously, we evaluated a screening panel representing nine of these families with BHD and reported the identification of one nonsense and two frameshift *BHD* mutations as well as five insertion/deletion mutations in the C_8 tract of exon 11. Exon 11 screening of the entire cohort of families revealed C_8 tract insertion/deletion mutations in probands from 22 of the 52 remaining families with BHD (Nickerson et al. 2002). In the present study, we have completed the mutation analysis of this large BHD cohort by screening, by direct sequence analysis, the remaining 30 families for mutations in the *BHD* gene. We have identified germline *BHD* mutations in affected members of 84% (51/61) of kindreds with BHD evaluated to date. In addition, we have collected phenotypic information on family members and have correlated phenotype with germline *BHD* mutation to evaluate possible genotype-phenotype associations.

Methods

Patient Recruitment

We recruited members of 61 BHD-affected families to our study at the NCI, from 1998 to 2001, through patient recruitment letters to dermatologists (55 families) and by referrals from urologic surgeons (6 families). All of the families with BHD were invited to participate in the study regardless of the number of affected individuals in the family or the presence or absence of associated health problems. A family was considered affected with BHD if it had (1) one or more members with 10 or more skin lesions that were clinically compatible with FFs and/or (2) a minimum of one histologically proven FF. Histologically, an FF was characterized by multiple anastomosing strands of 2–4 epithelial cells extending from a central hair follicle. Phenotypic expression of BHD skin papules can be variable among affected members of a family with BHD; therefore, once a proband with clinically positive or histologically proven FFs was identified in a BHD-affected family, other family members were screened and classified as affected for genotype-phenotype evaluation on the basis of (1) the presence of a histologically proven FF, (2) inheritance of the family's germline *BHD* mutation, (3) inheritance of the family's BHD-affected haplotype, or (4) obligate carrier status. We also included family 238 as affected with BHD, because multiple members were affected with bilateral, renal oncocytic hybrid neoplasms, a rare histologic variant uniquely associated with BHD. Participants in this study provided written informed consent. The protocol was approved by the institutional review boards of the NCI and the University of Manitoba.

Patient Evaluation

All members of families with BHD who were aged >20 years were evaluated at the NIH Clinical Center and/or in the field. Blood samples were obtained for DNA extraction and mutation analysis. Each patient received a detailed dermatologic examination, and biopsies were performed for lesions suspected to be FFs.

Family members seen at the NIH were evaluated for other phenotypic manifestations associated with BHD. Occult renal malignancies were detected by CT scan of the abdomen before and after administration of ~120 ml of Ioxilan 300 (Cook Imaging). The presence of lung cysts and evidence of spontaneous pneumothorax were evaluated by thoracic CT scan, by use of high-resolution sections (1 mm) through the chest at 10-mm intervals. Additional information was obtained from patient medical histories, outside medical records, and tissue specimens obtained for NIH pathology review.

Mutation Analysis of the BHD *Gene*

DNA was extracted from peripheral-blood leukocytes, in accordance with standard procedures. Exon/intron structure of the *BHD* gene was determined by BLAST alignment of two overlapping, uncharacterized, full-length transcripts from skin melanoma (GenBank accession numbers BC015725 and BC015687), against the BAC clone RP11-45M22 (GenBank accession number AC055811); intronic primers were designed to amplify 14 coding exons and splice junctions for sequencing, as described elsewhere (Nickerson et al. 2002). Subsequent analyses showed that this exon/intron structure matched the cloned full-length *BHD* transcript. PCR products were generated using standard conditions and were purified; double-stranded sequencing was performed using BigDye Terminators (Applied Biosystems), as described elsewhere (Nickerson et al. 2002). Sequence variants were examined for cosegregation with disease in their respective families by denaturing high-performance liquid chromatography or by single-stranded sequencing. Insertions and deletions were subcloned with Topo Cloning Kit (Invitrogen) and were sequenced. At least 160 unaffected individuals were examined for each disease-associated sequence variant.

BHD *Haplotype Carrier Analysis*

Family members were evaluated for inheritance of the BHD-affected haplotype in cases in which a *BHD* germline mutation was not identified in the proband. To determine if a family member inherited the BHD-affected haplotype, individuals were genotyped using seven microsatellite markers (*D17S953, D17S740,* [location of *BHD*] *D17S2196, D17S620, AGAT100, D17S805,* and *D17S1824*) that spanned an 8-cM distance flanking the *BHD* locus on chromosome 17p. Haplotypes were determined from the genotype order in which the least number of recombinants occurred. All members of BHD-affected families who presented with FFs inherited the family's BHD-affected haplotype.

Statistical Analysis

The percentage of BHD-affected individuals with renal tumors was calculated in two ways: (1) by dividing the number of BHD-affected individuals with renal tumors by the number of BHD-affected individuals seen at the NIH and in the field, and (2) by dividing the number of BHD-affected individuals who had renal tumors by the number of BHD-affected individuals who were screened by abdominal CT scan. To overcome selection bias, we assessed the frequency of renal tumors found in patients with BHD two ways. Generally, patients who were affected with BHD skin lesions and/or were symptomatic for renal tumor came to the NIH to be seen and screened. Some patients who were less severely affected did not come to the NIH and were seen only in the field and therefore did not undergo abdominal/pulmonary CT screening. Differences in frequency of renal tumors, pneumothorax, or lung cysts between the groups with exon 11 C-insertion and C-deletion mutations were tested with Fisher's exact test (two-sided) (see the Calculation of Fisher's Exact Test Web site). $P < .05$ was considered statistically significant.

Results

Description of Patients

For the present study, 219 individuals (110 females and 109 males) from 53 families (whose members inherited either a germline mutation or the affected haplotype) were classified as affected with BHD. Of those individuals, 187 were evaluated in the field or at the NIH Clinical Center. Data were available for 7 deceased individuals with obligate carrier status, 12 individuals were evaluated by outside dermatologists, and 10 individuals provided a blood sample for mutation analysis but did not undergo further medical evaluation at the NIH.

The number of affected individuals in a family ranged from 1 to 25. In the present study, the largest number (25) of affected family members in a family with BHD was found in the Canadian family with BHD, family 172, originally studied by Drs. Birt, Hogg, and Dubé (Birt et al. 1977). Twenty-four families had only one member affected with BHD.

Dermatologic Manifestations

The hallmark BHD cutaneous manifestation is a benign tumor (hamartoma) of the hair follicle, an FF. Of the 175 BHD-affected individuals whose skin papules were biopsied and evaluated histologically, 147 (84%) were diagnosed with a histologically proven FF. All families that carried a *BHD* mutation or inherited the affected haplotype contained individuals who developed BHD skin lesions, with the exception of one family, family 238, referred to the NCI by the proband's urologist, in which three sisters developed bilateral renal oncocytic hybrid neoplasms and lung cysts without evidence of FFs. In the present study, the cutaneous lesions were not found in patients aged <20 years.

Pulmonary Manifestations

A high percentage of patients with BHD develop air-filled lung cysts (Zbar et al. 2002) and have a 50-fold higher risk of developing spontaneous pneumothorax. In the present study, 64 (32%) of 198 BHD-affected individuals for whom medical history was available had a history of spontaneous pneumothorax. Of the 129

BHD-affected individuals who were screened by pulmonary CT scan, 110 (85%) were found to have one or more lung cysts consistent with the BHD phenotype. Forty-five (85%) of 53 families with *BHD* germline mutations or affected-haplotype carriers had members who developed lung cysts or spontaneous pneumothorax.

Renal Neoplasia in BHD

BHD is unique among inherited renal cancer syndromes because patients develop not one, but a variety of histologic types of renal tumors, including chromophobe RCC, renal oncocytoma, clear-cell RCC, and papillary RCC (Pavlovich et al. 2002, 2005). Most often, BHD-associated renal neoplasms are oncocytic hybrid tumors, comprising elements of both chromophobe and renal oncocytoma. Thirty-eight BHD-affected individuals representing 24 BHD-affected families developed renal tumors. Males developed renal tumors 2.5-fold more often than did females (27 males; 11 females). The median age at diagnosis was 48 years (range 31–71 years). Tumors developed both bilaterally with multiple foci and unilaterally with a single focus. The number of patients with renal neoplasia in a BHD-affected family ranged from one to three, most frequently one case per family. The frequency of renal tumor among BHD-affected individuals seen at the NIH or in the field was 20% (38/187). The frequency of renal tumor among BHD-affected individuals who were evaluated by CT scan was 29% (38/132). Overall, 45% (24/53) of BHD-affected families with germline *BHD* mutations or affected-haplotype carriers contained individuals who were affected with renal tumors.

Other Phenotypic Features Found in BHD-Affected Individuals

There are reports that describe a number of additional phenotypic manifestations in BHD-affected individuals, including colon polyps and colon carcinoma (Hornstein and Knickenberg 1975; Hornstein 1976; Rongioletti et al. 1989; Le Guyadec et al. 1998), lipomas (Chung et al. 1996; Toro et al. 1999), angiolipomas (Chung et al. 1996), parathyroid adenomas (Chung et al. 1996), and parotid oncocytomas (Liu et al. 2000). Among the 219 BHD-affected individuals in the present study, four parotid gland tumors were reported in 2 men (diagnosed at ages 20 and 39 years) and 2 women (diagnosed at ages 62 and 72 years). Three of the parotid tumors were classified as oncocytomas. Additionally, three individuals with lipomas and nine individuals with colon polyps/carcinoma were identified through medical history.

Variable Expression of Phenotypic Manifestations

BHD is characterized by FFs, lung cysts, spontaneous pneumothorax, and an increased risk of developing renal neoplasia. These manifestations may occur singly or in various combinations in a patient, and variable phenotypic expression may be observed among family members from the same BHD-affected family. Among the 53 families with BHD whose affected members had a *BHD* germline mutation or carried the BHD-affected haplotype, 22 (41.5%) of the families had skin, lung, and renal manifestations, 22 (41.5%) of the families had members with skin and lung phenotypic features, 1 (2%) of the families had renal and lung phenotypic features, 7 (13%) of the families had only skin papules, and 1 (2%) of the families had renal tumors and skin papules (table 1).

BHD-*Mutation Spectrum and Mutational Hotspot*

Elsewhere, we reported the identification of *BHD* germline mutations, by direct sequence analysis, in 30 of 61 families with BHD recruited to the NCI (Nickerson et al. 2002). In the present study, we have completed mutation analysis of the remaining 30 families and, to date, have identified germline *BHD* mutations in 51 (84%) of 61 families with BHD in the NCI cohort. Each family's mutation cosegregated with disease and was not found in at least 160 unaffected individuals. Altogether, 22 novel mutations have been identified (5 were reported elsewhere [Nickerson et al. 2002]), including 16 insertions or deletions that cause frameshifts leading to premature truncation of the protein, 3 nonsense mutations that encode early termination codons, and 3 putative splice-site mutations (table 1 and fig. 1). Of note, no germline missense *BHD* mutations were detected in these BHD-affected families.

A total of 53% (27/51) of families with a germline *BHD* mutation had a cytosine insertion (c.1733insC [18 families]) or deletion (c.1733delC [9 families]) in the mononucleotide tract of eight cytosines (c.1733–1740) in exon 11. This mutational hotspot has been identified by several laboratories (Khoo et al. 2002; Nickerson et al. 2002). Mononucleotide tracts are thought to be hypermutable due to slippage of the DNA polymerase during replication (Streisinger et al. 1966), which results in frameshift mutations leading to protein truncation. Although most of the mutations identified in the remaining 24 BHD-affected families were unique, 2 families had the same 28-bp duplication in exon 9 (c.1378–1405 dup), 3 families shared a nonsense mutation in exon 12 (c.1844C→G), and 2 families shared a putative splice-site mutation in intron 9 (IVS9+2T→G) (table 1 and fig. 1).

Genotype-Phenotype Correlation: Location within the BHD *Gene*

Mutations were identified in all translated exons (exons 4–14), with the exception of exons 8 and 10 (fig. 2). Exon 11 was the most frequent site of mutation in

Table 1

***BHD* Germline Mutations and Phenotypes of Families with BHD**

	Mutation Analysis				No. of Family Members with Phenotype				
Family	Exon	Nucleotide[a] Change	Codon[b] Location	Type[c] (aa→ter)	Total Affected	FF[d]	Renal Tumors	Lung Cysts[e]	PT[f]
220	4	c.513delT	F20	FS (34)	1	1[g]	0	ND	0
249	5	IVS4-1G→A	G84	SS	3	1	1	ND	2
8188	5	c.707delC	G84	FS (45)	2	2	0	2	0
209	5	c.751delA	D99	FS (30)	2	2	0	1	0
233	6	c.1036delG	G195	FS (27)	1	1	0	1	0
202	7	c.1087delAGinsC	E211	FS (11)	8	7	1	5	0
224	7	c.1092delT	F213	FS (9)	1	1	0	1	0
166	7	c.1126delCA	T224	FS (22)	4	4	3	4	0
217	9	c.1378-1405dup	T317	FS (79)	1	1	1	1	0
228	9	c.1378-1405dup	T317	FS (79)	12	11	2	7	4
231	9	c.1468delG	W338	FS (14)	2	2	0	2	1
225	9	c.1473delC	R341	FS (11)	1	1[g]	ND	ND	0
242	9	IVS9+1G→A	V355	SS	9	6	1	7	8
229	9	IVS9+2T→G	V355	SS	5	5	3	4	1
238	9	IVS9+2T→G	V355	SS	3	0	3	3	0
239	11	c.1733insC	H429	FS (26)	1	1	1	1	1
8244	11	c.1733insC	H429	FS (26)	1	1[g]	0	1	0
8319	11	c.1733insC	H429	FS (26)	1	1	0	1	0
7561	11	c.1733insC	H429	FS (26)	1	1[h]	ND	ND	0
187	11	c.1733insC	H429	FS (26)	1	1	1	1	0
7399	11	c.1733insC	H429	FS (26)	1	1	0	0	0
250	11	c.1733insC	H429	FS (26)	3	2	1	1	1
246	11	c.1733insC	H429	FS (26)	8	8[g]	0	0	2
191	11	c.1733insC	H429	FS (26)	1	1[h]	ND	ND	0
211	11	c.1733insC	H429	FS (26)	1	1	0	1	0
241	11	c.1733insC	H429	FS (26)	4	4	1	4	0
183	11	c.1733insC	H429	FS (26)	1	1	1	ND	1
208	11	c.1733insC	H429	FS (26)	1	1	0	1	0
167	11	c.1733insC	H429	FS (26)	3	1	2	3	2
210	11	c.1733insC	H429	FS (26)	11	6	0	2	6
174	11	c.1733insC	H429	FS (26)	10	8	3	9	0
216	11	c.1733insC	H429	FS (26)	16	11	2	8	8
200	11	c.1733insC	H429	FS (26)	7	3	1	2	4
232	11	c.1733delC	H429	FS (38)	5	4	0	4	0
248	11	c.1733delC	H429	FS (38)	3	2	ND	ND	1
234	11	c.1733delC	H429	FS (38)	2	2	0	2	2
176	11	c.1733delC	H429	FS (38)	1	1	0	1	1
226	11	c.1733delC	H429	FS (38)	1	1	0	0	0
175	11	c.1733delC	H429	FS (38)	1	1	0	1	0
184	11	c.1733delC	H429	FS (38)	1	1	1	1	0
201	11	c.1733delC	H429	FS (38)	6	5	0	4	0
185	11	c.1733delC	H429	FS (38)	7	3	ND	1	5
6932	12	c.1758delT	F435	FS (32)	1	1	1	1	1
7416	12	c.1834delTC	L460	FS (24)	1	1	0	1	0
230	12	c.1844C→G	Y463X	NS	9	7	1	2	2
188	12	c.1844C→G	Y463X	NS	2	2	0	2	1
245	12	c.1844C→G	Y463X	NS	2	2	0	ND	1
8015	12	c.1881insG	D476	FS (9)	1	1	1	ND	0
7707	12	c.1884C→T	R477X	NS	1	1[g]	ND	ND	1
7706	13	c.1945insCTGT	V497	FS (24)	1	1[g]	ND	ND	0
168	14	c.2034C→T	R527X	NS	5	1	3	3	1
172	NF[i]	*BHD* haplotype	NA	NA	25	17	1	10	6
240	NF[i]	*BHD* haplotype	NA	NA	17	8	2	4	1

Note.—ND = not determined or no CT scan available; NA = not applicable.

[a] Nucleotide numbering according to GenBank accession number AF517523. Nucleotide 456 corresponds to A of ATG initiation codon. In cases of ins/del in a mononucleotide tract, the first nucleotide of the tract is given.

[b] First codon affected by sequence variation. The codon for initiator methionine is codon 1.

[c] FS = frameshift (missense amino acids to predicted premature termination codon); SS = splice site; NS = nonsense.

[d] FF diagnosis based on histology, except where indicated.

[e] Diagnosis based on thoracic CT scan.

[f] PT = spontaneous pneumothorax episodes.

[g] FF diagnosis based on clinical evaluation only.

[h] Positive BHD diagnosis based on >80 trichodiscomas.

[i] NF = not found.

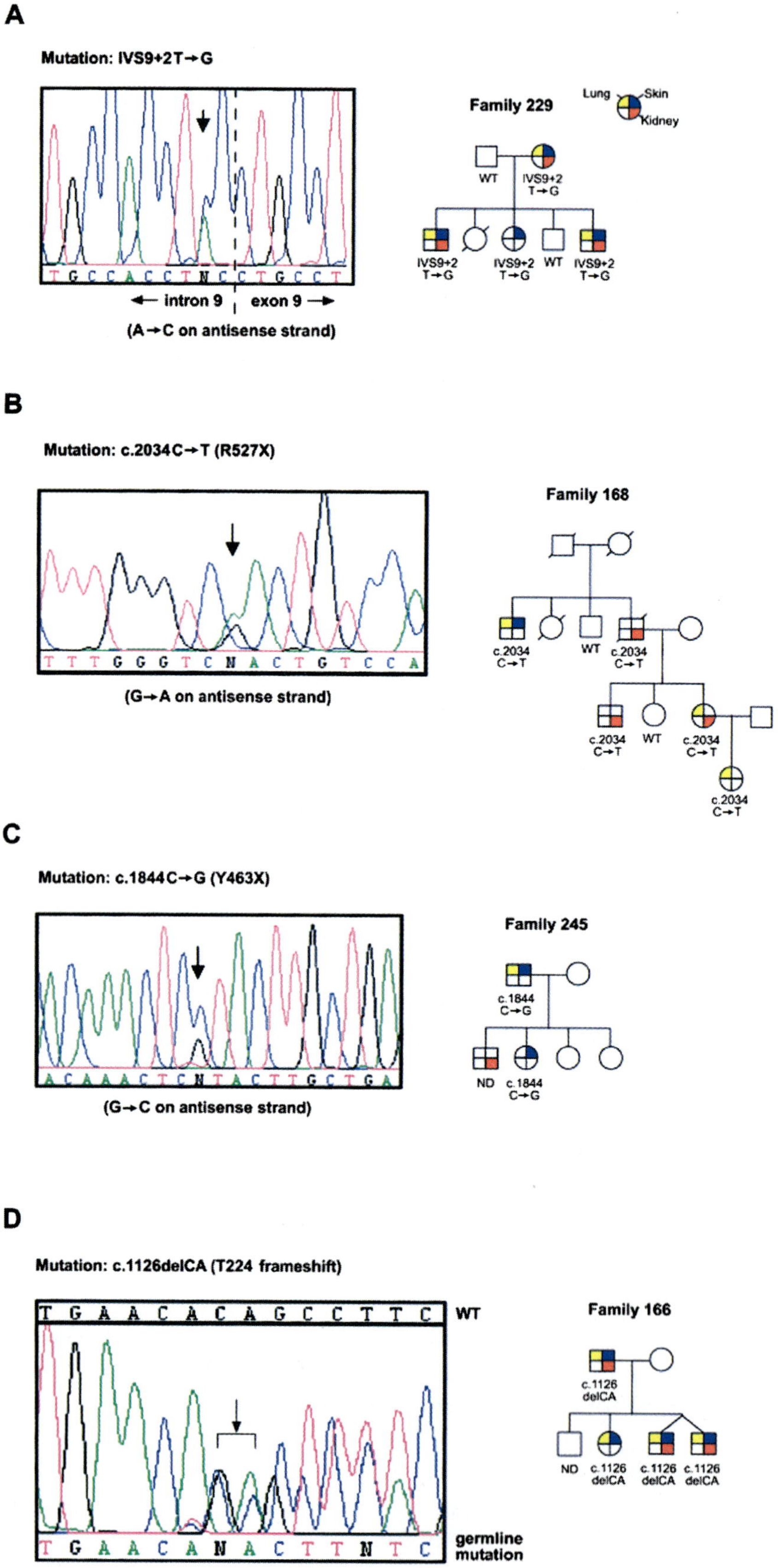
A
Mutation: IVS9+2T→G
T G C C A C C T N C C T G C C T
← intron 9
exon 9 →
(A→C on antisense strand)
Family 229
Lung
Skin
Kidney
WT
IVS9+2 T→G
IVS9+2 T→G
IVS9+2 T→G
WT
IVS9+2 T→G
B
Mutation: c.2034C→T (R527X)
T T T G G G T C N A C T G T C C A
(G→A on antisense strand)
Family 168
c.2034 C→T
WT
c.2034 C→T
c.2034 C→T
WT
c.2034 C→T
c.2034 C→T
C
Mutation: c.1844C→G (Y463X)
A C A A A C T C N T A C T T G C T G A
(G→C on antisense strand)
Family 245
c.1844 C→G
ND
c.1844 C→G
D
Mutation: c.1126delCA (T224 frameshift)
T G A A C A C A G C C T T C
WT
T G A A C A N A C T T N T C
germline mutation
Family 166
c.1126 delCA
ND
c.1126 delCA
c.1126 delCA
c.1126 delCA

the 51 BHD-affected families (27 families had the hotspot mutation), exons 9 and 12 were each the site of mutations in 7 families, and exons 5 and 7 were each the site of mutations in 3 families. Exons 4, 6, 13, and 14 were each the site of one unique mutation in a BHD-affected family. Eight (16%) of the families had mutations in the 5′ half, and 43 (84%) of the families had mutations in the 3′ half of the *BHD* gene.

The most 5′ mutation occurred at nt 513 (c.513delT) in exon 4 (20 aa from the initiation codon) in family 7306 (fig. 2). This frameshift mutation was predicted to truncate the protein 34 aa (missense) downstream. The affected individual in this family developed only BHD skin manifestations, without the other phenotypic features. The most 3′ mutation occurred at nt 2034 (c.2034 C→T) in exon 14 (family 168) and was predicted to produce a premature termination codon at codon 527, eliminating only 52 aa from the full-length protein (fig. 1*b*). Nonetheless, full expression of the BHD phenotype was observed in family 168; three affected members developed renal neoplasia and lung cysts, and one was diagnosed with FF. Interestingly, the other nonsense mutations predicted to produce premature termination codons were located in exon 12 (c.1844C→G and c.1884C→T), also near the 3′ end of the *BHD* gene.

Renal tumors were found in 5 (14%) of the mutation carriers with mutations in the 5′ half of the *BHD* gene and in 30 (86%) of the mutation carriers with mutations in the 3′ half of the *BHD* gene. Renal tumors were present in patients with frameshift mutations (insertion or deletion), nonsense mutations, and splice-site mutations in *BHD*. Of patients with spontaneous pneumothorax, 97% (55/57) inherited mutations in the 3′ half of the *BHD* gene (table 1), and frameshift, nonsense, and splice-junction mutations were represented among those affected individuals.

Genotype-Phenotype Correlation: Mutational Hotspot

The most frequently mutated site in *BHD* was a cytosine insertion or deletion in the C_8 tract of exon 11 (c.1733insC or c.1733delC), identified in 27 BHD-affected families. We estimated the frequency of developing FFs, lung cysts, spontaneous pneumothorax, or renal tumors in BHD-affected family members with the C-insertion mutation compared with those individuals with the C-deletion mutation (fig. 3). A total of 64 individuals carried the C-insertion mutation, and 27 individuals carried the C-deletion mutation. The frequency of histologically proven FFs among those individuals whose lesions were biopsied was similar among C-insertion–mutation carriers (83% [44/53]) and C-deletion–mutation carriers (87% [20/23]). The frequency of pneumothorax episodes was also similar between carriers of C-insertion (37% [23/62]) and C-deletion (35% [9/26]) mutations. Lung cysts were detected on thoracic CT scans in 88% (35/40) of C-insertion–mutation carriers, compared with 77% (13/17) of C-deletion–mutation carriers, which is not significantly different. However, we noted that renal tumors developed in significantly fewer C-deletion–mutation carriers than C-insertion–mutation carriers. Among C-deletion carriers, only 6% (1/16) of those who were evaluated by CT scan (4% [1/26] of those seen at the NIH or in the field) developed renal tumors. By comparison, 33% (13/40) of C-insertion–mutation carriers who were evaluated by CT scan (23% [13/56] of those seen at the NIH or in the field) developed renal tumors ($P = .03$) (fig. 3). The median age (46.5–50 years) of patients with BHD seen at the NIH was similar for men and women with the C-insertion and the C-deletion mutations, and the number of males and females in each mutation group was approximately equal.

Genotype-Phenotype Correlation: Putative Splice-Site Mutation in IVS9

Two apparently unrelated families were found to have a putative splice-site mutation in the *BHD* gene within intron 9, IVS9+2T→G (table 1 and fig. 1*a*). Renal-tumor frequency in the affected members of families 229 and 238 was 3/5 and 3/3, respectively, which raises the possibility that this splice-site mutation might be associated with a higher frequency of renal tumors. A third family (family 242) inherited a different nucleotide change in the same splice-donor site (IVS9+1G→A) and had a renal-tumor frequency of 1/9 (table 1).

Linkage to 17p11.2 without Detectable BHD *Mutation in Two Large Families with BHD*

We screened 61 families with BHD that were affected with histologically proven FFs, and we found germline *BHD* mutations in 51 families. Two additional families, however, showed linkage to chromosome 17p11.2 by

Figure 1 *BHD* mutations in affected families. Sequencing chromatograms of genomic DNA of patients with BHD are shown on the left (the arrow indicates position of nucleotide variation), and family pedigrees are shown on the right. Quadrants within pedigree symbols indicate presence of FFs (*blue*), lung cysts/pneumothorax (*yellow*), and/or renal tumor (*red*) in each family member. WT = wild-type BHD sequence; ND = not determined; diagonal line = deceased. *A,* Mutation in a splice-donor site in intron 9 (IVS9+2T→G) is predicted to cause exon skipping. *B* and *C,* Mutations at c.2034C→T and c.1844C→G encode premature termination codons predicted to truncate the BHD protein. *D,* A 2-bp deletion, c.1126delCA, will cause a shift in the reading frame and lead to a premature stop codon downstream, truncating the BHD protein.

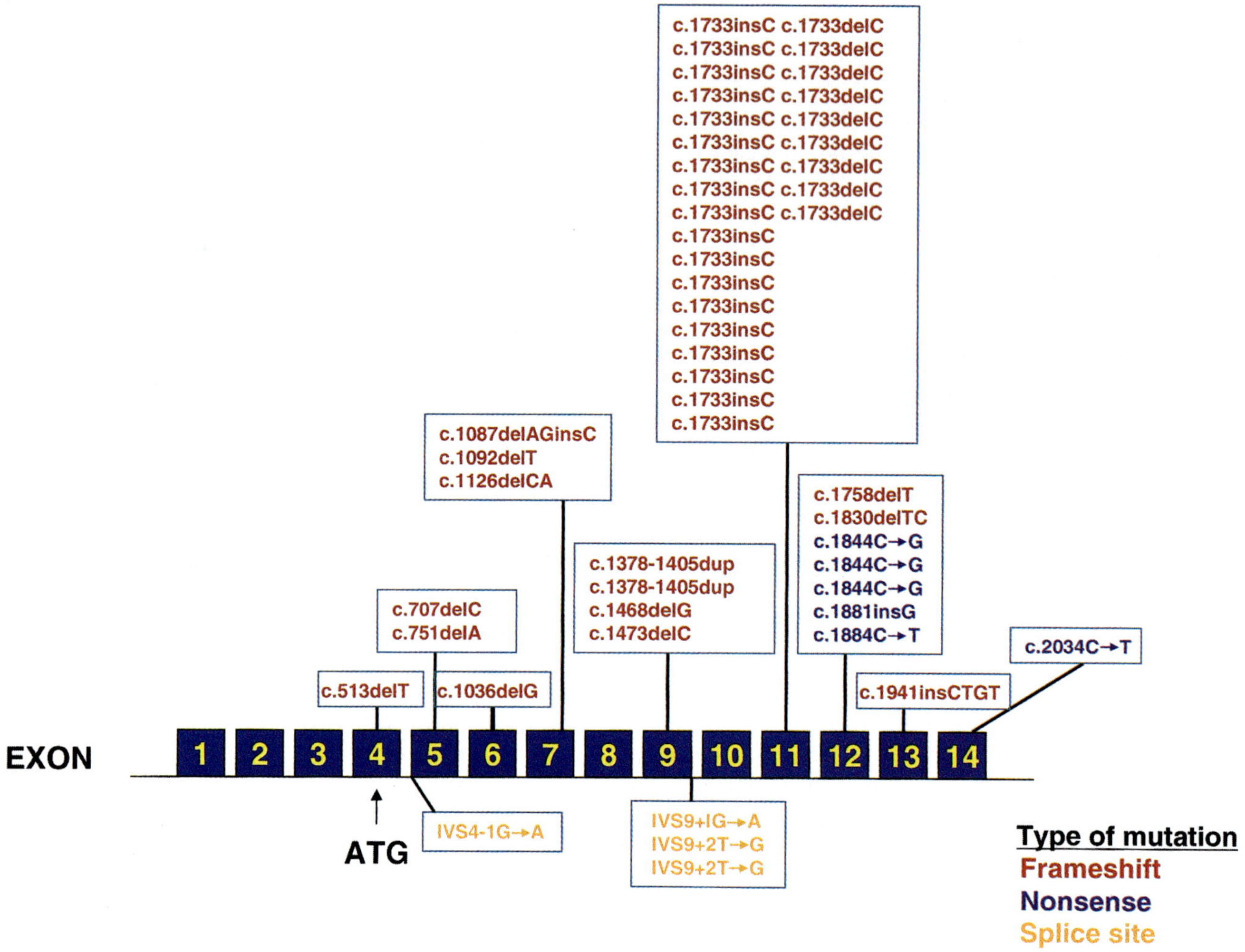

Figure 2 *BHD* exon-intron structure showing the location of germline mutations identified in 51 families with BHD. Frameshift (*red*) and nonsense (*blue*) mutations, predicted to prematurely truncate the BHD protein, were identified along the entire length of the coding region (exons 4–14). Splice-site (*yellow*) mutations predicted to cause exon skipping were identified in introns 4 and 9. The insertion or deletion of a cytosine in a C_8 tract in exon 11 was identified in 27 of 51 families with *BHD* mutations.

haplotype analysis with polymorphic microsatellite markers, but we were unable to detect a sequence variation in the *BHD* gene by direct sequence analysis. Evidence of heterozygosity at a number of informative SNP loci reduced the possibility of intragenic deletion in these families, although this deletion cannot be absolutely ruled out.

Family 172 is the original Canadian family described by Drs. Birt, Hogg, and Dubé (Birt et al. 1977) and was used in linkage analysis studies that identified the BHD-disease locus on 17p11.2 (LOD score 4.98 at marker *D17S740*; $\theta = 0$) (Schmidt et al. 2001). Twenty-five family members had the same BHD-affected haplotype over an 8.5-cM region of chromosome 17p11-12 (Schmidt et al. 2001). However, direct sequencing of the 14 coding exons revealed no *BHD* sequence variation in peripheral-blood DNA from affected members of family 172. All family members whose lesions were biopsied had at least one histologically proven FF; one affected family member developed a renal tumor, and six members had a history of pneumothorax (table 1).

In family 240, a large family with BHD recruited to the NCI study, eight family members were identified with histologically proven FFs (Lindor et al. 2001). Upon genotyping with six polymorphic microsatellite markers flanking the *BHD* locus, from *D17S953* to *D17S1824*, 17 members were found to inherit the BHD-affected haplotype on chromosome 17p11.2 (data not shown). One *BHD*-haplotype carrier had a history of pneumothorax, two developed renal tumors, and four were found, on thoracic CT scan, to have lung cysts (table

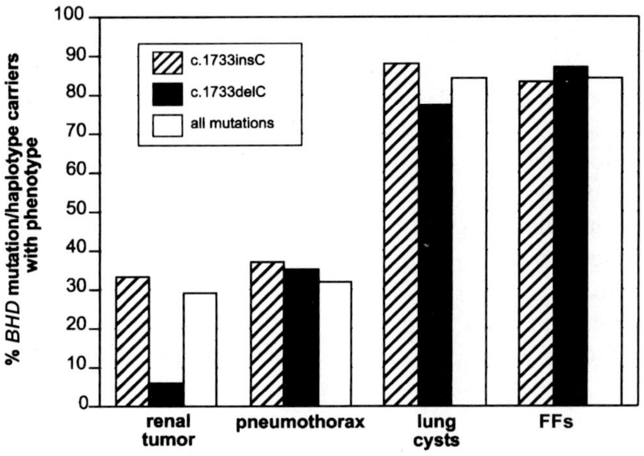

Figure 3 Frequency of BHD phenotypic manifestations in patients with the C-insertion mutation versus the C-deletion mutation in the C_8 tract of exon 11. Patients with the c.1733delC mutation developed renal tumors at a significantly lower frequency than did patients with the c.1733insC mutation ($P = .03$). Hatched bar indicates c.1733insC mutation carriers ($n = 64$); blackened bar indicates c.1733delC mutation carriers ($n = 27$); unblackened bar indicates all *BHD*-mutation/haplotype carriers ($n = 219$), included for comparison. Renal tumors were identified from medical histories, surgical reports, and abdominal CT scans. Spontaneous pneumothorax episodes were determined by patient history and thoracic CT scans. Lung cysts were identified by thoracic CT scans. Skin biopsies were evaluated by a dermatologist for FF-positive histology.

1). Complete sequencing of *BHD* in DNA from affected-haplotype carriers in family 240 did not reveal any sequence variation.

Discussion

In the present study, we completed *BHD*-mutation analysis, by direct sequencing, of 30 families with BHD that were recruited to the NCI. To date, we have identified mutations in 84% (51/61) of all families with BHD who were studied at the NCI, including 16 novel insertion/deletion mutations, 3 nonsense mutations, and 3 putative splice-site mutations. The majority of these mutations were predicted to prematurely terminate folliculin and to result in loss of function, suggesting that *BHD* may act as a tumor-suppressor gene.

These data support other lines of evidence that point to a tumor-suppressor role for *BHD*. The majority of germline *BHD* mutations reported to date are inactivating frameshift and nonsense mutations (Khoo et al. 2002; Nickerson et al. 2002; the present study). Loss of the wild-type *BHD* allele (loss of heterozygosity [LOH] 17%) or somatic frameshift second-hit mutations (53%) were confirmed in 77 BHD-associated renal tumors from kindreds with BHD (Vocke et al., in press), resulting in biallelic inactivation of *BHD*. A novel somatic mutation was identified in a BHD-related chromophobe RCC from an affected member of a family with BHD (Khoo et al. 2002). Additionally, two animal studies of BHD have been described that support a tumor-suppressor function for the BHD protein, the Nihon rat renal cancer model (Okimoto et al. 2000, 2004; Hino et al. 2001) and canine hereditary renal cystadenocarcinoma and nodular dermatofibrosis in the German shepherd (Lium and Moe 1985; Jonasdottir et al. 2000; Lingaas et al. 2003). Germline disease-cosegregating mutations have been identified in the *Bhd* rat and dog orthologs that lead to renal-tumor development in these animal models of BHD. The germline frameshift mutation in the Nihon rat *Bhd* ortholog is predicted to prematurely truncate the encoded protein.

We noted that, among the 53 BHD-affected families, no disease-associated missense mutations in the *BHD* gene were found. One possible explanation is that missense *BHD* mutations that lead to amino acid substitutions may have little or no effect on folliculin function, thereby producing either a mild (undetectable) phenotype or no phenotype at all.

No correlation between BHD phenotype and location of the mutation was found. We found disease-associated mutations along the entire length of the *BHD* gene, within 9 of the 11 coding exons. The location of the mutation did not affect the phenotypic expression of BHD. Renal tumors, lung cysts, spontaneous pneumothorax, and FFs developed in patients with mutations in both the 5′ half and the 3′ half of the gene. Since these mutations were predicted to introduce a premature termination codon, it is most likely that the mutant mRNA transcribed from the genomic DNA of these patients is degraded by nonsense-mediated decay (NMD) (Maquat 2004), a surveillance mechanism that eliminates mRNAs with premature termination codons in all but the last exon of a gene. If NMD effectively eliminates the *BHD* mutant mRNAs, then phenotypic variation among *BHD*-mutation carriers may reflect the efficiency of inactivation of the *BHD* wild-type allele by LOH or somatic mutation in tissues involved in the BHD phenotype. Additionally, genetic or environmental factors may contribute to the variability of BHD phenotypic expression. In support of this idea, the BHD phenotype in patients varies within and between families who harbor the same *BHD* germline mutation but who most likely have different genetic backgrounds and/or environmental exposures.

In an effort to identify genotype-phenotype correlations, we took advantage of the large number of individuals with the c.1733ins/delC mutation in *BHD* and compared the phenotype of patients who harbored the C insertion with patients who inherited the C deletion.

Interestingly, the frequency of renal tumors in C-insertion carriers was significantly greater than the frequency of renal tumors in C-deletion carriers. If mutant *BHD* mRNA were not completely degraded by NMD but were at least partially translated to mutant folliculin, the C-insertion and C-deletion mutations would produce very different aberrant BHD proteins. One could speculate that the residual mutant protein produced in patients with the C-insertion mutation might have a dominant-negative effect and interfere with the wild-type BHD protein function, leading to the development of renal tumors. Alternatively, the residual mutant protein encoded by the C-insertion mutation might predispose kidney cells to form a renal tumor by some as-yet-unknown mechanism.

Among the BHD-affected family members with putative splice-site mutations in intron 9 predicted to cause exon skipping, 7 (40%) of 17 developed renal tumors, a significantly higher frequency than the overall frequency of renal tumors seen in all mutation carriers. It is possible that the aberrant BHD protein produced by exon skipping might predispose to the development of renal tumors by interacting with the wild-type BHD protein and compromising its function. The identification of the incorrectly spliced mutant *BHD* gene product and the study of its functional properties will contribute to our understanding of how mutations in *BHD* lead to renal-tumor development.

Analysis of the *BHD* gene identified mutations in 51 of 53 NCI-study families with BHD who inherited the BHD-affected haplotype; however, we were unable to identify mutations in two of those families by direct sequencing. The BHD-affected haplotypes, which cosegregated with disease in families 172 and 240, were tightly linked to the *BHD* locus on chromosome 17p11.2, and the full BHD phenotype was seen in affected individuals from these two families. Although the entire coding sequence for *BHD* was screened, the 5′ and 3′ regulatory regions and intronic sequences of the gene were not examined for sequence variation that might affect *BHD* expression, and the possibility of a small intragenic deletion cannot be ruled out. Careful evaluation of *BHD* for deletions or sequence variants in regulatory regions of the gene in families 172 and 240 is in progress.

In conclusion, we have completed mutation analysis of the largest cohort of families with BHD reported to date and have identified 22 different germline *BHD* mutations in 84% (51/61) of families recruited to our study. The majority of mutations were predicted to truncate folliculin and most likely lead to a reduction in folliculin expression. Renal tumors, lung cysts, spontaneous pneumothorax, and FFs develop as part of the complex BHD phenotype, with no particular correlation with mutation type or location within the gene.

A mutational hotspot, a C insertion/deletion in exon 11, is frequently mutated in BHD-affected families. Renal tumors developed with a higher frequency in C-insertion carriers than in C-deletion carriers and also more frequently in individuals who inherited a putative splice-site mutation in intron 9. The mechanism by which *BHD* acts as a tumor suppressor and its role in the development of renal tumors, benign skin hamartomas, and lung-wall defects remains to be elucidated, which may not be possible until the BHD protein is characterized. BHD should be considered in the differential diagnosis for patients with renal tumors with or without skin papules and for patients with a family history of spontaneous pneumothorax.

Acknowledgments

We thank the families with BHD for their cooperation and willingness to participate in our study. This publication has been funded in whole or in part by federal funds from the NCI, NIH, under contract N01-C0-12400. The content of this publication does not necessarily reflect the views or policies of the Department of Health and Human Services, nor does mention of trade names, commercial products, or organizations imply endorsement by the U.S. Government.

Electronic-Database Information

Accession numbers and URLs for data presented herein are as follows:

Calculation of Fisher's Exact Test, http://www.unc.edu/~preacher/fisher/fisher.htm

GenBank, http://www.ncbi.nlm.nih.gov/Genbank/ (for *FLCN*, or *BHD* [accession number AF517523; Ref Seq NM_144997], skin melanoma [BC015725 and BC015687], and BAC clone RP11-45M22 [accession number AC055811])

Online Mendelian Inheritance in Man (OMIM), http://www.ncbi.nlm.nih.gov/Omim/ (for BHD and *FLCN*)

References

Binet O, Robin J, Vicart M, Ventura G, Beltzer-Garelly E (1986) Fibromes perfolliculaires, polypose colique familaile, pneumothorax spontanes familiaux. Ann Dermatol Venereol 113: 928–930

Birt AR, Hogg GR, Dubé WJ (1977) Hereditary multiple fibrofolliculomas with trichodiscomas and acrochordons. Arch Dermatol 113:1674–1677

Chung JY, Ramos-Caro FA, Beers B, Ford MJ, Flowers F (1996) Multiple lipomas, angiolipomas, and parathyroid adenomas in a patient with Birt-Hogg-Dubé syndrome. Int J Dermatol 35:365–367

Hino O, Okimoto K, Kouchi M, Sakurai J (2001) A novel renal carcinoma predisposing gene of the Nihon rat maps on chromosome 10. Jpn J Cancer Res 92:1147–1149

Hornstein OP (1976) Generalized dermal perifollicular fibroma with polyps of the colon. Hum Genet 33:193–197

Hornstein OP, Knickenberg M (1975) Perifollicular fibromatosis cutis with polyps of the colon-a cutaneo-intestinal syndrome *sui generis*. Arch Dermatol Res 253:161–175

Jonasdottir TJ, Mellersh CS, Moe L, Heggebo R, Gamlem H, Ostrander EA, Lingaas F (2000) Genetic mapping of a naturally occurring hereditary renal cancer syndrome in dogs. Proc Natl Acad Sci USA 97:4132–4137

Khoo SK, Bradley M, Wong FK, Hedblad M-A, Nordenskjold M, Teh B (2001) Birt-Hogg-Dubé syndrome: mapping of a novel hereditary neoplasia gene to chromosome 17p12-q11.2. Oncogene 20:5239–5242

Khoo SK, Giraud S, Kahnoski K, Chen J, Motorna O, Nickolov R, Binet O, Lambert D, Friedel J, Levy R, Ferlicot S, Wolkenstein P, Hammel P, Bergerheim U, Hedblad M-A, Bradley M, Teh BT, Nordenskjold M, Richard S (2002) Clinical and genetic studies of Birt-Hogg-Dubé syndrome. J Med Genet 39:906–912

Le Guyadec T, Dufau JP, Poulain JF, Vaylet F, Grossin M, Lanternier G (1998) Multiple trichodiscomas associated with colonic polyposis. Ann Dermatol Venereol 125:717–719

Lindor NM, Hand J, Burch PA, Gibson LE (2001) Birt-Hogg-Dubé syndrome: an autosomal dominant disorder with predisposition to cancers of the kidney, fibrofolliculomas, and focal cutaneous mucinosis. Int J Dermatol 40:653–656

Lingaas F, Comstock KE, Kirkness EF, Sorensen A, Aarskaug T, Hitte C, Nickerson ML, Moe L, Schmidt LS, Thomas R, Breen M, Galibert F, Zbar B, Ostrander EA (2003) A mutation in the canine *BHD* gene is associated with hereditary multifocal renal cystadenocarcinoma and nodular dermatofibrosis in the German shepherd dog. Hum Mol Genet 12: 3043–3053

Liu V, Kwan T, Page EH (2000) Parotid oncocytoma in the Birt-Hogg-Dubé syndrome. J Am Acad Dermatol 43:1120–1122

Lium B, Moe L (1985) Hereditary multifocal renal cystadenocarcinomas and nodular dermatofibrosis in the German shepherd dog: macroscopic and histopathologic changes. Vet Pathol 22:447–455

Maquat LE (2004) Nonsense-mediated mRNA decay: splicing, translation and mRNP dynamics. Nat Rev Mol Cell Biol 5: 89–99

Nickerson ML, Warren MB, Toro JR, Matrosova V, Glenn G, Turner ML, Duray P, Merino M, Choyke P, Pavlovich CP, Sharma N, Walther M, Munroe D, Hill R, Maher E, Greenberg C, Lerman MI, Linehan WM, Zbar B, Schmidt LS (2002) Mutations in a novel gene lead to kidney tumors, lung wall defects, and benign tumors of the hair follicle in patients with the Birt-Hogg-Dubé syndrome. Cancer Cell 2:157–164

Okimoto K, Kouchi M, Kikawa E, Toyosawa K, Koujitani T, Tanaka K, Matsuoka N, Sakurai J, Hino (2000) A novel "Nihon" rat model of a Mendelian dominantly inherited renal cell carcinoma. Jpn J Cancer Res 91:1096–1099

Okimoto K, Sakurai J, Kobayashi T, Mitani H, Hirayama Y, Nickerson ML, Warren MB, Zbar B, Schmidt LS, Hino O (2004) A germ-line insertion in the Birt-Hogg-Dubé (*BHD*) gene gives rise to the Nihon rat model of inherited renal cancer. Proc Natl Acad Sci USA 101:2023–2027

Pavlovich CP, Grubb RL 3rd, Hurley K, Glenn GM, Toro J, Schmidt LS, Torres-Cabala C, Merino MJ, Zbar B, Choyke P, Walther MM, Linehan WM (2005) Evaluation and management of renal tumors in the Birt-Hogg-Dubé syndrome. J Urol 173:1482–1486

Pavlovich CP, Walther MM, Eyler RA, Hewitt SM, Zbar B, Linehan WM, Merino MJ (2002) Renal tumors in the Birt-Hogg-Dubé syndrome. Am J Surg Pathol 26:1542–1552

Rongioletti F, Hazini R, Gianotti G, Rebora A (1989) Fibrofolliculomas, trichodiscomas and acrochordons (Birt-Hogg-Dubé) associated with intestinal polyposis. Clin Exp Dermatol 14:72–74

Roth JS, Rabinowitz AD, Benson M, Grossman ME (1993) Bilateral renal cell carcinoma in the Birt-Hogg-Dubé syndrome. J Am Acad Dermatol 29:1055–1056

Schmidt LS, Warren MB, Nickerson ML, Weirich G, Matrosova V, Toro JR, Turner ML, Duray P, Merino M, Hewitt S, Pavlovich CP, Glenn G, Greenberg CR, Linehan WM, Zbar B (2001) Birt-Hogg-Dubé syndrome, a genodermatosis associated with spontaneous pneumothorax and kidney neoplasia, maps to chromosome 17p11.2. Am J Hum Genet 69: 876–882

Streisinger G, Okada Y, Emrich J, Newton J, Tsugita A, Terzaghi E, Inouye M (1966) Frameshift mutations and the genetic code. Cold Spring Harbor Symp Quant Biol 31:77–86

Tickoo SK, Reuter VE, Amin MB, Srigley JR, Epstein JI, Min KW, Rubin MA, Ro JY (1999) Renal oncocytosis: a morphological study of fourteen cases. Am J Surg Pathol 23:1094–1101

Toro JR, Glenn G, Duray P, Darling T, Weirich G, Zbar B, Linehan WM, Turner ML (1999) Birt-Hogg-Dubé syndrome: a novel marker of kidney neoplasia. Arch Dermatol 135: 1195–1202

Vocke C, Yang Y, Pavlovich CP, Schmidt LS, Nickerson ML, Torres-Cabala CA, Merino MJ, Walther MM, Zbar B, Linehan WM. High frequency of somatic frameshift *BHD* gene mutations in Birt-Hogg-Dubé-associated renal tumors. J Natl Cancer Inst (in press)

Warren MB, Torres-Cabala CA, Turner ML, Merino MJ, Matrosova VY, Nickerson ML, Ma W, Linehan WM, Zbar B, Schmidt LS (2004) Expression of Birt-Hogg-Dubé mRNA in normal and neoplastic human tissues. Mod Pathol 17:998–1011

Zbar B, Alvord WG, Glenn G, Turner M, Pavlovich CP, Schmidt L, Walther M, Choyke P, Weirich G, Hewitt SM, Duray P, Gabril F, Greenberg C, Merino MJ, Toro J, Linehan WM (2002) Risk of renal and colonic neoplasms and spontaneous pneumothorax in the Birt-Hogg-Dubé syndrome. Cancer Epidemiol Biomarkers Prev 11:393–400

Am. J. Hum. Genet. 76:1034–1049, 2005

Fatal Congenital Heart Glycogenosis Caused by a Recurrent Activating R531Q Mutation in the γ2-Subunit of AMP-Activated Protein Kinase (*PRKAG2*), Not by Phosphorylase Kinase Deficiency

Barbara Burwinkel,[1,*] John W. Scott,[2] Christoph Bührer,[3,*] Frank K. H. van Landeghem,[4] Gerald F. Cox,[5,*] Callum J. Wilson,[6,*] D. Grahame Hardie,[2] and Manfred W. Kilimann[1,*]

[1]Institut für Physiologische Chemie, Medizinische Fakultät, Ruhr-Universität Bochum, Bochum, Germany; [2]Division of Molecular Physiology, Faculty of Life Sciences, Wellcome Trust Biocentre, University of Dundee, Dundee, United Kingdom; Departments of [3]Neonatology and [4]Neuropathology, Charité Virchow Medical Center, Berlin; [5]Clinical Genetics Program, Children's Hospital, Boston; and [6]Great Ormond Street Hospital for Children, University College London Medical School, London

Fatal congenital nonlysosomal cardiac glycogenosis has been attributed to a subtype of phosphorylase kinase deficiency, but the underlying genes and mutations have not been identified. Analyzing four sporadic, unrelated patients, we found no mutations either in the eight genes encoding phosphorylase kinase subunits or in the two genes encoding the muscle and brain isoforms of glycogen phosphorylase. However, in three of five patients, we identified identical heterozygous R531Q missense mutations of the *PRKAG2* gene, which encodes the γ2-subunit of AMP-activated protein kinase, a key regulator of energy balance. Biochemical characterization of the recombinant R531Q mutant protein showed >100-fold reduction of binding affinities for the regulatory nucleotides AMP and ATP but an enhanced basal activity and increased phosphorylation of the α-subunit. Other *PRKAG2* missense mutations were previously identified in patients with autosomal dominant hypertrophic cardiomyopathy with Wolff-Parkinson-White syndrome, characterized by juvenile-to-adult clinical onset, moderate cardiac glycogenosis, disturbed excitation conduction, risk of sudden cardiac death in midlife, and molecular perturbations that are similar to—but less severe than—those observed for the R531Q mutation. Thus, recurrent heterozygous R531Q missense mutations in *PRKAG2* give rise to a massive nonlysosomal cardiac glycogenosis of fetal symptomatic onset and rapidly fatal course, constituting a genotypically and clinically distinct variant of hypertrophic cardiomyopathy with Wolff-Parkinson-White syndrome. R531Q and other *PRKAG2* mutations enhance the basal activity and α-subunit phosphorylation of AMP-activated protein kinase, explaining the dominant nature of *PRKAG2* disease mutations. Since not all cases displayed *PRKAG2* mutations, fatal congenital nonlysosomal cardiac glycogenosis seems to be genetically heterogeneous. However, the existence of a heart-specific primary phosphorylase kinase deficiency is questionable, because no phosphorylase kinase mutations were found.

Introduction

Glycogen storage diseases (GSDs) with clinically prominent cardiac involvement can be caused by various gene defects. The lysosomal glycogenoses GSD II (Pompe disease [MIM #232300]) (with α-1,4-glucosidase deficiency) and GSD IIb (Danon disease [MIM #300257]) (with lysosome-associated membrane protein 2 [LAMP-2] deficiency) are systemic disorders that also affect either skeletal muscle, smooth muscle, and liver (GSD II) or skeletal muscle and the nervous system (GSD IIb). However, cardiac involvement usually dominates the clinical picture and is life limiting in GSD IIb and in the classic infantile form of GSD II, whereas the adolescent- and adult-onset forms of GSD II are typically governed by muscle involvement. The infantile form of GSD II has an autosomal recessive mode of inheritance, manifests perinatally, and leads to death within the 1st year of life (Hirschhorn and Reuser 2001), whereas GSD IIb can be X-linked dominant or recessive, has a juvenile or early-adult clinical onset, and leads to death, typically during the 2nd to 4th decades of life (Sugie et al. 2002; Arad et al. 2005). There appears to be a distinct third type of lysosomal cardiac and skeletal muscle GSD, with normal α-1,4-glucosidase and LAMP-2, an infantile-fatal course, and an unidentified gene defect (Yamamoto et al. 2001).

Among the nonlysosomal glycogenoses, GSD III (Cori or Forbes disease [MIM +232400]) (with debranching

Received January 31, 2005; accepted for publication April 8, 2005; electronically published May 2, 2005.

Address for correspondence and reprints: Dr. Manfred W. Kilimann, Department of Cell and Molecular Biology, Uppsala University, Box 596, S-75124 Uppsala, Sweden. E-mail: Manfred.kilimann@icm.uu.se

* Present affiliations: Division of Molecular Genetic Epidemiology, German Cancer Research Center (DKFZ), Heidelberg, Germany (B.B.); University Children's Hospital, Basel, Switzerland (C.B.); Genzyme Corporation, Cambridge, MA (G.F.C.); Starship Children's Hospital, Auckland, New Zealand (C.J.W.); and Department of Cell and Molecular Biology, Uppsala University, Uppsala, Sweden (M.W.K.).

0002-9297/2005/7606-0010$15.00

enzyme deficiency) and GSD IV (Andersen disease [MIM #232500]) (with branching enzyme deficiency) are also systemic disorders. Liver and/or (less frequently) muscle involvement usually dominates the clinical picture (Chen 2001). However, patients with prominent cardiac involvement (manifesting during the 1st or 2nd decade of life) have also been reported (Servidei et al. 1987; Lee et al. 1997; Ewert et al. 1999; Chen 2001).

Mutations in the *PRKAG2* gene, encoding the γ2-subunit isoform of AMP-activated protein kinase (AMPK), give rise to a moderate, essentially heart-specific, nonlysosomal glycogenosis with clinical onset typically in late adolescence or in the 3rd decade of life, ventricular preexcitation predisposing to supraventricular arrythmias, mild-to-severe cardiac hypertrophy, enhanced risk of sudden cardiac death in midlife, and autosomal dominant inheritance with full penetrance (familial hypertrophic cardiomyopathy with Wolff-Parkinson-White syndrome [FHC/WPWS {MIM #600858}]) (Blair et al. 2001; Gollob et al. 2001*a*, 2001*b*, 2002; Arad et al. 2002, 2005). The AMPK complex, which acts as a sensor of cellular energy status, is a heterotrimer comprising a catalytic α-subunit and regulatory β- and γ-subunits (Hardie 2003, 2004). The γ-subunits contain four tandem repeats of a sequence motif first recognized by Bateman (1997) and termed a "cystathionine β-synthase" (CBS) motif. These have recently been shown to act in pairs to form two binding sites (now termed "Bateman domains" [Kemp 2004]) for the regulatory nucleotides AMP and ATP (Scott et al. 2004). Binding of AMP (a signal of cellular energy deficiency [Hardie and Hawley 2001]) causes activation of the complex by triggering increased phosphorylation of a specific threonine residue (Thr-172) in the kinase domain on the α-subunit by a distinct upstream kinase, an effect antagonized by high concentrations of the inhibitory nucleotide ATP (Hawley et al. 1996). The major upstream kinase has recently been identified to be the tumor suppressor LKB1 (Hawley et al. 2003; Woods et al. 2003; Shaw et al. 2004). Once activated by cellular stresses that deplete ATP and raise the concentration of AMP, AMPK switches on various ATP-producing catabolic pathways (including glucose uptake and fatty-acid oxidation) and, conversely, down-regulates ATP-consuming processes (Hardie and Hawley 2001; Kemp 2004; Scott et al. 2004). All seven distinct FHC/WPWS mutations in the *PRKAG2* gene identified to date were either heterozygous missense mutations or an insertion of a single amino acid within the Bateman domain region. At least four of the seven mutations have been shown to interfere with binding of the regulatory nucleotides AMP and ATP (Scott et al. 2004) and with activation of the complex by AMP (Daniel and Carling 2002; Scott et al. 2004). However, since these are loss-of-function effects, it has been difficult to explain why these mutations are dominant in vivo.

Rare, sporadic cases of severe prenatal- or neonatal-onset nonlysosomal cardiac glycogenosis—which leads to death within a few weeks to a few months after birth, through heart failure and respiratory compromise—have been attributed to a heart-specific variant of phosphorylase kinase (Phk) deficiency (MIM 261740) (Mizuta et al. 1984; Eishi et al. 1985; Servidei et al. 1988; Elleder et al. 1993; Regalado et al. 1999; Bührer et al. 2003). Phk is a regulatory protein kinase that stimulates glycogen breakdown in response to neural and endocrine signals by phosphorylating and activating the main glycogen-catabolizing enzyme, glycogen phosphorylase. It is composed of four subunits in a hexadecameric complex, $(\alpha\beta\gamma\delta)_4$, in which the δ-subunit is calmodulin, and it exists in numerous isoforms and splice variants. Two distinct genes encoding muscle and liver isoforms occur for both α and γ, a single gene occurs for β, and three genes encode identical calmodulin polypeptides. Genetic deficiency of Phk underlies a group of GSDs that differ in mode of inheritance and tissue involvement, depending on the mutant subunit gene. α_M (*PHKA1*) mutations cause X-linked recessive muscle glycogenosis, α_L (*PHKA2*) mutations cause X-linked recessive liver glycogenosis, β (*PHKB*) mutations give rise to autosomal recessive glycogenosis of both liver and muscle but with an essentially liver-specific clinical phenotype, and γ_{TL} (*PHKG2*) mutations underlie autosomal recessive liver glycogenosis with a particularly severe phenotype and a higher risk of cirrhosis (Kilimann 1997; Chen 2001). No mutations have been identified yet in the γ_M (*PHKG1*) gene, but they would be anticipated to cause an autosomal recessive muscle glycogenosis. A molecular explanation for an infantile-fatal, heart-specific, nonlysosomal glycogenosis with low Phk activity, however, has been lacking. Unlike the other forms of Phk deficiency, in which the tissue specificity of expression of the subunit isoforms provided guidance to the identification of the affected genes, no Phk gene sequences expressed specifically in the heart are known. However, particular missense mutations or genetic backgrounds could give rise to phenotypes of unanticipated tissue specificity, even though more widely expressed gene sequences are affected, as observed in other GSDs (Servidei et al. 1987; Ewert et al. 1999; Ziemssen et al. 2000; Chen 2001).

Here, we report the molecular genetic analysis of a group of sporadic patients with fatal congenital nonlysosomal cardiac glycogenosis and a biochemical diagnosis of cardiac Phk deficiency. The complete coding sequences of all eight genes encoding Phk subunits (including calmodulin) and of the two genes for the muscle and brain isoforms of glycogen phosphorylase were analyzed. When we found no mutations in the Phk or phosphorylase genes, we also analyzed the *PRKAG2* gene. In three of five cases, the disease was associated with a unique, recurrent heterozygous R531Q missense mutation in *PRKAG2*. Biochemical analysis of the recombinant mutant protein revealed stronger perturbations of molecular properties than those of any other *PRKAG2* mutation characterized to date.

Subjects and Methods

Case Reports

Detailed accounts of patients A, B (Regalado et al. 1999), and E (Bührer et al. 2003) have been published elsewhere. In patient A (1200; case 1 in the study by Regalado et al. [1999]), a Hispanic American female, cardiomegaly was detected in utero by ultrasound and echocardiography, and worsening bradycardia prompted cesarean section at 31 wk of gestation. Shortly after birth, the infant developed cardiorespiratory problems requiring intubation. Electrocardiography (ECG) revealed a short PR interval, wide QRS, inverted T waves, and ST elevation. She experienced recurrent cardiac and respiratory complications throughout her hospital course and succumbed at age $2\frac{3}{4}$ mo to ventricular fibrillation. An autopsy 10 h postmortem showed massive cardiomegaly (136 g [normal 21 g]), with biventricular mural thickening and effacement of both chambers. Other notable features were macroglossia, faciocervical dysmorphism, enlarged and dysmorphic kidneys, and an increased number of pancreatic islets. Microscopically, periodic acid Schiff (PAS) stain–positive and amylase-sensitive vacuolar glycogen depositions were seen in heart tissue. Cardiac glycogen concentration was 3.3% (control 0.9%), and cardiac Phk activity was 0.001 U (control 0.34 U). Histological examination revealed no abnormal glycogen deposition in skeletal muscle, tongue, kidneys, spleen, or liver.

Patient B (1877; case 2 in the study by Regalado et al. [1999]), a white American male, was delivered by cesarean section because of breech presentation and nonreassuring heart rate at 37 wk of gestation. He remained ventilator dependent through most of his hospital course, which was characterized by progressive cardiac enlargement (first noted at day 4 by chest X-ray), secondary pulmonary compression, and oral feeding intolerance. Increasing respiratory distress led to death at age 2 mo. An autopsy at 11 h postmortem showed marked cardiomegaly (65 g [normal 24 g ± 5 g]), with biventricular mural thickening and effaced, slitlike chambers. Other notable features were macroglossia and facial dysmorphism, bilateral cataracts, enlarged kidneys, and hydrocephalus. Histological examination revealed abundant vacuolar, PAS-positive, amylase-sensitive glycogen deposition in the heart. Cardiac glycogen was 3.1% (control 0.7%), and cardiac Phk was 0.03 U (control 0.38 U). No histological or histochemical evidence of abnormal glycogen deposition was found in tissues other than the heart.

Patient C (JW), a white American male, was born at full term by cesarean section because of breech presentation. He developed cardiorespiratory failure within 30 min of life and required mechanical ventilation and, ultimately, extracorporeal membrane oxygenation. ECG showed a normal PR interval, no delta wave, low QRS voltages, and prominent ST wave elevations, consistent with ischemia and/or a lateral wall infarct. Echocardiogram revealed severe left ventricular dysfunction without hypertrophy or structural heart disease. His clinical course was complicated by renal failure secondary to hypotension. On day 10, he became less responsive and developed unusual movements. Electroencephalogram revealed a burst suppression pattern and seizure activity, indicating a dismal prognosis. Support was withdrawn, and he died on day 11. An autopsy at 2 h postmortem consisted of limited biopsies of heart, liver, lung, skeletal muscle, and kidney. Gross examination revealed no congenital malformations, but there was pulmonary congestion with bilateral pleural effusions, anasarca, ascites, a right occipital cephalohematoma, and incomplete, broad palmar creases. Light microscopy revealed diffuse vacuolization of the cardiac myofibers, but not of other tissues. Electron microscopy showed abundant non–membrane-bounded glycogen in cardiac myocytes and a slight increase in non–membrane-bounded glycogen in liver. Glycogen concentration was enhanced in the heart (3.2% [control 0.5%]) and was normal in skeletal muscle and liver. Phosphorylase kinase activity was 15% of the control value in heart and 50%–60% of control values in liver and skeletal muscle. Total phosphorylase and debranching enzyme activities were also ~50% of control values in all three tissues. Family history was notable for a previous sister who had died at several hours of life from respiratory failure, despite mechanical ventilation. She had a loud systolic murmur, but no echocardiogram could be obtained. She also had dysmorphic features (flattened occiput, epicanthal folds, and nuchal folds, as well as possible cystic hygroma, single palmar crease, and clinodactyly), hypotonia, and large adrenals (determined by ultrasound). Karyotype was normal, and autopsy was declined. The parents (nonconsanguineous) and two other siblings are unaffected.

Patient D (RB), a white British female, was delivered at 37 wk of gestation by cesarean section because of fetal bradycardia. The parents are nonconsanguineous, and there are two previous healthy children. The baby had problems with feeding, bradycardia, and recurrent apnea in the 1st wk of life. She was not dysmorphic and had normal peripheral power and tone and normal primitive reflexes. There was no hepatomegaly. ECG showed evidence of preventricular hypertrophy with a short PR interval and very large QRS voltages in all leads. Chest X-ray revealed massive cardiomegaly, and echocardiogram confirmed a severe hypertrophic cardiomyopathy.

Despite medical management, she developed progressive cardiac failure with pulmonary edema and hypotension and died at age 34 d. An autopsy at 6 h postmortem showed an extremely hypertrophic heart (124 g [normal 22 g]), which occupied the greater part of the thoracic cavity. The walls of both atria and ventricles appeared diffusely hypertrophic, smooth, and pale. The heart was otherwise anatomically normal. The lungs were edematous, and the liver was congested and focally hemorrhagic but not enlarged; the rest of the postmortem examination was unremarkable. Glycogen concentration was elevated both in heart (2.4%) and in skeletal muscle (2.9%). Phk was at 10% of the normal range mean in liver and at 1% of the normal range mean in muscle and was undetectable in heart, whereas total phosphorylase was in the normal range in all tissues. Branching enzyme was normal in liver and undetectable in muscle. α-Glucosidase in cultured fibroblasts was normal.

Patient E (Bührer et al. 2003), a white male, the first child of healthy nonconsanguineous German/Polish parents, was delivered at 28 wk of gestation by cesarean section after routine ultrasound examination detected persistent bradycardia. Heart rate remained between 90 and 120 beats per min, despite adequate oxygenation. An ECG revealed left-axis deviation, very short PQ intervals (0.06 s), enlarged QRS complexes with delta waves suggestive of WPWS, and depressed ST segments. Echocardiography showed atrial and biventricular hypertrophy without outflow obstruction and a small pericardial effusion. Respiratory distress necessitated mechanical ventilation nearly throughout the infant's life, with the need for supplemental oxygen rising to 100% at day 14. Progressive cardial and pleural effusions, ascites, and pulmonary and peripheral edemas led to death at day 21. An autopsy was performed at 3 h postmortem. Light microscopy demonstrated massive subplasmalemmal, non–membrane-bounded, PAS-positive, and amylase-sensitive glycogen deposits in all tissues analyzed (heart, diaphragm, vastus lateralis muscle, and liver). Biochemically determined glycogen was also enhanced markedly in heart (10.8%) and muscle (6.7%/9.9% [normal 0.5%–2.0%]), and moderately in liver (7.0% [normal 2.0%–6.0%]) and erythrocytes (15 mg/dl [normal 0–10 mg/dl]). Phk activity was undetectable in heart, normal in muscle, slightly below the normal range in liver, and slightly above the normal range in erythrocytes. Phosphorylase-a was moderately below the normal range in heart, muscle, and liver and was normal in white blood cells; total phosphorylase was normal in all samples. α-Glucosidase in leukocytes was normal.

Mutation Analysis

The study was approved by the ethics committee of the University of Bochum Medical School. The complete coding sequences of *PHKA1, PHKA2, PHKB, PHKG1* (except patient C), *CALM1-3,* and *PYGM* were amplified by RT-PCR from total RNA purified from heart or skeletal muscle autopsy samples from patients A–D. The differentially spliced *PHKA1* exons 27 and 28 (phosphorylation sites) and exon 19 ("α′ region") were amplified, together with their flanking intron sequences, from genomic DNA. The *PHKG1* promoter regions (~1 kb) of patients A–D, the coding exons and flanking intron sequences of the *PHKG1* gene of patient C, and the coding exons and flanking intron sequences of the *PHKG2* genes of patients A–D were amplified from genomic DNA. All PCR products were analyzed by direct cycle sequencing with Applied Biosystems reagents and instruments. In addition, the intact overall organization of the *PHKG1* genes of patients A–D was confirmed by bridging the four large introns by overlapping PCRs, and normal lengths of these PCR products were verified by agarose-gel electrophoresis. Mutation analysis of these genes has been described in more technical detail elsewhere: *PHKA1, PHKB, PHKG1, CALM1-3,* and *PYGM* (Burwinkel et al. 2003); *PHKA2* (Burwinkel et al. 1996); and *PHKG2* (Burwinkel et al. 1998). The *PYGB* coding sequences of patients A–D were amplified from total RNA (heart or skeletal muscle) in five overlapping intervals between −30 nt upstream of the start codon and +43 nt downstream of the stop codon. The *PRKAG2* coding sequences of patients A–E were amplified by RT-PCR from RNA (2 + 1 overlapping intervals for the long splice variant and 1 + 1 intervals for the short splice variant) as well as by PCR from genomic DNA, and the PCR products were sequenced. Mutations were independently confirmed from RNA and genomic DNA.

Expression and Mutagenesis of AMPK Domains and Subunits and Their Analysis

Isolated Bateman domains from AMPK-γ2 were expressed as glutathione-S-transferase (GST) fusions in bacteria, and heterotrimeric AMPK complexes were expressed in mammalian cells as described elsewhere (Scott et al. 2004). All mutations were created using the QuikChange Site-Directed Mutagenesis system (Stratagene). Binding of nucleotides and assays of AMPK were performed as described elsewhere (Scott et al. 2004). Phosphorylation of Thr-172 on AMPK-α and of the AMPK phosphorylation site on acetyl-CoA carboxylase (ACC) was monitored with phosphospecific antibodies by use of an infrared scanner, as described elsewhere (Hawley et al. 2003).

Results

No Mutations in Phk and Glycogen Phosphorylase Genes

No Phk isoform genes or differentially spliced exons are known to be specifically expressed in the heart. There-

Table 1

Mutation Analysis of Five Patients with Fatal Congenital Nonlysosomal Heart Glycogenosis and Low Phk Activity

	Variant(s) Found in Patient				
Gene	A[a]	B[b]	C[b]	D[a]	E[b]
PHKA1	...	...	...	...	NA
PHKA2	...	hemi. E38Q[c]	...	...	NA
PHKB	...	...	...	...	NA
PHKG1 + promoter	...	...	...	...	NA
PHKG2	...	...	...	...	NA
CALM1	...	...	...	...	NA
CALM2	...	...	...	...	NA
CALM3	...	...	...	...	NA
PYGM	het. G21S[d], het. R414G[e]	...	...	...	NA
PYGB	...	...	het. A303S[f], het. D502N[g]	het. A303S, het. D502N	NA
PRKAG2	het. R531Q[h]	...	...	het. R531Q[h]	het. R531Q[h]

Note.—Only nonsynonymous sequence variants are given. Numerous synonymous and intronic SNPs were also encountered; ellipses indicate that no nonsynonymous sequence variants were found; hemi. = hemizygous (*PHKA2* is X chromosomal); het. = heterozygous; NA = not analyzed.

[a] Female.

[b] Male.

[c] Polymorphism (GAG→CAG; 112G→C): frequency 0.025; three heterozygotes and one homozygote found in 200 mostly female control chromosomes (in the present study).

[d] Rare or unique sequence variant (GGC→AGC; 61G→A), not found in 200 control chromosomes analyzed (in the present study).

[e] Known polymorphism (CGG→GGG; 1240C→G) (dbSNP accession number rs11231866).

[f] Known polymorphism (GCC→TCC; 907G→T) (dbSNP accession number rs3818199).

[g] Known polymorphism (GAT→AAT; 1504G→A) (dbSNP accession number rs2227891); S303 and N502 seem to be on the same allele, since they cosegregate in family C with each other and with adjacent intronic polymorphisms and are also found in the same constellation in patient D.

[h] Identical in patients A, D, and E (CGG→CAG; 1592G→A).

fore, the mutation search could not be targeted directly to heart-specific Phk sequences. The muscle and liver isoform mRNAs of the α- and γ-subunits are coexpressed in comparable amounts in the heart, as are the three calmodulin genes (*CALM1-3*) and the muscle (*PYGM*) and brain (*PYGB*) isoforms of glycogen phosphorylase (Kilimann 1997). A search of the current genome and EST sequence databases, as well as our own experimental investigations (Burwinkel et al. 2003; the present study [data not shown]), did not indicate the existence of additional functional Phk subunit isoform genes or splice variants. To account for the possibility that, for example, certain missense mutations might affect the stability of—or functional interactions within—the cardiac isoform constellation of the Phk/phosphorylase protein complex in an unanticipated, heart-specific, and possibly dominant negative way, we analyzed the complete coding sequences of 10 candidate genes from patients A–D. However, we found no mutations or splicing abnormalities (table 1 [see the note to table 1 and the "Discussion" section for further comment]).

A Recurrent R531Q Mutation in the PRKAG2 *Gene of Three Patients*

FHC/WPWS is a cardiac glycogenosis with familial occurrence and a much less dramatic clinical manifestation than that of our patient group. However, to see whether our subjects might represent a particularly severe variant of FHC/WPWS that is possibly associated with a distinctive genotype, we analyzed the *PRKAG2* gene. In patients A and D, and in the newly recruited patient E, we found identical, heterozygous R531Q missense mutations (fig. 1). Parental DNA was available only for patient E, but the R531Q mutation could be detected in neither the mother nor the father, indicating that it was a de novo mutation. This sequence variant was not found in 190 control chromosomes.

Electron microscopy of cardiac tissue from the R531Q-mutation–positive patient E showed massive, subsarcolemmal, and intermyofibrillar deposition of nonlysosomal β-glycogen within enlarged myocytes (fig. 2). Glycogen rosettes (α particles) could not be detected. Sarcomeres were often multifocally destroyed, and some fibers were totally degenerated. However, large amylopectinlike polysaccharide aggregates, as reported in adult patients with FHC/WPWS and *PRKAG2* mutations (Arad et al. 2002), were not observed.

Biochemical Characterization of the Mutant Protein

The R531Q mutation severely impairs AMP and ATP binding by the γ2-subunit.—Among the previously characterized mutations, the most pronounced functional consequences—both molecular (Daniel and Carling 2002; Scott et al. 2004) and clinical—are associated with a dif-

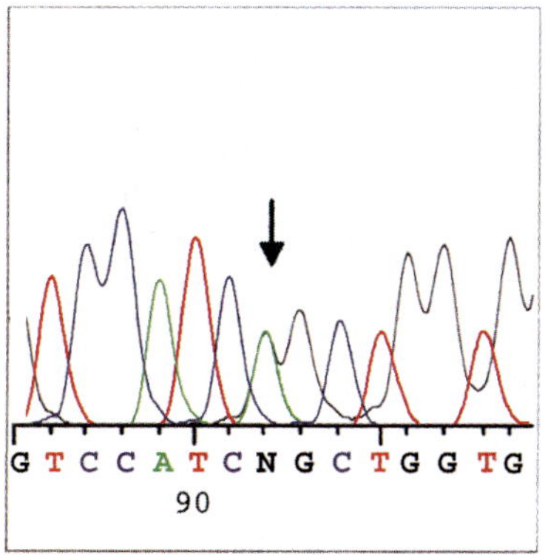

				531			
A	E	V	H	**R**	L	V	V
GCT	GAG	GTC	CAT	CGG	CTG	GTG	GTG
GCT	GAG	GTC	CAT	C**A**G	CTG	GTG	GTG
A	E	V	H	**Q**	L	V	V

Hs	PRKAG2	CBS4	RAEVH**R**LVVVNEAD
Hs	PRKAG1	CBS4	EAEVH**R**LVVVNEAD
Hs	PRKAG3	CBS4	REQVH**R**LVLVDETQ
Pig	PRKAG3	CBS4	REQVH**R**LVLVDETQ
Dros	Snf4A	CBS4	RAEVH**R**LVVVDENR
Yeast	Snf4	CBS4	KARVH**R**FFVVDDVG

Hs	PRKAG2	CBS4	RAEVH**R**LVVVNEAD	R531G	Gollob et al. 2001*b*
Hs	PRKAG2	CBS1	VANGV**R**AAPLWESK	R302Q	Gollob et al. 2001*a*
Hs	PRKAG2	CBS2	KNKI**HR**L-PVIDPI	H383R	Blair et al. 2001
Pig	PRKAG3	CBS1	VANGV**R**AAPLWDSK	R225Q	Milan et al. 2000

Figure 1 Heterozygous R531Q missense mutation underlying fatal congenital nonlysosomal heart glycogenosis. A typical sequencer readout is shown (*top*). The high conservation of the mutant R531 residue is illustrated (*middle*) by alignments with the corresponding partial sequences from CBS4 of the human ("Hs") $\gamma 1$ and $\gamma 3$ isoforms, pig $\gamma 3$, and the *Drosophila* ("Dros") and yeast AMPK paralogs. Alignments with partial sequences from other CBS domains of $\gamma 2$ and $\gamma 3$, in which mutations were identified in the corresponding arginine residues or the adjacent histidine residue, are shown (*bottom*). In the course of analysis of the *PRKAG2* gene and cDNA, the following additional sequence features were noted: (1) RT-PCR product sequences displayed partial deletion of codon 251 (apparently leaky splicing) at the beginning of exon 6 in all five patients and a normal control individual and (2) SNPs include CDS-26C→T (allele frequencies: C, 0.89; T, 0.11 [n = 190]), Ex6+36insA (allele frequency: A, 0.83 [n = 12]), and Ex10-42C→T (allele frequencies: C, 0.83; T, 0.17 [n = 12]).

ferent replacement in the same amino acid position (R531G), indicating that arginine 531 is of particular importance. The R531G-positive patient displayed severe arrhythmia since the age of 2 years but was still alive at age 43 years (Gollob et al. 2001*b*). We therefore employed the R531G mutant protein as an internal reference in the biochemical experiments of the present study.

Binding of AMP and ATP was measured in vitro to GST fusion proteins containing Bateman domains A and B (GST-A/B [residues 274–569, CBS motifs 1–4]) or Bateman domain B only (GST-B [residues 430–556, CBS motifs 3–4]) of human $\gamma 2$ (Scott et al. 2004), with either the normal arginine-531 residue, the R531Q mutation, or the R531G mutation (fig. 3 and table 2). The GST-B protein with the normal $\gamma 2$ sequence bound one molecule of the activating nucleotide, AMP, and the affinity was reduced 16-fold by the R531G mutation, confirming previous findings (Scott et al. 2004). The R531Q mutation reduced the affinity for AMP even further (66-fold). The mutations also reduced the affinity for the inhibitory nucleotide ATP, and again the effect of R531Q (23-fold) was stronger than that of R531G (4.5-fold). The wild-type fusion protein containing both Bateman domains (GST-A/B) bound two molecules of AMP with high affinity and strong positive cooperativity, as observed previously (Scott et al. 2004). When the data were fitted to a two-site Hill plot model, the concentration giving half-maximal binding ($B_{0.5}$) was 71 μM, and the Hill coefficient (h) was 1.8. The R531G mutant also bound two molecules of AMP with positive cooperativity but with a $B_{0.5}$ of 2.3 mM, 33-fold higher than that for the wild type. The effect of the R531Q mutation was even more extreme, with a >100-fold increase in $B_{0.5}$ and a loss of cooperativity (h = 0.7). The loss of cooperative binding is evident from the much lower slope of the semilogarithmic plot in figure 3C. The results for ATP binding were analogous. Whereas the R531G mutation caused a 6-fold increase in the $B_{0.5}$ for ATP but retained

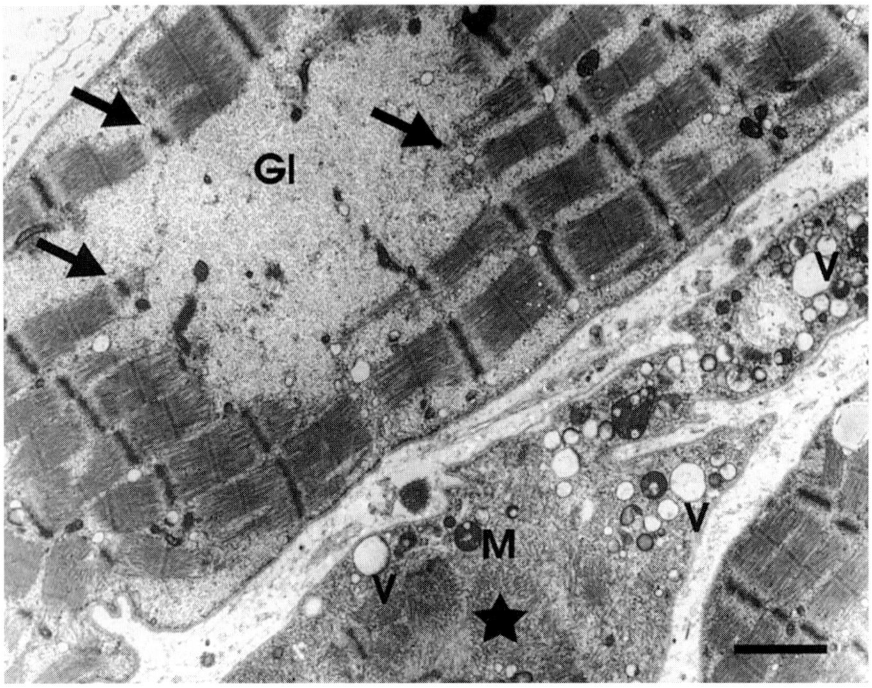

Figure 2 Image from electron microscopy of glycogen storage in myocardial fibers of R531Q-mutation–positive patient E. Large amounts of free monodispersed β-glycogen ("Gl") accumulate between the myofibrils and beneath the sarcolemma. Many sarcomeres appear to be destroyed (*arrows*), and some fibers are totally degenerated (*star*). In most mitochondria ("M"), solitary vacuoles and electron-dense, thickened, and disoriented cristae can be observed. Numerous endomembranaceous vacuoles ("V"), some of them containing lipid, are seen in fibers with advanced degeneration (*star*). The scale bar is 1 μm.

cooperativity, with the R531Q mutation, the effect was >200-fold, and cooperativity was lost.

The R531Q and R531G mutations abolish AMP activation of the holoenzyme.—To assess the effect of the R531Q mutation on AMP activation of the AMPK holoenzyme, we expressed the wild-type, R531G-mutant, and R531Q-mutant proteins of γ2 in HEK-293 cells, together with *myc*-tagged α1 and β1. The recombinant complexes were immunoprecipitated using anti-*myc* antibodies prior to assay. Extracts initially were made using a "slow lysis" procedure that involves scraping the cells off the culture plate, centrifuging them down, and resuspending them in lysis buffer. This procedure is known to cause maximal phosphorylation of Thr-172 on the α-subunit, because of undefined stresses occurring during the cell harvesting (Daniel and Carling 2002), and it allowed the effects of the mutations on allosteric activation by AMP to be observed independent of effects on phosphorylation. As observed elsewhere (Scott et al. 2004), the wild-type α1β1γ2 complex was activated 4-fold by AMP, with a half-maximal effect ($A_{0.5}$) at 19 μM ± 11 μM (fig. 4). However, neither the R531G nor the R531Q mutant was activated significantly by AMP up to the maximal concentration of 100 μM (fig. 4), consistent with the strongly reduced binding affinity of these mutants for AMP (fig. 3). Instead, both mutants were slightly inhibited by AMP, which may be due to competition of AMP with ATP at the catalytic site on the kinase domain. The higher AMP affinity of holoenzyme activation, as compared with AMP binding to the isolated Bateman domain construct GST-A/B, confirms previous findings (Scott et al. 2004) and suggests that the integration of the Bateman domains into the holoenzyme context enhances nucleotide affinity.

The R531Q and R531G mutations increase the basal phosphorylation and activity of AMPK.—We next compared the activities (in the absence of AMP) of recombinant α1β1γ2 complexes that were prepared from HEK-293 cells by the "rapid" and "slow" lysis procedures (fig. 5*A*). The rapid lysis procedure involves lysing the cells in situ on the culture plate, and we believe that it preserves the phosphorylation status of AMPK that existed in the intact cells better than does the slow lysis procedure (Daniel and Carling 2002). Compared with the wild type, there was a significant increase (2.3-fold) in the basal activity (measured after rapid lysis) of the R531G mutant and an even greater increase (3.5-fold) in that of the R531Q mutant. Both mutants were further activated by the slow lysis procedure, but relatively less so than the wild-type enzyme, such that, after slow lysis, the activities of all three were similar. The increased basal activities of the R531G and R531Q mutants, as well as

Table 2

Binding Parameters for AMP and ATP Measured with Wild-Type, R531G-Mutant, and R531Q-Mutant GST Fusion Proteins Containing Bateman Domain(s) B or A/B

Fusion Type and Protein	N^a	AMP K_d or $B_{0.5}$[b]	AMP h	ATP K_d or $B_{0.5}$[b]	ATP h
GST-B:					
WT	1	97 ± 7	...	396 ± 34	...
R531G	1	1,570 ± 120	...	1,790 ± 130	...
R531Q	1	6,400 ± 380	...	9,150 ± 140	
GST-A/B:					
WT	2	71 ± 5	1.8 ± .2	239 ± 12	1.8 ± .2
R531G	2	2,340 ± 220	1.4 ± .2	1,350 ± 66	2.9 ± .3
R531Q	2	7,320 ± 490	.7 ± .1	53,000 ± 15,000	.5 ± .1

NOTE.—WT = wild type.

[a] N = number of binding sites assumed per protein molecule.

[b] All values (in μM) are shown as mean ± SE of the mean. If a single binding site is assumed ($N = 1$), the data were fitted to a simple binding equation $Y = L/(K_d+L)$, where "Y" represents fractional saturation and "L" represents ligand concentration; the value given in this column is K_d. Where two binding sites are assumed ($N = 2$), the data were fitted to the Hill equation, $Y = 2 \times L^h/(B_{0.5}{}^h+L^h)$, and the value given in this column is $B_{0.5}$ (i.e., the concentration of ligand that gives half-maximal binding).

the further increase after slow lysis, correlated with an increased phosphorylation of Thr-172 on the α-subunit (fig. 5*B*) and an increased phosphorylation of the downstream target, ACC (fig. 5*C*).

Discussion

A Recurrent R531Q Missense Mutation in PRKAG2 *Causes a Severe Congenital, Rapidly Fatal, Nonlysosomal Heart Glycogenosis*

The present study identifies, for the first time, a molecular cause of congenital, rapidly fatal, nonlysosomal cardiac glycogenosis. Strikingly, we found three identical but independent heterozygous R531Q missense mutations in *PRKAG2,* in three of the five sporadic cases, all from diverse geographic origins. These findings extend the clinical spectrum of *PRKAG2* mutations toward a very severe manifestation characterized by fetal onset (prenatal bradycardia was noted in all three patients, prompting preterm delivery by cesarean section, and prenatal cardiomegaly was noted in one patient), extreme cardiomegaly, and an infantile-fatal outcome. The R531Q-positive patients died of hemodynamic and respiratory failure secondary to hypertrophic nonobstructive cardiomyopathy but also had WPWS-like conduction anomalies. In patients with classic juvenile-/adult-onset FHC/WPWS, arrhythmia usually dominates the clinical picture (also in the few reported patients with symptomatic onset in early childhood [Blair et al. 2001; Gollob et al. 2001*b*]), and these patients virtually always survive into reproductive age. It will be of interest to investigate whether other *PRKAG2* mutations associated with intermediate phenotypes can be found among children with hypertrophic cardiomyopathy and electrophysiological abnormalities (Strauss and Lock 2003; Arad et al. 2005). The phenotypes of the three R531Q-positive infants were very uniform, and there was no other *PRKAG2* mutation in our group of five patients. Conversely, the R531Q mutation has never been reported in patients with classic FHC/WPWS, despite its tendency to arise recurrently, like the R302Q mutation in classic FHC/WPWS (see below). In accordance with this strict, mutually exclusive correlation between genotype and clinical phenotype, the molecular abnormalities of the R531Q mutant protein are more pronounced than those of any other *PRKAG2* mutants characterized to date. Hence, the R531Q mutation by itself appears to be sufficient to cause the distinctive, very severe phenotype of its carriers, and neither the additional sequence variants (mostly polymorphisms) in the *PYGM* and *PYGB* genes of patients A and D (table 1) nor other, unidentified elements of genetic background need to be invoked.

All R531Q-positive infants were sporadic cases, and analysis of the parents of patient E showed that R531Q was a newly arisen mutation in this family (the only family available for analysis). Given the complete penetrance of *PRKAG2* mutations even in the less-severe, juvenile-/adult-onset FHC/WPWS, this suggests that R531Q mutations invariably cause an infantile-fatal disease, are therefore not passed on by their carriers, and always occur de novo. At the nucleotide level, these mutations are G→A replacements in a CpG context (fig. 1), which are known to occur at least 13-fold more frequently than other single-nucleotide replacements in the CG dinucleotide (Antonarakis et al. 2001). An identical replacement in the analogous position of the first CBS

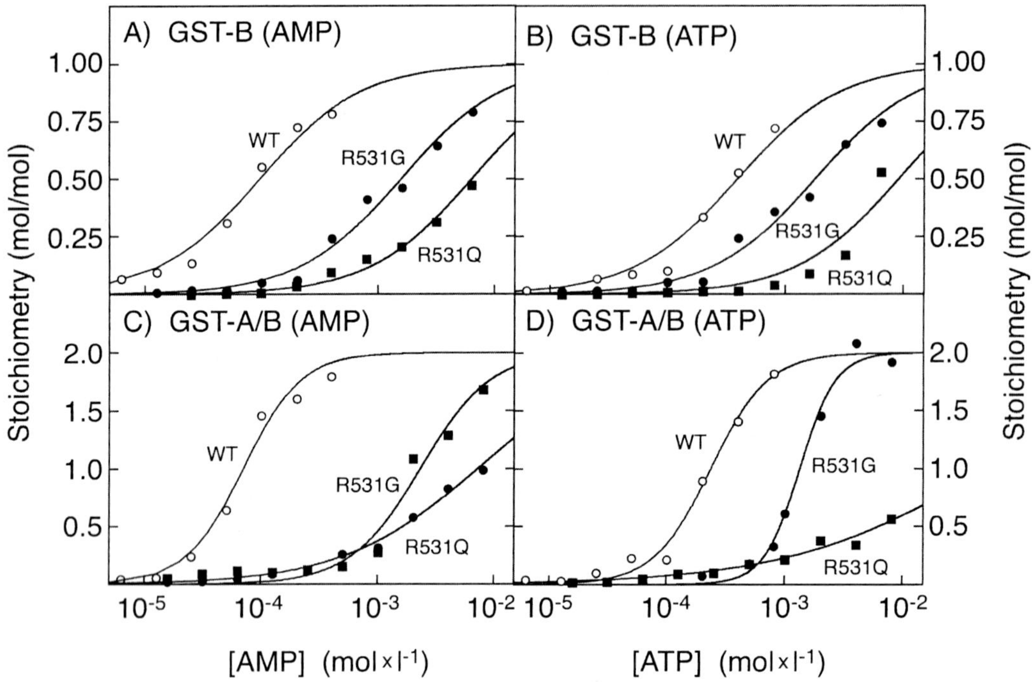

Figure 3 Binding of AMP (*panels A* and *C*) and ATP (*panels B* and *D*) by fusion proteins between GST and the Bateman domain B of γ2 ("GST-B" [*panels A* and *B*]) or between GST and both Bateman domains ("GST-A/B" [*panels C* and *D*]). In panels A and B, data were fitted to the binding model: $Y = L/(K_d+L)$. In panels C and D, data were fitted to a two-site Hill plot model: $Y = 2 \times L^h/(B_{0.5}{}^h + L^h)$. "$Y$" represents fractional saturation, "L" represents ligand concentration, "$B_{0.5}$" is the concentration of nucleotide that gives half-maximal binding, and "h" is the Hill coefficient. Best-fit parameters were estimated using GraphPad Prism (GraphPad software), and the curves were generated using the equation with those binding parameters.

motif (arginine 531 is in the fourth CBS motif), R302Q (fig. 1), is the most common *PRKAG2* mutation and has also arisen recurrently but is associated with milder clinical and molecular phenotypes (Gollob et al. 2001*a*, 2002; Arad et al. 2002; Daniel and Carling 2002; Scott et al. 2004). The occurrence of the R531Q mutation in a large proportion of cases with prenatal- or neonatal-onset severe nonlysosomal cardiac GSD offers a rapid, noninvasive diagnostic test in this fatal condition, and its apparently obligate de novo occurrence has corresponding implications for genetic counseling.

The clinical manifestation of *PRKAG2* mutations is restricted to the heart. However, the γ2-subunit of AMPK is expressed in many tissues, and, even in the heart, it does not appear to be the predominant isoform, at least in rodents (Cheung et al. 2000; Mahlapuu et al. 2003). In patients with the severe R531Q mutation, glycogen accumulation was indeed seen in tissues other than the heart (patients D and E [see the "Case Reports" section]). Detailed examination can also reveal glycogen accumulation in noncardiac tissues in adult patients with FHC/WPWS and with milder *PRKAG2* mutations (Murphy et al. 2005), and the systemic hypertension observed in two kindreds with FHC/WPWS (Gollob et al. 2001*a*, 2001*b*) may likewise be an extracardial manifestation. Specific aspects of the role of AMPK in cardiac metabolic physiology, however, may cause a particularly pronounced accumulation of glycogen in the heart.

The pronounced heart glycogenosis observed in patients with the R531Q mutation strengthens the view that glycogen storage is the primary pathological consequence of *PRKAG2* mutations and that the conduction defects are secondary to this. This was first proposed after histological investigation of heart tissues of patients with FHC/WPWS and was corroborated by studies of transgenic mice overexpressing the N488I mutant of γ2 (Arad et al. 2002, 2003). The mice displayed massive cardiac glycogen deposition, ventricular pre-excitation, and an infiltration of the annulus fibrosus, which normally insulates the atria from the ventricles, by glycogen-filled myocytes. It was proposed that this infiltration gives rise to microscopic atrioventricular connections and causes the conduction abnormalities in these mice, in human patients with *PRKAG2* mutations, and similarly also in patients with other cardiac glycogenoses (GSD II, GSD IIb, and GSD III) (Arad et al. 2002; Gollob et al. 2002).

The glycogen that accumulates in the cardiomyocytes of individuals with *PRKAG2* mutations may in part be of abnormal structure. In the hearts of five adult patients

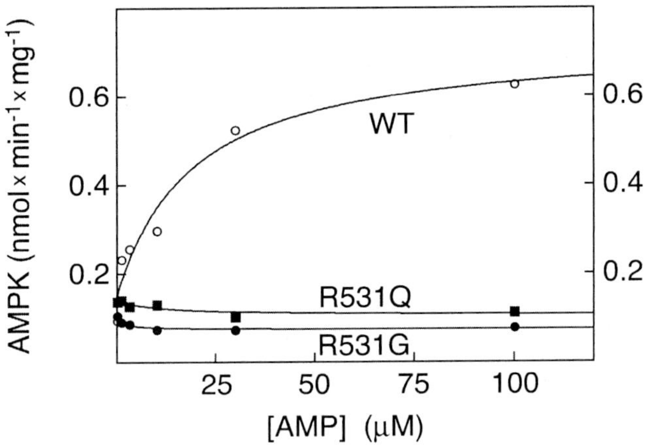

Figure 4 Activation of heterotrimeric $\alpha1\beta1\gamma2$ complexes expressed in HEK-293 cells, with extracts made using the slow lysis procedure that causes maximal phosphorylation (Hardie et al. 2000). The complexes contained either wild-type ("WT") $\gamma2$ or R531G and R531Q mutations of $\gamma2$ and were assayed in anti-*myc* immunoprecipitates at various concentrations of AMP. Data were fitted to the following equation: activity = basal + $\frac{[(\text{stimulation} \times \text{basal}) - \text{basal}] \times [\text{AMP}]}{A_{0.5}+[\text{AMP}]}$, where "basal" is the activity in the absence of AMP, "stimulation" is the maximal stimulation by AMP, and "$A_{0.5}$" is the concentration of AMP that gives half-maximal activation. Best-fit parameters were estimated, and curves were generated as for figure 3.

with three different *PRKAG2* mutations, Arad et al. (2002) found large, amorphous, amylase-resistant amylopectinlike polysaccharide aggregates, similar to those observed in patients with GSD IV. It is conceivable that the perturbation of AMPK function by these mutations directly or indirectly upsets the balance of the different enzyme activities that participate in glycogen synthesis and degradation and thus affects the structure of the branched glycogen polymer. However, in R531Q-mutation–positive patients A and E, the glycogen deposits were amylase sensitive (amylase was not applied in case D), and electron microscopy of the cardiac tissue of patient E (fig. 2) revealed normal glycogen β particles, with no evidence of the aggregates seen by Arad et al. (2002). Neither were abnormal polysaccharide aggregates reported in the hearts of transgenic mice overexpressing the FHC/WPWS mutation N488I, although these mice developed massive cardiac glycogenosis (Arad et al. 2003). The amylase-resistant molecular variant may be a minor side product, inert to physiological turnover, of the patients' perturbed glycogen metabolism. It may accumulate only over the course of years or decades, and therefore it may be apparent only in adult patients.

Genetic Heterogeneity of Fatal Congenital Nonlysosomal Heart Glycogenosis

No mutations were found in patients B and C, either in *PRKAG2* or in the Phk and phosphorylase genes. The hemizygous E38Q replacement in the *PHKA2* gene of patient B is a polymorphism also found in controls (in both hetero- and homozygous constellations), and the heterozygous A303S and D502N replacements in the *PYGB* gene of patient C are common polymorphisms also detectable in his healthy parents (see the note to table 1). It remains to be seen whether the two *PRKAG2* mutation–negative subjects are mutant in novel disease genes or whether they represent unusually severe manifestations of mutations in one of the other genes known to give rise to GSDs involving the heart. Their *PHKA2* and *PYGB* polymorphisms might have mild functional consequences that aggravate the manifestation of a principal defect in another gene or influence its tissue specificity (Hansen et al. 1995; Westphal et al. 2002).

When the phenotypes of the three R531Q-positive subjects are compared with each other, with the two mutation-negative subjects, and with the three first-published cases of infantile-fatal nonlysosomal heart glycogenosis with low Phk activity and undefined genotype (Mizuta et al. 1984; Eishi et al. 1985; Servidei et al. 1988; Elleder et al. 1993), they all appear very similar. All but patient C display extreme cardiomegaly (heart weights 2.7–6.5-fold greater than normal), onset of cardiac or respiratory distress from before birth to within the first weeks of life, and death between age 3 wk and age 5 mo. The R531Q-negative patient C is set apart by a particularly malignant course and short lifespan (11 d), neurological symptoms, no WPWS-like ECG features or cardiomegaly, and a family history suggestive of autosomal recessive inheritance, probably reflecting a different genetic etiology of his condition.

The Existence of a Heart-Specific Primary Phk Deficiency Is Doubtful

Low-to-zero Phk enzyme activities were determined in heart autopsy samples from all five patients studied here, leading to their tentative identification as heart-specific Phk deficiency, an entity described previously (Mizuta et al. 1984; Eishi et al. 1985; Servidei et al. 1988; Elleder et al. 1993). However, we found no mutations or splicing abnormalities in three of the four patients whose Phk genes were analyzed, and the hemizygous E38Q replacement in the *PHKA2* gene of the fourth patient is an innocuous polymorphism. We cannot exclude unusual mutation types not covered by our approach (such as a mutation in a transcription factor binding site affecting expression specifically in the heart), but it appears most likely that the low Phk activities in our patient group—and possibly in autopsy samples from infantile-fatal heart glycogenosis cases, in general—either are of secondary nature or are artifacts. AMPK is not believed to regulate Phk directly, but it is plausible that, in a metabolic status causing massive gly-

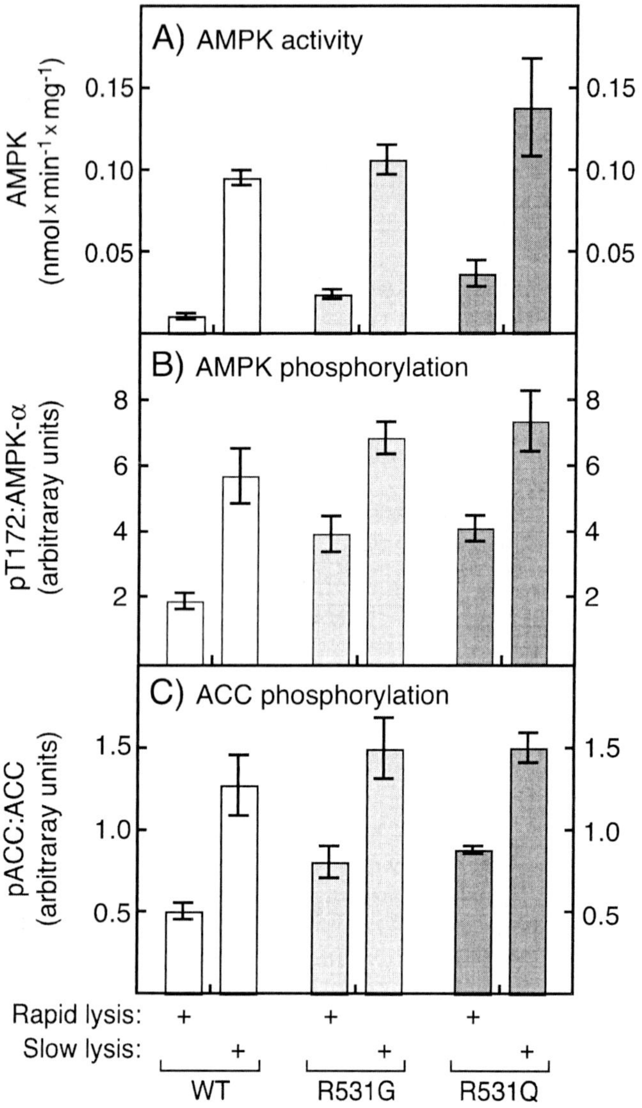

Figure 5 AMPK activity (*A*), phosphorylation of Thr-172 on the AMPK α-subunit (*B*), and phosphorylation of the downstream target ACC (*C*) in HEK-293 cells expressing heterotrimeric α1β1γ2 complexes, with or without γ2 mutations, as in figure 4. Cells were harvested by both the rapid and the slow lysis procedures, and AMPK activities were measured in anti-*myc* immunoprecipitates in the absence of AMP. Data are means ± SE of the mean, for results from duplicate culture plates.

cogen deposition, the activity or expression of Phk is down-regulated, so that low Phk activities in these cases may be authentic but secondary. It is noteworthy that, also in most patients with skeletal muscle glycogenosis and low Phk activity, we could not detect mutations either in Phk subunits or in PRKAG3 (the skeletal muscle isoform of the AMPK γ-subunit that is mutated in a mild muscle glycogenosis in pigs [Milan et al. 2000]) (Burwinkel et al. 2003). Phk is a notoriously unstable enzyme. In striated muscle tissues, it may be particularly sensitive to inactivation (e.g., by dephosphorylation or proteolysis). This could occur in vivo (i.e., in myopathic tissue chronically damaged by another primary defect) or after sampling (for further discussion, see the study by Burwinkel et al. [2003]). In the cardiac cases, in particular, samples were always obtained through autopsy several hours postmortem and would be particularly vulnerable to dephosphorylation or degradation.

The R531Q and R531G Mutations Reduce the AMP and ATP Affinities but Enhance the Basal Activity and Phosphorylation of AMPK

All seven previously identified mutations in the γ2 gene that cause FHC/WPWS occur in the Bateman domain region (Gollob et al. 2002; Oliveira et al. 2003). Three of them (R302Q, R531G, and H383R) affect residues in (R302Q and R531G) or adjacent to (H383R) equivalent positions in the first, second, and fourth CBS motifs (fig. 1). These, together with a fourth mutation (T400N), cause defects in the binding of AMP and ATP to isolated Bateman domains, as well as defects in activation of the α1β1γ2 complexes by AMP (Daniel and Carling 2002; Scott et al. 2004). A fifth mutation that inserts a leucine residue between the first and second CBS motif has only a weak effect, if any, on these parameters (Daniel and Carling 2002; Scott et al. 2004), and the remaining two (Y487H and N488I) have not yet been tested. On the basis of structural modeling of the Bateman domains from γ2, we have proposed that the basic residues affected by the mutations are involved with binding of the phosphate group of AMP (Scott et al. 2004). Of the five PRKAG2 mutants previously tested, the R531G mutation caused the most severe defect in the binding of AMP and ATP to the GST fusion containing both Bateman domains (Scott et al. 2004), as well as the most severe defect in AMP activation of the intact heterotrimeric complex (Daniel and Carling 2002; Scott et al. 2004). Here, we show that the R531Q mutation causes even more severe defects in the binding of AMP and, especially, ATP. Binding of AMP or ATP to the construct containing both Bateman domains is highly cooperative ($h = 2$), indicating that one of the sites is inaccessible to AMP until the nucleotide is bound to the other site. One explanation of the severe nature of mutations in Bateman domain B (R531G and R531Q) may be that this is the domain that binds the nucleotides first, so that mutations in this domain impair the binding of *both* molecules of the nucleotide. The R531Q mutation additionally reduces or abolishes the cooperative interactions between the two binding sites. The extension of our knowledge of Bateman domain mutations also has implications for the understanding of other Bateman domain–containing proteins, including several proteins involved in hereditary disorders, as well as for the design of drugs that target AMPK, for example, in type 2 diabetes (Kemp 2004; Scott et al. 2004).

Most, if not all, *PRKAG2* mutations impair or abolish activation of the AMPK complex by AMP (i.e., they cause a loss of function). However, a loss-of-function mechanism is hard to reconcile with the dominant nature of these mutations, especially given a background of one wild-type $\gamma2$ allele plus the coexpressed $\gamma1$ isoform (under the assumption that the AMPK holoenzyme is an $\alpha\beta\gamma$ heterotrimer with no potential for dominant negative interactions between mutant and wild-type γ-subunits within a single holoenzyme complex). Arad et al. (2002) suggested, on the basis of equivalent mutations in the budding yeast homologue of the AMPK γ-subunits (Snf4), that two of the mutations (T400N and N488I) caused constitutive activation of the AMPK complex. Direct analysis of γ mutant proteins in mammalian cells has yielded conflicting results. Coexpression of an R70Q mutant in $\gamma1$ (equivalent to the R302Q mutant in $\gamma2$) with $\alpha1$ and $\beta1$ in COS7 cells was reported to cause an increase in basal phosphorylation and activity of AMPK (Hamilton et al. 2001). Also, the coexpression of the R225Q mutant of $\gamma3$ (equivalent to R70Q in $\gamma1$ and to R302Q in $\gamma2$ [see fig. 1]) with $\alpha2$ and $\beta2$ in COS cells led to an increase in basal activity and α-subunit phosphorylation (Barnes et al. 2004). Results from studies of transgenic mice overexpressing either the R225Q mutant $\gamma3$-subunit in skeletal muscle (Barnes et al. 2004) or the N488I mutant γ-subunit in the heart (Arad et al. 2003) also indicated increases in the basal activities of the mutant, compared with the wild-type enzymes. In contrast to these results, analysis of four (Daniel and Carling 2002) or five (Scott et al. 2004) FHC/WPWS mutations in human $\gamma2$, which are coexpressed with $\alpha1$ and $\gamma1$ in CCL13 cells, exhibited reduced or absent activation by AMP but no evidence of an increase in the basal activity.

In the present study, we have reinvestigated the effect of the R531G mutation (as well as the R531Q mutation) on AMPK activity by studying expression in HEK-293, instead of CCL13, cells. Although the R531G and R531Q mutations both completely abolished AMP activation of the AMPK complex (fig. 4), they also caused an increase in the basal phosphorylation and activity of the heterotrimeric AMPK complex, determined using the rapid lysis method that we believe preserves the phosphorylation state (fig. 5). The latter was not observed in two previous studies of the R531G mutant (Daniel and Carling 2002; Scott et al. 2004), but this can now be ascribed to the use of CCL13 cells. Although originally derived from human liver (Chang 1954), the CCL13 cells available from the American Type Culture Collection are now thought to have resulted from contamination with HeLa cells (see the American Type Culture Collection Web site). Unlike HEK-293 cells, HeLa cells do not express the major upstream kinase for AMPK (i.e., LKB1) (Hawley et al. 2003), and we have now verified that CCL13 cells do not express LKB1 either (data not shown). We also confirmed (data not shown) that the increase in basal phosphorylation and activity, caused by the R531G and R531Q mutations when coexpressed with $\alpha1$ and $\beta1$ in HEK-293 cells, is not observed upon expression in HeLa cells. Thus, the increased basal phosphorylation is observed only in cells expressing LKB1.

How can an increase in basal AMPK activity lead to glycogen storage? Activation of AMPK increases glucose uptake by causing acute activation or translocation, as well as increased expression, of both GLUT1 and GLUT4 (Hayashi et al. 1998; Kurth-Kraczek et al. 1999; Barnes et al. 2002; Fryer et al. 2002) in several tissues, including the heart (Russell et al. 1999). Although AMPK also phosphorylates the muscle isoform of glycogen synthase both in cell-free assays (Carling and Hardie 1989) and in vivo (Jørgensen et al. 2004) at a site that causes inactivation of the enzyme (Flotow and Roach 1989), the inactivation caused by phosphorylation at this site is overridden by high concentrations of the allosteric activator, glucose-6-phosphate (Flotow and Roach 1989). Increased glucose uptake caused by an elevated basal activity of AMPK over an extended period, in the absence of a proportional increase in consumption of glucose, may cause increased intracellular glucose-6-phosphate, leading to persistent allosteric activation of glycogen synthase and inhibition of glycogen phosphorylase. Increased glycogen content in the hearts of transgenic mice overexpressing wild-type $\gamma2$ (Arad et al. 2003) and reduced glycogen resynthesis in skeletal muscles of $\gamma3$-knockout mice after exercise (Barnes et al. 2004) also indicate that AMPK activity enhances glycogen synthesis; these data support the view that *PRKAG2* disease mutations cause glycogen storage through basal activation of AMPK.

Correlations between Genotype, Molecular Properties, and Clinical Manifestation

The molecular properties of the mutant AMPK proteins can, in general terms, be correlated with their biological effects: the increase in the basal phosphorylation and activity of AMPK caused by disease mutations in *PRKAG2* explains the dominant, gain-of-function–like character of these mutations, and the R531Q mutation is associated with both the most severe clinical phenotype and the most severe molecular abnormalities of all known *PRKAG2* mutations. Yet, on closer inspection, we are left with paradoxes that indicate that we are still far from a coherent understanding of the molecular mechanisms of AMPK and of its physiology and pathophysiology in the heart; the particular severity of the R531Q mutation highlights these gaps in understanding.

Concerning the gain- versus loss-of-function issue, it remains striking that most disease-causing mutations have a specific impact on AMP and ATP affinity and occur very selectively—and even recurrently (R302Q and R531Q)—in strategic positions within the CBS motifs or in linker sequences between the motifs. In contrast, no mutations have been found in other parts of the γ-subunit or in the α- or β-subunits (Oliveira et al. 2003). This indicates a specific connection between nucleotide binding and the pathological effects of these mutations. However, it is believed that the phosphorylation of the α-subunit at Thr-172 occurs subsequent to AMP binding. It is therefore unclear how the observed increase of phosphorylation and basal activity in the rapid lysis cell culture system is brought about if the mutant proteins cannot bind AMP at physiological concentrations. This contradiction might be resolved if the mutations not only reduced nucleotide affinity but also simultaneously were "AMP-mimetic" (i.e., if they induced a more active conformation of the Bateman domains, even when no AMP is bound).

Of all the *PRKAG2* mutations characterized to date, R531Q has the strongest effect on nucleotide binding and basal activation, but there is no abrupt transition in the nature of the molecular impacts between the R531G and R531Q mutations (figs. 3, 4, and 5). In contrast, the clinical phenotype of patients with R531Q is dramatically more severe than that of patients with the other mutations associated with classic FHC/WPWS, including R531G. The two patient groups differ strikingly in terms of (1) age at onset, course, and outcome; (2) degree of cardiomegaly; (3) the fact that hemodynamic and respiratory failure, as opposed to arrhythmia and conduction anomalies, dominate the clinical picture; and (4) in sporadic versus familial occurrence reflecting the profound difference in survival. It is possible that the molecular parameter in which the R531Q protein differs most markedly from the other mutants—and which most faithfully correlates with the biological impact of *PRKAG2* mutations in general—has not yet been characterized. In this context, the R109insL mutation is also of interest, because it only slightly affects AMP binding (Scott et al. 2004) but still results in a severe adult phenotype (Blair et al. 2001); it may affect a mechanistic step between AMP binding and basal activation.

There are two known molecular effects in which R531Q is indeed unique among the *PRKAG2* mutations characterized to date: it abolishes the cooperativity of nucleotide binding, and it has a particularly large impact on ATP binding. The latter effect makes the R531Q mutant the only $\gamma2$ mutant protein that is probably unoccupied by either AMP or ATP under in vivo conditions, whereas the wild type and the other mutant $\gamma2$-subunits are predicted to be occupied by ATP under resting conditions. The R531Q-mutant $\gamma2$-subunit, unoccupied by ATP, might be in a partially active conformation. If this is correct, AMPK might be regarded an "ATP-inhibited" as much as an "AMP-activated" kinase. Another aspect that deserves consideration is the highly cooperative, "ultrasensitive" response of AMPK, through which a small increase in the AMP:ATP ratio over a critical range of concentrations can translate into a strong activation of AMPK (Hardie et al. 1999). Shifting this narrow "window of sensitivity" to different degrees by different mutations could thus lead to profoundly nonlinear consequences. Also, the overexpression of the wild type and the N488I mutant $\gamma2$-subunits at similar levels in transgenic mice led to a much more severe phenotype in the N488I mice (Arad et al. 2003). All these observations suggest that the underlying pathomechanism is a form of AMPK dysregulation specifically connected with its interaction with AMP and ATP, which subsequently leads to an increase of basal phosphorylation and activity by the upstream kinase. However, the detailed molecular mechanisms linking the two phenomena remain to be fully elucidated.

Acknowledgments

We thank J. J. Regalado (Miami) and V. Worthington, A. W. Bates, and J. V. Leonard (London), for their contributions to the procurement and analysis of human specimens, and D. Carling, for the original plasmids encoding AMPK subunits. This work was supported by grants from the Deutsche Forschungsgemeinschaft (Ki 324/11), the University of Bochum Medical School intramural research grant program (FoRUM), and the Fonds der Chemischen Industrie (to M.W.K.), as well as by Research and Technological Development contract QLG1-CT-2001-01488 from the European Commission and a program grant from the Wellcome Trust (to D.G.H.). Tissue samples from patients A and B were obtained from the University of Miami Brain and Tissue Bank for Developmental Disorders, which is funded by National Institutes of Health contract NO1-HD-8-3284.

Electronic-Database Information

Accession numbers and URLs for data presented herein are as follows:

American Type Culture Collection, http://www.atcc.org/

dbSNP, http://www.ncbi.nlm.nih.gov/SNP/ (for 1240C→G [accession number rs11231866], 907G→T [accession number rs3818199], and 1504G→A [accession number rs2227891])

Online Mendelian Inheritance in Man (OMIM), http://www.ncbi.nlm.nih.gov/Omim/ (for Pompe disease, Danon disease, Cori or Forbes disease, Andersen disease, FHC/WPWS, and Phk deficiency)

References

Antonarakis SE, Krawczak M, Cooper DN (2001) The nature and mechanisms of human gene mutation. In: Scriver CR, Beaudet AL, Sly WS, Valle D (eds) The metabolic and molecular bases of inherited disease, 8th ed. McGraw-Hill, New York, pp 343–377

Arad M, Benson DW, Perez-Atayde AR, McKenna WJ, Sparks EA, Kanter RJ, McGarry K, Seidman JG, Seidman CE (2002) Constitutively active AMP kinase mutations cause glycogen storage disease mimicking hypertrophic cardiomyopathy. J Clin Invest 109:357–362

Arad M, Maron BJ, Gorham JM, Johnson WH Jr, Saul JP, Perez-Atayde AR, Spirito P, Wright GB, Kanter RJ, Seidman CE, Seidman JG (2005) Glycogen storage diseases presenting as hypertrophic cardiomyopathy. N Engl J Med 352:362–372

Arad M, Moskowitz IP, Patel VV, Ahmad F, Perez-Atayde AR, Sawyer DB, Walter M, Li GH, Burgon PG, Maguire CT, Stapleton D, Schmitt JP, Guo XX, Pizard A, Kupershmidt S, Roden DM, Berul CI, Seidman CE, Seidman JG (2003) Transgenic mice overexpressing mutant PRKAG2 define the cause of Wolff-Parkinson-White syndrome in glycogen storage cardiomyopathy. Circulation 107:2850–2856

Barnes BR, Marklund S, Steiler TL, Walter M, Hjalm G, Amarger V, Mahlapuu M, Leng, Y, Johansson C, Galuska D, Lindgren K, Abrink M, Stapleton D, Zierath JR, Andersson L (2004) The 5′-AMP-activated protein kinase $\gamma 3$ isoform has a key role in carbohydrate and lipid metabolism in glycolytic skeletal muscle. J Biol Chem 279:38441–38447

Barnes K, Ingram JC, Porras OH, Barros LF, Hudson ER, Fryer LG, Foufelle F, Carling D, Hardie DG, Baldwin SA (2002) Activation of GLUT1 by metabolic and osmotic stress: potential involvement of AMP-activated protein kinase (AMPK). J Cell Sci 115:2433–2442

Bateman A (1997) The structure of a domain common to archaebacteria and the homocystinuria disease protein. Trends Biochem Sci 22:12–13

Blair E, Redwood C, Ashrafian H, Oliveira M, Broxholme J, Kerr B, Salmon A, Ostman-Smith I, Watkins H (2001) Mutations in the $\gamma 2$ subunit of AMP-activated protein kinase cause familial hypertrophic cardiomyopathy: evidence for the central role of energy compromise in disease pathogenesis. Hum Mol Genet 10:1215–1220

Bührer C, van Landeghem FKH, Felderhoff-Mueser U, Stadelmann C, Obladen M (2003) Fetal bradycardia at 28 weeks of gestation associated with cardiac glycogen phosphorylase b kinase deficiency. Acta Paediatr 92:1352–1353

Burwinkel B, Hu B, Schroers A, Clemens PR, Moses SW, Shin YS, Pongratz D, Vorgerd M, Kilimann MW (2003) Muscle glycogenosis with low phosphorylase kinase activity: mutations in *PHKA1, PHKG1* or six other candidate genes explain only a minority of cases. Eur J Hum Genet 11:516–526

Burwinkel B, Shin YS, Bakker HD, Deutsch J, Lozano MJ, Maire I, Kilimann MW (1996) Mutation hotspots in the *PHKA2* gene in X-linked liver glycogenosis due to phosphorylase kinase deficiency with atypical activity in blood cells (XLG2). Hum Mol Genet 5:653–658

Burwinkel B, Shiomi S, Al-Zaben A, Kilimann MW (1998) Liver glycogenosis due to phosphorylase kinase deficiency: *PHKG2* gene structure and mutations associated with cirrhosis. Hum Mol Genet 7:149–154

Carling D, Hardie DG (1989) The substrate and sequence specificity of the AMP-activated protein kinase: phosphorylation of glycogen synthase and phosphorylase kinase. Biochim Biophys Acta 1012:81–86

Chang RS (1954) Continuous subcultivation of epithelial-like cells from normal human tissues. Proc Soc Exp Biol Med 87:440–443

Chen YT (2001) Glycogen storage diseases. In: Scriver CR, Beaudet AL, Sly WS, Valle D (eds) The metabolic and molecular bases of inherited disease, 8th ed. McGraw-Hill, New York, pp 1521–1551

Cheung PCF, Salt IP, Davies SP, Hardie DG, Carling D (2000) Characterization of AMP-activated protein kinase γ subunit isoforms and their role in AMP binding. Biochem J 346: 659–669

Daniel TD, Carling D (2002) Functional analysis of mutations in the $\gamma 2$ subunit of AMP-activated protein kinase associated with cardiac hypertrophy and Wolff-Parkinson-White syndrome. J Biol Chem 277:51017–51024

Eishi Y, Takemura T, Sone R, Yamamura H, Narisawa K, Ichinohasama R, Tanaka M, Hatakeyama S (1985) Glycogen storage disease confined to the heart with deficient activity of cardiac phosphorylase kinase: a new type of glycogen storage disease. Hum Pathol 16:193–197

Elleder M, Shin YS, Zuntova A, Vojtovic P, Chalupecki V (1993) Fatal infantile hypertrophic cardiomyopathy secondary to deficiency of heart specific phosphorylase b kinase. Virchows Archiv A Pathol Anat 423:303–307

Ewert R, Gulijew A, Wensel R, Dandel M, Hummel M, Vogel M, Meyer R, Hetzer R (1999) Glycogenosis type IV as a seldom cause of cardiomyopathy. Z Kardiol 88:850–856

Flotow H, Roach PJ (1989) Synergistic phosphorylation of rabbit muscle glycogen synthase by cyclic AMP-dependent protein kinase and casein kinase I: implications for hormonal regulation of glycogen synthase. J Biol Chem 264: 9126–9128

Fryer LG, Foufelle F, Barnes K, Baldwin SA, Woods A, Carling D (2002) Characterization of the role of the AMP-activated protein kinase in the stimulation of glucose transport in skeletal muscle cells. Biochem J 363:167–174

Gollob MH, Green MS, Tang ASL, Gollob T, Karibe A, Hassan AS, Ahmad F, Lozado R, Shah G, Fananapazir L, Bachinski LL, Roberts R (2001*a*) Identification of a gene responsible for familial Wolff-Parkinson-White syndrome. N Engl J Med 344:1823–1831

Gollob MH, Green MS, Tang ASL, Roberts R (2002) PRKAG2 cardiac syndrome: familial ventricular preexcitation, conduction system disease, and cardiac hypertrophy. Curr Opin Cardiol 17:229–234

Gollob MH, Seger JJ, Gollob TN, Tapscott T, Gonzales O, Bachinski L, Roberts R (2001*b*) Novel PRKAG2 mutation responsible for the genetic syndrome of ventricular preexcitation and conduction system disease with childhood onset and absence of cardiac hypertrophy. Circulation 104:3030–3033

Hamilton SR, Stapleton D, O'Donnell JB, Kung JT, Dalal SR, Kemp BE, Witters LA (2001) An activating mutation in the γ1 subunit of the AMP-activated protein kinase. FEBS Lett 500:163–168

Hansen L, Hansen T, Vestergaard H, Björbaek C, Echwald SM, Clausen JO, Chen YH, Chen MX, Cohen PTW, Pedersen O (1995) A widespread amino acid polymorphism at codon 905 of the glycogen-associated regulatory subunit of protein phosphatase-1 is associated with insulin resistance and hypersecretion of insulin. Hum Mol Genet 4:1313–1320

Hardie DG (2003) Minireview: the AMP-activated protein kinase cascade: the key sensor of cellular energy status. Endocrinology 144:5179–5183

——— (2004) The AMP-activated protein kinase pathway—new players upstream and downstream. J Cell Sci 117:5479–5487

Hardie DG, Hawley SA (2001) AMP-activated protein kinase: the energy charge hypothesis revisited. BioEssays 23:1112–1119

Hardie DG, Salt IP, Davies SP (2000) Analysis of the role of the AMP-activated protein kinase in the response to cellular stress. Methods Mol Biol 99:63–75

Hardie DG, Salt IP, Hawley SA, Davies SP (1999) AMP-activated protein kinase: an ultrasensitive system for monitoring cellular energy charge. Biochem J 338:717–722

Hawley SA, Boudeau J, Reid JL, Mustard KJ, Udd L, Makela TP, Alessi DR, Hardie DG (2003) Complexes between the LKB1 tumor suppressor, STRADa/b and MO25a/b are upstream kinases in the AMP-activated protein kinase cascade. J Biol 2:28

Hawley SA, Davison M, Woods A, Davies SP, Beri RK, Carling D, Hardie DG (1996) Characterization of the AMP-activated protein kinase kinase from rat liver, and identification of threonine-172 as the major site at which it phosphorylates and activates AMP-activated protein kinase. J Biol Chem 271:27879–27887

Hayashi T, Hirshman MF, Kurth EJ, Winder WW, Goodyear LJ (1998) Evidence for 5′ AMP-activated protein kinase mediation of the effect of muscle contraction on glucose transport. Diabetes 47:1369–1373

Hirschhorn R, Reuser AJJ (2001) Glycogen storage disease type II: acid α-glucosidase (acid maltase) deficiency. In: Scriver CR, Beaudet AL, Sly WS, Valle D (eds) The metabolic and molecular bases of inherited disease, 8th ed. McGraw-Hill, New York, pp 3389–3420

Jørgensen SB, Nielsen JN, Birk JB, Olsen GS, Viollet B, Andreelli F, Schjerling P, Vaulont S, Hardie DG, Hansen BF, Richter EA, Wojtaszewski JF (2004) The α2-5′AMP-activated protein kinase is a site 2 skeletal muscle glycogen synthase kinase in skeletal muscle and is responsive to glucose loading. Diabetes 53:3074–3081

Kemp BE (2004) Bateman domains and adenosine derivatives form a binding contract. J Clin Invest 113:182–184

Kilimann MW (1997) Glycogen storage disease due to phosphorylase kinase deficiency. In: Swallow DM, Edwards YH (eds) Protein dysfunction in human genetic disease. Bios Scientific Publishers, Oxford, United Kingdom, pp 57–75

Kurth-Kraczek EJ, Hirshman MF, Goodyear LJ, Winder WW (1999) 5′ AMP-activated protein kinase activation causes GLUT4 translocation in skeletal muscle. Diabetes 48:1667–1671

Lee PJ, Deanfield JE, Burch M, Baig K, McKenna WJ, Leonard JV (1997) Comparison of the functional significance of left ventricular hypertrophy in hypertrophic cardiomyopathy and glycogenosis type III. Amer J Cardiol 79:834–838

Mahlapuu M, Johansson C, Lindgren K, Hjälm G, Barnes BR, Krook A, Zierath JR, Andersson L, Marklund S (2003) Expression profiling of the γ-subunit isoforms of AMP-activated protein kinase suggests a major role for γ3 in white skeletal muscle. Am J Physiol Endocrinol Metab 286:E194–E200

Milan D, Jeon JT, Looft C, Amarger V, Robic A, Thelander M, Rogel-Gaillard C, Paul S, Iannuccelli N, Rask L, Ronne H, Lundström K, Reinsch N, Gellin J, Kalm E, Roy PL, Chardon P, Andersson L (2000) A mutation in PRKAG3 associated with excess glycogen content in pig skeletal muscle. Science 288:1248–1251

Mizuta K, Hashimoto E, Tsutou A, Eishi Y, Takemura T, Narisawa K, Yamamura H (1984) A new type of glycogen storage disease caused by deficiency of cardiac phosphorylase kinase. Biochem Biophys Res Commun 119:582–587

Murphy RT, Mogensen J, McGarry K, Bahl A, Evans A, Osman E, Syrris P, Gorman G, Farrell M, Holton JL, Hanna MG, Hughes S, Elliot PM, Macrae CA, McKenna WJ (2005) Adenosine monophosphate-activated protein kinase disease mimicks hypertrophic cardiomyopathy and Wolff-Parkinson-White syndrome: natural history. J Am Coll Cardiol 45:922–930

Oliveira SMJ, Ehtisham J, Redwood CS, Ostman-Smith I, Blair EM, Watkins H (2003) Mutation analysis of AMP-activated protein kinase subunits in inherited cardiomyopathies: implications for kinase function and disease pathogenesis. J Mol Cell Cardiol 35:1251–1255.

Regalado JJ, Rodriguez MM, Ferrer PL (1999) Infantile hypertrophic cardiomyopathy of glycogenosis type IX: isolated cardiac phosphorylase kinase deficiency. Pediatr Cardiol 20: 304–307

Russell RR, Bergeron R, Shulman GI, Young LH (1999) Translocation of myocardial GLUT-4 and increased glucose uptake through activation of AMPK by AICAR. Am J Physiol 277:H643–H649

Scott JW, Hawley SA, Green KA, Anis M, Stewart G, Scullion GA, Norman DG, Hardie DG (2004) CBS domains form energy-sensing modules whose binding of adenosine ligands is disrupted by disease mutations. J Clin Invest 113:274–284

Servidei S, Metlay LA, Chodosh J, DiMauro S (1988) Fatal infantile cardiopathy caused by phosphorylase b kinase deficiency. J Pediatr 113:82–85

Servidei S, Riepe RE, Langston C, Tani LY, Bricker JT, Crisp-Lindgren N, Travers H, Armstrong D, DiMauro S (1987) Severe cardiopathy in branching enzyme deficiency. J Pediatr 111:51–56

Shaw RJ, Kosmatka M, Bardeesy N, Hurley RL, Witters LA, DePinho RA, Cantley LC (2004). The tumor suppressor LKB1 kinase directly activates AMP-activated kinase and regulates apoptosis in response to energy stress. Proc Natl Acad Sci USA 101:3329–3335

Strauss A, Lock JE (2003) Pediatric cardiomyopathy—a long way to go. N Engl J Med 348:1703–1705

Sugie K, Yamamoto A, Murayama K, Oh SJ, Takahashi M, Mora M, Riggs JE, Colomer J, Iturriaga C, Meloni A, Lamperti C, Saitoh S, Byrne E, DiMauro S, Nonaka I, Hirano

M, Nishino I (2002) Clinicopathological features of genetically confirmed Danon disease. Neurology 58:1773–1778

Westphal V, Kjaergaard S, Schollen E, Martens K, Grunewald S, Schwartz M, Matthijs G, Freeze HH (2002) A frequent mild mutation in ALG6 may exacerbate the clinical severity of patients with congenital disorder of glycosylation Ia (CDG-Ia) caused by phosphomannomutase deficiency. Hum Mol Genet 11:599–604

Woods A, Johnstone SR, Dickerson K, Leiper FC, Fryer LG, Neumann D, Schlattner U, Wallimann T, Carlson M, Carling D (2003) LKB1 is the upstream kinase in the AMP-activated protein kinase cascade. Curr Biol 13:2004–2008

Yamamoto A, Morisawa Y, Verloes A, Murakami N, Hirano M, Nonaka I, Nishino I (2001) Infantile autophagic vacuolar myopathy is distinct from Danon disease. Neurology 57:903–905

Ziemssen F, Sindern E, Schröder JM, Shin YS, Zange J, Kilimann MW, Malin JP, Vorgerd M (2000) Novel missense mutations in the glycogen-branching enzyme gene in adult polyglucosan body disease. Ann Neurol 47:536–540

Report

Replication of Autism Linkage: Fine-Mapping Peak at 17q21

Rita M. Cantor,[1,2,3] Naoko Kono,[1] Jackie A. Duvall,[1,3,4] Ana Alvarez-Retuerto,[3] Jennifer L. Stone,[1] Maricela Alarcón,[3,4,5] Stanley F. Nelson,[1,4] and Daniel H. Geschwind[3,4,5]

Departments of [1]Human Genetics and [2]Pediatrics, Centers for [3]Autism Research and [4]Neurobehavioral Genetics, Neuropsychiatric Institute, [5]Program in Neurogenetics, Department of Neurology, David Geffen School of Medicine, University of California at Los Angeles, Los Angeles

Autism is a heritable but genetically complex disorder characterized by deficits in language and in reciprocal social interactions, combined with repetitive and stereotypic behaviors. As with many genetically complex disorders, numerous genome scans reveal inconsistent results. A genome scan of 345 families from the Autism Genetic Resource Exchange (AGRE) (AGRE_1), gave the strongest evidence of linkage at 17q11-17q21 in families with no affected females. Here, we report a full-genome scan of an independent sample of 91 AGRE families with 109 affected sibling pairs (AGRE_2) that also shows the strongest evidence of linkage to 17q11-17q21 in families with no affected females. Taken together, these samples provide a replication of linkage to this chromosome region that is, to our knowledge, the first such replication in autism. Fine mapping at 2-centimorgan (cM) intervals in the combined sample of families with no affected females reveals a linkage peak at 66.85 cM, which places this locus at 17q21.

Autism (MIM 209850) is a lifelong neuropsychiatric condition with onset in early childhood. First described in 1943 (Kanner 1943), it is characterized by impairments in language and nonverbal communication, deficits in reciprocal social interactions, and the presence of restricted and repetitive behaviors. Cases of autism may occur in conjunction with chromosomal anomalies, such as duplications on the long arm of chromosome 15q11-13, Rett syndrome (MIM 300005), and fragile-X syndrome (MIM 309550). However, these recognized conditions explain only a small fraction of the observed prevalence of autism, currently estimated to be as high as 3 in 1,000 (Yeargin-Allsopp et al. 2003). Suggestions of a variety of environmental and genetic risk factors for idiopathic autism have resulted in inconsistent findings, and the specific etiologies remain unknown. An autism concordance rate of 92% in MZ twin pairs versus 10% in DZ twin pairs (Bailey et al. 1995) implies that there is a substantial genetic contribution to the risk. However, these very divergent concordance rates indicate that autism is likely to result from the interactive effects of multiple genes, making it genetically complex. Given this level of complexity, it is not surprising that the predisposing genes have thus far remained elusive.

To date, the results of eight independent full-genome scans analyzed for the autism phenotype have been reported (Barrett et al. 1999; Philippe et al. 1999; Risch et al. 1999; Buxbaum et al. 2001; International Molecular Genetic Study of Autism Consortium [IMGSAC] 2001; Auranen et al. 2002; Shao et al. 2002; Yonan et al. 2003). Multiple suggestive but not significant linked loci have emerged from each of these individual studies. A meta-analysis (Badner and Gershon 2002) of four of these autism genome scans (Barrett et al. 1999; Philippe et al. 1999; Risch et al. 1999; IMGSAC 2001) provided evidence of linkage to chromosome 7. Recently, an analysis that considered all eight independent genome scans and focused on detecting common linked regions applied criteria of a maximum LOD score (MLS) >1.5 and a distance of no more than 10 cM between linkage peaks (Smalley et al., in press). The region on chromosome 7 did not satisfy these criteria, and only one region, 17p11-17q11, was linked to autism in more than one of these studies (IMGSAC 2001; Yonan et al. 2003). The lack of consistent linkage results for genetically complex disorders such as autism is not surprising. This is likely due to study differences in such factors as family ascertainment, the instruments used to diagnose autism, the eth-

Received January 13, 2005; accepted for publication March 16, 2005; electronically published April 1, 2005.

Address for correspondence and reprints: Dr. Rita M. Cantor, Department of Human Genetics, David Geffen School of Medicine, University of California at Los Angeles, Los Angeles, CA 90095-7088. E-mail: rcantor@mednet.ucla.edu

0002-9297/2005/7606-0011$15.00

nicity of the sample, and the analytic methods employed. Genetic heterogeneity coupled with stochastic fluctuations among samples can also contribute to inconsistent linkage results.

Thus, given the likely genetic complexity of autism and the lack of replication, studies designed to confirm linkage in independent, well-matched samples are critical prior to extensive fine-mapping and association studies. Rules for confirming linkage, developed in the 1970s for Mendelian disorders, preclude the possibility of a replication if there is an overlap in personnel between two studies. These criteria may be too stringent for genetically complex disorders, and Vieland (2001) presents a strong argument for their reformulation. We suggest that an independent sample, from the same cohort, in which family ascertainment, methods of diagnosis, and analytic approaches are identical may be the best sample to use when testing for replication. However, autism cohorts that are large enough to contain independent samples are rare.

The Autism Genetic Resource Exchange (AGRE) cohort currently consists of ~500 nuclear families, each with a sibling pair that meets narrow, "not quite autism" (NQA), or broad definitions of autism (Geschwind et al. 2001). In these families, ascertained in the United States through a proband with autism spectrum disorder and a potentially affected sibling, the parents or caregivers of each child were queried using the Autism Diagnostic Interview-Revised (ADI-R) (Lord et al. 1994). The ADI-R is constructed to diagnose autism on the basis of the classifications of the International Statistical Classification of Diseases and Related Health Problems, 10th Revision (World Health Organization 1992), and the Diagnostic and Statistical Manual of Mental Disorders, 4th Edition (American Psychiatric Association 2000). The algorithms associated with the ADI-R are used by AGRE to classify the children into the categories of narrow autism, broad spectrum disorder, or NQA. The specific criteria for classification as NQA are listed on the AGRE Web site. Those who do not satisfy the criteria for narrow autism or NQA are classified as having broad spectrum disorder if they display patterns of impairment consistent with those of pervasive developmental disorders but do not meet the criteria for autism because of their age at onset. Nonidiopathic cases of autism—which include those having a premature birth, evidence of a perinatal insult, another diagnosed psychiatric disorder, a small nuclear ribonucleoprotein polypeptide N (SNRPN) chromosome 15 duplication, fragile-X syndrome, or an abnormal imaging or medical test—were omitted from these analyses. MZ twin pairs were omitted from the linkage analyses, although the DZ twin pairs were retained. AGRE has human subjects' approval from the Western Institutional Review Board, and the current study has the approval of the institutional review board of the University of California at Los Angeles (UCLA).

In a previously reported full-genome–scan linkage analysis of the first 345 families (AGRE_1) with at least broad spectrum disorder that were genotyped for 335 multiallelic markers with a sex-averaged map, an MLS of 2.04 ($P < .002$) was observed at 17q11 (Yonan et al. 2003). Additional 17q11 markers genotyped at intermarker distances of ~2 cM resulted in a multipoint MLS of 2.83 ($P < .00029$) at 52 cM. Since males predominate among autistic children, Stone and colleagues (2004) stratified this sample into 148 sibships with no affected females to explore the possibility that there are male-specific loci contributing to autism. This resulted in an MLS of 4.3, revealing evidence of significant linkage to 17q11 (Stone et al. 2004). In a subsequent analysis of a diagnostic subset of these data, the posterior-probability-of-linkage statistic, which allowed for different male and female recombination fractions and parent-of-origin effects, obtained a peak on chromosome 17 at 45 cM (Bartlett et al. 2005).

Here, we undertook a full-genome scan in an independent sample of 109 sibling pairs with at least broad spectrum disorder from the 91 families of AGRE_2 (table 1). The parents and affected offspring were genotyped for 401 multiallelic markers by the Center for Inherited Disease Research, by use of a marker panel different from the one genotyped in AGRE_1. There were 236 markers common to both scans. The markers had an average spacing of 9 cM, and no intermarker gap was >20 cM. A genotyping error rate of 0.02% was inferred by examination of ~11,000 repeat genotypes, and a 3.22% rate of missing data was observed in these pedigrees. Mendelian errors were identified using the GAS software, and the marker data were replaced with unknown genotypes for these families. Misspecifications

Table 1

Sibships in AGRE_2, Stratified by Sex

Sample and No. of Affected Siblings per Family	No. of Sibships	No. of Individuals	No. of Sib Pairs
AGRE_2:			
2	82	164	82
3	9	27	27
Total	91	191	109
Male[a]:			
2	44	88	44
3	4	12	12
Total	48	100	56
Mixed[b]:			
2	38	76	38
3	5	15	15
Total	43	91	53

[a] Sibships with only affected males.

[b] Sibships with at least one affected female.

The figure is available in its entirety in the online edition of *The American Journal of Human Genetics.*

Figure 1 MLS for a whole-genome scan, by chromosome, of 109 autistic sibling pairs in 91 families in AGRE_2. Those regions showing an MLS >1.0 have been identified with the name of the marker nearest the peak.

of family relationships were tested using the RELCHECK software (Boehnke and Cox 1997; Broman and Weber 1998), and a pair of MZ twins was identified and eliminated, resulting in 109 sib pairs for the analysis. The map order and sex-averaged intermarker distances were estimated using the Marshfield marker map (see Center for Medical Genetics Web site).

As in the original analysis of AGRE_1 (Yonan et al. 2003), multipoint MLSs were generated for AGRE_2, by the Genehunter software (Kruglyak et al. 1996), at 1-cM intervals along the chromosomes. No regions of significant linkage were observed for AGRE_2, and only two loci exhibited LOD scores exceeding the replication threshold of 1.4 ($P < .01$) posed by Lander and Kruglyak (1995). The complete results of this scan can be found in figure 1. A 12-cM region on 3p14-3p12 had a peak at 105 cM near *D3S2406,* with an MLS of 1.8, but there was no evidence of linkage to that chromosomal region in AGRE_1. However, a 25-cM region with all LOD scores >1.4 on 17q11-23 had a peak at 61 cM with an MLS of 1.9 near *D17S1299* (fig. 2). To assess whether the linkage signal was derived from the 48 families with no affected females (table 1), as seen in AGRE_1 (Stone et al. 2004), we applied the same strategy to AGRE_2 on chromosome 17. Strikingly, multipoint analyses of AGRE_2 stratified into the 56 sibling pairs from the sibships containing no affected females revealed an MLS of 4.1 with a linkage peak at 61 cM in 17q21. Figure 2 shows the MLS plots for AGRE_2 stratified into 56 pairs from the 48 sibships with no affected females, for the 53 pairs from the 43 sibships with at least one affected female, and for their combination of 109 pairs from the 91 sibships. These linked regions show a considerable overlap, and it is likely that the 9-cM separation between the peak LOD scores is due to the differences between the two samples in the distributions of markers in this region.

We examined the linkage evidence in detail to evaluate whether these study samples together provide a statistical replication of linkage to a single locus on 17q11-21, although we recognized that the replication would

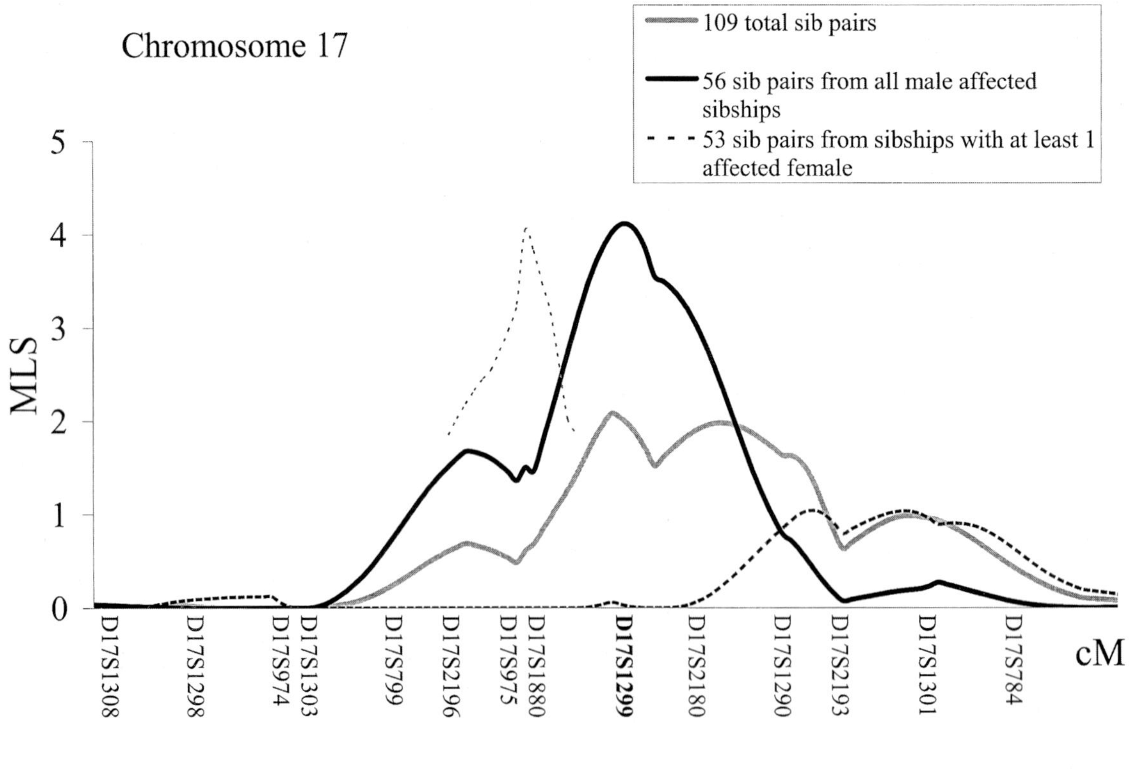

Figure 2 Chromosome 17 linkage-analysis MLSs of 109 autistic sibling pairs from AGRE_2 (*gray line*). MLSs obtained by stratifying the sibships into those with no autistic females are indicated by a black line. MLSs from sibships with at least one autistic female are indicated by a dashed line. The additional gray dashed peak represents the location and MLS plot from the analysis of AGRE_1 sibships with no affected females. The peak marker is in boldface type.

Table 2

Allele Sharing at 17p11-q21 in AGRE_1, Stratified by Sex

Position (cM)	Marker	Proportion of Alleles Shared IBD (*P*) for Total Sample	Male[a]
44		.54 (.007)	.57 (.003)
46		.55 (.005)	.58 (.002)
48	*D17S1871*	.55 (.003)	.58 (.001)
50	*D17S1824*	.56 (.002)	.58 (.001)
51	*D17S1294*	.56 (.002)	.58 (.001)
52	*D17S1800*	.56 (.002)	.59 (.0009)
53	*D17S798*	.55 (.005)	.59 (.0009)
54		.54 (.01)	.58 (.001)
56	*D17S1293*	.53 (.04)	.57 (.004)
58		***.53 (.05)***	***.56 (.008)***
60		.53[b]	.55 (.02)
62	*D17S1299*	.53[b]	.55 (.04)
64		.53[b]	.54 (.04)

NOTE.—Linkage at position 58 (shown in bold italics) is replicated in AGRE_1 and AGRE_2 families with only affected males.

[a] Sibships with no affected females.

[b] Not significant.

not occur at the linkage peak in either sample. We applied a formal criterion of significant linkage of $P < .000022$ in one sample and $P < .01$ in a second sample (Lander and Kruglyak 1995). Multipoint identical-by-descent (IBD) allele-sharing statistics and their *P* values were generated across the linked regions in AGRE_1 and AGRE_2 separately, through use of the GENIBD and SIBPAL programs of the Statistical Analysis for Genetic Epidemiology (SAGE) software. For the affected sibling pairs from AGRE_1, table 2 reports IBD allele-sharing estimates and their corresponding *P* values at 2-cM intervals and the genotyped markers for the total sample and for the sibships that have no affected females. For AGRE_2, table 3 reports the same information at 4-cM intervals and genotyped markers and includes the IBD allele-sharing estimates for the sibships that have at least one affected female. These statistics are reported for the regions with linkage, beginning at 44 cM, where AGRE_1 showed significant allele sharing ($P < .01$). Table 2 reports these statistics up to 64 cM, for comparison with the results at the peak marker in AGRE_2. Statistics in table 3 extend to 84 cM, beyond which the *P* value is >.01. At position 58 cM, the proportions of IBD allele sharing of .65 with $P = .00002$ and .56 with $P = .008$ in families with no affected females indicate that AGRE_2 linkage is replicated by AGRE_1 at the genomewide level of significance (tables 2 and 3).

Although linkage was replicated statistically, the peaks from the two samples did not coincide. To resolve this difference, we undertook additional fine mapping of 13 multiallelic markers in the combined AGRE samples. The original genome scans of the two samples used different marker sets with different and uneven distributions of intermarker distances. Those markers were excluded from these new analyses. The fine-mapping markers were selected using the criterion that any bias that could be introduced by their distribution or informativeness be minimized. The markers are between positions at 48 and 82 cM, have ~2–3-cM intervals, and have an expected multipoint information content of ⩾.70 or better in the combined sample. Two additional markers, at 24 and 100 cM, serve as anchors.

With use of the Genehunter software (Kruglyak et al. 1996), multipoint and single-point MLS scores were generated at 1-cM intervals across the region from 24 to 100 cM by use of a sex-averaged map of the separate and combined samples of the sibships containing no affected females. Plots of the multipoint MLSs in the separate and combined stratified samples are shown in figure 3. Whereas peaks seen in the original genome scans of AGRE_1 and AGRE_2 are observed at *D17S1294* at 51 cM and at *D17S1299* at 61 cM, respectively, in the present fine-mapping analysis, the most significant LOD score of 4.1 is at marker *D17S2180*, at a distance of 66.85 cM from the p telomere. A 1-LOD drop includes the peak from the second scan, with an MLS of 3.6 at *D17S1299*. The proportion of multipoint allele-sharing IBD in the combined sample estimated at *D17S2180* is .59 ($P = .00002$), by use of the SIBPAL software of the SAGE package. The analogous single-point estimate is .58 ($P = .00002$).

Some factors contributing to this successful stratification strategy have been discussed in detail by Stone et

Table 3

Allele Sharing at 17p11-q23 in AGRE_2, Stratified by Sex

Position (cM)	Marker	Proportion of Alleles Shared IBD (*P*) for Total Sample	Male[a]	Mixed[b]
44	*D17S2196*	.56 (.04)	.63 (.003)	.47
48		.55 (.05)	.62 (.004)	.47
52	*D17S1880*	.55 (.04)	.61 (.005)	.49
56		.57 (.008)	.64 (.0001)	.49
58		***.58 (.004)***	***.65 (.00002)***	***.49***
60		.59 (.003)	.67 (.00001)	.48
61	*D17S1299*[c]	.59 (.003)	.68 (.000009)	.48
64		.58 (.004)	.67 (.00001)	.47
66	*D17S2180*	.58 (.007)	.67 (.00004)	.47
68		.58 (.004)	.66 (.00006)	.48
72		.58 (.002)	.63 (.0003)	.51
76		.58 (.002)	.61 (.003)	.54
80		.59 (.003)	.59 (.02)	.57
81	*D17S1290*	.59 (.004)	.58 (.03)	.57
84		.57 (.007)	.56[d]	.57

NOTE.—Linkage at position 58 (shown in bold italics) is replicated in AGRE_1 and AGRE_2 families with only affected males.

[a] Sibships with no affected females.

[b] Sibships with at least one affected female.

[c] Peak marker.

[d] Not significant.

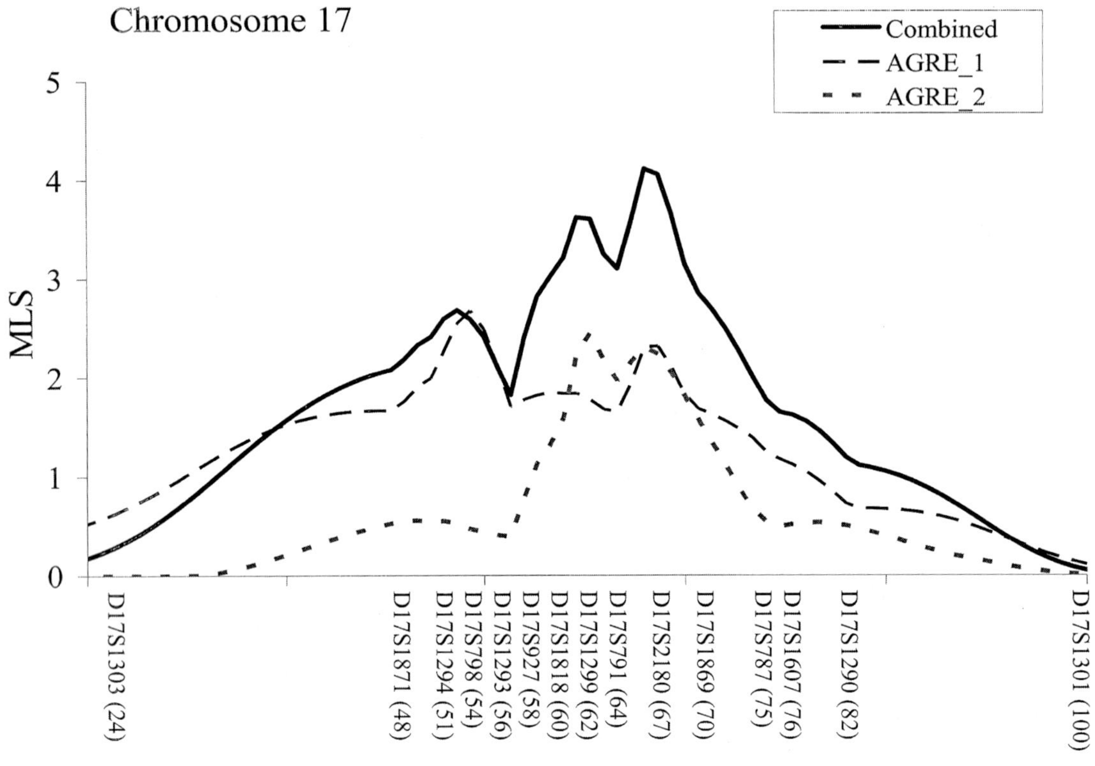

Figure 3 Chromosome 17q fine-mapping linkage-analysis MLSs of 220 autistic sibling pairs with no affected females from AGRE_1 and AGRE_2 separately (*black and gray dashed lines*, respectively) and combined (*solid black line*). Markers and their distances from the p telomere (in parentheses) appear on the horizontal axis.

al. (2004). They include the fact that male and female brains have different structures and function differently and that the incidences of autism and other neurodevelopmental disorders are different between males and females. Here, we turn to the reported analyses of other genetically complex diseases for additional insight. We first note that there have been similar sex-stratification analyses that resulted in positive sex-specific linkage and association findings for other complex traits. In a linkage and association analysis of the insertion-deletion polymorphism of the angiotensinogen-converting enzyme (*ACE*) gene, male-specific association and linkage findings were seen for blood pressure traits in humans (O'Donnell et al. 1998). In a complementary study, gene-targeting experiments in mice provided additional evidence that functional inactivation of the *ACE* gene contributes to blood-pressure levels in males but not in females (Krege et al. 1995). Loughlin and colleagues (2000) were able to remove heterogeneity from a linkage analysis of osteoarthritis and chromosome 2q by use of sex stratification, and the positive linkage signal was observed when the affected individuals were limited to males. In a study of the linkage of inflammatory bowel disease to the HLA region, sex stratification removed heterogeneity and improved the LOD score from 1.2 to 4.5 in the male-only sibships (Fisher et al. 2002). In each case, the mechanism by which the sex effect operates needs additional investigation.

For possible positional candidate genes, the serotonin transporter gene (*SLC6A4*), which codes for a protein controlling the reuptake of serotonin in the synapse (Murphy et al. 2004), is at 49 cM, under the original peak in AGRE_1. It has been investigated by association studies of the combined AGRE_1 and AGRE_2 samples. No evidence for allelic association was observed between the putative functional promoter variant (5-HTTLPR) and autism spectrum disorder; however, evidence of association was observed with two SNPs (A. Yonan and C. Gilliam, personal communication). Given the peak in the combined AGRE_1 and AGRE_2 samples, it is of interest that a recent report addressed the sex-specific genetic architecture of whole-blood serotonin levels in 806 Hutterites from a single pedigree (Weiss et al. 2005). This trait is sexually dimorphic, and a QTL for male serotonin levels was identified on 17q, with the linkage peak at 66 cM, very close to the one identified in the present study. An association with a SNP in the integrin *β3* (*ITGB3*) gene under the peak at 66 cM was reported by the same group (Weiss et al. 2004). *ITGB3* is a biologically plausible candidate for autism susceptibility because it is a cell-adhesion molecule involved in nervous system development, including the processes of cell proliferation, migration, differentiation, and synapse maturation (Sajid et al. 2002). This gene provides a good positional candidate for follow-up studies of the combined sex-stratified AGRE sample, since its disruption would clearly affect brain development and functioning, although potentially in a subtle manner.

In conclusion, linkage analyses of 109 autistic sibling pairs from 91 AGRE families in combination with analyses of those pairs from an independent sample of 345 families from the same cohort establish three points. First, stratification of families with autism into only those with affected males reveals significant linkage to 17q11-21 in both samples, supporting the value of this approach. Second, linkage to 17q11-21 is replicated at the genomewide level of significance; this provides the first formal replication of a locus for idiopathic autism. Third, the multipoint linkage evidence in the combined sample localizes the peak to 17q21.

Acknowledgments

We thank the AGRE families who participated in this study; the Cure Autism Now Foundation, for supporting the AGRE program; and the scientists who have provided oversight to the AGRE Consortium. Members of AGRE Consortium are D.H.G.; R.M.C.; S.F.N.; Maja Bucan, University of Pennsylvania, Philadelphia; W. Ted Brown, New York State Institute for Basic Research in Developmental Disabilities, Staten Island; Joseph D. Buxbaum, Mt. Sinai School of Medicine, New York; John N. Constantino, Washington University School of Medicine, St. Louis; T. Conrad Gilliam, University of Chicago, Chicago; David H. Ledbetter, Emory University, Atlanta; Gerard D. Schellenberg, University of Washington and Veterans Affairs Medical Center, Seattle; Carol A. Samango-Sprouse, George Washington University, Washington; and Rudolph E. Tanzi, Massachusetts General Hospital, Boston. This work was supported by National Institutes of Health (NIH) grant MH64547 (to D.H.G., R.M.C., and S.F.N.). Some of the results of this study were obtained by using the program package SAGE, which is supported by U.S. Public Health Service resource grant RR03655 from the National Center for Research Resources. Genotyping services were provided by the Center for Inherited Disease Research (CIDR). CIDR is fully funded through a federal contract from the NIH to The Johns Hopkins University, contract number N01-HG-65403.

Electronic-Database Information

The URLs for data presented herein are as follows:

AGRE, http://www.agre.org
Center for Inherited Disease Research, http://www.cidr.jhmi.edu/
Center for Medical Genetics, http://research.marshfieldclinic.org/genetics/ (for the Marshfield marker maps)
Online Mendelian Inheritance in Man (OMIM), http://www.ncbi.nlm.nih.gov/Omim/ (for autism, Rett syndrome, and fragile-X syndrome)

References

American Psychiatric Association (2000) Diagnostic and statistical manual of mental disorders, 4th ed. American Psychiatric Association, Washington, DC

Auranen M, Vanhala R, Varilo T, Ayers K, Kempas E, Ylisaukko-oja T, Sinsheimer JS, Peltonen L, Järvelä I (2002) A genomewide screen for autism-spectrum disorders: evidence for a major susceptibility locus on chromosome 3q25-27. Am J Hum Genet 71:777–790

Badner JA, Gershon ES (2002) Regional meta-analysis of published data supports linkage of autism with markers on chromosome 7. Mol Psychiatry 7:56–66

Bailey A, Le Couteur A, Gottesman I, Bolton P, Simonoff E, Yuzda E, Rutter M (1995) Autism as a strongly genetic disorder: evidence from a British twin study. Psychol Med 25: 63–77

Barrett S, Beck JC, Bernier R, Bisson E, Braun TA, Casavant TL, Childress D, et al (1999) An autosomal genomic screen for autism: collaborative linkage study of autism. Am J Med Genet 88:609–615

Bartlett CW, Goedken R, Vieland VJ (2005) Effects of updating linkage evidence across subsets of data: reanalysis of autism genetic resource exchange data set. Am J Hum Genet 76:688–695

Boehnke M, Cox NJ (1997) Accurate inference of relationships in sib-pair linkage studies. Am J Hum Genet 61:423–429

Broman KW, Weber JL (1998) Estimation of pairwise relationships in the presence of genotyping errors. Am J Hum Genet 63:1563–1564

Buxbaum JD, Silverman JM, Smith CJ, Kilifarski M, Reichert J, Hollander E, Lawlor BA, Fitzgerald M, Greenberg DA, Davis KL (2001) Evidence for a susceptibility gene for autism on chromosome 2 and for genetic heterogeneity. Am J Hum Genet 68:1514–1520

Fisher SA, Hampe J, Macpherson AJ, Forbes A, Lennard-Jones JE, Schreiber S, Curran ME, Mathew CG, Lewis CM (2002) Sex stratification of an inflammatory bowel disease genome search shows male-specific linkage to the HLA region of chromosome 6. Eur J Hum Genet 10:259–265

Geschwind DH, Sowinski J, Lord C, Iversen P, Shestack J, Jones P, Ducat L, Spence SJ, and the AGRE Steering Committee (2001) The Autism Genetic Resource Exchange: a resource for the study of autism and related neuropsychiatric conditions. Am J Hum Genet 69:463–466

International Molecular Genetic Study of Autism Consortium (IMGSAC) (2001) A genomewide screen for autism: strong evidence for linkage to chromosomes 2q, 7q, and 16p. Am J Hum Genet 69:570–581

Kanner L (1943) The original description of autism, with excellent case examples. Nervous Child 2:217–250

Krege JH, John SW, Langenbach LL, Hodgin JB, Hagaman JR, Bachman ES, Jennette JC, O'Brien DA, Smithies O (1995) Male-female differences in fertility and blood pressure in ACE-deficient mice. Nature 375:146–148

Kruglyak L, Daly MJ, Reeve-Daly MP, Lander ES (1996) Parametric and nonparametric linkage analysis: a unified multipoint approach. Am J Hum Genet 58:1347–1363

Lander E, Kruglyak L (1995) Genetic dissection of complex traits: guidelines for interpreting and reporting linkage results. Nat Genet 11:241–247

Lord C, Rutter M, Le Couteur A (1994) Autism Diagnostic Interview-Revised: a revised version of a diagnostic interview for caregivers of individuals with possible pervasive developmental disorders. J Autism Dev Disord 24:659–685

Loughlin J, Mustafa Z, Smith A, Irven C, Carr AJ, Clipsham K, Chitnavis J, Bloomfield VA, McCartney M, Cox O, Sinsheimer JS, Sykes B, Chapman KE (2000) Linkage analysis of chromosome 2q in osteoarthritis. Rheumatology (Oxford) 39:377–381

Murphy DL, Lerner A, Rudnick G, Lesch KP (2004) Serotonin transporter: gene, genetic disorders, and pharmacogenetics. Mol Interv 4:109–123

O'Donnell CJ, Lindpaintner K, Larson MG, Rao VS, Ordovas JM, Schaefer EJ, Myers RH, Levy D (1998) Evidence for association and genetic linkage of the angiotensin-converting enzyme locus with hypertension and blood pressure in men but not women in the Framingham Heart Study. Circulation 97:1766–1772

Philippe A, Martinez M, Guilloud-Bataille M, Gillberg C, Rastam M, Sponheim E, Coleman M, Zappella M, Aschauer H, Van Maldergem L, Penet C, Feingold J, Brice A, Leboyer M, and the Paris Autism Research International Sibpair Study (1999) Genome-wide scan for autism susceptibility genes. Hum Mol Genet 8:805–812

Risch N, Spiker D, Lotspeich L, Nouri N, Hinds D, Hallmayer J, Kalaydjieva L, et al (1999) A genomic screen of autism: evidence for a multilocus etiology. Am J Hum Genet 65:493–507

Sajid M, Vijayan KV, Souza S, Bray PF (2002) PlA polymorphism of integrin beta 3 differentially modulates cellular migration on extracellular matrix proteins. Arterioscler Thromb Vasc Biol 22:1984–1989

Shao Y, Wolpert CM, Raiford KL, Menold MM, Donnelly SL, Ravan SA, Bass MP, McClain C, von Wendt L, Vance JM, Abramson RH, Wright HH, Ashley-Koch A, Gilbert JR, DeLong RG, Cuccaro ML, Pericak-Vance MA (2002) Genomic screen and follow-up analysis for autistic disorder. Am J Med Genet 114:99–105

Smalley SL, Loo SK, Yang MH, Cantor RM. Toward localizing genes underlying cerebral asymmetry and mental health. Am J Med Genet (in press)

Stone JL, Merriman B, Cantor RM, Yonan AL, Gilliam TC, Geschwind DH, Nelson SF (2004) Evidence for sex-specific risk alleles in autism spectrum disorder. Am J Hum Genet 75:1117–1123

Vieland VJ (2001) The replication requirement. Nat Genet 29: 244–245

Weiss LA, Abney M, Cook EH Jr, Ober C (2005) Sex-specific genetic architecture of whole blood serotonin levels. Am J Hum Genet 76:33–41

Weiss LA, Veenstra-Vanderweele J, Newman DL, Kim SJ, Dytch H, McPeek MS, Cheng S, Ober C, Cook EH Jr, Abney M (2004) Genome-wide association study identifies ITGB3 as a QTL for whole blood serotonin. Eur J Hum Genet 12: 949–954

World Health Organization (1992) International statistical classification of diseases and related health problems, 10th revision. World Health Organization, Geneva

Yeargin-Allsopp M, Rice C, Karapurkar T, Doernberg N, Boyle C, Murphy C (2003) Prevalence of autism in a US metropolitan area. JAMA 289:49–55

Yonan AL, Alarcón M, Cheng R, Magnusson PKE, Spence SJ, Palmer AA, Grunn A, Hank Juo S-H, Terwilliger JD, Liu J, Cantor RM, Geschwind DH, Gilliam TC (2003) A genome-wide screen of 345 families for autism-susceptibility loci. Am J Hum Genet 73:886–897

Report

A Novel Linkage to Generalized Vitiligo on 4q13-q21 Identified in a Genomewide Linkage Analysis of Chinese Families

Jian-Jun Chen,[1,2,*] Wei Huang,[3,*] Jin-Ping Gui,[4] Sen Yang,[1,2] Fu-Sheng Zhou,[1,2] Quan-Geng Xiong,[4] Hong-Bo Wu,[4] Yong Cui,[1,2] Min Gao,[1,2] Wei Li,[1,2] Jin-Xian Li,[4] Kai-Lin Yan,[1,2] Wen-Tao Yuan,[3] Shi-Jie Xu,[3] Jian-Jun Liu,[1,2,5] and Xue-Jun Zhang[1,2]

[1]Institute of Dermatology and Department of Dermatology, First Affiliated Hospital, Anhui Medical University, and [2]Key Laboratory of Genome Research, Hefei, Anhui, China; [3]Chinese National Human Genome Center at Shanghai, Shanghai; [4]Vitiligo Clinic of the Railway Hospital, Xiangfan, Hubei, China; and [5]Genome Institute of Singapore, Singapore

Generalized vitiligo is a common, autoimmune, familial-clustering depigmentary disorder of the skin and hair that results from selective destruction of melanocytes. Generalized vitiligo is likely a heterogeneous disease, with five susceptibility loci reported so far—on chromosomes 1p31, 6p21, 7q, 8p, and 17p13—in white populations. To investigate vitiligo susceptibility loci in the Chinese population, we performed a genomewide linkage analysis in 57 multiplex Chinese families, each with at least two affected siblings, and we identified interesting linkage evidence on 1p36, 4q13-q21, 6p21-p22, 6q24-q25, 14q12-q13, and 22q12. Subsequently, to extract more linkage information, we investigated our initial genomewide linkage findings in a follow-up analysis of 49 new families and additional markers. Our initial genomewide linkage analysis and our subsequent follow-up analysis have identified a novel linkage to vitiligo on 4q13-q21, with highly significant linkage evidence (a nonparametic LOD score of 4.62 [*P* = .000003] and a heterogeneity LOD score of 4.01, under a recessive inheritance model), suggesting that 4q13-q21 likely harbors a major susceptibility locus for vitiligo in the Chinese population. We observed a minimal overlap between the linkage results of our current genomewide analysis in the Chinese population and the results of previous analyses in white populations, and we thus hypothesize that, as a polygenic disorder, vitiligo may be associated with great genetic heterogeneity and a substantial difference in its genetic basis between ethnic populations.

Generalized vitiligo (MIM 193200) is a common acquired autoimmune disorder of skin and hair that results from selective destruction of melanocytes (Cho et al. 2000). It is characterized by the appearance of sharply delimited patches of white skin overlying hair, oral mucosa, and occasionally the eyes, which are due to noninflammatory loss of pigment-forming melanocytes in affected areas. Vitiligo is associated with autoimmune disorders such as hypothyroidism, diabetes mellitus, chronic active hepatitis, pernicious anemia, and adrenal insufficiency (Kovacs 1998). The population prevalence of vitiligo ranges from 0.1% to 2% and shows a wide variability among ethnic groups (Bolognia et al. 1998; Hann and Nordlund 2000). For example, whereas the estimated population prevalence of vitiligo is ~0.38% for whites in the United States and northern Europe (Howitz et al. 1977), vitiligo affects only ~0.19% of the population in China (Xu et al. 2002).

Genetic risk for vitiligo is well supported by multiple lines of evidence. Vitiligo is frequently associated with familial clustering (Mehta et al. 1973; Carnevale et al. 1980; Goudie et al. 1983; Hafez et al. 1983; Das et al. 1985; Majumder et al. 1993; Alkhateeb et al. 2003), and ~20% of probands have at least one affected first-degree relative (Alkhateeb et al. 2003). The risk for first-degree relatives of patients with vitiligo to develop the disease is elevated by 7- to 10-fold (Nath et al. 1994) compared with the risk for the general population. Similarly, our recent study of the Chinese population indicated that ~1.8% of patients' first-degree relatives were

Received January 31, 2005; accepted for publication March 16, 2005; electronically published April 4, 2005.

Address for correspondence and reprints: Dr. Xue-Jun Zhang, Institute of Dermatology, Anhui Medical University, 69 Meishan Road, Hefei, Anhui 230032, China. E-mail: ayzxj@mail.hf.ah.cn

* These authors contributed equally to this work.

0002-9297/2005/7606-0012$15.00

Table 1

Summary of Analyses of Families

Analysis	Total No. of Families	Total No. of Affecteds	No. of Families by No. of Affecteds (Total No. of Affecteds): Two Affecteds	Three Affecteds	Four or More Affecteds
Initial genomewide scan	57	172	23 (46)	17 (51)	17 (75)
Follow-up	49	114	35 (70)	12 (36)	2 (8)
Combined	106	286	58 (116)	29 (87)	19 (83)

affected with vitiligo, which was 9-fold higher than the prevalence rate in general population (Zhang et al. 2004*b*). In addition, segregation analysis suggested that vitiligo is a multifactorial and polygenic disorder that likely results from multiple genetic and environmental factors (Arcos-Burgos et al. 2002; Alkhateeb et al. 2003; Zhang et al. 2004*b*). However, no disease genes have been identified for vitiligo so far.

Several genomewide linkage analyses of vitiligo have been performed in the past few years, and multiple linkages to vitiligo have been identified (Nath et al. 2001; Alkhateeb et al. 2002; Fain et al. 2003; Spritz et al. 2004). Using 16 European American pedigrees with cosegregation of systemic lupus erythematosus and vitiligo, Nath et al. (2001) performed the first genomewide linkage analysis of vitiligo and identified a significant linkage on 17p13. Shortly afterwards, Spritz and his colleagues performed a series of genomewide linkage analyses of vitiligo in white families. Their initial genomewide scan was done in a three-generation multiplex family with cosegregation of vitiligo and Hashimoto thyroiditis, and they identified a candidate gene with highly significant linkage at a locus (named "*AIS1*") on chromosome 1p32.2-p31.3 (Alkhateeb et al. 2002). Subsequently, they performed a follow-up genomewide linkage analysis by studying 70 additional white families (Fain et al. 2003). Their follow-up analysis confirmed the original linkage finding at the *AIS1* locus with highly significant linkage evidence (nonparametric LOD [NPL] score of 5.56) and identified additional linkage evidence on chromosomes 1, 7, 8, 11, 19, and 22. More recently, the group performed an extended genomewide linkage analysis, using 102 multiplex families (including the 70 families used in the previous genomewide scan) (Spritz et al. 2004). The linkage results from the 102 families reinforced the strong support for the *AIS1* locus and also confirmed the previously suggestive linkage findings on chromosomes 7q and 8p (*AIS2* and *AIS3*). The study also provided supporting evidence for a disease locus on chromosome 17, which likely corresponds to the *SLEV1* locus identified by Nath et al. (2001). Interestingly, by stratifying their 102 families into autoimmunity- and nonautoimmunity-associated groups, Spritz and colleagues (2004) found that, whereas the linkage evidence at the *AIS1*, *AIS2*, and *SLEV1* loci was mainly from the autoimmunity-associated families, the evidence at the *AIS3* locus was primarily from the nonautoimmunity-associated families, suggesting that generalized vitiligo might be divided into two distinct phenotypic subcategories that involve different disease loci or alleles. In addition to the genomewide linkage analyses, population-based association analyses were used to investigate several candidate genes for vitiligo—for example, *CTLA-4* (Kemp et al. 1999; Blomhoff et al. 2005), *CAT* and *TAP1* (Casp et al. 2002, 2003), *MC1R* and *ASIP* (Na et al. 2003), *ACE* (Jin et al. 2004), and *HLA* (Zamani et al. 2001; Tastan et al. 2004; Zhang et al. 2004*a*).

Here, we report the first genomewide linkage analysis of vitiligo in a Chinese population. Our family collection includes 106 Chinese multiplex families, each with at least two siblings affected with generalized vitiligo (table 1). All the families were recruited by experienced dermatologists from the Department of Dermatology at First Affiliated Hospital of Anhui Medical University at Hefei, Anhui, China, and from the Vitiligo Clinic of the Railway Hospital at Xiangfan, Hubei, China. The diagnosis of generalized vitiligo was made on the basis of the patient's history and the presence of typical clinical features (discrete, well-circumscribed depigmented patches). Phenotypes were carefully determined by history, lesion maps, and, in most cases, physical examination and/or photographs. Any individual whose phenotype was questionable was excluded from the study. Only patients with clear signs of acquired patches on the extremities, trunk, genitalia, central face, or other areas were scored as affected. The mean age at onset of the 286 affected individuals (148 male [51.7%] and 138 female [48.3%]) from the 106 families was 18.6 years (range 1–63 years). Of the 106 families, 57 families were used in an initial genomewide linkage analysis, and 49 families were used in a follow-up linkage analysis in which the initial linkage findings from the genomewide scan were further investigated by use of dense marker coverage (table 1). For each family, blood samples were collected from all affected individuals, their parents, and additional family members connecting affected individuals. Among the 106 families, blood samples were collected from both parents in 81 families and from one parent in 17 families. Eight families were missing samples from both parents of affected individuals. When samples from one or both parents of an affected individual were unavailable, a blood sample was collected from at least one additional unaffected sibling. Informed consent was obtained from each recruited subject. The study was approved by the Ethical Committee of the Chinese National Human Genome Center at Shanghai.

Genomic DNA was extracted from whole blood by use of a simple salting-out procedure, as described elsewhere (Miller et al. 1988). We performed a genomewide linkage analysis of vitiligo by genotyping 382 microsatellite markers from the ABI Prism Linkage Mapping Set (version 2) in 57 families. Average marker spacing is 8.85 cM (range 1–19 cM), and average marker information content is 0.72, on the basis of genotypes from the 57 families. All the marker positions were based on an interpolated genetic map that incorporates the information from a physical map (build 34.3) and from published deCODE and Marshfield genetic maps (see David Duffy's QIMR Homepage). All the markers were genotyped in multiplex PCR, in accordance with the manufacturer's guidelines (Applied Biosystems). Before being used in linkage analysis, all genotyping data were subjected to quality checking by use of the programs PedCheck (O'Connell and Weeks 1998) and MERLIN (Abecasis et al. 2002). Problematic genotypes either were corrected by rechecking original allele callings or were removed if allele status could not be reliably determined.

Both nonparametric and parametric linkage analyses were performed using the program GENEHUNTER 2.1 (Kruglyak et al. 1996). For nonparametric analysis, the NPL score was calculated using the S_{all} statistic to capture the information about allele sharing between all affected individuals in a pedigree. For parametric analysis, the heterogeneity LOD (HLOD) score was calculated by assuming a dominant or recessive inheritance of the disease allele and a disease-allele frequency of 0.01, consistent with the population prevalence of 0.19% in China (Xu et al. 2002). Moreover, to reduce the impact of the nonpenetrant disease allele on linkage analysis, genomewide parametric analysis was performed by using an "affecteds-only" approach, in which all normal individuals were treated as "unknown" instead of "unaffected," and by assuming a simple genetic model with high penetrance (0.99) and very low phenocopy rates (0.001). Marker-allele frequency was estimated on the basis of founders' genotypes of either 57 families (for the genomewide analysis) or 106 families (for the follow-up analysis) by use of the program Linkage 5.10 (Lathrop and Lalouel 1984).

Multipoint nonparametric analysis identified linkage signals on 1p36, 4q13-q21, 6p21-p22, 6q24-q25, 14q12-q13, and 22q12 (fig. 1). Of these, the highest NPL score was 3.05 (P = .0017), identified at the marker interval *D6S308–D6S441* on 6q24-q25; this was followed by NPL scores of 2.94 (P = .0021) at the marker interval *D4S1592–D4S1534* on 4q13-q21, 2.87 (P = .0023) at the marker interval *D22S280–D22S283* on 22q12, 2.83 (P = .0026) at the marker interval *D14S275–D14S70* on 14q12-13, 2.68 (P = .0044) at the marker interval *D6S422–D6S273* on 6p21-p22, and 2.67 (P = .0045) at the marker interval *D1S234–D1S2885* on 1p36. Multipoint parametric linkage analysis under a recessive model of inheritance identified suggestive evidence for linkage (HLOD score of 1.86 or higher) (Lander and Kruglyak 1995) on 4q12-q13, 5p15, 6q24-q25, and 8q24 (fig. 1). The most significant HLOD score under a recessive model was 2.99 (α = 36%) at the marker interval *D6S308–D6S441,* which was followed by multipoint HLOD scores of 2.48 (α = 34%) at the marker interval *D5S1981–D5S406,* 2.15 (α = 38%) at the marker interval *D8S284–D8S272,* and 1.94 (α = 28%) at the marker interval *D4S1592–D4S392.* Under a dominant model of inheritance, multipoint parametric analysis identified suggestive linkage evidence on 2q13, 6p21-p22, 14q12-q13, and 22q12 (fig. 1). The highest HLOD score of 2.28 (α = 59%) was identified at marker *D2S160,* which was followed by HLOD scores of 2.26 (α = 37%) at the marker interval *D6S422–D6S273,* 2.15 (α = 48%) at the marker interval *D14S275–D14S70,* and 2.07 (α = 46%) at the marker interval *D6S308–D6S441.* For both nonparametric and parametric genomewide linkage analyses, two-point LOD scores (data not shown) were consistent with the multipoint LOD scores but were generally lower.

Our genomewide linkage analysis of vitiligo in the 57 Chinese families identified interesting linkage signals in six genomic regions. The most significant evidence for linkage was on 6q24-q25 and was supported by a maximum multipoint NPL score of 3.05 and a recessive HLOD score of 2.99. The second-most significant evidence was on 4q13-q21, with a maximum multipoint NPL score of 2.94 and a recessive HLOD score of 1.94, which was followed by linkage evidence on 6p21-p22, with a maximum multipoint NPL score of 2.67 and a dominant HLOD score of 2.26. Linkage evidence was also identified on 1p36, 14q12-q13, and 22q12, but the evidence was less significant (table 2). To further investigate these initial linkage findings, we analyzed an additional 49 Chinese families recruited from the same clinics in a follow-up analysis in which additional markers were genotyped to extract more linkage information. Instead of using the "affecteds-only" approach, we performed the follow-up parametric analysis of the initial linkage findings by assuming a disease-allele frequency of 0.01, a variable penetrance rate (range 0.5–0.99), and a fixed phenotype rate of 0.001 and by using the inheritance model under which the initial linkage evidence was identified in the genomewide analysis. Changing the penetrance rate made almost no impact on HLOD score results (data not shown); therefore, only HLOD scores under the penetrance rate of 0.99 were reported.

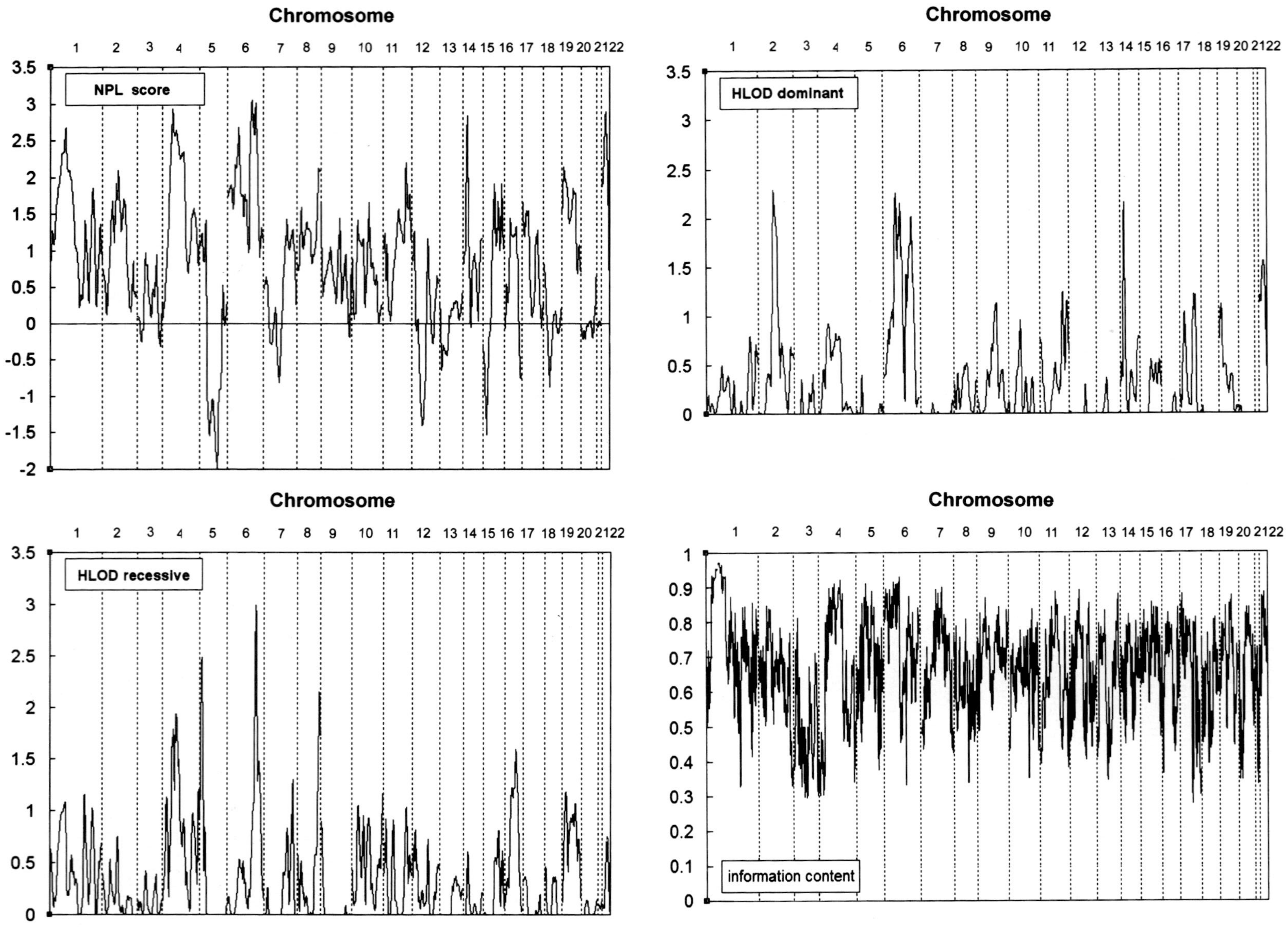

Figure 1 Summary plot of the multipoint NPL and HLOD scores on 22 chromosomes from the genomewide linkage analysis of 382 microsatellite markers in 57 Chinese multiplex families with vitiligo.

Table 2

Summary of the Multipoint LOD Scores from the Initial Genomewide and Follow-up Linkage Analyses

Chromosome	Marker or Interval	Initial Analysis[a]				Follow-Up Analysis[b]				Combined Analysis[c]				Genetic Model[d]
		NPL	*P*	HLOD	α (%)	NPL	*P*	HLOD	α (%)	NPL	*P*	HLOD	α (%)	
1p36	*D1S2674–D1S2885*	2.67	.0045	1.08	21	.98	.16	.09	4.5	2.37	.0093	1.17	11	Rec
4q13-q21	*D4S1592–D4S1534*	2.94	.0021	1.94	28	4.29	.00001	2.74	35	4.62	.000003	4.01	31	Rec
6p21-p22	*D6S289–D6S291*	2.68	.0044	2.26	37	2.17	.016	1.32	45	3.16	.00092	2.14	32	Dom
6q24-q25	*D6S308–D6S441*	3.05	.0017	2.99	36	1.27	.11	.31	11	2.98	.0016	1.37	16	Rec
14q12-q13	*D14S70*	2.83	.0026	2.15	48	.048	.48	0	0	2.17	.014	1.51	34	Dom
22q12	*D22S280–D22S283*	2.87	.0023	1.55	33	.47	.32	.0066	.038	1.75	.039	.72	19	Dom

[a] Performed by analyzing 382 microsatellite markers in 57 multiplex Chinese families.
[b] Performed by analyzing various numbers of markers in 49 multiplex Chinese families.
[c] Performed by analyzing various numbers of markers in 106 multiplex Chinese families.
[d] Rec = recessive inheritance; Dom = dominant inheritance.

The initial linkage finding on 4q13-q21 was further investigated by genotyping 12 new and 5 original microsatellite markers in 106 families, which increased the marker density to an average marker spacing of 3.3 cM. We first performed a joint linkage analysis of 106 families, including 57 original and 49 new families. Multipoint linkage analysis of 17 markers yielded a maximum NPL score of 4.62 ($P = .000003$) at the marker interval *D4S392–D4S3042* and a maximum HLOD score of 4.01 ($\alpha = 31\%$) at the adjacent marker interval *D4S3042–D4S2947*, under a recessive model of inheritance (fig. 2 and table 2). The multipoint LOD score results were supported by a two-point analysis that yielded a maximum two-point NPL score of 4.53 ($P = .000004$) and a recessive HLOD score of 5.97 ($\alpha = 42\%$) at the marker locus *D4S392*. Both nonparametric and parametric LOD scores of the joint linkage analysis of the 106 families on 4q13-q21 surpassed the suggested genomewide criteria for significant linkage evidence (Lander and Kruglyak 1995). In addition, we also performed an independent linkage analysis of the same 17 markers in 49 new families by using the same genetic model. The linkage analysis of the 49 new families provided independent supporting evidence for linkage, yielding a multipoint NPL score of 4.29 ($P = .00001$) and an HLOD score of 2.74 ($\alpha = 35\%$) at the same genetic position. Therefore, our initial genomewide and subsequent fine-mapping linkage analyses have identified a novel linkage to vitiligo on 4q13-q21.

The two-point HLOD score at *D4S392* is considerably higher than the multipoint HLOD score. This is not unexpected, because two-point linkage analysis is known to be more prone than multipoint analysis to inflated or deflated LOD scores. Marker information content at the *D4S392* locus is 0.61 in our families, which is much lower than the marker information content of ~0.9 that was achieved in our multipoint linkage analysis (fig. 2). A less informative marker, which is more likely to be present in two-point analysis than in multipoint analysis, can cause partial pedigrees to become uninformative at the marker locus. When partial linked or unlinked pedigrees become uninformative, the LOD score will be deflated or inflated, respectively. This problem is largely responsible for the phenomenon of having strong evidence for linkage to a single marker, without evidence, or with much weaker evidence, for the flanking markers.

The follow-up linkage analysis on 6p21-p22 was performed by analyzing nine new and six original markers in the 106 families and yielded a multipoint NPL score of 3.16 ($P = .00092$) at the marker interval *D6S422–D6S1660* and a parametric HLOD score of 2.14 ($\alpha = 32\%$) at the adjacent marker interval *D6S1584–D6S422*, under the dominant model of inheritance (table 2). Two-point nonparametric and parametric linkage analyses

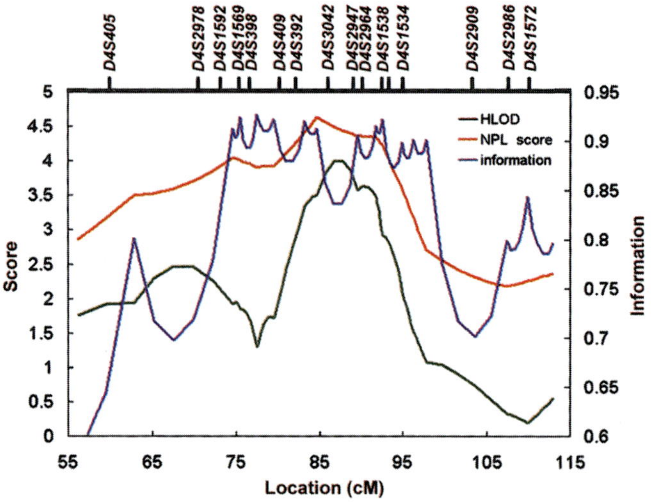

Figure 2 Multipoint LOD scores on 4q13-q21 from the joint linkage analysis of 106 families. Multipoint NPL scores (*red line*); multipoint HLOD scores, under a recessive model of inheritance (*black line*); and marker information content (*blue line*) are plotted.

also provided supporting evidence (data not shown). Therefore, the follow-up linkage analysis of additional families and markers increased the NPL score from 2.67 to 3.16, and the enhanced linkage evidence was only slightly below the genomewide criteria for "suggestive linkage" (Lander and Kruglyak 1995; Nyholt 2000).

Our linkage finding on 6p21-p22 is consistent with the suggested autoimmune pathogenesis of vitiligo and the involvement of the major histocompatibility complex (MHC) locus in genetic predisposition to vitiligo. Autoimmune pathogenesis of vitiligo has been suggested by both clinical and immunological observations (Kovacs 1998; Ongenae et al. 2003; Le Poole et al. 2004). For example, vitiligo is associated with other autoimmune disorders in many patients. Immunological studies also demonstrated that autoantibodies to melanocytes can be detected, and depigmentation of skin is often accompanied by T-cell infiltration to the skin in many patients with vitiligo (Wankowicz-Kalinska et al. 2003). Moreover, repigmenting therapies are often associated with an immunosuppressive effect. All of these observations provide direct and indirect supporting evidence for an autoimmunity-mediated pathogenesis of vitiligo. Because of the extensive pathogenic association of the MHC locus with a large number of autoimmune disorders (Horton et al. 2004), the involvement of the MHC genes in the pathogenesis of vitiligo was suspected and was intensively investigated by genetic association analysis. Candidate gene–based genetic association analyses of vitiligo in Chinese (Zhang et al. 2004*a*) and white populations (Venneker et al. 1992; Zamani et al. 2001; Arcos-Burgos et al. 2002; de Vijlder et al. 2004; Tastan et al. 2004) have revealed multiple evidence for association between alleles of the MHC genes and vitiligo. Therefore, our linkage finding on 6p21-p22 was probably not unexpected, and it provides additional linkage evidence for the involvement of the MHC region in genetic risk of vitiligo. Moreover, our result also supports the suggestion that vitiligo shares some genetic risk factors with other autoimmune disorders (Spritz et al. 2004).

The linkage signal on 1p36 from the genomewide analysis was further investigated by analyzing six new and five original markers in 106 families. The follow-up linkage analysis of the 106 families yielded a multipoint NPL score of 2.37 ($P = .009$) and a multipoint recessive HLOD score of 1.17 at the marker interval *D1S2734–D1S234* (table 2), which failed to strengthen the original linkage evidence on 1p36. Our moderate linkage evidence on chromosome 1p is at least 30 cM away from the *AIS1* locus that was identified in the white population (Alkhateeb et al. 2002; Fain et al. 2003; Spritz et al. 2004). Therefore, our linkage analysis in Chinese families did not provide supporting evidence for this previously identified linkage on 1p in the white population. The linkage findings on 6q24-q25, 14q12-q13, and 22q12 were also further investigated in the 106 families, but none of these linkage findings was enhanced by the follow-up analysis of additional families (table 2).

Our linkage findings in the Chinese population show a minimal overlap with the previous linkage findings in white populations. Except for the 6p21-p22 region, our findings (highly significant linkage on 4q13-q21 and moderate linkage on 1p36, 6q24-q25, 14q12-q13, and 22q12) are all novel and were not reported in previous genomewide linkage analyses of white populations. Furthermore, previously identified strong linkage evidence on 1p31 (*AIS1*) (Alkhateeb et al. 2002; Fain et al. 2003; Spritz et al. 2004), 7q (*AIS2*), and 8p (*AIS3*) (Spritz et al. 2004) in the white population received little, if any, supporting evidence from our current linkage analysis of Chinese families. Such little overlap between the linkage findings in Chinese and white populations is very intriguing and might suggest that vitiligo is associated with strong genetic heterogeneity and that it involves different genetic risk factors in different ethnic populations. Meanwhile, we still need to keep in mind that it is possible that the current and previous linkage findings are largely false positives, which could account for the small amount of overlap in linkage findings. However, considering the high statistical significance of our linkage finding on 4q13-q21 in Chinese families and the previous linkage findings on 1p31 (*AIS1*), 7q (*AIS2*), and 8p (*AIS3*) in white families, we reason that this possibility is unlikely, although it can not be totally ruled out. Moreover, we hypothesize that there may be a significant difference in the genetic basis of vitiligo between Chinese and white populations. Such a difference in linkage results between Chinese and white populations can also be seen in studies of psoriasis, another autoimmune skin disorder (Gudjonsson et al. 2004), in which the 4q28-q31 region was recently recognized as a strong candidate region for hosting a susceptibility gene for psoriasis (Bowcock 2004). Linkage to psoriasis on 4q28-q31 was identified with highly significant evidence in a genomewide linkage analysis of Chinese families (Zhang et al. 2002) but not in any of five previous genomewide linkage analyses of white families. Independent supporting evidence for this linkage emerged only after the five white population–based genomewide linkage studies were pooled together in a meta-analysis (Sagoo et al. 2004). This suggests that, although the as-yet-unidentified susceptibility gene within the 4q28-q31 region is a major susceptibility gene that contributes significantly to genetic risk of psoriasis in the Chinese population, it probably contributes much less in the white population and thus can only be detected by the analysis of a very large number of families. An interesting question is whether the same is true for the linkage to vitiligo on 4q13-q21. Additional linkage studies in Chinese and white populations will likely shed light on this question.

In summary, we have performed the first genomewide linkage study of vitiligo in a Chinese population. We have identified linkage evidence in several genomic regions, and the evidence on 4q13-q21 has been confirmed by our follow-up analysis of additional new families. Not only has the overall linkage evidence from the joint linkage analysis of the 106 families surpassed the genomewide criteria for "significant linkage," but the linkage results from the follow-up linkage analysis of the 49 new families also have provided independent evidence for linkage. Our linkage results strongly suggest that the 4q13-q21 region likely harbors a major susceptibility locus for vitiligo and should be targeted as a candidate for disease-gene discovery.

Acknowledgments

This work was funded by grants from the Chinese High Tech Program (863) (2003AA227030, 2002BA711A10, 2001AA227031, and 2001AA224021), the Shanghai Science and Technology Committee (03DJ14008), and the Chinese Ministry of Education (2003). We are grateful to all the families who participated in this study.

Electronic-Database Information

The URLs for data presented herein are as follows:

David Duffy's QIMR Homepage, http://www2.qimr.edu.au/davidD/

MERLIN, http://www.sph.umich.edu/csg/abecasis/Merlin/index.html

Online Mendelian Inheritance in Man (OMIM), http://www.ncbi.nlm.nih.gov/Omim/ (for vitiligo)

References

Abecasis GR, Cherny SS, Cookson WO, Cardon LR (2002) Merlin-rapid analysis of dense genetic maps using sparse gene flow trees. Nat Genet 30:97–101

Alkhateeb A, Fain PR, Thody T, Bennett DC, Spritz RA (2003) Vitiligo and associated autoimmune diseases in Caucasian probands and their families. Pigment Cell Res 16:208–214

Alkhateeb A, Stetler GL, Old W, Talbert J, Uhlhorn C, Taylor M, Fox A, Miller C, Dills DG, Ridgway EC, Bennett DC, Fain PR, Spritz RA (2002) Mapping of an autoimmunity susceptibility locus (*AIS1*) to chromosome 1p31.3-p32.2. Hum Mol Genet 11:661–667

Arcos-Burgos M, Parodi E, Salgar M, Bedoya E, Builes JJ, Jaramillo D, Ceballos G, Uribe A, Rivera N, Rivera D, Fonseca I, Camargo M, Palacio LG (2002) Vitiligo: complex segregation and linkage disequilibrium analyses with respect to microsatellite loci spanning the HLA. Hum Genet 110: 334–342

Blomhoff A, Helen Kemp E, Gawkrodger DJ, Weetman AP, Husebye ES, Akselsen HE, Lie BA, Undlien DE (2005) CTLA4 polymorphisms are associated with vitiligo, in patients with concomitant autoimmune diseases. Pigment Cell Res 18:55–58

Bolognia JL, Nordlund JJ, Ortonne J-P (1998) Vitiligo vulgaris. In: Nordlund JJ, Boissy RE, Hearing VJ, King RA, Ortonne J-P (eds) The pigmentary system. Oxford University Press, New York, pp 513–551

Bowcock AM (2004) Psoriasis genetics: the way forward. J Invest Dermatol 122:xv–xvii

Carnevale A, Zavala C, Castillo VD, Maldonado RR, Tamayo L (1980) Analisis genetico de 127 families con vitiligo. Rev Invest Clin 32:37–41

Casp CB, She JX, McCormack WT (2002) Genetic association of the catalase gene (CAT) with vitiligo susceptibility. Pigment Cell Res 15:62–66

——— (2003) Genes of the LMP/TAP cluster are associated with the human autoimmune disease vitiligo. Genes Immun 4:492–499

Cho S, Kang HC, Hahm JH (2000) Characteristics of vitiligo in Korean children. Pediatr Dermatol 17:189–193

Das SK, Majumder PP, Majumder TK, Haldar B (1985) Studies on vitiligo. II. Familial aggregation and genetics. Genet Epidemiol 2:255–262

de Vijlder HC, Westerhof W, Schreuder GM, de Lange P, Claas FH (2004) Difference in pathogenesis between vitiligo vulgaris and halo nevi associated with vitiligo is supported by an HLA association study. Pigment Cell Res 17:270–274

Fain PR, Gowan K, LaBerge GS, Alkhateeb A, Stetler GL, Talbert J, Bennett DC, Spritz RA (2003) A genomewide screen for generalized vitiligo: confirmation of *AIS1* on chromosome 1p31 and evidence for additional susceptibility loci. Am J Hum Genet 72:1560–1564

Goudie BM, Wilkinson C, Goudie RB (1983) A family study of vitiligo patterns. Scott Med J 28:338–342

Gudjonsson JE, Johnston A, Sigmundsdottir H, Valdimarsson H (2004) Immunopathogenic mechanisms in psoriasis. Clin Exp Immunol 135:1–8

Hafez M, Sharaf L, Abd el-Nabi SM (1983) The genetics of vitiligo. Acta Derm Venereol 63:249–251

Hann S-K, Nordlund J (2000) Vitiligo: a comprehensive monograph on basic and clinical science. Blackwell Science, Oxford, United Kingdom

Horton R, Wilming L, Rand V, Lovering RC, Bruford EA, Khodiyar VK, Lush MJ, Povey S, Talbot CC Jr, Wright MW, Wain HM, Trowsdale J, Ziegler A, Beck S (2004) Gene map of the extended human MHC. Nat Rev Genet 5:889–899

Howitz J, Brodthagen H, Schwartz M, Thompsen K (1977) Prevalence of vitiligo: epidemiological survey of the Isle of Bornholm, Denmark. Arch Dermatol 113:47–52

Jin SY, Park HH, Li GZ, Lee HJ, Hong MS, Hong SJ, Park HK, Chung JH, Lee MH (2004) Association of angiotensin converting enzyme gene I/D polymorphism of vitiligo in Korean population. Pigment Cell Res 17:84–86

Kemp EH, Ajjan RA, Waterman EA, Gawkrodger DJ, Cork MJ, Watson PF, Weetman AP (1999) Analysis of a microsatellite polymorphism of the cytotoxic T-lymphocyte antigen-4 gene in patients with vitiligo. Br J Dermatol 140:73–78

Kovacs SO (1998) Vitiligo. J Am Acad Dermatol 38:647–666

Kruglyak L, Daly MJ, Reeve-Daly, MP, Lander ES (1996) Parametric and nonparametric linkage analysis: a unified multipoint approach. Am J Hum Genet 58:1347–1363

Lander E, Kruglyak L (1995) Genetic dissection of complex traits: guidelines for interpreting and reporting linkage results. Nat Genet 11:241–247

Lathrop GM, Lalouel JM (1984) Easy calculations of lod scores and genetic risks on small computers. Am J Hum Genet 36:460–465

Le Poole IC, Wankowicz-Kalinska A, van den Wijngaard RM, Nickoloff BJ, Das PK (2004) Autoimmune aspects of depigmentation in vitiligo. J Investig Dermatol Symp Proc 9: 68–72

Majumder PP, Nordlund JJ, Nath SK (1993) Pattern of familial aggregation of vitiligo. Arch Dermatol 129:994–998

Mehta NR, Shah KC, Theodore C, Vyas VP, Patel AB (1973) Epidemiological study of vitiligo in Surat area. Indian J Med Res 61:145–154

Miller S, Dykes D, Polesky H (1988) A simple salting out procedure for extraction of high molecular weight DNA from human nucleated cells. Nucl Acids Res 16:1215

Na GY, Lee KH, Kim MK, Lee SJ, Kim do W, Kim JC (2003) Polymorphisms in the melanocortin-1 receptor (MC1R) and agouti signaling protein (ASIP) genes in Korean vitiligo patients. Pigment Cell Res 16:383–387

Nath SK, Kelly JA, Namjou B, Lam T, Bruner GR, Scofield RH, Aston CE, Harley JB (2001) Evidence for a susceptibility gene, *SLEV1,* on chromosome 17p13 in families with vitiligo-related systemic lupus erythematosus. Am J Hum Genet 69:1401–1406

Nath SK, Majumder PP, Nordlund JJ (1994) Genetic epidemiology of vitiligo: multilocus recessivity cross-validated. Am J Hum Genet 55:981–990

Nyholt DR (2000) All LODs are not created equal. Am J Hum Genet 67:282–288

O'Connell JR, Weeks DE (1998) PedCheck: a program for

identification of genotype incompatibilities in linkage analysis. Am J Hum Genet 63:259–266

Ongenae K, Van Geel N, Naeyaert JM (2003) Evidence for an autoimmune pathogenesis of vitiligo. Pigment Cell Res 16: 90–100

Sagoo GS, Tazi-Ahnini R, Barker JW, Elder JT, Nair RP, Samuelsson L, Traupe H, Trembath RC, Robinson DA, Iles MM (2004) Meta-analysis of genome-wide studies of psoriasis susceptibility reveals linkage to chromosomes 6p21 and 4q28-q31 in Caucasian and Chinese Hans population. J Invest Dermatol 122:1401–1405

Spritz RA, Gowan K, Bennett DC, Fain PR (2004) Novel vitiligo susceptibility loci on chromosomes 7 (*AIS2*) and 8 (*AIS3*), confirmation of *SLEV1* on chromosome 17, and their roles in an autoimmune diathesis. Am J Hum Genet 74:188–191

Tastan HB, Akar A, Orkunoglu FE, Arca E, Inal A (2004) Association of HLA class I antigens and HLA class II alleles with vitiligo in a Turkish population. Pigment Cell Res 17: 181–184

Venneker GT, Westerhof W, de Vries IJ (1992) Molecular heterogeneity of the fourth component of complement (C4) and its genes in vitiligo. J Invest Dermatol 99:853–858

Wankowicz-Kalinska A, van den Wijngaard RM, Tigges BJ, Westerhof W, Ogg GS, Cerundolo V, Storkus WJ, Das PK (2003) Immunopolarization of $CD4^+$ and $CD8^+$ T cells to type-1-like is associated with melanocyte loss in human vitiligo. Lab Invest 83:683–695

Xu YY, Ye DQ, Tong ZC, Hao JH, Jin J, Shen SF, Li CR, Zhang XJ (2002) An epidemiological survey for four skin diseases in Anhui [In Chinese]. Chin J Dermatol 35:406–407

Zamani M, Spaepen M, Sghar SS, Huang C, Westerhof W, Nieuweboer-Krobotova L, Cassiman JJ (2001) Linkage and association of HLA class II genes with vitiligo in a Dutch population. Br J Dermatol 145:90–94

Zhang XJ, He PP, Wang ZX, Zhang J, Li YB, Wang HY, Wei SC, Chen SY, Xu SJ, Jin L, Yang S, Huang W (2002) Evidence for a major psoriasis susceptibility locus at 6p21 (PSORS1) and a novel candidate region at 4q31 by genome-wide scan in Chinese Hans. J Invest Dermatol 119:1361–1366

Zhang XJ, Liu HS, Liang YH, Sun LD, Wang JY, Yang S, Liu JB, Gao M, He PP, Cui Y, Yang Q (2004*a*) Association of HLA class I alleles with vitiligo in Chinese Hans. J Dermatol Sci 35:165–168

Zhang XJ, Liu JB, Gui JP, Li M, Xiong QG, Wu HB, Li JX, Yang S, Wang HY, Gao M, Yang J, Yang Q (2004*b*) Characteristics of genetic epidemiology and genetic models for vitiligo. J Am Acad Dermatol 51:383–390

Am. J. Hum. Genet. 76:1066–1073, 2005

Report

In Silico Analysis of Disease-Association Mapping Strategies Using the Coalescent Process and Incorporating Ascertainment and Selection

Ying Wang and Bruce Rannala

Genome Center and Section of Evolution and Ecology, University of California Davis, Davis

We present a new method for simulating samples of marker haplotypes, genotypes, or diplotypes in case-control studies in which the markers are linked to a disease locus in any specified region of the genome. The method allows realistic features to be incorporated into the simulations, including selection acting on disease alleles, sample ascertainment of disease chromosomes and polymorphic markers, a genetic dominance model of disease expression that allows incomplete penetrance and phenocopies, and an accurate genetic map of recombination rates and hotspots for recombination in the human genome (or, alternatively, an improved method for simulating the distribution of hotspots). The new method uses an approach that combines simulation of the coalescent process for the sampled chromosomes with a diffusion process used to model the evolution of the disease-mutation frequency over time. Examples illustrate how the method may be used to study the expected power of a marker-disease association study.

Recent initiatives such as the International HapMap Project, as well as expanding databases of mapped SNPs (dbSNP) and microsatellite polymorphisms (Marshfield Center for Medical Genetics), have created opportunities for large-scale association studies to map human disease loci with the use of unrelated cases and controls. To examine the power of particular mapping strategies, a comprehensive simulation program is needed that allows samples of haplotypes, genotypes, or diplotypes to be generated under realistic conditions. Here, we present a new simulation methodology that has been developed for this purpose. The method combines a coalescent process (which is used for modeling the genealogy underlying a sample of chromosomes from cases and controls) and a diffusion process (which is used for modeling the evolutionary history of the frequency of a disease mutation), and it allows for the incorporation into simulation studies of additional features that are very important in human populations (and human disease studies) but that have been neglected by past simulation methodologies. New features include sample ascertainment of disease chromosomes and polymorphic markers, a genetic dominance model of disease expression that allows incomplete penetrance and phenocopies, and an accurate genetic map of recombination rates and hotspots for recombination in the human genome (or, alternatively, an improved method for simulating the distribution of hotspots).

Several programs have been developed recently to simulate samples of chromosomes under either a neutral Fisher-Wright model (Hudson 2002; Posada and Wiuf 2003) with recombination and genetic drift or a model with selection acting on a specified locus (Spencer and Coop 2004). These methods are perfectly adequate for simulating a random sample of chromosomes from a large population. However, in case-control association studies, linkage disequilibrium mapping studies, and other disease-gene mapping contexts, the sample is highly nonrandom. Ascertainment of individuals that exhibit a disease enriches the sample for an underlying disease mutation, increasing its frequency in the sample, relative either to that in the population or to that expected in a random sample. Zöllner and von Haeseler (2000) developed a method for simulating the joint coalescent structure for a neutral disease locus in cases and controls in which all cases have exclusively disease-mutation–bearing chromosomes and all controls have exclusively normal chromosomes. This is suitable for modeling a

Received March 15, 2005; accepted for publication March 23, 2005; electronically published April 7, 2005.

Address for correspondence and reprints: Dr. Bruce Rannala, Genome Center, One Shields Avenue, University of California Davis, Davis, CA 95616. E-mail: brannala@ucdavis.edu

0002-9297/2005/7606-0013$15.00

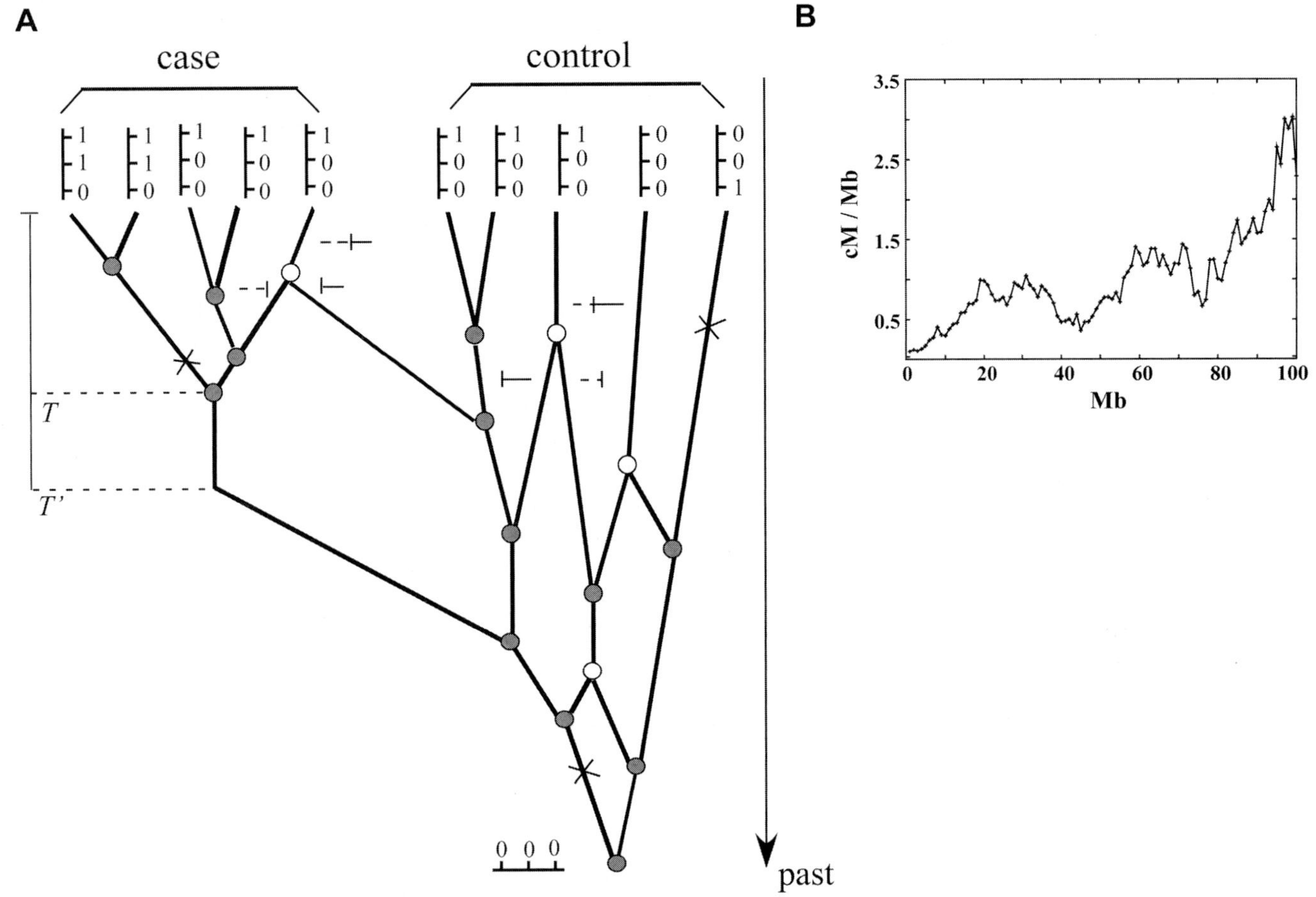

Figure 1 *A,* The structure of a coalescent model with recombination, between a chromosomal segment descended from a disease mutation at a given locus (*left*) and a sample of chromosomes not descended from the mutant (*right*). The alleles present at three diallelic marker loci are indicated by "0" and "1" for the sampled chromosomes that are represented as vertical lines at the top of the figure. Ancestral chromosomes involved in coalescence and recombination events are indicated by shaded and unshaded circles, respectively, on the ancestral recombination graph, and mutation events are represented as crosses. Segments of chromosomes transmitted to descendent lineages from each of the two ancestral lineages following a recombination event are represented as solid and broken horizontal lines. *B,* The distribution of recombination rates over a chromosome, generated by one instance of a GBM simulation.

sample of cases and controls for a rare recessive disease, for example. One drawback to their approach is that it assumes that the population frequency of the disease mutation has remained constant since it arose. Wang and Rannala (2004) used a diffusion process to model the evolution of the disease-allele frequency over time, thus relaxing the assumption of a constant disease-mutation frequency but retaining the assumption of a simple Mendelian inheritance pattern and a neutral disease locus. The objective of the present study is to extend the model of Wang and Rannala (2004) to allow both for a complex model of inheritance for a disease locus and for natural selection acting on the locus. We also incorporate more-realistic models of recombination hotspots into our simulation procedure. Our approach builds on earlier work by Kaplan et al. (1988) and Hudson and Kaplan (1988), who focused primarily on modeling the effects of deterministic selection on summary statistics (such as the number of segregating sites) for a random sample of chromosomes by use of a coalescent theory framework.

A unique (nonrecurrent) mutation is assumed to arise as a single copy at generation T' in the past (fig. 1*A*). A present-day sample of chromosomes is generated by fixing the age of the mutation (T') and then simulating the frequency of the mutation forward through time, conditional on nonextinction, where p_t is the frequency at generation t in the past. Our method also allows one to condition on the present-day allele frequency, p_0, via rejection sampling. For a neutral allele, the process of random drift of the allele frequency can be simulated by use of a diffusion approximation (e.g., Kimura and Takahata 1983). Given the sample path of the frequency of the disease allele over time, $\mathbf{p} = \{p_t, p_{t-1}, \ldots, p_0\}$,

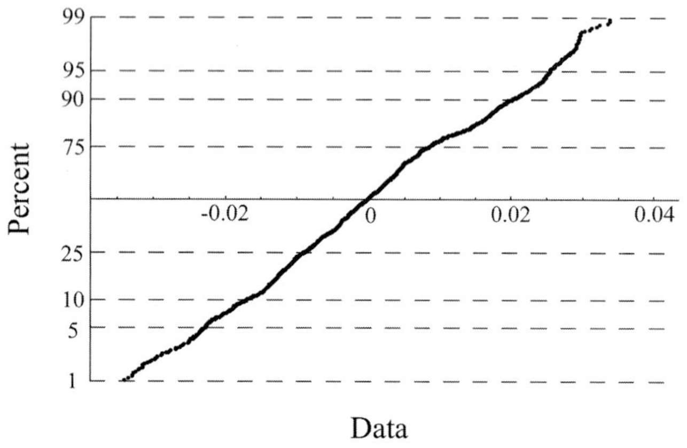

Figure 2 Normal probability plot, constructed by use of conditional distribution of normalized log recombination rates for the Icelandic map data of Kong et al. (2002). The plot is based on marker data obtained from the q arm of chromosome 2 in females. The more linear the appearance of the plot, the better the fit to the GBM model.

the coalescent process with recombination is simulated on the basis of an ancestral recombination graph with variable population size $2N_tp_t$ among chromosomes carrying the mutation and with variable population size $2N_t(1-p_t)$ among those not carrying the mutation (Wang and Rannala 2004). We assume a model of either constant population size or continuous exponential growth, but arbitrary population growth patterns can be readily incorporated.

The waiting time until a coalescent event occurs in the gene tree of either mutation-bearing chromosomes or normal chromosomes is simulated using a discrete-time model (with time measured in units of generations), rather than the more usual continuous-time model. To efficiently simulate the waiting times on a discrete-time scale, a recursion strategy is used (Wang and Rannala 2004). At times after the origin of the mutation, mutant chromosomes only coalesce with one another, as do the normal chromosomes. Recombination can occur both within and between genealogies of the mutant and normal chromosomes. If a homogeneous recombination model is used, then the recombination breakpoints are uniformly distributed along the chromosomal region. Otherwise, recombination rates along the region either are simulated using a geometric Brownian motion (GBM) model (described below) or are extracted from the Icelandic recombination map data (Kong et al. 2002).

After the genealogy of the sample of the disease and normal chromosomes is generated, mutations are superimposed on it. Given the size of the chromosomal interval and the mutation rate either for SNPs under a Jukes-Cantor model or for STRP (microsatellite) markers under a stepwise mutation model (Ohta and Kimura 1973; Valdes et al. 1993), the number of mutations that occur in the history of the sample at each site follows a Poisson distribution. The numbers and the positions of markers are treated as random variables, and the distribution of the positions of mutations on branches of the genealogy is uniform under a Poisson process model of mutation (see Hudson 1990). Only polymorphic sites are retained as potential markers. The evolution of the polymorphic sites is simulated forward in time. Because of recombination or relatively younger mutations at marker loci, some markers may be monomorphic or may have a low polymorphism level. The markers that comprise the sample are randomly chosen in accordance with a predefined polymorphism cutoff level.

If a disease locus is under selection, the sample path of the population frequency of the disease mutation is instead generated by use of a diffusion model with selection. The Kimura and Takahata (1983) procedure for simulation of the sample path under neutral drift can be modified to incorporate selection. The allele frequency at the next generation, given the current frequency, is normally distributed, with expectation and variance determined by the diffusion model. The average change of allele frequency per generation under selection (with selection coefficient $s>0$) is $M_{\delta p}=sp(1-p)$, in accordance with a diffusion approximation (with no dominance). If population size (N) is constant, the variance of the change in allele frequency ($\sigma^2_{\delta p}$) that results from random drift is $p(1-p)/(2N)$. If we assume that the population has grown exponentially with rate r to the current population size (N_0), then, at generation t in the past, $\sigma^2_{\delta p}=p(1-p)/(2N_0e^{-rt})$. Given the age and initial frequency, $1/(2N_0e^{-rT'})$, of the disease mutation, the change of frequency is simulated by generating a uniform random variable with mean $M_{\delta p}$ and variance $\sigma^2_{\delta p}$, conditional on nonextinction. If fewer than four copies of the disease allele are present in the population, the diffusion approximation is no longer accurate, and the number of alleles in the next generation is instead simulated as a Poisson random variable (with parameter pe^r) by use of the branching-process approximation for a rare allele (see Ewens 1979). The method can be extended to other selection models by simply replacing the average rate of change of allele frequency under a diffusion model.

Recent studies suggest that the human genome consists of haplotype blocks (Phillips et al. 2003). This haplotype-block structure is a consequence of population processes as well as recombination hotspots, and, to accurately model human haplotype structure, both processes should be incorporated into the model. Recent evidence suggests that recombination rates in humans are higher near the telomeres and lower near the centromeres. The Icelandic recombination map displays a

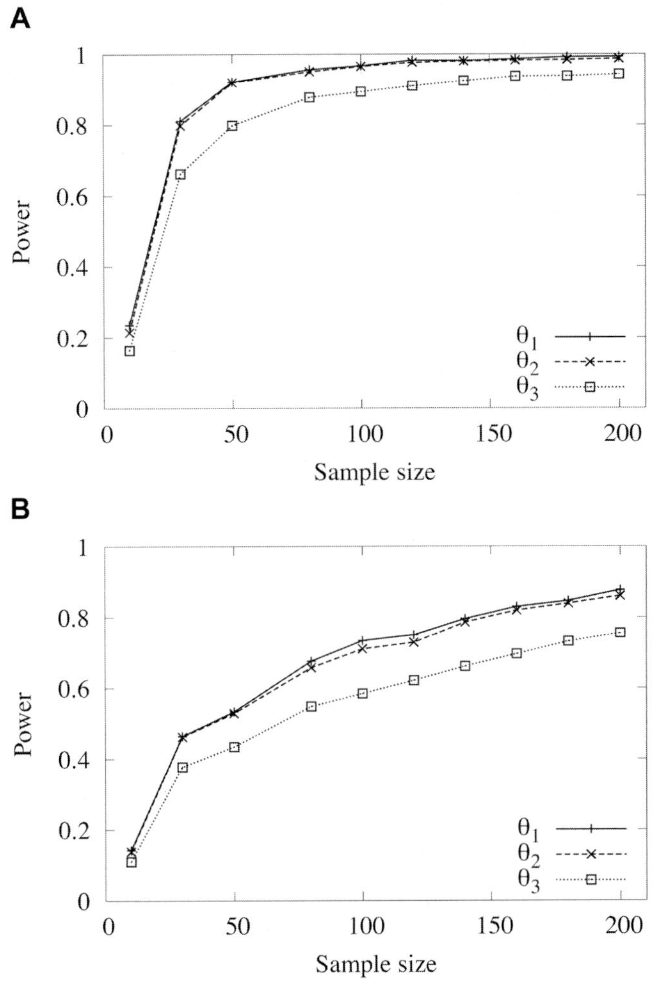

Figure 3 Expected power, as a function of sample size, of an association study to detect a disease locus with either purely recessive (*A*) or purely dominant (*B*) inheritance for markers positioned in three different chromosomal intervals, with average distances of 1 kb (θ_1), 10 kb (θ_2), or 100 kb (θ_3) from the disease locus. The parameters $N_0 = 10^6$, $r = 0.01$, and $s = 0$ were used for the simulations. The disease-mutation age $T = 840$ was chosen to satisfy $E(p) = 0.1$. A total of 5,000 replicate simulations were used to compute the expected power.

large number of recombination rate peaks and valleys distributed along each chromosome, with an increasing trend in rates from centromere to telomere (Kong et al. 2002). We propose a new method that uses a GBM model, with the recombination rate evolving over the length of the chromosome, to simulate the distribution of nonhomogeneous recombination rates along a chromosomal region. The GBM process, also called "log-normal growth," is a particularly attractive model of rate evolution because it assumes that changes of rate are random but that the magnitude of such changes is proportional to the current rate.

Under a GBM model, the log ratio of the recombination rate at one point on a chromosome, conditional on the rate at the preceding point, follows a normal distribution, with the mean and variance correlated with the physical distance between the two points. If a GBM model is used to simulate the distribution of recombination rates in this way, it implies that adjacent loci will tend to have similar crossover rates, yet there exists a stochastic deviation of rates between loci that depends on the diffusion coefficient (σ^2) in the GBM process and the physical distance between the two sites. If a GBM process with drift ($\mu > 0$) is assumed, if the initial recombination rate is set to a relatively small value, and if recombination rates are always simulated from centromere to telomere, then the process mimics the tendency for recombination to be high near the telomere and low near the centromere. An example of a simulated GBM process of the evolution of recombination hotspots on a chromosome is given in figure 1*B*.

The validity of the GBM model for the distribution of recombination rates along a chromosome was examined by fitting the conditional distribution of the normalized log rates at adjacent sites to a standard normal distribution via a normal probability plot applied to the data of Kong et al. (2002) (fig. 2). In the simulation program, the default drift (μ) and diffusion (σ^2) parameters are the average of the maximum-likelihood estimator (MLE) over all autosomal chromosomes (pooling females and males), calculated by using the data of Kong et al. (2002). The MLEs are $\mu = 3.074 \times 10^{-8}$ and $\sigma^2 = 2.503 \times 10^{-8}$, respectively. Other options included in the program are uniform rates of recombination (e.g., 1 cM = 1 Mb) and rates of recombination for any specified chromosomal interval obtained directly from the Icelandic map (Kong et al. 2002).

Phenocopies, low penetrance, and other factors may lead to a loss of power for identification of disease-mutation location by use of association methods. The effect of disease penetrance was incorporated into in our simulation procedure by using a standard three-parameter penetrance model. At the disease-mutation locus, the disease-causing allele is denoted by "D," and the alternative allele is denoted by "N." The probability that an individual has a certain genotype at the disease locus (e.g., genotype DN), given that the individual expresses the disease phenotype, is

$$f(\mathrm{DN}|\mathrm{affected}) = \frac{f_\mathrm{D}(\mathrm{DN})\ g(\mathrm{DN})}{\sum_X f_\mathrm{D}(X)\ g(X)}\ , \qquad (1)$$

where $f_\mathrm{D}(\cdot)$ represents the penetrance of a genotype at the disease locus and $g(\cdot)$ denotes the frequency of a genotype. If we assume Hardy-Weinberg equilibrium at

Table 1

Descriptions of Parameters and Variables Used in Simulation Studies

Parameter/Variable	Description
n_D and n_N	Numbers of affected and normal (control) individuals in the sample
N_0	Current population size
r	Exponential population growth rate
T'	Age (in generations) of the disease-susceptibility allele
p	Population frequency of the disease-susceptibility allele
E(p)	Expected population frequency of the disease-susceptibility allele
$\theta_{(\cdot)}$	Marker location (in Mb)
s	Selection coefficient
$f_{(\cdot)}$	Disease-penetrance parameter of a genotype
ϕ	Disease prevalence
$R_{(\cdot)}$	Genotype-specific disease risk relative to the homozygous (nonsusceptibility allele) genotype

the disease locus and if the population frequency (p) of the disease mutation is known, equation (1) becomes

$$f(\mathrm{DN}|\mathrm{affected}) = \frac{f_{\mathrm{D}}(\mathrm{DN})\ 2p(1-p)}{f_{\mathrm{D}}(\mathrm{DD})p^2 + f_{\mathrm{D}}(\mathrm{DN})2p(1-p) + f_{\mathrm{D}}(\mathrm{NN})(1-p)^2}\ . \tag{2}$$

Similarly, the probability that an individual has a certain genotype at the disease locus (e.g., genotype DN), given that the individual does not express the disease phenotype, denoted by "$f(\mathrm{DN}|\mathrm{unaffected})$," can be obtained by replacing $f_{\mathrm{D}}(\mathrm{DN})$ in $f(\mathrm{DN}|\mathrm{affected})$ with $1 - f_{\mathrm{D}}(\mathrm{DN})$. Conditional probabilities for other genotypes can be calculated using the above equation, by substituting the corresponding penetrance and frequency terms.

Given the above conditional probabilities for two categories (cases and controls) and the number of individuals in these two categories, the distribution of the counts of individuals in a sample with each genotype at the disease locus will follow a multinomial distribution. The distribution of the number of disease and normal chromosomes in a sample is therefore completely specified by this sampling model. Genotypes are simulated from the multinomial distribution defined by this model. For example, the distribution of genotypes among n_{A} affected individuals is

$$f(n_{\mathrm{DD}},n_{\mathrm{DN}},n_{\mathrm{NN}}|n_{\mathrm{A}}) = \binom{n_{\mathrm{A}}}{n_{\mathrm{DD}},n_{\mathrm{DN}},n_{\mathrm{NN}}} \times f(\mathrm{DD}|\mathrm{affected})^{n_{\mathrm{DD}}} \times f(\mathrm{DN}|\mathrm{affected})^{n_{\mathrm{DN}}} \times f(\mathrm{NN}|\mathrm{affected})^{n_{\mathrm{NN}}}\ , \tag{3}$$

where n_{DD}, for example, is the number of DD genotypes in a sample of n_{A} affected individuals. Given the numbers of disease-mutation–bearing chromosomes and normal chromosomes in the sample (a simple function of the genotype counts), the simulation methods discussed above are used to generate a sample of disease and normal chromosomes that have multiple linked markers.

Here, we provide several examples of how our program can be applied to examine the prospective power of association studies to detect a mutation that contributes to a disease. Power is measured as the proportion of replicate simulations for which the simulated case-control genotype data show a significant marker-disease association, as determined by a χ^2 test of association applied to genotypes, with the critical value set at $P = .05$. The parameters and variables used in the simulations are summarized in table 1.

Two penetrance models were considered in our simulation study: additive and multiplicative models. If, for convenience, we define ρ and α as two intermediate coefficients, then $f_{\mathrm{D}}(\mathrm{DD}) = 2\rho$, $f_{\mathrm{D}}(\mathrm{DN}) = \rho + \alpha$, and $f_{\mathrm{D}}(\mathrm{NN}) = 2\alpha$ for the additive model and $f_{\mathrm{D}}(\mathrm{DD}) = \rho^2$, $f_{\mathrm{D}}(\mathrm{DN}) = \rho\alpha$, and $f_{\mathrm{D}}(\mathrm{NN}) = \alpha^2$ for the multiplicative model. Given $\phi = f_{\mathrm{D}}(\mathrm{DD})p^2 + f_{\mathrm{D}}(\mathrm{DN})2p(1-p) + f_{\mathrm{D}}(\mathrm{NN})(1-p)^2$ and the relative disease risk for genotype DD (denoted as "R_{DD}" [we define the risk relative to genotype NN]), the parameters ρ and α in an additive penetrance model are

$$\rho = \frac{R_{\mathrm{DD}}\phi}{2(1-p+pR_{\mathrm{DD}})} \tag{4}$$

and

$$\alpha = \frac{\rho}{R_{\mathrm{DD}}}\ , \tag{5}$$

and the parameters ρ and α in a multiplicative model are

$$\rho = \sqrt{\frac{\phi}{p^2 + \sqrt{\frac{1}{R_{\mathrm{DD}}}}2p(1-p) + \frac{1}{R_{\mathrm{DD}}}(1-p)^2}} \tag{6}$$

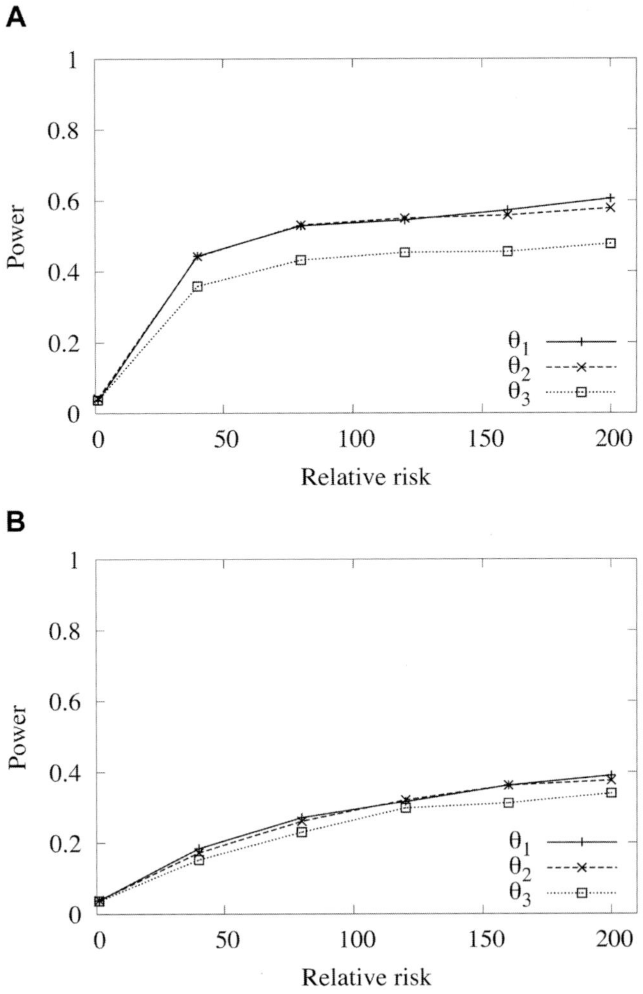

Figure 4 Expected power, as a function of genotype relative risk, of an association study to detect a neutral disease-associated mutation, computed by using markers positioned in three different chromosomal intervals, with average distances of 1 kb (θ_1), 10 kb (θ_2), or 100 kb (θ_3) from the disease locus. Power was estimated using simulated samples with $n_D = 100$ and $n_N = 100$. *A,* Expected power, with an average present-day population frequency of the disease mutation of $p = 0.1$ and a mutation age of 840 generations. *B,* Expected power, with an average present-day population frequency of the disease mutation of $p = 0.01$ and a mutation age of 600 generations.

and

$$\alpha = \rho\sqrt{\frac{1}{R_{DD}}} \; . \tag{7}$$

The results of our simulations will be presented in terms of relative risk, etc., rather than in terms of the parameters of the penetrance model, to make the interpretation more straightforward.

Simulation studies were performed to examine the power of marker-disease association studies for simple Mendelian disorders and for a range of more complex models of disease inheritance. In the case of a purely recessive disease ($f_{DD} = 1$, $f_{DN} = 0$, and $f_{NN} = 0$), the power of association methods to detect a disease locus is high, as expected, and is >0.9 when the sample size exceeds 50 for both cases and controls (fig. 3). For a purely dominant disease ($f_{DD} = 1$, $f_{DN} = 1$, and $f_{NN} = 0$), association studies are less powerful, but the power consistently increases with increasing sample sizes (fig. 3). For both sets of results shown in figure 3, the parameters $N_0 = 10^6$, $r = 0.01$, and $s = 0$ were used to perform the simulations, and $T' = 840$ was chosen to satisfy $E(p) = 0.1$. A total of 5,000 replicates were used to compute the expected power.

For more-general models of disease inheritance, given $E(p)$, ϕ, and R_{DD}, an additive model is assumed, and penetrance parameters are calculated using equation (2). The power of association studies is plotted against the relative risk of a disease. The parameters $N_0 = 10^6$, $r = 0.01$, $n_D = 100$, and $n_N = 100$ were used for the simulations. Two different average present-day population frequencies of a disease mutation were considered: a relatively high frequency of 0.1 and a relatively low frequency of 0.01. The age of the disease mutation was chosen such that the mean frequency would be equal to the present-day population frequency—either 840 or 600 generations (for frequencies of 0.1 and 0.01, respectively) for a neutral disease mutation (fig. 4) or 780 or 560 generations (for frequencies of 0.1 and 0.01, respectively) for a disease mutation under selection with $s = 0.001$ (results [not shown] are virtually identical to those shown in fig. 4). Figure 5 shows the results when the simulation parameters used to generate figure 4 are again used, but with a larger sample size ($n_D = 500$ and $n_N = 500$, instead of $n_D = 100$ and $n_N = 100$). For sample sizes of $n_D = 100$ and $n_N = 100$, the power to detect an association, computed by using the markers at three chromosomal intervals, is moderately higher for a more frequent disease than for a less frequent disease, and the power is similar, independent of whether markers in any of the three intervals are used, especially for a less frequent disease (fig. 4). Selection appeared to have little effect on the power. The results shown in figure 5 suggest that sample size can greatly affect the power of marker-disease association studies; much greater power is achieved if sample size is increased. This is true for both common and rare diseases.

The method we present focuses on a single disease locus. Allelic and locus heterogeneity are incorporated into the model in a vague manner through the phenocopy probability. It is straightforward to simulate two or more disease mutations of the same gene (allelic heterogeneity) with the use of our methodology by simulating multiple disease-locus genealogies. One could then use an expanded penetrance model (e.g., with six

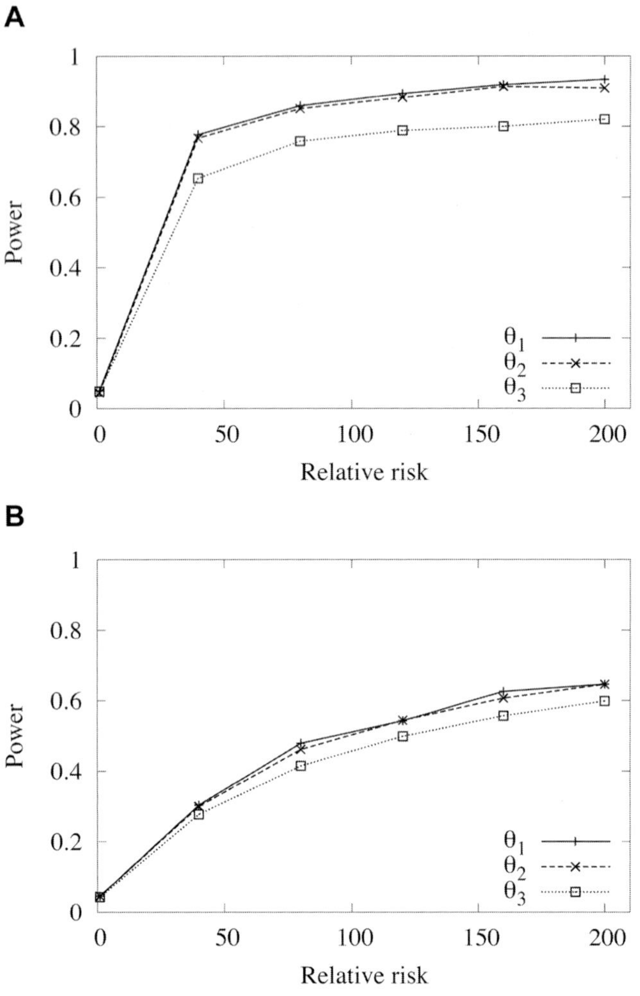

Figure 5 Expected power, as a function of genotype relative risk, of an association study to detect a neutral disease-associated mutation, computed by using markers positioned in three different chromosomal intervals, with average distances of 1 kb (θ_1), 10 kb (θ_2), or 100 kb (θ_3) from the disease locus. Power was estimated using simulated samples with $n_D = 500$ and $n_N = 500$. *A*, Expected power, with an average present-day population frequency of the disease mutation of $p = 0.1$ and a mutation age of 840 generations. *B*, Expected power, with an average present-day population frequency of the disease mutation of $p = 0.01$ and a mutation age of 600 generations.

parameters for two disease-risk alleles). Similarly, one could model disease-locus heterogeneity (for unlinked loci) by using a quantitative genetic model that allows for epistasis among two or more disease loci to obtain the probability distribution of multilocus genotypes in cases and controls and then by independently simulating each locus in cases and controls.

Another way the model could be extended would be to allow population genotype frequencies to deviate from Hardy-Weinberg equilibrium proportions by incorporating an inbreeding coefficient. This would be useful for simulating small populations with high levels of consanguineous matings, for example. Our method conditions on the disease-mutation age and then simulates the present-day frequency. To condition on frequency and age, we use rejection sampling; the user specifies an interval for the population frequency of the disease mutation, and only those simulated data sets for which the frequency is in this interval are accepted. Although technically correct, this can be computationally inefficient, and alternative approaches might instead either condition on frequency and generate random ages via the simulation or condition on both frequency and age. The simulation method of Spencer and Coop (2004) conditions on the frequency of the disease mutation and samples from the distribution of mutation ages, taking advantage of the reversibility property of the diffusion process (Griffiths 2003). The method assumes that population size is constant, however, and it cannot be easily extended to model growing populations.

A final problem in simulating case-control studies is how to correct for marker ascertainment bias. In many instances, markers are prescreened for polymorphisms by using a sample of unrelated normal individuals; a subset of these prescreened polymorphic markers is then screened in cases and controls. We modeled ascertainment bias by assuming that a random subset of markers is chosen in an interval from the total set of polymorphic markers in the interval (in sampled cases and controls). One could make this procedure slightly more realistic by assuming that the markers are chosen from those sites that are polymorphic in an expanded sample of "normal" chromosomes (rather than from the present sample of normal and disease chromosomes). In our opinion, power analyses based on computer simulations of population samples, such as those proposed here, are more reliable for predicting when a particular study design will have low power than for predicting when the design will have high power. This is because we expect important (and perhaps unidentified) factors that have not been included in the model to be more likely, a priori, to reduce the power than to increase it.

The program GeneArtisan, written in the C++ language, is available as either a command-line program or a crossplatform graphical interface program for Linux, Windows, and Mac OS X. The program can be downloaded from authors' Web site.

Acknowledgments

Support for this research was provided by Canadian Institutes of Health Research (CIHR) grant MOP 44064 and National Institutes of Health grant HG01988 (to B.R). Salary support for B.R. was provided by the Alberta Heritage Foundation for Medical Research and the CIHR/Peter Lougheed Scholar Award.

Electronic-Database Information

The URLs for data presented herein are as follows:

Authors' Web site, http://www.rannala.org/ (for the program GeneArtisan)
dbSNP, http://www.ncbi.nlm.nih.gov/SNP/
International HapMap Project, http://www.hapmap.org/
Marshfield Center for Medical Genetics, http://research.marshfieldclinic.org/genetics/

References

Ewens WJ (1979) Mathematical population genetics. Springer-Verlag, New York

Griffiths RC (2003) The frequency spectrum of a mutation, and its age, in a general diffusion model. Theor Popul Biol 64:241–251

Hudson RR (1990) Gene genealogies and the coalescent process. Oxf Surv Evol Biol 7:1–44

——— (2002) Generating samples under a Wright-Fisher neutral model of genetic variation. Bioinformatics 18:337–338

Hudson RR, Kaplan NL (1988) The coalescent process in models with selection and recombination. Genetics 120:831–840

Kaplan NL, Darden T, Hudson RR (1988) The coalescent process in models with selection. Genetics 120:819–829

Kimura M, Takahata N (1983) Selective constraint in protein polymorphism: study of the effectively neutral mutation model by using an improved pseudosampling method. Proc Natl Acad Sci USA 80:1048–1052

Kong A, Gudbjartsson DF, Sainz J, Jonsdottir GM, Gudjonsson SA, Richardsson B, Sigurdardottir S, et al (2002) A high-resolution recombination map of the human genome. Nat Genet 31:241–247

Ohta T, Kimura M (1973) The model of mutation appropriate to estimate the number of electrophoretically detectable alleles in a genetic population. Genet Res 22:201–204

Phillips MS, Lawrence R, Sachidanandam R, Morris AP, Balding DJ, Donaldson MA, Studebaker JF, et al (2003) Chromosome-wide distribution of haplotype blocks and the role of recombination hot spots. Nat Genet 33:382–387

Posada D, Wiuf C (2003) Simulating haplotype blocks in the human genome. Bioinformatics 19:289–290

Spencer CCA, Coop G (2004) SelSim: a program to simulate population genetic data with natural selection and recombination. Bioinformatics 20:3673–3675

Valdes AM, Slatkin M, Freimer NB (1993) Allele frequencies at microsatellite loci: the stepwise mutation model revisited. Genetics 133:737–749

Wang Y, Rannala B (2004) Simulating a coalescent process with recombination and ascertainment. Lect Notes Comp Sci 2983:84–95

Zöllner S, von Haeseler A (2000) A coalescent approach to study linkage disequilibrium between single-nucleotide polymorphisms. Am J Hum Genet 66:615–628

Report

Identification of FOXP2 Truncation as a Novel Cause of Developmental Speech and Language Deficits

Kay D. MacDermot,[1,2] Elena Bonora,[1,*] Nuala Sykes,[1] Anne-Marie Coupe,[1] Cecilia S. L. Lai,[1,†] Sonja C. Vernes,[1] Faraneh Vargha-Khadem,[3] Fiona McKenzie,[4] Robert L. Smith,[4] Anthony P. Monaco,[1] and Simon E. Fisher[1]

[1]Wellcome Trust Centre for Human Genetics, University of Oxford, Oxford, United Kingdom; [2]Department of Medical and Community Genetics, Imperial College, and [3]Developmental Cognitive Neuroscience Unit, Institute of Child Health, University College London, London; and [4]John Hunter Children's Hospital Genetics and Neurology, Waratah, Australia

FOXP2, the first gene to have been implicated in a developmental communication disorder, offers a unique entry point into neuromolecular mechanisms influencing human speech and language acquisition. In multiple members of the well-studied KE family, a heterozygous missense mutation in _FOXP2_ causes problems in sequencing muscle movements required for articulating speech (developmental verbal dyspraxia), accompanied by wider deficits in linguistic and grammatical processing. Chromosomal rearrangements involving this locus have also been identified. Analyses of _FOXP2_ coding sequence in typical forms of specific language impairment (SLI), autism, and dyslexia have not uncovered any etiological variants. However, no previous study has performed mutation screening of children with a primary diagnosis of verbal dyspraxia, the most overt feature of the disorder in affected members of the KE family. Here, we report investigations of the entire coding region of _FOXP2_, including alternatively spliced exons, in 49 probands affected with verbal dyspraxia. We detected variants that alter FOXP2 protein sequence in three probands. One such variant is a heterozygous nonsense mutation that yields a dramatically truncated protein product and cosegregates with speech and language difficulties in the proband, his affected sibling, and their mother. Our discovery of the first nonsense mutation in _FOXP2_ now opens the door for detailed investigations of neurodevelopment in people carrying different etiological variants of the gene. This endeavor will be crucial for gaining insight into the role of _FOXP2_ in human cognition.

The *FOXP2* gene (MIM 605317) has been implicated in a severe form of speech and language disorder (SPCH1 [MIM 602081]) found in a large multigenerational pedigree and in an independent chromosome translocation case (Lai et al. 2001). This discovery has had an impact on a range of fields, including genetics, neuroscience, clinical neurology, and evolutionary anthropology (for reviews, see Fisher et al. 2003; Marcus and Fisher 2003; Vargha-Khadem et al. 2005). *FOXP2*, located in band 7q31, encodes a transcription factor, containing polyglutamine tracts, a zinc finger, a leucine zipper motif, and a forkhead-box DNA-binding domain (Lai et al. 2001; Wang et al. 2003), and it is likely to regulate gene expression in defined areas of developing lung, cardiovascular, intestinal, and neural tissue (Shu et al. 2001; Lai et al. 2003). The available expression data are compatible with a conserved role (or roles) for this gene in regulating development of neural circuitry underlying motor control and sensory-motor integration in mammals and birds (Ferland et al. 2003; Lai et al. 2003; Takahashi et al. 2003; Haesler et al. 2004; Teramitsu et al. 2004). Notwithstanding the high conservation of *FoxP2* gene sequences and expression patterns in the different vertebrate species studied thus far, evolutionary analyses have demonstrated that the human version of the gene has been subject to positive selection within the past 200,000 years (Enard et al. 2002; Zhang et al. 2002). Thus, the relevant neurogenetic pathways may

Received February 21, 2005; accepted for publication April 7, 2005; electronically published April 22, 2005.

Address for correspondence and reprints: Dr. Simon E. Fisher, Wellcome Trust Centre for Human Genetics, University of Oxford, Roosevelt Drive, Oxford, OX3 7BN, United Kingdom. E-mail: simon.fisher@well.ox.ac.uk

* Present affiliation: Unità di Genetica Medica, Bologna, Italy.

† Present affiliation: Wolfson Institute for Biomedical Research, University College London, London, U.K.

0002-9297/2005/7606-0014$15.00

have undergone human-specific modifications at a time when spoken language was emerging (Enard et al. 2002; Zhang et al. 2002), although the precise nature of the putative mechanisms has yet to be determined.

FOXP2 represents a unique molecular entry point into the investigation of neuronal processes involved in speech and language. However, there has been considerable debate over whether sequence variation in this gene might have significance beyond the unusual case of the KE family. In this three-generation pedigree, a heterozygous missense mutation (Lai et al. 2001) cosegregates with deficits in sequencing the complex, coordinated orofacial movements required for speech (verbal dyspraxia), accompanied by a wide range of linguistic and grammatical deficits (Vargha-Khadem et al. 1998; Watkins et al. 2002). The mutation results in an arginine-to-histidine substitution (R553H) at a highly conserved residue within the DNA-binding domain (Lai et al. 2001). In vitro studies of the corresponding substitution in another forkhead-box protein (R127H in human FOXC1) suggest that the change can dramatically interfere with DNA-binding and transactivation capacity (Saleem et al. 2003), although this has not yet been demonstrated for FOXP2 itself. The *FOXP2* locus has also been found to be directly disrupted in an independent case of speech and language disorder (CS) associated with a de novo balanced translocation involving chromosomes 7 and 5 (Lai et al. 2001).

Following identification of the KE family mutation and CS translocation, many studies have carried out targeted linkage/association analyses of the 7q region or mutation screening of *FOXP2* in children with language-related disorders, including specific language impairment (SLI [MIM 606711]), autism (MIM 608636), and dyslexia (MIM 604254) (e.g., Newbury et al. 2002; Wassink et al. 2002; Gauthier et al. 2003; Kaminen et al. 2003; O'Brien et al. 2003). Despite such efforts, the missense mutation of the KE family remains the single reported case of an unambiguous etiological variant in *FOXP2* coding sequence in the literature. This places limits on what can be learned about the influences of *FOXP2* on human brain development, since, up to this point, all the relevant neuropsychological and neuroimaging investigations have necessarily been limited to just this one allelic variant (Vargha-Khadem et al. 1998; Watkins et al. 2002; Belton et al. 2003; Liégeois et al. 2003) or to gross chromosomal rearrangements that may involve effects of multiple additional genes (Liégeois et al. 2001).

Our current investigation was driven by the observation that, to date, no study had fully examined the sequence of *FOXP2* in children with a phenotypic profile which closely corresponds to that found in the KE family (or to that found in cases of chromosomal abnormality involving *FOXP2*). Although a broad range of language-related deficits are evident in these individuals, the most overt symptom of their disorder is a severe developmental verbal dyspraxia, and it is this feature that provides the most reliable indicator of affection status (Vargha-Khadem et al. 1998; Liégeois et al. 2001; Watkins et al. 2002). Notably, previous screening studies of the entire *FOXP2* ORF have focused on individuals affected with typical SLI, autism, or dyslexia (Newbury et al. 2002; Wassink et al. 2002; Gauthier et al. 2003; Kaminen et al. 2003). Verbal dyspraxia might indeed be present in a subset of such children, but it is not generally considered to be a core feature for any of these developmental disorders (World Health Organization 1993; American Psychiatric Association 1994) and may represent the defining symptom of a distinctive clinical entity (or entities) (Lewis et al. 2004). Given that *FOXP2* was the first known case of a gene to be implicated in impaired speech and language acquisition, it was appropriate for these previous investigations to assess its possible involvement in a variety of language-related disorders. Nevertheless, for the present study, we hypothesized that we might maximize the possibility of detecting further etiological variants by screening, for the first time, a panel of patients with a primary diagnosis of verbal dyspraxia.

After the publication by Lai et al. (2001), our department received many referrals of cases with unexplained speech and language deficits, requesting testing for *FOXP2* abnormalities. To more closely match the phenotype of the KE family, patients were selected for *FOXP2* screening only if they fulfilled the following criteria: presence of speech articulation problems diagnosed by a clinician (e.g., a pediatrician or neurologist), normal karyotype, absence of mental retardation and congenital abnormalities, normal hearing, and no other medical/genetic diagnosis. The study was approved by the Oxfordshire Clinical Research Ethics Committee. Patients were enrolled sequentially, with no preference given to those with a family history of language disorder. The referring doctors and parents filled in a questionnaire for the study, which contained confirmation of the phenotype and provided results of the karyotype, speech examination report, and family history. DNA samples were collected from 49 probands, of whom 10 had one (or more) affected siblings whose samples were also included in the study. All affected cases were white, were within the 4–12-year-old age group (except for one pair of siblings aged 30 and 33 years), and resided in Europe, Australia, or the United States.

We conducted mutation screening across all *FOXP2* exons identified by Lai et al. (2001) via denaturing high-performance liquid chromatography (DHPLC), followed by direct sequencing of fragments showing variant elution patterns, using identical protocols and primers to those described elsewhere by Newbury et al. (2002). We similarly analyzed additional alternatively spliced and 5′ UTR exons reported by Bruce and Margolis (2002) (see table A1 for sequences of all primers). All assays spanned entire exons, plus short stretches of flanking intronic sequence. Screening of our cohort of 49 probands revealed two 5′ UTR variants and six intronic changes (fig. 1). Five of these changes correspond to polymorphisms reported in earlier studies of *FOXP2* (Newbury et al. 2002), and two overlap with SNPs that are present in public databases (*rs17137124* and *rs10227893*). In support of the sensitivity of our DHPLC-based approach, the public databases contain no other validated SNPs in the regions of *FOXP2* investigated in this study.

Our screening of probands also identified three novel exonic allelic variants in the coding region, each of which is predicted to yield a change in FOXP2 protein sequence (fig. 1). Crucially, one of these coding changes was a heterozygous C→T transition in exon 7, yielding a stop codon at position 328 of the FOXP2 protein (R328X) (fig. 2). We directly sequenced exon 7 in 252 control chromosomes from Human Random Control panels (obtained from the European Collection of Cell Cultures [ECACC]) but did not detect any sequence alterations, indicating that the change observed in the proband is unlikely to represent a polymorphism, according to criteria suggested by Collins and Schwartz (2002). Moreover, this nonsense mutation was also found in the affected sibling of the proband, as well as their mother, who was known to have a history of speech problems, and it was absent in their father, who has normal speech. The R328X mutation is highly likely to have functional significance, since it leads to dramatic truncation of the predicted product, yielding a FOXP2 protein lacking critical functional domains—including the zinc-finger and leucine zipper, which mediate dimerization (Wang et al. 2003), and the characteristic forkhead DNA-binding domain, known to be critical for transcription factor function (fig. 2). It is also possible that this mutation could lead to nonsense-mediated mRNA decay of transcripts from the mutant allele.

The two remaining coding changes that we identified were a heterozygous A→T transversion in exon 2 in one proband, and a heterozygous insertion of the sequence CAGCAGCAACAA into the polyglutamine-encoding region of exon 5 in another. At the amino acid level, these changes are predicted to yield a glutamine-to-leucine change at residue 17 (Q17L) and a polyglutamine-tract expansion from 40 to 44 consecutive glutamines, respectively (fig. 2). Neither change was detected in screening of large numbers of chromosomes from Human Random Control panels (366 chromosomes screened for the Q17L change and 228 chromosomes screened for the polyglutamine expansion). However, in each case, the proband had a sibling who was diagnosed as affected but did not carry the relevant coding change. In addition, on the basis of current data and analyses of protein function using *in silico* methods (Ng and Henikoff 2001; Ramensky et al. 2002), it is not clear what the potential functional consequences of a Q17L change in FOXP2 might be. The substitution site lies in a region of unknown function close to the N-terminus of the protein but is conserved in the FOXP2 orthologues of all species thus far studied, including birds, rodents, and primates (Enard et al. 2002; Zhang et al. 2002; Webb and Zhang 2005), as well as in the closely related proteins FOXP1 and FOXP4 (Teufel et al. 2003). With regard to the polyglutamine change, although Wassink et al. (2002) previously detected small internal deletions in the Q_{40} tract in two families with autism, our study represents the first report of an expansion of this region in any individual. Newbury et al. (2002) previously identified a potential insertion of two CAGs within the smaller (Q_{10}) tract in a family with SLI, but this did not cosegregate with the disorder, and its location in a repetitive region at the intron/exon border of exon 6 suggested that it would not have any impact on FOXP2 protein sequence. The expansion from 40 to 44 residues of the longer FOXP2 polyglutamine tract in our proband with verbal dyspraxia is outside the normal intraspecies range observed for FOXP2 orthologues; the number of consecutive glutamines in the corresponding region in other species varies from 38 glutamines (in zebra finch, chicken, and gorilla) to a maximum of 41 glutamines (in chimpanzee) (Enard et al. 2002; Zhang et al. 2002; Webb and Zhang 2005).

Our discovery of an R328X variant cosegregating with speech deficits in a multiplex family gives an opportunity to compare the neurodevelopmental consequences of a *FOXP2* nonsense mutation to those of the missense mutation in the KE family. Recent clinical evaluation of cases carrying the R328X mutation suggests a similar phenotype to that associated with the R553H mutation of the KE family, where prominent difficulties in speech articulation are accompanied by more general problems with expressive and receptive language. The development of the children carrying the R328X mutation was assessed using the Griffiths (1970) Mental Development Scales, which evaluate overall development from birth to 8 years of age in six domains ("Locomotor," "Personal and Social," "Hearing and Speech," "Eye/Hand Coordination," "Performance," and "Practical Reasoning"), while the Preschool Language Scale-3 (Zimmerman et al. 1992) was used to formally measure receptive and expressive language skills. Assessment of the proband when he was 4 years old indicated developmental delays in the domains of speech and language, and social skills. He communicated mainly using single words and was unable to repeat multisyllabic words. Eye-hand coordination was satisfactory, but he had difficulty with activities in the Practical

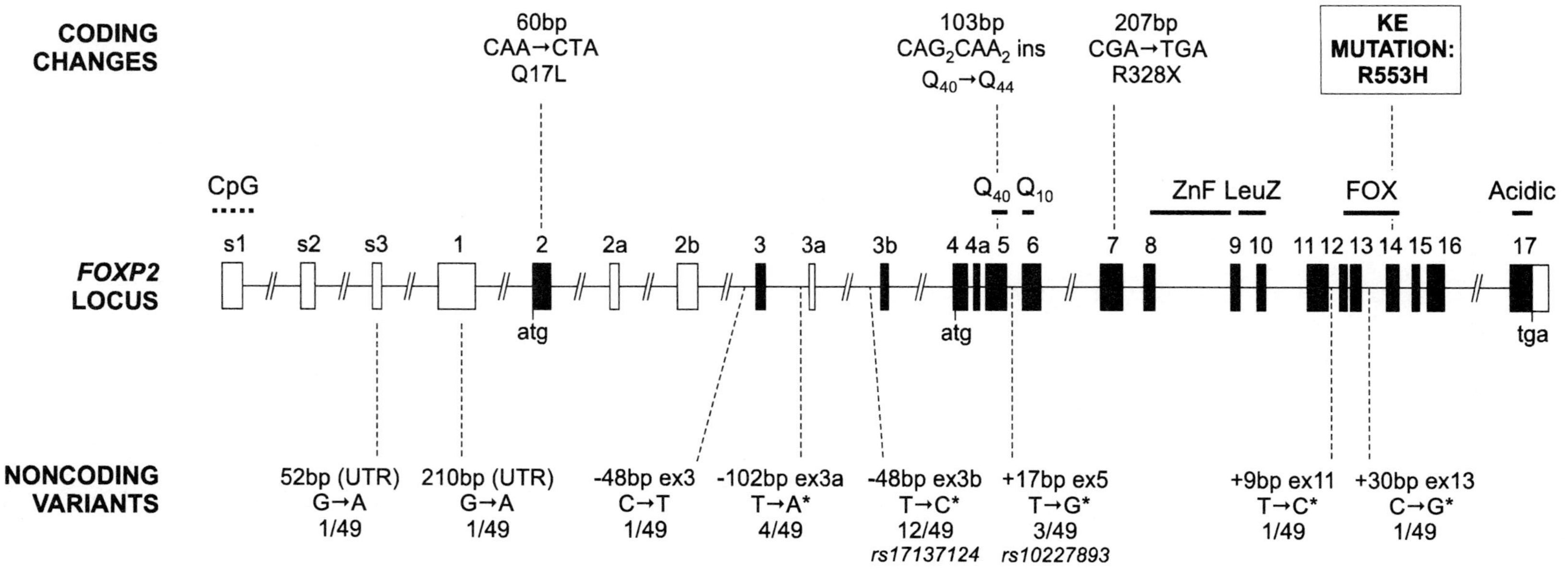

Figure 1 Schematic of the human *FOXP2* locus, which spans >600 kb of genomic DNA, showing sequence variants identified in subjects with verbal dyspraxia. Black shading indicates translated exons; "atg" and "tga" denote positions of initiation and termination codons. Known domains encoded by exons include polyglutamine tracts (Q_{40} and Q_{10}), a zinc-finger motif (ZnF), a leucine zipper (LeuZ), the forkhead domain (FOX), and an acidic C-terminus (Acidic). Exons 3b and 4a are alternatively spliced coding exons yielding amino acid insertions, whereas alternatively spliced exons 2a, 2b, and 3a are predicted to be noncoding. Exons s1–s3 and 1 represent alternative 5′ UTR regions that have not been found in the same human transcript; the position of the 5′ end of exon 1 is based on currently available EST data. For more information on splicing and isoforms, see Lai et al. (2001) and Bruce and Margolis (2002). All known exons were screened for mutations, with the exception of two noncoding exons: s1 (5′ CpG-rich UTR) and 2a (alternatively spliced and untranslated). Coding variants are shown above the locus, with resulting codon and amino acid changes indicated. For reference, the KE mutation is also included. Noncoding variants are shown below the locus, with information regarding relative position (with respect to the exon in question) and frequency in probands (number of heterozygous probands/total probands screened). An asterisk (*) denotes intronic variants that correspond to those previously detected by Newbury et al. (2002), and rs numbers are indicated for polymorphisms also present in dbSNP. Locus schematic is adapted from Fisher et al. (2003).

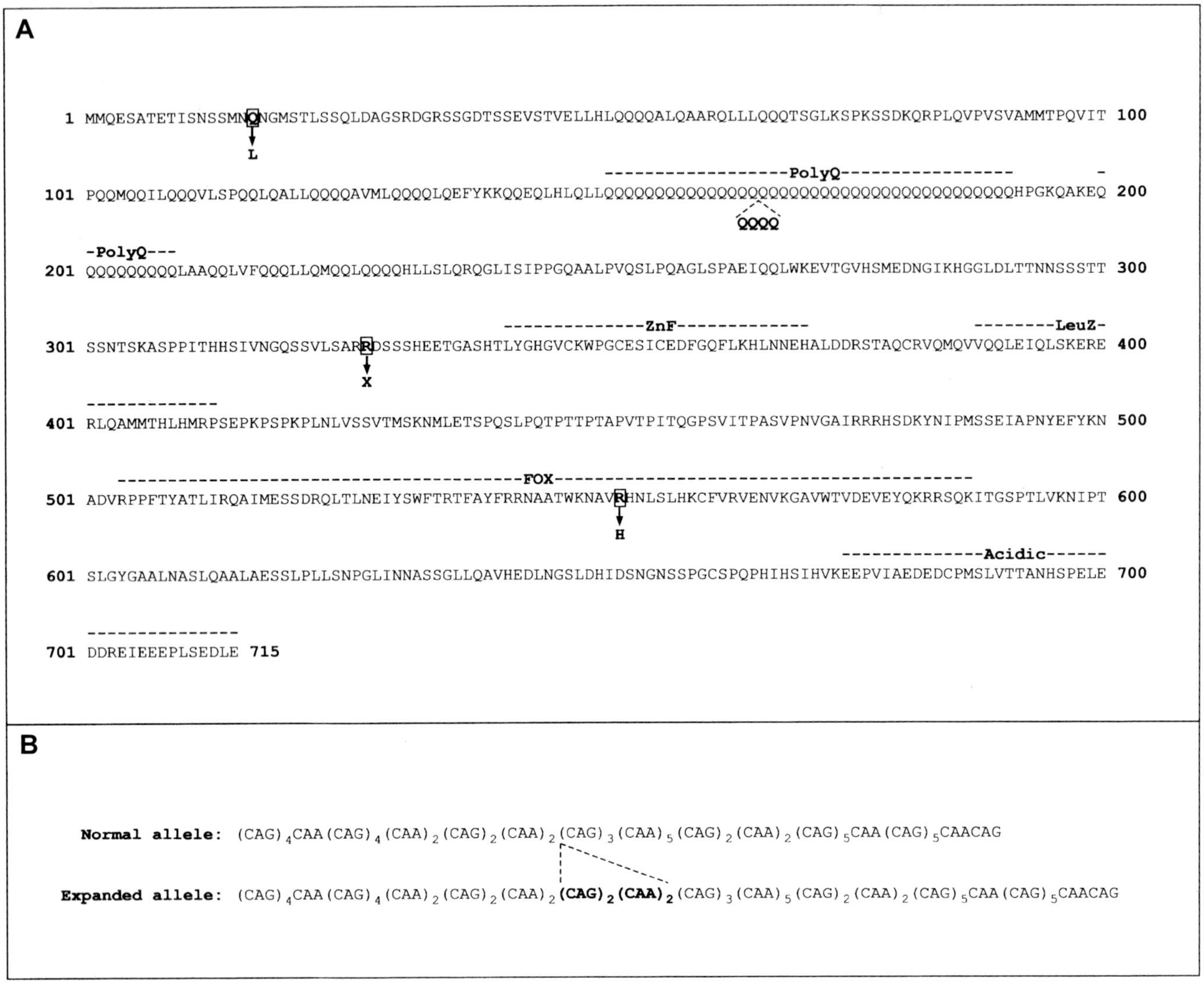

Figure 2 *A*, Amino acid sequence of main isoform of human FOXP2, showing all coding changes found thus far in individuals with developmental verbal dyspraxia (Lai et al. 2001; present study). Each change was absent from large numbers of control chromosomes, but only the R328X and R553H mutations are found in multiple affected members in families segregating developmental speech and language disorder. *B*, Nucleotide sequence of normal and expanded polyglutamine-encoding region identified in one of the probands in this study.

Reasoning domain. His receptive and expressive language scores were 55 and 54, respectively (mean standard score is 100, with an SD of 15; scores between 85 and 115 are considered within normal limits). Thus, his language skills were almost 3 standard deviations below the normative mean, equivalent to that of a child of 2 years 6 mo (~18 mo below chronological age). During informal assessment of articulation, he had difficulty in producing consonants at the beginning of words and became frustrated and significantly less intelligible during word repetition.

His younger sister has a history of motor and oropharyngeal dyspraxia, otitis media, and oesophageal reflux. On assessment using the Griffith Scales, at age 1 year 8 mo, she showed her poorest performance in the Hearing and Speech domain. She did not speak any words and could not identify objects, and her vocalization was poor. However, she was interested in puzzle-type toys and was able to put different shapes into form boards; her general motor skills at this age appeared normal. When she was subsequently assessed on the Preschool Language Scale-3 , at the age of 2 years and 11 mo, her receptive and expressive language scores were 71 and 73, respectively. Both scores were almost 2 standard deviations below the normative mean and were equivalent to the performance of an 11-mo-old child (i.e., 2 years below chronological age).

The mother, who also carried the R328X mutation,

reported a history of speech delay in childhood. At present, she has severe problems with communication. She volunteered to bring a relative to the consultations, because she could not understand the nuances of what was said and was afraid of misinterpretation. She had poor speech clarity and very simple grammatical constructions. Her speech had less varied cadence than most people's, but her vocabulary was satisfactory. Her receptive difficulties were compounded by performance anxiety. Formal speech and language assessment has been offered to her and will be reported separately.

Overall, the data from our screening of cases with verbal dyspraxia support a number of important conclusions. First, the evidence indicates that one of the coding changes detected in our patients (R328X) is of direct etiological significance, since it was not found in a large panel of control chromosomes, it cosegregates with the disorder in all three affected members of a multiplex family, and it is a nonsense mutation that yields a substantially truncated protein lacking key functional domains. Thus, this is the first report of an independent causative point mutation in *FOXP2* following the identification of the KE mutation by Lai et al. (2001), and the only known case of a nonsense mutation in this gene. The other coding changes (Q17L and $Q_{40}\rightarrow Q_{44}$), although similarly undetected in control chromosomes, were only found in probands, and so functional studies will be important to assess whether they have any impact on the behavior of FOXP2. Second, screening of *FOXP2* in <50 probands diagnosed on the basis of developmental verbal dyspraxia yielded a much higher frequency of protein sequence changes (~6.1%) than that previously found by studying the entire coding region in children with typical SLI (no unambiguous coding mutations in 43 probands) or with autism (<0.8%; two heterozygous poly-Q deletions in a total of 239 families) (Newbury et al. 2002; Wassink et al. 2002; Gauthier et al. 2003). The frequency of unequivocal etiological variants in our sample was ~2%. It is worth reiterating that we did not make familial clustering of the disorder a requirement when ascertaining our sample. These data suggest that a re-evaluation of the relevance of *FOXP2* for common cases of neurodevelopmental disorder is warranted, and that additional coding changes might be identified in individuals with an appropriate phenotypic profile. The situation could be comparable to that found for telomere abnormalities in idiopathic mental retardation, where the former account for a small (5.1%) but significant proportion of the many individuals affected with the disorder (Flint and Knight 2003). Third, our data caution against drawing conclusions about the influence of *FOXP2* from limited mutation searches that screen only small regions of the *FOXP2* coding region, such as that encoding the forkhead domain (see, e.g., O'Brien et al. 2003)—especially given that nonsense mutations, like the one identified here, might lie far from known functional domains but still have major consequences for protein function. Fourth, the observation of a heterozygous nonsense mutation that severely truncates FOXP2 in multiple cases with developmental verbal dyspraxia, gives independent support to the hypothesis that *FOXP2*-related disorder may result from a mechanism of reduced functional gene dosage in the developing CNS.

In conclusion, the present study indicates that, whereas the neurodevelopmental consequences of *FOXP2* disruption are complex, involving impairment of both speech and language skills, the presence of verbal dyspraxia is a key clinical aspect that identifies children most suitable for *FOXP2* mutation screening. The identification of an unambiguous causative mutation in a cohort of <50 probands (without prior selection for familial transmission) suggests that other etiological variants may be discovered in the future. Finally, the development of individuals carrying the R328X nonsense mutation can now be assessed using neuropsychological tests and neuroimaging paradigms identical to those employed for the intensive studies of the KE family conducted over the past 15 years (see, e.g., Watkins et al. 2002; Belton et al. 2003; Liégeois et al. 2003). Therefore, our work opens the door for the future integration of behavioral and neurological data from patients with different allelic variants of *FOXP2*, an endeavor that will be essential for understanding the role of this gene in human cognition.

Acknowledgments

We are very grateful to all the patients and their families who took part in this study and to the clinicians who referred them. Thanks to Toril Fagerheim for help with sequencing and to W. Wetherall for his support. This work was funded by the Royal Society and the Wellcome Trust. S.C.V. is supported by the Clarendon Fund and a Christopher Welch Scholarship. A.P.M. is a Wellcome Trust Principal Research Fellow. S.E.F. is a Royal Society Research Fellow.

Electronic-Database Information

The URLs for data presented herein are as follows:

dbSNP Home Page, http://www.ncbi.nlm.nih.gov/SNP/
Online Mendelian Inheritance in Man (OMIM), http://www.ncbi.nlm.nih.gov/Omim/

References

American Psychiatric Association (1994) Diagnostic and statistical manual of mental disorders (DSM-IV). American Psychiatric Association, Washington, DC

Belton E, Salmond CH, Watkins KE, Vargha-Khadem F, Gadian DG (2003) Bilateral brain abnormalities associated with dominantly inherited verbal and orofacial dyspraxia. Hum Brain Mapp 18:194–200

Bruce HA, Margolis RL (2002) *FOXP2*: novel exons, splice variants, and CAG repeat length stability. Hum Genet 111: 136–144

Collins JS, Schwartz CE (2002) Detecting polymorphisms and mutations in candidate genes. Am J Hum Genet 71:1251–1252

Enard W, Przeworski M, Fisher SE, Lai CSL, Wiebe V, Kitano T, Monaco AP, Pääbo S (2002) Molecular evolution of *FOXP2,* a gene involved in speech and language. Nature 418:869–872

Ferland RJ, Cherry TJ, Preware PO, Morrisey EE, Walsh CA (2003). Characterization of Foxp2 and Foxp1 mRNA and protein in the developing and mature brain. J Comp Neurol 460:266–279

Fisher SE, Lai CSL, Monaco AP (2003) Deciphering the genetic basis of speech and language disorders. Annu Rev Neurosci 26:57–80

Flint J, Knight S (2003) The use of telomere probes to investigate submicroscopic rearrangements associated with mental retardation. Curr Opin Genet Dev 13:310–316

Gauthier J, Joober R, Mottron L, Laurent S, Fuchs M, De Kimpe V, Rouleau GA (2003) Mutation screening of *FOXP2* in individuals diagnosed with autistic disorder Am J Med Genet 118A:172–175

Griffiths R (1970) The abilities of young children. Child Development Research Centre, London

Haesler S, Wada K, Nshdejan A, Morrisey EE, Lints T, Jarvis ED, Scharff C (2004) *FoxP2* expression in avian vocal learners and non-learners. J Neurosci 24:3164–3175

Kaminen N, Hannula-Jouppi K, Kestila M, Lahermo P, Muller K, Kaaranen M, Myllyluoma B, Voutilainen A, Lyytinen H, Nopola-Hemmi J, Kere J (2003) A genome scan for developmental dyslexia confirms linkage to chromosome 2p11 and suggests a new locus on 7q32. J Med Genet 40:340–345

Lai CSL, Fisher SE, Hurst JA, Vargha-Khadem F, Monaco AP (2001) A novel forkhead-domain gene is mutated in a severe speech and language disorder. Nature 413:519–523

Lai CSL, Gerrelli D, Monaco AP, Fisher SE, Copp AJ (2003) *FOXP2* expression during brain development coincides with sites of pathology in a severe speech and language disorder. Brain 126:2455–2462

Lewis BA, Freebairn LA, Hansen A, Gerry Taylor H, Iyengar S, Shriberg LD (2004) Family pedigrees of children with suspected childhood apraxia of speech. J Commun Disord 37:157–175.

Liégeois F, Baldeweg T, Connelly A, Gadian DG, Mishkin M, Vargha-Khadem F (2003) Language fMRI abnormalities associated with *FOXP2* gene mutation. Nature Neurosci 6: 1230–1237

Liégeois FJ, Lai CSL, Baldeweg T, Fisher SE, Monaco AP, Connelly A, Vargha-Khadem, F (2001) Behavioural and neuroimaging correlates of a chromosome 7q31 deletion containing the SPCH1 gene. Abstr Soc Neurosci 27:529.17

Marcus GF, Fisher SE (2003) *FOXP2* in focus: what can genes tell us about speech and language? Trends Cogn Sci 7:257–262

Newbury DF, Bonora E, Lamb JA, Fisher SE, Lai CSL, Baird G, Jannoun L, Slonims V, Stott CM, Merricks MJ, Bolton PF, Bailey A, Monaco AP, International Molecular Genetic Study of Autism Consortium (2002) *FOXP2* is not a major susceptibility gene for autism or specific language impairment. Am J Hum Genet 70:1318–1327

Ng PC, Henikoff S (2001) Predicting deleterious amino acid substitutions. Genome Res 11:863–874

O'Brien EK, Zhang X, Nishimura C, Tomblin JB, Murray JC (2003) Association of specific language impairment (SLI) to the region of 7q31. Am J Hum Genet 72:1536–1543

Ramensky V, Bork P, Sunyaev S (2002) Human non-synonymous SNPs: server and survey. Nucleic Acids Res 30:3894–3900

Saleem RA, Banerjee-Basu S, Berry FB, Baxevanis AD, Walter MA (2003) Structural and functional analyses of disease-causing missense mutations in the forkhead domain of FOXC1. Hum Mol Genet 12:2993–3005

Shu W, Yang H, Zhang L, Lu MM, Morrisey EE (2001) Characterization of a new subfamily of winged-helix/forkhead (Fox) genes that are expressed in the lung and act as transcriptional repressors. J Biol Chem 276:27488–27497

Takahashi K, Liu FC, Hirokawa K, Takahashi H (2003) Expression of *Foxp2,* a gene involved in speech and language, in the developing and adult striatum. J Neurosci Res 73:61–72

Teramitsu I, Kudo LC, London SE, Geschwind DH, White SA (2004) Parallel *FoxP1* and *FoxP2* expression in songbird and human brain predicts functional interaction. J Neurosci 24:3152–3163

Teufel A, Wong EA, Mukhopadhyay M, Malik N, Westphal H (2003) *FoxP4,* a novel forkhead transcription factor. Biochim Biophys Acta 1627:147–152

Vargha-Khadem F, Watkins KE, Price CJ, Ashburner J, Alcock KJ, Connelly A, Frackowiak RS, Friston KJ, Pembrey ME, Mishkin M, Gadian DG, Passingham RE (1998) Neural basis of an inherited speech and language disorder. Proc Natl Acad Sci USA 95:12695–12700

Vargha-Khadem F, Gadian DG, Copp A, Mishkin M (2005) *FOXP2* and the neuroanatomy of speech and language. Nat Rev Neurosci 6: 131–138

Wang B, Lin D, Li C, Tucker P (2003) Multiple domains define the expression and regulatory properties of Foxp1 forkhead transcriptional repressors. J Biol Chem 278:24259–24268

Wassink TH, Piven J, Vieland VJ, Pietila J, Goedken RJ, Folstein SE, Sheffield VC (2002) Evaluation of *FOXP2* as an autism susceptibility gene. Am J Med Genet 114:566–569

Watkins KE, Dronkers NF, Vargha-Khadem F (2002) Behavioural analysis of an inherited speech and language disorder: comparison with acquired aphasia. Brain 125:452–464

Webb DM, Zhang J (2005) *FoxP2* in song-learning birds and vocal-learning mammals. J Hered 96:212–216

World Health Organization (1993) The ICD-10 classification for mental and behavioural disorders: diagnostic criteria for research. World Health Organisation, Geneva

Zhang J, Webb DM, Podlaha O (2002) Accelerated protein evolution and origins of human-specific features: Foxp2 as an example. Genetics 162:1825–1835

Zimmerman IL, Steiner VC, Evatt Pond R (1992) The preschool language scale. Psychological Corporation, San Antonio

Am. J. Hum. Genet. 76:1081–1086, 2005

Report

Deficiency of the ADP-Forming Succinyl-CoA Synthase Activity Is Associated with Encephalomyopathy and Mitochondrial DNA Depletion

Orly Elpeleg,[1,2] Chaya Miller,[1] Eli Hershkovitz,[3] Maria Bitner-Glindzicz,[4] Gili Bondi-Rubinstein,[1] Shamima Rahman,[5] Alistair Pagnamenta,[5] Sharon Eshhar,[1] and Ann Saada[1]

[1]Metabolic Disease Unit, Shaare-Zedek Medical Center, and [2]Faculty of Medicine, the Hebrew University, Jerusalem; [3]Pediatric Department, Soroka Medical Center, Faculty of Medicine, Ben-Gurion University, Beer-Sheba, Israel; and [4]Clinical and Molecular Genetics Unit and [5]Biochemistry, Endocrinology and Metabolism Unit, Institute of Child Health, University College London, London

The mitochondrial DNA (mtDNA) depletion syndrome is a quantitative defect of mtDNA resulting from dysfunction of one of several nuclear-encoded factors responsible for maintenance of mitochondrial deoxyribonucleoside triphosphate (dNTP) pools or replication of mtDNA. Markedly decreased succinyl-CoA synthetase activity due to a deleterious mutation in *SUCLA2*, the gene encoding the β subunit of the ADP-forming succinyl-CoA synthetase ligase, was found in muscle mitochondria of patients with encephalomyopathy and mtDNA depletion. Succinyl-CoA synthetase is invariably in a complex with mitochondrial nucleotide diphosphate kinase; hence, we propose that a defect in the last step of mitochondrial dNTP salvage is a novel cause of the mtDNA depletion syndrome.

The oxidative phosphorylation (OXPHOS) system consists of 87 proteins that are assembled into five enzymatic complexes. Of the 87 subunits, 13 are encoded by mtDNA, which also encodes all mitochondrial tRNA and rRNA transcripts. mtDNA is constantly synthesized throughout the cell cycle, requiring a balanced supply of dNTPs within the mitochondria and a large number of factors, mostly nuclear encoded, that participate in the replication, transcription, and translation processes.

In the past decade, a growing number of patients with OXPHOS dysfunction due to depletion of mtDNA have been reported. The onset of symptoms usually occurs during the first months of life, and most patients die in early childhood. Clinical presentation is heterogeneous and includes progressive muscle weakness, liver failure, encephalopathy, cardiomyopathy, and renal disease, usually accompanied by lactic acidemia (Moraes et al. 1991; Tritschler et al. 1992; Vu et al. 1998; Ducluzeau et al. 1999; reviewed by Elpeleg 2003). Autosomal recessive inheritance was suspected in many cases, and no mutations were identified in the mtDNA molecule, which suggests that mtDNA depletion results from defects in nuclear factors involved in mtDNA replication. Four genes have previously been implicated in the pathogenesis of mtDNA depletion; mutations in the thymidine phosphorylase gene are associated with leukodystrophy and gastrointestinal disorder (Nishino et al. 1999); mutations in the deoxyguanosine kinase and mtDNA polymerase γ genes are associated with encephalopathy and fatal infantile liver disease (Mandel et al. 2001; Naviaux and Nguyen 2004); and mutations in the mitochondrial thymidine kinase gene result in progressive muscle disease with variable brain involvement (Saada et al. 2001).

We identified a small Muslim pedigree (fig. 1) with autosomal recessive encephalomyopathy associated with mtDNA depletion. Patient II-7 is a female, the second child born to consanguineous parents of Muslim origin. Her older sister died of neurodegenerative disease at age 7 mo, and her younger sister and brother are healthy. The pregnancy was uneventful, apart from a markedly elevated level of α-feto protein in maternal blood. The patient was born at term but was small for gestational age (weight 2,250 g, <3rd percentile). In early infancy, the patient was irritable, with inconsolable crying. Psychomotor development was severely retarded, with marked muscle hypotonia and impaired hearing. She had frequent respiratory infections, which were thought to

Received March 8, 2005; accepted for publication April 7, 2005; electronically published April 22, 2005.

Address for correspondence and reprints: Dr. Orly Elpeleg, Metabolic Disease Unit, Shaare-Zedek Medical Center, Jerusalem, 91031, Israel. E-mail: Elpeleg@cc.huji.ac.il

0002-9297/2005/7606-0015$15.00

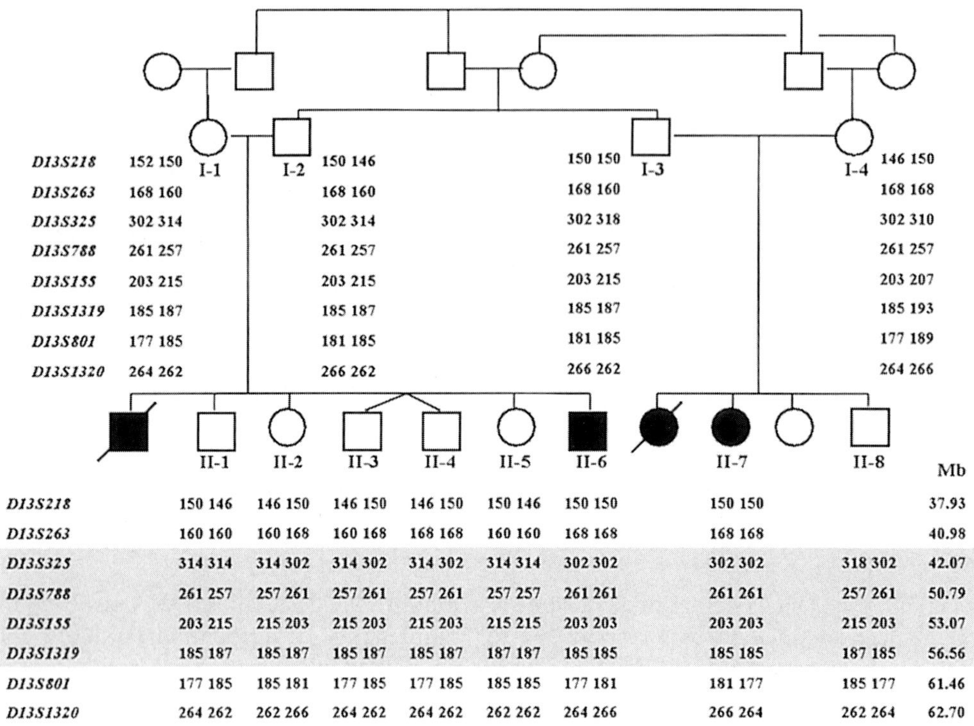

Figure 1 Family tree, with allele sizes of the microsatellite markers in the critical region on chromosome 13. Only those individuals whose DNA was available for analysis were annotated. The region of shared homozygosity is shaded. Markers are listed in the left column, and their physical locations on the chromosome are given (in Mb) in the right column.

be secondary to severe gastroesophageal reflux. Generalized seizures, first noted at age 1 year, were controlled by valproic acid. Brain MRI performed at age 18 mo was suggestive of Leigh syndrome, with high signal T2 intensity in the putamen bilaterally and moderate dilatation of the lateral ventricles and sulci, compatible with generalized atrophy. Physical examination at age 7 years revealed contractures at the knee and hip joints and dystonic posturing of the fingers. The patient was able to roll over but was unable to sit unsupported. At age 7 years, she recognized and greeted her relatives with a smile and cried when being scolded but had neither speech nor gestures. She had mild ptosis, but her vision appeared intact. The patient's hearing was impaired, but this condition was not assessed any further. Chronic microcytic anemia (hemoglobin level [Hb] 9.1 g/dl; mean corpuscular volume [MCV] 65 femtoliters [fl]) and an elevated lactate level in plasma (4.3 mM; normal level is <2.1 mM) were present. Liver and renal function tests, plasma creatine kinase level, abdominal ultrasound, electrocardiogram, and echocardiogram were normal.

Patient II-6 is the cousin of II-7 and is the seventh child born to consanguineous parents. An older brother had a cot death at age 4 mo. The patient was born at term but was small for gestational age (weight 2,180 g, <3rd percentile). At age 2 mo, he was found unresponsive and hypopneic. Electroencephalogram showed generalized slow activity, and CT scan of the brain revealed lacunar infarcts in the basal ganglia. The patient slowly regained consciousness and, after 2 d of assisted ventilation, started breathing spontaneously, but his subsequent development was poor. Echocardiogram was normal. At age 1 year, there was generalized muscle hypotonia, lack of voluntary movements, and bilateral hearing loss. A generalized seizure disorder, first noted at age 3 years, was controlled by clonazepam. At age 5 years, the patient's condition was unchanged, with severe psychomotor retardation and prominent muscle hypotonia. He had microcytic anemia (Hb 11.1 g/dl; MCV 65 fl) and an elevated lactate level in plasma (4–5 mM), but his liver and renal function tests and plasma creatine kinase level were normal.

The enzymatic activities of the OXPHOS complexes I–V in muscle mitochondria were determined by standard spectrophotometric methods (Hoppel and Cooper 1969; Dooijewaard and Slater 1976). The activities of complexes I and IV were significantly decreased, and complexes III and V were less affected, whereas complex II, the only complex that does not contain mtDNA-encoded proteins, was borderline normal (table 1). It is notable that the pathological and histochemical examinations of the muscle tissue from the two patients showed

Table 1

Activity of the Enzymatic Complexes of the Mitochondrial Respiratory Chain in Mitochondria Isolated from Muscle and Fibroblasts

Tissue and Subject(s)	Citrate Synthase Activity	Activity of Enzymatic Complex[a]					
		I	I+III	II+III	II	IV	V
Muscle mitochondria:							
Patient II-7	1,780	127 (52%)	148 (28%)	202 (72%)	255 (87%)	409 (35%)	501 (83%)
Patient II-6	1,790	107 (43%)	134 (25%)	181 (64%)	211 (72%)	307 (26%)	351 (58%)
Controls (n = 50):							
Mean ± SD	1,990 ± 370	274 ± 127	586 ± 234	312 ± 118	327 ± 52	1,326 ± 501	645 ± 203
Range	1,320–2,900	115–503	305–999	192–531	255–442	829–2,300	222–1,002
Fibroblast mitochondria:							
Patient II-7	199	23 (93%)	ND	82 (78%)	44 (59%)	335 (101%)	ND
Controls (n = 27):							
Mean ± SD	249 ± 97	31 ± 11	ND	131 ± 44	81 ± 31	412 ± 59	ND
Range	135–415	15–38	ND	63–204	50–101	203–586	ND

[a] Values are given in nmol/min/mg of protein. For patients, the percentage of the control mean normalized for citrate synthase activity is shown in parentheses. ND = not determined.

unremarkable results. The activities of all OXPHOS complexes were normal in mitochondria isolated from fibroblasts (table 1). The findings in muscle mitochondria suggested a defect in the synthesis of the mtDNA-encoded proteins. Sequence analysis of muscle mtDNA excluded mutations in the 22 mitochondrial tRNA genes in patient II-7. Southern blot analysis of muscle DNA, performed as described elsewhere (Saada et al. 2001), revealed a normal-size band of mtDNA in both patients, but the ratio of mtDNA to nuclear DNA, determined by real-time PCR, was reduced to 32% of the mean control value. The mtDNA:nuclear DNA ratio in fibroblasts was 95% of the mean control value.

Genomic DNA was extracted from blood samples from the two patients and 10 unaffected family members, after informed consent was obtained from the subjects or their guardians. To localize the mutated gene in this family, we performed a genomewide screen to search for homozygosity by using polymorphic microsatellite markers with an average intermarker distance of 10 cM (ABI PRISM Linkage Mapping Set MD10, version 2.0 [Applied Biosystems]). Genotypes were obtained for 402 markers, of which 21 were homozygous in both patients. Five of these markers were located successively on an ~50-Mb fragment of chromosome 13, bordered by markers *D13S175* and *D13S156*. Additional markers from other mapping sets and other selected polymorphic dinucleotide repeat markers were genotyped, which enabled us to exclude all other chromosomal regions and to narrow the shared homozygosity region to 20 Mb on chromosome 13, bordered by (but excluding) markers *D13S263* and *D13S801* (fig. 1). Mitochondrial localization was predicted (score >60) in only 3 of 113 ORFs in this region, by use of the MitoP2 prediction program: ORFs encoding the β chain of the ADP-forming succinyl-CoA ligase (*SUCLA2* [MIM 603921, NCBI accession number NM_003850]), a hypothetical protein FLJ25853, and the copper-transporting ATPase 2 (ATP7B) associated with Wilson disease (Andreoli et al. 2004). Sequence analysis of the 12 exons of the *SUCLA2* gene (*Homo sapiens* chromosome 13, nt 47414793–47473463 [NCBI accession number NC_000013.9]) and their exon-intron boundaries (primer sequences available on request) revealed a complex genomic rearrangement at the 3′ end of exon 6, with a homozygous deletion of 43 nt, encompassing the last 14 nt of exon 6 and the first 29 nt of IVS6, and an insertion of 5 nt (32720del43ins5) (fig. 2*A*). Analysis of the *SUCLA2* cDNA by use of primers cF1 (5′-TTCAAAAGATGTCTGATAAAGG-3′) and cR1 (5′-CGCATGATTCCTCCAAAAATGT-3′) resulted in two amplification products of nearly equal abundance, both of which skip exon 6 and one of which also lacks the first 74 bp of exon 7 (fig. 2*B*). Analysis of the genomic PCR products from the other family members, by use of exon/intron 6 primers 6F1 (5′-GTTGATTAGACATATG-CAAACTACCT-3′) and 6R2 (5′-AGGGAAGCATATTA-GAGAAATAAATG-3′), confirmed that all available relatives are heterozygous for the rearrangement, except for individual II-5, who is homozygous for the wild-type sequence. Using the same primer set, we analyzed 105 anonymous Muslim Arabs for the presence of the mutation and found no carriers.

The *SUCLA2* gene spans nearly 60 kb and encodes the 463 amino acids of the β subunit of the ADP-forming succinyl-CoA synthetase (SCS-A) (Allen and Ottaway 1986; Weitzman et al. 1986). This mitochondrial matrix enzyme catalyzes the formation of succinate and ATP from succinyl-CoA and ADP in the tricarboxylic acid (TCA) cycle in a reversible manner. SCS-A is a heterodimer that shares its α subunit with another mitochondrial matrix succinyl-CoA synthetase, SCS-G, which uses GDP (Sanadi et al. 1954). Thus, the two enzymes, SCS-G and SCS-A, catalyze a similar reaction by using different phosphate donors, with their β subunits deter-

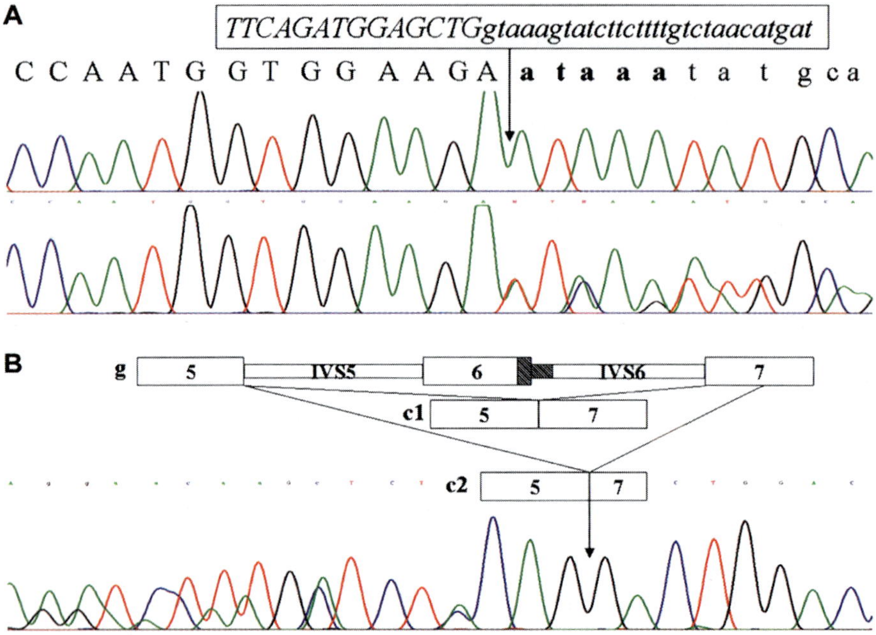

Figure 2 *A*, Genomic sequence of the exon 6–IVS6 junction of the *SUCLA2* gene in patient II-7 and her mother, I-4 (upper and lower chromatograms, respectively). The deleted 43 nt are shown in italics, and the 14 exonic nucleotides are also capitalized. The deletion start site is indicated by an arrow. The inserted 5 nt are shown in bold and are followed by the normal IVS6 sequence. *B*, *SUCLA2* cDNA sequence of patient II-7. A schematic representation (g) shows the exon-intron organization around the mutation site, which is shown in black. With the use of primers cF1 and cR1, two amplification products (c1 and c2) were seen, both of which skip exon 6, and transcript c2 also lacks the first 74 bp of exon 7. The splicing site of exon 5 with mid-exon 7 is indicated by an arrow.

mining the nucleotide specificity (Johnson et al. 1998*a*, 1998*b*). Notably, the activity of both SCS-G and SCS-A is considerable in mitochondria from rat liver, kidney, and heart, but SCS-A, the ADP-forming enzyme, predominates in the brain (Lambeth et al. 2004).

Exon 6 of the *SUCLA2* gene is composed of 139 nt and encodes 47 amino acids (residues 221–267) that form the ATP grasp domain of the protein. Skipping exon 6 is likely to result in the synthesis of the first 221 amino acids, followed by 50 residues of a different reading frame. Since the CoA-ligase domain is created by residues 305–441, truncated polypeptide chains are likely to adversely affect the catalytic activity. The shorter transcript, lacking exon 6 as well as the first part of exon 7, remains in-frame and is predicted to lead to the absence of 71 residues, starting at amino acid 221 but preserving the CoA-ligase domain. Accordingly, SCS-A activity in muscle mitochondria from patient II-6, determined in the direction of succinyl-CoA formation (Cha and Parks 1964), was decreased to 0.038 U per mg of mitochondrial protein (U/mg) (the average control value from six healthy children who underwent orthopedic surgery was 0.210 U/mg; range 0.18–0.25 U/mg). In contrast, the activity of SCS-G in the patient's muscle mitochondria was 0.408 U/mg (average control value 0.386 U/mg; range 0.31–0.41 U/mg; $n = 6$). Thus, the ratio of SCS-A to SCS-G activity in mitochondria isolated from the patient muscle was reduced to 17% of the control value. The activity of SCS-A was normal in mitochondria isolated from muscle of a patient with markedly decreased activities of complexes I and IV due to a high load of the A3243G mutation in the tRNALeu(UUR) gene, indicating that impaired OXPHOS activity does not perturb the function of SCS-A.

How does a mutation in the *SUCLA2* gene cause mtDNA depletion? The gene product of the *LSC1* gene, which is the yeast homologue of the *SUCLA1* gene, is a component of the yeast mtDNA nucleoid (Chen et al. 2005). Defects in some nucleoid proteins in humans, such as the mtDNA polymerase, the mitochondrial single-stranded DNA-binding protein, and the adenine nucleotide translocator 1, were associated with mtDNA depletion or multiple mtDNA deletions. However, the gene product of *LSC2*, the yeast homologue of *SUCLA2*, was not shown in nucleoids, and none of the succinyl-CoA synthase subunits was identified in the mtDNA nucleoids in higher eukaryotes (Bogenhagen et al. 2003).

A plausible explanation is offered by the finding that SCS-A copurifies and is tightly associated in a complex with nucleoside diphosphate kinase (NDPK) in both prokaryotes and eukaryotes (Kadrmas et al. 1991; Kavanaugh-Black et al. 1994; Kowluru et al. 2002). NDPKs are ubiquitous protein kinases that also catalyze the exchange of terminal phosphates between tri- and diphosphoribonucleosides and are crucial for maintaining the homeostasis of ribonucleotides and deoxyribonucleotides (Parks and Agarwal 1973). Specifically, mitochondrial deoxyribonucleotide diphosphates are phosphorylated by a mitochondrial NDPK, NM23-H4 (Milon et al. 2000). The importance of this salvage pathway step for mtDNA synthesis is underscored by the lack of de novo synthesis of dNTPs in this organelle and by the constant need for building blocks for mtDNA synthesis throughout the whole cell cycle (Bogenhagen and Clayton 1976; reviewed by Saada 2004).

Whereas the physical proximity of succinyl-CoA synthetase (SCS) and NDPK is indisputable, the functional significance of their coexistence in a complex is less clear. It was proposed that this proximity signals the involvement of NDPK in energy metabolism, possibly by directly activating the SCS by phosphorylation (Kowluru et al. 2002). Our data suggest that SCS activity is essential for mtDNA synthesis and that SCS deficiency results in mtDNA depletion, possibly because of secondary NDPK dysfunction. Whether such an interference involves the nucleotide triphosphate donation or a conformational change induced by the SCS protein is presently unknown. Regardless of the precise mechanism, the brain seems to be the most vulnerable tissue, not only because all of its SCS activity can be attributed to the SCS-A enzyme, but also because the mitochondrial NDPK is hardly expressed in the human brain (Milon et al. 1997) and because of the rate-limiting role of NDPK in mtDNA replication in postmitotic tissues (Bradshaw and Samuels 2005). The fact that other tissues, such as liver, kidney, and heart, are not affected in our patients suggests that the nature of the interaction between SCS and NDPK is not influenced by the specific phosphate donor.

Genetic defects of the TCA cycle are uncommon in humans, and the most severe defects are probably lethal in early gestation (Rustin et al. 1997). Deficiency of SCS-A in our patients is compatible with life, likely because of the presence of SCS-G, an enzyme with an overlapping activity. For some of the TCA cycle proteins, additional cellular roles beyond their catalytic activities in the cycle have been proposed (Jeffery 1999). For example, fumarase and succinate dehydrogenase act as tumor suppressors in humans (Baysal et al. 2000; Tomlinson et al. 2002). Our finding that SCS-A deficiency is associated with mtDNA depletion in humans parallels the essential role of aconitase in mtDNA maintenance in yeast (Chen et al. 2005), and both highlight yet another pathway in which TCA cycle enzymes are involved.

Acknowledgments

We gratefully acknowledge the collaboration of the patients' family; Dr. Mira Korner of the Center of Genomic Technologies, at the Hebrew University, Jerusalem; and Corinne Belaiche for OXPHOS analysis. We thank Dr. V. Tiranti, for helpful discussions, and Dr. O. Birk, for providing DNA samples. This work was supported in part by Israeli Academy of Sciences and Humanities grant 406/01-1; by Israeli Ministry of Health grant 5307; by Ministry of Science and Technology, Israel, grant 3–904; by the Ministry of Research, France; by the Hebrew University-Shaare-Zedek Joint Research Foundation; by the Child Health Research Appeal Trust; and by Children Living with Inherited Metabolic Diseases.

Electronic-Database Information

Accession numbers and URLs for data presented herein are as follows:

MitoP2, http://ihg.gsf.de/mitop2/start.jsp

NCBI, http://www.ncbi.nlm.nih.gov/ (for *Homo sapiens* chromosome 13 [accession number NC_000013.9], nt 47414793–47473463 [complement], and *Homo sapiens* succinate-CoA ligase, ADP-forming, β subunit [*SUCLA2*] mRNA [accession number NM_003850])

Online Mendelian Inheritance in Man (OMIM), http://www.ncbi.nlm.nih.gov/Omim/ (for *SUCLA2*)

References

Allen DA, Ottaway JH (1986) Succinate thiokinase in pigeon breast muscle mitochondria. FEBS Lett 194:171–175

Andreoli C, Prokisch H, Hortnagel K, Mueller JC, Munsterkotter M, Scharfe C, Meitinger T (2004) MitoP2, an integrated database on mitochondrial proteins in yeast and man. Nucleic Acids Res 32:D459–D462

Baysal BE, Ferrell RE, Willett-Brozick JE, Lawrence EC, Myssiorek D, Bosch A, van der Mey A, Taschner PE, Rubinstein WS, Myers EN, Richard CW, Cornelisse CJ, Devilee P, Devlin B (2000) Mutations in SDHD, a mitochondrial complex II gene, in hereditary paraganglioma. Science 287:848–851

Bogenhagen D, Clayton DA (1976) Thymidylate nucleotide supply for mitochondrial DNA synthesis in mouse L-cells: effect of 5-fluorodeoxyuridine and methotrexate in thymidine kinase plus and thymidine kinase minus cells. J Biol Chem 251:2938–2944

Bogenhagen DF, Wang Y, Shen EL, Kobayashi R (2003) Protein components of mitochondrial DNA nucleoids in higher eukaryotes. Mol Cell Proteomics 2:1205–1216

Bradshaw PC, Samuels DC (2005) A computational model of mitochondrial deoxynucleotide metabolism and DNA replication. Am J Physiol Cell Physiol, published online Jan 5

Cha S, Parks RE (1964) Succinic thiokinase. I. Purification of the enzyme from pig heart. J Biol Chem 239:1961–1967

Chen XJ, Wang X, Kaufman BA, Butow RA (2005) Aconitase couples metabolic regulation to mitochondrial DNA maintenance. Science 307:714–717

Dooijewaard G, Slater EC (1976) Steady state kinetics of high molecular weight (type I) NADH dehydrogenase. Biochem Biophys Acta 440:1–15

Ducluzeau PH, Lachaux A, Bouvier R, Streichenberger N, Stepien G, Mousson B (1999) Depletion of mitochondrial DNA associated with infantile cholestasis and progressive liver fibrosis. J Hepatol 30:149–155

Elpeleg O (2003) Inherited mitochondrial DNA depletion. Pediatr Res 54:153–159

Hoppel C, Cooper C (1969) An improved procedure for preparation of inner membrane vesicles from rat liver mitochondria by treatment with digitonin. Arch Biochem Biophys 135: 173–183

Jeffery CJ (1999) Moonlighting proteins. Trends Biochem Sci 24:8–11

Johnson JD, Mehus JG, Tews K, Milavetz BI, Lambeth DO (1998*a*) Genetic evidence for the expression of ATP- and GTP-specific succinyl-CoA synthetases in multicellular eucaryotes. J Biol Chem 273:27580–27586

Johnson JD, Muhonen WW, Lambeth DO (1998*b*) Characterization of the ATP- and GTP-specific succinyl-CoA synthetases in pigeon: the enzymes incorporate the same α-subunit. J Biol Chem 273:27573–27579

Kadrmas EF, Ray PD, Lambeth DO (1991) Apparent ATP-linked succinate thiokinase activity and its relation to nucleoside diphosphate kinase in mitochondrial matrix preparations from rabbit. Biochim Biophys Acta 1074:339–346

Kavanaugh-Black A, Connolly DM, Chugani SA, Chakrabarty AM (1994) Characterization of nucleoside-diphosphate kinase from *Pseudomonas aeruginosa*: complex formation with succinyl-CoA synthetase. Proc Natl Acad Sci USA 91: 5883–5887

Kowluru A, Tannous M, Chen HQ (2002) Localization and characterization of the mitochondrial isoform of the nucleoside diphosphate kinase in the pancreatic β cell: evidence for its complexation with mitochondrial succinyl-CoA synthetase. Arch Biochem Biophys 398:160–169

Lambeth DO, Tews KN, Adkins S, Frohlich D, Milavetz BI (2004) Expression of two succinyl-CoA synthetases with different nucleotide specificities in mammalian tissues. J Biol Chem 279:36621–36624

Mandel H, Szargel R, Labay V, Elpeleg O, Saada A, Shalata A, Anbinder Y, Berkowitz D, Hartman C, Barak M, Eriksson S, Cohen N (2001) The deoxyguanosine kinase gene is mutated in individuals with depleted hepatocerebral mitochondrial DNA. Nat Genet 29:337–341

Milon L, Meyer P, Chiadmi M, Munier A, Johansson M, Karlsson A, Lascu I, Capeau J, Janin J, Lacombe ML (2000) The human *nm23*-H4 gene product is a mitochondrial nucleoside diphosphate kinase. J Biol Chem 275:14264–14272

Milon L, Rousseau-Merck MF, Munier A, Erent M, Lascu I, Capeau J, Lacombe ML (1997) nm23-H4, a new member of the family of human nm23/nucleoside diphosphate kinase genes localized on chromosome 16p13. Hum Genet 99:550–557

Moraes CT, Shanske S, Tritschler HJ, Aprille JR, Andreetta F, Bonilla E, Schon EA, DiMauro S (1991) mtDNA depletion with variable tissue expression: a novel genetic abnormality in mitochondrial diseases. Am J Hum Genet 48:492–501

Naviaux RK, Nguyen KV (2004) POLG mutations associated with Alpers' syndrome and mitochondrial DNA depletion. Ann Neurol 55:706–712

Nishino I, Spinazzola A, Hirano M (1999) Thymidine phosphorylase gene mutations in MNGIE, a human mitochondrial disorder. Science 283:689–692

Parks RE, Agarwal RP (1973) Nucleoside diphosphokinases. In: Boyer PD (ed) The enzymes. Academic Press, New York, pp 307–333

Rustin P, Bourgeron T, Parfait B, Chretien D, Munnich A, Rotig A (1997) Inborn errors of the Krebs cycle: a group of unusual mitochondrial diseases in human. Biochim Biophys Acta 1361:185–197

Saada A (2004) Deoxyribonucleotides and disorders of mitochondrial DNA integrity. DNA Cell Biol 23:797–806

Saada A, Shaag A, Mandel H, Nevo Y, Eriksson S, Elpeleg O (2001) Mutant mitochondrial thymidine kinase in mitochondrial DNA depletion myopathy. Nat Genet 29:342–344

Sanadi DR, Gibson M, Ayengar P (1954) Guanosine triphosphate, the primary product of phosphorylation coupled to the breakdown of succinyl coenzyme A. Biochim Biophys Acta 14:434–436

Tomlinson IP, Alam NA, Rowan AJ, Barclay E, Jaeger EE, Kelsell D, Leigh I, et al (2002) Germline mutations in *FH* predispose to dominantly inherited uterine fibroids, skin leiomyomata and papillary renal cell cancer. Nat Genet 30: 406–410

Tritschler HJ, Andreetta F, Moraes CT, Bonilla E, Arnaudo E, Danon MJ, Glass S, Zelaya BM, Vamos E, Telerman-Toppet N (1992) Mitochondrial myopathy of childhood associated with depletion of mitochondrial DNA. Neurology 42:209–217

Vu TH, Sciacco M, Tanji K, Nichter C, Bonilla E, Chatkupt S, Maertens P, Shanske S, Mendell J, Koenigsberger MR, Sharer L, Schon EA, DiMauro S, DeVivo DC (1998) Clinical manifestations of mitochondrial DNA depletion. Neurology 50:1783–1790

Weitzman PD, Jenkins T, Else AJ, Holt RA (1986) Occurrence of two distinct succinate thiokinases in animal tissues. FEBS Lett 199:57–60

Book Reviews

Am. J. Hum. Genet. 76:0, 2005

Human Evolutionary Genetics: Origins, Peoples and Disease. By M. A. Jobling, M. E. Hurles, and C. Tyler-Smith. New York: Garland Science, 2004. Pp. 523. $59.95 paperback.

This is an absolutely superb book! I have been recommending it enthusiastically to professional colleagues, graduate students, and even the occasional highly motivated undergraduate student ever since it was published last year, and the response to the book has been overwhelmingly positive. Not only is the book unique in terms of topical coverage, but it is also extremely well executed. In fact, it is one of the best textbooks on any subject that I have read. It belongs on the shelves of everyone interested in the genetic aspects of human evolution. There is also much of value in it for paleoanthropologists, historical linguists, archaeologists, and human biologists (biological anthropologists), as well as for geneticists with various complementary specialties and interests.

The book's 15 chapters are organized around six focal questions: Why study human evolutionary genetics? (chapter 1), How do we study genome diversity? (chapters 2–4), How do we interpret genetic variation? (chapters 5 and 6), Where and when did humans originate? (chapters 7 and 8), How did humans colonize the world? (chapters 9–12), and How is an evolutionary perspective useful? (chapters 13–15). Chapter 1 sets the tone for what follows by discussing the limitations of human genetic data in terms of the kinds of questions that can be addressed effectively and those that cannot. Chapter 2 then presents a short overview of basic genetics, emphasizing molecular aspects of the human genome. Chapter 3 explains the various kinds of data that can be used to assess genomic diversity and discusses the genetic processes that produced the different classes of variants. Chapter 4 gives an overview of laboratory methods appropriate for molecular genetics data collection and concludes with some useful cautionary notes about ancient DNA. Chapter 5 focuses on the population genetics processes that originate and shape human genetic variation, whereas chapter 6 details the panoply of mathematical and statistical methods used to make inferences from molecular data.

The rest of the book is devoted to data presentation and interpretation. By use of a palimpsest metaphor, different chronological strata are successively encountered and are explicated by an analysis of human genetic-diversity data. For instance, chapter 7 explores human phylogenetic relationships, primarily within the order Primates. Chapter 8 reviews scenarios for the origin of our species by synthesizing paleoanthropological, archaeological, and genetic data. Prehistoric migrations that trace the dispersal of humans from Africa to Asia, Australia, Europe, the Americas, and the Pacific are covered in chapters 9–11. Chapter 12 concentrates on historic migrations and admixture phenomena. The genetics of human adaptation and disease are investigated in chapters 13 and 14. Chapter 15 concludes the book with a demonstration of how molecular genetic data can be usefully applied to genealogical studies and individual identification.

Overall, the text is clearly written, and the illustrations are excellent. The boxed supplementary text is especially informative, whether just explanatory information or an opinion piece by an outside expert. There is a real richness to the mtDNA and Y-chromosome data presented in a phylogenetic/phylogeographic framework in the three chapters on prehistoric range expansion and global colonization. Students have found chapters 3–6 (about genome diversity) quite helpful and have deemed the text's brief excursions into the realm of mathematics to be effectively presented and not overly technical. Appropriate Web sites are mentioned throughout the book, to foster independent research. I must confess that I learned something new (and important) from every chapter in the book!

As the authors opine, many of the interpretations, conclusions, and scenarios advocated in the book will serve as flash points of contention and disagreement. This is another positive attribute of the book. The ensuing discussions and debates can provide a didactic forum for helping students learn to sort through arguments and form opinions based on evidence when faced with conflicting interpretations and viewpoints. To wit, a few of the "big picture" questions I have successfully used for class discussion that were derived from statements and/or positions adopted by the authors include Are species *really* discrete units? (p. 374), Is anagenesis *really* a form of speciation? (p. 433), and Is genetic transmission *really* an exclusively vertical process? (p. 419).

Although the text is remarkably free of typographical errors (for a first edition), the occasional glitch did sneak through during the reviewing and proofing process (especially in the illustrations). For instance, the correct spelling of the generic name of the ~6-million-year-old possible human ancestor from Kenya is *Orrorin* (pp. 15, 237, 238, and 519). The terms "Platyrrhine" and "Catarrhine" should be reversed in figure 7.2 (p. 204), and figure 8.11 confuses geological "periods" and "epochs" (p. 246). Also, "skull" is not an exact synonym for the term "cranium" because the skull includes the mandible, whereas the cranium does not (p. 236). But enough nongenetic nits! It is far more accurate and appropriate to close this review on a resoundingly positive note.

Ten years elapsed between the publication of the magisterial tome of Cavalli-Sforza, Menozzi, and Piazza, *The History and*

Geography of Human Genes, which detailed our collective knowledge about the distribution of traditional serogenetic variation within a holistic anthropological framework, and the appearance of *Human Evolutionary Genetics*. This new compendium emphasizes the enormous explosion in knowledge derived from human haploid systems and molecular genetic markers, and, as such, it is a most worthy successor. It should quickly become *the* book to consult for genetic information pertinent to the evolution of our species. To the authors, I offer both a sincere thank you and a hearty congratulations for a job well done!

STEPHEN L. ZEGURA

Anthropology Department
The University of Arizona
Tucson

0002-9297/2005/7606-0016$15.00

Am. J. Hum. Genet. 76:1, 2005

Facioscapulohumeral Muscular Dystrophy: Clinical Medicine and Molecular Cell Biology. Edited by Meena Upadhyaya and David N. Cooper. New York: BIOS Scientific Publishers, 2004. Pp. 250. $149 hardcover.

Facioscapulohumeral muscular dystrophy (FSHD) is a fascinating disorder from both clinical and molecular standpoints. The molecular basis of FSHD is still being debated and refined, 15 years after it was localized by linkage to chromosome 4q and 13 years after the causative genetic rearrangement was identified. This book presents a comprehensive compendium of the state of knowledge about all aspects of FSHD as of approximately 2003, with chapters written by clinicians and investigators who have been intimately involved in contributing to this knowledge base.

For those interested in clinical aspects of FSHD, there are three chapters that discuss the typical and unusual clinical features of the disease and one devoted to the retinal changes seen in some patients. Genetic counseling for FSHD, which is often complex, is discussed in detail by two different clinicians in separate chapters, and a third chapter (on genotype-phenotype correlation) covers many of the same issues. These chapters address interpretation of genetic test results, clinical anticipation (which is suggested in some families but is not uniformly agreed on), and the effect of sex on disease severity. An additional chapter covers genetic mosaicism in FSHD. Clinicians who are interpreting reports of DNA testing for FSHD will also find the chapter entitled "Molecular Diagnosis of FSHD" extremely helpful. Finally, there is a brief chapter reviewing clinical management.

Most of the remainder of the book is devoted to the unfolding story of the molecular basis of this disorder, beginning with linkage analysis and identification of the subtelomeric deletion that is the basis of the clinical diagnostic test. Subsequent chapters present proposed mechanisms of disease, identification of candidate genes, and genomic analysis of the deletion. The evidence for a genetic derepression model of pathogenesis is detailed, along with gene expression profiling that suggests an alternative model.

This book is an ideal resource for someone who wishes to have an in-depth understanding of FSHD. This includes genetic counselors or clinicians who deal with many FSHD families, as well as researchers who are considering entering this field. The book conveys the current state of understanding, as well as the remaining questions to be answered and conflicts to be resolved.

KATHERINE D. MATHEWS

Division of Child Neurology
Department of Pediatrics
University of Iowa Carver College of Medicine
Iowa City

0002-9297/2005/7606-0017$15.00

Erratum

In the November 2004 issue of the *Journal,* in the article entitled "Functional Analysis of Genetic Variation in Catechol-O-Methyltransferase (*COMT*): Effects on mRNA, Protein, and Enzyme Activity in Postmortem Human Brain," by Chen et al. (75:807–821), in the last paragraph of the "Single SNP Has a Predominant Effect on Final COMT Activity" section (p. 818), "G alleles" should read "A alleles," "P2 promoter A" should read "P2 promoter G," and "P2A" should read "P2G."

Also, the label above bars in figure 8*A* should be "−17%." The authors regret the errors.

Announcements[1]

Employment Opportunities

Director.—The Department of Child Health at the University of Missouri–Columbia School of Medicine is seeking a full-time Director for the Division of Medical Genetics. Applicants must be board certified in medical genetics and pediatrics and must have a record of academic, medical, and leadership excellence. The Director will lead a faculty of board-certified geneticists and researchers, genetic counselors, and nurses, with interests in autism, dysmorphology, biochemical genetics, and teratology. He or she will direct clinical and research programs, as well as training programs accredited by the American Board of Medical Genetics and the Accreditation Council for Graduate Medical Education, and will be responsible for developing progressive programs that support the missions of the Division of Medical Genetics, the Department of Child Health, and the School of Medicine. Academic rank at the associate-professor or full-professor level on either the clinical or tenure track is expected. Please direct all inquiries—as well as your letters of reference and curriculum vitae—to Bert Bachrach, M.D., Assistant Professor, Department of Child Health, Columbia, MO 65212; e-mail: bachrachb@missouri.edu. We also invite you to visit our Web site (http://www.genetics.missouri.edu/). Columbia, MO, has a lot to offer you! Visit the Chamber of Commerce Web site (http://chamber.columbia.mo.us/visitors.html) for additional information. The University of Missouri is an equal opportunity employer and complies with the guidelines of the Americans with Disabilities Act (ADA) of 1990. The department welcomes applications from underrepresented physician groups. For ADA accommodations, please contact our ADA coordinator; telephone: (573) 884-8278.

1. Announcements are published free of charge for members of The American Society of Human Genetics (ASHG). Please e-mail announcements to ajhg@emory.edu. Submission must be received *at least 7 weeks* before the month of issue in which publication is requested. They must be double spaced with a $1\frac{1}{2}$-inch margin on all sides. The maximum length is *250 words*, excluding the address for correspondence. Please include a cover letter indicating the name of the sponsoring ASHG member.

Faculty Positions.—The Center for Human Genetics at the University of California, San Francisco (UCSF) invites applications for two tenure-track positions at the assistant-, associate-, or full-professor level. Expertise in population genetics, human evolution, comparative evolution, informatics/computational genetics, or statistical genetics—with an interest in the genetics of susceptibility to disease or variation in drug response (pharmacogenetics)—is desired. Candidates should have a doctoral degree and postdoctoral research experience. The new faculty members will be expected to teach in the Center and to establish an independent research program that will attract and maintain extramural funding. Please send a curriculum vitae, including a brief description of research interests, and the names of three references to Neil Risch, c/o Cory Fergus, UCSF, San Francisco, CA, 94143-0749; e-mail: fergusc@humgen.ucsf.edu. The University of California is an equal opportunity/affirmative action employer. All qualified applicants are encouraged to apply, including minorities and women.

Conferences

Jefferson Matrix Biology Days 2005.—The 12th International Symposium on Basement Membranes will be held at Jefferson Medical College in Philadelphia, PA, on June 15–18, 2005. The conference is sponsored by the Lennox K. Black International Prize for Excellence in Medicine, in memory of Rupert Timpl. A special Matrix Biology Symposium will be held to honor Darwin J. Prockop. For further information on the programs, topics, abstract submissions/deadlines, and hotel accommodations and to register for this event, please visit our Web site (http://www.jeffersonhospital.org/matrixbiology2005) or contact Eileen O'Shaughnessy, Executive Secretary; telephone: (215) 503-5786; fax: (215) 503-5788; e-mail: eileen.oshaughnessy@jefferson.edu

British Human Genetics Conference.—The British Human Genetics Conference will be held September 12–14, 2005, at the University of York in England. Symposium topics include "Diabetes/Obesity" (speakers: Professor Andrew Hattersley [Exeter], Dr. Jonathan Cohen [Dallas, TX], and Professor Steve O'Rahilly [Cambridge]), "Post Genome Technology and Medical Genetics" (speakers: Professor Stephen Pennington [Dublin], Dr. Roy Goodacre [Manchester], and Professor Han Brunner [Nijmegen, The Netherlands]), "Evaluating Genetic Services" (speakers: Dr. Nicholas Steel [Norwich], Dr. Mandy Collins [Southampton], Ms. Lesley Gren [CLIMB], Dr. Marion McAllister [NOWGEN], Ms. Sarah Sahman [TrentCOM], and Linda Davies [NOWGEN]), "Genome Variation and Evolution" (speakers: Dr. Evan Eichler [Seattle, WA], Dr. Stephen Scherer [Ontario], and Dr. Chris Tyler-Smith [Cambridge]), and "Chromatin Diseases" (speakers: Professor Wendy Bickmore [Edinburgh], Dr. Silvere van der Maarel [Leiden, The Netherlands], Professor Doug Higgs [Oxford], and Professor Angus Clarke [Cardiff]). The Carter Lecture on "Humanity's Genes" will be given by Professor Sydney Brenner, FRS, Nobel laureate. The topic for debate will be as follows: "This house believes that healthy carriers identified during neonatal screening should have their carrier status disclosed to their parents" (speakers to be confirmed). Workshops will include "Genetic Education and Practice for Non-Specialist Health Professionals" (speakers: Dale Lea [United States], Clara Gaff [Cardiff], Greta Westwood [Southampton], Glenda Augustine [Birmingham], and Maggie Kirk [NHS GEDC UK]), "Array Based Technologies: Copy Number Changes and Gene Expression in Acute Leukaemia" (speakers: Professor Bryan Young [London], Dr. Jon Strefford [Southampton], Dr. Jan Cools [Leuvan, Belgium], and Professor Torsten Haferlach [Munich]), "Molecular Genetics and Cancer Diagnosis" (speakers: Professor Ian Tomlinson [London], Francis Barany [New York], and Dr. Brian Clark [London]), and "Skeletal Dysplasias in the Clinic: A Practical Approach to Diagnosis and Management" (speakers: Professor Geert Mortier [Ghent], Professor Christine Hall [London], and Dr. Michael Wright [Newcastle]). Plenary and concurrent sessions will be drawn from submitted papers. Further information is available from The Conference Office, British Society for Human Genetics, Clinical Genetics Unit, Birmingham Women's Hospital, Edgbaston, Birmingham B15 2TG, United Kingdom; telephone: 0121 627 2634; fax: 0121 623 6971; e-mail: york2005@bshg.org.uk. Information is also available on the British Society for Human Genetics Web site (http://www.bshg.org.uk/). The registered charity number is 1058821.

Symposium

The 6th International Symposium on Familial Amyloidotic Polyneuropathy and Other Transthyretin Related Disorders and the 5th International Workshop on Liver Transplantation in Familial Amyloid Polyneuropathy.—The 6th International Symposium on Familial Amyloidotic Polyneuropathy and Other Transthyretin Related Disorders and the 5th International Workshop on Liver Transplantation in Familial Amyloid Polyneuropathy will be held August 24–26, 2005, in La Jolla, California. Registration and abstract-submission information is available on our Web site (http://www.scripps.edu/mem/rheum/index2.html). For further details, please contact Dr. Joel Buxbaum, The Scripps Research Institute, 10550 North Torrey Pines Road, MEM-230, La Jolla, CA 92037; telephone: (858) 784-8884; fax: (858) 784-8891; e-mail: michaelp@scripps.edu

THE AMERICAN JOURNAL OF HUMAN GENETICS

Volume 76

2005

Published Monthly for
THE AMERICAN SOCIETY OF HUMAN GENETICS
BY THE UNIVERSITY OF CHICAGO PRESS

THE AMERICAN SOCIETY OF HUMAN GENETICS

Contents of Volume 76

January 2005

i **This Month in the *Journal***
Kathryn Garber

Review Articles

1 **Prospects for Admixture Mapping of Complex Traits**
Paul M. McKeigue

8 **Long-Range Control of Gene Expression: Emerging Mechanisms and Disruption in Disease**
Dirk A. Kleinjan and Veronica van Heyningen

Articles

33 **Sex-Specific Genetic Architecture of Whole Blood Serotonin Levels**
Lauren A. Weiss, Mark Abney, Edwin H. Cook, Jr., and Carole Ober

42 **Mutations within the Programmed Cell Death 10 Gene Cause Cerebral Cavernous Malformations**
F. Bergametti, C. Denier, P. Labauge, M. Arnoult, S. Boetto, M. Clanet, P. Coubes, B. Echenne, R. Ibrahim, B. Irthum, G. Jacquet, M. Lonjon, J. J. Moreau, J. P. Neau, F. Parker, M. Tremoulet, E. Tournier-Lasserve, and Société Française de Neurochirurgie

52 **Identification of a 3.0-kb Major Recombination Hotspot in Patients with Sotos Syndrome Who Carry a Common 1.9-Mb Microdeletion**
Remco Visser, Osamu Shimokawa, Naoki Harada, Akira Kinoshita, Tohru Ohta, Norio Niikawa, and Naomichi Matsumoto

68 **Genetic Investigation of Quantitative Traits Related to Autism: Use of Multivariate Polygenic Models with Ascertainment Adjustment**
Yun Ju Sung, Geraldine Dawson, Jeffrey Munson, Annette Estes, Gerard D. Schellenberg, and Ellen M. Wijsman

82 **Systematic Evaluation of Genetic Variation at the Androgen Receptor Locus and Risk of Prostate Cancer in a Multiethnic Cohort Study**
Matthew L. Freedman, Celeste L. Pearce, Kathryn L. Penney, Joel N. Hirschhorn, Laurence N. Kolonel, Brian E. Henderson, and David Altshuler

91 **Association between Maternal Age and Meiotic Recombination for Trisomy 21**
Neil E. Lamb, Kai Yu, John Shaffer, Eleanor Feingold, and Stephanie L. Sherman

100 **A Whole-Genome Scan for 24-Hour Respiration Rate: A Major Locus at 10q26 Influences Respiration During Sleep**
E. J. C. de Geus, D. Posthuma, N. Kupper, M. van den Berg, G. Willemsen, A. L. Beem, P. E. Slagboom, and D. I. Boomsma

112 **Extreme Heterogeneity in the Molecular Events Leading to the Establishment of Chiasmata during Meiosis I in Human Oocytes**
Michelle L. Lenzi, Jenetta Smith, Timothy Snowden, Mimi Kim, Richard Fishel, Bradford K. Poulos, and Paula E. Cohen

128 **Robust Multipoint Identical-by-Descent Mapping for Affected Relative Pairs**
Daniel J. Schaid, Jason P. Sinnwell, and Stephen N. Thibodeau

Reports

139 **Malic Enzyme 2 May Underlie Susceptibility to Adolescent-Onset Idiopathic Generalized Epilepsy**
David A. Greenberg, Eftihia Cayanis, Lisa Strug, Sudhir Marathe, Martina Durner, Deb K. Pal, Gabriele B. Alvin, Irene Klotz, Elisa Dicker, Shlomo Shinnar, Edward B. Bromfield, Stanley Resor, Jeffrey Cohen, Solomon L. Moshe, Cynthia Harden, and Harriet Kang

147 **Mapping of a Major Locus that Determines Telomere Length in Humans**
Mariuca Vasa-Nicotera, Scott Brouilette, Massimo Mangino, John R. Thompson, Peter Braund, Jenny-Rebecca Clemitson, Andrea Mason, Clare L. Bodycote, Stuart M. Raleigh, Edward Louis, and Nilesh J. Samani

152 **Mathematical Assumptions versus Biological Reality: Myths in Affected Sib Pair Linkage Analysis**
Robert C. Elston, Danhong Song, and Sudha K. Iyengar

157 **Regression Mapping of Association between the Human Leukocyte Antigen Region and Graves Disease**
Matthew J. Simmonds, Joanna M. M. Howson, Joanne M. Heward, Heather J. Cordell, Helen Foxall, Jackie Carr-Smith, Sarah M. Gibson, Neil Walker, Yaron Tomer, Jayne A. Franklyn, John A. Todd, and Stephen C. L. Gough

164 **Mapping of the Major Psoriasis-Susceptibility Locus (*PSORS1*) in a 70-Kb Interval around the Corneodesmosin Gene (*CDSN*)**
Sandro Orrù, Erika Giuressi, Carlo Carcassi, Mirella Casula, and Licinio Contu

172 **Mapping a Mendelian Form of Intracranial Aneurysm to 1p34.3-p36.13**
Brian V. Nahed, Askin Seker, Bulent Guclu, Ali K. Ozturk, Karin Finberg, Abigail A. Hawkins, Michael L. DiLuna, Matthew State, Richard P. Lifton, and Murat Gunel

180 **Strong Evidence of Linkage Disequilibrium between Polymorphisms at the *IRF6* Locus and Nonsyndromic Cleft Lip With or Without Cleft Palate, in an Italian Population**
Luca Scapoli, Annalisa Palmieri, Marcella Martinelli, Furio Pezzetti, Paolo Carinci, Mauro Tognon, and Francesco Carinci

Letters to the Editor

184 **The R620W Polymorphism of the Protein Tyrosine Phosphatase PTPN22 Is Not Associated with Multiple Sclerosis**
Ann B. Begovich, Stacy J. Caillier, Heather C. Alexander, Joanne M. Penko, Stephen L. Hauser, Lisa F. Barcellos, and Jorge R. Oksenberg

187 **Corrections to the Parameterization of Constraints on Allele Sharing in Sibling Pairs Alter Covariate-Parameter Estimates but Not Sharing-Probability Estimates or Power of Tests for Linkage**
Celia M. T. Greenwood and Shelley B. Bull

Book Reviews

190 **Statistical Methods in Genetic Epidemiology**
Written by Duncan C. Thomas
Reviewed by Diego F. Wyszynski

190 **Examining the Farming/Language Dispersal Hypothesis**
Edited by Peter Bellwood and Colin Renfrew
Reviewed by David Glenn Smith

Announcements

193 **Conferences; Call for Papers; Employment Opportunities; Call for Submissions**

Errata

196 **CHEK2*1100delC and Susceptibility to Breast Cancer: A Collaborative Analysis Involving 10,860 Breast Cancer Cases and 9,065 Controls from 10 Studies**
The CHEK2 Breast Cancer Case-Control Consortium (June 2004 [74:1175–1182])

196 **Disrupted in Schizophrenia 1 (DISC1): Association with Schizophrenia, Schizoaffective Disorder, and Bipolar Disorder**
Hodgkinson et al. (November 2004 [75:862–872])

196 **Chronic and Recurrent Otitis Media: A Genome Scan for Susceptibility Loci**
Kathleen A. Daly et al. (December 2004 [75:988–997])

February 2005

i **This Month in the *Journal***
Kathryn Garber

197 **2004 Cotterman Award Winners**

2004 ASHG Presidential Address

198 **What Is Special about the "Human" in "Human Genetics"?**
Robert L. Nussbaum

2004 William Allan Award Address

203 **Introductory Speech for Louis Kunkel**
Jane Gitschier

205 **Cloning of the DMD Gene**
Louis M. Kunkel

2004 ASHG Award for Excellence in Human Genetics Education

215 **Introductory Speech for Robert J. Gorlin**
Judith G. Hall

216 **And the Band Played On...**
Robert J. Gorlin

2004 Curt Stern Award Address

219 **Introductory Speech for Neil Risch**
Leon E. Rosenberg

221 **The SNP Endgame: A Multidisciplinary Approach**
Neil Risch

Articles

227 **Mutations in the *JARID1C* Gene, Which Is Involved in Transcriptional Regulation and Chromatin Remodeling, Cause X-Linked Mental Retardation**
Lars Riff Jensen, Marion Amende, Ulf Gurok, Bettina Moser, Verena Gimmel, Andreas Tzschach, Andreas R. Janecke, Gholamali Tariverdian, Jamel Chelly, Jean-Pierre Fryns, Hilde Van Esch, Tjitske Kleefstra, Ben Hamel, Claude Moraine, Jozef Gécz, Gillian Turner, Richard Reinhardt, Vera M. Kalscheuer, Hans-Hilger Ropers, and Steffen Lenzner

237 **Genomewide Scan for Affective Disorder Susceptibility Loci in Families of a Northern Swedish Isolated Population**
Tine Venken, Stephan Claes, Samuël Sluijs, Andrew D. Paterson, Cornelia van Duijn, Rolf Adolfsson, Jurgen Del-Favero, and Christine Van Broeckhoven

249 **Parental Phenotypes in Family-Based Association Analysis**
Shaun Purcell, Pak Sham, and Mark J. Daly

260 **Dent Disease with Mutations in *OCRL1***
Richard R. Hoopes, Jr., Antony E. Shrimpton, Stephen J. Knohl, Paul Hueber, Bernd Hoppe, Janos Matyus, Ari Simckes, Velibor Tasic, Burkhard Toenshoff, Sharon F. Suchy, Robert L. Nussbaum, and Steven J. Scheinman

268 **Genetic Structure, Self-Identified Race/Ethnicity, and Confounding in Case-Control Association Studies**
Hua Tang, Tom Quertermous, Beatriz Rodriguez, Sharon L. R. Kardia, Xiaofeng Zhu, Andrew Brown, James S. Pankow, Michael A. Province, Steven C. Hunt, Eric Boerwinkle, Nicholas J. Schork, and Neil J. Risch

276 **Ethnicity and Human Genetic Linkage Maps**
Eric Jorgenson, Hua Tang, Maya Gadde, Mike Province, Mark Leppert, Sharon Kardia, Nicholas Schork, Richard Cooper, D. C. Rao, Eric Boerwinkle, and Neil Risch

291 **Contrasting Effects of Natural Selection on Human and Chimpanzee CC Chemokine Receptor 5**
Stephen Wooding, Anne C. Stone, Diane M. Dunn, Srinivas Mummidi, Lynn B. Jorde, Robert K. Weiss, Sunil Ahuja, and Michael J. Bamshad

302 **Role of Replication and CpG Methylation in Fragile X Syndrome CGG Deletions in Primate Cells**
Kerrie Nichol Edamura, Michelle R. Leonard, and Christopher E. Pearson

312 **High-Resolution Mapping of Genotype-Phenotype Relationships in Cri du Chat Syndrome Using Array Comparative Genomic Hybridization**
Xiaoxiao Zhang, Antoine Snijders, Richard Segraves, Xiuqing Zhang, Anita Niebuhr, Donna Albertson, Huanming Yang, Joe Gray, Erik Niebuhr, Lars Bolund, and Dan Pinkel

Reports

327 **A New Susceptibility Locus for Migraine with Aura in the 15q11-q13 Genomic Region Containing Three GABA-A Receptor Genes**
Luisa Russo, Paolo Mariotti, Eugenio Sangiorgi, Tiziana Giordano, Iolanda Ricci, Francesca Lupi, Rossella Chiera, Francesco Guzzetta, Giovanni Neri, and Fiorella Gurrieri

334 **Impaired Mitochondrial Glutamate Transport in Autosomal Recessive Neonatal Myoclonic Epilepsy**
Florence Molinari, Annick Raas-Rothschild, Marlène Rio, Giuseppe Fiermonte, Ferechté Encha-Razavi, Luigi Palmieri, Ferdinando Palmieri, Ziva Ben-Neriah, Noman Kadhom, Michel Vekemans, Tania Attié-Bitach, Arnold Munnich, Pierre Rustin, and Laurence Colleaux

340 Constitutional Rearrangement of the Architectural Factor *HMGA2*: A Novel Human Phenotype Including Overgrowth and Lipomas
Azra H. Ligon, Steven D. P. Moore, Melissa A. Parisi, Matthew E. Mealiffe, David J. Harris, Heather L. Ferguson, Bradley J. Quade, and Cynthia C. Morton

349 Fine Mapping and Positional Candidate Studies Identify *HLA-G* as an Asthma Susceptibility Gene on Chromosome 6p21
Dan Nicolae, Nancy J. Cox, Lucille A. Lester, Daniel Schneider, Zheng Tan, Christine Billstrand, Susan Kuldanek, Joseph Donfack, Paul Kogut, Nina M. Patel, Jeffrey Goodenbour, Timothy Howard, Raoul Wolf, Gerard H. Koppelman, Steven R. White, Rodney Parry, Dirkje S. Postma, Deborah Meyers, Eugene R. Bleecker, Joan S. Hunt, Julian Solway, and Carole Ober

358 Mutations in the D-2-Hydroxyglutarate Dehydrogenase Gene Cause D-2-Hydroxyglutaric Aciduria
Eduard A. Struys, Gajja S. Salomons, Younes Achouri, Emile Van Schaftingen, Salvatore Grosso, William J. Craigen, Nanda M. Verhoeven, and Cornelis Jakobs

361 Mutations that Cause Osteoglophonic Dysplasia Define Novel Roles for FGFR1 in Bone Elongation
Kenneth E. White, Jose M. Cabral, Siobhan I. Davis, Tonya Fishburn, Wayne E. Evans, Shoji Ichikawa, Joanna Fields, Xijie Yu, Nick J. Shaw, Neil J. McLellan, Carole McKeown, David FitzPatrick, Kai Yu, David M. Ornitz, and Michael J. Econs

Book Reviews

368 Inborn Errors of Development: The Molecular Basis of Clinical Disorders of Morphogenesis
Edited by Charles J. Epstein, Robert P. Erickson, and Anthony Wynshaw-Boris
Reviewed by Julie Ann Neidich

368 The Genetics of Renal Disease
Edited by Frances Flinter, Eamonn Maher, and Anand Saggar-Malik
Reviewed by Peter C. Harris

Announcements

370 Employment Opportunities; Call for Papers

Errata

373 A Combined Linkage-Physical Map of the Human Genome
Kong et al. (December 2004 [75:1143–1148])

373 Mapping of a Major Locus that Determines Telomere Length in Humans
Vasa-Nicotera et al. (January 2005 [76:147–151])

March 2005

i This Month in the *Journal*
Kathryn Garber

Review Article

375 The D4Z4 Repeat–Mediated Pathogenesis of Facioscapulohumeral Muscular Dystrophy
Silvère M. van der Maarel and Rune R. Frants

Articles

387 **Linkage Disequilibrium Patterns and tagSNP Transferability among European Populations**
Jakob C. Mueller, Elin Lõhmussaar, Reedik Mägi, Maido Remm, Thomas Bettecken, Peter Lichtner, Saskia Biskup, Thomas Illig, Arne Pfeufer, Jan Luedemann, Stefan Schreiber, Peter Pramstaller, Irene Pichler, Giovanni Romeo, Anthony Gaddi, Alessandra Testa, Heinz-Erich Wichmann, Andres Metspalu, and Thomas Meitinger

399 **Rapid Simulation of *P* Values for Product Methods and Multiple-Testing Adjustment in Association Studies**
S. R. Seaman and B. Müller-Myhsok

409 **Functional Consequences of *PRODH* Missense Mutations**
Hans-Ulrich Bender, Shlomo Almashanu, Gary Steel, Chien-An Hu, Wei-Wen Lin, Alecia Willis, Ann Pulver, and David Valle

421 ***PHOX2B* Genotype Allows for Prediction of Tumor Risk in Congenital Central Hypoventilation Syndrome**
Delphine Trochet, Louise M. O'Brien, David Gozal, Ha Trang, Agneta Nordenskjöld, Béatrice Laudier, Pär-Johan Svensson, Sabine Uhrig, Trevor Cole, Arnold Munnich, Claude Gaultier, Stanislas Lyonnet, and Jeanne Amiel

427 **Possible Genomic Imprinting of Three Human Obesity–Related Genetic Loci**
Chuanhui Dong, Wei-Dong Li, Frank Geller, Lei Lei, Ding Li, Olga Y. Gorlova, Johannes Hebebrand, Christopher I. Amos, Robert D. Nicholls, and R. Arlen Price

438 **Accuracy of Haplotype Reconstruction from Haplotype-Tagging Single-Nucleotide Polymorphisms**
Julian Forton, Dominic Kwiatkowski, Kirk Rockett, Gaia Luoni, Martin Kimber, and Jeremy Hull

449 **Accounting for Decay of Linkage Disequilibrium in Haplotype Inference and Missing-Data Imputation**
Matthew Stephens and Paul Scheet

463 **Population Structure, Admixture, and Aging-Related Phenotypes in African American Adults: The Cardiovascular Health Study**
Alexander P. Reiner, Elad Ziv, Denise L. Lind, Caroline M. Nievergelt, Nicholas J. Schork, Steven R. Cummings, Angie Phong, Esteban González Burchard, Tamara B. Harris, Bruce M. Psaty, and Pui-Yan Kwok

478 **Regulation of α-Synuclein Expression by Poly (ADP Ribose) Polymerase-1 (PARP-1) Binding to the NACP-Rep1 Polymorphic Site Upstream of the *SNCA* Gene**
Ornit Chiba-Falek, Jeffrey A. Kowalak, Mark E. Smulson, and Robert L. Nussbaum

493 **Antenatal Presentation of Bardet-Biedl Syndrome May Mimic Meckel Syndrome**
Houda Karmous-Benailly, Jelena Martinovic, Marie-Claire Gubler, Yoann Sirot, Laure Clech, Catherine Ozilou, Joëlle Augé, Nora Brahimi, Heather Etchevers, Eric Detrait, Chantal Esculpavit, Sophie Audollent, Géraldine Goudefroye, Marie Gonzales, Julia Tantau, Philippe Loget, Madeleine Joubert, Dominique Gaillard, Corinne Jeanne-Pasquier, Anne-Lise Delezoide, Marie-Odile Peter, Ghislaine Plessis, Brigitte Simon-Bouy, Hélène Dollfus, Martine Le Merrer, Arnold Munnich, Férechté Encha-Razavi, Michel Vekemans, and Tania Attié-Bitach

Reports

505 **Association between the Gene Encoding 5-Lipoxygenase–Activating Protein and Stroke Replicated in a Scottish Population**
A. Helgadottir, S. Gretarsdottir, D. St. Clair, A. Manolescu, J. Cheung, G. Thorleifsson, A. Pasdar, S. F. A. Grant, L. J. Whalley, H. Hakonarson, U. Thorsteinsdottir, A. Kong, J. Gulcher K. Stefansson, and M. J. MacLeod

510 **Identification of *C7orf11* (*TTDN1*) Gene Mutations and Genetic Heterogeneity in Nonphotosensitive Trichothiodystrophy**
Kazuhiko Nakabayashi, Daniela Amann, Yan Ren, Ulpu Saarialho-Kere, Nili Avidan, Simone Gentles, Jeffrey R. MacDonald, Erik G. Puffenberger, Angela M. Christiano, Amalia Martinez-Mir, Julio C. Salas-Alanis, Renata Rizzo, Esther Vamos, Anja Raams, Clifford Les, Eric Seboun, Nicolaas G. J. Jaspers, Jacques S. Beckmann, Charles E. Jackson, and Stephen W. Scherer

517 **No Evidence of Association or Interaction between the IL4RA, IL4, and IL13 Genes in Type 1 Diabetes**
Lisa M. Maier, Juliet Chapman, Joanna M. M. Howson, David G. Clayton, Rebecca Pask, David P. Strachan, Wendy L. McArdle, Rebecca C. J. Twells, and John A. Todd

522 **A 4-bp Deletion in the Birt-Hogg-Dubé Gene (*FLCN*) Causes Dominantly Inherited Spontaneous Pneumothorax**
Jodie N. Painter, Hanna Tapanainen, Mirja Somer, Pentti Tukiainen, and Kristiina Aittomäki

528 **Polymorphisms in the Tyrosine Kinase 2 and Interferon Regulatory Factor 5 Genes Are Associated with Systemic Lupus Erythematosus**
Snaevar Sigurdsson, Gunnel Nordmark, Harald H. H. Göring, Katarina Lindroos, Ann-Christin Wiman, Gunnar Sturfelt, Andreas Jönsen, Solbritt Rantapää-Dahlqvist, Bozena Möller, Juha Kere, Sari Koskenmies, Elisabeth Widén, Maija-Leena Eloranta, Heikki Julkunen, Helga Kristjansdottir, Kristjan Steinsson, Gunnar Alm, Lars Rönnblom, and Ann-Christine Syvänen

538 **Association Testing in a Linked Region Using Large Pedigrees**
Rita M. Cantor, Gary K. Chen, Päivi Pajukanta, and Kenneth Lange

Book Review

543 **The Principles of Clinical Cytogenetics, second edition**
Edited by Steven L. Gersen and Martha B. Keagle
Reviewed by Gail Stetten

Announcements

544 **Employment Opportunity; Call for Papers; Conferences; Postdoctoral Positions**

April 2005

i **This Month in the *Journal***
Kathryn Garber

Editorial

547 **Embracing Our Duty**
Susanne B. Haga

Articles

548 **Population Genetics of *CAPN10* and *GPR35:* Implications for the Evolution of Type 2 Diabetes Variants**
J. Vander Molen, L. M. Frisse, S. M. Fullerton, Y. Qian, L. del Bosque-Plata, R. R. Hudson, and A. Di Rienzo

561 Analysis of Families in the Multiple Autoimmune Disease Genetics Consortium (MADGC) Collection: the *PTPN22* 620W Allele Associates with Multiple Autoimmune Phenotypes
Lindsey A. Criswell, Kirsten A. Pfeiffer, Raymond F. Lum, Bonnie Gonzales, Jill Novitzke, Marlena Kern, Kathy L. Moser, Ann B. Begovich, Victoria E. H. Carlton, Wentian Li, Annette T. Lee, Ward Ortmann, Timothy W. Behrens, and Peter K. Gregersen

572 Genetic Heterogeneity in Rubinstein-Taybi Syndrome: Mutations in Both the *CBP* and *EP300* Genes Cause Disease
Jeroen H. Roelfsema, Stefan J. White, Yavuz Ariyürek, Deborah Bartholdi, Dunja Niedrist, Francesco Papadia, Carlos A. Bacino, Johan T. den Dunnen, Gert-Jan B. van Ommen, Martijn H. Breuning, Raoul C. Hennekam, and Dorien J. M. Peters

581 Strong Evidence That *KIAA0319* on Chromosome 6p Is a Susceptibility Gene for Developmental Dyslexia
Natalie Cope, Denise Harold, Gary Hill, Valentina Moskvina, Jim Stevenson, Peter Holmans, Michael J. Owen, Michael C. O'Donovan, and Julie Williams

592 Genetic Association Analysis Using Data from Triads and Unrelated Subjects
Michael P. Epstein, Colin D. Veal, Richard C. Trembath, Jonathan N. W. N. Barker, Chun Li, and Glen A. Satten

609 Molecular and Clinical Analyses of Greig Cephalopolysyndactyly and Pallister-Hall Syndromes: Robust Phenotype Prediction from the Type and Position of *GLI3* Mutations
Jennifer J. Johnston, Isabelle Olivos-Glander, Christina Killoran, Emma Elson, Joyce T. Turner, Kathryn F. Peters, Margaret H. Abbott, David J. Aughton, Arthur S. Aylsworth, Michael J. Bamshad, Carol Booth, Cynthia J. Curry, Albert David, Mary Beth Dinulos, David B. Flannery, Michelle A. Fox, John M. Graham Jr., Dorothy K. Grange, Alan E. Guttmacher, Mark C. Hannibal, Wolfram Henn, Raoul C. M. Hennekam, Lewis B. Holmes, H. Eugene Hoyme, Kathleen A. Leppig, Angela E. Lin, Patrick MacLeod, David K. Manchester, Carlo Marcelis, Laura Mazzanti, Emma McCann, Marie T. McDonald, Nancy J. Mendelsohn, John B. Moeschler, Billur Moghaddam, Giovanni Neri, Ruth Newbury-Ecob, Roberta A. Pagon, John A. Phillips III, Laurie S. Sadler, Joan M. Stoler, David Tilstra, Catherine M. Walsh Vockley, Elaine H. Zackai, Touran M. Zadeh, Louise Brueton, Graeme Charles M. Black, and Leslie G. Biesecker

623 Variation in Antiviral 2′,5′-Oligoadenylate Synthetase (2′5′AS) Enzyme Activity Is Controlled by a Single-Nucleotide Polymorphism at a Splice-Acceptor Site in the *OAS1* Gene
Vagn Bonnevie-Nielsen, L. Leigh Field, Shao Lu, Dong-Jun Zheng, Min Li, Pia M. Martensen, Thomas B. Nielsen, Henning Beck-Nielsen, Yu-Lung Lau, and Flemming Pociot

634 A High-Resolution Linkage-Disequilibrium Map of the Human Major Histocompatibility Complex and First Generation of Tag Single-Nucleotide Polymorphisms
Marcos M. Miretti, Emily C. Walsh, Xiayi Ke, Marcos Delgado, Mark Griffiths, Sarah Hunt, Jonathan Morrison, Pamela Whittaker, Eric S. Lander, Lon R. Cardon, David R. Bentley, John D. Rioux, Stephan Beck, and Panos Deloukas

Reports

647 Genomewide Significant Linkage to Stuttering on Chromosome 12
Naveeda Riaz, Stacy Steinberg, Jamil Ahmad, Anna Pluzhnikov, Sheikh Riazuddin, Nancy J. Cox, and Dennis Drayna

652 Position Effects Due to Chromosome Breakpoints that Map ~900 Kb Upstream and ~1.3 Mb Downstream of *SOX9* in Two Patients with Campomelic Dysplasia
Gopalrao V. N. Velagaleti, Gabriel A. Bien-Willner, Jill K. Northup, Lillian H. Lockhart, Judy C. Hawkins, Syed M. Jalal, Marjorie Withers, James R. Lupski, and Pawel Stankiewicz

663 **Fine Mapping of Chromosome 17 Translocation Breakpoints ≥900 Kb Upstream of *SOX9* in Acampomelic Campomelic Dysplasia and a Mild, Familial Skeletal Dysplasia**
Katherine L. Hill-Harfe, Lee Kaplan, Heather J. Stalker, Roberto T. Zori, Ramona Pop, Gerd Scherer, and Margaret R. Wallace

672 **Identification of a Novel *LRRK2* Mutation Linked to Autosomal Dominant Parkinsonism: Evidence of a Common Founder across European Populations**
Jennifer Kachergus, Ignacio F. Mata, Mary Hulihan, Julie P. Taylor, Sarah Lincoln, Jan Aasly, J. Mark Gibson, Owen A. Ross, Timothy Lynch, Joseph Wiley, Haydeh Payami, John Nutt, Demetrius M. Maraganore, Krzysztof Czyzewski, Maria Styczynska, Zbigniew K. Wszolek, Matthew J. Farrer, and Mathias Toft

681 **A Comparison of Linkage Disequilibrium Patterns and Estimated Population Recombination Rates across Multiple Populations**
David M. Evans and Lon R. Cardon

688 **Effects of Updating Linkage Evidence across Subsets of Data: Reanalysis of the Autism Genetic Resource Exchange Data Set**
Christopher W. Bartlett, Rhinda Goedken, and Veronica J. Vieland

696 **Gene-Environment Interaction Effects on the Development of Immune Responses in the 1st Year of Life**
Sabine Hoffjan, Dan Nicolae, Irina Ostrovnaya, Kathy Roberg, Michael Evans, Daniel B. Mirel, Lori Steiner, Karen Walker, Peter Shult, Ronald E. Gangnon, James E. Gern, Fernando D. Martinez, Robert F. Lemanske, Jr., and Carole Ober

Letters to the Editor

705 **No Convincing Evidence of Linkage for Restless Legs Syndrome on Chromosome 9p**
1Amrita Ray and Daniel E. Weeks

707 **Reply to Ray and Weeks: Linkage for Restless Legs Syndrome on Chromosome 9p Is Significant**
Shenghan Chen, Lin Li, Shaoqi Rao, William G. Ondo, and Qing Wang

Book Review

711 **The X in Sex: How the X Chromosome Controls our Lives**
Written by David Bainbridge
Reviewed by Barbara Migeon

Announcements

713 **Employment Opportunities; Samples Available; Database Available**

Errata

715 **Localization of a Gene for Migraine without Aura to Chromosome 4q21**
Björnsson et al. (November 2003 [73:986–993])

715 **Contrasting Effects of Natural Selection on Human and Chimpanzee CC Chemokine Receptor 5**
Wooding et al. (February 2005 [76:291–301])

715 ***PHOX2B* Genotype Allows for Prediction of Tumor Risk in Congenital Central Hypoventilation Syndrome**
Trochet et al. (March 2005 [76:421–426])

May 2005

i **This Month in the *Journal***
Kathryn Garber

Review Article

717 **Autosomal Recessive Primary Microcephaly (MCPH): A Review of Clinical, Molecular, and Evolutionary Findings**
C. Geoffrey Woods, Jacquelyn Bond, and Wolfgang Enard

Articles

729 **Diversity and Function of Mutations in P450 Oxidoreductase in Patients with Antley-Bixler Syndrome and Disordered Steroidogenesis**
Ningwu Huang, Amit V. Pandey, Vishal Agrawal, William Reardon, Pablo D. Lapunzina, David Mowat, Ethylin Wang Jabs, Guy Van Vliet, Joseph Sack, Christa E. Flück, and Walter L. Miller

750 **Exon Array CGH: Detection of Copy-Number Changes at the Resolution of Individual Exons in the Human Genome**
Pawandeep Dhami, Alison J. Coffey, Stephen Abbs, Joris R. Vermeesch, Jan P. Dumanski, Karen J. Woodward, Robert M. Andrews, Cordelia Langford, and David Vetrie

763 **Increased Level of Linkage Disequilibrium in Rural Compared with Urban Communities: A Factor to Consider in Association-Study Design**
Veronique Vitart, Andrew D. Carothers, Caroline Hayward, Peter Teague, Nicholas D. Hastie, Harry Campbell, and Alan F. Wright

773 **Localization of a Type 1 Diabetes Locus in the *IL2RA/CD25* Region by Use of Tag Single-Nucleotide Polymorphisms**
Adrian Vella, Jason D. Cooper, Christopher E. Lowe, Neil Walker, Sarah Nutland, Barry Widmer, Richard Jones, Susan M. Ring, Wendy McArdle, Marcus E. Pembrey, David P. Strachan, David B. Dunger, Rebecca C. J. Twells, David G. Clayton, and John A. Todd

780 **Nonparametric Tests of Association of Multiple Genes with Human Disease**
Daniel J. Schaid, Shannon K. McDonnell, Scott J. Hebbring, Julie M. Cunningham, and Stephen N. Thibodeau

794 **Mutations in *ABCA12* Underlie the Severe Congenital Skin Disease Harlequin Ichthyosis**
David P. Kelsell, Elizabeth E. Norgett, Harriet Unsworth, Muy-Teck Teh, Thomas Cullup, Charles A. Mein, Patricia J. Dopping-Hepenstal, Beverly A. Dale, Gianluca Tadini, Philip Fleckman, Karen G. Stephens, Virginia P. Sybert, Susan B. Mallory, Bernard V. North, David R. Witt, Eli Sprecher, Aileen E. M. Taylor, Andrew Ilchyshyn, Cameron T. Kennedy, Helen Goodyear, Celia Moss, David Paige, John I. Harper, Bryan D. Young, Irene M. Leigh, Robin A. J. Eady, and Edel A. O'Toole

804 **A Novel *STX16* Deletion in Autosomal Dominant Pseudohypoparathyroidism Type Ib Redefines the Boundaries of a *cis*-Acting Imprinting Control Element of *GNAS***
Agnès Linglart, Robert C. Gensure, Robert C. Olney, Harald Jüppner, and Murat Bastepe

815 **Quantitative Founder-Effect Analysis of French Canadian Families Identifies Specific Loci Contributing to Metabolic Phenotypes of Hypertension**
P. Hamet, E. Merlo, O. Šeda, U. Broeckel, J. Tremblay, M. Kaldunski, D. Gaudet, G. Bouchard, B. Deslauriers, F. Gagnon, G. Antoniol, Z. Pausová, M. Labuda, M. Jomphe, F. Gossard, G. Tremblay, R. Kirova, P. Tonellato, S. N. Orlov, J. Pintos, J. Platko, T. J. Hudson, J. D. Rioux, T. A. Kotchen, and A. W. Cowley Jr.

833 **Over- and Underdosage of *SOX3* Is Associated with Infundibular Hypoplasia and Hypopituitarism**
Kathryn S. Woods, Maria Cundall, James Turton, Karine Rizotti, Ameeta Mehta, Rodger Palmer, Jacqueline Wong, W. K. Chong, Mahmoud Al-Zyoud, Maryam El-Ali, Timo Otonkoski, Juan-Pedro Martinez-Barbera, Paul Q. Thomas, Iain C. Robinson, Robin Lovell-Badge, Karen J. Woodward, and Mehul T. Dattani

Reports

850 **Identifying Candidate Hirschsprung Disease–Associated *RET* Variants**
Grzegorz M. Burzynski, Ilja M. Nolte, Agnes Bronda, Krista K. Bos, Jan Osinga, Ivan Plaza Menacho, Bas Twigt, Saskia Maas, Alice S. Brooks, Joke B. G. M. Verheij, Charles H. C. M. Buys, and Robert M. W. Hofstra

859 **Single- and Multilocus Allelic Variants within the $GABA_B$ Receptor Subunit 2 (*GABAB2*) Gene Are Significantly Associated with Nicotine Dependence**
Joke Beuten, Jennie Z. Ma, Thomas J. Payne, Randolph T. Dupont, Karen M. Crews, Grant Somes, Nancy J. Williams, Robert C. Elston, and Ming D. Li

865 **Microduplication and Triplication of 22q11.2: A Highly Variable Syndrome**
Twila M. Yobb, Martin J. Somerville, Lionel Willatt, Helen V. Firth, Karen Harrison, Jennifer MacKenzie, Natasha Gallo, Bernice E. Morrow, Lisa G. Shaffer, Melanie Babcock, Judy Chernos, Francois Bernier, Kathy Sprysak, Jesse Christiansen, Shelagh Haase, Basil Elyas, Margaret Lilley, Steven Bamforth, and Heather E. McDermid

877 **Congenital Diaphragmatic Hernia and Chromosome 15q26: Determination of a Candidate Region by Use of Fluorescent In Situ Hybridization and Array-Based Comparative Genomic Hybridization**
M. Klaassens, M. van Dooren, H. J. Eussen, H. Douben, A. T. den Dekker, C. Lee, P. K. Donahoe, R. J. Galjaard, N. Goemaere, R. R. de Krijger, C. Wouters, J. Wauters, B. A. Oostra, D. Tibboel, and A. de Klein

883 **Saami and Berbers—An Unexpected Mitochondrial DNA Link**
Alessandro Achilli, Chiara Rengo, Vincenza Battaglia, Maria Pala, Anna Olivieri, Simona Fornarino, Chiara Magri, Rosaria Scozzari, Nora Babudri, A. Silvana Santachiara-Benerecetti, Hans-Jürgen Bandelt, Ornella Semino, and Antonio Torroni

887 **A Note on Exact Tests of Hardy-Weinberg Equilibrium**
Janis E. Wigginton, David J. Cutler, and Gonçalo R. Abecasis

894 **The Dual Origin of the Malagasy in Island Southeast Asia and East Africa: Evidence from Maternal and Paternal Lineages**
Matthew E. Hurles, Bryan C. Sykes, Mark A. Jobling, and Peter Forster

902 **The *Epsin 4* Gene on Chromosome 5q, Which Encodes the Clathrin-Associated Protein Enthoprotin, Is Involved in the Genetic Susceptibility to Schizophrenia**
Jonathan Pimm, Andrew McQuillin, Srinivasa Thirumalai, Jacob Lawrence, Digby Quested, Nicholas Bass, Graham Lamb, Helen Moorey, Susmita R. Datta, Gursharan Kalsi, Allison Badacsonyi, Katie Kelly, Jenny Morgan, Bhaskar Punukollu, David Curtis, and Hugh Gurling

Announcements

908 **Employment Opportunities; Conference**

June 2005

i **This Month in the *Journal***
Kathryn Garber

Review Article

911 **Single-Gene Disorders: What Role Could Moonlighting Enzymes Play?**
Ganesh Sriram, Julian A. Martinez, Edward R. B. McCabe, James C. Liao, and Katrina M. Dipple

Articles

925 **A Genomewide Exploration Suggests a New Candidate Gene at Chromosome 11q23 as the Major Determinant of Plasma Homocysteine Levels: Results from the GAIT Project**
Juan Carlos Souto Francisco Blanco-Vaca, José Manuel Soria, Alfonso Buil, Laura Almasy, Jordi Ordoñez-Llanos, Jesús Mª Martín-Campos, Mark Lathrop, William Stone, John Blangero, and Jordi Fontcuberta

934 **Joint Modeling of Linkage and Association: Identifying SNPs Responsible for a Linkage Signal**
Mingyao Li, Michael Boehnke, and Gonçalo R. Abecasis

950 **Candidate-Gene Screening and Association Analysis at the Autism-Susceptibility Locus on Chromosome 16p: Evidence of Association at *GRIN2A* and *ABAT***
Gabrielle Barnby, Aaron Abbott, Nuala Sykes, Andrew Morris, Daniel E. Weeks, Richard Mott, Janine Lamb, Anthony J. Bailey, Anthony P. Monaco, and the International Molecular Genetics Study of Autism Consortium (IMGSAC)

967 **Rational Inferences about Departures from Hardy-Weinberg Equilibrium**
Jacqueline K. Wittke-Thompson, Anna Pluzhnikov, and Nancy J. Cox

987 **Alternative Splicing Suggests Extended Function of *PEX26* in Peroxisome Biogenesis**
Sabine Weller, Ivelisse Cajigas, James Morrell, Cassandra Obie, Gary Steel, Stephen J. Gould, and David Valle

1008 **Heterozygous Mutations of *OTX2* Cause Severe Ocular Malformations**
Nicola K. Ragge, Alison G. Brown, Charlotte M. Poloschek, Birgit Lorenz, R. Alex Henderson, Michael P. Clarke, Isabelle Russell-Eggitt, Alistair Fielder, Dianne Gerrelli, Juan Pedro Martinez-Barbera, Piers Ruddle, Jane Hurst, J. Richard O. Collin, Alison Salt, Simon T. Cooper, Pamela J. Thompson, Sanjay M. Sisodiya, Kathleen A. Williamson, David R. FitzPatrick, Veronica van Heyningen, and Isabel M. Hanson

1023 **Germline *BHD*-Mutation Spectrum and Phenotype Analysis of a Large Cohort of Families with Birt-Hogg-Dubé Syndrome**
Laura S. Schmidt, Michael L. Nickerson, Michelle B. Warren, Gladys M. Glenn, Jorge R. Toro, Maria J. Merino, Maria L. Turner, Peter L. Choyke, Nirmala Sharma, James Peterson, Patrick Morrison, Eamonn R. Maher, McClellan M. Walther Berton Zbar, and W. Marston Linehan

1034 **Fatal Congenital Heart Glycogenosis Caused by a Recurrent Activating R531Q Mutation in the γ2-Subunit of AMP-Activated Protein Kinase (*PRKAG2*), Not by Phosphorylase Kinase Deficiency**
Barbara Burwinkel, John W. Scott, Christoph Bührer, Frank K. H. van Landeghem, Gerald F. Cox, Callum J. Wilson, D. Grahame Hardie, and Manfred W. Kilimann

Reports

1050 **Replication of Autism Linkage: Fine-Mapping Peak at 17q21**
Rita M. Cantor, Naoko Kono, Jackie A. Duvall, Ana Alvarez-Retuerto, Jennifer L. Stone, Maricela Alarcón, Stanley F. Nelson, and Daniel H. Geschwind

1057 **A Novel Linkage to Generalized Vitiligo on 4q13-q21 Identified in a Genomewide Linkage Analysis of Chinese Families**
Jian-Jun Chen, Wei Huang, Jin-Ping Gui, Sen Yang, Fu-Sheng Zhou, Quan-Geng Xiong, Hong-Bo Wu, Yong Cui, Min Gao, Wei Li, Jin-Xian Li, Kai-Lin Yan, Wen-Tao Yuan, Shi-Jie Xu, Jian-Jun Liu, and Xue-Jun Zhang

1066 ***In Silico* Analysis of Disease-Association Mapping Strategies Using the Coalescent Process and Incorporating Ascertainment and Selection**
Ying Wang and Bruce Rannala

1074 **Identification of FOXP2 Truncation as a Novel Cause of Developmental Speech and Language Deficits**
Kay D. MacDermot, Elena Bonora, Nuala Sykes, Anne-Marie Coupe, Cecilia S. L. Lai, Sonja C. Vernes, Faraneh Vargha-Khadem, Fiona McKenzie, Robert L. Smith, Anthony P. Monaco, and Simon E. Fisher

1081 **Deficiency of the ADP-Forming Succinyl-CoA Synthase Activity Is Associated with Encephalomyopathy and Mitochondrial DNA Depletion**
Orly Elpeleg, Chaya Miller, Eli Hershkovitz, Maria Bitner-Glindzicz, Gili Bondi-Rubinstein, Shamima Rahman, Alistair Pagnamenta, Sharon Eshhar, and Ann Saada

Book Reviews

1087 **Human Evolutionary Genetics: Origins, Peoples, and Disease**
Written by M. A. Jobling, M. E. Hurles, and C. Tyler-Smith
Reviewed by Stephen L. Zegura

1088 **Facioscapulohumeral Muscular Dystrophy: Clinical Medicine and Molecular Cell Biology**
Edited by Meena Upadhyaya and David N. Cooper
Reviewed by Katherine D. Mathews

Erratum

1089 **Functional Analysis of Genetic Variation in Catechol-O-Methyltransferase (*COMT*): Effects on mRNA, Protein, and Enzyme Activity in Postmortem Human Brain**
Chen et al. (November 2004 [75:807-821])

Announcements

1090 Employment Opportunities; Conferences; Symposium

Information for Contributors

Information for Contributors

Postal address: **Stephen T. Warren, Ph.D., Editor, The American Journal of Human Genetics, Department of Human Genetics, Emory University School of Medicine, 615 Michael Street, Room 301, Atlanta, GA 30322-3050.** Telephone: (404) 712-9980. Fax: (404) 712-9984. E-mail: ajhg@emory.edu. Web page: http://www.ajhg.org/.

The American Journal of Human Genetics is a record of research and review relating to heredity in humans; to the applications of genetic principles in medicine, psychology, anthropology, and social services; and to areas of molecular and cell biology relevant to human genetics. It is published monthly. The *Journal* is owned and controlled by The American Society of Human Genetics and is edited, in conjunction with the publisher, by a staff appointed by the Board of Directors of the Society.

Electronic Edition

The entire content of the *Journal* is published electronically on the World Wide Web, at http://www.ajhg.org/. The full text is available to subscribers, as is material supplemental to the print version, including video and archival databases. Articles will be posted as they are ready for publication. Approximately 2 weeks before publication of the hard copy, the table of contents for that issue will be posted with final pagination, along with editorials and other material.

Editorial Policy

The *Journal* welcomes submissions of articles and reports on timely subjects concerning all aspects of human genetics, including studies of model organisms that are of direct relevance to human genetics. Letters commenting on material previously published in the *Journal* are also welcome. Review articles, editorials, and book reviews usually are solicited by the editor. The *Journal* does not publish reports of either single mutations or mutational surveys of previously identified loci unless they have unusual significance and substantial insight. Descriptions of new linkage assignments will be considered only if they are of unusual interest and significance. Reports of negative data, without substantial insight and interest, will not normally be considered. Membership in The American Society of Human Genetics is not a prerequisite for publication in the *Journal.* Papers will be considered for publication on condition that they are not currently under consideration by any other publication and that no portion of them has been published elsewhere.

- *Review process.* Manuscripts will be considered for appropriateness to the *Journal* by the editor in conjunction with the editorial board. Those considered appropriate will be reviewed by two or more external reviewers or by members of the editorial board, and those not considered appropriate will be returned to the authors. Authors are requested to suggest appropriate referees. Manuscripts will be judged on their value as original contributions to the field and on their overall presentation. Authors whose manuscripts are returned without external review may appeal by writing the editor.
- *Return of figures.* For manuscripts that are reviewed but not accepted, all figures submitted as glossy prints will be returned whenever possible.
- *Editing.* Manuscripts will be edited to conform to *Journal* style, to correct spelling and grammar where necessary, and to improve conciseness, clarity, and precision of expression. Significant editorial changes will be identified on the page proofs.
- *Publication costs.* For papers published—except for invited contributions and Letters to the Editor—authors will be charged $50.00 per printed *Journal* page or portion thereof. Each *Journal* page contains ~800 words. If authors wish, they may instead pay a single publication fee of $5,000 for an article or $2,700 for a report, to make their work freely and immediately available to all readers at publication, rather than after the usual 6-month delay for nonsubscribers. All authors will also be charged for printing of color figures (see Illustrations, below).
- *Copyright agreement.* All authors of all manuscripts accepted for publication (except U.S. government employees) must sign an agreement transferring copyright to The American Society of Human Genetics. Corresponding authors must assume responsibility for obtaining the signatures of all coauthors. Material published in the *Journal* may not be reproduced or published elsewhere without written consent of the Society and the publisher. Requests for such permission should be addressed to the publisher: Copyright, University of Chicago Press, 1427 East 60th Street, Chicago, IL 60637. Fax: (773) 702-9756.
- *Research materials.* It is assumed that authors whose research is published in the *Journal* will make cell lines, antibodies, cloned DNA sequences, and similar materials available to other investigators in noncommercial institutions, so as to permit replication of the reported work.
- *Page proofs.* Page proofs will be sent to the corresponding author for correction of typographical errors only. Corresponding authors are responsible for the return of corrected page proofs to the publisher by the designated deadline.
- *Reprints.* The corresponding author will receive an order form for reprints, along with the page proofs.

Manuscript Submission

Manuscripts should now be submitted via the *AJHG* Web Peer Review System at http://mss.uchicago.edu/AJHG. Basic instructions for submission via the WPR system can be found at the Web site (http://mss.uchicago.edu/AJHG/auth_msprep_AJHG.epl), and detailed instructions are given below.

Manuscript Preparation

Manuscripts must be written in English. MS Word, Rich Text, or LaTeX formats are acceptable. All components of the text (including references and figure legends but not tables) must

be typed double spaced in 12-point type. Tables must be single spaced. *Manuscripts that are not double spaced throughout will not be sent out for review.* Use a 1-inch margin on all four sides of each page, and do not justify the right margin. Begin each manuscript component on a separate page, and arrange components in the following order: title page, Summary (abstract), text (articles separated into Introduction, Material and Methods, Results, and Discussion), Acknowledgments, appendices (if any), Electronic-Database Information, References, tables, and figure legends. Number all pages consecutively in the upper-right-hand corner, beginning with the title page.

Cover letter. Include a letter from the author who will be responsible for correspondence regarding the manuscript as well as for communications among authors in regard to revisions, publication agreements, and approval of proofs. This letter should indicate the category of manuscript being submitted (e.g., article, report, letter, review) and highlight the significance of the manuscript in a few sentences. It should also disclose the source of funding and any affiliations with or involvement in any companies, trade associations, unions, litigants, or other groups with a direct financial interest in the subject matter or materials discussed in the manuscript by any authors and/or their immediate family within the last 5 years. Also indicate whether the first author is a student or postdoctoral fellow and a member of The American Society of Human Genetics (to be eligible for the Cotterman awards, presented at the ASHG's annual meeting).

Please indicate the category of your manuscript in the cover letter:

Articles are full-length, original research articles.

Reports are short (approximately four *Journal* pages, 800 words per page) scientific correspondence with a brief abstract but without further subdivision of the manuscript. This category is designed for timely publication of original findings that may substantially impact their field.

Letters to the Editor are brief commentaries (less than one printed page) concerning articles published in the *Journal* within the past 2 months. They may also present new data. Also included in this section are short general news items of interest to the Society. Any letter concerning a previously published article will first be sent for external review, to determine whether it meets an appropriate level of significance for publication in the *Journal*. If the letter achieves this basic level of significance, it will then be sent to the corresponding author of the pertinent article, who will be given an opportunity to submit a response. This response will be provided to the corresponding author of the letter to the editor. After considering the response, the authors may choose to withdraw their letter or to proceed with publication without further revision.

Fast-track review. If circumstances so warrant, you may request in the cover letter a fast-track review of your paper. At the editor's discretion, a 24- to 48-hour fast-track review is available to expedite manuscripts that deserve rapid review and publication.

Related manuscripts. Please submit a copy of any related papers, by any of the authors, that have been submitted but not published elsewhere or that are in press. For citation of such manuscripts, see "*Work submitted to a publication but not yet accepted, personal communications, and unpublished data*," below.

All papers should adhere to the guidelines that follow, with two exceptions:

1) *Reports* should contain a brief summary of five sentences or fewer, but the remainder of the text should not be divided into sections.

2) *Letters to the Editor* do not contain a summary, nor should the text be divided into sections.

Otherwise, please prepare all submissions according to the following directives:

Title page. This page should contain a concise title; a running title of no more than 40 characters (including spaces); the names and institutional affiliations of all authors at the time of the study (and present affiliations, if different); and the corresponding author's name, complete current mailing address, telephone number, fax number, and e-mail address. Each paper can be assigned only one corresponding author. Joint authorship is permitted only for the first author position, with a maximum of two individuals being given this designation.

Summary (abstract). The Summary should state the purpose of the study, the basic procedures and analytical methods, the findings, and the principal conclusions. The Summary must not exceed 275 words.

Text. The text should be as concise as possible and should be organized into the following sections: Introduction, Material and Methods (or Subjects and Methods), Results, and Discussion. Some manuscripts may require different formats appropriate to their content. Brief subheadings may be used where necessary.

The Introduction should summarize the rationale for the study, without reviewing the subject extensively. Using the past tense, describe the selection of subjects and identify the methods, apparatus, and procedures in detail. Provide references for established methods and brief descriptions of those that are not well known. Describe any new or modified methods used, including reasons for their use and evaluations of their limitations.

Present results in logical sequence in the text, tables, and illustrations. Do not repeat in the text all the data that appear in the tables and illustrations. Detailed results of statistical analyses may be presented as an appendix.

Electronic-Database Information. Please provide accession numbers along with the URL of any genome or locus-specific database in which information has been deposited. (This is required for establishing links in the electronic edition of the *Journal*.) Place this information in the text and in a separate section entitled "Electronic-Database Information," following the Acknowledgments. Please do not include URLs in the text or in the References.

MIM numbers should be listed in the text after the first mention of the relevant disorder or gene. Example: adrenal hypoplasia congenita (AHC [MIM 300200]). In the Electronic-Database Information section, only the URL for the OMIM database, and not the individual MIM numbers, should be noted. Example: Online Mendelian Inheritance in Man (OMIM), http://www.ncbi.nlm.nih.gov/Omim/.

Human subjects. If the manuscript reports results of studies of either human subjects or materials obtained from human subjects, state in the Material and Methods section that the study was approved by the appropriate institutional review board and/or that appropriate informed consent was obtained from human subjects. Copies of signed consent forms from identifiable persons appearing in any photographs submitted with the manuscript must be faxed to the *AJHG* office at the time of submission: (404) 712-9984. To avoid violation of HIPAA regulations, this consent form should state that the subject understands that his or her identity (but not his or her medical records) will be divulged to the *Journal* office by the transmission of the signed consent form. Alternatively, a letter from a member of your institutional review board (IRB) can be sent to us confirming that signed consent forms have been obtained from the individuals pictured in the manuscript without naming these individuals. Your manuscript cannot be processed until we receive these consent forms or a letter from your IRB.

Acknowledgments. Acknowledge those who have made substantive contributions to the study reported, as well as the institution(s) or grant sponsor(s) that supported the research.

Reference citations. Authors must assume responsibility for the accuracy of reference citations. Reference citations in the text, tables, or figure legends should be in parentheses and include author surname(s) and year of publication. When citing a work by two authors, provide both authors' names joined by "and." When citing a work by three or more authors, provide the first author's name followed by "et al." When the author name(s) and the year of publication are identical for two or more works, distinguish between the works by appending a lowercase italic letter to the year, to match the order in which the works appear in the References section. Examples: (Charlesworth 2001), (Peters and Sandkuijl 1992), (Devriendt et al. 1997), (Stack et al. 1995*a*). List two or more works in the same citation in chronological order, separated by semicolons. When two or more works in a citation were published in the same year, arrange them alphabetically by the first author's surname. When the same author name(s) are used for two or more works in the same citation, group those works together in chronological order, with the years separated by commas. If such a group occurs in a citation that includes other works, place the group chronologically within the citation according to the first year in the group, using semicolons between the group and the other works cited. Examples: (Erdmann 1994; Braverman et al. 1997; Purdue et al. 1997), (Hellsten 1995; Redding et al. 1996*a*, 1996*b*, 2000; Kessler et al. 1997).

References section. References should be arranged alphabetically by author surname(s). References by the same author(s) should be arranged chronologically. References by the same author(s) for which the year of publication is also the same should be arranged alphabetically by title. List the names of up to 25 authors; if more than 25, list the first 7 plus "et al." Use standard abbreviations for journal titles. Do not use excess punctuation.

References examples:

Journal: Devriendt K, Matthijs G, Legius E, Schollen E, Blockmans D, van Geet C, Degreef H, Cassiman J-J, Fryns J-P (1997) Skewed X-chromosome inactivation in female carriers of dyskeratosis congenita. Am J Hum Genet 60:581–587

Chapter: Peters DJM, Sandkuijl LA (1992) Genetic heterogeneity of polycystic kidney disease in Europe. In: Breuning MH, Devoto M, Romeo G (eds) Contributions to nephrology 97: polycystic kidney disease. Karger, Basel, pp 128–139

Entire volume: Dayhoff MV (ed) (1978) Atlas of protein sequence and structure. Vol 5, suppl 3. National Biomedical Research Foundation, Washington, DC

Meeting paper: Kessler S (1997) Transcripts of genetic counseling sessions: exercises in missed opportunities. Paper presented at Talking Human Genetics: Verbal Communication, Knowledge and Genetic Makeup. Hamburg, April 24–27

Thesis/dissertation: Hellsten E (1995) Positional cloning of the infantile ceroid lipofuscinosis gene. PhD thesis, National Public Health Institute, Helsinki

Computer software: SAS Institute (1997) SAS release 6.12, Cary, NC

Work "in press": Jones TM, Peterson RW. Ethical issues in screening for genetic diseases. Am J Hum Genet (in press)

Work submitted to a publication but not yet accepted, personal communications, and unpublished data: Do not list in References. Cite in the text as "personal communication" (if none of the individuals cited are authors of the manuscript being submitted) or "unpublished data" (if at least one of the individuals cited is also an author of the manuscript being submitted). List the names (including first initials) of all individuals responsible for the unpublished data or personal communication, and include letters of authorization from the individuals named.

Tables. Each table should appear on a separate page and should be single spaced. Whenever possible, construct exceptionally large tables and pedigree diagrams in sections. Number tables consecutively and give each a brief title. Give each column a short heading. Use footnotes to explain all abbreviations that are used in each table, and denote them by letter. Titles and footnotes should be included on the same page with the tables themselves. Use the table editor of a word-processing program to create tables. Do not use tabs or spaces, and omit vertical and horizontal lines from tables. Each row of data must be in a separate row of table cells. Do not submit tables as photographs. For more detailed instructions about tables, see "Special Instructions for Tables" at the *AJHG* homepage. For further guidelines, see *Scientific Style and Format: The CBE Manual for Authors, Editors, and Publishers* and *The Chicago Manual of Style* (cited in Style Guidelines, below).

Illustrations (figures). For complete instructions on preparing figures, please refer to http://www.ajhg.org/artguide.html. Design and prepare the figures carefully; they are the visual presentation of the scientific findings and will be carefully evaluated by the reviewers and editors. Figures should be saved as Encapsulated Postscript (EPS) files or Tagged Image File Format (TIF) files. Common Web formats, such as GIF or JPEG, are not acceptable; neither are proprietary application

formats, such as PowerPoint. Most figures will be set as single column (80 mm), some as double column (175 mm), and some broadside on a page (230 mm). Prepare the figures in publication size or larger (the lettering must be large enough so that the smallest letter will be at least 2.0 mm in height when the figure is reduced to publication size).

Use patterns, such as diagonal lines, rather than shading, which does not reproduce evenly. For pedigree construction, follow the guidelines described in Bennett et al.'s "Recommendations for Standardized Human Pedigree Nomenclature" (Am J Hum Genet 56:745–752, 1995). Include the key (explanation of symbols) within the figure. For micrographs, indicate magnification either by means of a micron bar or in the legend.

Use Helvetica lettering throughout the figure. Insert uppercase letters, in a larger font size, to designate panels.

For initial submission, we require that all figures and tables be included in the main text file. The figures may be converted to the file format of the main text file, since they are being used only for evaluation purposes. External reviewers are only permitted access to the main text file, so they will see only figures and tables included in that file. Thus, it is preferable that you include supplementary materials in the main text file as well. However, if including the supplementary materials makes the main text file too large to upload on our server, they may be uploaded separately.

In submission of revised manuscripts, the figure files should be uploaded as separate files in the appropriate format (EPS or TIFF) but should also be included in the main text file, as they were in the original submission, in case your paper is sent for further external review. Hard copies of figures are required for publication, but, if you wish, you may wait to send them until acceptance of the manuscript.

Color illustrations. Authors must sign an agreement to pay the costs of production of color figures when a manuscript with color figures is accepted. Each page containing a color figure will incur a charge of $450 for the first figure or separate part of a figure, plus $200 for each additional figure.

Figure legends. These should be double spaced, beginning on a separate page. The legend should begin with a brief phrase describing the figure content. The legend should describe the illustration so that it can be understood apart from the text and should explain any labels or symbols that are not included in a key.

Supplemental material. Authors may submit additional data, at the discretion of the editor, as a supplement to the *AJHG* electronic edition.

Supplemental clinical data. For manuscripts containing clinical information, it is important that as much clinical detail as possible be provided for others to verify the conclusions drawn. Photographs, radiographs, and imaging data as well as other laboratory, historical, and clinical data outside the immediate scope of the manuscript may be included as a supplement to the *AJHG* electronic edition.

Style Guidelines

For questions of grammar, punctuation, abbreviation, and scientific style, refer to *The Chicago Manual of Style* (15th ed., University of Chicago Press, Chicago) and *Scientific Style and Format: The CBE Manual for Authors, Editors, and Publishers* (6th ed., Cambridge University Press, Cambridge, UK). The preferred or first spelling of a word in *Merriam-Webster's Collegiate Dictionary* (11th ed., Merriam-Webster, Springfield, MA) is used by the *Journal.* Mathematical equations must be typed and spaced as they should appear in print. Use metric or other internationally accepted units for all quantitative measurements.

Genetic nomenclature and notation. For human genes, use genetic notation and symbols approved by the Human Gene Mapping Workshop. Approved gene symbols may be obtained, prior to submission, from Dr. Sue Povey of the HUGO Gene Nomenclature Committee (HGNC), Department of Biology, University College London, Wolfson House, 4 Stephenson Way, London NW1 2HE, United Kingdom (telephone: 44-20-7679-7410; fax: 44-20-7387-3496; e-mail: nome@galton.ucl.ac.uk). Nomenclature guidelines are available and the Gene Name Proposal form may be completed on the HGNC Web page: http://www.gene.ucl.ac.uk/nomenclature/. See Wain et al.'s "Guidelines for Human Gene Nomenclature" (Genomics 79:464470, 2002). Use ISCN nomenclature for cytogenetic notation (see Mitelman F [ed] ISCN 1995: an international system for human cytogenetic nomenclature. S. Karger, Basel). Human gene names and loci should be written in italicized capital letters and Arabic numerals. Protein product names are not italicized. For human-mutation nomenclature, see Antonarakis et al.'s "Recommendations for a Nomenclature System for Human Gene Mutations" (Hum Mutat 11:1-3, 1998) (http://www3.interscience.wiley.com/cgi-bin/fulltext/5001291/PDFSTART).

Approved mouse nomenclature may be obtained, prior to submission, from Lois Maltais, The Jackson Laboratory, Bar Harbor, ME 04609-0800; telephone: (207) 288-6429; fax: (207) 288-6132; e-mail: nomen@informatics.jax.org; Web page: http://www.informatics.jax.org/mgihome/nomen. For other organisms, consult the appropriate authorities.

Nucleotide sequence deposition. New nucleotide data must be submitted to and deposited in the DNA Data Bank of Japan (DDBJ)/European Molecular Biology Laboratory (EMBL)/GenBank databases, and accession number(s) must be obtained before the paper can be accepted for publication. Submission to any one of the three collaborating databases is sufficient to ensure data entry in all. The accession number(s) should be included in the manuscript's Electronic-Database Information section, and the following footnote should appear on the title page: "Nucleotide sequence data reported herein are available in the DDBJ/EMBL/GenBank databases; for details, see the Electronic-Database Information section of this article." The database will withhold release of data until publication, at authors' request. The most convenient method for submission of sequence data is by World Wide Web: DDBJ, via SAKURA (http://sakura.ddbj.nig.ac.jp/); EMBL, via WEBIN (http://www.ebi.ac.uk/embl/Submission/webin.html); or GenBank, via BankIt (http://www.ncbi.nlm.nih.gov/Sequin/).

Single-nucleotide polymorphisms. Newly described single-nucleotide polymorphisms (SNPs) should be submitted to an appropriate database such as dbSNP (http://www.ncbi.nlm

.nih.gov/SNP/) prior to submission of revised manuscripts. The identification numbers should be included in the "Electronic-Database Information" section of the manuscript.

Microarray data. All newly generated microarray data referred to in the text must be submitted for publication as a supplement to the *AJHG* electronic edition. Tables of quantitated raw data and processed data are acceptable, as outlined in guidelines proposed by the Microarray Gene Expression Data Society (for full details, see http://www.mged.org/Workgroups/MIAME/miame_checklist.html). For submission, please save the tables as tab-delimited ASCII text files and submit an electronic copy (no hard copies are necessary).

Computer programs. Authors of manuscripts that describe a novel computer program must make the relevant program publicly available by the time the manuscript is published.

Manuscript-Preparation Checklist

○ Cover letter
○ Copies of signed consent forms for all identifiable photographs of patients
○ Manuscript and figures
○ All pages of text and References *fully double spaced*
○ 1-inch margin on all four sides of each page
○ Title and running title
○ Order of manuscript elements: title page, Summary, text (Introduction, Material and Methods, Results, Discussion), Acknowledgments, appendixes, Electronic-Database Information, References, tables, figure legends
○ Summary: no more than 275 words
○ Acknowledgments: all sources of support and those who have made substantive contributions to the work reported
○ References: accurate, complete, and proper style in text and reference list; up to 25 authors' names included (if more than 25, list the first 7 plus "et al.")
○ Tables: *single spaced, no vertical lines, created with the table editor of a word-processing program, not with tabs;* title and footnotes included with table
○ Figures: all guidelines followed; figure legends on a separate page, double spaced
○ A copy of related manuscripts submitted or in press

Additional Components Required at Revision

○ Permission to reproduce previously published material
○ Letters of authorization from sources of personal communications and unpublished data

Submission via the Web Peer Review System

Formatting Electronic Files

Please follow the manuscript preparation requirements above to submit a new or revised manuscript via this system. The system relies on automated processing to create an Adobe Acrobat (PDF) file from your submission. If you do not follow these instructions, your submission cannot be processed automatically and will not be received by the journal office.

The following file formats are acceptable:

- Microsoft Word (.doc; any version that can be read by Word 2000 for Windows)
- Rich Text Format (.rtf)
- Adobe Acrobat (.pdf)
- LaTeX (see special instructions below)

File contents. For initial submission, manuscripts should be submitted as single files, in one of the formats listed above, with all figures, tables, and images embedded (inserted) directly into the document. We also request that supplementary materials be included in the same file, if possible. The figures may be converted to the file format of the main text file, since they are being used only for evaluation purposes. Only materials included in the main text file (and separate supplementary files, if necessary) will be examined by external reviewers.

If we request a revision, in addition to the main text file containing all figures and tables, each figure should be uploaded separately in EPS or TIFF format. Consult your word processing program's "Help" documentation for instructions on how to embed tables and figures. You must also submit in a second file, in one of the acceptable formats, a cover letter that includes your responses to reviewer comments.

Filename requirements. All filenames must be lowercase. (All file processing by the Web Peer Review system is done on Unix machines, where filenames are case-sensitive.)

File compression and archives. Although your manuscript itself must be provided in one file that includes the tables and figures, you will have at least two files to upload into our system (i.e. the cover letter, manuscript file, and any related manuscripts). Therefore, we strongly recommend that you combine these files into an archive so that you can upload a single file for submission. Applications for Mac OS (such as StuffIt) and Windows (such as WinZip) can create this archive.

The following archive formats may be used:

- Windows or Unix zip (e.g., "archiv.zip")
- Unix tar (e.g., "archive.tar" or compressed with gzip as "archive.tar.gz" or "archive.tgz")

If you cannot create archives in these formats, you may still compress individual files to shorten upload time:

- Unix compress (e.g., "ms.tex.Z")

Electronic File Specifications

Program	Main Text File	Cover Letter	Figures	Tables
Word	ms.doc	cover_letter.doc or cover_letter.txt	[embedded in main file]	[embedded in main file]
RTF	ms.rtf	cover_letter.rtf or cover_letter.txt	[embedded in main file]	[embedded in main file]
Acrobat	ms.pdf	cover_letter.pdf or cover_letter.txt	[embedded in main file]	[embedded in main file]
LaTeX	ms.tex	cover_letter.txt	f1.eps, f2.eps, etc.	tb1.tex, tb2.tex, etc.

- Unix gzip (e.g., "ms.tex.gz")

Revisions. If you are submitting a revised manuscript and have a response to the reviewers' comments, include your response as part of the cover letter file. When submitting a revised manuscript with figures, include all the figures even if they have not changed since the previous version.

Online Submission Instructions

Preparing the manuscript file. The preferred format for submitting manuscripts online is Microsoft Word (.doc files). If you are unable to submit a Microsoft Word file, the Web Peer Review system will also accept manuscripts in Acrobat (.pdf), Rich Text Format (.rtf) or LaTeX (.tex). We have provided a drop box in the "File format" area in which to indicate the document type.

As mentioned above, manuscripts should be submitted as single files with all figures, tables, and images embedded (inserted) directly into the document. Embedded figures must be in EPS or TIF format, as these formats result in the best overall outcome when manuscripts are converted to PDF. Please note that authors whose manuscripts are accepted for publication may be required by the publisher to submit high-resolution hard copies (e.g., glossy prints) after the review process is complete and press production is about to begin.

Special instructions for LaTeX. LaTeX files prepared with the AASTeX macro package are preferred. This package uses the "natbib" style for references. If you submit a LaTeX file, figures and tables may be kept in external files, as long as they are referenced within the main "ms.tex" file.

Submission Checklist

Please have the following items readily available before beginning the online submission process:

- Your manuscript as a MS Word, Acrobat (pdf), Rich Text, or LaTeX file including all tables, figures and images embedded in the document
- Cover letter
- Information from your title page for entry into the peer review database, including the title, running title, list of contributing authors and affiliations, word count, and contact information for the corresponding author
- A list of recommended reviewers and their e-mail addresses
- Related papers, by any of the authors, that have been submitted elsewhere or that are in press.
- Copies of signed consent forms for all identifiable photographs of patients (these should be faxed to the AJHG office at [404] 712-9984 at the time of submission).

Navigating the Peer Review Web Site

Step one: describing your manuscript. Go to the *AJHG* Peer Review Web site at http://mss.uchicago.edu/AJHG/. A username and password are required to enter the site. If you already have a username and password, click on "Login/See current tasks" to view the status of your account. If you are new to the site, click on "Create account" to register. After completing your login, click on the "Begin submission" button.

Once you have logged in, fill in the fields describing your manuscript. To move from one field to the next, press the "tab" key. When all the information is complete and you are sure it is correct, click "Ready to upload files" to proceed to step two.

Step two: uploading your file(s). Click the "Browse" button to locate a file on your local system. Once a file is specified in the field, click "Upload this file" to send the file to the Web Peer Review system. You must name your manuscript file "ms," using lowercase type. (All file processing by the Web Peer Review system is done on Unix machines, where filenames are case-sensitive.) The system will assign an ID number to your manuscript during the upload.

As previously mentioned, your manuscript file must contain all figures and tables as well as the text. Remember that if you have multiple files (such as if you are providing a manuscript "in press" for the reviewers), you can compress all of them into a single archive and upload just one file. We recommend that you make an archive of all the files for your submission and then upload the single archive file.

Check your results. Only files listed in the box labeled "Files uploaded so far" have been uploaded successfully. If you need to delete a file, click the file name in the box to select it, and then click the "Delete selected file" button.

When you have uploaded all the files for your submission, click "Process uploaded files" to proceed. The system will attempt to make a PDF version of your file. The conversion to PDF reduces the size of the file and makes it easier for editors and reviewers to read. PDF files can be viewed with Adobe Acrobat Reader version 3 or higher (available free at http://www.adobe.com) or with Ghostscript 5.1 or higher compiled with PDF support turned on (available free at http://www.cs.wisc.edu/~ghost). If successful, there will be a link to the PDF on the next Web page that appears.

If you want to delete all the uploaded files and make no submission, click "Cancel submission" instead.

Step three: submitting your information. After your file has been converted to a PDF file, view the file that was generated from your submission by clicking on "ms.pdf" (a link that will be provided on the next Web page that appears). Only the manuscript file, not the cover letter or related manuscript files, will be viewable at this time. After you finish viewing the manuscript PDF file, indicate how you would like to proceed.

If you select "Approve and submit now," you assert that you have viewed the PDF file via the link provided and that the file accurately shows your manuscript as reviewers should see it. If you select "Fix and resubmit later," the files you have already uploaded will be saved (for 30 days) so that you can return later and upload new or corrected files to make a new PDF file. If you wish to return later to upload other files, please make note of the file upload ID number.

Click "Finish" to complete the final process. Click "Cancel" if you wish to abort the submission.

If your manuscript has been successfully submitted to the *AJHG* Web Peer Review system, a confirmation screen, which includes your assigned manuscript number, will appear. Please carefully note this number and use it in all future correspondence with the *AJHG* editorial office. An e-mail message confirming your submission will be sent to you.

If you do not receive either a manuscript number or confirmation e-mail message, your manuscript was not success-

fully submitted to the journal and thus cannot be sent on to peer review. Please try again or contact ajhg-help@mss.uchicago.edu for assistance.

Announcements

Announcements are posted to the electronic edition of the *Journal* as soon as they are accepted, and they are published in the earliest possible print issue. They may also be viewed at http://www.journals.uchicago.edu/AJHG/journal/announce.html. Announcements are published free of charge for members of The American Society of Human Genetics. They should be submitted via e-mail (ajhg@emory.edu). For publication in print, announcements must be received at least 7 weeks before the month of issue in which publication is desired.

2005 MEMBERSHIP APPLICATION • THE AMERICAN SOCIETY OF HUMAN GENETICS

9650 Rockville Pike • Bethesda, Maryland 20814-3998 • (301) 634-7300 • Fax: (301) 634-7079 • Toll free: (1-866) HUMGENE
E-mail: babbott@ashg.org • http://www.ashg.org/

Please keep information page for description of membership categories and discount subscriptions. Mail completed application, including profile form, and remittance to the above address. ***Type or print****. Use the URL above to apply online!*

Name ______________________________ Degree(s) ______________
Last First Middle

Department ______________________________

Institution ______________________________

Street address ______________________________

City, state, zip, country ______________________________

Telephone ( ) ______________ Fax ( ) ______________ E-mail Address ______________
Area code Area code

Signature and membership start date: I, the undersigned, wish my membership in The American Society of Human Genetics to begin (check one): _________January 1, 2005 or_________January 1, 2006. Applications for 2006 will be accepted after September 1, 2005.

I will receive all applicable subscriptions beginning in January of the calendar year indicated above.

______________________________ ______________
Applicant's signature *Date*

We will acknowledge receipt of application and send it through the process established by the Board of Directors. Notification of the Board's action is usually sent in April or November. In the interim, you will be accorded all rights and privileges of a member in good standing, except that prior to Board approval you may not vote in ASHG elections.

DUES PAYMENT (Dues include 12 monthly issues of *The American Journal of Human Genetics* and are payable on a calendar year basis.)

1. Check one box and enter dues payment on line 1 .... $ __________ 1
   ☐ $130 Regular ☐ $65 Trainee with Journal ☐ $70 Overseas Trainee
   ☐ $135 Overseas Affiliate ☐ $25 Trainee without Journal ☐ $190 Husband/Wife

2. Optional air mail postage for *AJHG* outside the United States .... $ __________ 2
   ☐ $40 Canada, Mexico, Central America ☐ $70 all other areas

☐ Check here if you do not want to receive commercial mailings
☐ Check here if you do not wish to receive the printed Journal.

DISCOUNT SUBSCRIPTIONS

3. $650 North America, $850 elsewhere (print only) for ***American Journal of Medical Genetics*** .... $ __________ 3
   $530 North America, $690 elsewhere (print only) for ***AJMG without Neuropsychiatric Genetics***
4. $120 (print & online); $110 (online only) for ***BioEssays*** .... $ __________ 4
5. $115 North America, $195 elsewhere (print & online); $104 (online only) for ***Birth Defects Research: Clinical and Molecular Teratology*** .... $ __________ 5
6. $115 North America, $165 elsewhere (print & online); $104 (online only) for ***Birth Defects Research: Developmental and Reproductive Toxicology*** .... $ __________ 6
7. $799 for ***Cancer Genetics and Cytogenetics*** .... $ __________ 7
8. $159 Europe, $163 elsewhere for ***Clinical Dysmorphology*** .... $ __________ 8
9. $258 US/elsewhere not otherwise specified (online only), $271 (print & online); $276 Canada (online only), $290 (print & online); $271 Europe (online only), $285 (print & online) for ***Clinical Genetics*** .... $ __________ 9
10. $114 Europe, $117 elsewhere (print & online); $83 (online only) for ***Community Genetics*** .... $ __________ 10
11. $125 US, $134 Canada, $186 elsewhere for ***Current Biology*** .... $ __________ 11
12. $231 for ***Current Opinion in Cell Biology*** .... $ __________ 12
13. $231 for ***Current Opinion in Genetics & Development*** .... $ __________ 13
14. $623 Europe, $626 elsewhere (print & online); $557 (online only) for ***Cytogenetic and Genome Research*** .... $ __________ 14
15. $165 for ***European Journal of Human Genetics*** (includes membership in ESHG) .... $ __________ 15
    $500 (print only); $550 (print & online) for ***European Journal of Human Genetics***
16. $330 North America, $390 elsewhere (print & online); $300 North America (online only) for ***Genes, Chromosomes, and Cancer*** .... $ __________ 16
17. $105 US, $189 Canada, Mexico; $225 elsewhere for ***Genes & Development*** .... $ __________ 17
18. $160 North America, $200 elsewhere (print & online); $145 (online only) for ***Genetic Epidemiology*** .... $ __________ 18
19. $316 for ***Genetics in Medicine*** .... $ __________ 19
20. $179 US, $258 elsewhere (print only); $213 US, $292 elsewhere (print & online); $179 (online only) for ***Genetic Testing*** .... $ __________ 20
21. $98 US, $154 Canada, Mexico; $178 elsewhere for ***Genome Research*** .... $ __________ 21
22. $124 for ***Genomics*** .... $ __________ 22
23. $336 US, $395 elsewhere (print only); $402 US, $462 elsewhere (print & online); $336 (online only) for ***Human Gene Therapy*** .... $ __________ 23
24. $495 for ***Human Genetics*** .... $ __________ 24
25. $394 Europe, $397 elsewhere (print & online), $356 (online only) for ***Human Heredity*** .... $ __________ 25
26. $369 US/elsewhere (print & online); $307 (online only); $394 Canada (print & online); $328 (online only) for ***Human Molecular Genetics*** (not available Europe) .... $ __________ 26
27. $280 North America, $340 elsewhere (print & online); $255 North America (online only) for ***Human Mutation*** .... $ __________ 27
28. $459 (print only) for ***Journal of Human Genetics*** .... $ __________ 28
29. $289 (print & online), $130 (online only) for ***Journal of Medical Genetics*** .... $ __________ 29
30. $113 for ***Molecular Genetics and Metabolism*** .... $ __________ 30
31. $169 US, Canada, Mexico; $215 elsewhere for ***Nature Genetics*** (not available: Japan, Korea, & China) .... $ __________ 31
32. $169 US, Canada, Mexico; $215 elsewhere for ***Nature Medicine*** (not available: Japan, Korea, & China) .... $ __________ 32
33. $169 US, Canada, Mexico; $215 elsewhere for ***Nature Reviews Genetics*** (not available: Japan, Korea, & China) .... $ __________ 33
34. $247 Europe, $254 elsewhere for ***Pharmacogenetics and Genomics*** .... $ __________ 34
35. $157 for ***Trends in Genetics*** .... $ __________ 35
36. Identify ***Annual Reviews*** by title, volume, year and price: Member price $72 per year US, $77 per year elsewhere

______________ ________ ________ $ __________
Title Vol. Year Price

California and Indiana residents add state sales tax for ***Annual Reviews***: $ __________
Canadian residents add 7% GST for ***Annual Reviews***: $ __________

Enter total payment for ***Annual Reviews*** .... $ __________ 36

37. Optional contribution to ASHG general fund: $25 ____ $50 ____ $75 ____ $100 ____ other ____ .... $ __________ 37
38. **TOTAL REMITTANCE ENCLOSED** .... $ __________ 38

PLEASE RETURN THIS NOTICE WITH YOUR REMITTANCE (U.S. currency only). See reverse for credit card information.

METHOD OF PAYMENT - 2005 ASHG MEMBER DUES

Payment may be made via money order; a check drawn on a U.S. bank, in U.S. currency only, and made payable to The American Society of Human Genetics; MasterCard, Visa, American Express (AMEX) or Discover credit card. Checks drawn on foreign banks cannot be accepted. Persons in countries with currency restrictions may apply to the Administrative Office for assistance.

For credit card remittance, please supply the following information:

Signature ______________________________

Cardholder name ______________________________
(please print)

Circle type of card: MasterCard VISA AMEX Discover
(no other cards accepted).

Credit card number ______________________________ [ ]

VISA only: Supply final 3 digits on reverse of card

Expiration date ______________________________

Please note: ASHG is qualified as a 501(C) (3) organization. Dues and contributions are deductible as allowed by law. Dues payment includes $60 for a calendar year subscription to *The American Journal of Human Genetics.*

Member Profile Form

Name: ______________________________

Please type or print.

PRIMARY AFFILIATION *Check one:*

MEDICAL SCHOOL DEPTS.

A. ___ Genetics
B. ___ Pediatrics
C. ___ Pathology
D. ___ Psychiatry/Psychology
E. ___ Medicine
F. ___ Ob/Gyn
G. ___ Repro. Med.
H. ___ Neurology
I. ___ Family Medicine
J. ___ Internal Medicine

OTHER

K. ___ Hospitals and Clinics
L. ___ HMO
M. ___ Dental Schools
N. ___ Pub Hlth & Grad School
O. ___ College or University
P. ___ Nursing School
Q. ___ Veterinary School
R. ___ Priv Practice/Consultant
S. ___ Commercial Company
T. ___ Institutes/Foundations
U. ___ Federal Government
V. ___ State/Local Government
W. ___ Retired
X. ___ Other
Y. ___ Consultant

See box at right for codes:

Earned Degrees ☐☐☐☐ **Academic Rank** ☐ **Position** ☐☐

MAJOR TYPE OF WORK *Check one that accounts for more than 50% of your time:*

A.___ Research B.___ Teaching C.___ Administration D.___ Clinical E.___ Counseling

SECONDARY TYPE OF WORK *Check one if it represents a significant portion of time and is different from your major type of work*:

A.___ Research B.___ Teaching C.___ Administration D.___ Clinical E.___ Counseling

LABORATORY SETTING *If you are primarily in a laboratory setting, indicate focus:*

A.___ private diagnostic/reference lab
B.___ univ affiliated diagnostic/reference lab
C.___ gov't affiliated research lab
D.___ private research lab
E.___ univ affiliated research lab

SPECIAL INTEREST AREAS *Do not check more than two:*

A. ___ cancer genetics
B. ___ cytogenetics
C. ___ DNA forensics
D. ___ differentiation & development
E. ___ dysmorphology
F. ___ ethics/social/legal/policy issues
G. ___ gene structure & function
H. ___ inborn errors/biochemical genetics
I. ___ late onset/adult genetic disorders
J. ___ linkage mapping & polymorphisms
K. ___ molecular genetics
L. ___ pediatric genetics
M. ___ physical mapping
N. ___ population genetics/epidemiology
O. ___ prenatal/perinatal genetics
P. ___ genomics
Q. ___ model systems
R. ___ informatics
S. ___ neurogenetics/behavorial genetics
T. ___ public health genetics

CURRENT GRANT SUPPORT *Check all that apply (US and Canadian members only):*

A. ___ NSF (NSERC in Canada)
B. ___ NIH (CIHR) training grant
C. ___ private industry
D. ___ NIH (CIHR in Canada)
E. ___ postdoc fellowship
F. ___ private foundation or charity
G. ___ state
H. ___ province
I. ___ institutional
J. ___ other national agencies
K. ___ HHMI

DESIGNATIONS(S) FOR YOUR RESEARCH
You may check more than one:

A. ___ Applied clinical research
B. ___ Applied lab research
C. ___ Applied mathematical research
D. ___ Basic clinical research
E. ___ Basic lab research
F. ___ Basic mathematical research
G. ___ Other

Degree Code

A. MD
B. PhD
C. MSW
D. DVM
E. SCD
F. DDS/DMD
G. EDD
H. MS
I. MA
J. MSN
K. JD
L. MPH
M. RN
N. BSN
O. BS/BA
P. Other

Academic Rank Code

A. Professor
B. Associate Professor
C. Assistant Professor
D. Instructor
E. Nonfaculty

Position Code

A. Dean
B. Department Chair
C. Division Chief
D. Institute Center Director
E. Laboratory Director
F. Training Program Director
G. Research Program Director
H. Program Coordinator/Administrator
I. Senior Research Associate
J. Research Associate
K. Research Assistant
L. Genetic Counselor
M. Postdoctoral Research Fellow
N. Postdoctoral Clinical Fellow
O. Resident
P. Graduate Student
Q. Private Practice
R. Corporate Executive
S. Consultant
T. Other
U. Principal Investigator/Professor

OPTIONAL:
Year of Birth: _____
Gender: F ☐ M ☐

Check Box(es):
A. ☐ American Indian, Eskimo and Aleut
B. ☐ Asian, Pacific Islander
C. ☐ Black
D. ☐ White
E. ☐ Other
F. ☐ Mixed
Hispanic (Yes ☐ No ☐)

2005 ASHG MEMBERSHIP AND SUBSCRIPTIONS INFORMATION
Please keep this page for your reference.

Line 1. MEMBERSHIP CATEGORIES

Regular Membership is open to any resident of the Americas (U.S., Canada, Mexico, Caribbean, Central and South America) who is interested in research in human genetics or in issues pertaining to human genetics.

Overseas Affiliate Status is open to individuals residing outside the Americas (U.S., Canada, Mexico, Caribbean, Central and South America).

Husband/Wife Membership is open to couples who are both Regular members, but who receive only one Journal subscription. Please fill out one membership application for each person.

Trainee Membership is open to postdoctoral fellows and bona fide students enrolled in degree-granting programs at institutions in the Americas (U.S., Canada, Mexico, Caribbean, Central and South America).

Overseas Trainee Membership is open to postdoctoral fellows and bona fide students enrolled in degree-granting programs at institutions outside the Americas.

Please note: ASHG is qualified as a 501(C) (3) organization. Dues and contributions are deductible as allowed by law. Dues payment includes $60 for a calendar year subscription to *The American Journal of Human Genetics.*

Line 2. OPTIONAL AIR MAIL POSTAGE OUTSIDE THE U.S.

For those who would like to receive *The American Journal of Human Genetics* via airmail, note additional postage on line 2.

DISCOUNT SUBSCRIPTIONS

To obtain these discounts, orders must be placed through the ASHG Administrative Office. It is understood that these orders are intended for personal use only. Standing orders are not available through ASHG. Typically, the publisher will begin mailing issues one or two months after your order is received in the Administrative Office. *Annual Reviews* will be mailed at the book rate in the month of issue.

Line 3. ***American Journal of Medical Genetics,*** 40 issues, list price $685, **member price $650 North America,** list price $855, **$850 elsewhere** (print only) ***AJMG without Neuropsychiatric Genetics,*** 32 issues, list price $565, **member price $530 North America,** list price $707, **$690 elsewhere** (print only)
Line 4. ***BioEssays, Volume 27,*** 12 issues, list price $170, **member price $120** (print & online); **$110** (online only)
Line 5. ***Birth Defects Research: Clinical & Molecular Teratology,*** 16 issues, **member price $115 North America, $195 elsewhere** (print & online); **$104** (online only)
Line 6. ***Birth Defects Research: Developmental & Reproductive Toxicology,*** 10 issues, **member price $115 North America, $165 elsewhere** (print & online); **$104** (online only)
Line 7. ***Cancer Genetics and Cytogenetics,*** 16 issues, list price $3,169 US, **member price $799**
Line 8. ***Clinical Dysmorphology,*** 4 issues, **member price $159 Europe, $163 elsewhere**
Line 9. ***Clinical Genetics***, 12 issues, list price $371 US/elsewhere not otherwise specified, **member price $258** (online only), **$271** (print & online); **$276 Canada** (online only), **$290** (print & online); **$271 Europe** (online only), **$285** (print & online)
Line 10. ***Community Genetics***, 4 issues, list price $147 US, **member price $114 Europe, $117 elsewhere** (print & online), **$83** (online only)
Line 11. ***Current Biology,*** 24 issues, list price $165, **member price $125 US, $134 Canada,** list price $249, **$186 elsewhere**
Line 12. ***Current Opinion in Cell Biology,*** 6 issues, list price $271, **member price $231**
Line 13. ***Current Opinion in Genetics & Development,*** 6 issues, list price $271, **member price $231**
Line 14. ***Cytogenetic and Genome Research,*** 16 issues, list price $1,841, **member price $623 Europe, $626 elsewhere** (print & online)**; $557** (online only)
Line 15. ***European Journal of Human Genetics,*** 12 issues, $165 (includes membership in ESHG); **member price $500** (print only); **$550** (print & online)
Line 16. ***Genes, Chromosomes, and Cancer,*** 12 issues, list price $365, **member price $330 North America, $390 elsewhere** (print & online); **$300 North America** (online only)
Line 17. ***Genes & Development,*** 24 issues, list price $140, **member price $105 US;** list price $260, **$189 Canada, Mexico; $225 elsewhere**
Line 18. ***Genetic Epidemiology,*** 8 issues, **member price $160 North America, $200 elsewhere** (print & online); **$145** (online only)
Line 19. ***Genetics in Medicine,*** 9 issues, list price $366, **member price $316**
Line 20. ***Genetic Testing,*** 4 issues, **member price $179 US, $258 elsewhere** (print only); **$213 US, $292 elsewhere** (print & online); **$179** (online only)
Line 21. ***Genome Research***, 12 issues, list price $123, **member price $98 US;** list price $179, **$154 Canada, Mexico,** list price $203, **$178 elsewhere**
Line 22. ***Genomics,*** 12 issues, list price $458, **member price $124**
Line 23. ***Human Gene Therapy***, 18 issues, **member price $336 US, $395 elsewhere** (print only); **$402 US, $462 elsewhere** (print & online); **$336** (online only)
Line 24. ***Human Genetics,*** 12 issues, list price $3,799 Europe, **member price $495**
Line 25. ***Human Heredity,*** 8 issues, list price $746 US, **member price $394 Europe, $397 elsewhere** (print & online); **$356** (online only)
Line 26. ***Human Molecular Genetics,*** 26 issues, list price $391, **member price $369 US/elsewhere** (print & online); **$307 US/elsewhere** (online only); **$394 Canada** (print & online); **$328 Canada** (online only) **(not available Europe)**
Line 27. ***Human Mutation,*** 12 issues, **member price $280 North America, $340 elsewhere** (print & online); **$255 North America** (online only)
Line 28. ***Journal of Human Genetics,*** list price $544, **member price $459** (print only)
Line 29. ***Journal of Medical Genetics,*** 12 issues, list price $478, **member price $289** (print & online); **$130** (online only)
Line 30. ***Molecular Genetics and Metabolism,*** 12 issues, list price $430, **member price $113**
Line 31. ***Nature Genetics,*** 12 issues, list price $199 US, **member price $169 US, Canada, Mexico; $215 elsewhere (not available: Japan, Korea & China)**
Line 32. ***Nature Medicine,*** 12 issues, list price $199 US, **member price $169 US, Canada, Mexico; $215 elsewhere (not available: Japan, Korea & China)**
Line 33. ***Nature Reviews Genetics,*** 12 issues, list price $199 US, **member price $169 US, Canada, Mexico; $215 elsewhere (not available: Japan, Korea & China)**
Line 34. ***Pharmacogenetics and Genomics,*** 12 issues, **member price $247 Europe, $254 elsewhere**
Line 35. ***Trends in Genetics,*** 12 issues, list price $182, **member price $157**
Line 36. ***Annual Reviews,*** **member price $72* per year US, $77* per year elsewhere**

Annual Review of:	*Genetics*	*Microbiol*	*Cell & Dev Biol*	*Ecol & Sys*	*Immunology*	*Medicine*	*Public Hlth*	*Biochem*	*Genomics & HG*
2003 Volumes	Vol. 37	Vol. 57	Vol. 19	Vol. 34	Vol. 21	Vol. 54	Vol. 24	Vol. 72	Vol. 4
2004 Volumes	Vol. 38	Vol. 58	Vol. 20	Vol. 35	Vol. 22	Vol. 55	Vol. 25	Vol. 73	Vol. 5
2005 Volumes	Available late 2005, will be offered on 2006 dues notice				Vol. 23	Vol. 56	Vol. 26	Vol. 74	Vol. 6
Month of Publication	Dec.	Oct.	Nov.	Dec.	April	February	May	July	Sept.

***California and Indiana residents add applicable sales tax. Canadian residents add 7% GST on total.**

Line 37: OPTIONAL CONTRIBUTIONS Optional contributions to the general fund are welcome. Contributions received will support projects designed to attract more young people to the field of human genetics and are tax deductible to the extent permitted by law.

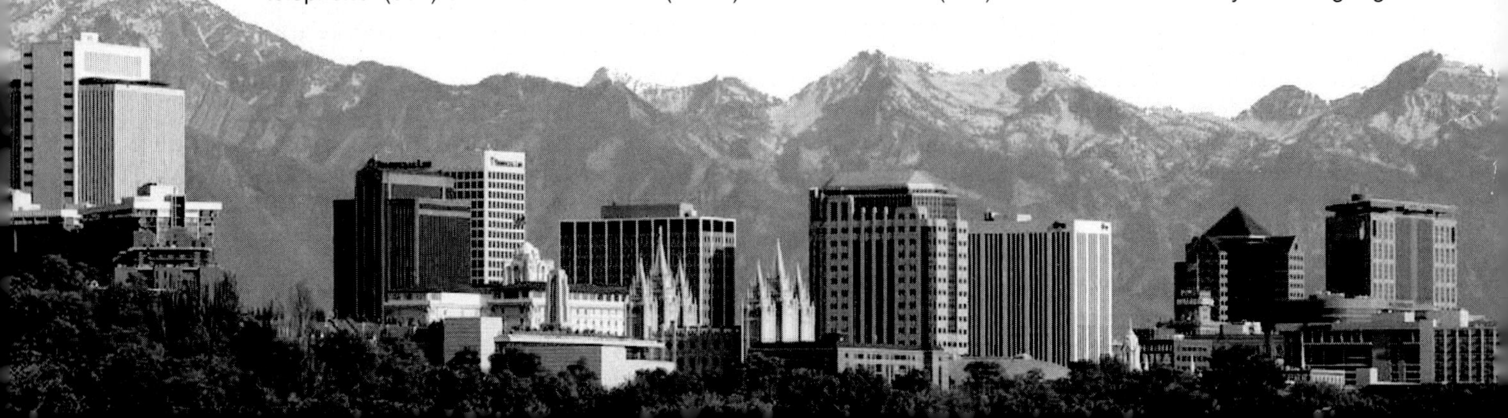

THE AMERICAN SOCIETY OF HUMAN GENETICS

was organized in 1948. Its purpose is to encourage and integrate research, scholarship and education in all areas of human genetics, to bring into close contact investigators in the many general fields of research that involve human genetics, and to encourage discourse on applications of human genetics to society at large.

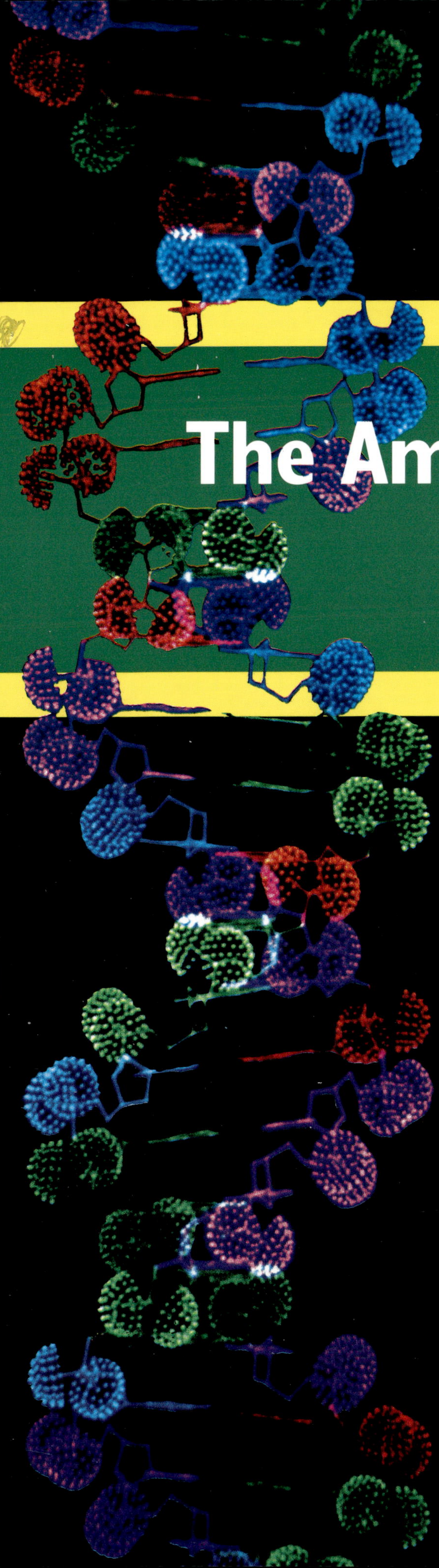

The American Journal of Human Genetics

VOLUME 77 NUMBER 1 JULY 2005

THE AMERICAN SOCIETY OF HUMAN GENETICS

Published for The American Society of Human Genetics by The University of Chicago Press

DIRECT INQUIRIES AND SUBMISSIONS TO

The American Journal of Human Genetics
Department of Human Genetics
Emory University School of Medicine
615 Michael Street, Room 301
Atlanta, GA 30322-3050

Telephone: (404) 712-9980
Fax: (404) 712-9984
E-mail: ajhg@emory.edu
Web page: http://www.ajhg.org

Subscription orders and correspondence should be addressed to the University of Chicago Press, P.O. Box 37005, Chicago, IL 60637. Checks should be made out to the University of Chicago Press. All orders must be in U.S. currency. Telephone: (8:00 A.M.–5:00 P.M. Central Standard Time, Monday–Friday) U.S. & Canada toll free, (877) 705-1878; Rest of World, (773) 753-3347. Fax: U.S. & Canada toll free, (877) 705-1879; Rest of World, (773) 753-0811. E-mail: subscriptions@press.uchicago.edu; Web site: http://www.journals.uchicago.edu. Remittance for nonmember subscription is payable to the publisher on a calendar-year basis. For domestic nonmember individuals and institutions, the single-copy rate is $88.00 and the calendar-year rate is $995.00; for foreign nonmember individuals and institutions, the single-copy rate is $88.00 (U.S. currency) and the calendar-year rate is $1050.00 (U.S. currency); the calendar-year rate for Canadian citizens, which includes GST, is $1088.65 (U.S. currency). All rates above include International Surface Airlift (ISAL) delivery to addresses outside the U.S. Subscription agent for Japan: Kinokuniya Company, Ltd. Individuals have the option to order directly from the University of Chicago Press.

Memberships.—A membership application and dues schedule appear at the back of each issue of the *Journal.*

The American Journal of Human Genetics (ISSN 0002-9297) is published monthly at 1427 East 60th Street, Chicago, IL 60637. Periodicals postage is paid at Chicago, IL, and at additional mailing offices by the American Society of Human Genetics. All rights reserved.

Postmaster: send address changes to *The American Journal of Human Genetics,* The University of Chicago Press, Journals Division, P.O. Box 37005, Chicago, IL 60637.

The American Journal of Human Genetics

Volume 77 Number 1 July 2005

i **This Month in the *Journal***
Kathryn Garber

Review Article

1 **Identifying Novel Genes for Atherosclerosis through Mouse-Human Comparative Genetics**
Xiaosong Wang, Naoki Ishimori, Ron Korstanje, Jarod Rollins, and Beverly Paigen

Articles

16 **Biotin-Responsive Basal Ganglia Disease Maps to 2q36.3 and Is Due to Mutations in *SLC19A3***
Wen-Qi Zeng, Eiman Al-Yamani, James S. Acierno, Jr., Susan Slaugenhaupt, Tammy Gillis, Marcy E. MacDonald, Pinar T. Ozand, and James F. Gusella

27 **An Entropy-Based Statistic for Genomewide Association Studies**
Jinying Zhao, Eric Boerwinkle, and Momiao Xiong

41 **Allan-Herndon-Dudley Syndrome and the Monocarboxylate Transporter 8 (*MCT8*) Gene**
Charles E. Schwartz, Melanie M. May, Nancy J. Carpenter, R. Curtis Rogers, Judith Martin, Martin G. Bialer, Jewell Ward, Javier Sanabria, Silvana Marsa, James A. Lewis, Roberto Echeverri, Herbert A. Lubs, Kytja Voeller, Richard J. Simensen, and Roger E. Stevenson

54 **Mutations in *PIP5K3* Are Associated with François-Neetens Mouchetée Fleck Corneal Dystrophy**
Shouling Li, Leila Tiab, Xiaodong Jiao, Francis L. Munier, Leonidas Zografos,Béatrice E. Frueh, Yuri Sergeev, Janine Smith, Benjamin Rubin, Mario A. Meallet, Richard K. Forster, J. Fielding Hejtmancik, and Daniel F. Schorderet

64 **Polymorphisms within the C-Reactive Protein (CRP) Promoter Region Are Associated with Plasma CRP Levels**
Christopher S. Carlson, Shelley Force Aldred, Philip K. Lee, Russell P. Tracy, Stephen M. Schwartz, Mark Rieder, Kiang Liu, O. Dale Williams, Carlos Iribarren, E. Cora Lewis, Myriam Fornage, Eric Boerwinkle, Myron Gross, Cashell Jaquish, Deborah A. Nickerson, Richard M. Myers, David S. Siscovick, and Alexander P. Reiner

78 **Segmental Duplications and Copy-Number Variation in the Human Genome**
Andrew J. Sharp, Devin P. Locke, Sean D. McGrath, Ze Cheng, Jeffrey A. Bailey, Rhea U. Vallente, Lisa M. Pertz, Royden A. Clark, Stuart Schwartz, Rick Segraves, Vanessa V. Oseroff, Donna G. Albertson, Daniel Pinkel, and Evan E. Eichler

89 **Identification of a Major Recombination Hotspot in Patients with Short Stature and *SHOX* Deficiency**
Katja U. Schneider, Nitin Sabherwal, Karin Jantz, Ralph Röth, Nadja Muncke, Werner F. Blum, Gordon B. Cutler, Jr., and Gudrun Rappold

97 **A Powerful and Robust Method for Mapping Quantitative Trait Loci in General Pedigrees**
G. Diao and D. Y. Lin

Reports

112 **Germline Susceptibility to Colorectal Cancer Due to Base-Excision Repair Gene Defects**
Susan M. Farrington, Albert Tenesa, Rebecca Barnetson, Alice Wiltshire, James Prendergast, Mary Porteous, Harry Campbell, and Malcolm G. Dunlop

120 Homozygous Nonsense Mutations in *KIAA1279* Are Associated with Malformations of the Central and Enteric Nervous Systems
Alice S. Brooks, Aida M. Bertoli-Avella, Grzegorz M. Burzynski, Guido J. Breedveld, Jan Osinga, Ludolf G. Boven, Jane A. Hurst, Grazia M. S. Mancini, Maarten H. Lequin, Rene F. de Coo, Ivana Matera, Esther de Graaff, Carel Meijers, Patrick J. Willems, Dick Tibboel, Ben A. Oostra, and Robert M. W. Hofstra

127 Disentangling Fetal and Maternal Susceptibility for Pre-Eclampsia: A British Multicenter Candidate-Gene Study
The GOPEC Consortium

132 Mapping of a Single Locus Capable of Complementing the Defective Heterochromatin Phenotype of Roberts Syndrome Cells
Lisa D. McDaniel, Darrell J. Tomkins, Eric J. Stanbridge, Martin J. Somerville, Errol C. Friedberg, and Roger A. Schultz

140 Genetic Variation in the Human Androgen Receptor Gene Is the Major Determinant of Common Early-Onset Androgenetic Alopecia
Axel M. Hillmer, Sandra Hanneken, Sibylle Ritzmann, Tim Becker, Jan Freudenberg, Felix F. Brockschmidt, Antonia Flaquer, Yun Freudenberg-Hua, Rami Abou Jamra, Christine Metzen, Uwe Heyn, Nadine Schweiger, Regina C. Betz, Bettina Blaumeiser, Jochen Hampe, Stefan Schreiber, Thomas G. Schulze, Hans Christian Hennies, Johannes Schumacher, Peter Propping, Thomas Ruzicka, Sven Cichon, Thomas F. Wienker, Roland Kruse, and Markus M. Nöthen

149 Strong Association of the Y402H Variant in Complement Factor H at 1q32 with Susceptibility to Age-Related Macular Degeneration
Sepideh Zareparsi, Kari E. H. Branham, Mingyao Li, Sapna Shah, Robert J. Klein, Jurg Ott, Josephine Hoh, Gonçalo R. Abecasis, and Anand Swaroop

154 3q29 Microdeletion Syndrome: Clinical and Molecular Characterization of a New Syndrome
Lionel Willatt, James Cox, John Barber, Elisabet Dachs Cabanas, Amanda Collins, Dian Donnai, David R. FitzPatrick, Eddy Maher, Howard Martin, Josep Parnau, Lesley Pindar, Jacqueline Ramsay, Charles Shaw-Smith, Erik A. Sistermans, Michael Tettenborn, Dorothy Trump, Bert B. A. de Vries, Kate Walker, and F. Lucy Raymond

161 Characterization of a New Syndrome That Associates Craniosynostosis, Delayed Fontanel Closure, Parietal Foramina, Imperforate Anus, and Skin Eruption: CDAGS
Roberto Mendoza-Londono, Edward Lammer, Rosemarie Watson, John Harper, Atsushi Hatamochi, Saori Hatamochi-Hayashi, Dobrawa Napierala, Pia Hermanns, Sinead Collins, Benjamin B. Roa, Madhuri R. Hedge, Keiko Wakui, Diep Nguyen, David W. Stockton, and Brendan Lee

Announcements

169 Conferences

Information for Contributors

This Month in the *Journal*

This month in the *Journal,* Wang et al. describe how mouse-human comparative genetics can be used to identify human genes associated with a complex trait, specifically atherosclerosis. There are at least 27 unique human QTLs for atherosclerosis, but few genes have been reliably associated with this trait. However, about half of the QTLs found in mouse models of atherosclerosis have concordant human QTLs. Wang et al. explain how this overlap can be used to identify the causative genes within these QTLs and the types of mouse crosses that will facilitate gene identification. In fact, the authors have successfully used the general approach they describe to identify the *TNFSF4* gene as being associated with the risk of heart attack and coronary artery disease in humans.

Mutations in* SLC19A3 *Cause BBGD, *by Zeng et al. (p. 16)*

In this issue of the *Journal,* two articles report transporter defects that are associated with neurological phenotypes. The first, by Zeng et al., is an investigation of biotin-responsive basal ganglia disease (BBGD). This disorder first appears in children as a subacute encephalopathy, with confusion and vomiting. It progresses to acute encephalopathy, with speech difficulties, inability to swallow, seizures, and partial or complete paralysis. These symptoms can be completely reversed if treatment with high doses of biotin is started at an early stage; without continuous treatment, there is progressive encephalopathy and, ultimately, death. The dramatic improvements with treatment placed biotin metabolism as a key player in this disorder. Unfortunately, no defects in the enzymes that require biotin were found. Linkage analysis placed the critical region on chromosome 2, and Zeng et al. focused on *SLC19A3* as a candidate gene because it belongs to a family of transporter proteins. They found mutations in *SLC19A3* in all four families they examined. Because BBGD is so effectively treated with biotin, the authors speculate that *SLC19A3* encodes a biotin transporter, a hypothesis supported by the recent finding that people with induced biotin deficiency have reductions in *SLC19A3* mRNA levels in their blood. Curiously, the presentation of BBGD seems to have neurological specificity. Affected individuals do not have evidence of a generalized biotin deficiency; therefore, the biotin insufficiency appears to be limited to the brain.

0002-9297/2005/7701-0001$15.00

Allan-Herndon-Dudley Syndrome, *by Schwartz et al. (p. 41)*

The second article that reports a transporter defect is by Schwartz et al., who found a transporter defect in Allan-Herndon-Dudley syndrome. This is a severe form of X-linked mental retardation that is associated with hypotonia, delayed motor development, and muscle hypoplasia. Linkage studies had placed the candidate gene in the region of Xq13–Xq21. Schwartz et al. realized that *MCT8* was a good candidate gene in this region because mutations in this gene have recently been reported in males with mental retardation, hypotonia, and thyroid abnormalities. Schwartz et al. studied six kindreds and found that some of the affected individuals did, in fact, have thyroid abnormalities, and all of them had mutations in *MCT8*. This gene encodes the monocarboxylate transporter 8, which has recently been shown to be a thyroid-hormone transporter. The association with thyroid abnormalities could help to prioritize individuals with X-linked mental retardation for *MCT8* mutation screening. As with the *SLC19A3* mutations above, there is specificity for the presentation of the transporter defect, because individuals with *MCT8* mutations don't show the effects of a general thyroid disturbance. Dumitrescu et al. (74:168–175) speculated that the severe neurological phenotype coupled with mild evidence of a thyroid disturbance in people with *MCT8* mutations could suggest a brain-specific function for MCT8 beyond its action as a hormone transporter.

Segmental Duplication Array CGH, *by Sharp et al. (p. 78)*

Segmental duplications have been associated with several recurrent genomic disorders and are thought to be prone to instability. With recent reports that there is normal copy-number variation in the human genome, it seemed likely that segmental duplications might also mediate the generation of some of this variation. To test this hypothesis, Sharp et al. developed a microarray of BACs containing regions of segmental duplication and analyzed the DNA of 47 individuals from different populations to assess normal copy-number polymorphism (CNP) in these genetic regions. This approach was certainly successful in identifying CNPs; 119 regions of CNP were found, 73 of them novel. Compared with control BACs, CNPs were enriched in regions that were flanked by or contained segmental duplications, supporting the theory that these duplications mediate the generation of normal genetic variation. Not only did these duplications seem to generate CNPs, but they were also often variant in copy number themselves. Sharp et al. have created a Web-based database that includes their results and that they hope will serve as a resource for facilitating further studies of structural polymorphisms.

AR *Is the Major Determinant of AGA,* *by Hillmer et al.* (*p. 140*)

Hillmer et al. report that a major determinant of male-pattern baldness (androgenetic alopecia) is the androgen receptor (*AR*) gene. In a sample of families with at least two affected brothers, they found linkage to the X chromosome in a region containing *AR*. This finding led the authors to do an association study of markers in the area, and they report a 1-Mb region that is strongly associated with baldness in both a case-control and a family-based association analysis. The only known gene within this region is *AR*, and a GGN repeat is the only specific feature in this gene that shows a strong association with baldness. Previously, it was shown that there is allele-specific variation in protein and activity levels for the GGN repeat, so this association may have functional significance. Alternatively, the GGN repeat could instead be in linkage disequilibrium with the actual but as-yet-undetected causal variation. Although it appears to contribute significantly to male-pattern baldness, *AR* is obviously not the whole story behind this phenotype, because its location on the X chromosome cannot explain the fact that many sons resemble their fathers in terms of baldness.

KATHRYN GARBER
Deputy Editor

REVIEW ARTICLE
Identifying Novel Genes for Atherosclerosis through Mouse-Human Comparative Genetics

Xiaosong Wang,[1] Naoki Ishimori,[2] Ron Korstanje,[3] Jarod Rollins,[1] and Beverly Paigen[1]

[1]The Jackson Laboratory, Bar Harbor, ME; [2]Department of Cardiovascular Medicine, Hokkaido University Graduate School of Medicine, Sapporo, Japan; and [3]Department of Pathology and Laboratory Medicine, Medical Biology Section, University of Groningen and University Medical Centre Groningen, Groningen, The Netherlands

Susceptibility to atherosclerosis is determined by both environmental and genetic factors. Its genetic determinants have been studied by use of quantitative-trait–locus (QTL) analysis. So far, 21 atherosclerosis QTLs have been identified in the mouse: 7 in a high-fat–diet model only, 9 in a sensitized model (apolipoprotein E– or LDL [low-density lipoprotein] receptor–deficient mice) only, and 5 in both models, suggesting that different gene sets operate in each model and that a subset operates in both. Among the 27 human atherosclerosis QTLs reported, 17 (63%) are located in regions homologous (concordant) to mouse QTLs, suggesting that these mouse and human atherosclerosis QTLs have the same underlying genes. Therefore, genes regulating human atherosclerosis will be found most efficiently by first finding their orthologs in concordant mouse QTLs. Novel mouse QTL genes will be found most efficiently by using a combination of the following strategies: identifying QTLs in new crosses performed with previously unused parental strains; inducing mutations in large-scale, high-throughput mutagenesis screens; and using new genomic and bioinformatics tools. Once QTL genes are identified in mice, they can be tested in human association studies for their relevance in human atherosclerotic disease.

Introduction

Atherosclerosis is the pathological basis of ischemic coronary artery disease (CAD), the leading cause of death in industrialized nations. It is characterized by accumulation of plasma lipids, fibrous tissues, and cell components (mostly macrophages, smooth-muscle cells, and lymphocytes) in large arteries. Atherosclerosis is a complex disease caused by both genetic (with ~50% heritability) and environmental (mostly diet) factors. The underlying genes have been studied through genotype- and phenotype-driven approaches. In the genotype-driven approach, a gene suspected of contributing to atherosclerosis is tested for a pathological role either in atherogenesis, by use of transgenic/knockout animal models, or in rare Mendelian forms of human atherosclerosis. Studies with mouse models have identified >80 atherosclerosis-regulating genes, and some of their human orthologs have confirmed polymorphisms associated with human atherosclerotic diseases, including genes encoding the angiotensin-converting enzyme (*ACE* [MIM 106180]); adrenergic receptor, beta 2 (*ADRB2* [MIM 109690]); 5-lipoxygenase–activating protein (*ALOX5AP* [MIM 603700]); apolipoprotein E (*APOE* [MIM 107741]); coagulation factor VII (*F7* [MIM 227500]); fibrinogen, B beta polypeptide (*FGB* [MIM 134830]); glycoprotein 1b, alpha polypeptide (*GP1BA* [MIM 606672]); matrix metalloproteinase 3 (*MMP3* [MIM 185250]); matrix metalloproteinase 9 (*MMP9* [MIM 120361]); 5,10-methylenetetrahydrofolate reductase (*MTHFR* [MIM 607093]); nitric oxide synthase 3, endothelial cell (*NOS3* [MIM 163729]); serum paraoxonase (*PON1* [MIM 168820]); transforming growth factor, beta 1 (*TGFB1* [MIM 190180]); thrombospondin 2 (*THBS2* [MIM 188061]); thrombospondin 4 (*THBS4* [MIM 600715]); toll-like receptor 4 (*TLR4* [MIM 603030]) (Agah and Topol 2002; Humphries and Morgan 2004; Lusis et al. 2004; Manolio et al. 2004; McCarthy et al. 2004); and tumor necrosis factor (ligand) superfamily, member 4 (*TNFSF4* [MIM 603594]) (Wang et al. 2005*b*). In the phenotype-driven approach, no assumption is made as to which genes cause a disease phenotype, and atherosclerosis is linked to chromosome locations, QTLs, in a genomewide scan. This approach has the advantage of finding novel atherosclerosis-susceptibility genes. Two reviews summarize some of these QTLs (Allayee et al. 2003; Smith 2003).

Here, we present an updated review of atherosclerosis QTLs found in mice and humans, compare atherosclerosis QTLs found in the two most commonly used

Received April 14, 2005; accepted for publication May 4, 2005; electronically published May 19, 2005.

Address for correspondence and reprints: Dr. Xiaosong Wang, The Jackson Laboratory, 600 Main Street, Bar Harbor, ME 04509. E-mail: xw@jax.org

0002-9297/2005/7701-0002$15.00

mouse models (diet-induced and sensitized), and comment on their concordance with human atherosclerosis QTLs. Finally, we propose future strategies for finding novel genes regulating human atherosclerosis.

QTLs for Atherosclerotic Diseases in Humans

So far, nine genomewide scans have been reported for human atherosclerotic diseases, including myocardial infarction (MI), CAD, acute coronary syndrome (ACS; acute MI and unstable angina), and carotid artery intimal-medial thickness (CIMT) (table 1). Thirty-one individual QTLs (those found in different populations, regardless of whether they are at the same chromosomal locations) have been identified. They are distributed on 27 chromosome locations, and four of them—on chromosomes 2, 3, 12, and 13—are found in two populations, so there are 27 unique QTLs (fig. 1). Six genes that have confirmed association with the risk of atherosclerotic diseases in at least two independent populations lie in 6 of the 27 QTLs. Analyses consistently indicate that *ALOX5AP* underlies the MI and stroke QTL on proximal chromosome 13 (Ben-Asher and Lancet 2004; Helgadottir et al. 2004; Lohmussaar et al. 2005). The R353Q polymorphism in *F7* is significantly associated with MI (McCarthy et al. 2004), so it is a candidate for the MI QTL on distal chromosome 13q. The C-1252T polymorphism in the promoter region of *MMP9* is associated with the size of complicated lesions and the stenosis of coronary arteries (Zhang et al. 1999; Pollanen et al. 2001), suggesting that it is the gene underlying the ACS QTL on chromosome 20q. The *C677T* SNP in *MTHFR* is significantly associated with CIMT in a Chinese population and a Japanese population (Humphries and Morgan 2004), making it a candidate for the top chromosome 1p QTL. More than two dozen studies indicate that the Q192R polymorphism of *PON1* underlies the CAD QTL on chromosome 7q (Durrington et al. 2001; Agah and Topol 2002), although a recent meta-analysis revealed only a weak relative risk of 1.12 (95% CI 1.07–1.16) (Wheeler et al. 2004). Association studies in two groups of patients with MI revealed that a polymorphism in the first intron of *TNFSF4* is associated with the risk of MI and CAD, suggesting that it underlies the CAD QTL on chromosome 1q (Wang et al. 2005*b*). In addition, it is highly likely that *MEF2A* (encoding myocyte enhancer factor 2A [MIM 600660]) is the gene underlying the chromosome 15q MI QTL, because there is a 7-aa deletion in MEF2A in all 13 of the patients with MI but not from the 8 normal individuals from a family (Wang et al. 2003*a*), and three novel mutations in exon 7 of *MEF2A* are present in 4 of the 207 study patients with CAD/MI but not in 191 control subjects (Bhagavatula et al. 2004).

Of the >80 genes shown to influence atherosclerosis in either gene-knockout or transgenic mouse models—and at least 17 genes having confirmed polymorphisms associated with human atherosclerotic diseases—only about a quarter of them fall within human atherosclerosis QTLs, as indicated in fig. 1. Half of the human atherosclerosis QTLs have no obvious candidate genes, which suggests that their genetic determinants are unknown.

QTLs for Atherosclerosis in Mice

Atherosclerosis QTLs in mice have been identified in two models: (1) a high-fat–diet model, in which a diet containing 15% fat, 1.25% cholesterol, and 0.5% cholic acid is used to induce atherosclerosis, and (2) the sensitized model, in which mice deficient in *Apoe*—or low-density lipoprotein receptor (*Ldlr*)—are used (Jawien et al. 2004; Meir and Leitersdorf 2004). *Apoe*-deficient mice develop atherosclerosis spontaneously when fed a chow diet; their lesions develop faster when they are fed a Western diet (containing 21% fat and 0.15% cholesterol) and more so when they are fed the high-fat diet described above. *Ldlr*-deficient mice also develop atherosclerotic lesions when fed the chow diet, but the lesions are very small and take considerable time to develop; feeding these mice a Western diet or the high-fat diet described above accelerates their lesion formation.

A total of 15 studies using mouse models of atherosclerosis detected 35 individual QTLs. Among them, there are 21 unique QTLs (QTLs identified in different crosses but at the same chromosomal location are counted as one unique QTL because they may have the same underlying gene [table 2 and fig. 2]). Of the 21 QTLs, 7 are revealed only in the high-fat–diet model, 9 only in the sensitized model, and 5 in both models (fig. 3). Of the 21 QTLs, 12 are replicated in more than one cross, which enables the use of haplotype analysis to narrow these QTLs (Wang and Paigen 2005*b*). The causal genes underlying 2 of the 21 mouse atherosclerosis QTLs have been identified: *Tnfsf4* (*Ox40l*) for *Ath1* (atherosclerosis susceptibility 1) on chromosome 1 (Wang et al. 2005*b*) and *Alox5* for *Artles* on chromosome 6 (Mehrabian et al. 2002). Additionally, *Angptl3* is probably one gene underlying a complex locus, *Ath8*, on chromosome 4, which may contain more than one QTL (Korstanje et al. 2004).

Concordance of Human and Mouse Atherosclerosis QTLs

The term "concordance" refers to the fact that QTLs for the same trait but from different species map to homologous genomic regions. It was first used to describe hypertension QTLs that map to homologous regions in rats, mice, and humans (Stoll et al. 2000; Sugiyama et

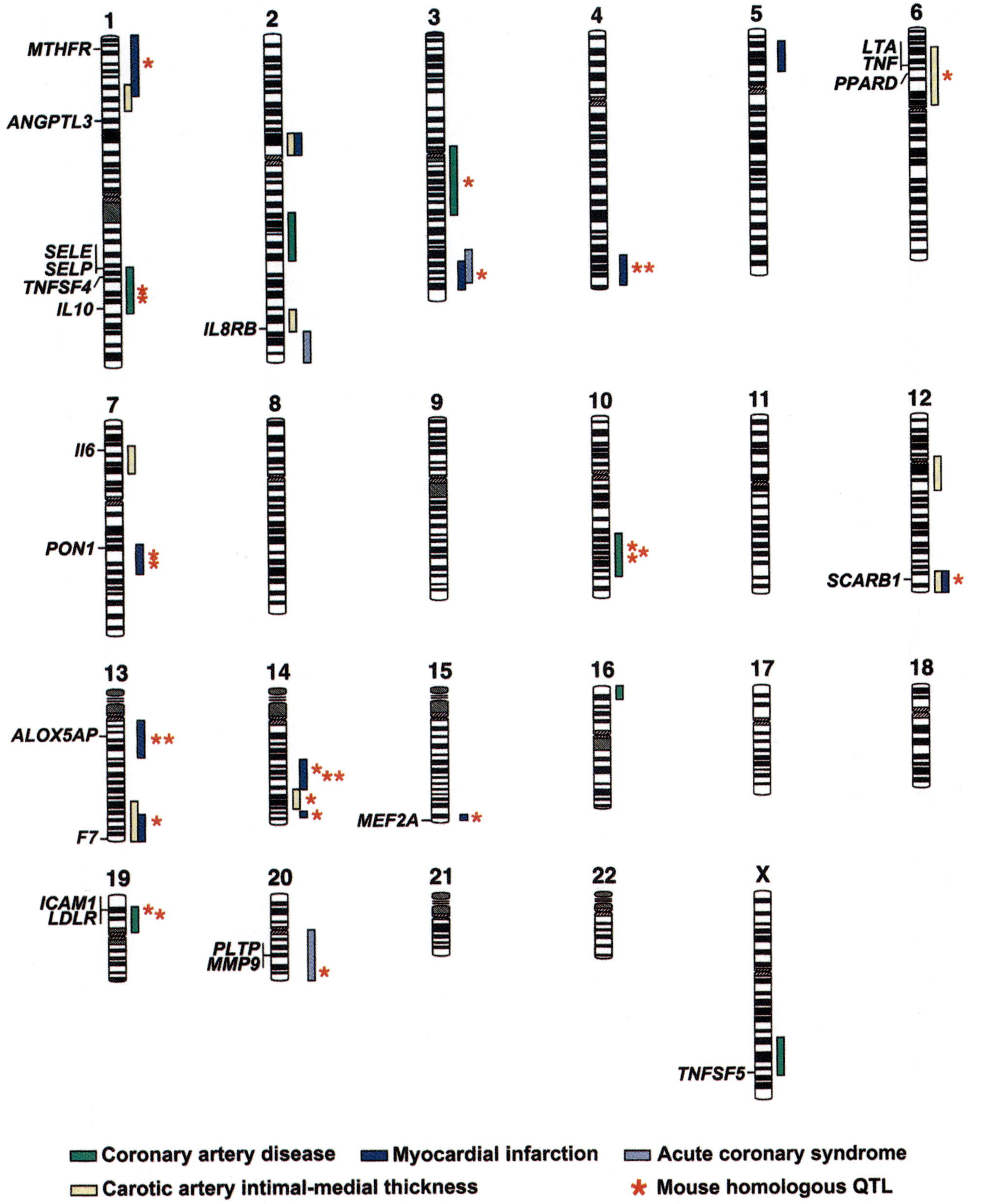

Figure 1 Chromosome map of human QTLs for atherosclerotic diseases. Chromosomes are drawn to scale, on the basis of the length of each from the Ensembl Human Genome Browser. Each bar to the right of a chromosome represents a human atherosclerosis QTL from one population (see table 1). The size of the QTL is determined either as a 1.5-LOD CI or as ±10 Mb on either side of the peak marker when the information on CI is unavailable. Candidate genes are listed to the left of the chromosomes. Human homologous regions of mouse QTLs that fall within the human QTLs are represented by red stars.

Table 1

QTLs for Atherosclerotic Diseases in Humans

Chromosome and Cytogenetic Band Peak[a] (95% CI[b])	Peak (cM)[c]	Peak, in Mb[d] (95% CI[b])	Nearest Marker	LOD	Mouse Homologous Regions[e] and Chromosome Peak, in cM (95% CI)	Disease	Population[f]	Reference
1:								
1p36.1 (p36-34)	47	21 (0–41)	*D1S3669*	11.7	4–66 (50–83)[g]	MI	U.S., 1,613/428	Wang et al. 2004*a*
1p33 (p34.3-32.2)	76	48	*D1S2134*	2.4	4–55 (49–61)	CIMT	U.S., 1,242/311	Fox et al. 2004
1q31.1 (q24.2-1q32.1)	202	184 (164–200)	*D1S518*	2.2	1–82 (69–85)[g]	CAD	International, 1,168/438	Hauser et al. 2004
2:								
2p11.2 (p12-11.2)	103	85	*D2S1790*	3.3	6–31	MI	U.S., 1,613/428	Wang et al. 2004*a*
2p11.2 (p12-11.2)	103	85	*D2S1790*	1.6	6–31	CIMT	U.S., 1,242/311	Fox et al. 2004
2q22.1 (q21.2-24.3)	150	142 (134–168)	*D2S129*	3.2	2–34 (30–38), 1–67	CAD	Finnish, 364/156	Pajukanta et al. 2000
2q34 (q33.3-35)	210	214 (205–221)	*D2S2944*	3.1	1–36 (30–44)	CIMT	Mexican Americans, 274/91	Wang et al. 2005*a*
2q36-37.3	250	...	...	2.6	1- (41–59)	ACS	61 Australian sib pairs	Harrap et al. 2002
3:								
3q13.31 (p12.1-3q22.1)	140	119 (86–134)	*D3S2460*	3.5	16–23 (21–44)[g], 6–38, 9–56	CAD	International, 1,168/438	Hauser et al. 2004
3q27.2 (q26.31-28)	199	187 (175–191)	*D3S1571-3686*	2.4	16–14 (14–22)[g], 3–13	MI	Indo-Mauritian, 535/99	Francke et al. 2001
3q26-27	...	...	...	1.8	16- (14–21)[g], 3- (11–15)	ACS	61 Australian sib pairs	Harrap et al. 2002
4:								
4q34.1 (q32.3-35.1)	176	175	*D4S2431*	4.4	8–31[g]	MI	U.S., 1,613/428	Wang et al. 2004*a*
5:								
5p14.3 (p15.2-13.3)	36	22	*D5S2845*	3.7	15–5	MI	U.S., 1,613/428	Wang et al. 2004*a*
6:								
6p22.1 (p22.3-12)	44	29 (19–65)	*D6S1022*	2.2	13–12 (9–28), 17- (11–30), 9–42[g]	CIMT	Mexican Americans, 274/91	Wang et al. 2005*a*
7:								
7p14.3 (p15.3-14.1)	50	31	*D7S817*	1.6	6–27 (23–29), 13–9	CIMT	U.S., 1,242/311	Fox et al. 2004
7q22.2 (q21.3-31.1)	114	104	*D7S1799*	3.6	5–78, 12–15[g]	MI	U.S., 1,613/428	Wang et al. 2004*a*
10:								
10q23.33 (q23.2-26.11)	116	95 (86–119)	*D10S185*	2.1	19–48 (35–55)[g], 14–16[g]	CAD	Indo-Mauritian, 535/99	Francke et al. 2001

12:								
12q12 (p11.21-q13.13)	56	42	*D12S1301*	1.7	15–55 (53–62)	CIMT	U.S., 1,242/311	Fox et al. 2004
12q24.33 (q24.23-24.33)	161	129	*D12S1045*	4.4	5–65, 10- (42–49)[g]	MI	U.S., 1,613/428	Wang et al. 2004*a*
12q24.33 (q24.23-24.33)	161	129	*D12S1045*	4.1	5–65, 10- (42–49)[g]	CIMT	U.S., 1,242/311	Fox et al. 2004
13:								
13q12.3 (q12.11-14.11)	24	30	*D13S289*	2.5	5–84 (82–88), 14-(20–30)[g], 3–29	MI	Iceland, 713/296	Helgadottir et al. 2004
13q33.3 (q31.1-34)	94	107 (80–109)	*D13S796*	1.3	8–2 (1–10)[g], 14- (51–68)	CIMT	Mexican Americans, 274/91	Wang et al. 2005*a*
13q33.3 (q32.1-34)	94	107	*D13S796*	3.6	8–5[g]	MI	U.S., 1,613/428	Wang et al. 2004*a*
14:								
14q23.1 (q22.1-24.2)	67	60	*D14S592*	4.2	12–31[g], 14–18[g]	MI	U.S., 1,613/428	Wang et al. 2004*a*
14q31.2 (q24.3-32.12)	92	83	*D14S606*	1.8	12–48 (37–57)[g]	CIMT	U.S., 1,242/311	Fox et al. 2004
14q32.2 (q32.2-32.31)	126	100 (98–101)	*D14S1426*	3.9	12–53 (52–57)[g]	MI	German, 1,406/513	Broeckel et al. 2002
15:								
15q26.3 (q26.2-26.3)	113	97 (96–99)	*D15S120*	4.2	7- (29–41)[g]	CAD/MI	U.S., 21/1	Wang et al. 2003*a*
16:								
16p13.3 (p13.3-13.2)	9	4 (0–8)	*D16S3027*	3.1	16–2 (1–7), 17–11 (8–16), 11–16	CAD	Indo-Mauritian, 535/99	Francke et al. 2001
19:								
19p13.12 (p13.2-12)	44	16	*D19S252*	1.7	8–34[g], 10–42[g], 17–20	CAD	International, 1,168/438	Hauser et al. 2004
20:								
20q11-13	...	...	...	1.6	2- (83–108)[g]	ACS	61 Australian sib pairs	Harrap et al. 2002
X:								
Xq25 (q23-26)	82	129 (109–137)	*DX1047*	3.5	X-16 (13–18), X-65	CAD	Finnish, 364/156	Pajukanta et al. 2000

[a] Peak cytogenetic bands were retrieved from the Ensembl database (release 26.35.1), according the positions of the peak markers.

[b] CIs were determined either by the 1.5-LOD drop method when LOD score curves and markers were available (found in LOD score tables) or by use of ±10 Mb around the peak marker in the absence of the above information.

[c] cM positions were retrieved from the genetic map at the Center for Medical Genetics Web site, by use of the markers named in the references.

[d] Mb are based on Ensembl release 26.35.1. CIs, in Mb, are shown only if CIs of cytogenetic bands were available from the references.

[e] Mouse homologous chromosome regions of the human cytogenetic bands were determined by use of the Mammalian Orthology Query Form (MGI). The ranges of the positions were derived either from CIs of cytogenetic bands if the data were available or from the mouse homologous regions of the peak cytogenetic bands if CIs of cytogenic bands were not available.

[f] Number of individuals/families.

[g] Mouse homologous regions of the human QTLs that fall within atherosclerosis QTLs (marker with peak LOD ± 10 cM) from mouse crosses shown in table 2.

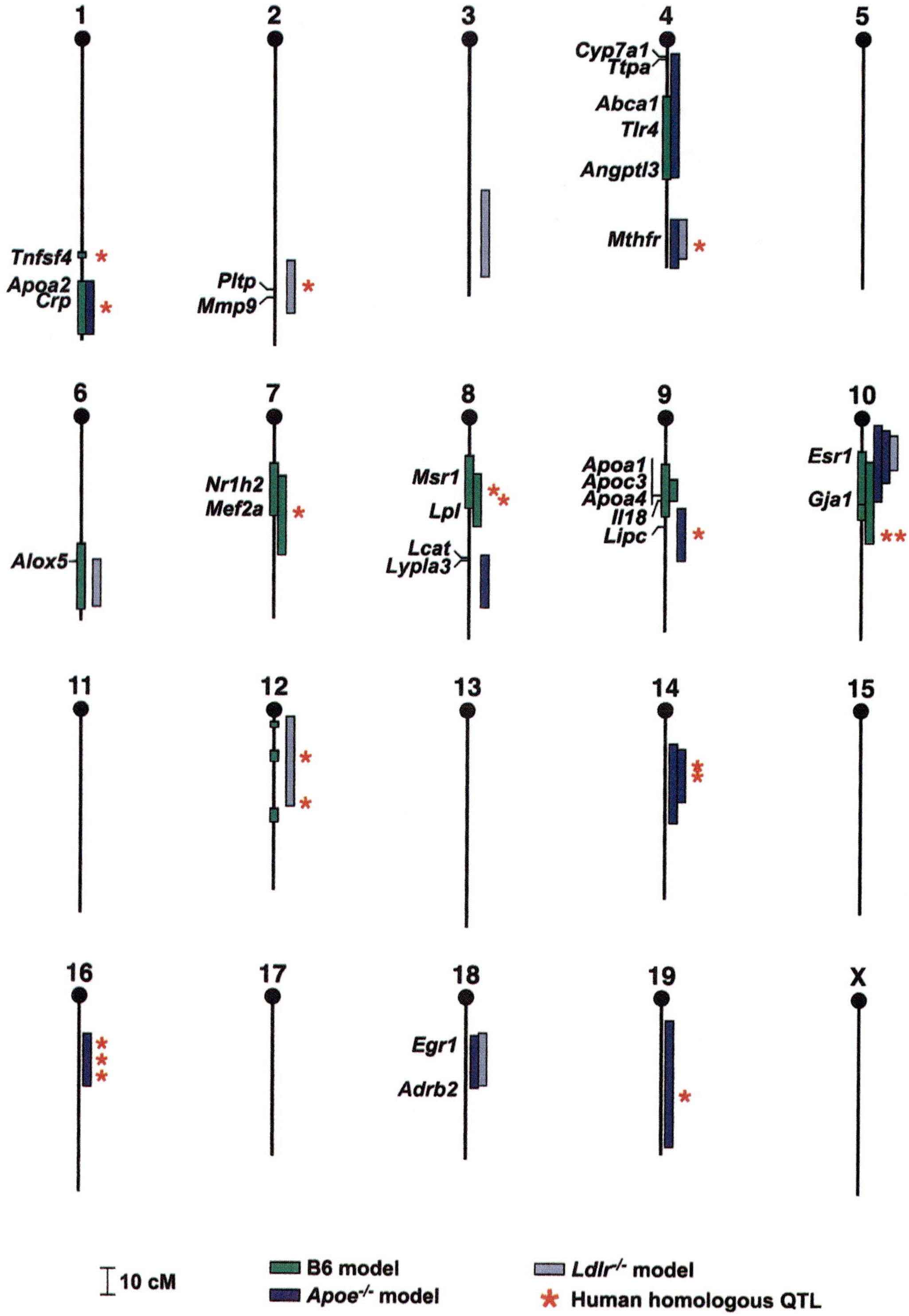

Figure 2 Chromosome map of mouse atherosclerosis QTLs. Each chromosome is represented by a vertical line (centromeres at the top). Genetic distances (in cM) from the centromere are drawn to scale (scale shown at lower left of the figure. Chromosomes are drawn to scale, on the basis of the estimated cM position of the most distally mapped locus on the Mouse Genome Informatics (MGI) Web site. Mouse atherosclerosis QTLs are represented by the bars to the right of each chromosome (interacting QTLs are not shown). Each bar represents a QTL from one cross (sharing the same parental strains, regardless of the breeding strategy) in the specified mouse model (see table 2). The size of the QTL is determined either as a 95% CI or as ±10 cM on either side of the LOD score peak when the information on CI is unavailable. Candidate genes are listed to the left of the chromosomes. Mouse homologous regions of human QTLs that fall within mouse QTLs are represented by red stars.

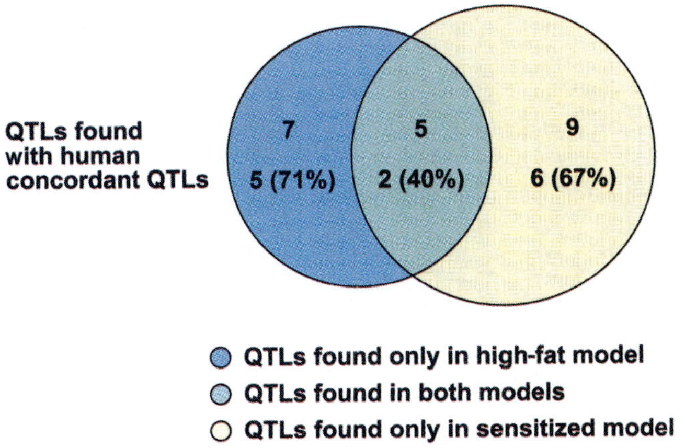

Figure 3 Comparison of mouse atherosclerosis QTLs found in high-fat and sensitized models (*Apoe*$^{-/-}$ and *Ldlr*$^{-/-}$ mice), shown in different colors. The number of QTLs concordant with human QTLs is also shown.

al. 2001). It has since been observed for kidney disease (Korstanje and DiPetrillo 2004) and plasma levels of high-density lipoprotein (HDL) (Wang and Paigen 2005*a*), low-density lipoprotein, and triglycerides (Wang and Paigen 2005*b*). For atherosclerosis, 13 (62%) of the 21 mouse QTLs are concordant with human QTLs, and 17 (63%) of the 27 human QTLs are concordant with mouse QTLs (figs. 1 and 2), suggesting that more than half of the mouse and human atherosclerosis QTLs have the same underlying genes. Thus, identifying them in one species should greatly facilitate identifying them in the other.

Concordant QTLs are found for five (71%) of the seven mouse atherosclerosis QTLs in the high-fat model, six (67%) of the nine in a sensitized model, and two (40%) of the five in both models (fig. 3). Altogether, more than half of the QTLs found in each model have concordant human QTLs, so it cannot be said that one model is more relevant to human atherosclerotic disease than the other. Three reasons may explain why some of the human QTLs do not have concordant mouse QTLs. First, not enough mouse crosses have been made. Second, and perhaps more important, C57BL/6 (B6) mice were used as the susceptible parental strain in 11 of the 13 crosses made so far to detect mouse atherosclerosis QTLs. Use of different susceptible strains may detect different QTLs that are concordant with human QTLs. Third, the size of atherosclerotic lesions in mice (used as the phenotype in all the QTL studies in mice so far) only partially corresponds to the incidence of human atherosclerotic diseases. In fact, the incidence of human ACS is determined not only by lesion size but also, more importantly, by plaque stability. Thus, future mouse QTL studies that include plaque stability as a phenotype may identify additional QTLs that are concordant with human atherosclerosis QTLs.

Strategies for Finding Novel Genes Regulating Human Atherosclerosis

Using the Mouse-to-Human Strategy

Finding QTL genes in mice is much more cost-effective, less time consuming, and less fraught with ethical issues than is finding them first in humans, especially now that many new genetic, genomic, and bioinformatics tools for the mouse are available (discussed in the "Integrating Traditional Genetic Approaches with New Genetic, Genomic, and Bioinformatic Resources and Tools" section). After a QTL gene is identified in the mouse, it can be tested in human association studies for its role in human diseases. The completion of the human HapMap project will greatly simplify such studies by facilitating the selection of representative SNPs of a haplotype block. In addition, dense SNPs throughout the human genome have made possible whole-genome association studies, whereby the candidacy of all the genes in human diseases are systematically studied (Ozaki et al. 2002; Carlson et al. 2004).

This mouse-to-human strategy has been successfully used to identify *POMC* (encoding pro-opiomelanocortin-alpha [MIM 176830]) as a gene influencing obesity (Krude et al. 1998; Hixson et al. 1999); *CTLA4* (encoding cytotoxic T-lymphocyte-associated protein 4 [MIM 123890]) as a gene contributing to autoimmune disorders, including Graves disease, autoimmune hypothyroidism, and type 1 diabetes (Ueda et al. 2003); and *EN2* (encoding engrailed 2 [MIM 131310]) as a gene for autism-spectrum disorder (Gharani et al. 2004). This strategy has also been used to identify an atherosclerosis-susceptibility gene in humans. *Ath1* is a QTL on chromosome 1 that makes B6 mice more susceptible to atherosclerosis than C3H mice (Paigen et al. 1987*a*, 1987*b*). By using congenic strains, we narrowed *Ath1* to a 0.66-cM region containing 11 genes (Phelan et al. 2002). Three of the 11 genes could be involved in atherosclerosis: *Prdx6* (peroxiredoxin 6 [also called "antioxidant protein 2"]) encodes an antioxidant (Steinberg and Witztum 2002), *Tnfsf4* encodes a membrane protein on lymphocytes and endothelial cells (Hansson et al. 2002), and *Fasl* (Fas ligand) is important for apoptosis (Geng 2001). After analyzing atherosclerosis susceptibility in mouse mutants for each of these genes, we found that only *Tnfsf4*-targeted mutants were significantly less susceptible to diet-induced atherosclerosis than were wild-type controls and that mice overexpressing *Tnfsf4* were more susceptible to atherosclerosis than were wild-type controls. We then tested SNPs in *TNFSF4* as well as in the nearby genes in human association studies, and we

Table 2

QTL for Atherosclerosis in Inbred Mouse Crosses

Chromosome, Locus, and Marker[a]	Peak cM (95% CI)[b]	LOD	Cross[c]	Sex[d]	High Allele (inheritance)[e]	Variance (%)	Human Ortholog Region[f]	Reference(s)
1:								
Ath1:								
D1Mit159	82	…	B × H and C × B RI lines	F	B6		1q25.1[g]	Paigen et al. 1987*b*; Phelan et al. 2002
1–169 Mb	100	3.4	(B6 × A) F_2	F	B6 (dom)		1q22-41[g]	N. Ishimori and B. Paigen, unpublished data
Ath9:								
D1Mit359	100	3.3	(B6.129-*Apoe*$^{-/-}$ × FVB.129-*Apoe*$^{-/-}$) F_2	F+M		7	1q22-41[g]	Dansky et al. 2002
2:								
D2Mit504	92	2.8	(PERA × B6.129-*Ldlr*$^{-/-}$) × B6.129-*Ldlr*$^{-/-}$)	M/	B6	16	20q11-13[g]	Seidelmann et al. 2005
3:								
D3Mit45	79 (55–88)	4.5	(B6.129-*Ldlr*$^{-/-}$ × FVB.129-*Ldlr*$^{-/-}$) F_2	F/	B6 (add)		1p13-31	Teupser and Breslow 2003
4:								
D4Mit111	22 (3–50)	3.0	(B6.129-*Apoe*$^{-/-}$ × C3H.129-*Apoe*$^{-/-}$) F_2	F	B6 (add)		9q22-33	Wang et al. 2003*b*
Ath8:								
D4Mit44	29 (18–51)	3.6	(SM × NZB) F_2	F	SM (rec)		9q22-33	Korstanje et al. 2004
4–135 Mb	76	4.6	(A × B6.129-*Apoe*$^{-/-}$) F_2	F	A (add)		1p35-36[g]	N. Ishimori and B. Paigen, unpublished data
Athsq1:								
D4Mit127	78 (66–81)	6.2	(MOLF × B6-*Ldlr*$^{-/-}$) × B6-*Ldlr*$^{-/-}$	F/	MOLF	32	1p35-36[g]	Welch et al. 2001
6:								
Artles:								
D6Mit256	61 (46–71)	6.7	(CAST × B6) F_2	F+M	B6 (rec)		12p13, 10q11, 3p25	Mehrabian et al. 2001, 2002
Athsq2:								
D6Mit110	64 (52–70)	6.7	(MOLF × B6-*Ldlr*$^{-/-}$) × B6-*Ldlr*$^{-/-}$	F, M	B6	16	12p13, 10q11, 3p25	Welch et al. 2001
7:								
D7Mit193	25	3.7	(B6 × DBA/2) F_2	F	DBA (add)	10	19q13, 11p15, 15q11, 15q26[g]	Colinayo et al. 2003
Ath3:								
Tyr	44 (20–50)	…	A × B and B × A RI lines	F+M	B6		11p15-q14, 15q24-26[g]	Stewart-Phillips et al. 1989
8:								
8–54 Mb	22	2.8	(B6 × A) F_2	F	A (add)		4q31-35[g], 8p22-23, 19p12-13[g], 13q34[g]	N. Ishimori and B. Paigen, unpublished data
D8Mit41	29	3.4	(B6 × DBA/2) F_2	F	B6 (add)	9	4q31-35[g], 8p22-23, 19p12-13[g], 16q12	Colinayo et al. 2003
8–109 Mb	60	2.0	(A × B6.129-*Apoe*$^{-/-}$) F_2	F	A (rec)		16q22-24, 1q42	N. Ishimori and B. Paigen, unpublished data
9:								
9–48 Mb	25	4.1	(B6 × A) F_2	F	B6 (add)		11q22-24, 15q21-24	N. Ishimori and B. Paigen, unpublished data
D9Mit330	26		SWR (SWR × SJL)	F	SJL		11q22-24, 15q21-24	Svenson and Paigen, unpublished data
9–64 Mb	42	3.7	(A × B6.129-*Apoe*$^{-/-}$) F_2	F	A (dom)		6p12-q13[g], 15q21-24	N. Ishimori and B. Paigen, unpublished data
10:								
Ath20[h]:								
D10Mit213	10 (5–40)	…	(B6 × 129) F_2	F	…	5	6q21-24, 10q21-22	Ishimori et al. 2004
Ath11:								
D10Mit213	11 (0–29)	5.1	(B6.129-*Apoe*$^{-/-}$ × FVB.129-*Apoe*$^{-/-}$) F_2	F, M	FVB (rec)	21	6q21-24, 10q21-22	Dansky et al. 2002

10–27 Mb	12	2.8	(A × B6.129-*Apoe*$^{-/-}$) F_2	F	A (dom)		6q21-24, 10q21-22	N. Ishimori and B. Paigen, unpublished data
D10Mit16	16 (4–17)	12.9	(B6.129-*Ldlr*$^{-/-}$ × FVB.129-*Ldlr*$^{-/-}$) F_2	F, M	FVB (rec)		6q21-24, 10q21-22	Teupser and Breslow 2003
10–27 Mb	20	3.9	(B6 × A) F_2	F	A (add)		6q21-24, 10q21-22	N. Ishimori and B. Paigen, unpublished data
Artles2:								
D10Mit42	30 (14–45)	4.5	(B6 × DBA/2) F_2	F	DBA (add)	11	6q21-22, 10q21-22, 12q24[g], 19p13[g], 21q22	Colinayo et al. 2003
Ath17:								
D10Mit31	34 (30–36)	6.6	(B6 × 129) F_2	F	129	10	6q21-22, 10q21-22, 12q24[g], 19p13[g], 21q22	Ishimori et al. 2004
11:								
Ath19[h]:								
D11Mit333	60 (55–70)	...	(B6 × 129) F_2	F	...	4	17q21-25	Ishimori et al. 2004
12:								
Ath6:								
D12Mit49	3 (2–4)	2.5	(B6-*db/db* × BKS) F_2	F	BKS		2p23-25	Mu et al. 1999; Purcell et al. 2001
Ath18:								
D12Mit243	16 (13–17)	3.7	(B6 × 129) F_2	F	B6 or 129	6	7q22-31[g], 2p25	Ishimori et al. 2004
D12Mit222	18 (0–34)	3.7	(B6.129-*Ldlr*$^{-/-}$ × FVB.129-*Ldlr*$^{-/-}$) F_2	F, M	B6 (add)		7q22-31[g], 2p23-25, 14q12-24[g]	Teupser and Breslow 2003
Ath7:								
D12Mit158	38 (35–40)		SWR × (SWR × SJL), SWR × SJL RI	F	SWR		14q23-31[g]	Svenson and Paigen, unpublished data
Ath21[h]:								
D12Mit7	50 (10–70)	...	(B6 × 129) F_2	F	...	5	14q23-32[g], 7q36	Ishimori et al. 2004
14:								
Ath13:								
D14Mit60	15 (10–40)	2.5	(B6.129-*Apoe*$^{-/-}$ × FVB.129-*Apoe*$^{-/-}$) F_2	M/	B6 (dom)	10	14q11-22[g], 10q21-23[g], 8p21, 13q12, 3p21	Dansky et al. 2002
14–52 Mb	22	2.6	(A × B6.129-*Apoe*$^{-/-}$) F_2	F	B6 (add)		14q11-22[g], 10q21-23[g], 8p21, 13q12, 3p21	N. Ishimori and B. Paigen, unpublished data
16:								
D16Mit103	22	2.5	(B6.129-*Apoe*$^{-/-}$ × FVB.129-*Apoe*$^{-/-}$) F_2	F+M		6	3q27-29[g], 3q13[g]	Dansky et al. 2002
18:								
D18Mit23	21	3.1	(B6.129-*Ldlr*$^{-/-}$ × FVB.129-*Ldlr*$^{-/-}$) F_2	F, M	B6		5q23-31, 18q12	Teupser and Breslow 2003
18–52 Mb	22	2.5	(A × B6.129-*Apoe*$^{-/-}$) F_2	F	B6 (add)		5q23-31, 18q12	N. Ishimori and B. Paigen, unpublished data
19:								
Ath16:								
D19Mit120	41 (6–54)	3.8	(B6.129-*Apoe*$^{-/-}$ × FVB.129-*Apoe*$^{-/-}$) F_2	M/	FVB (dom)	16	10q23-25[g]	Dansky et al. 2002
Unknown:								
Ath2:		...	A × B RI, B × A RI					Paigen 1995

[a] Peak marker. The non-MIT markers are all SNP markers with their positions (e.g., 1–169 Mb denotes a SNP on chromosome 1 at 169 Mb).
[b] Genetic distances were retrieved from MGI.
[c] RI strains; F2, intercross.
[d] F = only females were studied; M = only males were studied; F/ (M/) = mice of both sexes were studied, and QTLs were found in only in females (males); F, M = QTLs were detected in both female and male mice; F+M = data from both females and males were used in the same analysis.
[e] add = additive; dom = dominant; rec = recessive.
[f] Human homologous regions of the peak cM of mouse QTLs were retrieved from MGI Whole Genome Orthology Map.
[g] Falls within a QTL for either MI, CAD, ACS, or CIMT in humans (see table 1).
[h] Interacting QTL.

found that only a polymorphism of *TNFSF4* was significantly associated with the risk of MI and CAD in humans (Wang et al. 2005*b*). We therefore identified a human atherosclerosis gene from a mouse QTL.

Making More Mouse Crosses

Although 21 mouse atherosclerosis QTLs have been revealed, additional mouse crosses will expedite finding genes that regulate atherosclerosis, for the following reasons. First, among the 25 individual mouse atherosclerosis QTLs published since 2003, 14 are new, and only 11 are replicates of QTLs found before, suggesting that the mouse QTL map has not been saturated and that new QTLs will be identified in new crosses. Second, additional mouse crosses may confirm previously found QTLs (nearly half of the mouse QTLs are found in only one cross) and may provide more strains for haplotype analysis (Wang et al. 2004*b*; Wang and Paigen 2005*b*). Third, 11 of the 13 crosses use B6 as the susceptible parent. Using different susceptible strains—such as SM/J, SWR/J, and NON/LtJ—may reveal different QTLs. Fourth, there are 27 human and only 21 mouse QTLs, and 10 of the 27 human ones have no concordant mouse QTL. Additional mouse crosses may reveal QTLs concordant with these human QTLs and may expedite finding their underlying genes with the mouse-to-human strategy.

Including Plaque Stability and Coronary Atherosclerosis as Phenotypes

Effective treatment of human atherosclerosis should include stabilizing plaque as well as reducing the accumulation of plasma lipids, and consequently the formation of fibrolipid cores in the arterial wall. So far, the only atherosclerosis phenotype used in mouse genomewide-scan studies is the size of the lipid-staining lesions. Thus, some of the genes identified may regulate intimal lipid deposition but not plaque stability. The latter may be more relevant to clinical events of human atherosclerosis, because ACS is usually caused by plaque rupture and the subsequently formed thrombi that obstruct coronary arteries rather than increased plaque size. Thus, future genomewide scans should include phenotypes that reflect stability of atherosclerotic plaques, such as thickness and rupture of fibrous cap and formation of intraplaque hemorrhage, thrombus, and buried fibrous cap. Plaque rupture has been observed in B6 mice with deficiency of *Apoe* when mice are fed either chow (Rosenfeld et al. 2000) or a diet with high-cholesterol content (Johnson and Jackson 2001; Williams et al. 2002; Johnson et al. 2005). The most frequently observed site of rupture is the innominate (brachiocephalic) artery, as shown in the studies just cited, and genes controlling atherosclerosis in the innominate artery and aortic root may be different (Reardon et al. 2003; Teupser et al. 2004). The vessels most relevant to human atherosclerotic diseases are, of course, the coronary arteries. Advanced atherosclerotic lesions do occur in mouse coronary arteries when mice are deficient in either *Apoe, Ldlr,* both *Apoe* and *Ldlr,* or *Scarb1* (encoding scavenger receptor class B, member 1) and when they are fed either chow (Braun et al. 2002) or a diet with high-cholesterol content (Caligiuri et al. 1999; Calara et al. 2001). Thus, future genomewide scans in mice perhaps should include coronary atherosclerosis as a phenotype.

Finding Genes Regulating Human Atherosclerosis by Studying QTLs for Both Atherosclerosis and HDL

So far, 37 mouse and 30 human HDL-regulating QTLs have been identified (Wang and Paigen 2005*a*). Some of the genes underlying these QTLs may also regulate atherogenesis, given the compelling evidence that HDL protects against atherosclerosis (Brewer 2004; Gotto and Brinton 2004). Thus, human atherosclerosis-regulating genes can be identified by either (1) finding the gene underlying a mouse atherosclerosis QTL and then testing it for a role in human atherosclerosis or (2) finding the gene underlying a mouse HDL QTL and then testing whether it regulates HDL levels and atherosclerosis in humans.

Integrating Traditional Genetic Approaches with New Genetic, Genomic, and Bioinformatic Resources and Tools

A QTL interval is usually large and typically contains hundreds of genes. The first step toward finding a causal gene is to narrow the QTL. QTL-narrowing strategies that take advantage of recombinations in mouse crosses include one or more of the following: (1) interval-specific congenic strains, (2) advanced intercross lines, (3) heterogeneous stocks, (4) recombinant inbred (RI) segregation test, (5) recombinant progeny testing, (6) selective phenotyping, (7) yin-yang cross, and (8) collaborative cross.

Interval-specific congenic strains.—Mice that are recombinant in the QTL region are crossed for several generations with the background parental strain to eliminate alleles from the donor parental strain at all QTLs affecting the trait (other than the QTL being mapped). Animals are then intercrossed, and homozygotes for the recombinant haplotype are selected to establish one congenic strain. Several congenic strains with overlapping regions can differentiate which region contains the QTL gene (Darvasi 1998). Recently, two sets of mice with overlapping congenic regions, covering the whole genome, were generated; one set is B6.DBA/2, the other is B6.CAST. These sets will facilitate narrowing QTLs from B6 × DBA/2 and B6 × CAST crosses (Iakoubova et al. 2001).

Advanced intercross lines.—Mice from two inbred progenitor strains are crossed to yield F1 offspring, which are intercrossed to produce F2 offspring. Fifty F2 × F2 matings are made (avoiding brother-sister matings) to produce F3 offspring, and fifty F3 × F3 matings are made (avoiding brother-sister and cousin matings) to produce F4 offspring, and so on, until the desired advanced intercross (F5, F6, and so on) is attained. Thus, the many recombinations required to narrow a QTL accumulate in a relatively small final population (Darvasi 1998).

Heterogeneous stocks.—Heterogeneous stocks are derived from multiple inbred strains (eight strains in current stocks) through continued intercrossing. They are essentially advanced intercross lines made from multiple strains instead of two (Mott et al. 2000).

RI segregation test.—This strategy requires an existing set of RI strains and takes advantage of the high mapping resolution of RI strains and applies it to QTL mapping. An RI strain with a recombinant haplotype in the region of interest is crossed with both parental strains to produce two separate F1 populations. Intercrossing these F1 individuals then produces F2 mice. By analysis of the F2 populations, a QTL can be located relative to the recombination point, because the QTL previously mapped to this region will segregate in only one of the two F2 populations (Darvasi 1998).

Recombinant progeny testing.—Mice carrying a recombinant chromosome in the QTL region are crossed with one of the parental strains, and their progeny are phenotyped to determine the location of the QTL relative to the recombination point (Darvasi 1998).

Selective phenotyping.—In a large intercross or backcross population, only individuals recombinant at an interval previously found to contain a QTL are phenotyped, because only those individuals contribute to further mapping accuracy (Darvasi 1998).

Yin-yang cross.—Yin-yang cross is a generalization of the RI segregation test that uses inbred strains as if they are RI lines (Shifman and Darvasi 2005). This method is based on the observation that the many inbred laboratory mice are derived from a limited number of founder populations, so the large number of recombination events accumulated in inbred strains since their origin can be used to fine map a QTL to a very small region. The statistical analysis of a yin-yang cross depends on the knowledge of the SNPs of the strains used and is actually similar to haplotype analysis of multiple crosses (Hitzemann et al. 2002; Park et al. 2003; Manenti et al. 2004; Wang et al. 2004*b*).

Collaborative cross.—The collaborative cross is not an existing resource, but it has been recently proposed (Churchill et al. 2004). It is a panel of 1,000 RI strains derived from eight inbred strains. With an estimated 135,000 unique recombination events and known genotypes in the whole panel, QTLs can be mapped to a very small interval without making any crosses.

However, all these approaches require many recombinant animals, which makes the analyses slow, labor intensive, and sometimes difficult to generate because of the existence of recombination hotspots (Kelmenson et al. 2005). In addition to the above strategies, new genetic and genomic resources, especially mouse and human genome sequences, have led to new strategies in narrowing a QTL and even in identifying its underlying gene by analysis of combined cross data, comparison of mouse and human homologous QTLs, analysis of SNPs and haplotypes in multiple strains, and detection of *in silico* QTLs, as discussed by Wang and Paigen (2005*b*). It should be cautioned that successfully identifying a QTL gene from haplotype analysis and *in silico* QTL mapping depends in large part on detailed genome sequence/SNP information in many strains, which is only partly available now. A complete sequence of more mouse strains is likely to fully empower haplotype analysis and *in silico* QTL mapping, as reviewed by Flint et al. (2005). Once a QTL is narrowed with the above approaches, candidate genes can be tested for sequence and expression difference between parental strains (Wang and Paigen 2005*b*). To study the genetics of gene expression, Jansen and Nap proposed a genomewide scan using gene-expression data as phenotypes that can be obtained from microarray analysis (Jansen and Nap 2001); chromosome segments thus obtained are called "expression QTLs" (eQTLs). Because the vast majority of eQTL genes are *cis*-regulated (Bystrykh et al. 2005; Chesler et al. 2005; Hubner et al. 2005), candidate genes of a physiological QTL (pQTL) (with use of clinical traits as phenotype) can be identified by overlapping such a pQTL with eQTLs: differentially expressed genes in a pQTL region could be good candidates (Schadt et al. 2003; Chesler et al. 2005; Hubner et al. 2005).

Using Mutagenesis as a Complementary Approach

Although the QTL approach takes advantage of spontaneous mutations that had accumulated in the past and had been fixed in the various inbred strains of laboratory mice (Lander and Botstein 1989), a mutagenesis approach is capable of generating, in a short time, large numbers of mutations across the genome (Balling 2001). Very efficient at low toxicity, ENU is an alkylating mutagen that induces $\sim 1 \times 10^{-3}$ random point mutations per locus. It affects germ cells, particularly spermatogonial stem cells. Once adult mice are mutagenized, they are bred, and offspring abnormalities are detected in high-throughput phenotyping screens. Deviants are tested for heritability (Balling 2001). The large-scale and high-throughput features of mutagenesis can potentially generate mutations in every gene. Some of these mutations will help us understand a gene's functions. The HLB Mutagenesis Program at The Jackson Laboratory is using ENU mutagenesis to identify genes regulating a wide range of cardiovascular phenotypes (Svenson et al. 2003). Atherosclerosis in mutagenized mice cannot be screened with either cross-sectional (Paigen et al. 1987*c*) or *en face* analysis (Palinski et al. 1994), because deviant mice need to be kept for breeding. Instead, noninvasive methods should be used. Magnetic resonance imaging (MRI) provides high-resolution images on not only lesion size (Fayad et al. 1998; Choudhury et al. 2002; Hockings et al. 2002) but also its components (lipid core and cap) (McAteer et al. 2004; Schneider et al. 2004). MRI could be used for an atherosclerosis screen in mutagenized mice if the throughput could be increased.

Summary

The most efficient way to find atherosclerosis-regulating genes in humans is to first find orthologs underlying concordant QTLs, preferably replicate ones, in the mouse. Such QTLs will increase in numbers as new mouse crosses are performed, and they can be rapidly narrowed by analysis of combined cross data, *in silico* QTL analyses, and haplotype analyses. Because replicated QTLs are likely caused by conserved ancestral alleles, causal genes within the narrowed region should exhibit sequence and/or expression differences consistent with their allele effects in all parental strains. These candidate genes, if associated with atherosclerotic diseases in humans, can then be tested, positively identified, and their functions studied in transgenic and/or knockout mice.

Acknowledgments

This work was supported by National Institutes of Health grants HL66611 and HL77796 (to B.P.) and HL70486 (to X.W.) and from American Heart Association grant AHA430381N (to X.W.). We thank Michael Marion and Ray Lambert, for helping to prepare the manuscript; Jennifer L. Torrance, for helping to prepare the graphics; and Dr. Keith DiPetrillo, for critically reviewing the manuscript.

Web Resources

The URLs for data presented herein are as follows:

Center for Medical Genetics, http://research.marshfieldclinic.org/genetics/
Ensembl Human Genome Browser, http://www.ensembl.org/Homo_sapiens/
MGI, http://www.informatics.jax.org/
MGI Whole Genome Orthology Map, http://www.informatics.jax.org/reports/homologymap/mouse_human.shtml
Online Mendelian Inheritance in Man (OMIM), http://www.ncbi.nlm.nih.gov/Omim/ (for *ACE, ADRB2, ALOX5AP, APOE, F7, FGB, GP1BA, MMP3, MMP9, MTHFR, NOS3, PON1, TGFB1, THBS2, THBS4, TLR4, TNFSF4, MEF2A, POMC, CTLA4,* and *EN2*)

References

Agah R, Topol EJ (2002) Genetic testing for coronary heart disease: the approaching frontier. Expert Rev Mol Diagn 2: 448–460
Allayee H, Ghazalpour A, Lusis AJ (2003) Using mice to dissect genetic factors in atherosclerosis. Arterioscler Thromb Vasc Biol 23:1501–1509
Balling R (2001) ENU mutagenesis: analyzing gene function in mice. Annu Rev Genomics Hum Genet 2:463–492
Ben-Asher E, Lancet D (2004) 5-Lipoxygenase activating protein (ALOX5AP): association with cardiovascular infarction and stroke. Isr Med Assoc J 6:318–319
Bhagavatula MR, Fan C, Shen GQ, Cassano J, Plow EF, Topol EJ, Wang Q (2004) Transcription factor MEF2A mutations in patients with coronary artery disease. Hum Mol Genet 13: 3181–3188
Braun A, Trigatti BL, Post MJ, Sato K, Simons M, Edelberg JM, Rosenberg RD, Schrenzel M, Krieger M (2002) Loss of SR-BI expression leads to the early onset of occlusive atherosclerotic coronary artery disease, spontaneous myocardial infarctions, severe cardiac dysfunction, and premature death in apolipoprotein E-deficient mice. Circ Res 90:270–276
Brewer HB Jr (2004) High-density lipoproteins: a new potential therapeutic target for the prevention of cardiovascular disease. Arterioscler Thromb Vasc Biol 24:387–391
Broeckel U, Hengstenberg C, Mayer B, Holmer S, Martin LJ, Comuzzie AG, Blangero J, Nurnberg P, Reis A, Riegger GA, Jacob HJ, Schunkert H (2002) A comprehensive linkage analysis for myocardial infarction and its related risk factors. Nat Genet 30:210–214
Bystrykh L, Weersing E, Dontje B, Sutton S, Pletcher MT, Wiltshire T, Su AI, Vellenga E, Wang J, Manly KF, Lu L, Chesler EJ, Alberts R, Jansen RC, Williams RW, Cooke MP, de Haan G (2005) Uncovering regulatory pathways that affect hematopoietic stem cell function using "genetical genomics." Nat Genet 37:225–232
Calara F, Silvestre M, Casanada F, Yuan N, Napoli C, Palinski W (2001) Spontaneous plaque rupture and secondary thrombosis in apolipoprotein E-deficient and LDL receptor-deficient mice. J Pathol 195:257–263
Caligiuri G, Levy B, Pernow J, Thoren P, Hansson GK (1999) Myocardial infarction mediated by endothelin receptor signaling in hypercholesterolemic mice. Proc Natl Acad Sci USA 96:6920–6924
Carlson CS, Eberle MA, Kruglyak L, Nickerson DA (2004) Mapping complex disease loci in whole-genome association studies. Nature 429:446–452
Chesler EJ, Lu L, Shou S, Qu Y, Gu J, Wang J, Hsu HC, Mountz JD, Baldwin NE, Langston MA, Threadgill DW, Manly KF, Williams RW (2005) Complex trait analysis of gene expression uncovers polygenic and pleiotropic networks that modulate nervous system function. Nat Genet 37:233–242
Choudhury RP, Aguinaldo JG, Rong JX, Kulak JL, Kulak AR, Reis ED, Fallon JT, Fuster V, Fisher EA, Fayad ZA (2002) Atherosclerotic lesions in genetically modified mice quanti-

fied in vivo by non-invasive high-resolution magnetic resonance microscopy. Atherosclerosis 162:315–321

Churchill GA, Airey DC, Allayee H, Angel JM, Attie AD, Beatty J, Beavis WD, et al (2004) The Collaborative Cross, a community resource for the genetic analysis of complex traits. Nat Genet 36:1133–1137

Colinayo VV, Qiao JH, Wang X, Krass KL, Schadt E, Lusis AJ, Drake TA (2003) Genetic loci for diet-induced atherosclerosis lesions and plasma lipids in mice. Mamm Genome 14:464–471

Dansky HM, Shu P, Donavan M, Montagno J, Nagle DL, Smutko JS, Roy N, Whiteing S, Barrios J, McBride TJ, Smith JD, Duyk G, Breslow JL, Moore KJ (2002) A phenotype-sensitizing Apoe-deficient genetic background reveals novel atherosclerosis predisposition loci in the mouse. Genetics 160: 1599–1608

Darvasi A (1998) Experimental strategies for the genetic dissection of complex traits in animal models. Nat Genet 18: 19–24

Durrington PN, Mackness B, Mackness MI (2001) Paraoxonase and atherosclerosis. Arterioscler Thromb Vasc Biol 21: 473–480

Fayad ZA, Fallon JT, Shinnar M, Wehrli S, Dansky HM, Poon M, Badimon JJ, Charlton SA, Fisher EA, Breslow JL, Fuster V (1998) Noninvasive in vivo high-resolution magnetic resonance imaging of atherosclerotic lesions in genetically engineered mice. Circulation 98:1541–1547

Flint J, Valdar W, Shifman S, Mott R (2005) Strategies for mapping and cloning quantitative trait genes in rodents. Nat Rev Genet 6:271–286

Fox CS, Cupples LA, Chazaro I, Polak JF, Wolf PA, D'Agostino RB, Ordovas JM, O'Donnell CJ (2004) Genomewide linkage analysis for internal carotid artery intimal medial thickness: evidence for linkage to chromosome 12. Am J Hum Genet 74:253–261

Francke S, Manraj M, Lacquemant C, Lecoeur C, Lepretre F, Passa P, Hebe A, Corset L, Yan SL, Lahmidi S, Jankee S, Gunness TK, Ramjuttun US, Balgobin V, Dina C, Froguel P (2001) A genome-wide scan for coronary heart disease suggests in Indo-Mauritians a susceptibility locus on chromosome 16p13 and replicates linkage with the metabolic syndrome on 3q27. Hum Mol Genet 10:2751–2765

Geng YJ (2001) Biologic effect and molecular regulation of vascular apoptosis in atherosclerosis. Curr Atheroscler Rep 3:234–242

Gharani N, Benayed R, Mancuso V, Brzustowicz LM, Millonig JH (2004) Association of the homeobox transcription factor, ENGRAILED 2, 3, with autism spectrum disorder. Mol Psychiatry 9:474–484

Gotto AM Jr, Brinton EA (2004) Assessing low levels of high-density lipoprotein cholesterol as a risk factor in coronary heart disease: a working group report and update. J Am Coll Cardiol 43:717–724

Hansson GK, Libby P, Schonbeck U, Yan ZQ (2002) Innate and adaptive immunity in the pathogenesis of atherosclerosis. Circ Res 91:281–291

Harrap SB, Zammit KS, Wong ZY, Williams FM, Bahlo M, Tonkin AM, Anderson ST (2002) Genome-wide linkage analysis of the acute coronary syndrome suggests a locus on chromosome 2. Arterioscler Thromb Vasc Biol 22:874–878

Hauser ER, Crossman DC, Granger CB, Haines JL, Jones CJH, Mooser V, McAdam B, et al (2004) A genomewide scan for early-onset coronary artery disease in 438 families: the GENECARD Study. Am J Hum Genet 75:436–447

Helgadottir A, Manolescu A, Thorleifsson G, Gretarsdottir S, Jonsdottir H, Thorsteinsdottir U, Samani NJ, et al (2004) The gene encoding 5-lipoxygenase activating protein confers risk of myocardial infarction and stroke. Nat Genet 36:233–239

Hitzemann R, Malmanger B, Cooper S, Coulombe S, Reed C, Demarest K, Koyner J, Cipp L, Flint J, Talbot C, Rademacher B, Buck K, McCaughran J Jr (2002) Multiple cross mapping (MCM) markedly improves the localization of a QTL for ethanol-induced activation. Genes Brain Behav 1: 214–222

Hixson JE, Almasy L, Cole S, Birnbaum S, Mitchell BD, Mahaney MC, Stern MP, MacCluer JW, Blangero J, Comuzzie AG (1999) Normal variation in leptin levels in associated with polymorphisms in the proopiomelanocortin gene, *POMC*. J Clin Endocrinol Metab 84:3187–3191

Hockings PD, Roberts T, Galloway GJ, Reid DG, Harris DA, Vidgeon-Hart M, Groot PH, Suckling KE, Benson GM (2002) Repeated three-dimensional magnetic resonance imaging of atherosclerosis development in innominate arteries of low-density lipoprotein receptor-knockout mice. Circulation 106: 1716–1721

Hubner N, Wallace CA, Zimdahl H, Petretto E, Schulz H, Maciver F, Mueller M, Hummel O, Monti J, Zidek V, Musilova A, Kren V, Causton H, Game L, Born G, Schmidt S, Muller A, Cook SA, Kurtz TW, Whittaker J, Pravenec M, Aitman TJ (2005) Integrated transcriptional profiling and linkage analysis for identification of genes underlying disease. Nat Genet 37:243–253

Humphries SE, Morgan L (2004) Genetic risk factors for stroke and carotid atherosclerosis: insights into pathophysiology from candidate gene approaches. Lancet Neurol 3:227–235

Iakoubova OA, Olsson CL, Dains KM, Ross DA, Andalibi A, Lau K, Choi J, Kalcheva I, Cunanan M, Louie J, Nimon V, Machrus M, Bentley LG, Beauheim C, Silvey S, Cavalcoli J, Lusis AJ, West DB (2001) Genome-tagged mice (GTM): two sets of genome-wide congenic strains. Genomics 74:89–104

Ishimori N, Li R, Kelmenson PM, Korstanje R, Walsh KA, Churchill GA, Forsman-Semb K, Paigen B (2004) Quantitative trait loci analysis for plasma HDL-cholesterol concentrations and atherosclerosis susceptibility between inbred mouse strains C57BL/6J and 129S1/SvImJ. Arterioscler Thromb Vasc Biol 24:161–166

Jansen RC, Nap JP (2001) Genetical genomics: the added value from segregation. Trends Genet 17:388–391

Jawien J, Nastalek P, Korbut R (2004) Mouse models of experimental atherosclerosis. J Physiol Pharmacol 55:503–517

Johnson J, Carson K, Williams H, Karanam S, Newby A, Angelini G, George S, Jackson C (2005) Plaque rupture after short periods of fat feeding in the apolipoprotein E-knockout mouse: model characterization and effects of pravastatin treatment. Circulation 111:1422–1430

Johnson JL, Jackson CL (2001) Atherosclerotic plaque rupture in the apolipoprotein E knockout mouse. Atherosclerosis 154: 399–406

Kelmenson PM, Petkov P, Wang X, Higgins DC, Paigen BJ, Paigen K (2005) A torrid zone on mouse chromosome 1 containing a cluster of recombinational hotspots. Genetics 169: 833–841

Korstanje R, DiPetrillo K (2004) Unraveling the genetics of chronic kidney disease using animal models. Am J Physiol Renal Physiol 287:F347–F352

Korstanje R, Eriksson P, Samnegard A, Olsson PG, Forsman-Semb K, Sen S, Churchill GA, Rollins J, Harris S, Hamsten A, Paigen B (2004) Locating *Ath8,* a locus for murine atherosclerosis susceptibility and testing several of its candidate genes in mice and humans. Atherosclerosis 177:443–450

Krude H, Biebermann H, Luck W, Horn R, Brabant G, Gruters A (1998) Severe early-onset obesity, adrenal insufficiency and red hair pigmentation caused by *POMC* mutations in humans. Nat Genet 19:155–157

Lander ES, Botstein D (1989) Mapping Mendelian factors underlying quantitative traits using RFLP linkage maps. Genetics 121:185–199

Lohmussaar E, Gschwendtner A, Mueller JC, Org T, Wichmann E, Hamann G, Meitinger T, Dichgans M (2005) *ALOX5AP* gene and the *PDE4D* gene in a central European population of stroke patients. Stroke 36:731–736

Lusis AJ, Mar R, Pajukanta P (2004) Genetics of atherosclerosis. Annu Rev Genomics Hum Genet 5:189–218

Manenti G, Galbiati F, Gianni-Barrera R, Pettinicchio A, Acevedo A, Dragani TA (2004) Haplotype sharing suggests that a genomic segment containing six genes accounts for the pulmonary adenoma susceptibility 1 (*Pas1*) locus activity in mice. Oncogene 23:4495–4504

Manolio TA, Boerwinkle E, O'Donnell CJ, Wilson AF (2004) Genetics of ultrasonographic carotid atherosclerosis. Arterioscler Thromb Vasc Biol 24:1567–1577

McAteer MA, Schneider JE, Clarke K, Neubauer S, Channon KM, Choudhury RP (2004) Quantification and 3D reconstruction of atherosclerotic plaque components in apolipoprotein E knockout mice using ex vivo high-resolution MRI. Arterioscler Thromb Vasc Biol 24:2384–2390

McCarthy JJ, Parker A, Salem R, Moliterno DJ, Wang Q, Plow EF, Rao S, Shen G, Rogers WJ, Newby LK, Cannata R, Glatt K, Topol EJ (2004) Large scale association analysis for identification of genes underlying premature coronary heart disease: cumulative perspective from analysis of 111 candidate genes. J Med Genet 41:334–341

Mehrabian M, Allayee H, Wong J, Shi W, Wang XP, Shaposhnik Z, Funk CD, Lusis AJ, Shih W (2002) Identification of 5-lipoxygenase as a major gene contributing to atherosclerosis susceptibility in mice. Circ Res 91:120–126

Mehrabian M, Wong J, Wang X, Jiang Z, Shi W, Fogelman AM, Lusis AJ (2001) Genetic locus in mice that blocks development of atherosclerosis despite extreme hyperlipidemia. Circ Res 89:125–130

Meir KS, Leitersdorf E (2004) Atherosclerosis in the apolipoprotein-E-deficient mouse: a decade of progress. Arterioscler Thromb Vasc Biol 24:1006–1014

Mott R, Talbot CJ, Turri MG, Collins AC, Flint J (2000) A new method for fine mapping quantitative trait loci in outbred animal stocks. Proc Natl Acad Sci USA 97:12649–12654

Mu JL, Naggert JK, Svenson KL, Collin GB, Kim JH, McFarland C, Nishina PM, Levine DM, Williams KJ, Paigen B (1999) Quantitative trait loci analysis for the differences in susceptibility to atherosclerosis and diabetes between inbred mouse strains C57BL/6J and C57BLKS/J. J Lipid Res 40: 1328–1335

Ozaki K, Ohnishi Y, Iida A, Sekine A, Yamada R, Tsunoda T, Sato H, Sato H, Hori M, Nakamura Y, Tanaka T (2002) Functional SNPs in the lymphotoxin-α gene that are associated with susceptibility to myocardial infarction. Nat Genet 32:650–654

Paigen B (1995) Genetics of responsiveness to high-fat and high-cholesterol diets in the mouse. Am J Clin Nutr 62:458S–462S

Paigen B, Albee D, Holmes PA, Mitchell D (1987*a*) Genetic analysis of murine strains C57BL/6J and C3H/HeJ to confirm the map position of *Ath-1,* a gene determining atherosclerosis susceptibility. Biochem Genet 25:501–511

Paigen B, Mitchell D, Reue K, Morrow A, Lusis AJ, LeBoeuf RC (1987*b*) *Ath-1,* a gene determining atherosclerosis susceptibility and high density lipoprotein levels in mice. Proc Natl Acad Sci USA 84:3763–3767

Paigen B, Morrow A, Holmes PA, Mitchell D, Williams RA (1987*c*) Quantitative assessment of atherosclerotic lesions in mice. Atherosclerosis 68:231–240

Pajukanta P, Cargill M, Viitanen L, Nuotio I, Kareinen A, Perola M, Terwilliger JD, Kempas E, Daly M, Lilja H, Rioux JD, Brettin T, Viikari JSA, Rönnemaa T, Laakso M, Lander ES, Peltonen L (2000) Two loci on chromosomes 2 and X for premature coronary heart disease identified in early- and late-settlement populations of Finland. Am J Hum Genet 67:1481–1493

Palinski W, Ord VA, Plump AS, Breslow JL, Steinberg D, Witztum JL (1994) ApoE-deficient mice are a model of lipoprotein oxidation in atherogenesis: demonstration of oxidation-specific epitopes in lesions and high titers of autoantibodies to malondialdehyde-lysine in serum. Arterioscler Thromb 14: 605–616

Park YG, Clifford R, Buetow KH, Hunter KW (2003) Multiple cross and inbred strain haplotype mapping of complex-trait candidate genes. Genome Res 13:118–121

Phelan SA, Beier DR, Higgins DC, Paigen B (2002) Confirmation and high resolution mapping of an atherosclerosis susceptibility gene in mice on Chromosome 1. Mamm Genome 13:548–553

Pollanen PJ, Karhunen PJ, Mikkelsson J, Laippala P, Perola M, Penttila A, Mattila KM, Koivula T, Lehtimaki T (2001) Coronary artery complicated lesion area is related to functional polymorphism of matrix metalloproteinase 9 gene: an autopsy study. Arterioscler Thromb Vasc Biol 21:1446–1450

Purcell MK, Mu JL, Higgins DC, Elango R, Whitmore H, Harris S, Paigen B (2001) Fine mapping of *Ath6,* a quantitative trait locus for atherosclerosis in mice. Mamm Genome 12:495–500

Reardon CA, Blachowicz L, Lukens J, Nissenbaum M, Getz GS (2003) Genetic background selectively influences innominate artery atherosclerosis: immune system deficiency as a probe. Arterioscler Thromb Vasc Biol 23:1449–1454

Rosenfeld ME, Polinsky P, Virmani R, Kauser K, Rubanyi G, Schwartz SM (2000) Advanced atherosclerotic lesions in the innominate artery of the ApoE knockout mouse. Arterioscler Thromb Vasc Biol 20:2587–2592

Schadt EE, Monks SA, Drake TA, Lusis AJ, Che N, Colinayo V, Ruff TG, Milligan SB, Lamb JR, Cavet G, Linsley PS, Mao M, Stoughton RB, Friend SH (2003) Genetics of gene expression surveyed in maize, mouse and man. Nature 422: 297–302

Schneider JE, McAteer MA, Tyler DJ, Clarke K, Channon KM, Choudhury RP, Neubauer S (2004) High-resolution, multi-contrast three-dimensional-MRI characterizes atherosclerotic plaque composition in ApoE$^{-/-}$ mice ex vivo. J Magn Reson Imaging 20:981–989

Seidelmann SB, De Luca C, Leibel RL, Breslow JL, Tall AR, Welch CL (2005) Quantitative trait locus mapping of genetic modifiers of metabolic syndrome and atherosclerosis in low-density lipoprotein receptor-deficient mice: identification of a locus for metabolic syndrome and increased atherosclerosis on chromosome 4. Arterioscler Thromb Vasc Biol 25: 204–210

Shifman S, Darvasi A (2005) Mouse inbred strain sequence information and yin-yang crosses for quantitative trait locus fine mapping. Genetics 169:849–854

Smith J (2003) Quantitative trait locus mapping for atherosclerosis susceptibility. Curr Opin Lipidol 14:499–504

Steinberg D, Witztum JL (2002) Is the oxidative modification hypothesis relevant to human atherosclerosis? Do the antioxidant trials conducted to date refute the hypothesis? Circulation 105:2107–2111

Stewart-Phillips JL, Lough J, Skamene E (1989) ATH-3, a new gene for atherosclerosis in the mouse. Clin Invest Med 12: 121–126

Stoll M, Kwitek-Black AE, Cowley AW Jr, Harris EL, Harrap SB, Krieger JE, Printz MP, Provoost AP, Sassard J, Jacob HJ (2000) New target regions for human hypertension via comparative genomics. Genome Res 10:473–482

Sugiyama F, Churchill GA, Higgins DC, Johns C, Makaritsis KP, Gavras H, Paigen B (2001) Concordance of murine quantitative trait loci for salt-induced hypertension with rat and human loci. Genomics 71:70–77

Svenson KL, Bogue MA, Peters LL (2003) Invited review: identifying new mouse models of cardiovascular disease: a review of high-throughput screens of mutagenized and inbred strains. J Appl Physiol 94:1650–1659

Teupser D, Breslow JL (2003) Quantitative trait locus mapping of atherosclerotic lesions in a cross between B6.129-*Ldlr*$^{-/-}$ and FVB.129-*Ldlr*$^{-/-}$ mice. Paper presented at the 5th Annual Conference on Arteriosclerosis, Thrombosis and Vascular Biology, San Francisco, May 6–8, 2004

Teupser D, Pavlides S, Tan M, Gutierrez-Ramos JC, Kolbeck R, Breslow JL (2004) Major reduction of atherosclerosis in fractalkine (CX3CL1)-deficient mice is at the brachiocephalic artery, not the aortic root. Proc Natl Acad Sci USA 101: 17795–17800

Ueda H, Howson JM, Esposito L, Heward J, Snook H, Chamberlain G, Rainbow DB, et al (2003) Association of the T-cell regulatory gene CTLA4 with susceptibility to autoimmune disease. Nature 423:506–511

Wang D, Yang H, Quinones MJ, Bulnes-Enriquez I, Jimenez X, De La Rosa R, Modilevsky T, Yu K, Li Y, Taylor KD, Hsueh WA, Hodis HN, Rotter JI (2005*a*) A genome-wide scan for carotid artery intima-media thickness: the Mexican-American Coronary Artery Disease family study. Stroke 36: 540–545

Wang L, Fan C, Topol SE, Topol EJ, Wang Q (2003*a*) Mutation of MEF2A in an inherited disorder with features of coronary artery disease. Science 302:1578–1581

Wang Q, Rao S, Shen G-Q, Li L, Moliterno DJ, Newby LK, Rogers WJ, Cannata R, Zirzow E, Elston RC, Topol EJ (2004*a*) Premature myocardial infarction novel susceptibility locus on chromosome 1p34-36 identified by genomewide linkage analysis. Am J Hum Genet 74:262–271

Wang S, Shi W, Wang X, Lusis AJ (2003*b*) Identification of a locus in mice that influences aortic aneurysm formation. Circulation 108:IV–177

Wang X, Korstanje R, Higgins D, Paigen B (2004*b*) Haplotype analysis in multiple crosses to identify a QTL gene. Genome Res 14:1767–1772

Wang X, Paigen B (2005*a*) Genetics of variation in HDL cholesterol in humans and mice. Circ Res 96:27–42

——— (2005*b*) Genome-wide search for new genes controlling plasma lipid concentrations in mice and humans. Curr Opin Lipidol 16:127–137

Wang X, Ria M, Kelmenson PM, Eriksson P, Higgins DC, Samnegard A, Petros C, Rollins J, Bennet AM, Wiman B, de Faire U, Wennberg C, Olsson PG, Ishii N, Sugamura K, Hamsten A, Forsman-Semb K, Lagercrantz J, Paigen B (2005*b*) Positional identification of *TNFSF4,* encoding OX40 ligand, as a gene that influences atherosclerosis susceptibility. Nat Genet 37:365–372

Welch CL, Bretschger S, Latib N, Bezouevski M, Guo Y, Pleskac N, Liang CP, Barlow C, Dansky H, Breslow JL, Tall AR (2001) Localization of atherosclerosis susceptibility loci to chromosomes 4 and 6 using the Ldlr knockout mouse model. Proc Natl Acad Sci USA 98:7946–7951

Wheeler JG, Keavney BD, Watkins H, Collins R, Danesh J (2004) Four paraoxonase gene polymorphisms in 11 212 cases of coronary heart disease and 12 786 controls: meta-analysis of 43 studies. Lancet 363:689–695

Williams H, Johnson JL, Carson KG, Jackson CL (2002) Characteristics of intact and ruptured atherosclerotic plaques in brachiocephalic arteries of apolipoprotein E knockout mice. Arterioscler Thromb Vasc Biol 22:788–792

Zhang B, Ye S, Herrmann SM, Eriksson P, de Maat M, Evans A, Arveiler D, Luc G, Cambien F, Hamsten A, Watkins H, Henney AM (1999) Functional polymorphism in the regulatory region of gelatinase B gene in relation to severity of coronary atherosclerosis. Circulation 99:1788–1794

Biotin-Responsive Basal Ganglia Disease Maps to 2q36.3 and Is Due to Mutations in *SLC19A3*

Wen-Qi Zeng,[1,*] Eiman Al-Yamani,[1,2,*] James S. Acierno, Jr.,[1,†] Susan Slaugenhaupt,[1] Tammy Gillis,[1] Marcy E. MacDonald,[1] Pinar T. Ozand,[2] and James F. Gusella[1]

[1]Molecular Neurogenetics Unit, Center for Human Genetic Research, Massachusetts General Hospital, Charlestown; and [2]King Faisal Specialist Hospital and Research Centre, Riyadh, Saudi Arabia

Biotin-responsive basal ganglia disease (BBGD) is a recessive disorder with childhood onset that presents as a subacute encephalopathy, with confusion, dysarthria, and dysphagia, and that progresses to severe cogwheel rigidity, dystonia, quadriparesis, and eventual death, if left untreated. BBGD symptoms disappear within a few days with the administration of high doses of biotin (5–10 mg/kg/d). On brain magnetic resonance imaging examination, patients display central bilateral necrosis in the head of the caudate, with complete or partial involvement of the putamen. All patients diagnosed to date are of Saudi, Syrian, or Yemeni ancestry, and all have consanguineous parents. Using linkage analysis in four families, we mapped the genetic defect near marker *D2S2158* in 2q36.3 (LOD = 5.9; $\theta = 0.0$) to a minimum candidate region (~2 Mb) between *D2S2354* and *D2S1256*, on the basis of complete homozygosity. In this segment, each family displayed one of two different missense mutations that altered the coding sequence of *SLC19A3*, the gene for a transporter related to the reduced-folate (encoded by *SLC19A1*) and thiamin (encoded by *SLC19A2*) transporters.

Introduction

Biotin-responsive basal ganglia disease (BBGD [MIM 607483]) was first described in 1998 in a number of families in Saudi Arabia (Ozand et al. 1998). Patients presented in childhood with a subacute encephalopathic picture of undefined origin, including confusion, vomiting, and a vague history of febrile illness. They progressed to acute encephalopathy, with sudden loss of developmental milestones; inability to swallow; loss of speech (or slurred speech); loss of motor function, with development of quadriparesis or quadriplegia; and seizures. Left untreated, the disorder results in a chronic or slowly progressive encephalopathy, with an akinetic mute state, permanent loss of speech and comprehension, and eventual death. Magnetic resonance imaging (MRI) examination of patients with BBGD revealed specific bilateral necrosis in the head of the caudate nucleus and in the putamen. However, results of tests to uncover evidence of infection, storage or mitochondrial diseases, or toxicological damage were all negative. Since all affected individuals had consanguineous parents, it was concluded that BBGD is likely due to a recessive genetic defect. Fortunately, administration of high doses of biotin (5–10 mg/kg/d) early in the disorder was found to eliminate the symptoms of BBGD within a few days, with no recurrence unless biotin treatment was discontinued. In the latter circumstance, symptoms returned within a month. Treatment later in the disorder left residual paraparesis, mild mental retardation, or dystonia. Even when biotin administration resolved the clinical symptoms of BBGD, the abnormal MRI findings remained but showed no further progression.

Biotin is essential for the activity of a number of critical carboxylases, including propionyl coenzyme A (CoA), acetyl CoA, 3-methylcrotonyl CoA, and pyruvate carboxylases (Moss and Lane 1971). These are converted from apoenzymes to active holoenzymes by transfer of biotin from holocarboxylase synthetase. Specific carboxylase deficiencies have been described that are due to mutations in the corresponding structural genes. Mutation in the holocarboxylase synthetase gene leads to multiple carboxylase deficiency (Suzuki et al. 1994; Aoki et al. 1995; Dupuis et al. 1996; Narisawa et al. 1996), which may, in some cases, be biotin responsive (Wolf and Feldman 1982). Since biotin is not synthesized de novo in humans, multiple carboxylase deficiency may also result from mutation in biotinidase (Pomponio et al. 1995), which is essential for recycling endogenous biotin. The patients with BBGD did not display deficiency of any of

Received February 14, 2005; accepted for publication April 14, 2005; electronically published May 3, 2005.

Address for correspondence and reprints: Dr. James F. Gusella, Molecular Neurogenetic Unit, Center for Human Genetic Research, Massachusetts General Hospital East, Room 6214, 149 13th Street, Charlestown, MA 02129-2000. E-mail: gusella@helix.mgh.harvard.edu

* These two authors contributed equally to this work.

† Present affiliation: Illumina, Inc., San Diego.

0002-9297/2005/7701-0003$15.00

these enzymes, indicating that their genetic defect lay in some additional component of biotin metabolism. We have used linkage mapping and positional cloning to identify mutations in the transporter gene *SLC19A3* as the cause of BBGD in four families.

Material and Methods

Families with BBGD

Four families with seven affected members are shown in figure 1. After institutional review board approval, informed consent to participate and blood samples were obtained from patients and family members; standard methods were used for extraction of DNA. Families 11, 30, and 44 are of Saudi origin; these families each involve a first-cousin mating, and they each comprise affected individuals described in the study by Ozand et al. (1998) (patients 1 [patient 1103 in the present study], 2 [1102], 3 [4407], 4 [4408], and 7 [3003]). Related kindreds 12 and 14 are of Yemeni origin. Affected individual 1403 was described as "patient 6" in the study by Ozand et al. (1998). Affected individual 1203 is a previously undescribed affected family member with features of BBGD; this individual has an affected sibling not available for the present study.

Genotyping

PCR was performed in a total volume of 7.5 μl, with 30 ng/μl of genomic DNA, 0.1–1.0 μl (of a 5-μM concentration) of each dye-labeled primer pair (PerkinElmer/Applied Biosystems and Research Genetics), 0.06 μl (of a 5-U/μl concentration) Ampli*Taq* Gold DNA polymerase (PerkinElmer/Applied Biosystems), 0.75 μl 10 × GeneAmp PCR buffer II (PerkinElmer/Applied Biosystems), 0.75 μl GeneAmp dNTP mix (2.5 mM [PerkinElmer]), 0.75 μl $MgCl_2$ (25 mM), and sufficient dH_2O to bring the final volume to 7.5 μl. PCR was performed in the MJ Research DNA Engine tetrad with the following conditions: initial denaturation at 95°C for 12 min; 10 cycles at 94°C for 30 s, 58°C for 30 s, and 72°C for 60 s; 25 cycles at 89°C for 30 s, 55°C for 30 s, and 72°C for 60 s; and 1 cycle at 72°C for 40 min. Analysis of marker *D2S1256* used reagents as stated above, except for the final $MgCl_2$ concentration, which was 1.0 mM, not 2.5 mM. The PCR conditions were also different: initial denaturation at 95°C for 15 min; 35 cycles at 94°C for 30 s, 60°C for 30 s, and 72°C for 45 s; and 1 cycle at 72°C for 10 min. PCR products were run on a 4.5% acrylamide gel (4.5% AutoPAGE Plus [Sigma]) on the ABI 377XL DNA Sequencer (PerkinElmer/Applied Biosystems) for 2 h, with a size standard (GS350 TAMRA or GS500 TAMRA [PerkinElmer/Applied Biosystems]) run in each lane to ensure lane-to-lane and gel-to-gel size-calling consistency. The data from the gels were analyzed with ABI GeneScan, version 3.1, and Genotyper, version 2.1, software. The genome scan used 302 highly polymorphic di-, tri-, and tetranucleotide repeat microsatellite markers from the ABI Linkage Mapping Set, versions 1 and 2 (PerkinElmer), and from the Weber Human Screening Set, version 9 (Research Genetics). After 2q36-37 was implicated in the genome scan, we chose additional markers in this vicinity using the Human Genome Database and the UCSC Genome Browser. Sequences for primers used for markers in figure 1 are listed in table 1. Allele sizes were related to previous typing on the CEPH panel by regenotyping CEPH individual 133101 (Fondation Jean Dausset CEPH Web Server). Alleles were numbered in figure 1, consistent with the allele designations given in the Human Genome Database, except for the following alleles: alleles 1–9 of *D2S1344* were 280–304 bp, differing by 3 bp; alleles 1–11 of *D2S1256* were 285–325 bp, differing by 4 bp; and alleles 1 and 2 of *D2S260* were 269 bp and 267 bp, respectively.

Two microsatellite markers, *D19S596* and *D19S867* (table 1), flanking the 1.2-Mb critical region in 19q13 that was defined for infantile bilateral striatal necrosis, were specifically genotyped to exclude this genomic segment. PCR cycling conditions were the same as for genome scan markers, except that the second set of cycles was performed 21 times and 23 times, respectively, for *D19S596* and *D19S867*. These products were analyzed on Applied Biosystems 3730xl DNA Analyzer, with size standard GS500 LIZ. The data were analyzed with GeneMapper, version 3.5 (Applied Biosystems).

Statistical Analysis

Two-point LOD scores between the disease locus and the individual markers in our screening set were calculated using the MLINK program of the FASTLINK 3.0P software package (Lathrop and Lalouel 1984; Lathrop et al. 1984, 1986; Cottingham et al. 1993; Schaffer et al. 1994; Schaffer 1996). Haplotypes were constructed manually through visual inspection of the markers under consideration. Fine mapping of the markers in our linked region was accomplished by consulting known linkage and physical maps.

Mutation Scanning

From patient genomic DNA, we amplified coding exons of *SLC19A3*; three exons of a neighboring hypothetical gene, *DKFZp547H025* (GenBank accession number NM_020161); and two other related sequences, named "alt3" and "alt4" (see the "Results" section and fig. 2), and, with primers located in flanking intron and UTR sequences, we performed standard 30-μl PCR (in 10 mM Tris [pH 8.9], 50 mM KCl, 1.5–2.5 mM $MgCl_2$, 10 pmol of each primer, and 200 μM of each dNTP, including 50–

100 ng DNA and 1 U *Taq* polymerase [Invitrogen]). The oligonucleotide primers were designed using Primer3 and are available on request. The PCR products were assessed by SSCP analysis; when an abnormal band shift was observed, the sample was analyzed by direct sequencing by using the BigDye Terminator Cycle Sequencing Kit (Applied Biosystems) on an ABI 377XL DNA Sequencer (PerkinElmer). Screening of controls was performed by PCR-SSCP analysis of the *SLC19A3* 68G→T/G23V mutation: the 219-bp exon 2 product was amplified with primers 5′-TCAGCCATGGATTGTTACAGA-3′ and 5′-TCCTTGTTCAAGTCCCATAAAA-3′ for 30 cycles at 94°C for 45 s, 58°C for 45 s, and 72°C for 1 min and a final 10-min extension at 72°C. The PCR product was labeled by incorporation of [^{32}P]-dGTP, was displayed on 8% nondenaturing polyacrylamide gels containing 10% glycerol, and was then detected by autoradiography with the use of XAR film (Kodak). Screening of controls was performed by PCR-RFLP analysis of the *SLC19A3* exon 5 1264A→G/T422A mutation: a 291-bp PCR product was amplified with primers 5′-CCCTGTGGCCAATATGTTCT-3′ and 5′-TTGCTTGTTGTAAGGTTGAGAAA-3′ for 30 cycles at 94°C for 45 s, 57°C for 45 s, and 72°C

Table 1

Primers Sequences Used for Markers on Chromosomes 2 and 19

The table is available in its entirety in the online edition of *The American Journal of Human Genetics.*

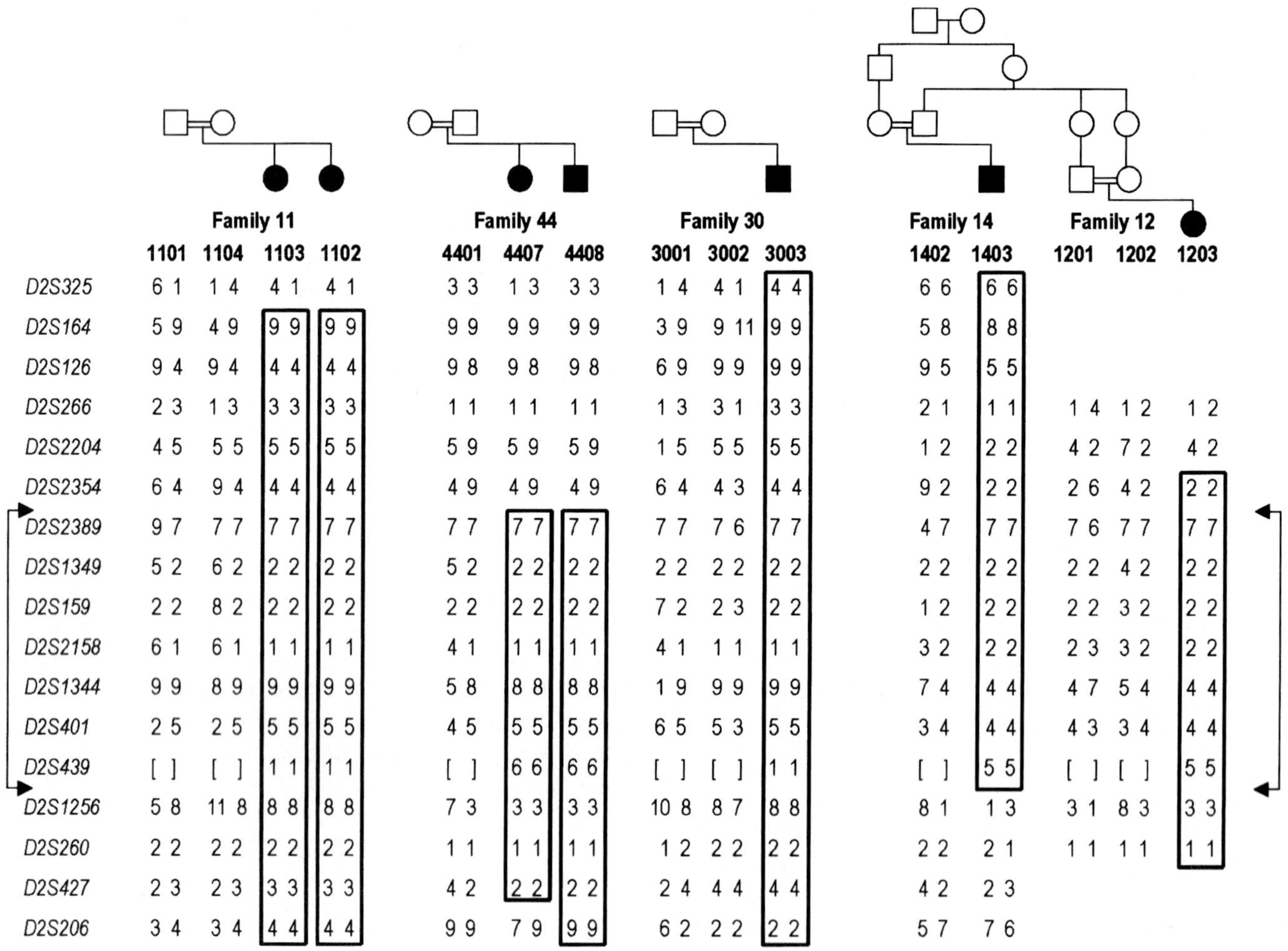

Figure 1 Homozygosity mapping and 2q haplotypes in four consanguineous families with BBGD. Blackened symbols indicate patients; unblackened symbols indicate unaffected individuals. Marker alleles, numbered as described in the "Material and Methods" section, are given for seven affected individuals and eight parents within four families with BBGD. Boxes highlight regions of complete homozygosity in affected individuals, indicating disease-chromosome haplotypes. Borders of the minimum candidate interval are denoted by the connected arrows. Genotypes that were not determined are shown by square brackets. Not shown, for confidentiality, are seven unaffected siblings in three of the families who were genotyped and included in the LOD score calculations. None of these samples showed homozygosity for the candidate region. On the basis of the results of mutation analysis, the first three families (11, 20, and 44), all of which involve first-cousin matings, likely share a common ancestor, with the difference in the allele for *D2S1344* in family 44 likely being due to a change in the microsatellite marker repeat.

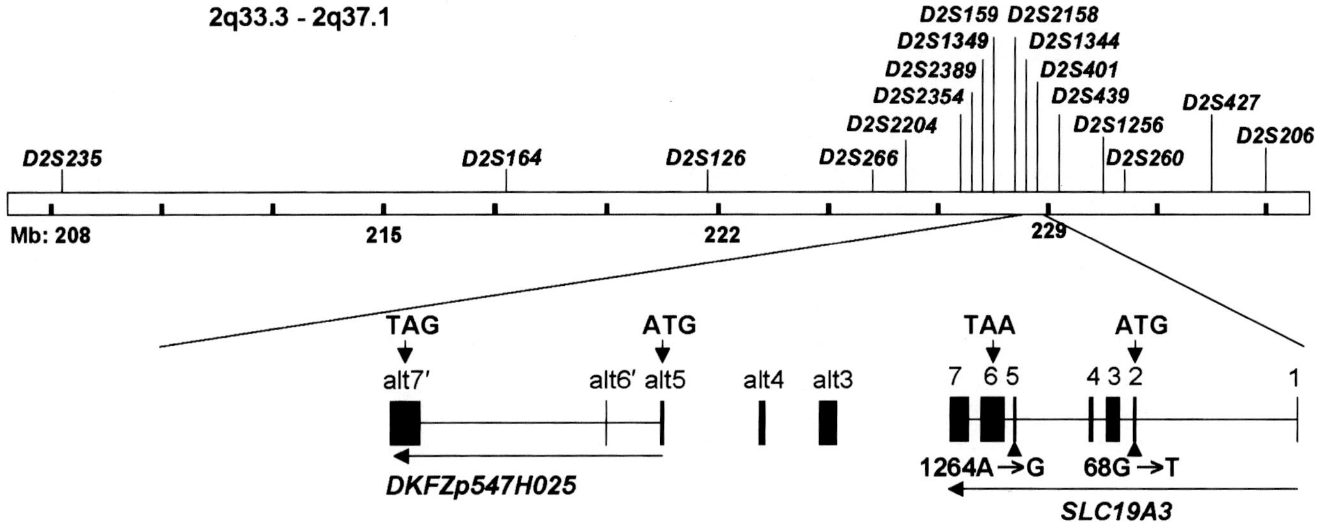

Figure 2 *SLC19A3* genomic region, gene structure, and BBGD point mutations. Locations of the microsatellite markers used for the linkage study of the 2q33.3-2q37.1 region and the corresponding gene region for *SLC19A3* and *DKFZp547H025* are shown. The human *SLC19A3* gene is located in 2q36.3, spans 32.91 kb of genomic DNA, and consists of seven exons with a start codon in exon 2 and a TAA stop codon in exon 6. The *SLC19A3* cDNA includes a predicted 1,488-bp ORF encoding a 496-aa protein of 55.6 kDa molecular weight. One mutation, 68 G→T, was identified in exon 2, and another mutation, 1264 A→G, was found in exon 5. Sequences alt3, alt4, and alt5 were detected by TBLASTN search (see the BLAST Web site) and were found to be similar to *SLC19A3* exons 3, 4, and 5, respectively. The nearby hypothetical protein DKFZp547H025, which is based on a sequenced cDNA, contains three exons (alt5, along with sequences designated "alt6′" and "alt7′," which are unrelated to *SLC19A3*), with start and stop codons indicated by arrows. Nine novel SNPs were identified in the 5′ UTR, alt3, alt6′, and alt7′ in *SLC19A3* and *DKFZp547H025*; the SNPs were submitted to dbSNP and were assigned accession numbers 32476166–32476174.

for 1 min and a final 10-min extension at 72°C. The PCR product was digested with *Bsp*HI to produce fragments of 170 bp and 121 bp (wild type) and 291 bp (mutant) and was resolved by electrophoresis on 2% agarose gels (Invitrogen). White control chromosomes were from 162 unrelated grandparents or parents from the extended CEPH pedigrees (Fondation Jean Dausset CEPH Web Server). Arab control chromosomes were from the Coriell Cell Repositories (two panels of 10 individuals each [catalog IDs HD05 and HD27]) and from 42 unrelated members of other Arab disease pedigrees collected for mapping/polymorphism studies.

Hydrophobicity Predictions

Hydrophobicity plots in figure 3 were determined using HMMTOP 2.0 (Tusnady and Simon 1998, 2001). SLC19A3 (National Center for Biotechnology Information [NCBI] Entrez Protein accession number NP_079519) was submitted for analysis.

Results

Genome Scan

For our initial genome scan, we genotyped 12 individuals, including 6 affected subjects, from four families with 302 markers (fig. 1 [excluding family 12]). On the basis of initial positive LOD scores on the long arm of chromosome 2, we added additional markers to saturate this region, genotyping all 22 available samples: the 12 original individuals, 3 members of family 12, and 7 unaffected siblings in these families (not shown, for confidentiality). Marker *D2S2158* demonstrated significant linkage, with a maximum LOD score of 5.9 at $\theta = 0.0$ (table 2). In each family, the affected individuals were homozygous for the region surrounding *D2S2158*, consistent with the known consanguinity and recessive inheritance pattern (fig. 1). The minimum region of complete homozygosity was between *D2S2354* and *D2S1256*, a segment of ~2 Mb. The families did not share identical haplotypes across the entire minimum candidate region, indicating either that more than one founder mutation was represented or that a single-founder defect could be further localized by examining regions of identity in all seven affected individuals.

Analysis of the Candidate Region

We examined the region for known gene candidates using the UCSC Genome Browser, as well as using 20-kb chunks of genomic BAC sequence in BLASTX searches (see the BLAST Web site) of GenBank, to identify additional conserved sequences. The candidate region contained genes for the insulin-receptor substrate (*IRS1*), collagens 4A3 and 4A4 (*COL4A3* and *COL4A4*), a nu-

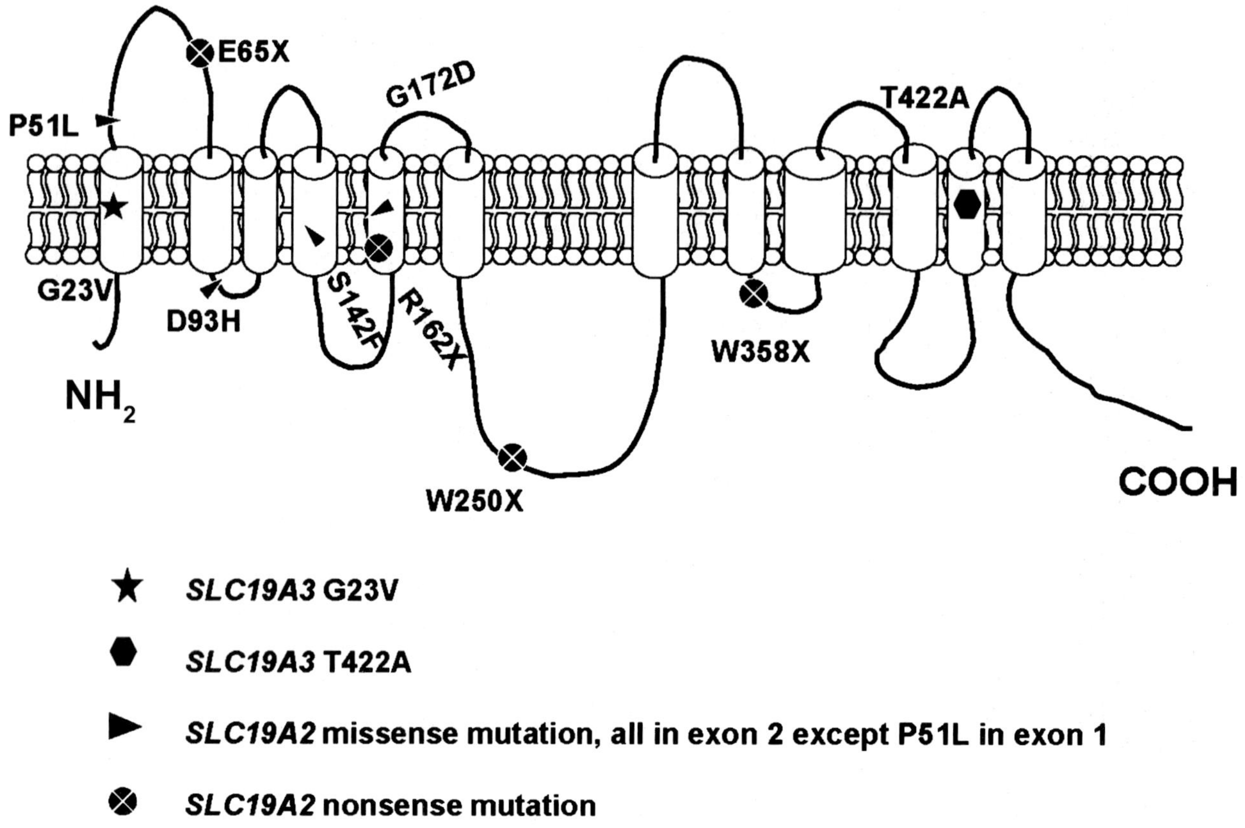

Figure 3 Schematic model of the reduced-folate transporter family. *SLC19A3* encodes a predicted protein containing 12 putative transmembrane domains. The relative positions of the mutations identified in *SLC19A3* in patients with BBGD and of the missense and nonsense mutations in *SLC19A2*, reported in patients with Rogers syndrome, are shown (Diaz et al. 1999; Labay et al. 1999; Raz et al. 2000; Scharfe et al. 2000; Lagarde et al. 2004). The positions of mutations in *SLC19A2* were assigned in accordance with hydrophobicity plots that were determined by HMMTOP 2.0 (Tusnady and Simon 1998, 2001). SLC19A2 and SLC19A3 (NCBI accession numbers NP_008927 and NP_079519) were used for analysis.

cleoporin family member (*HRB*), chemokine ligand 20 (*CCL20*), several anonymous cDNAs, and SLC19A3. We first focused on the latter, since it is related to THTR-1 (encoded by *SLC19A2*), the high-affinity transporter for thiamin, another water-soluble vitamin. Mutations in *SLC19A2* underlie thiamin-responsive megaloblastic anemia (or "Rogers syndrome") (Diaz et al. 1999; Fleming et al. 1999; Labay et al. 1999).

SLC19A3 is predicted to comprise seven exons spanning 32.9 kb in 2q36.3, with the coding sequence confined to exons 2–6 (fig. 2). To ensure that we identified all *SLC19A3*-related potential coding sequences in the vicinity, we used the THTR-1 protein sequence and the predicted *SLC19A3* coding sequence to search the candidate region with TBLASTN (see the BLAST Web site). This search identified another set of related sequences, which begin ∼40 kb 3′ to the gene and correspond to sequences related to exons 3, 4, and 5; we designated these sequences as "alt3," "alt4," and "alt5," respectively. The latter two represent ORFs encoding amino acids that are 68% identical to those encoded by the equivalent segment of *SLC19A3*. However, alt3 predicts 71% identity but has two separate stop codons that interrupt the ORF. No reported human ESTs connect alt3, alt4, and alt5 in a cDNA. However, the cDNA *DKFZp547H025* has been reported to encode a hypothetical protein of 140 aa that begins from the ORF of alt5 and continues into two additional exons with ORFs unrelated to *SLC19A3*. We designated these putative coding exons "alt6′" and "alt7′." Since *SLC19A3* and the other potential exons are all in the same orientation, it is conceivable that alternative splicing could produce a hybrid transcript. Consequently, to search for the BBGD defect, we performed mutation scanning of exons 1–6 of *SLC19A3*, as well as alt3, alt4, alt5, alt6′, and alt7′.

Mutations in SLC19A3

Two putative mutations were identified in the four families, and both of these mutations predicted missense changes in the protein structure, as shown in figure 4.

Table 2

LOD Scores for Linkage of BBGD to 2q36-37

Marker	Location[a] (Mb)	LOD at $\theta=$ 0	.01	.05	.1	.2	.3	.4
D2S325	208.096	$-\infty$	−.06	.85	.93	.62	.28	.08
D2S164	217.786	4.43	4.30	3.78	3.15	1.98	1.03	.38
D2S126	221.843	1.47	1.88	2.08	1.89	1.28	.67	.22
D2S266	225.111	.89	2.20	2.38	2.08	1.30	.64	.20
D2S2204	226.302	−1.01	.99	1.85	1.91	1.48	.88	.36
D2S2354	227.175	3.29	3.66	3.68	3.28	2.24	1.25	.49
D2S2389	227.372	3.52	3.42	3.03	2.55	1.65	.91	.36
D2S1349	227.636	4.04	3.91	3.43	2.85	1.77	.90	.31
D2S159	227.649	4.20	4.08	3.62	3.04	1.97	1.07	.41
D2S2158	227.886	***5.90***	5.74	5.10	4.30	2.76	1.43	.48
D2S1344	227.912	4.94	4.80	4.27	3.60	2.34	1.26	.47
D2S401	228.084	5.66	5.50	4.86	4.06	2.55	1.29	.42
D2S439	229.006	4.39	4.26	3.75	3.13	2.00	1.06	.40
D2S1256	229.241	1.36	2.84	2.98	2.62	1.69	.88	.33
D2S260	230.090	−1.78	−.22	.24	.30	.20	.11	.04
D2S427	232.032	1.06	1.59	1.83	1.67	1.13	.58	.17
D2S206	233.534	$-\infty$	.23	1.17	1.29	1.00	.58	.20

NOTE.—The peak LOD score is shown in bold italics.

[a] Marker location is based on the May 2004 human genome assembly (UCSC Genome Browser).

The mutation in exon 2 was found in two patients (1203 and 1403) from a Yemeni family. Sequence analysis disclosed a homozygous G→T change at nucleotide 68, which is predicted to alter a highly conserved glycine at codon 23 to valine (c.68G→T; p.G23V) (fig. 2). An equivalent glycine residue is present at this position in mouse Slc19a3 and in both SLC19A2 and SLC19A1, the two other members of this transporter family in humans. This putative mutation is predicted to alter the first transmembrane domain (fig. 3) of the SLC19A3 protein.

In the three other families, all of Saudi origin, we identified an A→G missense mutation at nucleotide position 1264 in exon 5, that alters a *Bsp*HI restriction site (fig. 4). This sequence change predicts a substitution of the threonine at codon 422 of the SLC19A3 protein with alanine (c.1264A→G, p.T422A) (fig. 2). The equivalent threonine is also present in the penultimate transmembrane domain of the *SLC19A1*- and *SLC19A2*-encoded proteins (fig. 3).

BLASTP analysis (see the BLAST Web site) of *Drosophila melanogaster* and *Caenorhabditis elegans* proteins with any of the human SLC19A1, SLC19A2, or SLC19A3 proteins detects three related genes in each species: *CG6574, CG14694,* and *CG17036* in *D. melanogaster* and *5D352, 5L621,* and *5I82* in *C. elegans.* These appear to be the only three members of the reduced-folate carrier transporter family in each organism, and they are comparable to the three genes found in mammals. However, since the transporters show greater sequence identity within a species than across species, it is not possible to conclusively assign an orthologue for each of the human tranporters by sequence comparison. For example, the SLC19A3 protein shows 33%, 33%, and 35% identity with the three *Drosophila* proteins, respectively, whereas the SLC19A2 protein shows 35%, 34%, and 34% identity with these same proteins. Interestingly, however, all three members of this gene family, in both *D. melanogaster* and *C. elegans,* display conserved glycine and threonine residues at positions comparable to the sites in SLC19A3 that are altered in the families with BBGD (fig. 4).

To establish that these two alterations do not represent benign polymorphisms, we examined 364 chromosomes from unrelated whites in the extended CEPH collection (Fondation Jean Dausset CEPH Web Server) and 124 chromosomes from unrelated individuals of Arab ancestry. None of these 488 control chromosomes possessed either alteration, arguing strongly that these missense alterations cause BBGD in these families. Unfortunately, since we do not have access to cell lines from these subjects, we have not been able to determine whether these mutations have any effect on *SLC19A3* mRNA splicing in addition to their direct effect on the protein sequence.

Discussion

SLC19A1, SLC19A2, and *SLC19A3* are genes on chromosomes 21q22.3, 1q24.2, and 2q36.3, respectively, encoding closely related proteins, termed the "reduced-folate carrier family of transporters" on the basis of the function of the SLC19A1 protein. The SLC19A2 protein is a thiamin transporter that is defective in thiamin-responsive megaloblastic anemia (Rogers syndrome) (Diaz et al. 1999; Fleming et al. 1999; Labay et al. 1999). The SLC19A3 protein shares 39% identity and 56% similarity with SLC19A1 and 48% identity and 64% similarity with SLC19A2, including a single reduced-folate carrier–related domain (aa 11–439) (Eudy et al. 2000). Hydrophobicity analysis of all three proteins reveals a predicted topology with 12 putative transmembrane domains (fig. 3), which is consistent with a transporter function. Northern blot and RT-PCR analyses have showed the presence of 3.5-, 2.6-, and 2.0-kb *SLC19A3* transcripts in many tissues, including brain, but with greatest abundance in placenta, kidney, and liver. Interestingly, in the mouse, a single *Slc19a3* mRNA species is seen and is relatively more abundant in the mouse brain than has been reported for humans (Eudy et al. 2000). Our RT-PCR analysis of the *SLC19A3* transcript indicates that both exon 2 and exon 5 are expressed in the transcript in both brain and peripheral tissues (data not shown), suggesting that the brain-specific pathology of BBGD is not due to alternative splicing in peripheral tissues and that the differences in mRNA size detected by northern blot are not due to differences in the coding region. Refined expression studies in human intestinal

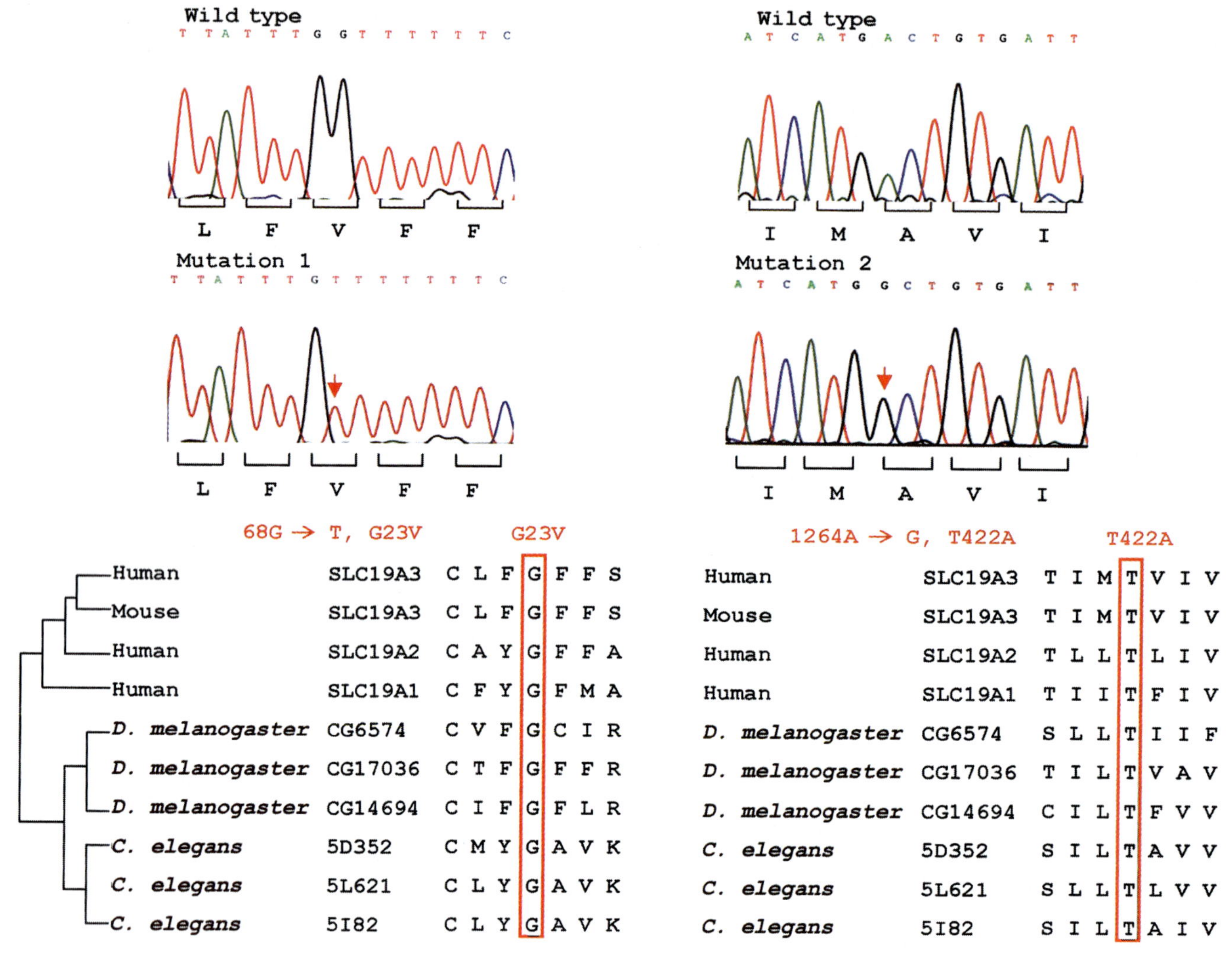

Figure 4 *SLC19A3* point mutations at sites conserved in the reduced-folate transporter family. Sequence chromatograms of the two missense mutations and the corresponding wild-type alleles are shown in the upper panel. These mutations altered glycine ("Mutation 1") and threonine ("Mutation 2") residues at codon 23 and codon 422, respectively, that are highly conserved in related transporters in humans, mouse, and lower organisms (*lower panel*).

epithelial cells have shown SLC19A3 protein to be expressed at the brush-border membrane but not at the basolateral membrane (Said et al. 2004), consistent with a transporter function.

Our detection—in four families with BBGD, representing two different disease haplotypes—of two different missense changes that segregate with the disorder but are not found on 488 control chromosomes implicates *SLC19A3* as the disease gene. Furthermore, these mutations alter amino acid residues that are identical in all of the similar transporters in humans, mouse, and lower organisms, suggesting a strong functional pressure for evolutionary conservation. The c.68G→T mutation (p.G23V), found in a family of Yemeni origin, substitutes a hydrophobic valine residue for a more flexible glycine residue in the first transmembrane domain (fig. 3). A missense mutation that changes glycine to aspartic acid at codon 172 of *SLC19A2* has also been reported in patients with Rogers syndrome (Labay et al. 1999; Raz et al. 2000), and two recent studies showed that the mutant protein failed in normal-cell targeting to the plasma membrane, with consequent loss of the thiamin transporter activity (Balamurugan and Said 2002; Baron et al. 2002). Indeed, the *SLC19A3* G23V mutations and the clustering of Rogers syndrome mutations in exon 2 of *SLC19A2* support the view that this exon encodes a region that is critical for successful transport function (Diaz et al. 1999; Fleming et al. 1999; Labay et al. 1999; Raz et al. 2000; Scharfe et al. 2000; Gritli et al. 2001; Lagarde et al. 2004). The other BBGD mutation, c.1264A→G, found in three families of Saudi origin, also alters a transmembrane domain, substituting an alanine residue for the hydrophilic threonine at position 422 (p.T422A). Again, the extreme evolutionary conservation of this threonine residue suggests that it is critical for SLC19A3 function.

Since the symptoms of BBGD may be reversed by high doses of biotin therapy, it is reasonable to suspect that SLC19A3 may act normally as a biotin transporter. Humans lack the ability to synthesize biotin and therefore depend entirely on dietary sources (Combs 1992). Biotinidase can recycle endogenous biotin so that most of the biotin can be preserved in the body, but biotinidase activity is low in human brain and central spinal fluid, restricting the recycling of biotin in the CNS (Suchy et al. 1985; Fois et al. 1986). Normal carboxylase and biotinidase values in patients with BBGD are consistent with the disorder being caused by a defect in the biotin transporter system, possibly across cerebral capillaries at the blood-brain barrier or, alternatively, in the neuronal cells themselves (Ozand et al. 1998). The caudate neurodegeneration evident in patients with BBGD suggests that striatal neurons may be particularly susceptible to a lack of adequate biotin. The high dosage of biotin used to treat BBGD may then act simply by increasing passive diffusion, making sufficient biotin available to the caudate nucleus (Spector and Mock 1987). Recently, investigation of humans with induced marginal biotin deficiency has shown a much greater reduction in levels of *SLC19A3* mRNA in blood leukocytes than of mRNAs for 10 known biotin-related genes (Vlasova et al. 2005). These findings implicate SLC19A3 in biotin metabolism and indicate that it is a more sensitive indicator of biotin deficiency than the known biotin carboxylases, holocarboxylase synthetase, biotinidase, and the sodium-dependent multivitamin transporter.

In seeming contradiction with this hypothesis, SLC19A3 has recently been reported to be a second thiamin transporter (Rajgopal et al. 2001), like SLC19A2. These investigators used HeLa cells that were transiently transfected with *SLC19A3* cDNA to assess the transport activity for radiolabeled thiamin, folic acid, and methotrexate, but they did not test biotin. To date, the genes encoding the putative pyridoxine (vitamin B6) and niacin transporters also have not been identified. An uptake assay to reveal a novel transporter function should include those micronutrients to also test for the possibility of multivitamin transport via the same protein. Interestingly, Na^+-dependent multivitamin transporter, the intestinal biotin transporter, is also used by two other micronutrients, pantothenic acid and lipoate (Prasad et al. 1998, 1999; Wang et al. 1999). Additional work is required to establish whether SLC19A3 is capable of transporting biotin in addition to thiamin or, alternatively, whether the positive effect of biotin therapy in BBGD acts indirectly to rescue the effects of altered SLC19A3 transport of thiamin or another micronutrient.

In either of the above circumstances, explaining the brain-specific effects in patients with BBGD may require a fuller delineation and understanding of the options for biotin and thiamin transport, of the relative cellular distributions of the various transporters, of the specific requirements of different cells and tissues for these vitamins, and of the specific roles of biotin in different cells. Notably, global biotin deficiency produces many symptoms not seen in patients with BBGD, such as dry skin, seborrheic dermatitis, fungal infections, erythematous periorifacial macular rashes, nausea, and anorexia. The absence of these symptoms in patients with BBGD suggests that sufficient biotin is available in all regions except the brain. Moreover, the brain MRI findings in patients with biotinidase deficiency and those with multiple carboxylase deficiency are also different from the findings observed in patients with BBGD, implying that biotin may have other potential roles in the striatum beyond that of cofactor for carboxylases (McMahon 2002). Interestingly, several studies suggest that biotin may be involved directly or indirectly in the regulation of gene expression (Rodriguez-Melendez and Zempleni 2003), raising another option for the mechanism by which *SLC19A3* mutation may lead to the basal ganglia necrosis of BBGD.

As a result of the wider use of advanced brain imaging technologies such as MRI and CT, bilateral striatal necrosis has been recognized in a number of disorders (Fujita et al. 1994; Okiyama et al. 1994; Sola Martinez et al. 1994). Extrapyramidal symptoms are the main clinical correlates of striatal necrosis and can be observed in mitochondrial encephalopathies (Martin et al. 1988; Medina et al. 1990; Leuzzi et al. 1992; Thyagarajan et al. 1995), glutaric acidemia type I, 3-methylglutaconic academia (Gascon et al. 1994), Huntington disease (Finch 1980; Buck et al. 1981), Wilson disease (Sener 1993), and CNS infection (Larsen and Crisp 1996; Zambrino et al. 2000). Detailed clinical evidence excluded those diagnoses in patients with BBGD who were described elsewhere (Ozand et al. 1998). However, since the description of BBGD, this pathology has been described in patients with a novel disorder, infantile bilateral striatal necrosis (IBSN), in which symmetric degeneration of the caudate and putamen was observed. Interestingly, three patients were reported to have moderate response to biotin (Straussberg et al. 2002). In one Israeli Bedouin kindred showing an autosomal recessive inheritance pattern, linkage analysis refined the critical candidate region on 19q13 (Basel-Vanagaite et al. 2004). In view of the similarity of IBSN to BBGD, we specifically tested the IBSN locus–flanking markers *D19S596* and *D19S867*, to examine the possible involvement of this locus in BBGD. Linkage of BBGD to 19q13 was specifically excluded, indicating that these similar disorders are not allelic. However, careful comparison of these disorders and their degree of response to biotin may reveal new information concerning the role that biotin plays in the striatum. Similarly, the mechanism of striatal necrosis in IBSN and BBGD may indicate that an assessment of the potential participation of biotin metabolism in other neurodegenerative disorders of the striatum, such as Huntington disease, should be considered.

Although we identified the BBGD gene using Arab kindreds, it is likely that this disorder exists in other populations but that it may not have been recognized because it has only recently been formally described. Identification of mutations in the *SLC19A3* gene will help to differentiate and confirm the clinical diagnosis of BBGD and will open an avenue for prenatal and presymptomatic diagnosis. Early molecular diagnosis of BBGD is particularly important to prevent basal ganglia damage, since the progression of the pathology and of the clinical course of symptoms can be prevented simply by the administration of biotin. It is important to assess whether patients with phenotypic similarilites to those with BBGD are known within the neurogenetics community in the United States and elsewhere, since identification of such patients will permit their effective treatment and will prevent unnecessary debilitation and premature death.

Acknowledgments

We are grateful to the families with BBGD who participated in this study, as well as to the clinicians at the King Faisal Specialist Hospital and Research Centre. We would also like to thank Jianmin Chen and the Massachusetts General Hospital Genomics Core Facility, for their assistance in genotyping services; Dr. Tony Castelli, for technical advice; and Dr. Mei Sun, for help with northern blot. This work was supported by the King Faisal Specialist Hospital and Research Centre, National Institutes of Health grant NS16367, and the Huntington's Disease Society of America's Coalition for the Cure. W.Q.Z. was the recipient of a fellowship from the Harvard Center for Neurodegeneration and Repair.

Web Resources

Accession numbers and URLs for data presented herein are as follows:

BLAST, http://www.ncbi.nlm.nih.gov/blast/ (for BLASTX, TBLASTN, and BLASTP)

dbSNP, http://www.ncbi.nlm.nih.gov/SNP/ (for nine novel SNPs in the 5′ UTR, alt3, alt6′, and alt7′ of *SLC19A3* and *DKFZp547H025* [accession numbers 32476166–32476174])

Fondation Jean Dausset CEPH Web Server, http://www.cephb.fr/ (for CEPH family genotypes used in map construction)

HMMTOP 2.0, http://www.enzim.hu/hmmtop/index.html

Human Genome Database, http://www.gdb.org

GenBank, http://www.ncbi.nlm.nih.gov/Genbank/ (for *DKFZp547H025* mRNA [accession number NM_020161])

NCBI Entrez Protein Database, http://www.ncbi.nlm.nih.gov/entrez/query.fcgi?db=protein&cmd=search&term= (for SLC19A3 [accession number NP_079519])

Online Mendelian Inheritance in Man (OMIM), http://www.ncbi.nlm.nih.gov/Omim/ (for BBGD)

Primer3, http://frodo.wi.mit.edu/cgi-bin/primer3/primer3_www.cgi

UCSC Genome Browser, http://genome.ucsc.edu/

References

Aoki Y, Suzuki Y, Sakamoto O, Li X, Takahashi K, Ohtake A, Sakuta R, Ohura T, Miyabayashi S, Narisawa K (1995) Molecular analysis of holocarboxylase synthetase deficiency: a missense mutation and a single base deletion are predominant in Japanese patients. Biochim Biophys Acta 1272:168–174

Balamurugan K, Said HM (2002) Functional role of specific amino acid residues in human thiamine transporter *SLC19A2*: mutational analysis. Am J Physiol Gastrointest Liver Physiol 283:G37–G43

Baron D, Assaraf YG, Cohen N, Aronheim A (2002) Lack of plasma membrane targeting of a G172D mutant thiamine transporter derived from Rogers syndrome family. Mol Med 8:462–474

Basel-Vanagaite L, Straussberg R, Ovadia H, Kaplan A, Magal N, Shorer Z, Shalev H, Walsh C, Shohat M (2004) Infantile bilateral striatal necrosis maps to chromosome 19q. Neurology 62:87–90

Buck SH, Burks TF, Brown MR, Yamamura HI (1981) Reduction in basal ganglia and substantia nigra substance P levels in Huntington's disease. Brain Res 209:464–469

Combs GF (1992) Biotin. In: The vitamins: rundamental aspects in nutrition and health. Academic, San Diego, pp 329–343

Cottingham RW Jr, Idury RM, Schaffer AA (1993) Faster sequential genetic linkage computations. Am J Hum Genet 53: 252–263

Diaz GA, Banikazemi M, Oishi K, Desnick RJ, Gelb BD (1999) Mutations in a new gene encoding a thiamine transporter cause thiamine-responsive megaloblastic anaemia syndrome. Nat Genet 22:309–312

Dupuis L, Leon-Del-Rio A, Leclerc D, Campeau E, Sweetman L, Saudubray JM, Herman G, Gibson KM, Gravel RA (1996) Clustering of mutations in the biotin-binding region of holocarboxylase synthetase in biotin-responsive multiple carboxylase deficiency. Hum Mol Genet 5:1011–1016

Eudy JD, Spiegelstein O, Barber RC, Wlodarczyk BJ, Talbot J, Finnell RH (2000) Identification and characterization of the human and mouse *SLC19A3* gene: a novel member of the reduced folate family of micronutrient transporter genes. Mol Genet Metab 71:581–590

Finch CE (1980) The relationships of aging changes in the basal ganglia to manifestations of Huntington's chorea. Ann Neurol 7:406–411

Fleming JC, Tartaglini E, Steinkamp MP, Schorderet DF, Cohen N, Neufeld EJ (1999) The gene mutated in thiamine-responsive anaemia with diabetes and deafness (TRMA) encodes a functional thiamine transporter. Nat Genet 22:305–308

Fois A, Cioni M, Balestri P, Bartalini G, Baumgartner R, Bachmann C (1986) Biotinidase deficiency: metabolites in CSF. J Inherit Metab Dis 9:284–285

Fujita K, Takeuchi Y, Nishimura A, Takada H, Sawada T (1994) Serial MRI in infantile bilateral striatal necrosis. Pediatr Neurol 10:157–160

Gascon GG, Ozand PT, Brismar J (1994) Movement disorders in childhood organic acidurias: clinical, neuroimaging, and biochemical correlations. Brain Dev Suppl 16:94–103

Gritli S, Omar S, Tartaglini E, Guannouni S, Fleming JC, Steinkamp MP, Berul CI, Hafsia R, Jilani SB, Belhani A, Hamdi M, Neufeld EJ (2001) A novel mutation in the *SLC19A2* gene in a Tunisian family with thiamine-responsive megaloblastic anaemia, diabetes and deafness syndrome. Br J Haematol 113: 508–513

Labay V, Raz T, Baron D, Mandel H, Williams H, Barrett T, Szargel R, McDonald L, Shalata A, Nosaka K, Gregory S, Cohen N (1999) Mutations in *SLC19A2* cause thiamine-responsive megaloblastic anaemia associated with diabetes mellitus and deafness. Nat Genet 22:300–304

Lagarde WH, Underwood LE, Moats-Staats BM, Calikoglu AS (2004) Novel mutation in the *SLC19A2* gene in an African-American female with thiamine-responsive megaloblastic anemia syndrome. Am J Med Genet A 125:299–305

Larsen PD, Crisp D (1996) Acute bilateral striatal necrosis associated with *Mycoplasma pneumoniae* infection. Pediatr Infect Dis J 15:1124–1126

Lathrop GM, Lalouel JM (1984) Easy calculations of LOD scores and genetic risks on small computers. Am J Hum Genet 36:460–465

Lathrop GM, Lalouel JM, Julier C, Ott J (1984) Strategies for multilocus linkage analysis in humans. Proc Natl Acad Sci USA 81:3443–3446

Lathrop GM, Lalouel JM, White RL (1986) Construction of human linkage maps: likelihood calculations for multilocus linkage analysis. Genet Epidemiol 3:39–52

Leuzzi V, Bertini E, De Negri AM, Gallucci M, Garavaglia B (1992) Bilateral striatal necrosis, dystonia and optic atrophy in two siblings. J Neurol Neurosurg Psychiatry 55:16–19

Martin JJ, Van de Vyver FL, Scholte HR, Roodhooft AM, Ceuterick C, Martin L, Luyt-Houwen IE (1988) Defect in succinate oxidation by isolated muscle mitochondria in a patient with symmetrical lesions in the basal ganglia. J Neurol Sci 84:189–200

McMahon RJ (2002) Biotin in metabolism and molecular biology. Annu Rev Nutr 22:221–239

Medina L, Chi TL, DeVivo DC, Hilal SK (1990) MR findings in patients with subacute necrotizing encephalomyelopathy (Leigh syndrome): correlation with biochemical defect. Am J Neuroradiol 11:379–384

Moss J, Lane MD (1971) The biotin-dependent enzymes. Adv Enzymol Relat Areas Mol Biol 35:321–442

Narisawa K, Suzuki Y, Aoki Y (1996) [Cloning of the holocarboxylase synthetase cDNA and identification of mutations prevalent in Japanese HCS-deficient patients.] Nippon Rinsho 54:259–267

Okiyama R, Mitani M, Hayashi H, Tanabe H (1994) [Acute encephalopathy with symmetrical lesions of the thalamus, the putamen and the cerebellum on magnetic resonance imaging.] No To Shinkei 46:579–583

Ozand PT, Gascon GG, Al Essa M, Joshi S, Al Jishi E, Bakheet S, Al Watban J, Al-Kawi MZ, Dabbagh O (1998) Biotin-responsive basal ganglia disease: a novel entity. Brain 121: 1267–1279

Pomponio RJ, Reynolds TR, Cole H, Buck GA, Wolf B (1995) Mutational hotspot in the human biotinidase gene causes profound biotinidase deficiency. Nat Genet 11:96–98

Prasad PD, Wang H, Huang W, Fei YJ, Leibach FH, Devoe LD, Ganapathy V (1999) Molecular and functional characterization of the intestinal Na^+-dependent multivitamin transporter. Arch Biochem Biophys 366:95–106

Prasad PD, Wang H, Kekuda R, Fujita T, Fei YJ, Devoe LD, Leibach FH, Ganapathy V (1998) Cloning and functional expression of a cDNA encoding a mammalian sodium-dependent vitamin transporter mediating the uptake of pantothenate, biotin, and lipoate. J Biol Chem 273:7501–7506

Rajgopal A, Edmondnson A, Goldman ID, Zhao R (2001) *SLC19A3* encodes a second thiamine transporter ThTr2. Biochim Biophys Acta 1537:175–178

Raz T, Labay V, Baron D, Szargel R, Anbinder Y, Barrett T, Rabl W, Viana MB, Mandel H, Baruchel A, Cayuela JM, Cohen N (2000) The spectrum of mutations, including four novel ones, in the thiamine-responsive megaloblastic anemia gene *SLC19A2* of eight families. Hum Mutat 16:37–42

Rodriguez-Melendez R, Zempleni J (2003) Regulation of gene expression by biotin (review). J Nutr Biochem 14:680–690

Said HM, Balamurugan K, Subramanian VS, Marchant JS (2004) Expression and functional contribution of hTHTR-2 in thiamin absorption in human intestine. Am J Physiol Gastrointest Liver Physiol 286:G491–G498

Schaffer AA (1996) Faster linkage analysis computations for pedigrees with loops or unused alleles. Hum Hered 46:226–235

Schaffer AA, Gupta SK, Shriram K, Cottingham RW Jr (1994) Avoiding recomputation in linkage analysis. Hum Hered 44: 225–237

Scharfe C, Hauschild M, Klopstock T, Janssen AJ, Heidemann PH, Meitinger T, Jaksch M (2000) A novel mutation in the thiamine responsive megaloblastic anaemia gene *SLC19A2* in a patient with deficiency of respiratory chain complex I. J Med Genet 37:669–673

Sener RN (1993) Wilson's disease: MRI demonstration of cavitations in basal ganglia and thalami. Pediatr Radiol 23:157

Sola Martinez MT, Pierot L, Noseda G, Martin-Duverneuil N, Harpey JP, Roy C, Chiras J (1994) Acute bilateral striatal necrosis in an infant: CT and MRI. Neuroradiology 36:245–246

Spector R, Mock D (1987) Biotin transport through the blood-brain barrier. J Neurochem 48:400–404

Straussberg R, Shorer Z, Weitz R, Basel L, Kornreich L, Corie CI, Harel L, Djaldetti R, Amir J (2002) Familial infantile bilateral striatal necrosis: clinical features and response to biotin treatment. Neurology 59:983–989

Suchy SF, McVoy JS, Wolf B (1985) Neurologic symptoms of biotinidase deficiency: possible explanation. Neurology 35: 1510–1511

Suzuki Y, Aoki Y, Ishida Y, Chiba Y, Iwamatsu A, Kishino T, Niikawa N, Matsubara Y, Narisawa K (1994) Isolation and characterization of mutations in the human holocarboxylase synthetase cDNA. Nat Genet 8:122–128

Thyagarajan D, Shanske S, Vazquez-Memije M, De Vivo D, DiMauro S (1995) A novel mitochondrial ATPase 6 point mutation in familial bilateral striatal necrosis. Ann Neurol 38:468–472
Tusnady GE, Simon I (1998) Principles governing amino acid composition of integral membrane proteins: application to topology prediction. J Mol Biol 283:489–506
——— (2001) The HMMTOP transmembrane topology prediction server. Bioinformatics 17:849–850
Vlasova TI, Stratton SL, Wells AM, Mock NI, Mock DM (2005) Biotin deficiency reduces expression of *SLC19A3*, a potential biotin transporter, in leukocytes from human blood. J Nutr 135:42–47
Wang H, Huang W, Fei YJ, Xia H, Yang-Feng TL, Leibach FH, Devoe LD, Ganapathy V, Prasad PD (1999) Human placental Na^{+}-dependent multivitamin transporter: cloning, functional expression, gene structure, and chromosomal localization. J Biol Chem 274:14875–14883
Wolf B, Feldman GL (1982) The biotin-dependent carboxylase deficiencies. Am J Hum Genet 34:699–716
Zambrino CA, Zorzi G, Lanzi G, Uggetti C, Egitto MG (2000) Bilateral striatal necrosis associated with *Mycoplasma pneumoniae* infection in an adolescent: clinical and neuroradiologic follow up. Mov Disord 15:1023–1026

Am. J. Hum. Genet. 77:27–40, 2005

An Entropy-Based Statistic for Genomewide Association Studies

Jinying Zhao,[1] Eric Boerwinkle,[1] and Momiao Xiong[1,2]

[1]Human Genetic Center, University of Texas, Health Science Center at Houston, Houston; and [2]Laboratory of Theoretical Systems Biology, School of Life Science, Fudan University, Shanghai, China

Efficient genotyping methods and the availability of a large collection of single-nucleotide polymorphisms provide valuable tools for genetic studies of human disease. The standard χ^2 statistic for case-control studies, which uses a linear function of allele frequencies, has limited power when the number of marker loci is large. We introduce a novel test statistic for genetic association studies that uses Shannon entropy and a nonlinear function of allele frequencies to amplify the differences in allele and haplotype frequencies to maintain statistical power with large numbers of marker loci. We investigate the relationship between the entropy-based test statistic and the standard χ^2 statistic and show that, in most cases, the power of the entropy-based statistic is greater than that of the standard χ^2 statistic. The distribution of the entropy-based statistic and the type I error rates are validated using simulation studies. Finally, we apply the new entropy-based test statistic to two real data sets, one for the COMT gene and schizophrenia and one for the MMP-2 gene and esophageal carcinoma, to evaluate the performance of the new method for genetic association studies. The results show that the entropy-based statistic obtained smaller *P* values than did the standard χ^2 statistic.

Introduction

Genomewide association studies are emerging as a promising tool for genetic analysis of complex diseases (Risch and Merikangas 1996; Stumpf and Goldstein 2003; Carlson et al. 2004; Neale and Sham 2004). Such association studies depend on linkage disequilibrium (LD). However, population histories and evolutionary forces may generate aberrant LD patterns across marker loci and important differences in allele frequencies and LD patterns across populations (Morton and Collins 1998; Pritchard and Przeworsk 2001; Stephens et al. 2001; Freedman et al. 2004). An allele may show strong LD with the functional variants in one population but exhibit very weak LD in other populations (Carlson et al. 2004) or may show strong LD with one marker but exhibit weak LD with other nearby markers, even in the same population. These phenomena make it difficult to replicate genetic associations among populations and to obtain consistent results within a genomic region in the same population.

There are two ways to alleviate aberrant LD patterns, improve the power of association studies, and increase the probability of replications. One way is to construct haplotype blocks by studying LD patterns across the genome and to optimally select a set of robust tagSNPs such that all common variants are either directly genotyped or in strong LD with the genotyped tagSNPs (Goldstein 2001; Johnson et al. 2001; Stephens et al. 2001; Gabriel et al. 2002; Zhang et al. 2002, 2003*a*; Ke and Cardon 2003; Xiong et al. 2003). However, it is unclear whether the haplotype block patterns and tagSNPs are consistent among populations or among repeated sampling from within a population. Another way is to develop novel statistical methods for association studies. Currently, the two major statistical methods for association studies are to compare haplotype frequencies between affected and unaffected individuals (Chapman and Wijsman 1998; Akey et al. 2001), which is often referred to as the standard χ^2 test, and to compare haplotype similarities between affected and unaffected individuals (de Vries et al. 1996; van der Meulen and te Meerman 1997; Bourgain et al. 2000, 2001, 2002; Tzeng et al. 2003; Zhang et al. 2003*b*; Yu et al. 2004*b*). As Tzeng et al. (2003) pointed out, none of these frequency- or sharing-based methods is uniformly the most powerful.

The standard χ^2 statistic compares allele (or haplotype) frequencies—or linear transformations of allele (or haplotype) frequencies—and partially considers the variance-covariance structure of the allele or haplotype frequencies. Therefore, the standard χ^2 test statistic is not uniformly the most powerful (Tzeng et al. 2003). Amplifying the difference in allele (or haplotype) frequencies between cases and controls is key to increasing the power of current test statistics for association studies.

Received December 1, 2004; accepted for publication April 19, 2005; electronically published May 9, 2005.

Address for correspondence and reprints: Dr. Momiao Xiong, Human Genetics Center, University of Texas–Houston, P.O. Box 20334, Houston, TX 77225. E-mail: Momiao.Xiong@uth.tmc.edu

0002-9297/2005/7701-0004$15.00

One way to amplify the difference in allele (or haplotype) frequencies between cases and controls is to use nonlinear transformations of allele or haplotype frequencies, $f(P^A)$ and $f(P)$, where P^A is the frequency of the allele (or haplotype) in cases and P is the frequency in controls, and to construct new test statistics such that the statistics based on $f(P^A) - f(P)$ are larger than the statistics based on the difference in allele or haplotype frequencies, $P^A - P$. The nonlinear transformations of allele or haplotype frequencies should have the feature that the magnitude of the amplified difference in allele or haplotype frequencies will increase as the difference in allele or haplotype frequencies increases.

A typical nonlinear function of frequencies is Shannon entropy. Shannon entropy, originally defined in information theory (Shannon 1948), is used to measure the uncertainty removed or the information gained by performing an experiment. When it is applied to characterize DNA variation, entropy measures genetic diversity and extracts the maximal amount of information for a set of SNP markers (Hampe et al. 2003). Conditional entropy measures the average information gained, given the occurrence of specific events. Entropy of a genomic region carried by affected individuals or unaffected individuals is conditional entropy. The difference between affected and unaffected individuals in entropy of the SNP markers is a measure of the association of the markers with disease.

In this article, we first define the entropy of a set of SNP markers at a genomic region of interest and the partial entropy of a haplotype. We then define the conditional entropy and the partial entropy of the markers in affected individuals and describe the relationship between conditional entropy and LD. We present a novel statistic that is based on the concept of entropy, to test the association between SNP markers and disease, including a test of the association of marker alleles, haplotypes, multiple-marker loci, and haplotype blocks. The relationship between the entropy-based test statistic and the standard χ^2 test statistic is discussed.

Entropy and the Overall Measure of Multilocus LD

Entropy, proposed by Shannon (1948), measures the uncertainty of random variables or the degree of nonstructure of a system (Nothnagel et al. 2003). The entropy of a random variable X is defined as

$$S(X) = E[-\log P(X)] = -\sum_i P(x_i)\log P(x_i) \ ,$$

where $P(x_i)$ denotes the probability that the random variable X assumes the value x_i.

The concept of entropy can be used to study DNA variation at a marker locus and patterns of LD. First, we consider two marker loci, M_1 and M_2, with two alleles each. Assume locus M_1 has alleles A and a with frequencies P_A and P_a, respectively. Locus M_2 has alleles B and b with frequencies P_B and P_b, respectively. The frequencies of haplotypes AB, Ab, aB, and ab are denoted by P_{AB}, P_{Ab}, P_{aB}, and P_{ab}, respectively. Let δ denote the measure of LD between two loci and be defined as

$$\delta = P_{AB} - P_A P_B \ .$$

The entropy of the marker is defined as

$$S_{M_1} = -P_A\log P_A - P_a\log P_a \ ,$$

and the entropy of the haplotypes at two marker loci is defined as

$$S_{M_1M_2} = -P_{AB}\log P_{AB} - P_{Ab}\log P_{Ab} \\ -P_{aB}\log_{aB} P - P_{ab}\log P_{ab} \ .$$

For convenience of presentation, a component of the entropy of the haplotypes at two marker loci is referred to as "partial entropy" of the specific haplotype. Let the partial entropy of haplotype AB, S_{AB}, be equal to $-P_{AB}\log P_{AB}$. In appendix A, we show that

$$S_{AB} \approx -P_A P_B\log(P_A P_B) \\ -\delta(\log P_A + \log P_B + 1) - \frac{\delta^2}{2P_A P_B} \ .$$

The entropy of the haplotypes at marker loci M_1 and M_2 is given by

$$S_{M_1M_2} \approx S_{M_1} + S_{M_2} - \frac{\delta^2}{2P_A P_a P_B P_b}$$

(see appendix A), where the entropies of the alleles at marker loci M_1 and M_2 are $S_{M_1} = -P_A\log P_A - P_a\log P_a$ and $S_{M_2} = -P_B\log P_B - P_b\log P_b$, respectively.

Next, we consider multiple loci. Suppose that there are K marker loci that generate m haplotypes. Let $P_{H_{j_1\cdots j_k}}$ be the population frequency of haplotype $H_{j_1\cdots j_k}$ with a sequence of alleles $M_{j_1}\ldots M_{j_k}$, where the allele M_{j_i} at the ith locus is either allele 1 or allele 2. Let $P_{M_{j_i}}$ be the frequency of allele M_{j_i} in the population. Define an overall measure of the haplotype LD at the K loci as

$$\delta_{j_1\cdots j_k} = P_{H_{j_1\cdots j_k}} - P_{M_{j_1}}\cdots P_{M_{j_k}} \qquad (1)$$

(Xiong et al. 2003). The partial entropy of haplotype

$H_{j_1 \ldots j_k}$ is defined as $S_{H_{j_1 \ldots j_k}} = -P_{H_{j_1 \ldots j_k}} \log P_{H_{j_1 \ldots j_k}}$, and the entropy of the haplotype at K marker loci is defined as

$$S_k = -\sum_{j_1}\sum_{j_2}\cdots\sum_{j_k} P_{H_{j_1 \ldots j_k}} \log P_{H_{j_1 \ldots j_k}} = \sum_{j_1}\cdots\sum_{j_k} S_{H_{j_1 \ldots j_k}} .$$

In appendix A, we show that the partial entropy $S_{H_{j_1 \ldots j_k}}$ and the entropy of the haplotype at K marker loci, S_k, can be approximated by

$$S_{H_{j_1 \ldots j_k}} \approx -P_{M_{j_1}} \cdots P_{M_{j_k}} \log\left(P_{M_{j_1}} \cdots P_{M_{j_k}}\right) + \left[1 + \log\left(P_{M_{j_1}} \cdots P_{M_{j_k}}\right)\right]\delta_{j_1 \ldots j_k} - \frac{\delta^2_{j_1 \ldots j_k}}{2P_{M_{j_1}} \cdots P_{M_{j_k}}}$$

and

$$S_k \approx \sum_{i=1}^{k} S_{M_i} - \frac{1}{2}\sum_{j_1}\cdots\sum_{j_k} \frac{\delta^2_{j_1 \ldots j_k}}{P_{M_{j_1}} \cdots P_{M_{j_k}}} ,$$

where $S_{M_i} = -\sum_{j=1}^{2} P_{M_{j_i}} \log P_{M_{j_i}}$ is the entropy of marker M_i. This shows that the entropy of the haplotype at K marker loci is the approximation of the sum of the entropies of all K marker loci and a function of the overall measures of all haplotypes.

Entropy in Affected Individuals

If the marker allele or haplotype is in LD with the disease locus, the frequency of the marker allele or haplotype in affected individuals and unaffected individuals will be different. The entropy of the haplotypes in affected individuals and unaffected individuals will also be different, and the difference can quantify the level of LD between the marker and the disease locus.

Let H_i be one of the m haplotypes at K marker loci. Let P_{H_i} and $P^A_{H_i}$ be the frequency of haplotype H_i in unaffected individuals and affected individuals, respectively. Let S_{H_i} and $S^A_{H_i}$ be the partial entropy of haplotype H_i in unaffected individuals and affected individuals, respectively. Then, we have

$$S_{H_i} = -P_{H_i} \log P_{H_i} \text{ and } S^A_{H_i} = -P^A_{H_i} \log P^A_{H_i} .$$

In appendix B, we show that $S^A_{H_i}$ can be approximated by

$$S^A_{H_i} \approx S_{H_i} - b\delta_{H_iD}(1 + \log P_{H_i}) - \frac{b^2\delta^2_{H_iD}}{2P_{H_i}} ,$$

where δ_{H_iD} is the overall measure of LD between haplotype H_i and disease allele D.

Therefore, the difference in the partial entropy of the haplotype between the affected and unaffected individuals is given by

$$\Delta S_{H_i} = S_{H_i} - S^A_{H_i} \approx b\delta_{H_iD}(1 + \log P_{H_i}) + \frac{b^2\delta^2_{H_iD}}{2P_{H_i}} . \quad (2)$$

Clearly, the gain in information about the association of the haplotype with disease is a function of the overall measure of LD between the haplotype and the disease locus. If the haplotype or marker loci are in linkage equilibrium with the disease allele, then the difference in the partial entropy of the haplotype (ΔS_{H_i}) between affected and unaffected individuals will be zero.

The Entropy-Based Statistic for Association Tests

In this section, we present an entropy-based statistic for case-control association studies. We begin with an introduction of notation. The first partial derivatives of the partial entropy of haplotype H_i with respect to the frequency of haplotype H_j, denoted by b_{ij}, is given as

$$b_{ii} = \frac{\partial S_{H_i}}{\partial P_{H_i}} = -1 - \log P_{H_i}$$

and

$$b_{ij} = \frac{\partial S_{H_i}}{\partial P_{H_j}} = 0 \ (i \neq j) .$$

The $m \times m$ dimensional matrix of the first partial derivatives is denoted by $B = (b_{ij})_{m \times m}$, where m is the number of haplotypes, as defined above. The number of haplotypes follows a multinomial distribution, and the variance-covariance matrix is given by $2n_G\Sigma$, where n_G is the number of unaffected individuals, $\Sigma = (\sigma_{ij})_{m \times m}$, $\sigma_{ii} = P_{H_i}(1 - P_{H_i})$, and $\sigma_{ij} = -P_{H_i}P_{H_j}$ $(i \neq j)$.

The above quantities can be similarly defined for the affected individuals and will be denoted by the additional superscript "A" in the corresponding quantities—that is,

$$b^A_{ii} = -1 - \log P^A_{H_i} , \quad b^A_{ij} = 0 \ (i \neq j) ,$$

and $B^A = (b^A_{ij})_{m \times m}$. Likewise, $\sigma^A_{ii} = P^A_{H_i}(1 - P^A_{H_i})$, $\sigma^A_{ij} = -P^A_{H_i}P^A_{H_j}$ $(i \neq j)$, and $\Sigma^A = (\sigma^A_{ij})_{m \times m}$.

Let $S = [S_{H_1} \ldots S_{H_m}]^T$, $S^A = [S^A_{H_1} \ldots S^A_{H_m}]^T$, $W = B\Sigma B^T$, and $W^A = B^A\Sigma^A(B^A)^T$, where $S^A_{H_i}$ is defined as in the previous section.

Let $\hat{S}$, $\hat{S}^A$, $\hat{W}$, and $\hat{W}^A$ be the estimators of S, S^A, W, and W^A, respectively. The partial entropy–based statistic for an association test, denoted by T_{PE}, is defined as

$$T_{PE} = (\hat{S} - \hat{S}^A)^T \left(\frac{\hat{W}^A}{2n_A} + \frac{\hat{W}}{2n_G}\right)^{-1} (\hat{S} - \hat{S}^A) ,$$

where n_A and n_G are the number of affected and unaffected individuals, respectively. Because the matrix

$$\left(\frac{\hat{W}^A}{2n_A} + \frac{\hat{W}}{2n_G}\right)$$

may not be of full rank, the generalized inverse of the matrix will be used in situations where the inverse of the matrix does not exist.

We can show that, under the null hypothesis of no association between the K marker loci and disease, when the frequencies of the haplotypes are not zero, T_{PE} is asymptotically distributed as a central $\chi^2_{(m-1)}$ distribution (appendix C). Because application of theorem 1.9 in Lehmann (1983, p. 344) requires that entropy be continuously differentiable with respect to the frequencies of the haplotypes, theorem 1.9 cannot be applied when the frequency of the haplotype is zero. If the frequency of the haplotype in either cases or controls is zero, then the haplotype needs to be grouped with other haplotypes. For example, rare haplotypes can be grouped with the most similar haplotype. Under the alternative hypothesis that there is an association between the K marker loci and the disease locus, T_{PE} is asymptotically distributed as a noncentral $\chi^2_{(m-1)}$ distribution with the following noncentrality parameter:

$$\lambda_{PE} = (S - S^A)^T \left(\frac{W^A}{2n_A} + \frac{W}{2n_G}\right)^{-1} (S - S^A) .$$

By invoking the relationship between the partial entropy of the haplotypes and the measure of LD discussed in the previous section, the noncentrality parameter λ_{PE} can be further reduced to

$$\lambda_{PE} \approx b^2 \delta_1^T \Sigma_0^{-1} \delta_1 + R_{PE}$$

(see appendix C), where

$$b = \frac{P_D(f_{11} - f_{12}) + P_d(f_{12} - f_{22})}{P(A)} ,$$

$$P(A) = P_D^2 f_{11} + 2P_D P_d f_{12} + P_d^2 f_{22} ,$$

$$\Sigma_0 = \frac{\Sigma}{2n_G} + \frac{\Sigma^A}{2n_A} ,$$

$$\delta_1 = [\delta_{H_1D} \ldots \delta_{H_mD}]^T ,$$

and other parameters are as given in appendix C.

Relationship between the Entropy-Based Statistic and the Standard χ^2 Test Statistic

Entropy-based statistics have a close relationship with the standard χ^2 test statistic. To see this, we first derive the standard χ^2 statistic using theorem 1.9 in Lehmann (1983, p. 344), which leads to an entropy-based statistic. Let $f_i(\hat{P}_{H_1} \ldots \hat{P}_{H_m}) = \hat{P}_{H_i}$. Then, the matrix

$$B = \left(\frac{\partial f_i}{\partial P_{H_j}}\right)_{m \times m} = I .$$

The variance-covariance matrix of the haplotype frequencies is given by $(1/n_G)\Sigma$, where

$$\Sigma = \begin{bmatrix} P_{H_1}(1 - P_{H_1}) & -P_{H_1}P_{H_2} & \cdots & -P_{H_1}P_{H_m} \\ \vdots & \vdots & & \vdots \\ -P_{H_m}P_{H_1} & -P_{H_m}P_{H_2} & \cdots & P_{H_m}(1 - P_{H_m}) \end{bmatrix} .$$

If we ignore the terms $-P_{H_i}^2$ and $-P_{H_i}P_{H_j}(i,j = 1,\ldots,m)$ in the elements of matrix Σ, then the variance-covariance matrix Σ is reduced to

$$\Sigma \approx \begin{bmatrix} P_{H_1} & 0 & \cdots & 0 \\ 0 & P_{H_2} & \cdots & 0 \\ \vdots & \vdots & \ddots & \vdots \\ 0 & 0 & \cdots & P_{H_m} \end{bmatrix} = \text{diag}(P_{H_i}) .$$

Similarly, we have $\Sigma^A \approx \text{diag}(P_{H_i}^A)$ for the affected individuals. Let $P = [P_{H_1} \ldots P_{H_m}]^T$, and $P^A = [P_{H_1}^A \ldots P_{H_m}^A]^T$. Define the test statistic T as

$$T = (P - P^A)^T \left(\frac{\Sigma}{2n_G} + \frac{\Sigma^A}{2n_A}\right)^{-1} (P - P^A) ,$$

which can be reduced to

$$T = \sum_{i=1}^{m} \frac{(P_{H_i} - P_{H_i}^{A})^2}{\dfrac{P_{H_i}}{2n_G} + \dfrac{P_{H_i}^{A}}{2n_A}} .$$

If we assume that the numbers of affected and unaffected individuals are equal (i.e., that $n_A = n_G = n$), then the χ^2 test statistic T can be further reduced to

$$T = 2n \sum_{i=1}^{m} \frac{(P_{H_i} - P_{H_i}^{A})^2}{P_{H_i} + P_{H_i}^{A}} ,$$

which is exactly the formula of the standard χ^2 test statistic (Chapman and Wijsman 1998).

Applying theorem 1.9 (Lehman 1983, p. 344) with the function form $f_i(\hat{P}_{H_1} \dots \hat{P}_{H_m}) = -P_{H_i} \log P_{H_i}$ will yield the test statistic T_{PE}. Therefore, the difference between the standard χ^2 test statistic and the entropy-based statistic is that the χ^2 test statistic uses a linear function of haplotype frequencies, whereas the entropy-based test statistic uses a nonlinear function of haplotype frequencies. The difference between these two test statistics lies in the different mathematical forms of the haplotype frequencies when theorem 1.9 is used to construct the statistics.

In appendix C, we show that the noncentrality parameter λ_T of the standard χ^2 test statistic is given by $\lambda_T = b^2 \delta_1^T \Sigma_0^{-1} \delta_1$. This is the first term in the noncentrality parameter λ_{PE} of the test statistic based on partial entropy of the haplotypes.

Results

Distribution of the Entropy-Based Statistic

In the previous sections, we have shown that when the sample size is large enough to apply large-sample theory, the distribution of the entropy-based statistic under the null hypothesis of no association is asymptotically a central χ^2 distribution. To examine the validity of this statement, we performed a series of simulation studies. The computer program SNaP (Nothnagel 2002) was used to generate haplotypes of the sample individuals. Two data sets with a single haplotype block each were simulated. The first data set has two marker loci that generated four haplotypes with frequencies 0.2952, 0.2562, 0.1957, and 0.2529. The second data set has six marker loci that generated eight haplotypes with frequencies 0.1820, 0.1461, 0.1406, 0.1291, 0.1211, 0.1107, 0.0817, and 0.0887. For each data set, 20,000 individuals who were divided into equal groups of cases and controls were generated in the general population.

To examine whether the asymptotic results of the entropy-based test statistic still hold for a small sample size under the null hypothesis of no association, 200 individuals each were randomly sampled from the cases and controls. A total of 10,000 simulations were performed. In each simulation, the entropy-based test statistic T_{PE} was calculated. Figure 1*A* and 1*B* plot the histograms of the test statistic T_{PE} with the use of two-SNP haplotypes and six-SNP haplotypes, respectively. It can be seen that the distributions of T_{PE} are similar to the theoretical central χ^2 distributions, even under the scenario of a smaller sample size. Table 1 summarizes the type I error rates of the test statistic T_{PE} for sample sizes from 100 to 500 individuals with the use of two-SNP and six-SNP haplotypes. Table 1 shows that the estimated type I error rates of the entropy-based test statistic were not ap-

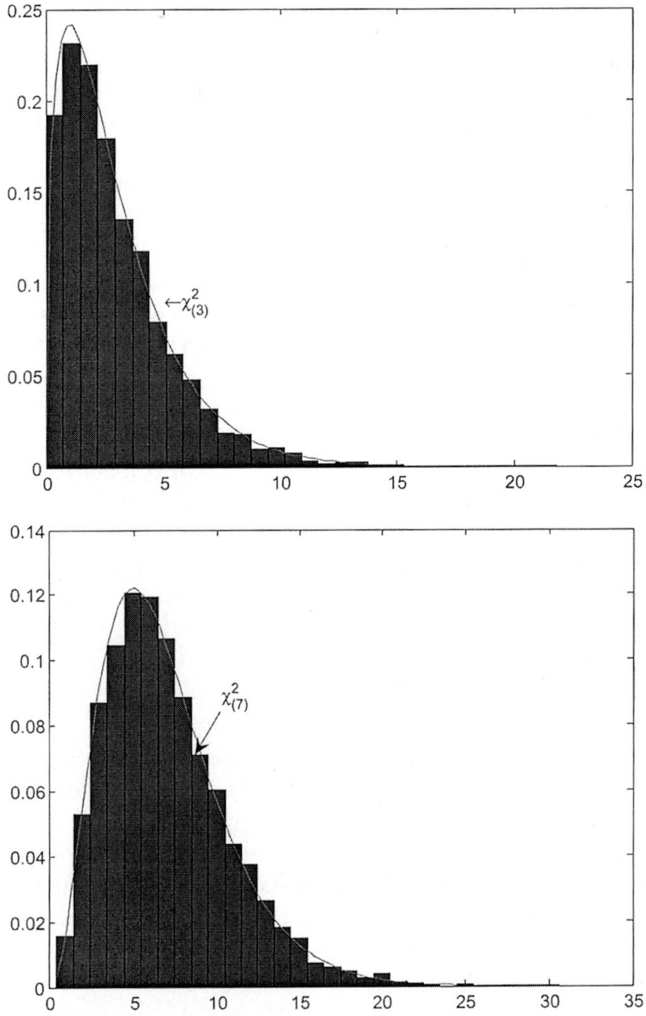

Figure 1 Distribution of the test statistic T_{PE} with the use of two-SNP haplotypes (*A*) and six-SNP haplotypes (*B*). $\chi^2_{(3)}$ and $\chi^2_{(7)}$ indicate χ^2 distribution with 3 df and 7 df, respectively.

Am. J. Hum. Genet. 77:27–40, 2005

Table 1

Estimated Type I Error Rates of the Test Statistic T_{PE} for 10,000 Simulations

Sample Size	Estimated Type I Error Rate for Two-SNP Haplotypes $\alpha = .05$	$\alpha = .01$	$\alpha = .001$	Six-SNP Haplotypes $\alpha = .05$	$\alpha = .01$	$\alpha = .001$
100	.0460	.0078	.0006	.0542	.0112	.0008
200	.0480	.0088	.0012	.0488	.0106	.0010
300	.0460	.0103	.0011	.0512	.0092	.0014
400	.0478	.0100	.0008	.0542	.0102	.0008
500	.0478	.0084	.0008	.0488	.0098	.0012

preciably different from the nominal levels $\alpha = 0.05$, $\alpha = 0.01$, and $\alpha = 0.001$.

Power of the Entropy-Based Test Statistic and the Standard χ^2 Test Statistic

The power of an association test statistic depends on a number of parameters, such as the measure of LD between haplotypes and disease alleles, the sample size, and the model of disease inheritance. We compared the power of the entropy-based test statistic with that of the standard χ^2 test statistic. The markers are assumed to be biallelic (i.e., SNPs). Specifically, we considered two marker loci and a disease locus that is located in the middle of two markers. We considered three disease models: recessive, dominant, and genotype relative-risk models, in which the genotype relative risk for genotypes *Dd* and *DD* is r and r^2 times greater, respectively, than that of the genotype *dd* (Risch and Merikangas 1996).

Exact analytical methods were used for calculation of power. The average haplotype frequencies in the affected and unaffected individuals were calculated by equations (1) and (4) from Akey et al. (2001). The power of the entropy-based statistic and the standard χ^2 statistic (Chapman and Wijsman 1998) ($\alpha = 0.001$), with the use of four haplotypes generated by two marker loci as a function of the genetic distance between the disease locus and its flanking marker loci for recessive, dominant, and genotype relative-risk models are shown in figure 2*A*, 2*B*, and 2*C*, respectively. The data demonstrate that the power of the entropy-based statistic for all three disease models is higher than the power of the standard χ^2 statistic. In appendix C, we show that the noncentrality parameter of the entropy-based statistic is approximately equal to the summation of the noncentrality parameter of the standard χ^2 test statistic and R_{PE}. But, R_{PE} is not always positive, and the entropy-based statistic does not monotonically increase with increasing allele-frequency differences, which implies that the entropy-based statistic is not uniformly more powerful than the standard χ^2 test. In fact, when the difference in allele frequencies is very large (i.e., when $|P^A - P| > 0.7$), the χ^2 test is more powerful than the entropy-based statistic proposed here.

Application to Real-Data Examples

To evaluate its performance, we applied the entropy-based test to two real data sets. The first example is a test of association between the catechol-O-methyltransferase (COMT) gene and schizophrenia (Shifman et al. 2002). The COMT gene plays an important biochemical function in the metabolism of catecholamine neurotransmitters and is being increasingly recognized as a contributor to velocardiofacial syndrome, which is associated with a high rate of psychosis (Shifman et al. 2002). The data were from a large case-control study of schizophrenia in the Ashkenazi Jewish population. Three SNPs within the COMT gene were typed. In table 2, we present the *P* values of the entropy-based statistic for testing the association of two-SNP haplotypes (generated from two SNP markers) and three-SNP haplotypes (generated from three SNP markers) with schizophrenia. For comparison, table 2 also includes the results of Shifman et al. (2002) that were obtained by the usual χ^2 test. It is evident that *P* values of the entropy-based test are smaller than those of the χ^2 test.

The second example studied the association between functional haplotypes in the promoter of the matrix metalloproteinase-2 (MMP-2) gene and esophageal squamous cell carcinoma in the Chinese Han population (Yu et al. 2004*a*). Two SNPs (−1306C/T and −735C/T) in the MMP-2 gene were typed in 527 patients with esophageal cancer and 777 controls. Frequencies of two-SNP haplotypes and *P* values obtained by the entropy-based test and standard χ^2 test are given in table 3. Again, the entropy-based test obtained a smaller *P* value compared with that obtained by the standard χ^2 test.

Discussion

Completion of the International HapMap Project will provide a powerful tool for identifying genes that contribute to complex disease (Collins 2004). To efficiently use DNA variants for genetic studies of complex diseases, the field of human genetics needs to accomplish two tasks: choose suitable marker sets and develop robust methods of statistical analysis (Wall and Pritchard 2003). The purpose of this report is to present an analytical method of assessing the relationship between DNA variation and disease in case-control association studies.

The standard χ^2 statistic is based on a linear function of haplotype or allele frequencies. Its drawback is a decrease in power as the number of degrees of freedom increases, which arises as a consequence of using a dense set of SNPs. There are two ways to increase the power

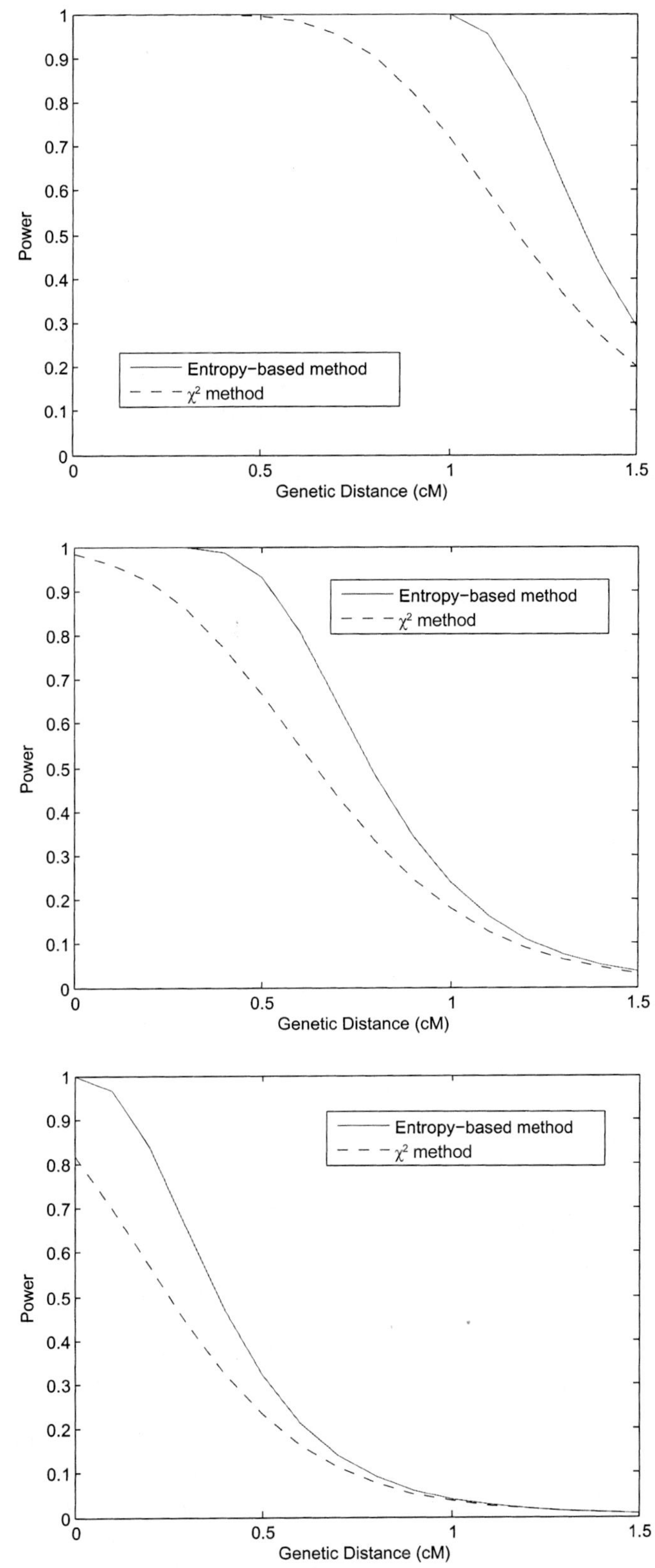

Figure 2 *A*, Power of the entropy-based test statistic and the standard χ^2 test statistic with a significance level of $\alpha = 0.001$, as a function of the genetic distance between the marker and disease loci, for a recessive disease (*A*) and a dominant disease (*B*) under the assumption that $N = 100$, $t = 100$ generations, the frequencies of the minor alleles at both of the marker loci are equal to 0.1, and $P_D = 0.1$. *C*, Power of the entropy-based test statistic and the standard χ^2 test statistic with a significance level of $\alpha = 0.001$ for a disease with genotype relative risk $r = 4$, as a function of the genetic distance between the marker and disease loci, under the assumption that $N = 200$, $t = 100$ generations, the frequencies of the minor alleles at the first and second marker loci are equal to 0.4 and 0.1, respectively, and $P_D = 0.2$.

Table 2

Tests of Association between COMT Haplotypes and Schizophrenia

Haplotype Size and Markers	*P* Value for χ^2			*P* Value for Entropy		
	Males	Females	All	Males	Females	All
Two-SNP haplotype						
rs737865, rs165599	.0093	.0014	.00014	.00012	1.5×10^{-6}	1.9×10^{-9}
rs737865, rs165688	.017	.046	.0057	.00018	.012	2.7×10^{-6}
rs165599, rs165688	.096	.0012	.0011	.0035	2.7×10^{-5}	2.9×10^{-6}
Three-SNP haplotype						
rs165688, rs737865, rs165599	.0084	.0069	.00045	8.4×10^{-9}	5.7×10^{-6}	1.5×10^{-12}

of an association test statistic. One is to find appropriate mathematical forms of the haplotype or allele frequencies that can be used to develop test statistics with higher power. Another is to reduce the degrees of freedom. Most publications in this field have focused on reducing the degrees of freedom. This report focuses on developing new entropy-based statistics to amplify the difference in allele or haplotype frequencies to increase power.

At its most fundamental level, the case-control study design provides a forum to compare allele frequencies or the transformation of allele frequencies between groups. Although the usual χ^2 test statistic is a quadratic function of the difference in allele frequencies, the difference represents a linear function of allele frequencies. There are two ways to amplify the difference in allele frequencies. One way is to make a nonlinear transformation of allele frequencies. Another way is to make a nonlinear transformation of the difference in allele frequencies between cases and controls. Although the second way can amplify the difference between allele frequencies, under the null hypothesis of zero difference, the entropy of the difference between allele frequencies is no longer differentiable at zero. Therefore, asymptotic theory of the nonlinear transformation of normal random variables cannot be applied to such statistics. The entropy-based statistic compares the difference in values of a nonlinear function of allele frequencies between cases and controls, in the hope that the difference will be larger than that of a linear function of allele frequencies between cases and controls.

Entropy measures the information contained in a stochastic process and can be used to measure haplotype diversity. In this report, we show that differences in the entropy of haplotypes between affected and unaffected individuals quantify the overall level of LD between the marker, haplotypes, and the disease locus. We note that the entropy of the observed haplotypes is a nonlinear function of haplotype frequencies. The entropy of haplotypes at *K* marker loci quantifies the information of all haplotypes generated at the *K* marker loci. The calculated entropy of the haplotypes depends on the choice of mathematical functions of the haplotype frequencies. We introduced the concept of partial entropy of a haplotype. If we compare the difference between affected and unaffected individuals in the partial entropy of a haplotype, we can test the association of that particular haplotype with disease. We can also test the association of a set of haplotypes or multiple marker loci by comparing differences in the partial entropy of the set between affected and unaffected individuals.

To use an entropy-based statistic to test the association of haplotypes with disease, we first need to study the distribution of the test statistic under the null hypothesis of no association. By simulation, we show that the distribution of the entropy-based test statistic is close to a χ^2 distribution, even for small sample sizes. To validate the test statistic and to estimate the false-positive rate, we calculated the type I error rates of the entropy-based statistic by simulation. The results showed that the type I error rates were close to the nominal significance levels, which implies that the test for association is valid for a single homogeneous population.

An important property of a test statistic for genetic association studies is power. We show, by analytical methods, that the power of the entropy-based statistic is higher than the power of the standard χ^2 statistic in most cases. The power gap between these two test statistics increases as the number of haplotypes increases (data not shown). However, the entropy-based statis-

Table 3

Tests of Association between MMP-2 Haplotypes and Esophageal Cancer

Haplotype −1306	Haplotype −735	Frequency in Cases	Frequency in Controls
T	T	.0057	.0335
T	C	.1120	.1313
C	T	.2116	.2181
C	C	.6708	.6171

Note.—Overall *P* value is 7.03×10^{-6} for the χ^2 statistic and 3.24×10^{-8} for the entropy-based statistic.

tic is not more powerful in all situations. When the difference in allele frequencies is very large, that is, $|P^A - P| > 0.7$, the χ^2 statistic is more powerful than the entropy-based statistic. However, such differences in allele frequencies between cases and controls are practically unheard of in real-world studies of common human diseases. The entropy-based statistic was applied to real data to test the association between COMT haplotypes and schizophrenia and the association between the MMP-2 gene and esophageal squamous cell carcinoma. The results of real-data analyses demonstrated that, for case-control studies, P values of the entropy-based statistic are smaller than those of the standard χ^2 test.

Asymptotical theory for nonlinear transformation of normal variables requires that entropy be continuously differentiable with respect to the frequencies of the haplotype. When the frequency of the haplotype in either cases or controls is zero, entropy is no longer continuously differentiable. In this case, the haplotype needs to be grouped with other haplotypes. However, such grouping may result in loss of statistical power, depending on the haplotype effects of the grouped haplotypes.

The entropy of a haplotype is a nonlinear function of haplotype frequencies. Other mathematical functions of haplotype frequencies should be investigated for designing novel test statistics in the future. This will open new ways of developing more powerful statistics for tests of association. The completion of the International HapMap Project and advances in genotyping technologies bode well for large-scale whole-genome association studies. Development of robust methods for relating considerable genomic information to risk of disease is urgently needed.

Acknowledgments

We thank Dr. Sagiv Shifman and Dr. Ariel Darvasi, for providing the detailed data for schizophrenic haplotype analyses. We also thank two anonymous reviewers for helpful comments on the manuscript, which led to much improvement of the article. M.X. is supported by National Institutes of Health–National Institute of Arthritis and Musculoskeletal and Skin Diseases (NIH-NIAMS) grant IP50AR44888, grant HL74735, and NIH grant ES09912. J.Z. is supported by NIH grant ES09912. E.B. is supported by a grant from the National Heart, Lung and Blood Institute.

Appendix A

First, we consider the partial entropy of a haplotype at two marker loci. By definition, the partial entropy of haplotype AB is

$$S_{AB} = -P_{AB}\log P_{AB} \ . \tag{A1}$$

But,

$$P_{AB} = P_A P_B + \delta \ . \tag{A2}$$

Substituting P_{AB} from equation (A2) into equation (A1) yields

$$S_{AB} = -(P_A P_B + \delta)\log(P_A P_B + \delta) \ ,$$

which can be simplified to

$$\begin{aligned} S_{AB} &= -(P_A P_B + \delta)\log(P_A P_B) - (P_A P_B + \delta)\log\left(1 + \frac{\delta}{P_A P_B}\right) \\ &\approx -P_A P_B(\log P_A + \log P_B) - \delta(\log P_A + \log P_B) - (P_A P_B + \delta)\left(\frac{\delta}{P_A P_B} - \frac{\delta^2}{2P_A^2 P_B^2}\right) \\ &\quad \left[\text{by } \log(1+x) \approx x - \frac{x^2}{2}\right] \\ &\approx -P_A P_B(\log P_A + \log P_B) - \delta(\log P_A + \log P_B + 1) - \frac{\delta^2}{2P_A P_B} \ . \end{aligned}$$

The above formula is derived by Taylor expansion of the logarithm function. The assumption for Taylor expansion of the logarithm function is that the argument x should be small. When the frequencies of alleles are small, δ/P_AP_B may be large. This will violate the assumption of the Taylor expansion and makes approximation inaccurate.

Similarly, we have

$$S_{Ab} \approx -P_AP_b(\log P_A + \log P_b) + \delta(\log P_A + \log P_b + 1) - \frac{\delta^2}{2P_AP_b} ,$$

$$S_{aB} \approx -P_aP_B(\log P_a + \log P_B) + \delta(\log P_a + \log P_B + 1) - \frac{\delta^2}{2P_aP_B} , \text{ and}$$

$$S_{ab} \approx -P_aP_b(\log P_a + \log P_b) - \delta(\log P_a + \log P_b + 1) - \frac{\delta^2}{2P_aP_b} .$$

The entropy of the haplotypes at marker loci M_1 and M_2 is equal to

$$S_{M_1M_2} \approx -P_A\log P_A - P_a\log P_a - P_B\log P_B - P_b\log P_b - \frac{\delta^2}{2}\left(\frac{1}{P_AP_B}+\frac{1}{P_AP_b}+\frac{1}{P_aP_B}+\frac{1}{P_aP_b}\right)$$

$$= S_{M_1}+S_{M_2} - \frac{\delta^2}{2P_AP_aP_BP_b} ,$$

where S_{M_1} and S_{M_2} are the entropies of marker loci M_1 and M_2, respectively.

Next, we consider the partial entropy of a haplotype at multiple marker loci. By definition, partial entropy of haplotype $H_{j_1\ldots j_k}$ is defined as

$$S_{H_{j_1\ldots j_k}} = -P_{H_{j_1\ldots j_k}}\log P_{H_{j_1\ldots j_k}} .$$

But, from equation (1), we have

$$S_{H_{j_1\ldots j_k}} = -(P_{M_{j_1}}\cdots P_{M_{j_k}} + \delta_{j_1\ldots j_k})\log(P_{M_{j_1}}\cdots P_{M_{j_k}} + \delta_{j_1\ldots j_k})$$

$$= -(P_{M_{j_1}}\cdots P_{M_{j_k}} + \delta_{j_1\ldots j_k})\log(P_{M_{j_1}}\cdots P_{M_{j_k}}) - (P_{M_{j_1}}\cdots P_{M_{j_k}} + \delta_{j_1\ldots j_k})\log\left(1+\frac{\delta_{j_1\ldots j_k}}{P_{M_{j_1}}\cdots P_{M_{j_k}}}\right)$$

$$\approx -P_{M_{j_1}}\cdots P_{M_{j_k}}\log(P_{M_{j_1}}\cdots P_{M_{j_k}}) - \delta_{j_1\ldots j_k}\left[\log(P_{M_{j_1}}\cdots P_{M_{j_k}})+1\right] - \frac{\delta^2_{j_1\ldots j_k}}{2P_{M_{j_1}}\cdots P_{M_{j_k}}} .$$

Summarizing $S_{H_{j_1\ldots j_k}}$ over all possible $j_1\ldots j_k$ yields

$$S_K \approx \sum_{i=1}^{K} S_{M_i} - \frac{1}{2}\sum_{j_1}\cdots\sum_{j_k}\frac{\delta^2_{j_1\ldots j_k}}{P_{M_{j_1}}\cdots P_{M_{j_k}}}$$

(note that $\sum_{j_1}\cdots\sum_{j_k}\delta_{j_1\ldots j_k} = 0$), where $S_{M_i} = -\sum_{j=1}^{2} P_{M_{j_i}}\log P_{M_{j_i}}$ is the entropy of marker M_i.

Appendix B

By definition,

$$S^A_{H_i} = -P^A_{H_i}\log P^A_{H_i} , \text{ where } P^A_{H_i} = \frac{P(H_i,A)}{P(A)} . \quad \text{(B1)}$$

If we assume Hardy-Weinberg equilibrium, then the prevalence of disease $P(A) = P_D^2f_{11} + 2P_DP_df_{12} + P_d^2f_{22}$, where

P_D and P_d denote the frequencies of alleles D and d at disease locus, respectively, and f_{11}, f_{12}, and f_{22} are the penetrances of genotype DD, Dd, and dd, respectively.

By theorem of total probability (Ross 1997),

$$\begin{aligned} P(H_i,A) &= P(H_i,DD,A) + P(H_i,Dd,A) + P(H_i,dd,A) \\ &= P_{H_iD}P_Df_{11} + (P_{H_iD}P_d + P_{H_id}P_D)f_{12} + P_{H_id}P_df_{22} \,. \end{aligned}$$

Therefore,

$$P^A_{H_i} = a_1P_{H_iD} + a_2P_{H_id} \,, \tag{B2}$$

where

$$a_1 = \frac{P_Df_{11} + P_df_{12}}{P(A)} \quad \text{and} \quad a_2 = \frac{P_Df_{12} + P_df_{22}}{P(A)} \,.$$

Note that

$$P_{H_iD} = P_{H_i}P_D + \delta_{H_iD} \quad \text{and} \quad P_{H_id} = P_{H_i}P_d + \delta_{H_id} \tag{B3}$$

(Xiong et al. 2003), where δ_{H_iD} and δ_{H_id} are the overall measure of LD between haplotype H_i and disease allele D and between haplotype H_i and allele d, respectively. Substituting P_{H_iD} and P_{H_id} from equation (B3) into equation (B2) leads to

$$\begin{aligned} P^A_{H_i} &= a_1(P_{H_i}P_D + \delta_{H_iD}) + a_2(P_{H_i}P_d + \delta_{H_id}) \\ &= P_{H_i}(a_1P_D + a_2P_d) + a_1\delta_{H_iD} + a_2\delta_{H_id} \,. \end{aligned} \tag{B4}$$

Since $a_1P_D + a_2P_d = 1$ and $\delta_{H_id} = -\delta_{H_iD}$, the above equation (B4) is simplified to

$$P^A_{H_i} = P_{H_i} + (a_1 - a_2)\delta_{H_iD} = P_{H_i} + b\delta_{H_iD} \,, \tag{B5}$$

where $b = a_1 - a_2$. Substituting $P^A_{H_i}$ from equation (B5) into equation (B1) yields

$$\begin{aligned} S^A = S^A_{H_i} &= -(P_{H_i} + b\delta_{H_iD})\log(P_{H_i} + b\delta_{H_iD}) \\ &= -(P_{H_i} + b\delta_{H_iD})\log\left[P_{H_i}\left(1 + \frac{b\delta_{H_iD}}{P_{H_i}}\right)\right] \\ &= -(P_{H_i} + b\delta_{H_iD})\log P_{H_i} - (P_{H_i} + b\delta_{H_iD})\log\left(1 + \frac{b\delta_{H_iD}}{P_{H_i}}\right) \\ &\approx -P_{H_i}\log P_{H_i} - b\delta_{H_iD}\log P_{H_i} - (P_{H_i} + b\delta_{H_iD})\left(\frac{b\delta_{H_iD}}{P_{H_i}} - \frac{b^2\delta^2_{H_iD}}{2P^2_{H_i}}\right) \\ &= -P_{H_i}\log P_{H_i} - b\delta_{H_iD}(1 + \log P_{H_i}) - \frac{b^2\delta^2_{H_iD}}{2P_{H_i}} \\ &= S_{H_i} - b\delta_{H_iD}(1 + \log P_{H_i}) - \frac{b^2\delta^2_{H_iD}}{2P_{H_i}} \,. \end{aligned}$$

Appendix C

Recall that

$$S = [S_{H_1} \ldots S_{H_m}]^T \text{ and } S^A = [S^A_{H_1} \ldots S^A_{H_m}]^T .$$

From equation (2), we have

$$S - S^A \approx U , \tag{C1}$$

where $U = [U_1 \ldots U_m]^T$ and $U_i = b(\log P_{H_i} + 1)\delta_{H_iD} + b^2\delta^2_{H_iD}/2P_{H_i}$. Next, we calculate the Jacobian matrix B^A. By definition,

$$\begin{aligned} b^A_{ii} &= \frac{\partial S^A_{H_i}}{\partial P^A_{H_i}} \\ &= -1 - \log P^A_{H_i} \\ &= -1 - \log (P_{H_i} + b\delta_{H_iD}) \\ &\approx -1 - \log P_{H_i} - \frac{b\delta_{H_iD}}{P_{H_i}} \quad [\text{by } \log(1+x) \approx x] \\ &= b_{ii} - \frac{b\delta_{H_iD}}{P_{H_i}} , \end{aligned}$$

where $b_{ii} = -1 - \log P_{H_i}$. Let $G_i = -b\delta_{H_iD}/P_{H_i}$ and $G = \text{diag}(G_1 \ldots G_m)$. Then, we have

$$B^A \approx B + G . \tag{C2}$$

Next, we study the relationship between covariance matrix Σ^A in the affected individuals and covariance matrix Σ in the unaffected individuals. Note that

$$P^A_{H_i}(1 - P^A_{H_i}) = (P_{H_i} + b\delta_{H_iD})(1 - P_{H_i} - b\delta_{H_iD}) \approx P_{H_i}(1 - P_{H_i}) + b(1 - 2P_{H_i})\delta_{H_iD}$$

and

$$-P^A_{H_i}P^A_{H_j} = -(P_{H_i} + b\delta_{H_iD})(P_{H_j} + b\delta_{H_jD}) \approx -P_{H_i}P_{H_j} - b(P_{H_i}\delta_{H_jD} + P_{H_j}\delta_{H_iD}) .$$

Thus, we have $\Sigma^A \approx \Sigma + bD$, where

$$D = \begin{bmatrix} (1-2P_{H_1})\delta_{H_1D} & -(P_{H_1}\delta_{H_2D} + P_{H_2}\delta_{H_1D}) & \cdots & -(P_{H_1}\delta_{H_mD} + P_{H_m}\delta_{H_1D}) \\ \vdots & \vdots & \cdots & \vdots \\ -(P_{H_m}\delta_{H_1D} + P_{H_1}\delta_{H_mD}) & -(P_{H_m}\delta_{H_2D} + P_{H_2}\delta_{H_mD}) & \cdots & (1-2P_{H_m})\delta_{H_mD} \end{bmatrix} .$$

Now we are ready to calculate the quantity $\frac{W}{2n_G} + \frac{W^A}{2n_A}$. With the definition of W^A and equation (C2), we have

$$W^A = B^A\Sigma^A(B^A)^T \approx (B+G)\Sigma^A(B+G)^T = B\Sigma^AB^T + R ,$$

where $R = B\Sigma^A G^T + G\Sigma^A B^T + G\Sigma^A G^T$. Thus,

$$\frac{W}{2n_G} + \frac{W^A}{2n_A} \approx \frac{1}{2n_G} B\Sigma B^T + \frac{1}{2n_A} B\Sigma^A B^T + \frac{1}{2n_A} R$$

$$= B\left(\frac{\Sigma}{2n_G} + \frac{\Sigma^A}{2n_A}\right) B^T + \frac{1}{2n_A} R$$

$$= W_0 + \frac{1}{2n_A} R ,$$

where $\Sigma_0 = \frac{\Sigma}{2n_G} + \frac{\Sigma^A}{2n_A}$ and $W_0 = B\Sigma_0 B^T$. But,

$$\left(W_0 + \frac{1}{2n_A} R\right)^{-1} = W_0^{-1} - W_0^{-1}(W_0^{-1} + 2n_A R^{-1})^{-1} W_0^{-1}$$

(Anderson 1984). Then, the noncentrality parameter λ_{PE} can be expressed as

$$\lambda_{PE} \approx (S - S^A)^T [W_0^{-1} - W_0^{-1}(W_0^{-1} + 2n_A R^{-1})^{-1} W_0^{-1}](S - S^A) . \qquad (C3)$$

Substituting $S - S^A \approx U$ from equation (C1) into the above equation (C3) yields

$$\lambda_{PE} \approx U^T [W_0^{-1} - W_0^{-1}(W_0^{-1} + 2n_A R^{-1})^{-1} W_0^{-1}] U$$

$$= U^T W_0^{-1} U - U^T W_0^{-1}(W_0^{-1} + 2n_A R^{-1})^{-1} W_0^{-1} U . \qquad (C4)$$

But,

$$U^T W_0^{-1} U = U^T (B^{-1})^T \Sigma_0^{-1} B^{-1} U$$

$$= (B^{-1} U)^T \Sigma_0^{-1} B^{-1} U$$

$$= (b\delta_1 + b^2\delta_2)^T \Sigma_0^{-1} (b\delta_1 + b^2\delta_2) , \qquad (C5)$$

where $\delta_1 = [\delta_{H_1 D} \ldots \delta_{H_m D}]^T$ and

$$\delta_2 = \left[\frac{\delta^2_{H_1 D}}{2(1 + \log P_{H_1}) P_{H_1}} \cdots \frac{\delta^2_{H_m D}}{2(1 + \log P_{H_m}) P_{H_m}}\right]^T .$$

Substituting equation (C5) into equation (C4) yields $\lambda_{PE} \approx b^2 \delta_1^T \Sigma_0^{-1} \delta_1 + R_{PE}$, where

$$R_{PE} = 2b^3 \delta_1^T \Sigma_0^{-1} \delta_2 + b^4 \delta_2^T \Sigma_0^{-1} \delta_2 - (b\delta_1 + b^2\delta_2)^T \Sigma_0^{-1} B^{-1} (W_0^{-1} + 2n_A R^{-1})^{-1} B^{-1} \Sigma_0^{-1} (b\delta_1 + b^2\delta_2) .$$

Then, we derive the noncentrality parameter λ_T of the standard χ^2 test statistic T. From equation (C5), we know

$$\lambda_T = (P - P^A)^T \left(\frac{\Sigma}{2n_G} + \frac{\Sigma^A}{2n_A}\right)^{-1} (P - P^A) = (P - P^A)^T \Sigma_0^{-1} (P - P^A) .$$

But, from equation (B5), we have $P^A - P = b\delta_1$. Therefore, $\lambda_T = b^2 \delta_1^T \Sigma_0^{-1} \delta_1$.

References

Akey J, Jin L, Xiong M (2001) Haplotypes vs single marker linkage disequilibrium tests: what do we gain? Eur J Hum Genet 9:291–300

Anderson TW (1984) An introduction to multivariate statistical analysis. John Wiley & Sons, New York

Bourgain C, Genin E, Margaritte-Jeannin P, Clerget-Darpoux F (2001) Maximum identity length contrast: a powerful method for susceptibility gene detection in isolated populations. Genet Epidemiol Suppl 21:S560–S564

Bourgain C, Genin E, Ober C, Clerget-Darpoux F (2002) Missing data in haplotype analysis: a study on the MILC method. Ann Hum Genet 66:99–108

Bourgain C, Genin E, Quesneville H, Clerget-Darpoux F (2000) Search for multifactorial disease susceptibility genes in founder populations. Ann Hum Genet 64:255–265

Carlson CS, Eberle MA, Kruglyak L, Nickerson DA (2004) Mapping complex disease loci in whole-genome association studies. Nature 429:446–452

Chapman NH, Wijsman EM (1998) Genome screens using linkage disequilibrium tests: optimal marker characteristics and feasibility. Am J Hum Genet 63:1872–1885

Collins FS (2004) The case for a US prospective cohort study of genes and environment. Nature 429:475–477

de Vries HG, van der Meulen MA, Rozen R, Halley DJ, Scheffer H, ten Kate LP, Buys CH, te Meerman GJ (1996) Haplotype identity between individuals who share a CFTR mutation allele "identical by descent": demonstration of the usefulness of the haplotype-sharing concept for gene mapping in real populations. Hum Genet 98:304–309

Freedman ML, Reich D, Penney KL, McDonald GJ, Mignault AA, Patterson N, Gabriel SB, Topol EJ, Smoller JW, Pato CN, Pato MT, Petryshen TL, Kolonel LN, Lander ES, Sklar P, Henderson B, Hirschhorn JN, Altshuler D (2004) Assessing the impact of population stratification on genetic association studies. Nat Genet 36:388–393

Gabriel SB, Schaffner SF, Nguyen H, Moore JM, Roy J, Blumenstiel B, Higgins J, DeFelice M, Lochner A, Faggart M, Liu-Cordero SN, Rotimi C, Adeyemo A, Cooper R, Ward R, Lander ES, Daly MJ, Altshuler D (2002) The structure of haplotype blocks in the human genome. Science 296:2225–2229

Goldstein DB (2001) Islands of linkage disequilibrium. Nat Genet 29:109–111

Hampe J, Schreiber S, Krawczak M (2003) Entropy-based SNP selection for genetic association studies. Hum Genet 114: 36–43

Johnson GC, Esposito L, Barratt BJ, Smith AN, Heward J, Di Genova G, Ueda H, Cordell HJ, Eaves IA, Dudbridge F, Twells RC, Payne F, Hughes W, Nutland S, Stevens H, Carr P, Tuomilehto-Wolf E, Tuomilehto J, Gough SC, Clayton DG, Todd JA (2001) Haplotype tagging for the identification of common disease genes. Nat Genet 29:233–237

Ke X, Cardon LR (2003) Efficient selective screening of haplotype tag SNPs. Bioinformatics 19:287–288

Lehmann EL (1983) Theory of point estimation. John Wiley & Sons, New York

Morton NE, Collins A (1998) Tests and estimates of allelic association in complex inheritance. PNAS 95:11389–11393

Neale BM, Sham PC (2004) The future of association studies: gene-based analysis and replication. Am J Hum Genet 75: 353–362

Nothnagel M (2002) Simulation of LD block-structured SNP haplotype data and its use for the analysis of case-control data by supervised learning methods. Am J Hum Genet Suppl 71:A2363

Nothnagel M, Furst R, Rohde K (2002) Entropy as a measure for linkage disequilibrium over multilocus haplotype blocks. Hum Hered 54:186–198

Pritchard JK, Przeworski M (2001) Linkage disequilibrium in humans: models and data. Am J Hum Genet 69:1–14

Risch N, Merikangas K (1996) The future of genetic studies of complex human diseases. Science 273:1516–1517

Ross SM (1997) Introduction to probability models. Academic Press, New York

Shannon CE (1948) A mathematical theory of communication. Bell Systems Tech J 27:379–423

Shifman S, Bronstein M, Sternfeld M, Pisante-Shalom A, Lev-Lehman E, Weizman A, Reznik I, Spivak B, Grisaru N, Karp L, Schiffer R, Kotler M, Strous RD, Swartz-Vanetik M, Knobler HY, Shinar E, Beckmann JS, Yakir B, Risch N, Zak NB, Darvasi A (2002) A highly significant association between a COMT haplotype and schizophrenia. Am J Hum Genet 71:1296–1302

Stephens JC, Schneider JA, Tanguay DA, Choi J, Acharya T, Stanley SE, Jiang R, et al (2001) Haplotype variation and linkage disequilibrium in 313 human genes. Science 293:489–493

Stumpf MP, Goldstein DB (2003) Demography, recombination hotspot intensity, and the block structure of linkage disequilibrium. Curr Biol 13:1–8

Tzeng JY, Devlin B, Wasserman L, Roeder K (2003) On the identification of disease mutations by the analysis of haplotype similarity and goodness of fit. Am J Hum Genet 72:891–902

van der Meulen MA, te Meerman GJ (1997) Haplotype sharing analysis in affected individuals from nuclear families with at least one affected offspring. Genet Epidemiol 14:915–920

Wall JD, Pritchard JK (2003) Haplotype blocks and linkage disequilibrium in the human genome. Nat Rev Genet 4:587–597

Xiong M, Zhao J, Boerwinkle E (2003) Haplotype block linkage disequilibrium mapping. Front Biosci 8:a85–a93

Yu C, Zhou Y, Miao X, Xiong P, Tan W, Lin D (2004*a*) Functional haplotypes in the promoter of matrix metalloproteinase-2 predict risk of the occurrence and metastasis of esophageal cancer. Cancer Res 64:7622–7628

Yu K, Gu CC, Province M, Xiong CJ, Rao DC (2004*b*) Genetic association mapping under founder heterogeneity via weighted haplotype similarity analysis in candidate genes. Genet Epidemiol 27:182–191

Zhang K, Calabrese P, Nordborg M, Sun F (2002) Haplotype block structure and its applications to association studies: power and study designs. Am J Hum Genet 71:1386–1394

Zhang K, Sun F, Waterman MS, Chen T (2003*a*) Haplotype block partition with limited resources and applications to human chromosome 21 haplotype data. Am J Hum Genet 73:63–73

Zhang S, Sha Q, Chen HS, Dong J, Jiang R (2003*b*) Transmission/disequilibrium test based on haplotype sharing for tightly linked markers. Am J Hum Genet 73:566–579

Am. J. Hum. Genet. 77:41–53, 2005

Allan-Herndon-Dudley Syndrome and the Monocarboxylate Transporter 8 (*MCT8*) Gene

Charles E. Schwartz,[1] Melanie M. May,[1] Nancy J. Carpenter,[2] R. Curtis Rogers,[1] Judith Martin,[3] Martin G. Bialer,[4] Jewell Ward,[5] Javier Sanabria,[6] Silvana Marsa,[6] James A. Lewis,[7] Roberto Echeverri,[1,8] Herbert A. Lubs,[1,8] Kytja Voeller,[1] Richard J. Simensen,[1] and Roger E. Stevenson[1]

[1]JC Self Research Institute of Human Genetics, Greenwood Genetic Center, Greenwood, SC; [2]Center for Genetic Testing, Tulsa, OK; [3]Inland NW Genetics Clinic, Spokane, WA; [4]Division of Medical Genetics, North Shore Long Island Jewish Health System, University Hospital, Manhasset, NY; [5]Division of Medical Genetics, Department of Pediatrics, University of Tennessee Health Science Center, Memphis; [6]Facultad de Química Bioquímica y Farmacia, Universidad Nacional de San Luis, San Luis, Argentina; [7]W. W. Hastings Indian Hospital, Talequah, OK; and [8]University of Miami, Miami

Allan-Herndon-Dudley syndrome was among the first of the X-linked mental retardation syndromes to be described (in 1944) and among the first to be regionally mapped on the X chromosome (in 1990). Six large families with the syndrome have been identified, and linkage studies have placed the gene locus in Xq13.2. Mutations in the monocarboxylate transporter 8 gene (*MCT8*) have been found in each of the six families. One essential function of the protein encoded by this gene appears to be the transport of triiodothyronine into neurons. Abnormal transporter function is reflected in elevated free triiodothyronine and lowered free thyroxine levels in the blood. Infancy and childhood in the Allan-Herndon-Dudley syndrome are marked by hypotonia, weakness, reduced muscle mass, and delay of developmental milestones. Facial manifestations are not distinctive, but the face tends to be elongated with bifrontal narrowing, and the ears are often simply formed or cupped. Some patients have myopathic facies. Generalized weakness is manifested by excessive drooling, forward positioning of the head and neck, failure to ambulate independently, or ataxia in those who do ambulate. Speech is dysarthric or absent altogether. Hypotonia gives way in adult life to spasticity. The hands exhibit dystonic and athetoid posturing and fisting. Cognitive development is severely impaired. No major malformations occur, intrauterine growth is not impaired, and head circumference and genital development are usually normal. Behavior tends to be passive, with little evidence of aggressive or disruptive behavior. Although clinical signs of thyroid dysfunction are usually absent in affected males, the disturbances in blood levels of thyroid hormones suggest the possibility of systematic detection through screening of high-risk populations.

Introduction

Progress in the identification of genes and gene loci on the X chromosome that are responsible for mental retardation has greatly outpaced the search for autosomal genes that cause mental retardation. This is a result, in great part, of the power of hemizygosity of the X chromosome in males to clinically expose gene defects and the identification of large numbers of families that could be subjected to linkage studies, positional cloning, and other molecular technologies (Stevenson and Schwartz 2002). The experience with Allan-Herndon-Dudley syndrome (MIM 309600) is typical. Multigenerational families, beginning with the one reported in 1944 by Allan, Herndon, and Dudley, have been identified on the basis of childhood hypotonia, dysarthria, athetoid or other distal limb movements, muscle hypoplasia, and severe mental retardation (Allan et al. 1944; Bialer et al. 1992; Zorick et al. 2004). Linkage studies in several of these families placed the gene in the interval Xq13-q21 (Schwartz et al. 1990; Bialer et al. 1992; Zorick et al. 2004). Identification of mutations in the monocarboxylate transporter 8 gene (*MCT8*) in males with hypotonia, involuntary movements, and mental retardation made this gene an attractive candidate for Allan-Herndon-Dudley syndrome (Dumitrescu et al. 2004; Friesema et al. 2004; Lenzner et al. 2004). Mutational analysis, reported here for six families with Allan-Herndon-Dudley syndrome, identified one truncating mutation, one in-frame deletion, and four missense mutations in the gene.

Received March 16, 2005; accepted for publication April 20, 2005; electronically published May 11, 2005.

Address for correspondence and reprints: Dr. Roger E. Stevenson, Greenwood Genetic Center, 1 Gregor Mendel Circle, Greenwood, SC 29646. E-mail: res@ggc.org

0002-9297/2005/7701-0005$15.00

Case Reports

Clinical findings for two families with Allan-Herndon-Dudley syndrome have been reported elsewhere (kindred 8005 [K8005] by Allan et al. [1944] and Stevenson et al. [1990] and K8090 by Davis et al. [1981] and Bialer et al. [1992]). Clinical findings for K8225, K8900, K9248, and K9251 are summarized below and in table 1. Pedigrees of the six kindreds are shown in figure 1. K8005 had lived for many generations in North Carolina and considered itself to be of Western European white ancestry, K8090 was of Irish ancestry, K8225 was white of uncertain ancestry, K8900 had lived for many generations in Mississippi and was presumed to be of Western European white ancestry, K9248 had mixed American Indian (Cherokee) and Irish ancestry, and K9251 was of Hispanic ancestry. High-resolution chromosome analysis results, molecular *FMR1* analysis results, and plasma amino acid levels were normal for at least one affected male in each kindred. Results of clinical testing of thyroid function are given in figure 2. Although affected males were not frankly hypothyroid, many did exhibit weakness, pale and cool skin, dry hair, and constipation. None had prolonged neonatal jaundice, macroglossia, umbilical hernia, or myxedema. Two individuals (one in K8005 and one in K8900) had prominent eyes. Among 16 carrier mothers, 4 had thyroid disturbances: 3 had thyroid nodules in adult life, and 1 required treatment in adult life for hypothyroidism. With the exception of one carrier female (III-2 in K8225) with borderline low free thyroxine (T4) levels, the thyroid hormone levels in carrier females ($n = 8$), noncarrier females ($n = 3$), and nonaffected males ($n = 3$) were normal (table 2). Neuropsychological evaluation showed all affected males to have severe cognitive impairment. Adaptive skills were also severely impaired (table 3). Carrier females have normal growth, appearance, and intellectual function.

K8225

Five males from four generations of this family were affected (fig. 1). The four living males, three obligate female carriers, and six nonaffected males were evaluated. Affected males are briefly described below, and findings are summarized in table 1. Nonaffected males and obligate female carriers had normal appearance, normal muscle mass, and normal intellectual function. Linkage analysis localized the syndrome between *DXS983* (Xp11.3) and *DXS101* (Xq22), with a maximum LOD score of 2.6 at *DXS566* and *DXS995* in Xq13-q21 (data not shown).

IV-1 was evaluated at age 1 year. The pregnancy had been complicated by maternal insulin-dependent diabetes mellitus. Delivery occurred at 39 wk, with a birth weight of 3.8 kg (80th percentile) and length of 53.3 cm (90th percentile). Respiratory and urinary tract infections occurred during the early months of life. Concern arose regarding his development at age 6 mo, by which time he showed poor feeding, general irritability, and poor muscle tone and strength. At 1 year of age, his measurements included a head circumference of 45.5 cm (10th percentile), length of 75 cm (30th percentile), and weight of 8.0 kg (<3rd percentile). The facies appeared normal (fig. 3*A*). Neuromuscular findings included inadequate head control, decreased muscle tone and strength, fisting, asymmetry of the thighs, eversion of the feet, increased deep tendon reflexes at the knees, Babinski signs, and exaggerated startle reflex.

III-3 was evaluated at age 28 years. His birth weight was 3.2 kg (40th percentile), and his birth length was 53.3 cm (80th percentile). Development was always delayed; he never walked and had no speech. Examination showed a head circumference of 54.7 cm (10th percentile), height with scoliosis of 155 cm (<3rd percentile), and weight of 30.8 kg (<3rd percentile). He was generally asthenic, and the head was held in a forward posture. The malar areas appeared prominent. Synophrys and vertical furrowing of the brow were present (fig. 3*C*). The upper helices were excessively folded. Testes were descended and of normal size. The hands were held in a clubbed position with clasped thumb. Elbow movement was restricted, scoliosis was present, and the halluces appeared long. Deep tendon reflexes in all four limbs were increased, and ankle clonus was present.

II-8 was evaluated at age 39 years. Birth weight was 3.6 kg (60th percentile). Development had always been severely impaired. Examination showed a head circumference of 57 cm (55th percentile), height of 165 cm (5th percentile), and weight of 49.5 kg (<3rd percentile). The facies appeared elongated, with prominent malar areas (fig. 3*D*). Pectus excavatum was present. Testes were not palpable. The hands were held in a clubbed position but were not contracted. There was a general reduction of muscle mass, and contractures were present at the knees.

III-11 was evaluated at age 14 years. His birth weight was 4.1 kg (85 percentile), and his length was 53.3 cm (80th percentile). Development was always severely delayed; he never walked or spoke. Seizures began at age 3 mo. His muscle mass was always poor. Examination showed a head circumference of 53.5 cm (20th percentile), length with contractures of 142 cm (<3rd percentile), and weight of 21.4 kg (<3rd percentile). The face appeared elongated and relatively expressionless (fig. 3*B*), and the palate was high. The right elbow was severely contracted, and the left elbow was minimally contracted. The right thumb was flexed, and the lower limbs were held in valgus positioning, with contractures at the knees and eversion of the feet. There was generalized

Table 1

Summary of Clinical Findings for Six Families with Allan-Herndon-Dudley Syndrome

	Clinical Finding for Family[a]						
Trait	K8005[b]	K8090[b]	K8225	K8900	K9248	K9251	Totals
Age range of individuals evaluated	25–71 y	30–76 y	1–39 y	2–16 y	22 mo–40 y	13–25 y	...
No. of affecteds (no. of affecteds evaluated)	28 (12)	9 (8)	5 (4)	4 (2)	10 (4)	6 (2)	62 (32)
Head circumference <3rd percentile	0/12	0/8	0/4	1/2	2/4	NA	3/30 (10%)
Height <3rd percentile	0/6	0/8	2/4	2/2	0/4	NA	4/24 (17%)
Weight <3rd percentile	6/11	3/8	4/4	2/2	4/4	NA	19/29 (66%)
Hypotonia	12/12	8/8	2/2	1/1	4/4	2/2	29/29 (100%)
Asthenic build/muscle hypoplasia	9/12	7/8	4/4	2/2	4/4	2/2	28/32 (88%)
Narrow, long face	6/12	8/8	4/4	2/2	2/4	2/2	24/32 (75%)
Myopathic appearance	1/12	0/8	1/4	1/2	0/4	0/2	3/32 (9%)
Cupped/simple ears	5/12	4/8	1/4	1/2	1/4	0/2	12/32 (38%)
Scoliosis	2/12	7/8	3/4	1/2	2/4	2/2	17/32 (53%)
Pectus excavatum	NA	6/8	1/4	0/1	2/4	2/2	11/19 (58%)
Contractures	7/12	4/8	3/4	1/2	2/4	2/2	19/32 (59%)
Hyperreflexia/clonus	12/12	7/8	3/4	2/2	4/4	2/2	30/32 (94%)
Dysarthria/limited speech	12/12	6/8	0/4	0/2	4/4	0/2	22/32 (69%)
Absent speech	0/12	2/8	4/4	2/2	0/4	2/2	10/32 (31%)
Nystagmus	0/10	0/4	0/4	0/2	0/4	0/2	0/26 (0%)
Ataxia and awkward gait	11/12	7/8	...	...	0/4	...	18/30 (60%)
Never walked	1/12	1/8	4/4	2/2	4/4	0/2	12/32 (38%)
Valgus/everted feet	NA	6/7	3/4	NA	NA	1/2	10/13 (77%)
Abnormal hand positioning	10/12	6/8	4/4	1/2	4/4	1/2	26/32 (81%)
Undescended testes	0/9	0/7	1/3	0/2	1/4	NA	2/25 (8%)
Testis volume <10 ml	0/8	2/7	0/1	...[c]	1/1	NA	3/17 (18%)
Seizures	1/11	2/7	1/1	1/2	0/4	0/2	5/27 (19%)

[a] Data are no. of individuals with trait/total no. of individuals in kindred, unless otherwise specified. NA = data not available; y = years.

[b] Clinical findings for K8005 were reported by Stevenson et al. (1990) and those for K8090 were reported by Bialer et al. (1992).

[c] Prepubertal at time of exam.

decreased muscle mass, increased bicep reflexes, and ankle clonus.

K8900

Two of the four affected males, four obligate carrier females, and one nonaffected male from this family were available for evaluation. Linkage analysis placed the gene locus between *DXS993* (Xp11.4) and *DXS1002* (Xq21.31), with maximum LOD scores of 2.1 at *DXS1003* in Xp11.3, 2.0 at *AR* in Xq12, and 2.0 at *DXS986* in Xq21 (data not shown). Although initially suspected of having thyroid-binding globulin (TBG) deficiency, the TBG locus was excluded by these linkage findings. By report from an older sister, II-6 and II-7 were severely disabled and never walked or spoke. They had poor musculature and, in their later years, had "twisting" of the hands and feet. They experienced difficulty swallowing, had little fine or gross motor control, and had seizures. They appeared to see and hear; the eyes were described as having a "wild and scared" appearance. II-6 died in his twenties, and II-7 died in his thirties.

IV-3 weighed 3.6 kg (60th percentile) and was 52 cm long (60th percentile) at birth. The pregnancy was notable for decreased fetal movement for a brief period at 7 mo. Cesarean delivery was performed because of breech presentation. He appeared hypotonic and, by age 2 years, could not sit unassisted, crawl, or pull up. Examination showed generalized hypotonia, myopathic face, asthenic build, broad and proximally placed thumbs, transverse crease on the left hand, hyperreflexia, and clonus. The serum T4 level was reported to be low, but the specific value was not available. He died in his sleep at age 7 years.

V-2 weighed 3.6 kg (60th percentile) at full-term birth. Pregnancy was complicated by pneumonia and bronchiectasis. At age 1 h, he became cyanotic below the neck for unknown reasons. Cranial CT at age 3 mo showed ventricular enlargement with subdural fluid in the frontal regions, findings considered to represent brain atrophy. Seizures began at age 5 mo, and hypothyroidism was diagnosed at age 9 mo. He sustained several fractures attributed to osteoporosis. Examination at age 16.5 years showed a head circumference of 53.8 cm (10th percentile), weight of 28 kg (<3rd percentile), length with contractures of 127 cm (<3rd percentile), inner canthal measurement of 2.8 cm (25th percentile), and interpupillary measurement of 5.8 cm (50th percentile). He was alert and appeared to have some nonverbal interaction with the examiner. He followed lights

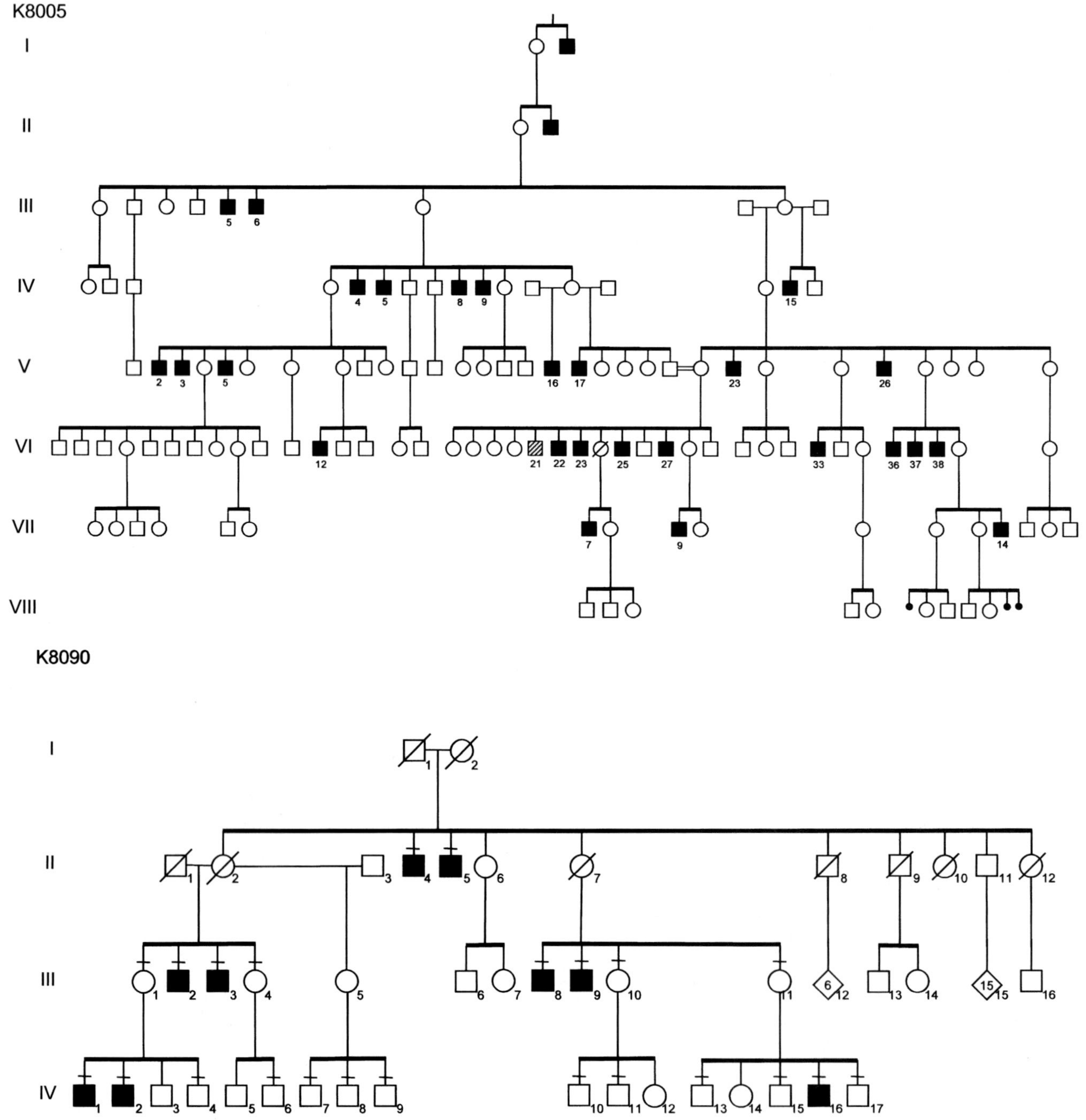

Figure 1 Partial pedigrees of six kindreds with Allan-Herndon-Dudley syndrome. Blackened squares indicate affected males, and hatched squares indicate males with unrelated neurodevelopmental disorders.

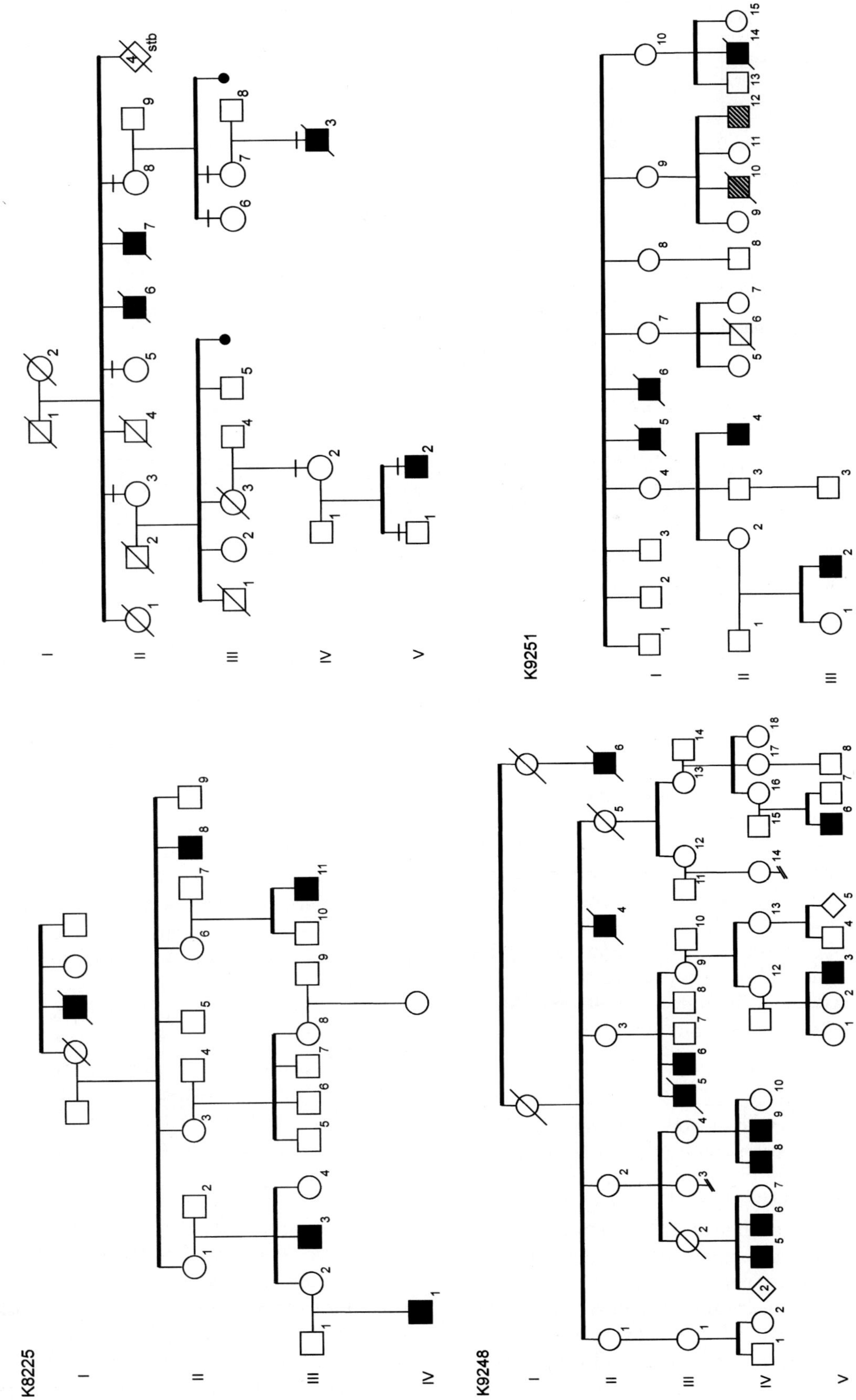
K8225
K8900
K9248
K9251

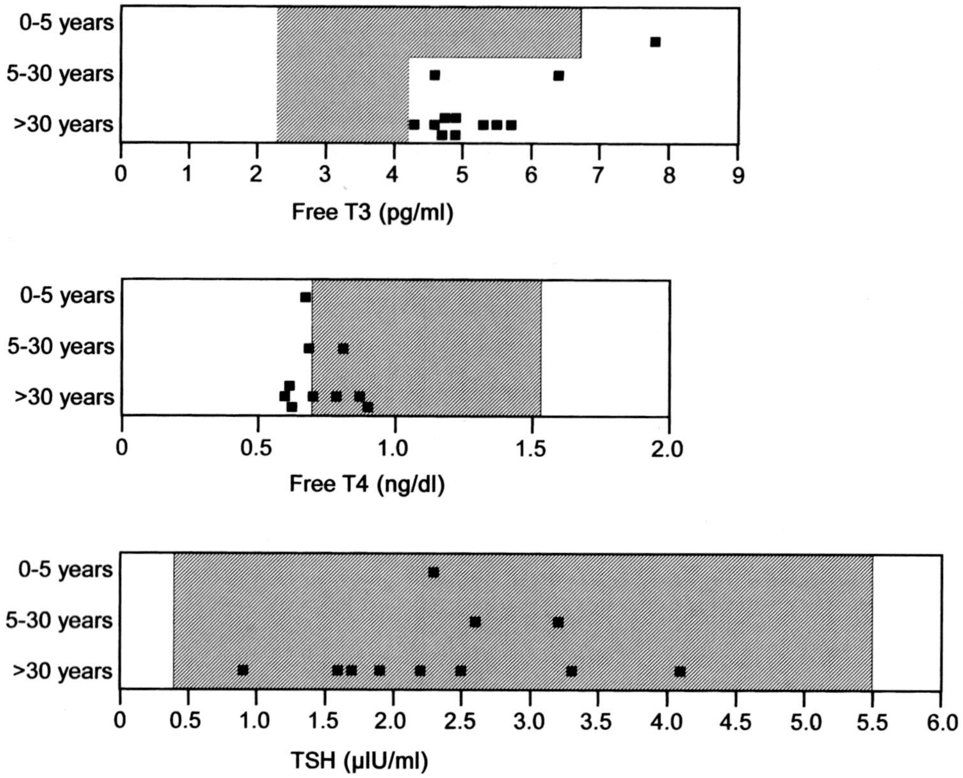

Figure 2 Serum levels of free T3 (*top panel*), free T4 (*middle panel*), and TSH (*bottom panel*) in affected males aged 0–5 years, 5–30 years, or >30 years from five of the six kindreds with Allan-Herndon-Dudley syndrome

and objects, but his capacity for hearing could not be determined. His eyes were prominent but not proptotic. Pinnae were simply formed, without folding of the superior helices. A gastrostomy feeding tube was in place. The limbs were poorly muscled, with contractures of the lower limbs and increased deep tendon reflexes at the left knee. The toes were held in clawed position, and the hands in clubbed position, with intermittent limb hyperextension and limb athetoid movements. Genitalia were prepubertal, and the testes were undescended. V-2 died at age 22 years of aspiration pneumonia.

K9248

Ten males with severe mental retardation, childhood hypotonia, and spastic paraplegia were from four generations of this white American Indian family. Four affected males, five obligate female carriers, and one nonaffected male were examined. Affected males appeared normal in growth and appearance at birth. Concerns arose during the latter part of the first 6 mo, because of failure to reach for objects and poor head control. Thereafter, the developmental lag became more obvious, as all motor and language milestones failed to occur on schedule. Except for one carrier female who suffered perinatal injury, all carrier females had normal intelligence and normal growth, including head circumference, and none had involuntary movements, hyperreflexia, or other neurological signs. One affected individual died of leukemia at 9 mo, one of pneumonia at age 32 years, and one of unknown cause in early adult life. Linkage analysis placed the gene locus distal to *DXS453* in Xq13, with no further recombination observed down to marker *DXS990* in Xq21.3, the most distal marker tested (data not shown).

IV-5 was developmentally delayed from birth. He developed speech that was limited to a few words or phrases, beginning at age 2–3 years, and he never walked. Examination at age 40 years showed a head circumference of 54.3 cm (5th percentile), length with contractures of 185 cm (90th percentile), and weight of 58 kg (<3rd percentile). The face was elongated, with midface hypoplasia, narrow high palate, anteverted nares, spaced teeth, and square face (fig. 4*D*). The chest wall was asymmetric. Testes were undescended. Muscle tone and deep tendon reflexes were increased, more so in the lower limbs than in the upper limbs. Dysarthria, scoliosis, lower-limb scissoring, knee contractures, wrist flexion, and athetoid posturing of the hands were present.

IV-6 never walked and developed only limited speech. At age 38 years, his head circumference was 55.4 cm

Table 2

Thyroid Hormone Levels in Carrier Females, Noncarrier Females, and Nonaffected Males

Subjects, Kindred, and Individual	Total T4 (mcg/dl)	Free T4 (ng/dl)	Total T3 (ng/dl)	Free T3 (pg/dl)	TSH (μIU/ml)
Carrier females:					
K8090:					
III-4	...	1.08	...	320	1.5
K8225:					
III-2	...	.8	...	286	1.5
K8900:					
II-3	...	1.1	114	...	...
II-8	...	.9	110	...	...
III-7	...	1.0	134	...	...
IV-2	...	1.2	126	...	...
K9248:					
IV-12	5.88	1.01	...	310	1.6
IV-16	8.07	1.02	...	290	1.8
Noncarrier females:					
K8900:					
NS[a]	...	1.0	114	...	...
II-5	...	1.1	94	...	...
III-6	...	1.0	106	...	...
Nonaffected males:					
K8005:					
VI-26	5.9	.86	...	...	2.6
K8900:					
V-1	...	1.2	154	...	...
K9248:					
V-7	10.3	1.23	...	410	1.2

NOTE.—Normal ranges are as follows: total T4, 4.5–12.5 mcg/dl; free T4, 0.8–1.8 ng/dl; total T3, 60–181 ng/dl; free T3, 230–420 pg/dl; and TSH, 0.4–5.5 μIU/ml.

[a] Noncarrier female not shown in abbreviated pedigree of K8900 in figure 1.

(20th percentile), height with contractures was 177 cm (60th percentile), and weight was 45 kg (<3rd percentile). A widow's peak was present, and the midface was hypoplastic, with high and narrow palate, widely spaced teeth, and square jaw (fig. 4*C*). Truncal hypotonia, pectus excavatum, scoliosis, decreased lower-limb musculature, increased limb muscle tone and deep tendon reflexes, knee contractures, wrist flexion, and hand athetoid posturing were present.

V-6 weighed 3.4 kg (45th percentile), measured 51 cm in length (50th percentile), and had a head circumference of 34.6 cm (40th percentile) at term birth. Hypotonia and poor head control were obvious by age 6 mo. He rolled over at age 3 years and, by age 5 years, could not sit, pull up, or walk and had speech limited to 3–6 words. Examination at age 5 years showed a head circumference of 48.2 cm (<3rd percentile), length of 108 cm (50th percentile), and weight of 14.8 kg (<3rd percentile). He has amblyopia and myopia, cupped ears, anteverted nares, tenting of the upper lip, narrow tall palate, normal prepubertal genitalia, and a straight spine (fig. 4*B*). He also has truncal hypotonia, poor head control, increased limb tone and deep tendon reflexes, intermittent internal rotation of the arms, elbow hyperextension, and ankle clonus.

V-3 had a weight of 3.5 kg (50th percentile), length of 48 cm (10th percentile), and head circumference of 35.5 cm (55th percentile) at birth. At ~6 mo of age, he was noted to have poor muscle tone, poor head control, and limited use of hands. He began rolling over at age 3–4 months but, at age 22 mo, could not sit, pull up, or crawl. Athetoid hand posturing was noted at age 5 mo. Although he said his first words at age 1 year, further speech development has been very limited. At age 22 mo, he had a head circumference of 46.5 cm (<3rd percentile), length of 84 cm (25th percentile), and weight of 9.7 kg (<3rd percentile). Facial features included depressed nasal bridge, anteverted nares, short philtrum, tented upper lip, and low-set and posteriorly rotated ears (fig. 4*A*). He had truncal hypotonia, limb hypertonia and hyperreflexia, upper-limb athetoid posturing, and lower-limb scissoring. Genitalia appeared normal.

K9251

Five males were affected in three generations of this family from Argentina. Three of those presumed to be

Table 3

Cognitive Function and Adaptive Behaviors

Kindred and Individual	Age	IQ[a,b]	Adaptive Skill Level[b] (years/mo) Communication	Daily Living	Socialization
K8225:					
II-8	51 years	<20	0/11	1/1	0/11
III-3	28 years	<20	...	NA	...
III-11	14 years	<20	...	NA	...
IV-1	13 years	NA	1/5	1/6	2/3
K8900:					
V-2	13 years	<20	0/11	0/10	0/11
K9248:					
IV-5	40 years	<20	1/3	1/56	1/2
IV-6	38 years	<20	0/11	1/4	0/8
V-6	5 years	24	1/0	0/11	0/9
V-3	22 mo	NA	0/6	0/9	0/9
K9251:					
II-4	25 years	<30	...	NA	...
III-2	13 years	<30	...	NA	...

[a] IQ scores are based on testing with the Stanford-Binet. IQ test results for K8005 and K8090 were reported by Stevenson et al. (1990) and Bialer et al. (1992), respectively.

[b] NA = information not available.

affected were deceased. I-5 and I-6 were diagnosed with hypotonic cerebral palsy. II-14 died at age 7 mo, with global developmental delay. Because the phenotype was consistent with Allan-Herndon-Dudley syndrome, linkage analysis was omitted, and mutational analysis of *MCT8* was pursued.

II-4 had lifelong global delay, truncal hypotonia, poor head control, and limited motor skills. He had facial elongation, pectus excavatum, scoliosis, hyperreflexia, cavus feet, and contractures of the fingers, knees, and ankles. He has severe mental retardation and cannot walk or speak.

III-2 was born at term by Cesarean delivery and weighed 4.3 kg (90th percentile). Fetal movements were diminished during the last months of pregnancy. From birth, he exhibited truncal hypotonia and delayed development. At age 13 years, he showed poor control of the head and trunk, elongation of the face, mental retardation, and absence of speech and independent ambulation. He had scoliosis and dorsal kyphosis, pectus excavatum, contractures at the knees and ankles, and hyperreflexia. Nerve conduction; findings of electromyography, electroencephalography, muscle biopsy, and brain MRI; and levels of creatine kinase, plasma amino acids, and urine oligosaccharides and mucopolysaccharides were normal. Cranial CT showed cortical and subcortical atrophy.

II-12 is considered to have an unrelated neuromotor disorder, having no symptoms until age 15 years, when he developed difficulty in running and walking up stairs. He lost fine and gross motor skills and, at age 27 years, had distal muscle atrophy, cavus feet, and hyperreflexia. His mother had normal results for *MCT8* mutational analysis.

Methods

Consent

Informed consent was obtained from the parent(s) or guardian(s) of the affected individuals by use of the consent form approved by the Self Regional Healthcare Institutional Review Committee.

Preparation of DNA

Genomic DNA was prepared using a high-salt precipitation method with peripheral blood (Schwartz et al. 1990). The purified genomic DNA was diluted to 105 μg/ml and was stored at 4°C.

PCR

All exons were amplified individually. The primers, sizes, and annealing temperatures are available in table 4. All primers were tailed with M13 primers to facilitate sequencing. All exons were amplified using a PTC-200 thermocycler (MJ Research), with a total volume of 60 μl containing 1 × PCR buffer with 1 μM of each primer, 0.08 mM dNTPs, and 0.02 U of GoTaq DNA polymerase (Promega).

Sequencing Analysis

PCR fragments for each exon were sequenced in both directions on the MegaBACE (Amersham Biosciences)

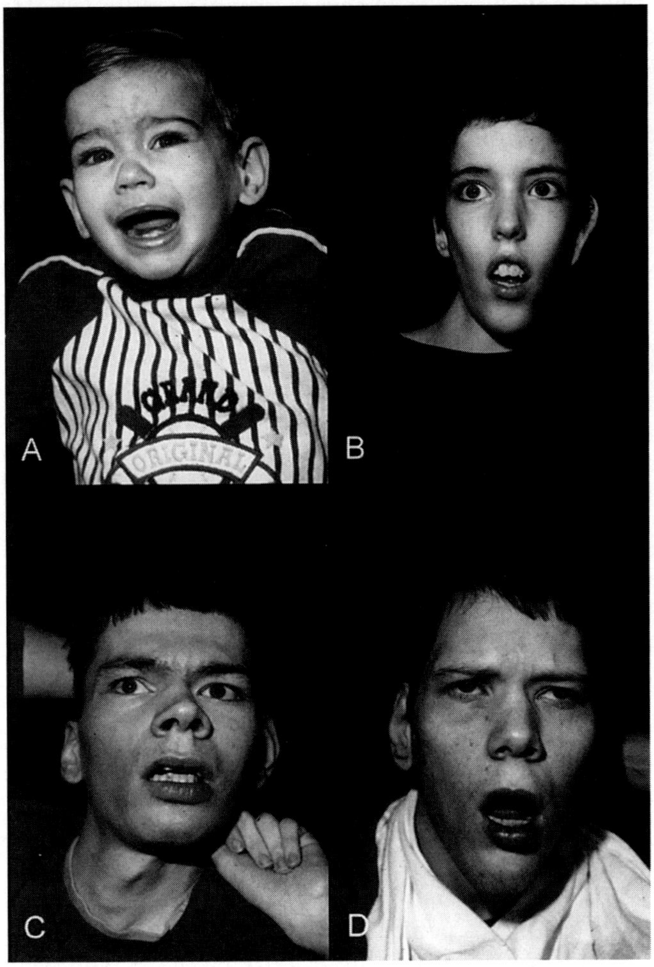

Figure 3 Appearance of four affected males in K8225. *A*, IV-1 at age 1 year, showing a normal face. *B*, III-11 at age 14 years, showing an elongated and myopathic face. *C*, III-3 at age 28 years, showing synophrys and prominence of the lower lip. *D*, II-8 at age 39 years, showing an elongated face with prominence of malar areas and an open mouth.

by use of the M13 forward and reverse primers, in accordance with the manufacturer's protocol. The alignment and analysis of the sequences were done using the DNASTAR program (Lasergene).

Denaturing High-Pressure Liquid Chromatography Analysis

Mutations in exons 1, 2, and 4 were subjected to heteroduplex analysis for segregation studies in the families and for screening in a cohort of normal males. To ensure proper formation of duplex DNA, the PCR product obtained from the proband or family member was mixed with an equal volume of PCR product from a control individual. The samples were denatured at 95°C for 12 min and were allowed to renature for 45 min by decreasing the temperature from 95°C to 25°C. For the normal male cohort, pools of four individuals were created for analysis after PCR amplification of each individual. Amplicons were analyzed on the WAVE DNA fragment analysis system equipped with DNA Sep column (Transgenomic), at the following temperatures: exon 1, 61°C; exon 2, 60°C and 63°C; and exon 4, 59.7°C and 60.5°C.

Ear*1 Digestion of Exon 6 Amplicon*

The mutation that was found in exon 6 destroyed an *Ear*1 restriction site. Digestion was performed using 10 μl of a PCR product generated using primers for exon 6 in a total reaction volume of 20 μl. The reaction mix contained 1 × NEBuffer 1, 1 × spermidine, and 0.25 μl *Ear*1 enzyme (NEB). The digestion occurred overnight at 37°C, and the products were analyzed on a 2% agarose gel. *Ear*1 digested the 395-bp product from the proband of K8005 into 2 fragments of 328 bp and 67 bp. A normal individual has three fragments after *Ear*1 digestion: 155 bp, 173 bp, and 67 bp.

Computational Analysis of Altered MCT8 Proteins

Estimation of the effect of a mutation in *MCT8* at the protein level was done using the Protean software available in DNASTAR (Lasergene).

Results

Direct genomic sequencing of the six exons of *MCT8*, plus 80 bp of flanking sequence on either side of the exons, detected alterations in all six kindreds with Allan-Herndon-Dudley syndrome (table 5). One mutation was truncating, one was an in-frame deletion, and four were missense. In K8900, a truncating mutation (p.S448X) was identified. The creation of the novel stop codon results in the protein missing the last four transmembrane domains (TMDs) as well as the carboxyl cytoplasmic end of the protein. K9251 was found to have an in-frame 3-bp deletion, c.683delTCT, which removes a phenylalanine at position 230 (delF230). This residue is the first of two phenylalanines in the middle of the second TMD and is highly conserved. In K8225, base substitution c.703G→A causes missense mutation p.V235M in the second TMD. This valine is highly conserved when compared to mouse and rat. Additionally, the presence of this methionine may create a novel initiation site. However, this possibility could not be ex-

Table 4

Sequences, Sizes, and Annealing Temperatures of Primers Used to Analyze the Exons and Adjacent Intron Sequences of *MCT8*

The table is available in its entirety in the online edition of *The American Journal of Human Genetics.*

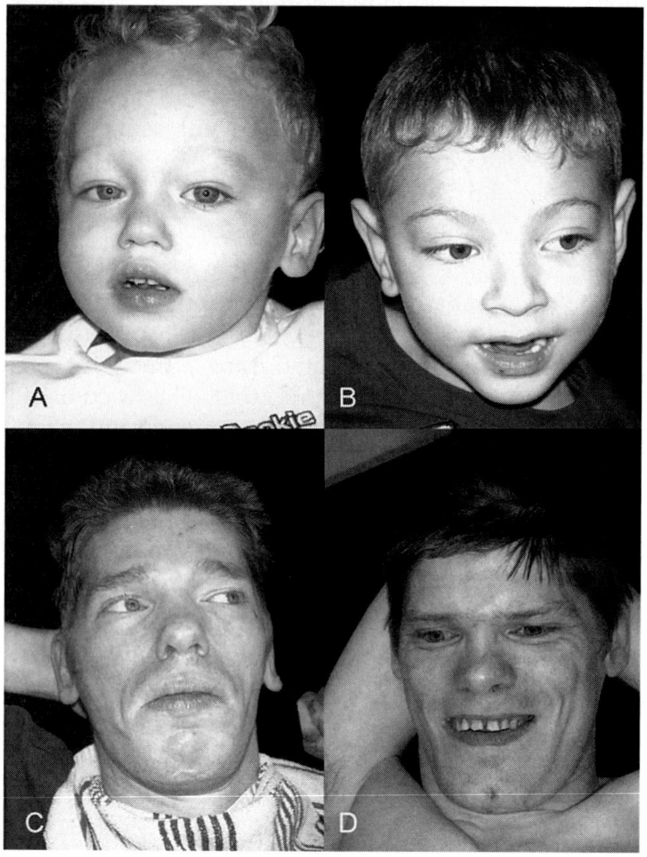

Figure 4 Appearance of four affected males in K9248. *A*, V-3 at age 22 mo, showing a cupped left ear, depressed nasal bridge, widely anteverted nares, and tenting of the upper lip with short philtrum. *B*, V-6 at age 5 years, showing incomplete folding of superior helices and short philtrum. *C*, IV-6 at age 38 years, showing elongated face with widow's peak, flattening of midface, and square jaw. *D*, IV-5 at age 40 years, showing a long face with short philtrum.

amined further, because *MCT8* is not transcribed in lymphocytes, the only tissue available for analysis. The second missense mutation, p.L434W in K8090, occurs in the eighth TMD. This leucine is highly conserved when compared to mouse and rat. In K8005, a c.1703T→C substitution produces missense mutation p.L568P. As with the p.L434W missense mutation, a highly conserved leucine residue is altered, this time in the twelfth TMD. The fourth missense mutation was found in K9248, resulting in a S194F change in the first extracellular domain between the first and second TMDs. None of these six mutations in *MCT8* was found in 470 normal male controls.

Discussion

Spastic paraplegia is among the more common of the clinical findings that co-occur with X-linked mental retardation. Spastic paraplegia 1 is part of the X-linked hydrocephaly spectrum caused by mutations in *L1CAM* (Vits et al. 1994). Spastic paraplegia 2 is the dominant clinical presentation of Pelizaeus-Merzbacher syndrome, caused by mutations in *PLP* (Saugier-Veber et al. 1994). In addition, spastic paraplegia is a prominent finding in 23 other X-linked mental retardation (XLMR) syndromes (Stevenson et al. 2000) (table 6). The progression to spastic paraplegia in the Allan-Herndon-Dudley syndrome is notable. From infancy into early childhood, hypotonia and decreased muscle mass dominate the neuromuscular findings. Hypotonia and weakness is particularly notable in the neck muscles. Truncal hypotonia persists into adult life. There is a transition in childhood to spasticity manifested by hyperreflexia at the large joints, clonus, and Babinski signs. Contractures commonly occur. Involuntary movements of the distal limbs, dystonic and/or athetoid in nature, occur in most affected individuals. Virtually all affected males become wheelchair bound in adult life, although many had achieved independent but delayed and unsteady ambulation.

In all affected males with available records, intrauterine growth was normal. In early childhood, weight typically fell below the 3rd percentile and remained there. Length during childhood was usually normal; measurement of adult length was compromised by scoliosis and contractures, commonly measuring <3rd percentile. Occipitofrontal head circumference usually fell below average, but in only two instances were measurements <3rd percentile recorded (table 1).

The development of all 32 affected males who were evaluated was severely impaired from birth. None developed normal speech: 10 had no speech, and 22 had limited and/or severely dysarthric speech. Twelve males never ambulated independently. Ambulation was markedly delayed among those who learned to walk and was lost by adult life.

Compatibility with longevity was evident by the 8 affected males, of the 32 evaluated, who lived beyond 70 years. This notwithstanding, the family histories indicated that three affected males died before age 10 years, one died during the teen years, two died during their twenties, and four died during their thirties.

Table 5

***MCT8* Mutations in Allan-Herndon-Dudley Syndrome**

Kindred	Mutation	Amino Acid Change
K8005	c.1703T→C (exon 6)	L568P
K8090	c.1301T→G (exon 4)	L434W
K8225	c.703G→A (exon 2)	V235M
K8900	c.1343C→A (exon 4)	S448X
K9248	c.581C→T (exon 1)	S194F
K9251	c.683delTCT (exon 2)	delF230

Table 6

X-Linked Syndromes with Spastic Paraplegia as a Major Phenotypic Manifestation

Syndrome	Gene Locus[a]	Gene (If Known)
Adrenoleukodystrophy	Xq28	*ABCD1*
Allan-Herndon-Dudley	Xq21	*MCT8*
Apak ataxia–spastic paraplegia (cerebellar ataxia 2)	Xp11.21-q21.3	
Arena	Xq22–25	
Ataxia-deafness (Schmidley)	NL	
Brooks-Wisniewski-Brown	NL	
Christianson	Xq24-q27.3	
Fitzsimmons	NL	
Gustavsson	Xq26	
Kang	NL	
Lesch-Nyhan	Xq26-q27.2	*HPRT1*
Miles-Carpenter	Xq13-q22	
Mohr-Tranebjaerg (Jensen)	Xq22	*TIMM8A*
Paine-Seemanova	NL	
Pallister W	NL	
Pelizaeus-Merzbacher (spastic paraplegia, type 2)	Xq22	*PLP1*
Pettigrew	Xq25-Xq27	
Psychosis–pyramidal signs–macroorchidism, X-linked	Xq28	*MECP2*
Proud	Xp22	*ARX*
Rett	Xq28	*MECP2*
Schimke	NL	
X-linked hydrocephalus spectrum (spastic paraplegia, type 1)	Xq28	*L1CAM*
X-linked lissencephaly	Xq22.3-q23	*DCX*
XLMR-blindness-seizures-spasticity (Hamel)	Xp11.3-q12	
XLMR-hydrocephaly–basal ganglia calcifications (Fried)	Xp22	
XLMR-hypotonia–recurrent infections (Lubs)	Xq28	

[a] NL = not localized.

Cognitive impairment in affected males was severe. Since most affected males were unable to meet the baseline of standardized cognitive tests, the precise level of mental retardation could not be determined (table 3). There was no evidence of an unusual cognitive strength—the neuropsychological profile was generally flat, except for the fact that the subjects were remarkably affable and tuned into social interactions, which was even more remarkable because of the significant motor and cognitive handicaps. Because of the severity of cognitive impairment, some patients were evaluated with only the Vineland Adaptive Behavior Scale–Interview Edition (table 3).

The pattern of findings in these families with Allan-Herndon-Dudley syndrome is the same as that in 10 other individuals/families with the *MCT8* mutation reported by Dumitrescu et al. (2004), Friesema et al. (2004), and Lenzner et al. (2004). Hypotonia in infancy and early childhood was accompanied by motor, speech, and mental delays and was followed by development of spasticity, dystonia, and other involuntary distal hand movements. Dumitrescu et al. (2004) reported rotary nystagmus, disconjugate eye movements, and feeding difficulties in two affected boys from different kindreds, findings that were not noted in the other reports or in the families with Allan-Herndon-Dudley syndrome.

Assessments of thyroid function in males with Allan-Herndon-Dudley syndrome showed, in most cases, high free triiodothyronine (T3) and low free T4 levels in serum (fig. 2). Serum TSH levels were normal. The alterations in free T3 and free T4 levels provide a convenient method of selecting males for *MCT8* mutational studies. Since an elevated free T3 level in serum is found more consistently than is a low free T4 level (fig. 2), measurement of serum free T3 levels would be the preferred method for screening high-risk populations, such as children with developmental delay and hypotonia.

The paucity of findings that suggest a disturbance in thyroid metabolism is perplexing. Specifically, affected males fail to show the somatic findings typical of hypothyroidism, such as prolonged neonatal jaundice, myxedematous skin changes, macroglossia, hoarseness, and umbilical hernias. Statural growth may be stunted but not as notably as in hypothyroidism. The overall weakness, pale cool skin, dry hair, and constipation in a number of affected males may be related to decreased thyroid-hormone availability to some tissues. Two affected males had prominent eyes, a finding suggestive of endocrine ophthalmopathy or thyrotoxicosis. Although the repertoire of molecules transported by the monocarboxylate transporter 8 is not known, the abnormal transport of another molecule essential to neurons cannot be ruled out as the disease-causing event (Friesema et al. 2005). Nonetheless, the perturbations in T3 and T4 levels may serve as useful biomarkers to screen for Allan-Herndon-Dudley syndrome.

It is tempting to speculate that dietary supplementation with T4 or T3 might be beneficial. To date, attempts at therapy with thyroxine administrated during infancy in two cases were unsuccessful in ameliorating the neurological signs (Dumitrescu et al. 2004).

Among the six novel mutations in *MCT8* reported here, one (p.S448X) truncates the protein near the end of the eighth TMD, removing the last four TMDs and the cytoplasmic region at the carboxy end of the protein. Another mutation was an in-frame deletion of 3 bp resulting in the removal of one of two adjacent phenylalanines (del F230) in the second TMD. This is predicted to remove a turn region and extend a β-sheet region.

Three missense mutations (V235M, L434W, and L568P) occur in other TMDs of the MCT8 protein. Each alters a highly conserved residue in their respective TMD. The V235M missense alteration is predicted to substitute a coil region and an alpha helix where a turn region would normally exist in the second TMD. The L434W missense mutation in the eighth TMD shortens a prominent β-sheet region and lengthens a coil region. The L568P missense mutation in the last TMD results in the formation of a small beta amphipathic region followed by a small alpha amphipatic region near the cytoplasmic region of the TMD and the removal of a short coil section at the end of the TMD. A fourth missense mutation, S194F, occurs within the first extracellular region of the protein, between the first and second TMDs. This alteration would appear to eliminate a β-sheet region, forming a coiled region instead.

The prevalence of *MCT8* mutations as a cause of XLMR is not known. With the rapid identification of mutations in 16 families (Dumitrescu et al. 2004; Friesema et al. 2004: Lenzner et al. 2004; the present study), it is possible that *MCT8* mutations may number among the more prevalent mutations on the X chromosome (e.g., mutations in *FMR1*, *MECP2*, *RSK2*, *ARX*, and *L1CAM*) that cause mental retardation. Studies of other families with XLMR linked to Xq13.2 and sporadic males with mental retardation will be necessary to determine the prevalence.

Expression in females is doubtful but has not been studied systematically or longitudinally. Dumitrescu et al. (2004) noted that some carrier females have abnormal thyroid hormone tests. Four of 16 carrier females in the six families with Allan-Herndon-Dudley syndrome reported a history of thyroid disease. Three had thyroid nodules in adult life, and one had hypothyroidism. Both thyroid nodules and hypothyroidism are common thyroid-related findings in adults. One carrier female (III-2 in K8225) had borderline low free T4 levels, and seven other carrier females had normal thyroid hormone levels (table 2). X-inactivation studies in 20 female gene carriers, aged 18–78 years, from the six kindreds with Allan-Herndon-Dudley syndrome showed no consistent pattern. Only one carrier had markedly skewed X-inactivation (>90% of cells having the same X chromosome active).

With the identification of mutations in *MCT8* as responsible for Allan-Herndon-Dudley syndrome, the gene defects have been found for all XLMR syndromes described before fragile X syndrome (Lubs 1969). Three of the early reports were descriptions of fragile X syndrome mutation in *FMR1*, as later confirmed by cytogenetic and molecular testing in each of these families (Martin and Bell 1943; Losowsky 1961; Dunn et al. 1962–1963). Other XLMR syndromes described between 1868 and 1969 for which the gene defect is known include Duchenne muscular dystrophy (*DMD*), Pelizaeus-Merzbacher syndrome (*PLD*), dyskeratosis congenita (*DKC*), Hunter syndrome (*IDS*), incontinentia pigmenti (*NEMO*), Norrie panophthalmia syndrome (*NDP*), X-linked hydrocephaly spectrum (*L1CAM*), Renpenning syndrome (*PQBP1*), and Snyder-Robinson syndrome (*SMS*). This is indicative of the progress in the molecular delineation of XLMR syndromes. Among 165 XLMR syndromes, the responsible gene has been identified in 78 syndromes, regional mapping has been achieved for an additional 53 syndromes, and 34 syndromes have not been mapped.

Acknowledgments

Foremost, we thank the members of all the families for their cooperation, with special appreciation for K8005, the family originally described in 1944 by William Allan, Nash Herndon, and Florence Dudley. Their continued interest in the efforts of doctors and researchers to identify the gene for Allan-Herndon-Dudley syndrome has spanned 60 years. We thank Cindy Skinner for coordinating the sample collection, Tonya Moss for the tissue-culture work, Dana Shultz for assisting with sequence analysis, and all the fellows and technologists who contributed to the project since 1990. This work was supported by grant HD 26202 from the National Institute of Child Health and Human Development (to C.E.S.) and in part by a grant from the South Carolina Department of Disabilities and Special Needs. Dedicated to the memory of Ethan Frances Schwartz, 1996–1998.

Web Resources

The URL for data presented herein is as follows:

Online Mendelian Inheritance in Man (OMIM), http://www.ncbi.nlm.nih.gov/Omim/ (for Allan-Herndon-Dudley syndrome)

References

Allan W, Herndon CN, Dudley FC (1944) Some examples of the inheritance of mental deficiency: apparently sex-linked idiocy and microcephaly. Am J Ment Defic 48:325–334

Bialer MG, Lawrence L, Stevenson RE, Silverberg G, Williams MK, Arena JF, Lubs HA, Schwartz CE (1992) Allan-Herndon-Dudley syndrome: clinical and linkage studies on a second family. Am J Med Genet 43:491–497

Davis JG, Silverberg G, Williams MK, Spiro A, Shapiro LR (1981) A new X-linked recessive mental retardation syndrome with progressive spastic quadriparesis. Am J Hum Genet Suppl 33:A75

Dumitrescu AM, Liao X-H, Best TB, Brockmann K, Refetoff S (2004) A novel syndrome combining thyroid and neurological abnormalities is associated with mutations in a monocarboxylate transporter gene. Am J Hum Genet 74: 168–175

Dunn HG, Renpenning H, Gerrard JW, Miller JR, Tabata T, Federoff S (1962–1963) Mental retardation as a sex-linked defect. Am J Ment Defic 67:827–848

Friesema ECH, Grueters A, Biebermann H, Krude H, von Moers A, Reeser M, Barrett TG, Mancilla EE, Svensson J, Kester MH, Kuiper GG, Balkassmi S, Uitterlinden AG, Koehrle J, Rodien P, Halestrap AP, Visser TJ (2004) Association between mutations in a thyroid hormone transporter and severe X-linked psychomotor retardation. Lancet 364: 1435–1437

Friesema ECH, Jansen J, Visser TJ (2005) Thyroid hormone transporters. Biochem Soc Trans 33:228–232

Lenzner S, Rosenkranz MD, Grueters A, Biebermann H, Chelly J, Moraine C, Frijns J, van Bokhoven H, Visser T, Ropers H (2004) Severe X-linked mental retardation caused by mutations in the gene for the thyroid hormone transporter MCT8. Paper presented at the European Society of Human Genetics Concurrent Symposia, Munich, June 12–15

Losowsky MS (1961) Hereditary mental defect showing the pattern of sex influence. J Ment Defic Res 5:60–62

Lubs HA (1969) A marker X chromosome. Am J Hum Genet 21:231–244

Martin JP, Bell J (1943) A pedigree of mental defect showing sex-linkage. J Neurol Psychiatr 6:154–157

Saugier-Veber P, Munnich A, Bonneau D, Rozet JM, Le Merrer M, Gil R, Boespflug-Tanguy O (1994) X-linked spastic paraplegia and Pelizaeus-Merzbacher disease are allelic disorders at the proteolipid protein locus. Nat Genet 6:257–262

Schwartz CE, Ulmer J, Brown A, Pancoast I, Goodman HO, Stevenson RE (1990) Allan-Herndon syndrome. II. Linkage to DNA markers in Xq21. Am J Hum Genet 47:454–458

Stevenson RE, Goodman HO, Schwartz CE, Simensen RJ, McLean WT Jr, Herndon CN (1990) Allan-Herndon syndrome. I. Clinical studies. Am J Hum Genet 47:446–453

Stevenson RE, Schwartz CE (2002) Clinical and molecular contributions to the understanding of X-linked mental retardation. Cytogenet Genome Res 99:265–275

Stevenson RE, Schwartz CE, Schroer RJ (2000) X-linked mental retardation. Oxford University Press, New York

Vits L, Van Camp G, Coucke P, Fransen E, De Boulle K, Reyniers E, Korn B, Poustka A, Wilson G, Schrander-Stumpel C, Winter RM, Schwartz C, Willems PJ (1994) MASA syndrome is due to mutations in the neural cell adhesion gene *L1CAM*. Nat Genet 7:408–413

Zorick TS, Kleimann S, Sertié A, Zatz M, Rosenberg S, Passos-Bueno MR (2004) Fine mapping and clinical reevaluation of a Brazilian pedigree with a severe form of X-linked mental retardation associated with other neurological dysfunction. Am J Med Genet 127A:321–332

Mutations in *PIP5K3* Are Associated with François-Neetens Mouchetée Fleck Corneal Dystrophy

Shouling Li,[1,*] Leila Tiab,[3,*] Xiaodong Jiao,[1] Francis L. Munier,[4] Leonidas Zografos,[4] Béatrice E. Frueh,[5] Yuri Sergeev,[1] Janine Smith,[2] Benjamin Rubin,[1] Mario A. Meallet,[6] Richard K. Forster,[7] J. Fielding Hejtmancik,[1] and Daniel F. Schorderet[3,4]

[1]Ophthalmic Genetics and Clinical Services Branch and [2]Office of the Clinical Director, National Eye Institute, Bethesda, MD; [3]Institut de Recherche en Ophtalmologie, Sion, Switzerland; [4]Jules Gonin Eye Hospital, Lausanne, Switzerland; [5]Department of Ophthalmology, Inselspital, Bern, Switzerland; [6]LA County and USC Medical Center/Doheny Eye Institute, Los Angeles; and [7]Department of Ophthalmology, Bascom Palmer Eye Institute, University of Miami School of Medicine, Miami

François-Neetens fleck corneal dystrophy (CFD) is a rare, autosomal dominant corneal dystrophy characterized by numerous small white flecks scattered in all layers of the stroma. Linkage analysis localized CFD to a 24-cM (18-Mb) interval of chromosome 2q35 flanked by *D2S2289* and *D2S126* and containing *PIP5K3*. PIP5K3 is a member of the phosphoinositide 3-kinase family and regulates the sorting and traffic of peripheral endosomes that contain lysosomally directed fluid phase cargo, by controlling the morphogenesis and function of multivesicular bodies. Sequencing analysis disclosed missense, frameshift, and/or protein-truncating mutations in 8 of 10 families with CFD that were studied, including 2256delA, 2274delCT, 2709C→T (R851X), 3120C→T (Q988X), IVS19-1G→C, 3246G→T (E1030X), 3270C→T (R1038X), and 3466A→G (K1103R). The histological and clinical characteristics of patients with CFD are consistent with biochemical studies of PIP5K3 that indicate a role in endosomal sorting.

Introduction

François-Neetens fleck corneal dystrophy (CFD [MIM 121850]) is an autosomal dominant corneal dystrophy characterized by numerous small white flecks scattered in all layers of the stroma. François and Neetens described this disorder for the first time in 1957, calling it "hérédodystrophie mouchetée" (François and Neetens 1957). Typically, the stroma in between the flecks is clear, and the endothelium, epithelium, Bowman layer, and Descemet membrane are normal. Except for an occasional patient with minor photophobia, patients are usually asymptomatic and have normal vision; the disease is most often found at routine examination. The corneal flecks appear to not progress significantly throughout life (Patten et al. 1976; Akova et al. 1994). In vivo confocal microscopy examination has made the clinical diagnosis more straightforward, with CFD evident by small bright deposits around keratocyte nuclei throughout the stroma.

The flecks in CFD may appear as early as at 2 years of age or even at birth, but generally they are reported not to progress significantly throughout life. However, individual 15 in family 50003 showed no signs of CFD on slit-lamp examination at age 2 years, but, at age 6 years, it was observed that two stromal lesions in the left eye and one in the right eye had developed (Jiao et al. 2003). Although CFD is thought to be rare, specific incidence figures are difficult to obtain. It has been suggested that, because of its subtle presentation, CFD might be much more common than has been appreciated in the literature (Streeten and Falls 1961; Birndorf and Ginsberg 1972; Patten et al. 1976; Goldberg et al. 1977).

On histological examination, the corneal flecks appear to correspond to abnormal keratocytes swollen with membrane-limited intracytoplasmic vesicles containing complex lipids and acid mucopolysaccharides. There are no extracellular abnormalities (Nicholson et al. 1977; Purcell et al. 1977), and laboratory screening has shown no systemic metabolic abnormalities (Patten et al. 1976). Thus, it was thought that this dystrophy might represent a dominantly inherited metabolic disorder confined to the cornea (Nicholson et al. 1977). CFD was previously mapped to a 27.9-cM region of chromosome 2q35 flanked by *D2S117* and *D2S126*, with the highest LOD scores shown at *D2S2289* ($Z_{max} = 4.46$; $\theta = 0$), *D2S325* ($Z_{max} = 3.28$; $\theta = 0$), *D2S317* ($Z_{max} = 3.1$; $\theta = 0$), *D2S143* ($Z_{max} = 3.8$; $\theta = 0.03$), and *D2S2382* ($Z_{max} = 5.0$; $\theta = 0$). Multipoint analysis confirmed linkage to the region between *D2S117* and *D2S126*, with a maximum multipoint

Received March 7, 2005; accepted for publication April 25, 2005; electronically published May 18, 2005.

Address for correspondence and reprints: Dr. Daniel F. Schorderet, Institut de Recherche en Ophtalmologie, Avenue du Grand-Champ sec 64, 1950 Sion, Switzerland. E-mail: daniel.schorderet@iro.vsnet.ch

* These two authors contributed equally to this work.

0002-9297/2005/7701-0006$15.00

Table 1

PCR Primers for 41 Exons and cDNA of *PIP5K3*

The table is available in its entirety in the online edition of *The American Journal of Human Genetics.*

LOD score of 5.0 located midway between *D2S2289* and *D2S325*. Analysis of CFD in the same families with the assumption of 90% penetrance increased the maximum LOD score to 6.28 at *D2S157* (Jiao et al. 2003).

The present study was performed with 10 families, including the original 4 families studied by Jiao et al. (2003), and refined the linked region to a 24-cM interval flanked by *D2S2289* and *D2S126* and containing ~18 Mb. Sequencing of numerous candidate genes in this region in affected members from 8 of 10 families showed mutations in *PIP5K3,* which encodes a widely expressed 2,089-aa phosphoinositide 3-kinase family member active in post-Golgi vesicular sorting.

Material and Methods

Patients and Clinical Findings

Ten unrelated families of European origin that contain 69 individuals, including 32 affected individuals, 27 unaffected individuals, and 10 unaffected spouses, were enrolled in this study. Families 50001 and 50007 are of mixed European origin (American), family 50002 is of Italian origin, family 50004 is of Yugoslavian origin, and the remaining families are of Swiss origin. Control individuals were of mixed European origin (from the United States, Italy, and Switzerland). The diagnosis of CFD was based on the presence of typical small white flecks throughout the corneal stroma. Both affected and unaffected family members underwent a complete ophthalmological examination. In affected individuals, the corneal epithelium and endothelial layer showed no abnormalities. The corneal stroma showed the presence of typical hyperreflective dots throughout but was otherwise normal. Confocal microscopy findings for family 5005 also showed hyperreflective inclusions associated with the basal nerves (Frueh and Bohnke 1999). Detailed ocular, medical, and family histories were obtained for each available family member. This project was approved by the institutional review board of the National Eye Institute and by the Ethics Committee of the Faculty of Medicine, University of Lausanne. The patients admitted to this study gave their informed consent, and the study adhered to the tenets of the Declaration of Helsinki.

Genotyping and Linkage Analyses

DNA was extracted either directly from blood or from transformed lymphoblastoid cell lines, by use of standard phenol-chloroform protocols (Smith et al. 1989). Two-point linkage analysis was performed using the FASTLINK version (Schaffer et al. 1994) of MLINK from the LINKAGE program package (Lathrop and Lalouel 1984; Cottingham et al. 1993). Maximum LOD scores were calculated using ILINK. CFD was initially analyzed as a fully penetrant, autosomal dominant trait. The gene frequency of CFD was set at 0.0001, and an equal allele frequency was used for all markers.

Candidate-Gene Analysis

Candidate genes were chosen in the 24-cM CFD-linked interval flanked by *D2S2289* and *D2S126* on chromosome 2q35, estimated to contain >300 genes or potential genes. To confirm that the candidate genes are expressed in the human cornea, human corneal total RNA was extracted with an RNeasy Fibrous Tissue Mini kit (QIAGEN), corneal cDNA was made using RT-PCR with the use of SuperScriptTM III First-Strand Synthesis System (Invitrogen), and direct PCR amplification of the cDNA was performed. Expression of *PIP5K3* was tested by PCR analysis of corneal cDNA with the use of exon 1 forward and exon 3 reverse primers (table 1).

Denaturing High-Pressure Liquid Chromatography (DHPLC) and Sequence Analysis

Coding exons and adjacent intronic sequences of *PIP5K3* were amplified from genomic DNA by use of the primers shown in table 1. PCR amplification of each of the 41 exons was performed in 20-μl reactions involving 2.5 U of AmpliTaq Gold (ABI), 2 μl of 10 × AmpliTaq Gold Buffer, 1.9 mM $MgCl_2$, 0.25 mM dNTPs, 0.25 mM of primers, and 40 g of genomic DNA. PCR cycling conditions consisted of an initial 10-min denaturation step at 95°C for 5 min; 32 cycles at 94°C for 40 s, 55°C for 30 s (61°C for exon 19b), and 72°C for 40 s; and a final elongation step at 72°C for 7 min. PCR products were screened by DHPLC on a WAVE system (Transgenomics). Buffer A contained 0.1 M triethylammonium acetate (TEAA [Transgenomics]). Buffer B contained 0.1 M TEAA and 25% acetonitrile, HPLC grade (Sigma-Aldrich). The flow rate was set at 0.9 ml/min, and the buffer B gradient increased by 2% per min for 4 min. The optimum temperature was determined for each DNA fragment by Wavemaker software (Transgenomics). When multiple melting domains were established, each domain was analyzed at the appropriate temperature. Initial buffer B concentrations

Table 2

Conditions for DHPLC of *PIP5K3* Exons

The table is available in its entirety in the online edition of *The American Journal of Human Genetics.*

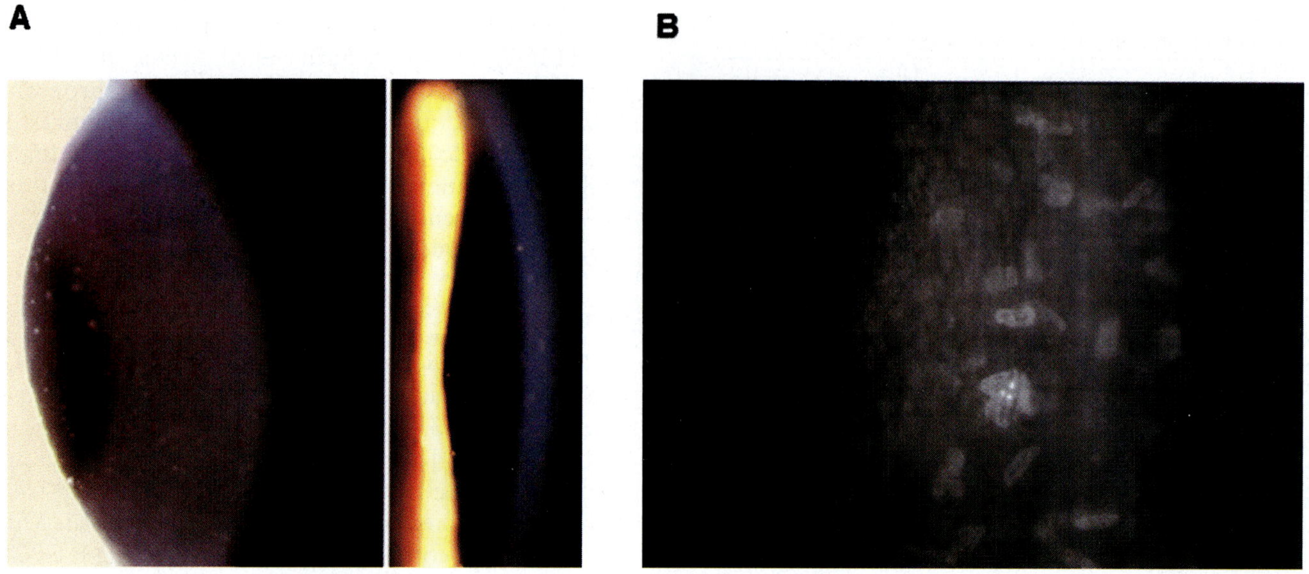

Figure 1 Slit-lamp image (*A*) and confocal microscopy image (*B*) of the cornea in a patient with CFD

and temperatures for each fragment are listed in table 2. PCR products were purified using Millipore Montage PCRμ96 plates or QIAquick PCR purification kits. The PCR templates were sequenced using ABI Dye Terminator, version 1 or 3, in a final reaction volume of 10 μl. Products of the sequencing reactions were purified using the Edge Biosystems Performa TM DTR gel-filtration system and were run on a 3100 ABI genetic analyzer. Sequences were aligned using the Seqman program of the DNASTAR package (DNASTAR) or Chromas, version 2.23 (Technelysium). The reference genomic sequence is available from NCBI (accession number NM_015040).

Protein Analysis

Structural motifs of the lipoprotein lipid attachment site were localized in the phosphatidylinositol-4-phosphate 5-kinase type III sequence (PIP5K3) by use of PROSITE. The search for spectrin sequence repeats was performed using rapid automatic detection and alignment of repeats (RADAR), and a search for structural motifs was performed using the simple modular architecture research tool (SMART), the Superfamily 1.65 HMM library and genome assignment service, the NIH homology alert service Whales, and the protein families database (PFAM) (see Web Resources). Sequence alignment was performed using the GCG-Lite+ ClustalW 1.74 multiple sequence alignment program (see Web Resources).

The chaperone-like domain structure of PIP5K3 was derived by homology modeling, with the crystal coordinates of protein database (PDB) file 1a6d as the structural template (Abola et al. 1987). For each model, amino acid sequences were aligned using the method of Needleman and Wunsch (1970). The three-dimensional structure was built using the program Look, version 3.5.2 (Lee and Subbiah 1991; Lee 1994), followed by 500 cycles of nonbound energy minimization. The conformation of mutant proteins was refined by 500 cycles of self-consistent ensemble optimization (Lee 1994). The geometry of the predicted structures was tested with the Procheck program (Laskowski et al. 1993).

Results

Patient Ascertainment

Individuals were diagnosed as affected on the basis of the typical appearance of corneal flecks on slit-lamp examination and, in some individuals, in vivo confocal microscopy (fig. 1). Of the 10 families investigated here, 4 (families 50001, 50002, 50003, and 50004) were previously studied by Jiao et al. (2003) and are described more fully in that study. Additional individuals and families 50005, 50006, 50008, 50009, and 50010 showed classical CFD and were asymptomatic, whereas affected individuals from family 50007 showed photophobia, which was severe enough in individual 5 (see pedigree in fig. 2) to result in blepharospasm and facial spasm, requiring multiple botulinum toxin injections to control the spasms. Family 50005 and one affected individual from family 50006 were reported elsewhere (Frueh and Bohnke 1999).

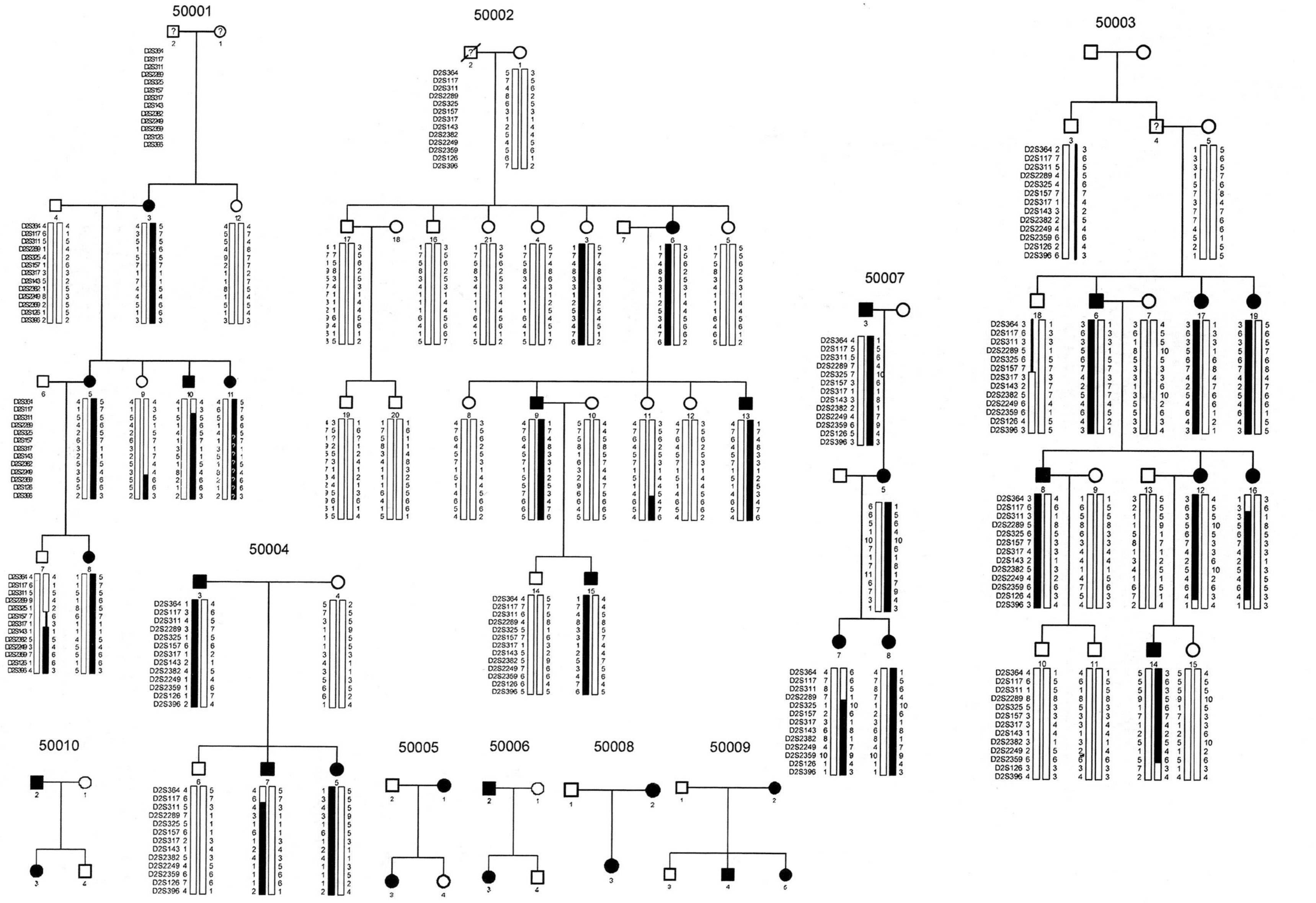

Figure 2 Pedigrees of families, with haplotypes for markers in the CFD region of chromosome 2 in the families used for linkage analysis. Blackened bars indicate the risk haplotype inherited by all affected individuals in a family.

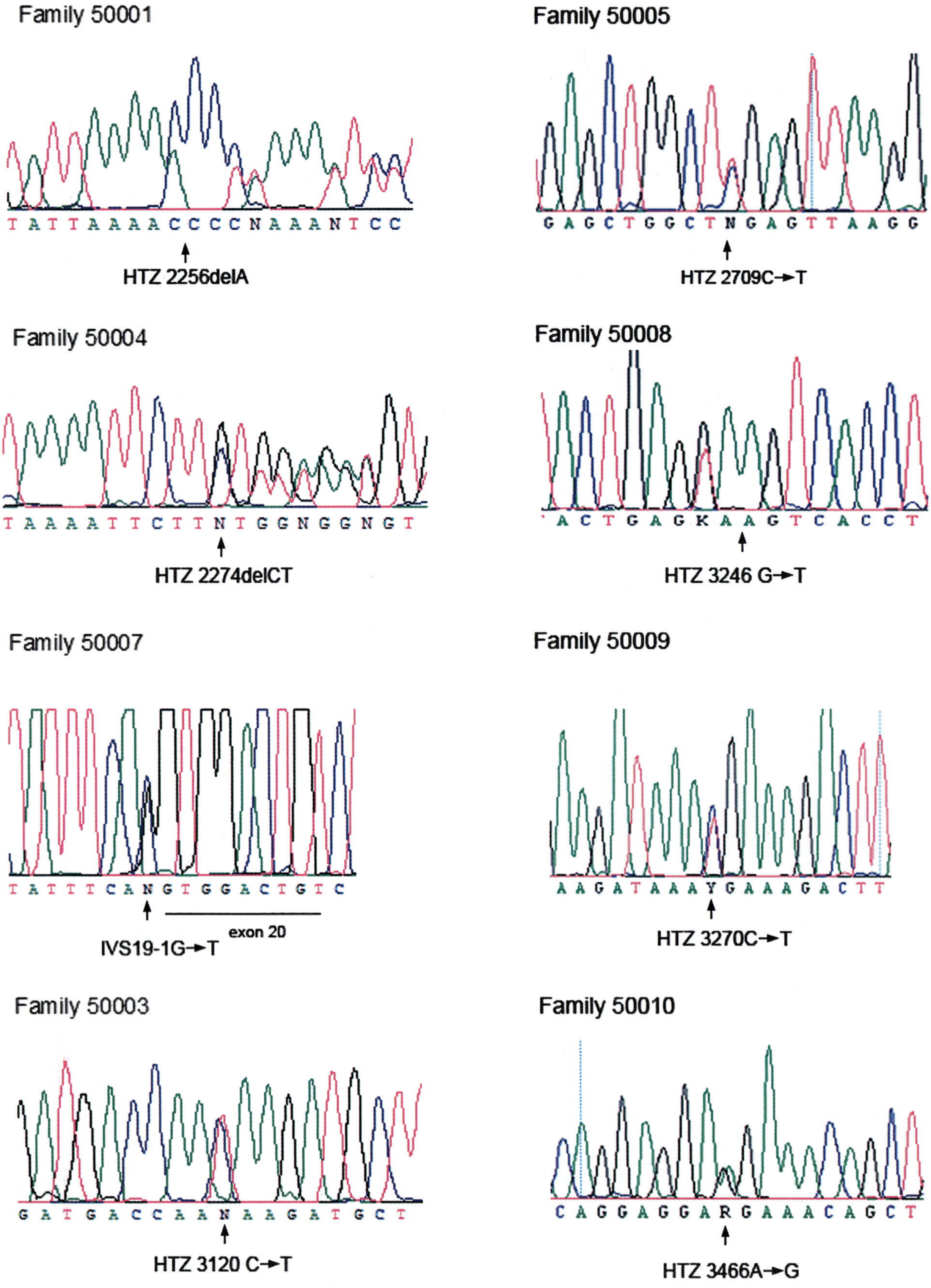

Figure 3 Sequence analysis for representative affected individuals from families with CFD. HTZ = heterozygous.

Linkage Analysis

Two-point linkage analysis suggested that the CFD locus is linked to a 12-cM region flanked by *D2S2289* and *D2S143* (table 3). This region includes markers *D2S325* ($Z_{max} = 4.64$; $\theta = 0$) and *D2S317* ($Z_{max} = 3.67$; $\theta = 0$). Significant LOD scores were also seen with other markers in the region, including *D2S2289* ($Z_{max} = 4.7$; $\theta = 0.03$), *D2S143* ($Z_{max} = 4.83$; $\theta = 0.05$), *D2S2382* ($Z_{max} = 5.27$; $\theta = 0.3$), and *D2S2249* ($Z_{max} = 4.54$; $\theta = 0.04$), although these markers showed obligate recombinants.

Haplotype analysis confirmed the critical interval (fig. 2). A recombination event in affected individual 7 of family 50007 set the centromeric boundary at *D2S2289,* and other centromeric obligate recombination events took place between *D2S117* and *D2S311* in individual 10 of family 50001, individual 16 of family 50003, and individual 7 of family 50004. Telomeric obligate recombination events took place between *D2S126* and *D2S396* in affected individuals 12 and 16 of family 50003, and the recombination in affected individual 14 of family 50003 set the telomeric boundary at *D2S126.* In addition, unaffected individual 9 of family 50001 showed a recombination event at *D2S2359,* and unaffected individual 7 of family 50001 showed an obligate recombination at *D2S143.* Thus, the CFD locus is linked to chromosome 2 between *D2S2289* and *D2S126,* and—on the basis of recombination events in unaffected individuals in whom the gene might not, in fact, be penetrant—the locus is probably between *D2S2289* and *D2S143.* In family 50003, unaffected individuals 3 and 18 share part of the risk haplotype, although individuals 1, 2, and 4 (through whom individuals 3 and 18 are connected to the affected individuals in this family) were not available for genotyping and examination.

DHPLC and Mutation Analysis

The interval contains *PIP5K3,* which has 41 coding exons spanning >89 kb and encodes a 2,098-aa protein. PCR amplification and DHPLC, followed by direct sequencing of the putative exons and intron-exon boundaries, showed mutations in 8 of 10 families studied (fig. 3). Mutations were confirmed in all available affected family members.

Screening of exon 16 revealed two significant sequence variations. Family 50001 showed mutation 2256delA, which causes a shift of the reading frame and the generation of an early stop codon after 6 aa, removing the final 1,392 aa. Family 50004 showed 2274delCT, which also causes a shift of the ORF and an early truncation after 5 aa. Five other families exhibit mutations in exon 19. Nonsense mutation 2962C→T (Q988X) was observed in family 50003; 2709C→T (R851X) in family 50005; 3246G→T (E1030X) in family 50008; and 3270C→T (R1038X) in family 50009. Family 50010 displays the only missense mutation observed to date. Nucleotide A at position 3466 was mutated to G, changing the lysine codon at position 1103 to arginine. In family 50007, the splice-acceptor site of exon 20 shows an IVS19-1 G→C transversion. This is predicted to cause skipping of exon 20, with a resultant frame shift and an early truncation after 10 additional amino acids. All these mutations were observed in a heterozygous state and were not observed in 100 control individuals (200 control individuals for mutation K1103R) of similar (European) ethnic background. In two families, 50002 and 50006, the complete screening of the coding regions of *PIP5K3* revealed neither point mutations nor small insertions and deletions. In family 50002, a single base insertion (IVS15-82insA) was observed in intron 15, as well as the 13-bp deletion IVS15+11→24. Both these

Table 3

Two-Point Linkage Results for Markers in the CFD Region of Chromosome 2q35

Marker	Position		LOD Score at θ =								
	cM	Mb	0	.01	.05	0.1	.02	.03	.04	Z_{max}	$\hat{\theta}$
D2S364	192.90	182.86	−∞	−1.32	1.14	1.89	2.05	1.57	.82	2.05	.2
D2S117	201.40	195.44	−∞	−3.90	−1.22	−.21	.48	.53	.30	.53	.3
D2S311	203.10	197.39	−∞	1.75	2.87	3.04	2.60	1.75	.75	3	.07
D2S2289	205.40	203.49	−∞	4.42	4.74	4.53	3.66	2.48	1.16	4.7	.03
D2S325	210.90	208.10	4.64	4.60	4.36	3.99	3.11	2.08	.98	4.64	0
D2S157	212.60	211.03	1.32	1.55	1.91	2.00	1.79	1.31	.69	2	.1
D2S317	215.10	213.33	3.67	3.61	3.38	3.05	2.29	1.45	.63	3.67	0
D2S143	217.00	214.70	−∞	3.87	4.83	4.82	4.02	2.75	1.25	4.83	.05
D2S2382	220.70	216.87	−∞	5.01	5.25	4.94	3.90	2.57	1.12	5.27	.3
D2S2249	223.10	218.54	−∞	4.18	4.51	4.30	3.46	2.34	1.06	4.54	.04
D2S2359	225.60	220.77	−∞	−1.16	.49	1.05	1.18	.85	.40	1.18	.2
D2S126	228.80	221.84	−∞	−1.75	1.26	2.13	2.26	1.65	.77	2.26	.2
D2S396	240.20	230.51	−∞	−6.20	−2.25	−.79	.20	.32	.12	.32	.3

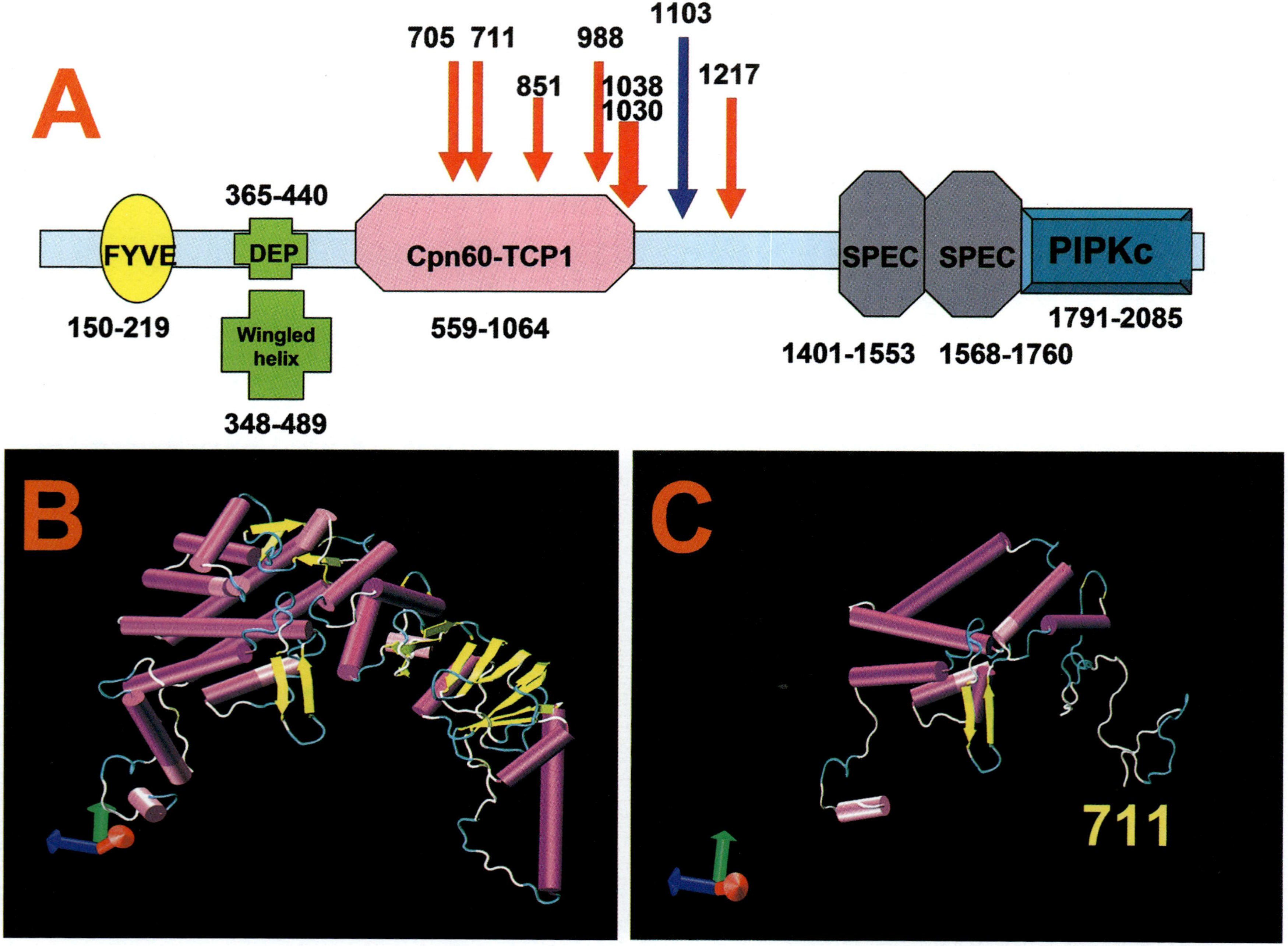
A
705 711
851
988
1038
1030
1103
1217
FYVE
150-219
365-440
DEP
Wingled
helix
348-489
Cpn60-TCP1
559-1064
SPEC
SPEC
PIPKc
1401-1553
1568-1760
1791-2085
B
C
711

sequence variants are observed in control individuals in a homozygous state and are not considered pathogenic.

PIP5K3 Molecular Organization

A schematic diagram of the PIP5K3 protein structure is shown in figure 4*A*. Homology to several structural fragments from the PDB was found. First, homology to a zinc finger–containing phosphoinositide kinase (FYVE [PDB: 1dvp]) is located at positions 150–219 (*E* value = 5.9e−18), with eight cysteines, at positions 160, 164, 167, 180, 183, 188, 191, and 192, that are potentially able to coordinate two zinc atoms. Second, a structural motif shows similarity to a DEP domain (Disheveled, EGL-10, plextrin homology domains of ~70 aa that are present in numerous signaling proteins [PDB: 1fsh]) of unknown function found in secreted proteins (positions 365–440; *E* value = 8.3e−27). A search with Superfamily 1.65 localizes a cytosolic chaperone CCTγ apical domain–like motif (PDB: 1gml) at position 677 through 843 of the PIP5K3 protein (*E* value = 1.3e−27), with a sequence identity of 29.8% and a similarity of 58.5%. The 1791–2085 region of the last C-terminal fragment is similar to that of the common kinase core found in the type IIβ phosphatidylinositol-4-phosphate 5-kinase (PDB: 1bo1) (Rao et al. 1998). The location of these four motifs agrees with that published previously (Shisheva et al. 2001). In addition, a small β-sheet "winged helix" DNA/RNA–binding motif at positions 348–489 (*E* value = 3.8e−18) and two spectrin repeats at positions 1490–1538 and 1679–1729 were found. Spectrin repeats form a three-helix bundle (PDB: 1quu) and are found in several proteins involved in cytoskeletal structure.

A search using the SMART method shows homology to the archaeal chaperonin thermosome structure (PDB: 1a6d), with an *E* value of 7.0e−14. The sequence of this protein is 36% identical to the CCTγ apical domain (Ditzel et al. 1998), containing ~170 overlapping residues. ClustalW 1.74 sequence alignment of the thermosome 1a6d and PIP5K3 (residues 462–1026) sequences have shown 20.2% identity and 50% similarity, suggesting that the structure of thermosome is suitable for use as a template for building an atomic model of this sequence fragment. The model of the three-dimensional structure of the domain similar to Cpn60-TCP1 was obtained using the thermosome 1a6d structure, as shown in figure 4*B*.

CFD nonsense mutations interrupt the PIP4K3 protein sequence at positions 705, 711, 951, 988, 1030, 1038, and 1217. All these mutations affect the C-terminal part of the PIP5K3 sequence, eliminating both the spectrin repeats and the PIPKc sequence. In addition, the two mutations at positions 705 and 711 remove almost half of the C-terminal domain (fig. 4C), destroying the polar surface of the central cavity of the protein domain possibly involved in protein folding (Ditzel et al. 1998), and are predicted to eliminate the chaperone-like domain of the protein.

Discussion

The CFD locus has been mapped in five unrelated families of European origin to a 24-cM (18-Mb) region of chromosome 2q35 flanked by *D2S2289* and *D2S126*, and CFD has been associated with mutations in PIP5K3, a protein which is important for post-Golgi vesicle processing. Mutations were identified in 8 of 10 families in the present study. All but one of these are protein-truncating mutations, predicted to cause termination of the peptide chain before the PIP5K3 structure is formed and to result in loss of activity.

No mutation was identified in family 50002 or 50006. Affected individuals in both of these families have typical CFD and could not be differentiated clinically from affected individuals from other families in the study. Although family 50006 is small and was not included in the linkage study, family 50002 is linked to the *PIP5K3* region, with a LOD score of 1.74, which is consistent with involvement of *PIP5K3* or a nearby gene, although unaffected individual 3 also inherited the risk haplotype specific for this family. This suggests, but does not prove, that affected individuals in family 50002 may have an intronic or noncoding regulatory mutation that has not yet been identified. Although these will be further investigated as additional families are studied, identification of noncoding mutations can be difficult and may require functional studies of splicing or promoter activity.

A K1103R missense mutation was observed in family 50010. Since most mutations reported here are nonsense mutations, the causative role of this variant may

Figure 4 Schematic diagram of PIP5K3, showing the locations and effect of the dominant mutations. *A*, Domain structure of PIP5K3. FYVE represents the FYVE zinc-finger domain; DEP represents the Disheveled, EGL-10, plextrin homology domain; Cpn60-TCP1 represents the chaperone-like Cpn-60-TCP1 domain; SPEC represents the two spectrin repeats; and PIPKc represents the domain with phosphatidylinositol-4-phosphate 5-kinase activity. Red arrows show the positions of the truncation mutations associated with CFD, and the blue arrow shows the missense mutation K1103R. *B*, Molecular structure of the Cpn60-TCP1 domain of PIP5K3, as predicted by homology modeling with the thermosome structure (PDB: 1a6d) as a structural template. The α helices (*cylinders*) and β strands (*ribbons*) are shown. C, Effect of dominant mutations in position 711 or 705 on the structure of the Cpn60-TCP1 domain.

be questionable. Several lines of evidence suggest that K1103R is a mutation. This variant segregated in all affected individuals and was not observed in >400 control chromosomes. A search of dbSNP indicated a total of 15 SNPs in the coding region of *PIP5K3*, 8 of which are nonsynonymous. Position 1103 is not among them. In addition, K1103 is conserved in various species as divergent as mouse, *Xenopus*, and *Fugu*. Confirmation of the causative role of this mutation awaits functional assays or studies of additional families with the same base change.

PIP5K3, a large gene comprising 41 exons that span >89 kb, encodes a predicted 2,098-aa protein. The PIP5K3 protein is a member of the phosphoinositide 3-kinase family, which comprises dual-specificity enzymes possessing an intrinsic protein kinase activity inseparable from a lipid kinase activity. These can generate and relay protein phosphorylation signals to regulate the formation and intracellular location of lipid products (Sbrissa et al. 2000). Both maintenance of mammalian cell morphology and endocytic membrane homeostasis require enzymatically active phosphoinositide 5-kinase PIKfyve (Ikonomov et al. 2001; Shisheva et al. 2001). Cultured mammalian cells transiently transfected with a kinase-deficient point mutant, PIKfyve K1831E, show dilation of PIKfyve-containing vesicles and progressive accumulation of multiple swollen lucent endosomal vacuoles, initially in the perinuclear cytoplasm and later in the cell periphery. This indicates that active PIKfyve enzyme must be present in a distinct set of late endocytic membranes for normal cell morphology (Ikonomov et al. 2001). The formation of enormously dilated late endocytic structures upon transfection of enzymatically inactive PIKfyve suggests a role for PIP5K3 in the endosome-to-*trans*-Golgi network (Ikonomov et al. 2003*b*).

It has been suggested that PIP5K3 selectively regulates the sorting and traffic of peripheral endosomes containing lysosomally directed fluid phase cargo by controlling the morphogenesis and function of multivesicular bodies (Ikonomov et al. 2003*a*). This role is entirely consistent with the clinical and histological findings for CFD, in which the corneal flecks appear to be abnormally swollen keratocytes with membrane-limited intracytoplasmic vacuoles containing complex lipids and glycosaminoglycans (Nicholson et al. 1977). Although the clinical findings for CFD are confined to the cornea, only limited studies of other tissues have been done, and the presence of a subset of abnormal cells in most tissues might not result in clinical symptoms.

In summary, the present study describes both the mapping of the CFD locus in 10 unrelated families of European origin to a 24-cM (18-Mb) region of chromosome 2q35 flanked by *D2S2289* and *D2S126* and the association of CFD with mutations in the PIP5K3 protein, which is important for post-Golgi vesicle processing. Mutations were identified in 8 of 10 families studied. All but one of these mutations are predicted to result in truncation of the PIP5K3 protein before the protein structure is formed, resulting in the loss of activity. Enzymatic studies of the PIP5K3 enzyme in affected individuals should further elucidate the role of this enzyme in CFD and in normal cellular metabolism.

Acknowledgments

We thank the members of the families, for their participation in this study, and Céline Agosti, Tatiana Favez, and Sylviane Métrailler, for their technical assistance. We acknowledge support from the Swiss National Science Foundation (grant 32-065250.01).

Web Resources

The accession number and URLs for data presented herein are as follows:

GCG-Lite+ ClustalW 1.74 multiple sequence alignment program, http://www.ebi.ac.uk/clustalw/
NCBI, http://www.ncbi.nlm.nih.gov/ (for reference genomic sequence [accession number NM_015040])
Online Mendelian Inheritance in Man (OMIM), http://www.ncbi.nlm.nih.gov/Omim/ (for CFD)
PFAM, http://www.sanger.ac.uk/Software/Pfam/
ScanProsite, tool to search the PROSITE database, http://us.expasy.org/tools/scanprosite/
RADAR, http://www.ebi.ac.uk/Radar/
SMART at European Laboratory of Molecular Biology, http://smart.embl-heidelberg.de/
Superfamily 1.65, HMM library and genome assignment service, http://supfam.mrc-lmb.cam.ac.uk/

References

Abola E, Bernstein FC, Bryant SH, Koetzle TF, Weng J (1987) Protein data bank. In: Allen FH, Bergerhoff G, Sievers R (eds) Crystallographic databases—information content, software systems, scientific applications. Data Comission of the International Union of Crystallography, Cambridge, United Kingdom, pp 107–132
Akova YA, Unlu N, Duman S (1994) Fleck dystrophy of the cornea: a report of cases from three generations of a family. Eur J Ophthalmol 4:123–125
Birndorf LA, Ginsberg SP (1972) Hereditary fleck dystrophy associated with decreased corneal sensitivity. Am J Ophthalmol 73:670–672
Cottingham RW, Idury RM, Schaffer AA (1993) Faster sequential genetic linkage computations. Am J Hum Genet 53: 252–263
Ditzel L, Lowe J, Stock D, Stetter KO, Huber H, Huber R, Steinbacher S (1998) Crystal structure of the thermosome, the archaeal chaperonin and homolog of CCT. Cell 93:125–138
François J, Neetens A (1957) Nouvelle dystrophie hérédofam-

iliale du parenchyme corneen (hérédo-dystrophie mouchetée). Bull Soc Belge Ophtalmol 114:641–646

Frueh BE, Bohnke M (1999) In vivo confocal microscopy of fleck dystrophy. Cornea 18:658–660

Goldberg MF, Krimmer B, Sugar J, Sewell J, Wong P (1977) Variable expression in flecked (speckled) dystrophy of the cornea. Ann Ophthalmol 9:889–896

Ikonomov OC, Sbrissa D, Foti M, Carpentier JL, Shisheva A (2003*a*) PIKfyve controls fluid phase endocytosis but not recycling/degradation of endocytosed receptors or sorting of procathepsin D by regulating multivesicular body morphogenesis. Mol Biol Cell 14:4581–4591

Ikonomov OC, Sbrissa D, Mlak K, Deeb R, Fligger J, Soans A, Finley RL Jr, Shisheva A (2003*b*) Active PIKfyve associates with and promotes the membrane attachment of the late endosome-to-*trans*-Golgi network transport factor Rab9 effector p40. J Biol Chem 278:50863–50871

Ikonomov OC, Sbrissa D, Shisheva A (2001) Mammalian cell morphology and endocytic membrane homeostasis require enzymatically active phosphoinositide 5-kinase PIKfyve. J Biol Chem 276:26141–26147

Jiao X, Munier FL, Schorderet DF, Zografos L, Smith J, Rubin B, Hejtmancik JF (2003) Genetic linkage of Francois-Neetens fleck (mouchetée) corneal dystrophy to chromosome 2q35. Hum Genet 112:593–599

Laskowski RA, MacArthur MW, Moss DS, Thornton JM (1993) PROCHECK: a program to check the stereochemical quality of protein structures. J Appl Cryst 26:283–291

Lathrop GM, Lalouel JM (1984) Easy calculations of lod scores and genetic risks on small computers. Am J Hum Genet 36:460–465

Lee C (1994) Predicting protein mutant energetics by self-consistent ensemble optimization. J Mol Biol 236:918–939

Lee C, Subbiah S (1991) Prediction of protein side-chain conformation by packing optimization. J Mol Biol 217:373–388

Needleman SB, Wunsch CD (1970) A general method applicable to the search for similarities in the amino acid sequence of two proteins. J Mol Biol 48:443–453

Nicholson DH, Green WR, Cross HE, Kenyon KR, Massof D (1977) A clinical and histopathological study of Francois-Neetens speckled corneal dystrophy. Am J Ophthalmol 83:554–560

Patten JT, Hyndiuk RA, Donaldson DD, Herman SJ, Ostler HB (1976) Fleck (mouchetee) dystrophy of the cornea. Ann Ophthalmol 8:25–32

Purcell JJ Jr, Krachmer JH, Weingeist TA (1977) Fleck corneal dystrophy. Arch Ophthalmol 95:440–444

Rao VD, Misra S, Boronenkov IV, Anderson RA, Hurley JH (1998) Structure of type II$^{\beta}$ phosphatidylinositol phosphate kinase: a protein kinase fold flattened for interfacial phosphorylation. Cell 94:829–839

Sbrissa D, Ikonomov OC, Shisheva A (2000) PIKfyve lipid kinase is a protein kinase: downregulation of 5′-phosphoinositide product formation by autophosphorylation. Biochemistry 39:15980–15989

Schaffer AA, Gupta SK, Shriram K, Cottingham RW (1994) Avoiding recomputation in genetic linkage analysis. Hum Hered 44:225–237

Shisheva A, Rusin B, Ikonomov OC, DeMarco C, Sbrissa D (2001) Localization and insulin-regulated relocation of phosphoinositide 5-kinase PIKfyve in 3T3-L1 adipocytes. J Biol Chem 276:11859–11869

Smith RJH, Holcomb JD, Daiger SP, Caskey CT, Pelias MZ, Alford BR, Fontenot DD, Hejtmancik JF (1989) Exclusion of Usher syndrome gene from much of chromosome 4. Cytogenet Cell Genet 50:102–106

Streeten BW, Falls HF (1961) Hereditary fleck dystrophy of the cornea. Am J Ophthalmol 51:275–281

Polymorphisms within the C-Reactive Protein (CRP) Promoter Region Are Associated with Plasma CRP Levels

Christopher S. Carlson,[1] Shelley Force Aldred,[3] Philip K. Lee,[1] Russell P. Tracy,[4] Stephen M. Schwartz,[2] Mark Rieder,[1] Kiang Liu,[5] O. Dale Williams,[6] Carlos Iribarren,[7] E. Cora Lewis,[6] Myriam Fornage,[8] Eric Boerwinkle,[8] Myron Gross,[9] Cashell Jaquish,[10] Deborah A. Nickerson,[1] Richard M. Myers,[3] David S. Siscovick,[2] and Alexander P. Reiner[2]

[1]Department of Genome Sciences and [2]Cardiovascular Health Research Unit, University of Washington, Seattle; [3]Department of Genetics, Stanford University, Stanford; [4]University of Vermont, Burlington; [5]Northwestern University, Chicago; [6]Division of Preventive Medicine, University of Alabama at Birmingham, Birmingham; [7]Kaiser Permanente Division of Research, Oakland; [8]University of Texas, Houston; [9]University of Minnesota, Minneapolis; and [10]National Heart, Lung, and Blood Institute (NHLBI), Bethesda

Elevated plasma levels of C-reactive protein (CRP), an inflammation-sensitive marker, have emerged as an important predictor of future cardiovascular disease and metabolic abnormalities in apparently healthy men and women. Here, we performed a systematic survey of common nucleotide variation across the genomic region encompassing the CRP gene locus. Of the common single-nucleotide polymorphisms (SNPs) identified, several in the CRP promoter region are strongly associated with CRP levels in a large cohort study of cardiovascular risk in European American and African American young adults. We also demonstrate the functional importance of these SNPs in vitro.

Introduction

C-reactive protein (CRP) was initially defined as a protein in serum that binds to the C polysaccharide of *Streptococcus pneumoniae* (Tillet and Francis 1930) and is the prototypical protein up-regulated as part of the acute phase response in humans (Abernathy and Avery 1941). More recently, elevated CRP has been identified as a biomarker for cardiovascular disease (CVD) risk, supplementary to traditional risk factors such as BMI, smoking, diabetes, and cholesterol levels (Ridker et al. 1997, 2000, 2005; Danesh et al. 2000, 2004; Hackam and Anand 2003). Family and twin studies suggest that additive genetic factors account for as much as 40% of the variance in plasma CRP levels (Pankow et al. 2001; Retterstol et al. 2003; MacGregor et al. 2004), but the specific genetic determinants remain poorly characterized.

Human genetic association studies of CRP include several that have assessed the relationship between genotype and plasma CRP levels (Szalai et al. 2002; Zee and Ridker 2002; Brull et al. 2003; Russell et al. 2004) or disease risk (Zee and Ridker 2002; Wolford et al. 2003; Russell et al. 2004). These generally have suffered from lack of functional data on DNA-sequence variation. Polymorphisms reported elsewhere as being associated with CRP levels include a polymorphism in the promoter region (Kovacs et al. 2005), a synonymous polymorphism in exon 2 (Russell et al. 2004; Suk et al. 2005), a polymorphism in the 3′ UTR (Brull et al. 2003), and a second polymorphism in the 3′ UTR (Russell et al. 2004). These studies have been restricted to a small number of polymorphisms within the CRP gene locus, without consideration of the patterns of variation across the locus as a whole. Thus, although the reported associations suggest that variation at the CRP locus is significantly correlated with basal CRP levels, it remains possible that the observed associations were attributable to other polymorphisms in strong linkage disequilibrium (LD) with the reported polymorphisms, because none of the prior work demonstrated functional differences between alleles. Prior analyses have also been largely restricted to European populations, with no prior study including >100 African Americans (AAs).

To explore whether common genetic variants at the human CRP gene locus influence plasma CRP, we used an approach that starts with genomic resequencing to identify all common patterns of nucleotide diversity and to define common haplotypes in the European American (EA) and AA populations. We then genotyped a set of polymorphisms representative of the patterns of common variation identified in a much larger population-based study sample, and we identified associations with specific haplotypes. Lastly, we experimentally validated the observed associations with polymorphisms in the promoter region, using in vitro CRP promoter analysis in a human hepatocyte cell line.

Received January 24, 2005; accepted for publication April 26, 2005; electronically published May 16, 2005.

Address for correspondence and reprints: Dr. Christopher Carlson, Health Sciences Center, University of Washington, Room K-322, 1705 NE Pacific Street, Seattle, WA 98195-7730. E-mail: csc47@u.washington.edu

0002-9297/2005/7701-0007$15.00

Table 1

***Taq*Man Primer and Probe Sequences**

The table is available in its entirety in the online edition of *The American Journal of Human Genetics.*

Material and Methods

SNP Discovery, tagSNP Selection, and Genotyping

Polymorphic sites were identified by resequencing of PCR products tiled across the CRP gene region by use of standard BigDye Terminator v3.1 chemistry from Applied Biosystems (ABI). The gene and flanking region were resequenced in 47 samples: 24 unrelated AAs from the Coriell AA100 panel and 23 unrelated EAs from the CEPH pedigrees. Coriell sample identifiers are available at the Web site of the SeattleSNPs Program for Genomic Applications. We resequenced 6,800 bp in each sample, covering the two exons, the intervening intron, and 1.7 kbp 5′ and 2.8 kbp 3′ of the gene. SNP numbering is based on the GenBank accession number AF449713. Bins of common SNPs (minor-allele frequency [MAF] >10%) in strong LD, as defined by $r^2 > 0.64$, were identified within each population by use of LDselect v1.0 (Carlson et al. 2004). Seven tagSNPs were selected for coverage of all bins in the two sequenced populations. Relative to AF449713, the seven tagSNPs positions were 790 (dbSNP *rs3093058*), 1440 (*rs3091244*), 1919 (*rs1417938*), 2667 (*rs1800947*), 3006 (*rs3093066*), 3872 (*rs1205*), and 5237 (*rs2808630*).

The previous literature has generally used a nomenclature for polymorphism positions relative to the ATG codon. Thus, the previously reported promoter polymorphism has been referred to as −286 (Kovacs et al. 2005), the synonymous polymorphism in exon 2 has been referred to as +1059 (Russell et al. 2004; Suk et al. 2005), and the polymorphisms in the 3′ UTR have been referred to as +1444 (Brull et al. 2003) and +2147 (Russell et al. 2004). Because our resequencing efforts identified several insertion/deletion polymorphisms in the CRP gene region, numbering relative to an origin such as the ATG codon would be ambiguous, so we have chosen to refer to each polymorphism relative to its position in GenBank accession number AF449713, which details the results of our polymorphism-discovery survey. For convenience, here is a brief list of pseudonyms for polymorphisms reported elsewhere: −717 is 1009 (*rs2794521*), −286 is 1440 (*rs3091244*), +1059 is 2667 (*rs1800847*), +1444 is 3014 (*rs1130864*), and +2147 is 3872 (*rs1205*).

tagSNPs were genotyped using *Taq*Man Assays By Design (ABI) under standard conditions, with the exception of the triallelic tagSNP (detailed below). Probe and primer sequences for each assay are listed in table 1. End-point fluorescence values were genotyped manually within the SDS software (ABI) for tagSNPs 790, 3872, and 5237. Threshold cycle (Ct) values from real-time reads were exported to Excel (Microsoft) and were used to cluster and manually score genotypes for 1919, 2667, and 3006. The triallelic SNP (1440) was genotyped in a single tube assay, by use of reagents, at the following final concentrations in a 5-μl reaction: three *Taq*Man probes at 0.2 μM each, two PCR primers at 1 μM each, 1 × Universal Mastermix (ABI), 1 M betaine (Sigma-Aldrich), and 1 ng/μl genomic DNA. Thermal cycling reactions were performed as follows: 50° for 2 min, 95° for 10 min, and then 45 cycles at 95° for 15 s, 53° for 30 s, and 60° for 1 min. Real-time data were acquired on the ABI 7900HT instrument. Ct values from real-time data for all three probes were exported from the SDS 2.1 software (ABI) and were used to visualize and manually call genotypes in Excel. Haplotypes for cladistic analysis were inferred using PHASE v2.0 (Stephens and Donnelly 2003).

CARDIA Population Study Sample

The Coronary Artery Risk Development in Young Adults (CARDIA) study is a population-based study, initiated in 1985, to investigate the evolution of cardiovascular risk factors in a large, biracial cohort of young adults (Hughes et al. 1987; Friedman et al. 1988). Participants aged 18–30 years were recruited from four geographic locations by community-based sampling (Birmingham, AL; Chicago; and Minneapolis) and through the membership of a large prepaid health plan (Oakland). In 1985–1986, baseline examinations of 5,115 participants, or 51% of the eligible persons contacted, were performed. Participants were contacted every 6 mo and were re-examined at five follow-up examinations (year 2 in 1987–1988, year 5 in 1990–1991, year 7 in 1992–1993, year 10 in 1995–1996, and year 15 in 2000–2001).

The initial study population was approximately balanced with respect to age (45% were aged 18–24 years; 55% were aged 25–30 years), sex (46% men; 54% women), race (52% AA; 48% EA), and education (40% had completed ⩽12 years of education; 60% had completed >12 years). Overall retention rates for follow-up examinations among surviving participants were 91% at year 2, 86% at year 5, 81% at year 7, 79% at year 10, and 74% at year 15. The CARDIA database includes repeated measures of lifestyle, physiologic, and metabolic risk factors, including smoking, obesity, and physical

Table 2

CARDIA Participant Characteristics at Year 15, by Race and Sex

The table is available in its entirety in the online edition of *The American Journal of Human Genetics.*

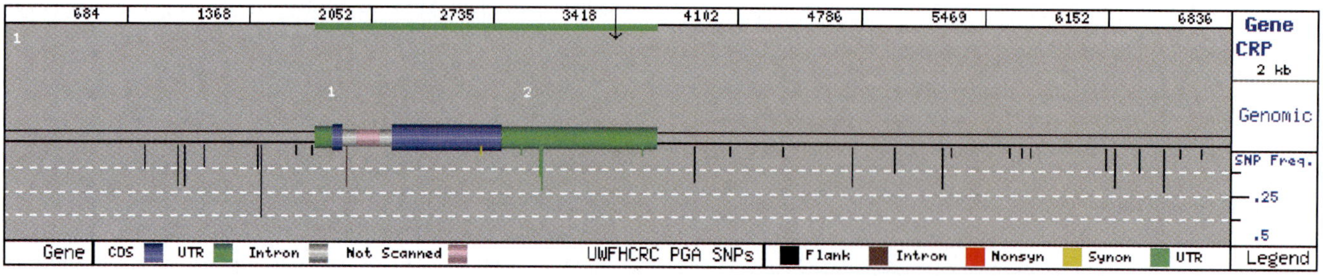

Figure 1 A GeneSNPs image of CRP, showing the region scanned for polymorphism. Coding regions of exons are shown in blue, and the UTR is shown in green. Polymorphic positions are indicated with ticks below the axis, and the length of the tick represents MAF in the combined population. A highly repetitive region of the intron (shown in pink) could not be screened for polymorphism by resequencing. Nonsyn = nonsynonymous; Synon = synonymous; CDS - coding sequence.

activity. Participants eligible for the current study included those who consented to isolation of genomic DNA from peripheral-blood leukocytes obtained at the year 10 examination and for which an adequate DNA sample was available ($n = 3,790$).

Phenotypic Measurements and Statistical Analysis

Plasma CRP levels were assayed using BNII immunonephelometry (BNII Nephelometer 100 Analyzer [Dade Behring]) on plasma, stored at year 7, from 3,382 returning CARDIA participants who also consented to DNA testing and on plasma from 3,146 consenting participants who returned at year 15. The latter number represents 86% of the 3,672 original CARDIA subjects who attended the year 15 examination. Two CRP measurements were available at year 15, BNII and ELISA. BNII is a more sensitive assay than ELISA (Wener et al. 2000), so only the results of analysis of the BNII data are presented, although results from an analysis of the ELISA data at year 15 were consistent (data not shown). BNII plasma CRP measurements had a range of 0–333 mg/liter. Samples with ELISA-based CRP >10 mg/liter have been suggested to represent acute illness, stress, or infection (Shine et al. 1981; Pearson et al. 2003); 48 such samples were observed at year 15, comparable to the 50 samples with BNII CRP >18 mg/liter at year 15. Exclusion of samples with BNII >18 mg/liter had negligible impact on results at either year 7 or year 15 (data not shown). Plasma-CRP measurements at years 7 and 15 were significantly correlated for samples above this threshold, so samples with high CRP measurements were not removed from the analysis.

Stepwise linear regression was run in the R statistics program v2.0.1, with ln(plasma CRP) (the natural log of plasma CRP) at year 7, ln(plasma CRP) at year 15, or change in ln(plasma CRP) between years 7 and 15 as the dependent variable. The following phenotypic measures were allowed to enter the model as independent variables: ln(BMI), age, sex, ethnicity, systolic blood pressure, diastolic blood pressure, ln(glucose), ln(insulin), ln(total cholesterol), ln(HDL), ln(LDL), and ln(insulin/glucose). The Bayesian information criterion (Hastie et al. 2001), a measure of how well each model fits the data that is penalized for the number of parameters in the model, was used for all model comparisons.

For each of the dependent variables (CRP at year 7 and CRP at year 15), independent variables retained in the best-fit model at both time points were included as covariables in an analysis of the effects of haplotype on ln(plasma CRP). Analyses were run using the haplo.stats package for R (Lake et al. 2003), a generalized linear-regression framework that incorporates haplotype phase uncertainty by inferring a probability matrix of haplotype likelihoods for each individual by use of the expectation-maximization (EM) haplotype-inference algorithm rather than by assignment of a most likely haplotype phase resolution to each sample. Haplo.stats analysis was performed on the complete CARDIA cohort, with race and sex included as covariables, as well as on subsets of the CARDIA cohort stratified by sex and race. Haplo.stats analysis was restricted to haplotypes with an inferred frequency >1%, representing ~33 chromosomes in this cohort.

In Vitro Promoter-Variant Vector Construction

PCR products from the CRP promoter region representing several haplotypes were cloned into a modified

The figure is available in its entirety in the online edition of *The American Journal of Human Genetics.*

Figure 2 Visual genotype diagram of patterns of common variation at the CRP locus. Each row corresponds to an individual DNA sample in the polymorphism-discovery panel; E001–E023 are EAs, and D001–D040 are AAs. Each column corresponds to a polymorphic site. Sites are ordered by LD, not position along the chromosome, with sites showing similar patterns of genotype shown adjacent to one another. Site numbers are relative to GenBank accession number AF449713. Selected tagSNPs are indicated with arrows.

Haplotype Phylogenetic Tree

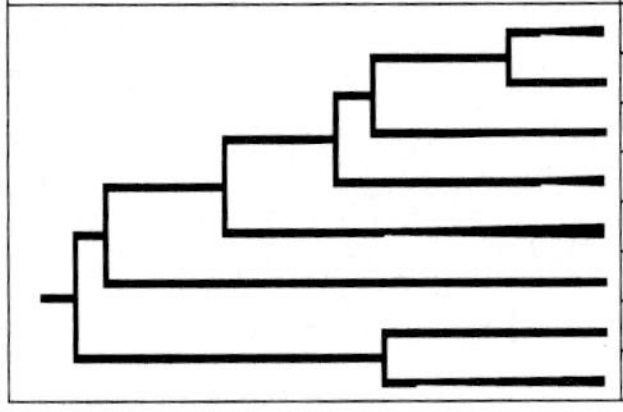

Haplotype	790	1440	1919	2667	3006	3872	5237
H1	A	C	A	C	C	A	A
H2	A	C	A	G	C	A	A
H3	A	C	A	G	C	G	A
H4	A	C	A	G	C	G	G
H5	A	T	T	G	C	G	A
H6	T	T	A	G	C	G	A
H7	A	A	A	G	C	G	A
H8	A	A	A	G	A	G	A

Figure 3 Phylogeny of common CRP haplotypes. Haplotypes were inferred for all 18 common SNPs (MAF >10% in either AA or EA sequenced samples) by use of PHASE v 2.0. A neighbor-joining phylogenetic tree of the major CRP haplotypes resolved using the seven selected tagSNPs is shown, with branch lengths representing evolutionary distance as the proportion of alleles shared at all 18 common SNPs. The tagSNP alleles associated with each resolved haplotype are shown.

pGL3-basic luciferase expression vector (Promega). Short and extended clones of the native promoter represent bps 540–1726 and bps 1023–1726, respectively, relative to GenBank AF449713 (corresponding to positions −1186 to +1 and −703 to +1, relative to the transcription start site (TSS) discussed by Li et al. [1990]). To reduce interleukin 6 (IL6) dependence, the proximal CRP promoter (−107 to +1, relative to TSS) was replaced with the SV40 minimal promoter (bps 2349–2513 of pDsRed2-C1 [Promega]). Construct sequences were verified by standard fluorescent resequencing, and all construct sequences have been deposited into GenBank. Maxipreps of each construct were made (Plasmid Maxi Kit, part #12162 [QIAGEN]) and were diluted to a concentration of 200 ng/μl by UV densitometry, verified by ethidium bromide staining of serial dilutions in agarose gels.

Luciferase Assays

Transient transfection assays were conducted in a human liver hepatoma cell line (PLC/PRF/5 cells from ATCC [Manassas]) in 24-well plates, with 24 replicate wells per construct per experiment. Cells were seeded in serum-containing media. After 24 h, cells were transfected in serum-free media (so that transfection time also served as serum-starvation time). In each well, 200 ng of plasmid was transfected, with Fugene 6 transfection reagent (Roche Diagnostics), per protocols provided with the reagent. After 18 h, transfection media was removed, and cells either were induced with 200 U/ml human IL6 (Stem Cell Technologies) in serum-free media or were mock induced with non-IL6–containing serum-free media. Cell lysates were prepared 24 h later, and luciferase activity was assayed in a Wallac plate luminometer, per protocols of the Luciferase Assay System (Promega).

For each 24-well data set, the two highest and the two lowest values were dropped to remove outliers possibly related to variation in transfection efficiency. For the remaining data, luciferase values were normalized to the average activity of the promoter-less empty vector in native promoter experiments or to the SV40 minimal promoter alone in replacement promoter experiments, to yield data reflecting fold-activity increase over baseline levels for each CRP promoter construct. Standard error measurements and two-tailed student's t tests were used to assess the significance of differences between haplotype constructs.

Results

SNP Discovery and Selection of CRP Gene tagSNPs

Polymorphisms in the CRP gene region were identified by direct resequencing of 47 individuals: 24 AAs and 23 EAs. We identified 31 SNPs overall, 30 polymorphic in AAs and 13 polymorphic in EAs (fig. 1). No amino acid–changing SNPs were identified in either population. There were 18 common SNPs (i.e., SNPs with a relative MAF >10% in at least one of the two populations). Ten unique CRP haplotypes were inferred from the 18 common SNPs by use of a Bayesian statistical method for haplotype reconstruction (PHASE v2.0) (Stephens et al. 2001).

We next used an LD-based tagSNP-selection algorithm (LDselect) (Carlson et al. 2004) at a threshold of $r^2 >$

Table 3

tagSNP Allele Frequencies in SNP Discovery and CARDIA Populations

			Allele Frequencies (%) in			
			AA		EA	
SNP	dbSNP Number	Alleles	Sequenced Samples (n = 24)	CARDIA Cohort (n = 1,557)	Sequenced Samples (n = 23)	CARDIA Cohort (n = 1,820)
790	*rs309358*	A/T	77/23	83/17	100/0	100/0
1440	*rs3091244*	A/C/T	33/26/41	26/45/29	5/62/33	7/64/30
1919	*rs1417938*	A/T	83/17	88/12	70/30	70/30
2667	*rs1800947*	C/G	2/98	1/99	4/96	6/94
3006	*rs3093066*	A/C	29/71	23/77	0/100	0/100
3872	*rs1205*	A/G	15/85	19/81	25/75	34/66
5237	*rs2808630*	A/G	94/6	82/18	65/35	72/28

Table 4

tagSNP Haplotype Frequencies in SNP Discovery and CARDIA Populations

The table is available in its entirety in the online edition of *The American Journal of Human Genetics.*

0.64, and we identified five tagSNPs that summarize common patterns of variation across the CRP gene in the sequenced samples (fig. 2). Two additional SNPs—a common triallelic SNP from the promoter region and a rare, synonymous SNP that previously was associated with CRP level (Zee and Ridker 2002)—were selected for analysis independent of the LDselect results. The seven tagSNPs resolved the 10 unique haplotypes observed in the sequenced samples as eight clades of related haplotypes (fig. 3), with each tagSNP allele tagging either a specific haplotype (SNPs 790, 1919, 2667, 3006, and 5237) or a clade of evolutionarily related haplotypes (SNP 1440 and 3872).

CRP Genotype-Phenotype Association Study

We subsequently genotyped the seven selected tagSNPs in 3,790 U.S. adults recruited as part of the CARDIA study (Hughes et al. 1987; Friedman et al. 1988). The subjects, who were aged 18–30 years at baseline, have been followed prospectively for 15 years and have undergone serial assessment for various cardiovascular risk factors (table 2). Allele frequencies at all tagSNPs were consistent between the sequenced samples and the CARDIA cohort (table 3), although tagSNP allele frequencies differed significantly between AAs and EAs. Inferred haplotype frequencies were also similar between the sequenced samples and the CARDIA cohort (table 4).

Stepwise linear regression of log-transformed CRP values on selected clinical, demographic, and lifestyle measurements identified six statistically significant predictors at both year 7 and year 15—BMI, race, sex, triglycerides, insulin level, and current smoking—as well as two significant interactions on CRP level, between sex and triglycerides ($P < .0001$) and between sex and smoking ($P < .0001$). Best-fit models at each time point are shown in table 5 (year 7) and table 6 (year 15). At both time points, the interaction between sex and triglycerides reflects a strong association with triglyceride levels in women and a weak association in men, and the interaction between sex and smoking reflects a strong association with smoking in men but not in women (data not shown).

There was significant variation in CRP level among CRP haplotypes ($P < 10^{-6}$), and the patterns of association were similar at both time points (fig. 4 and tables 7 and 8) as well as in analyses stratified by sex and race (data not shown). The results of a similar analysis without covariables were also consistent (data not shown). Haplotype 1 (H1) (tagged by SNP 2667) was associated with significantly reduced CRP levels relative to H2, the referent, at both time points. In addition, the clade of H1–H4, which carry the C allele of the triallelic SNP 1440, was associated with lower CRP levels than was the clade of H5–H8. Of the latter group, H6 (tagged by SNP 790) was associated with the highest CRP levels relative to all other haplotypes. The results of a similar analysis without covariables were also consistent (data not shown). Models fitted under the assumption of allelic independence showed a better fit than did recessive or dominant models at any of the loci (data not shown). Models fitted without interactions between haplotype and phenotypic variables other than race showed a better fit than did models including such interactions (data not shown). Exclusion of the 48 subjects with BNII CRP values >18 mg/liter did not alter these results. Similarly, exclusion of the upper and lower 5% of CRP values did not alter the results, so it is unlikely that the observed associations were attributable to a small number of influential data points. Comparison of the residual variance of the full model with the residual variance of models excluding single predictors demonstrated that only BMI explained a greater proportion of variance than did the tagSNPs at both time points (table 9). Results were similar for analyses stratified by race (data not shown).

The availability of high-sensitivity BNII CRP measurements at time points 8 years apart allowed us to assess the potential influence of CRP genotype on the temporal change in CRP level. Overall, the intrasubject correlation in ln(CRP) between years 7 and 15 was $r = 0.60$ ($P \ll .001$). On average, there was a 0.33 mg/liter, or 11.6%, increase during the 8-year interval. Although change in BMI and change in triglycerides were significantly correlated with change in CRP level, there were no significant associations between CRP haplotype and change in level (data not shown).

Contribution of CRP Genotype to Population Differences in CRP Levels

Median CRP levels were 1.0 mg/liter among EAs and 2.0 mg/liter among AAs ($P < 10^{-6}$ by t test on log-transformed data). Since the low-level CRP variant (H1) was more common among EAs and the high-level variant (H6) was more common among AAs, we assessed the extent to which CRP genotype or other known predictors accounted for variation in CRP levels between AAs and EAs in our population sample. To this end, we analyzed

Table 5

Best-Fit Model Predictors of ln(plasma CRP) Level at Year 7, in All Subjects ($N = 3,051$)

The table is available in its entirety in the online edition of *The American Journal of Human Genetics.*

Table 6

Best-Fit Model Predictors of ln(plasma CRP) Level at Year 15, in All Subjects (N = 2,995)

The table is available in its entirety in the online edition of *The American Journal of Human Genetics.*

a series of nested, multivariable regression models that variably included or excluded terms for race/ethnicity, sex, BMI, triglycerides, insulin level, smoking status, and CRP haplotypes or tagSNP genotypes. The non-genotypic covariables sex, triglycerides, insulin level, and smoking status all contributed relatively little to the mean difference in CRP level between racial groups, estimated from the regression model—mean difference in ln(CRP) level = 0.55 ± 0.04 unadjusted; 0.43 ± 0.04 adjusted for sex, triglycerides, insulin level, and smoking status. The further addition of BMI to the regression model had a more substantial effect—mean difference in ln(CRP) level = 0.20 ± 0.04—suggesting that more than half of the difference in CRP levels between ethnic groups was attributable to differences in BMI between AAs and EAs. The addition of CRP genotypes to the model resulted in an even greater reduction in the coefficient for ethnicity (e.g., mean difference in ln(CRP) level = −0.04 ± 0.05 at year 15 [table 8]), to the point where there was no longer a statistically significant difference between racial groups at either time point (P = .51 [table 7]; P = .41 [table 8]).

CRP Promoter Analysis In Silico

Comparison of the human and mouse genomic sequence of the CRP locus (Mayor et al. 2000) showed a strongly conserved promoter region 5′ of the exons (fig. 5, *upper panel*) that contains response elements for several hepatic transcription factor families (HNF, C/EBP, and NFKB) involved in induction of CRP by IL6 (Li et al. 1990). Two SNPs map to the 5′ edge of this region, tagSNP 1440 and a SNP perfectly associated with tagSNP 790, 1421. A transcription factor–motif analysis of the region (TFSEARCH; Heinemeyer et al. 1998) identified two upstream stimulating factor 1 (USF1)–binding motifs altered by SNPs 1421 and 1440 (fig. 5, *lower panel*). Only two other USF1-binding motifs were predicted within the CRP transcript or upstream region, at 1630 and 2650.

In Vitro Gene-Reporter Assays

In light of the observed associations between promoter-region polymorphism and CRP levels, as well as the *in silico* promoter analysis, in vitro assays were generated to explore the variation identified in promoter polymorphisms in CRP. Each of the five unique promoter-region haplotypes was cloned into a luciferase-reporter plasmid for in vitro analysis. Promoter activity in the native promoter constructs was weak without IL6 induction (fig. 6). Therefore, we also analyzed each promoter haplotype with the native TSS replaced by the SV40 TSS to generate detectable signal without IL6 induction (fig. 7). The IL6-induced native H7/H8 constructs showed elevated promoter activity relative to H1–H3 (fig. 6) but not in the SV40-replacement constructs (fig. 7), suggesting that the elevated CRP levels associated with H7/H8 require the proximal IL6 responsive element. By comparison, in the native promoter, there was no evidence of increased IL6-induced promoter activity from H5 or H6.

Dramatically stronger uninduced expression was observed in the SV40-replacement constructs, and significant variation was observed between haplotypes (fig. 7). Consistent with the CRP genotype-phenotype association observed in the population study, the H6 promoter showed the highest activity, and the promoter activity associated with the H5 construct was also significantly increased. Interestingly, the magnitude of the difference between H5/H6 and H1–H4 SV40-replacement promoter activities was similar both with and without IL6 induction, suggesting that, although the H5 and H6 promoter haplotypes associate with elevated CRP levels, this association is not IL6-dependent but, rather, reflects a change in basal promoter activity.

Discussion

To determine how common genetic variants at the human CRP gene locus influence plasma CRP, we used a three-stage experimental design. In the first phase, all common genetic variation across the gene region was defined by resequencing the region in a multiethnic variation discovery panel, and tagSNPs representative of all common patterns in each ethnicity were selected for genotyping in a larger panel of clinically phenotyped samples. Seven tagSNPs were selected for genotyping, and these defined eight common haplotypes (fig. 3). In the second phase, associations between haplotypes of tagSNPs and CRP levels were investigated using standard regression models, and significant associations were identified for several SNPs in the putative promoter region. In the third phase, the observed associations were experimentally validated by in vitro CRP promoter analysis in human hepatocytes.

The results from our large population sample suggest that CRP haplotypes can be grouped into four categories on the basis of associated CRP level: lowest (H1), low (H2–H4), high (H5, H7, and H8), and highest (H6) (fig. 4). These results were consistent between year 7 and year 15. Relative to the covariable-adjusted population mean of 3.1 mg/liter at year 15, the haplotype associated with the lowest levels (H1) decreased plasma

Table 7

Association of CRP Haplotypes with Plasma CRP Level at Year 7

Variable	tagSNP Alleles	Haplotype Frequency[a]	Coefficient	SE	*t*	*P*
Intercept	...	...	−8.0161	.0703	...	...
EA	...	...	−.0332	.0502	−.661	.509
Male	...	...	−1.0083	.1817	−5.549	<.00001
ln(BMI)	...	...	2.4367	.1008	24.18	<.00001
ln(insulin)	...	...	.1963	.0511	3.845	.00012
ln(triglycerides)	...	...	−.2996	.0722	−4.151	.00003
Current smoker	...	...	.7819	.1406	5.561	<.00001
H1	ACACCAA	.0381	−.1262	.0728	−1.734	.0831
H2	ACAGCAA	.2306	Referent	...	...	...
H3	ACAGCGA	.0398	.1387	.0725	1.912	.056
H4	ACAGCGG	.2215	.0563	.0393	1.432	.152
H5	ATTGCGA	.2053	.2818	.0398	7.085	<.00001
H6	TTAGCGA	.0717	.4498	.0592	7.602	<.00001
H7	AAAGCGA	.0481	.3128	.0669	4.677	<.00001
H8	AAAGAGA	.0948	.1749	.054	3.236	.00122
Other[b]	...	.0502	.1908	.0705	2.706	.00685
Sex × ln(triglycerides)	...	...	.367	.0441	8.324	<.00001
Sex × smoking	...	...	−.3587	.0877	−4.091	.00004

NOTE.—*t* statistics and *P* values were calculated from the coefficients and SEs within the best-fit multivariate model by the haplo.glm function of the haplo.stats R package.

[a] Haplotype frequencies were inferred using the EM algorithm within the haplo.stats package.

[b] Haplotypes with frequency <1% were pooled as "Other."

CRP an average of 1.5 mg/liter per copy, whereas the haplotype associated with the highest levels (H6) increased plasma CRP 1.5 mg/liter per copy.

An advantage of using tag SNPs defined on the basis of detailed sequence variation and LD data is that mapping the observed haplotype associations to potentially functional polymorphisms (or combinations thereof) can be straightforward. For example, the synonymous SNP at 2667 was the only observed difference between H1 and H2 in the SNP discovery samples. Therefore, it is likely that this polymorphism directly influences CRP levels, consistent with previous reports (Szalai et al. 2002; Zee and Ridker 2002; Brull et al. 2003; Russell et al. 2004), although the mechanism for a direct effect is

Table 8

Association of CRP Haplotypes with Plasma CRP Level at Year 15

Variable	tagSNP alleles	Haplotype Frequency[a]	Coefficient	SE	*t*	*P*
Intercept	...	...	−7.1203	.0745	...	...
EA	...	...	−.0405	.0495	−.819	.413
Male	...	...	−1.69	.1824	−9.265	<.00001
ln(BMI)	...	...	2.4717	.0963	25.657	<.00001
ln(insulin)	...	...	.2016	.0438	4.605	<.00001
ln(triglycerides)	...	...	−.4544	.0671	−6.771	<.00001
Current smoker	...	...	.7411	.1456	5.09	<.00001
H1	ACACCAA	.0378	−.2275	.0717	−3.172	.00153
H2	ACAGCAA	.2262	Referent			
H3	ACAGCGA	.0414	−.0335	.0706	−.475	.635
H4	ACAGCGG	.2231	.0534	.0386	1.381	.167
H5	ATTGCGA	.205	.2125	.0391	5.437	<.00001
H6	TTAGCGA	.0733	.5219	.0573	9.107	<.00001
H7	AAAGCGA	.0475	.3152	.066	4.778	<.00001
H8	AAAGAGA	.096	.2044	.0531	3.851	.00012
Other[b]	...	.0496	.1552	.0725	2.142	.0323
Sex × ln(triglycerides)	...	...	.4801	.0418	11.487	<.00001
Sex × smoking	...	...	−.3583	.0914	−3.918	.00009

NOTE.—*t* statistics and *P* values were calculated from the coefficients and SEs within the best-fit multivariate model by the haplo.glm function of the haplo.stats R package.

[a] Haplotype frequencies were inferred using the EM algorithm within the haplo.stats package.

[b] Haplotypes with frequency <1% were pooled as "Other."

Table 9

Proportion of Variance Explained

The table is available in its entirety in the online edition of *The American Journal of Human Genetics.*

unclear, so it remains possible that 2667 is in strong LD with a polymorphism in a distal regulatory element not within the region scanned for polymorphisms. Similarly, the sole consistent difference between the clade of haplotypes associated with low CRP levels (H1–H4) and the clade of haplotypes associated with higher CRP levels (H5–H8) appears to be the genotype at the triallelic promoter SNP 1440 (fig. 1); the low clade is associated with the C allele and the high clade with A or T alleles. Finally, the rare alleles at five SNPs (tagSNP 790 and unassayed SNPs 1123, 1421, 4741, and 6333) are restricted to the haplotype associated with highest CRP levels (H6), so the observed effect of this haplotype could be attributable to a haplotype of several of these SNPs.

Interestingly, stepwise regression analysis with phenotype and tagSNP genotype as independent variables identified exactly the same set of tagSNPs as being functionally important, because the functionally important haplotypes were uniquely associated with the rare allele of a single tagSNP. A haplotype-based analysis would have proven advantageous only if one of the haplotypes without such a tagSNP (H2, H3, or H7) showed a significant effect on CRP. In this case, haplotype analysis could even be considered a disadvantage because of the effort required to map the observed haplotype effects to specific tagSNPs, whereas direct tagSNP analysis immediately identified the key tagSNPs. Haplotype analysis may prove more powerful in genes with more complex recombination histories or when haplotype-tagging SNPs have not been comprehensively described, but our example demonstrates that haplotype-based analysis is not necessarily superior to direct tagSNP analyses.

To address the possibility that SNPs in the upstream region are functionally important in regulation of the CRP gene, haplotypes of the minimal (−703 to +1, rela-

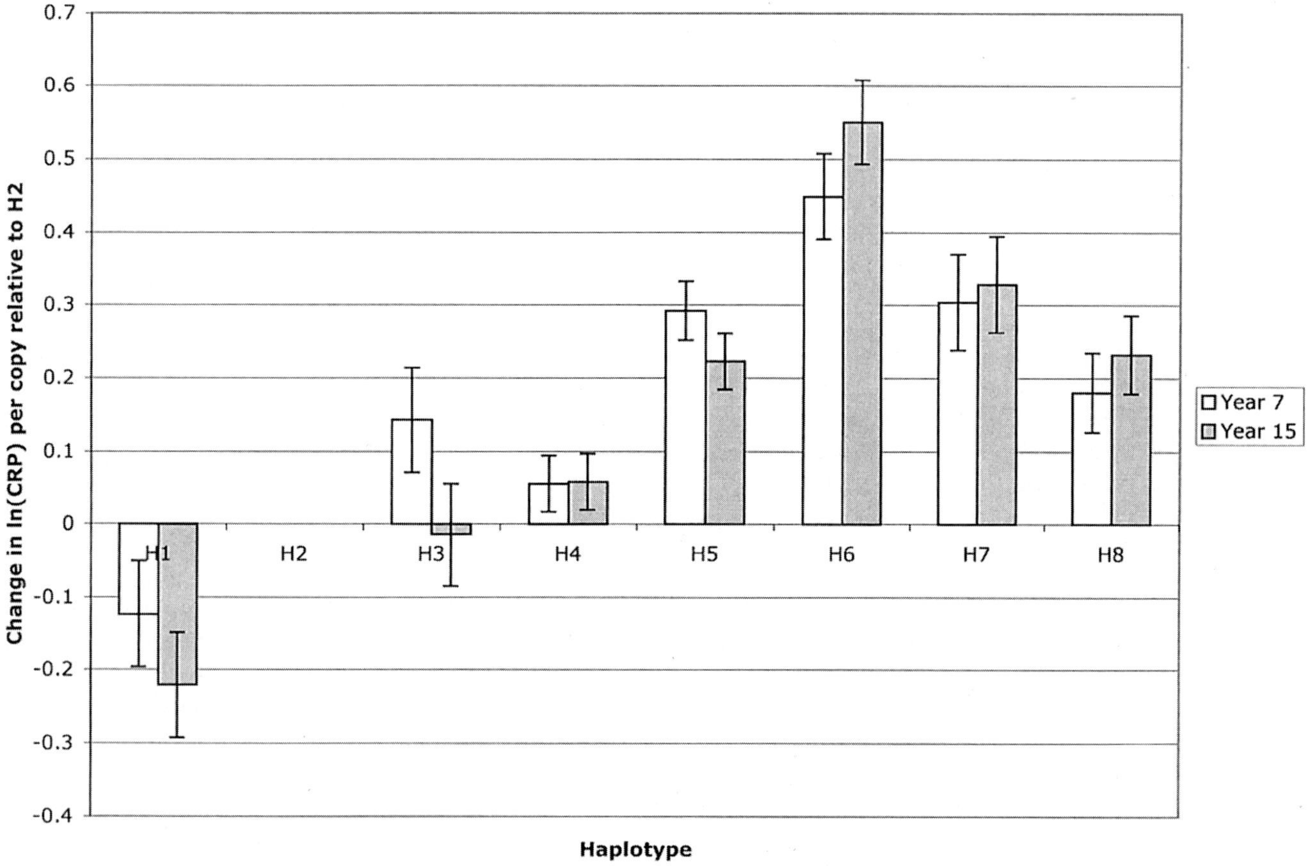

Figure 4 Relative effects of tagSNP haplotypes on ln(CRP). Regression coefficients from haplo.glm analysis were estimated for each haplotype, with phenotypic variables included as covariables. Coefficients reflect difference in mean ln(CRP) per copy relative to H2, the most frequent haplotype. H1 was significantly lower than H2, and H5–H8 were significantly higher (see *P* values in tables 7 and 8).

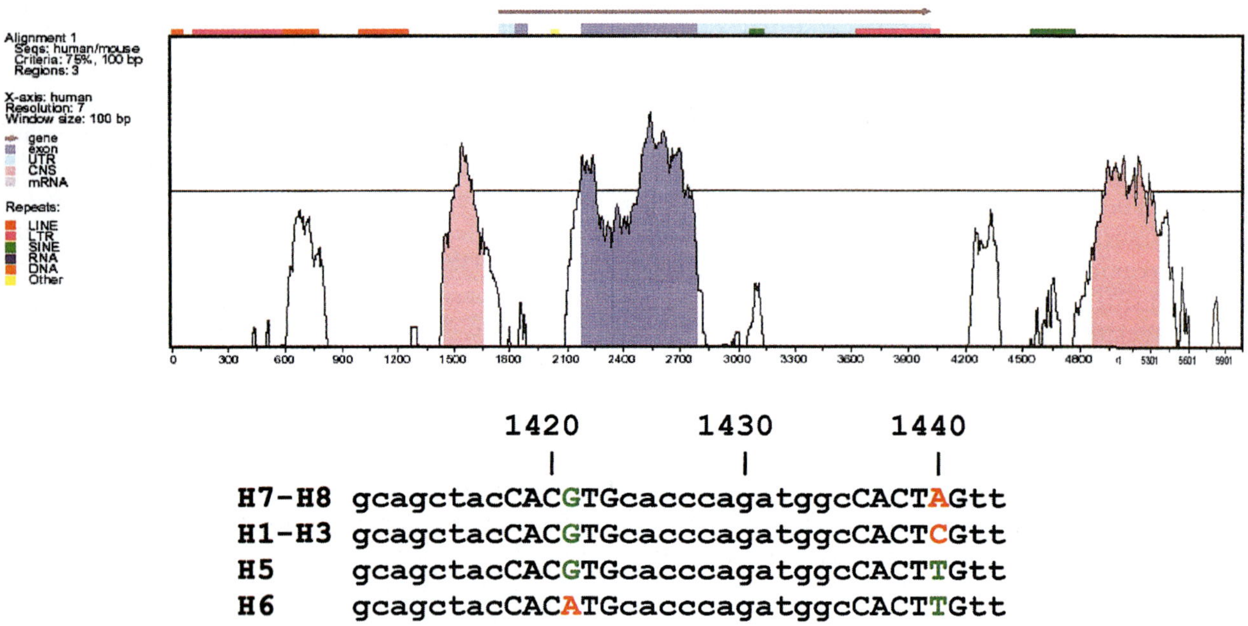

Figure 5 CRP promoter and predicted USF1 sites. *Upper panel,* A vista plot (Mayor et al. 2000) of mouse homology across the human CRP locus. The CRP transcript and repeat elements are annotated across the top of the plot (see key at left), and strong evolutionary conservation of the coding region in the second exon is apparent as the shaded blue peak. A putative promoter region (75% conserved) is visible as a pink peak stretching from 1444 to 1650; the two putatively functionally polymorphic USF1 sites (1421 and 1440) are on the edge of this region. *Lower panel,* Haplotypes of the polymorphisms at 1421 and 1440, with the putative USF1-binding sites indicated in uppercase letters. Alleles predicted to disrupt USF1 binding are shown in red, and alleles predicted to retain USF1 binding are shown in green. H1–H3 represents the ancestral haplotype, as inferred from the chimpanzee alleles at these SNPs. LINE = long interspersed nuclear element; LTR = long terminal repeat; SINE = short interspersed nuclear element.

tive to the TSS) and (−1186 to +1) extended promoter region were cloned into a luciferase-reporter plasmid for promoter-activity analysis. Some of the tagSNP haplotypes across the CRP region did not differ in the promoter region (e.g., H1–H3), so a single promoter construct represented these haplotypes. The relative basal and IL6-induced expression from each of the five unique promoter haplotypes was assessed in cultured human hepatoma cells. Basal expression levels for the native CRP promoter revealed no clear trend, because basal expression was quite weak (fig. 6). However, IL6-induced promoter activity from the H7/H8 constructs (tagged by the 1440 A allele) was marginally higher than all other haplotype constructs ($P < .05$ [uncorrected for multiple tests]). These results are consistent with the higher CRP levels associated with H7/H8 observed in the human population data. IL6-induced activity is a better model for CRP levels during an acute phase response than are basal CRP levels. Nonetheless, over time, we did not observe any apparent influence of H7/H8 on change in CRP levels.

The weak constitutive activity of the CRP promoter appears to be due to a negative regulatory element located within the proximal promoter region (Li et al. 1990). Therefore, we performed additional experiments in which we replaced the 107 bp adjacent to the TSS (including the proximal IL6-responsive elements present within the CRP promoter region) with the SV40 minimal promoter. As expected, the SV40-replacement promoter construct showed dramatically higher activity (fig. 7). For some haplotype comparisons, it was possible to assign the functional difference to a single SNP, because the constructs differed at only one SNP. For example, the significant difference observed between the H5 and H1–H3 constructs (fig. 7) is entirely attributable to the allele at SNP 1440 (C vs. T), which was the only sequence difference between these constructs. Similarly, the significant difference between the H4 and H1–H3 constructs is entirely attributable to SNP 1009. Thus, the marginally significant trend toward higher CRP levels that we observed for H4 in our population sample (fig. 3) may truly represent a functional effect of the H4-associated SNP 1009, as suggested elsewhere (Wolford et al. 2003). The significant difference observed between the H6 and H5 constructs might be attributable to any one of several polymorphic sites, but data from the shorter SV40-replacement constructs suggest that this difference is attributable to either 1123 or 1421 (fig. 7).

Of particular interest are the short replacement promoter constructs that reveal significantly different tran-

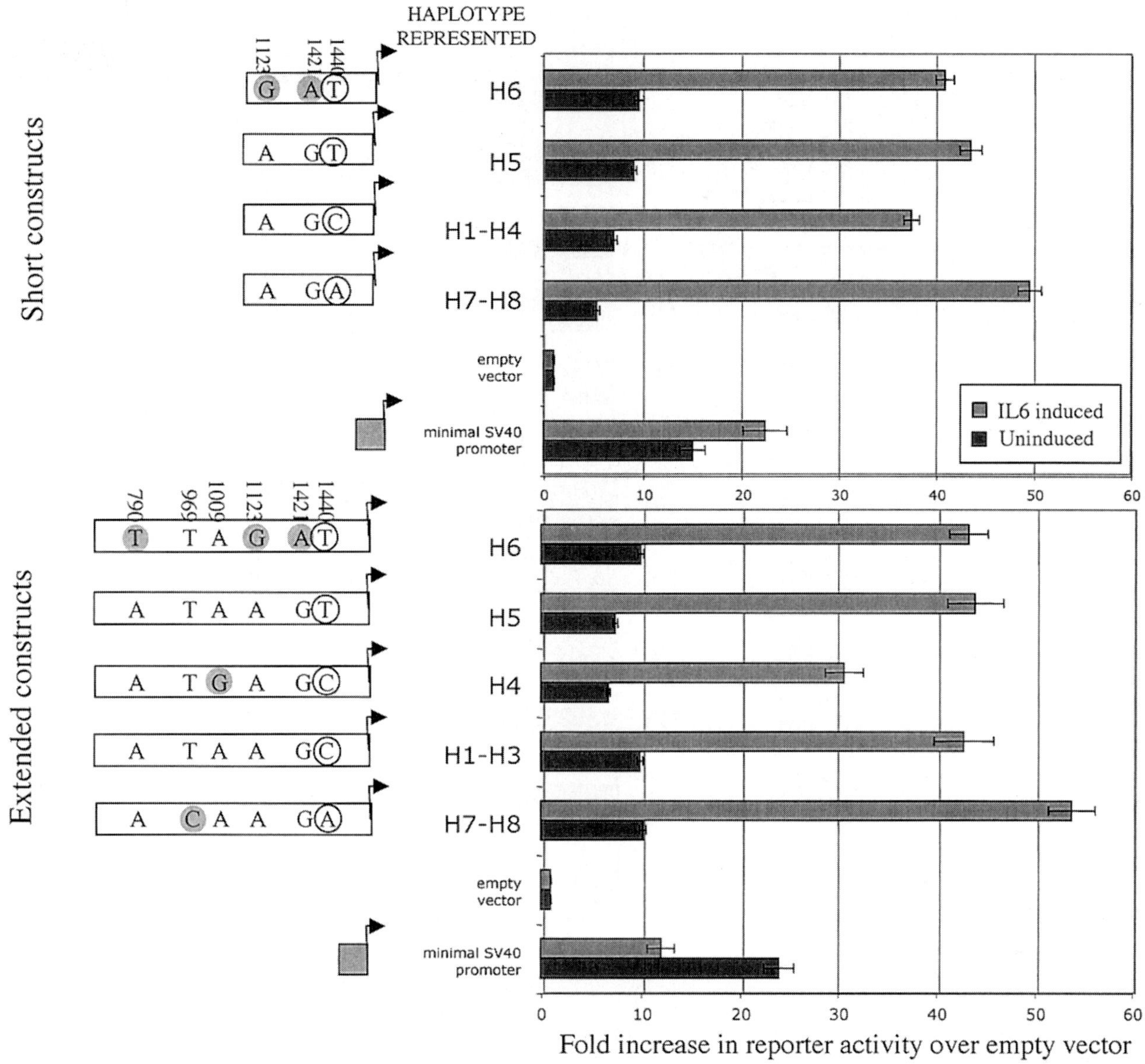

Figure 6 Native promoter construct activity. Short (−703 to +1, relative to TSS) and extended (−1186 to +1) versions of the CRP promoter region were cloned into a luciferase-reporter–gene plasmid. Transient transfection data show the increase in transcription levels for each construct over that of the plasmid-lacking promoter in both uninduced and IL6-induced environments. Shaded circles identify minor alleles at a given SNP. Unshaded circles identify one of the triallelic SNP variants at bp 1440. Error bars reflect SEM in 20 replicate experiments. The short construct group of H1–H4 is divided into two categories of long clones on the basis of the unique 1009 SNP in H4 that is not included in the short-clone constructs. Within the IL6-induced extended constructs, *t* tests show that H4 activity is significantly reduced, whereas H7–H8 activity is significantly increased ($P < .05$), consistent with the induced short constructs in which *t* tests show that H1–H4 activity is significantly reduced, whereas H7–H8 activity is significantly increased ($P < .05$). Uninduced activities showed similar trends, but the signal was relatively weak.

scriptional activity that is based solely on the allele at triallelic SNP position 1440. Previous reports of increased CRP levels associated with SNP 3014, which is restricted to H5 in Europeans (Brull et al. 2003; Russell et al. 2004), might reflect LD with the functional 1440T allele, although the 3014 polymorphism could conceivably be functional in addition to the demonstrated functional changes at 1440, because it is in the 3′ UTR and might affect RNA structure or turnover.

In contrast to the H5 and H6 results, in which the in vitro assays lend strong support to the hypothesis that the observed association between these haplotypes is largely attributable to functional polymorphisms within the promoter region, the in vitro results for H7 and

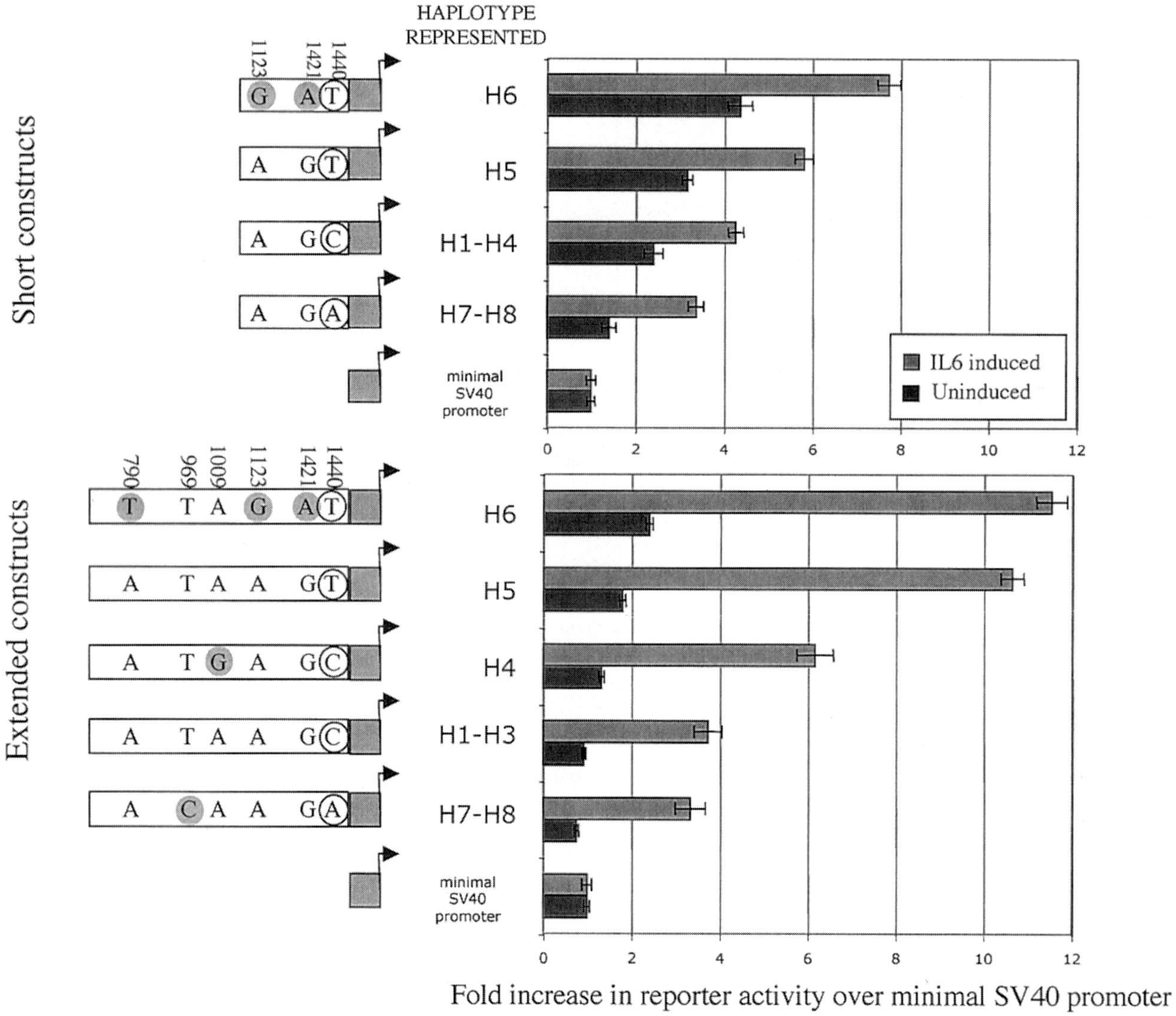

Figure 7 SV40-replacement promoter construct activity. To increase the level of uninduced expression, an IL6-responsive negative regulatory element in the proximal segment of the CRP promoter (−107 to +1) was replaced with the SV40 minimal promoter. Transient transfection data shows the increase in transcription levels for each construct over that of the SV40 minimal promoter alone. Shaded circles identify minor alleles at a given SNP. Unshaded circles identify one of the triallelic SNP variants at bp 1440. Error bars reflect SE measurements. Within each combination of construct length and induction condition, *t* tests show that all differences between haplotypes' behavior are significant ($P < .05$), except for H1–H3 versus H7–H8 in IL6-induced extended constructs.

H8 provide, at best, weak support for the observed associations. This might reflect one of several possibilities: the 1440A allele may indeed be functionally different from the 1440C allele but not under the conditions assayed. That is, in addition to IL6, IL1B and tumor necrosis factor α are known to regulate CRP, and H7 and H8 may behave differentially in response to these or other as-yet-unidentified signals but not in the basal activity assay or under IL6 induction. Alternatively, the association for these haplotypes may be the result of a polymorphism that is in strong LD with the 1440 A allele but falls outside of the region assayed for promoter activity. Curiously, there were only four SNP alleles restricted to H7 and H8: 969C, 1440A, 6192A, and 6469G. The first two were within the analyzed promoter region for the long clones, whereas the latter two SNPs are >2,000 bp past the polyadenylation site of the transcript and do not appear to lie in regions of strong evolutionary conservation that would suggest a distal regulatory element. Thus, at this time, we have not identified a good candidate SNP outside of the promoter region to account for the elevated activities of H7 and H8.

These experimental results support the hypothesis that

the CRP haplotype-phenotype associations observed in the CARDIA cohort are at least partially attributable to functional changes at promoter sites 1421 and 1440, each of which is also predicted to alter binding motifs for the transcription factor USF1. The clustering of USF1 sites in the promoter region (fig. 5) suggests that USF1 may play an important role in regulation of the CRP gene. The increased promoter activities associated with H5–H8 are particularly interesting in light of recent publications highlighting the potential importance of USF1 as a regulator of glucose and lipid-metabolism genes (Pajukanta et al. 2004).

African-descent populations have higher average CRP levels than do European-descent populations (Wener et al. 2000), although there is broad overlap in the range of levels across ethnic groups. Self-reported ethnicity in the United States is also associated with differences in morbidity and mortality from CVD and metabolic diseases, for a variety of medical, social, behavioral, and economic reasons (Watkins 2004). Thus, the genetic portion of the interethnic variance appeared to be attributable to frequency differences at three CRP SNPs (790, 1440, and 2667), in which the allele associated with lower CRP levels (790A, 1440C, and 2667C) was more frequent in EAs than in AAs. These results confirm recent observations that metabolic factors such as obesity account for a large portion of the variation in CRP levels associated with race/ethnicity (Albert et al. 2004; Anand et al. 2004) and suggest that the majority of the remaining variation in CRP levels associated with race/ethnicity in young adults is accounted for by genetic variants within the CRP locus.

It remains unclear whether CRP is a risk marker for inflammatory processes or is causally involved in the pathogenesis of CVD. The strong associations between CRP genotype and plasma-CRP level described here do not resolve this question directly but may prove useful in testing the hypothesis that CRP levels play a causal role in CVD pathogenesis. The functional CRP promoter variants appear to alter CRP levels independent of other CRP correlates, particularly BMI, and do so consistently within individuals over time. Thus, we expect that if CRP is causally involved in disease pathogenesis, then alleles associated with high CRP levels should be associated with greater risk of CVD. Currently, the average age in the CARDIA cohort is 42 years, so the number of incident CVD events is as yet insufficient to test this hypothesis. However, large, multiethnic human studies of older adults that assess atherosclerotic disease progression or occurrence of clinical cardiovascular events (such as myocardial infarction) can be used to address this important question. Such studies are currently in progress. Commonly prescribed cholesterol-lowering drugs, such as statins and PPARα activators, may additionally reduce cardiovascular risk through anti-inflammatory effects, including attenuation of constitutive and induced CRP gene expression (Kleemann et al. 2004; Ridker et al. 2005). Therefore, further characterization of the influence and interaction of common *cis*-acting nucleotide substitutions on transcriptional regulation of the CRP gene could have broad implications for the treatment and prevention of cardiovascular, metabolic, and related inflammatory disorders.

Note added in proof.—Functional associations between the 1440 and 1421 promoter SNPs and basal CRP levels have been confirmed in an independent study by Szalai et al. (in press).

Acknowledgments

This work was supported by Inflammatory Genomics and Atherosclerosis Prevention ancillary CARDIA grant HL71017 (to D.S.), by CARDIA contracts N01-HC-95095, N01-HC-48047, N01-HC-48048, N01-HC-48049, N01-HC-48050, N01-HC-45134, and N01-HC-05187 from NHLBI, and by NHLBI Program for Genomic Applications grants HL66682 and HL66642 (to D.N. and M.R.).

Web Resources

Accession numbers and URLs for data presented herein are as follows:

dbSNP Home Page, http://www.ncbi.nlm.nih.gov/SNP/index.html (for tagSNPs 790 [*rs3093058*], 1440 [*rs3091244*], 1919 [*rs1417938*], 2667 [*rs1800947*], 3006 [*rs3093066*], 3872 [*rs1205*], and 5237 [*rs2808630*])

GenBank, http://www.ncbi.nlm.nih.gov/Genbank/ (for the CRP gene [accession number AF449713])

SeattleSNPs Program for Genomic Applications, http://pga.gs.washington.edu/protocols/dnapanel_protocol.html

TFSEARCH, http://www.cbrc.jp/research/db/TFSEARCH.html

References

Abernathy TJ, Avery OT (1941) The occurrence during acute infections of a protein not normally present in the blood. I. Distribution of the reactive protein in patient's sera and the effect of calcium on the flocculation reaction with C-polysaccharide of pneumococcus. J Exp Med 73:173–182

Albert MA, Glynn RJ, Buring J, Ridker PM (2004) C-reactive protein levels among women of various ethnic groups living in the United States (from the Women's Health Study). Am J Cardiol 93:1238–1242

Anand SS, Razak F, Yi Q, Davis B, Jacobs R, Vuksan V, Lonn E, Teo K, McQueen M, Yusuf S (2004) C-reactive protein as a screening test for cardiovascular risk in a multiethnic population. Arterioscler Thromb Vasc Biol 24:1509–1515

Brull DJ, Serrano N, Zito F, Jones L, Montgomery HE, Rumley A, Sharma P, Lowe GD, World MJ, Humphries SE, Hingorani AD (2003) Human CRP gene polymorphism influences CRP levels: implications for the prediction and pathogenesis of coronary heart disease. Arterioscler Thromb Vasc Biol 23:2063–2069

Carlson CS, Eberle MA, Rieder MJ, Yi Q, Kruglyak L, Nickerson DA (2004) Selecting a maximally informative set of single-nucleotide polymorphisms for association analyses using linkage disequilibrium. Am J Hum Genet 74:106–120
Danesh J, Wheeler JG, Hirschfield GM, Eda S, Eiriksdottir G, Rumley A, Lowe GD, Pepys MB, Gudnason V (2004) C-reactive protein and other circulating markers of inflammation in the prediction of coronary heart disease. N Engl J Med 350:1387–1397
Danesh J, Whincup P, Walker M, Lennon L, Thomson A, Appleby P, Gallimore JR, Pepys MB (2000) Low grade inflammation and coronary heart disease: prospective study and updated meta-analyses. BMJ 321:199–204
Friedman GD, Cutter GR, Donahue RP, Hughes GH, Hulley SB, Jacobs DR Jr, Liu K, Savage PJ (1988) CARDIA: study design, recruitment, and some characteristics of the examined subjects. J Clin Epidemiol 41:1105–1116
Hackam DG, Anand SS (2003) Emerging risk factors for atherosclerotic vascular disease: a critical review of the evidence. JAMA 290:932–940
Hastie T, Tibshirani R, Friedman J (2001) The elements of statistical learning: data mining, inference and prediction. Springer-Verlag, New York
Heinemeyer T, Wingender E, Reuter I, Hermjakob H, Kel AE, Kel OV, Ignatieva EV, Ananko EA, Podkolodnaya OA, Kolpakov FA, Podkolodny NL, Kolchanov NA (1998) Databases on transcriptional regulation: TRANSFAC, TRRD and COMPEL. Nucleic Acids Res 26:362–367
Hughes GH, Cutter G, Donahue R, Friedman GD, Hulley S, Hunkeler E, Jacobs DR Jr, Liu K, Orden S, Pirie P, Tucker B, Wagenknecht L (1987) Recruitment in the Coronary Artery Disease Risk Development in Young Adults (CARDIA) Study. Control Clin Trials 8:68S–73S
Kleemann R, Verschuren L, de Rooij BJ, Lindeman J, de Maat MM, Szalai AJ, Princen HM, Kooistra T (2004) Evidence for anti-inflammatory activity of statins and PPARα activators in human C-reactive protein transgenic mice in vivo and in cultured human hepatocytes in vitro. Blood 103:4188–4194
Kovacs A, Green F, Hansson LO, Lundman P, Samnegard A, Boquist S, Ericsson CG, Watkins H, Hamsten A, Tornvall P (2005) A novel common single nucleotide polymorphism in the promoter region of the C-reactive protein gene associated with the plasma concentration of C-reactive protein. Atherosclerosis 178:193–198
Lake SL, Lyon H, Tantisira K, Silverman EK, Weiss ST, Laird NM, Schaid DJ (2003) Estimation and tests of haplotype-environment interaction when linkage phase is ambiguous. Hum Hered 55:56–65
Li SP, Liu TY, Goldman ND (1990) *cis*-acting elements responsible for interleukin-6 inducible C-reactive protein gene expression. J Biol Chem 265:4136–4142
MacGregor AJ, Gallimore JR, Spector TD, Pepys MB (2004) Genetic effects on baseline values of C-reactive protein and serum amyloid A protein: a comparison of monozygotic and dizygotic twins. Clin Chem 50:130–134
Mayor C, Brudno M, Schwartz JR, Poliakov A, Rubin EM, Frazer KA, Pachter LS, Dubchak I (2000) VISTA: visualizing global DNA sequence alignments of arbitrary length. Bioinformatics 16:1046–1047
Pajukanta P, Lilja HE, Sinsheimer JS, Cantor RM, Lusis AJ, Gentile M, Duan XJ, Soro-Paavonen A, Naukkarinen J, Saarela J, Laakso M, Ehnholm C, Taskinen MR, Peltonen L (2004) Familial combined hyperlipidemia is associated with upstream transcription factor 1 (USF1). Nat Genet 36:371–376
Pankow JS, Folsom AR, Cushman M, Borecki IB, Hopkins PN, Eckfeldt JH, Tracy RP (2001) Familial and genetic determinants of systemic markers of inflammation: the NHLBI family heart study. Atherosclerosis 154:681–689
Pearson TA, Mensah GA, Alexander RW, Anderson JL, Cannon RO 3rd, Criqui M, Fadl YY, Fortmann SP, Hong Y, Myers GL, Rifai N, Smith SC Jr, Taubert K, Tracy RP, Vinicor F (2003) Markers of inflammation and cardiovascular disease: application to clinical and public health practice: a statement for healthcare professionals from the Centers for Disease Control and Prevention and the American Heart Association. Circulation 107:499–511
Retterstol L, Eikvar L, Berg K (2003) A twin study of C-reactive protein compared to other risk factors for coronary heart disease. Atherosclerosis 169:279–282
Ridker PM, Cannon CP, Morrow D, Rifai N, Rose LM, McCabe CH, Pfeffer MA, Braunwald E (2005) C-reactive protein levels and outcomes after statin therapy. N Engl J Med 352: 20–28
Ridker PM, Cushman M, Stampfer MJ, Tracy RP, Hennekens CH (1997) Inflammation, aspirin, and the risk of cardiovascular disease in apparently healthy men. N Engl J Med 336: 973–979
Ridker PM, Hennekens CH, Buring JE, Rifai N (2000) C-reactive protein and other markers of inflammation in the prediction of cardiovascular disease in women. N Engl J Med 342:836–843
Russell AI, Cunninghame Graham DS, Shepherd C, Roberton CA, Whittaker J, Meeks J, Powell RJ, Isenberg DA, Walport MJ, Vyse TJ (2004) Polymorphism at the C-reactive protein locus influences gene expression and predisposes to systemic lupus erythematosus. Hum Mol Genet 13:137–147
Shine B, de Beer FC, Pepys MB (1981) Solid phase radioimmunoassays for human C-reactive protein. Clin Chim Acta 117: 13–23
Stephens M, Donnelly P (2003) A comparison of Bayesian methods for haplotype reconstruction from population genotype data. Am J Hum Genet 73:1162–1169
Stephens M, Smith NJ, Donnelly P (2001) A new statistical method for haplotype reconstruction from population data. Am J Hum Genet 68:978–989
Suk HJ, Ridker PM, Cook NR, Zee RY (2005) Relation of polymorphism within the C-reactive protein gene and plasma CRP levels. Atherosclerosis 178:139–145
Szalai AJ, McCrory MA, Cooper GS, Wu J, Kimberly RP (2002) Association between baseline levels of C-reactive protein (CRP) and a dinucleotide repeat polymorphism in the intron of the CRP gene. Genes Immun 3:14–19
Szalai AJ, Wu J, Lange EM, McCrory MA, Langefeld CD, Williams A, Zakharkin SO, George V, Allison DB, Cooper GS, Xie F, Fan Z, Edberg JC, Kimberly RP. Single-nucleotide polymorphisms in the C-reactive protein (CRP) gene promoter that affect transcription factor binding, alter transcriptional activity, and associate with differences in baseline serum CRP level. J Mol Med (in press)
Tillet W, Francis T (1930) Serologic reactions in pneumonia

with a non-protein somatic fraction of pneumococcus. J Exp Med 52:561–571
Watkins LO (2004) Perspectives on coronary heart disease in African Americans. Rev Cardiovasc Med (Suppl 3) 5:S3–S13
Wener MH, Daum PR, McQuillan GM (2000) The influence of age, sex, and race on the upper reference limit of serum C-reactive protein concentration. J Rheumatol 27:2351–2359
Wolford JK, Gruber JD, Ossowski VM, Vozarova B, Antonio Tataranni P, Bogardus C, Hanson RL (2003) A C-reactive protein promoter polymorphism is associated with type 2 diabetes mellitus in Pima Indians. Mol Genet Metab 78:136–144
Zee RY, Ridker PM (2002) Polymorphism in the human C-reactive protein (CRP) gene, plasma concentrations of CRP, and the risk of future arterial thrombosis. Atherosclerosis 162:217–219

Am. J. Hum. Genet. 77:78–88, 2005

Segmental Duplications and Copy-Number Variation in the Human Genome

Andrew J. Sharp,[1,*] Devin P. Locke,[1,*] Sean D. McGrath,[1] Ze Cheng,[1] Jeffrey A. Bailey,[2] Rhea U. Vallente,[4] Lisa M. Pertz,[3] Royden A. Clark,[3] Stuart Schwartz,[3] Rick Segraves,[5] Vanessa V. Oseroff,[5] Donna G. Albertson,[5] Daniel Pinkel,[5] and Evan E. Eichler[1]

[1]Department of Genome Sciences, University of Washington School of Medicine, Seattle; Departments of [2]Pathology and [3]Genetics, Case Western Reserve University, Cleveland; [4]Washington State University School of Molecular Biosciences, Pullman; and [5]Comprehensive Cancer Center, University of California–San Francisco (UCSF), San Francisco

The human genome contains numerous blocks of highly homologous duplicated sequence. This higher-order architecture provides a substrate for recombination and recurrent chromosomal rearrangement associated with genomic disease. However, an assessment of the role of segmental duplications in normal variation has not yet been made. On the basis of the duplication architecture of the human genome, we defined a set of 130 potential rearrangement hotspots and constructed a targeted bacterial artificial chromosome (BAC) microarray (with 2,194 BACs) to assess copy-number variation in these regions by array comparative genomic hybridization. Using our segmental duplication BAC microarray, we screened a panel of 47 normal individuals, who represented populations from four continents, and we identified 119 regions of copy-number polymorphism (CNP), 73 of which were previously unreported. We observed an equal frequency of duplications and deletions, as well as a 4-fold enrichment of CNPs within hotspot regions, compared with control BACs ($P < .000001$), which suggests that segmental duplications are a major catalyst of large-scale variation in the human genome. Importantly, segmental duplications themselves were also significantly enriched >4-fold within regions of CNP. Almost without exception, CNPs were not confined to a single population, suggesting that these either are recurrent events, having occurred independently in multiple founders, or were present in early human populations. Our study demonstrates that segmental duplications define hotspots of chromosomal rearrangement, likely acting as mediators of normal variation as well as genomic disease, and it suggests that the consideration of genomic architecture can significantly improve the ascertainment of large-scale rearrangements. Our specialized segmental duplication BAC microarray and associated database of structural polymorphisms will provide an important resource for the future characterization of human genomic disorders.

Introduction

Segmental duplications (also termed "low-copy repeats") are blocks of DNA that range from 1 to 400 kb in length, occur at more than one site within the genome, and typically share a high level of (>90%) sequence identity (reviewed by Eichler [2001]). Both in situ hybridization and *in silico* analyses have shown that ~5% of the human genome is composed of duplicated sequence (Cheung et al. 2001; Bailey et al. 2002; Cheung et al. 2003; She et al. 2004*a*), and many studies have noted a significant association between the location of segmental duplications and regions of chromosomal instability or evolutionary rearrangement (Ji et al. 2000; Samonte and Eichler 2002; Armengol et al. 2003; Locke et al. 2003*a*, 2003*b*; Bailey et al. 2004). Indeed, segmental duplications have been implicated as the probable mediators of >25 recurrent genomic disorders (reviewed by Stankiewicz and Lupski [2002]). Molecular studies have shown that the presence of large, highly homologous flanking repeats predisposes these regions to recurrent rearrangement by nonallelic homologous recombination, resulting in deletion, duplication, or inversion of the intervening sequence (Chance et al. 1994; Shaw et al. 2002).

A growing body of evidence now suggests that the duplication architecture of the genome may also mediate normal variation. The existence of large genomic polymorphisms, originally termed "heteromorphisms" or "euchromatic variants," has been recognized since the advent of high-resolution cytogenetic banding techniques (summarized at the Chromosome Anomaly Register Web site). With the use of more-targeted molecular analyses, a number of submicroscopic polymorphic re-

Received February 21, 2005; accepted for publication May 4, 2005; electronically published May 25, 2005.

Address for correspondence and reprints: Dr. Evan Eichler, Department of Genome Sciences, University of Washington, 1705 NE Pacific Street, Seattle, WA 98195. E-mail: eee@gs.washington.edu

* These two authors contributed equally to this work.

0002-9297/2005/7701-0008$15.00

arrangements between homologous blocks of sequence have been identified in the normal population (Siniscalco et al. 2000; Sprenger et al. 2000; Giglio et al. 2001; Osborne et al. 2001; Gimelli et al. 2003; Skaletsky et al. 2003). Recently, the use of methods such as array comparative genomic hybridization (array CGH) and representational oligonucleotide microarray analysis (ROMA) have revealed the presence of numerous copy-number polymorphisms (CNPs) in the human genome and have suggested an enrichment of segmental duplications associated with these variants (Iafrate et al. 2004; Sebat et al. 2004). However, these studies used arrays with either limited genomic coverage or limited resolution with respect to regions of segmental duplication, and even current tiling-path arrays with >30,000 BAC clones (Ishkanian et al. 2004) do not achieve complete coverage of regions rich in segmental duplications (Z.C. and E.E.E., unpublished data).

Because regions flanked by segmental duplications are susceptible to rearrangement by nonallelic homologous recombination, we hypothesized that these regions represent potential hotspots of genomic instability that are prone to copy-number variation. It has been shown that several factors—including the length, sequence identity, and orientation of and the distance between duplications—influence the probability of meiotic misalignment (Stankiewicz and Lupski 2002). Most of the blocks of duplicated sequence that have been implicated in known genomic disorders are large (10–400 kb in size) and have >96% sequence identity. This level of sequence sharing between intrachromosomal sites provides ample substrate for aberrant recombination, on the basis of the estimated minimal efficient-processing segment length (Waldman and Liskay 1988). In general, the larger and more homologous the block of duplicated sequence is, the more frequently sporadic segmental aneusomy events occur. For example, the most frequently occurring microdeletion syndrome (velocardiofacial and DiGeorge syndromes; frequency 1/3,000) occurs between blocks of duplications that are in excess of 300 kb in length and that share 99.7% sequence identity (Edelmann et al. 1999; Shaikh et al. 2000).

Thus, a review of the recurrent genomic disorders characterized to date suggests a strategy for the identification of novel regions of genomic instability. With a focus on regions flanked by intrachromosomal duplications that are >10 kb in length, share >95% sequence identity, and span from 50 kb to 10 Mb of intervening sequence (Stankiewicz and Lupski 2002), novel sites of genomic variation may be uncovered. On the basis of these criteria, *in silico* analysis of the human genome defines a map of potential rearrangement hotspots (Bailey et al. 2002). In total, 130 regions—covering 274 Mb, or ~10% of the entire genome—are flanked by intrachromosomal duplications whose characteristics suggest a potential predisposition to genomic instability. Whereas 25 of these regions are associated with known genomic disorders, the remainder represent novel sites whose genomic architecture is susceptible to either polymorphic or disease-causing rearrangement. We have constructed a custom BAC array, termed the "segmental duplication microarray" (SD microarray), specifically targeted to these rearrangement hotspots, and we used it to investigate copy-number variation in a panel of ethnically diverse normal individuals. We report the discovery of numerous novel CNPs distributed throughout the human population and demonstrate an enrichment of copy-number variation in regions of the genome flanked by segmental duplications.

Material and Methods

A total of 130 nonredundant regions of potential genomic instability (termed "rearrangement hotspots") were defined by the presence of intrachromosomal duplications >10 kb in length, with >95% similarity and flanking 50 kb to 10 Mb of intervening sequence in the July 2003 build of the human genome (Bailey et al. 2002; She et al. 2004*b*). A total of 1,986 nonredundant BACs (mean insert size 164 kb) were ultimately selected from the RPCI-11, CTC, and CTD libraries to encompass each rearrangement hotspot and were processed for construction of a microarray in accordance with protocols established elsewhere (Snijders et al. 2004) (table A1 in appendix A [online only]). When possible, three classes of BAC were selected: (1) BACs that were contained entirely within each rearrangement hotspot, (2) BACs overlapping the segmental duplications, and (3) flanking BACs in the peripheral unique sequence (as a local control) (fig. 1). During the design of this microarray, we confirmed the identity and location of all BACs by end-sequencing and by alignment of the end sequences against the human genome reference (builds 33 and 34). During our first-pass analysis, ~93% of all selected clones were confirmed. A second round of surrogate BAC selection resulted in a total of 1,986 identity-confirmed BACs. Of these, 1,206 overlapped a rearrangement hotspot, and 760 were contained within segmental duplications. As a control, an additional 192 randomly selected single-copy clones that had been extensively tested elsewhere (Snijders et al. 2001) were incorporated into the array. In total, our BAC array consisted of 2,194 confirmed BACs. All BAC DNA was amplified by ligation-mediated PCR (Snijders et al. 2004), and each BAC was printed in triplicate on GAPS II glass slides (Corning), with a spot diameter of 80 μm and 130-μm spacing.

DNA was extracted from 47 lymphoblastoid cell lines (NIGMS Cell Repository), representing seven ethnici-

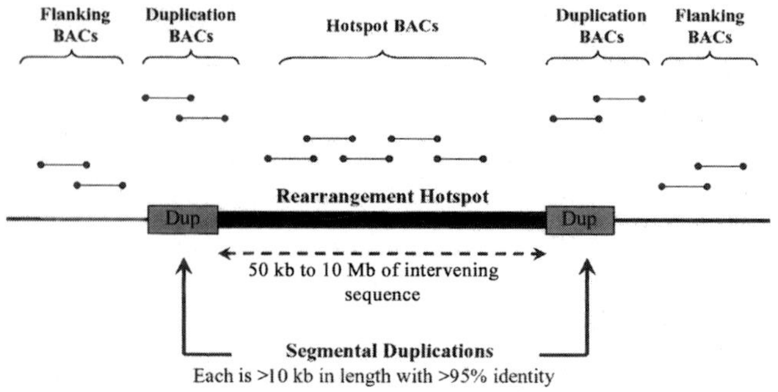

Figure 1 Targeted design strategy for choosing BACs for array CGH on the basis of genomic architecture. We hypothesized that the presence of large, highly homologous segmental duplications predisposes certain regions of the genome to microdeletion and/or microduplication by nonallelic homologous recombination (Bailey et al. 2002). Termed "rearrangement hotspots," these are defined by the presence of flanking intrachromosomal duplications >10 kb in length with >95% similarity and separated by 50 kb to 10 Mb of intervening sequence. For each region, we selected BACs that were contained entirely within each rearrangement hotspot, BACs that overlapped the segmental duplications, and BACs in the peripheral unique sequence for microarray manufacture. The SD microarray comprised a total of 2,194 BACs.

ties from Asia, Europe, sub-Saharan Africa, and South America. This collection comprised 8 Chinese, 4 Japanese, 10 Czech, 2 Druze, 7 Biaka, 9 Mbuti, and 7 American Indian samples (table A1 in appendix A [online only]). All hybridizations were performed in duplicate—once with test and reference DNAs labeled with Cy3 and Cy5, respectively, and a second time with the fluorochrome dyes reversed. All hybridizations used reference DNA isolated from blood lymphocytes from a single anonymous male donor of unknown ethnicity. A single reference genome was analyzed, as opposed to a pool of normal individuals, to increase signal-to-noise ratios over sites of polymorphic variation. In cases in which the reference sample represented the rare allele (i.e., the majority of individuals showed a change in the fluorescence intensity ratio), we classified the CNPs as minor-allele variants.

Test and reference DNAs were labeled with Cy3 or Cy5 (Amersham Biosciences) by random prime labeling (Bioprime DNA Labeling System [Invitrogen]) and were mixed and purified using Sephadex G-50 Spin Columns (Roche). Labeled DNA was coprecipitated with 75 μg of COT DNA (Roche), was resuspended in 50 μl of hybridization mix (50% formamide, 10% dextran sulfate, 2 × saline sodium citrate [SSC], and 4% SDS), was denatured, and was prehybridized at 37°C for 1 h to allow blocking of repetitive sequences. Array hybridizations were performed in a humid chamber at 37°C for 40 h in open rubber-cement wells on a gently rocking platform, to allow circulation of hybridization solution over the array (Snijders et al. 2004). Hybridization solution was removed under a stream of buffer (0.1 M Na_2HPO_4 and 0.1% Nonidet P-40; pH 8.0), and slides were washed for 15 min at 45°C in 50% formamide and 2 × SSC, were rinsed in buffer, and were mounted (in 90% glycerol, 10% PBS, and 1 μM 4′,6-diamidino-2-phenylindole) under a glass cover slip before being scanned with a custom-built CCD system.

Array image analysis and normalization were performed using UCSF Spot and Sproc software (Jain et al. 2002). BACs for which only one of the triplicates printed on the array yielded data, or for which the standard deviation of $\log_2$ ratio for the triplicates was >0.2, were removed from final analysis. Furthermore, we discarded BACs that failed to yield data in <20% of cases. For each hybridization experiment, we established a threshold $\log_2$ ratio of 2 SDs from the mean of all autosomal clones, and BACs that exceeded this threshold in both independent dye-swap experiments were classified as variant.

For comparison, we also hybridized a subset of our samples to a genomewide BAC microarray containing clones selected to minimize segmental-duplication content, spaced at an average resolution of ~1.4 Mb throughout the genome (Snijders et al. 2001). For these experiments, we used an identical protocol, except for the use of a different reference DNA (from GM15724, a male Czech). Verification of array CGH results by FISH was performed on the lymphoblastoid cell lines derived from the individuals used for array profiling, in accordance with standard procedures, by use of isolated BAC DNA as a probe source (Nucleobond [BD Biosciences]) (Pinkel et al. 1986).

Results

Initial Array Validation

To assess the performance of the SD microarray and to establish appropriate thresholds for the detection of copy-number changes, we performed a series of test hybridizations. First, we analyzed three previously characterized individuals possessing one, four, or six copies of the 15q11-q13 region (Locke et al. 2004). There was a strong correlation ($r^2 = 0.945$) between copy number and relative fluorescence ratios yielded by BACs within the variant region, which demonstrates the ability of our array to detect bona fide rearrangements and to reliably distinguish deletions, duplications, and triplications. Second, to determine the false-positive rate, we performed four self-versus-self hybridizations. Results indicated that the use of the threshold of $\log_2$ hybridization ratios deviating >2 SDs from the mean in both replicates of an experiment yields a false-positive rate of ~3 per 4,000 clones, or ~0.08% (table A1 in appendix A [online only]). As has been reported elsewhere (Vissers et al. 2003), we found that, by performing all hybridizations in duplicate and incorporating a dye reversal, we significantly reduced the false-positive rate.

Assessment of CNPs in the Human Population

Using the SD microarray, we analyzed a diverse panel of 47 unrelated humans representing four continental groups. On the basis of our conservative criteria, we identified 160 variant BACs among these 47 individuals. We identified 27 regions where neighboring or overlapping clones yielded concordant results, which suggested that some copy-number variations extended over regions of several hundred kilobases. Under the assumption that concordantly variant neighboring clones separated by <250 kb represent the same copy-number variation, the 160 variant clones correspond to 119 nonredundant regions. Whereas 66 of these 119 regions were polymorphic in multiple individuals, 53 were observed in only a single individual (fig. 2 and table A2 in appendix A [online only]). Conversely, 38 regions were variant in >10% of the individuals studied (fig. 2). The proportions of gains and losses were approximately equal (table 1).

Validation of CNPs Detected by Array CGH

Two analyses were performed to assess the validity of our hybridization results. First, we compared sites of copy-number variation with those identified recently in two other studies (Iafrate et al. 2004; Sebat et al. 2004). Of the sites we detected, 39% (46 of 119) had been reported elsewhere (within a 250-kb overlap), which thus validates the ability of our array to detect known copy-number alterations and which indicates that 73 of the 119 genomic regions we identified in the present study are novel. A comparison of our set of CNPs with those detected in a similar study that used ROMA (Sebat et al. 2004) revealed excellent concordance (table 1). Of the 31 CNPs detected by ROMA that were represented on the SD microarray, we detected 22 (71%). Seven of the nine variations that we did not detect were observed by Sebat et al. (2004) in only one individual, and therefore those variations probably represent rare polymorphisms that were not represented in our sample population. We also identified many other previously reported copy-number changes—for example, the β-defensin gene cluster at 8p23.1 (Hollox et al. 2003), the *IGHG1* gene cluster at 14q32.33 (Sasso et al. 1995), and the *IGVH/SLC6A8/CDM* pseudogene cluster at 16p11.2 (Barber et al. 1999) (fig. 3*A*). Figure 4 shows an example of the pattern of copy-number variation detected on chromosome 15 by use of the SD microarray. A genomewide map showing all 119 CNPs detected is shown in figure 5.

Second, we selected 11 BACs that showed putative duplication or deletion by array CGH for use as FISH probes (fig. 3 and table A2 in appendix A [online only]). Although multiple signals were evident in some cases, as a result of the presence of segmental duplications in the BAC probe, the results in metaphase and/or interphase nuclei for 7 of the 11 BACs were consistent with copy-number changes at these loci. For two loci, copy number could not be reliably determined because of the high segmental-duplication content; thus, results were ambiguous. For the remaining two loci, FISH results did not support the presence of CNPs. However, at one of these loci (*CTD-3185D7*), results by array CGH showed copy-number variation in seven of the individuals we tested, and, in addition, this same locus was independently reported in another study (Iafrate et al. 2004). Thus, it seems unlikely that this represents a false-positive result, and this structural variation simply may not be easily resolved by FISH. For the remaining BAC (RP11-325E8), only 1 of the 47 individuals analyzed by array CGH showed a $\log_2$ ratio >2 SDs from the mean for this locus, which suggests that this is a potential false-positive result.

Analysis of variation with respect to ethnicity revealed very little population stratification. Almost all of the CNPs detected were present in multiple ethnic groups, with no apparent clustering with respect to geographic origin. Among the 50 regions that were polymorphic in more than two individuals, only two CNPs (in regions 12 and 91) were confined to a single ethnicity, being present specifically in sub-Saharan Africans (table A2 in appendix A [online only]). It is surprising, however, that the African population did not show significantly more variation than any other continental group (table 1 and fig. 2).

Analysis of CNPs

Analysis of the sequence properties of structurally variant regions revealed some important trends. We observed a significant enrichment of copy-number variation within rearrangement hotspots (defined by the presence of flanking intrachromosomal duplications >10 kb in length, with >95% similarity and separated by 50 kb to 10 Mb of intervening sequence [fig. 1]), when those regions were compared with the control loci (Bailey et al. 2002). Of the 718 BACs that were contained within rearrangement-hotspot regions, 113 (15.7%) were variant, compared with 46 (4.1%) of the 1,110 BACs that were located outside of hotspot regions (3.8-fold enrichment; $\chi^2 = 73.8$; $P < .000001$). There was also an enrichment of rearrangement-hotspot sequence within the more frequent CNPs. The 96 BACs that were variant in multiple individuals contained an average of 76.4% hotspot sequence, compared with an average of 50.8% hotspot sequence in the 64 BACs that were variant in

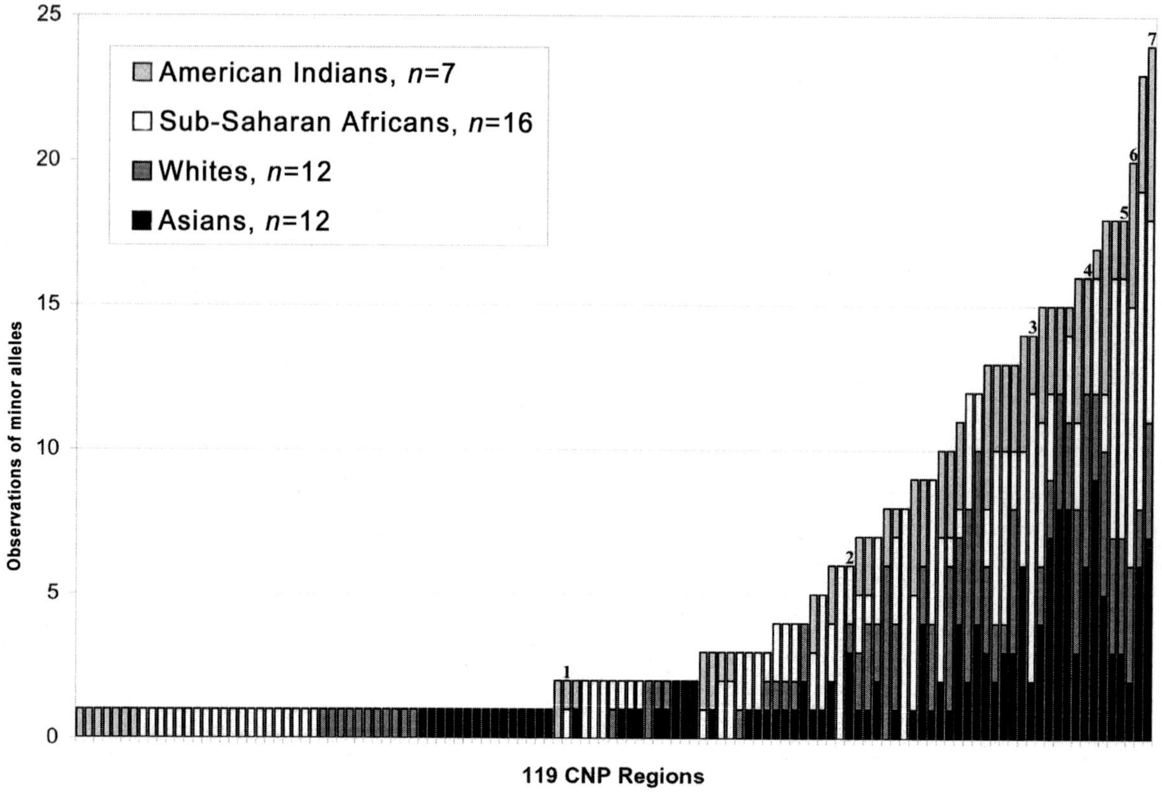

Figure 2 Observations of minor alleles in CNP regions. The 47 samples were categorized as American Indian, sub-Saharan African (Biaka and Mbuti), white (Czech and Druze), and Asian (Chinese and Japanese), and the 119 CNPs identified were plotted (see table A2 in appendix A [online only]). In cases in which the reference sample represented the rare allele (i.e., the majority of individuals showed a change in fluorescence intensity ratio), we classified the CNPs as minor-allele variants. Some previously identified CNPs are indicated by numerals above the bars: 1 = *CHRNA7/CHRFAM7A* at 15q13.3 (Riley et al. 2002); 2 = *IGVH/SLC6A8/CDM* pseudogene cluster at 16p11.2 (Barber et al. 1999); 3 = *CCL3-L1/CCL4-L1* at 17q12 (Townson et al. 2002); 4 = *IGHG1* gene cluster at 14q32.33 (Sasso et al. 1995); 5 = *IGL* gene cluster at 22q11.22 (van der Burg et al. 2002); 6 = *NF1/IGVH/GABRA5* pseudogene amplification at 15q11.2-q13 (Fantes et al. 2002); and 7 = β-defensin gene cluster at 8p23.1 (Hollox et al. 2003).

only a single individual. In total, CNPs were identified in 51 (39%) of 130 rearrangement hotspots.

It is interesting that both intrachromosomal and interchromosomal segmental duplications showed an association with copy-number variation. Variant BACs contained an average of 52.1% intrachromosomal duplication, compared with 12.0% in nonvariant BACs (4.3-fold enrichment). Similarly, interchromosomal duplications comprised 28.8% of variant BACs, compared with 5.9% of nonvariant BACs (4.9-fold enrichment). However, despite the accumulation of segmental duplications within pericentromeric and subtelomeric regions (Bailey et al. 2002), we observed no significant bias for copy-number variations within these regions of the genome.

Regions showing evidence of copy-number variation were not particularly gene poor. The 160 BACs exhibiting copy-number variation completely encompass a total of 108 genes and partially overlap a further 33 coding regions (table A3 in appendix A [online only]). This includes numerous gene families, consistent with the observed enrichment of segmental duplications with CNPs.

Hybridizations to a Genomewide Array

A subset of the samples were also hybridized to a second BAC microarray containing clones spaced at an average resolution of ~1.4 Mb throughout the genome (Snijders et al. 2001). With the use of this nontargeted array, only 8 (0.3%) of 2,460 BACs were variant in the eight individuals analyzed (table A4 in appendix A [online only]), compared with 82 (3.7%) of 2,194 BACs that were analyzed using the SD microarray, which represents an 11.5-fold difference. Two of the eight BACs that were classified as variant on the genomewide array overlapped clones on the SD microarray that were also classified as variant, thus yielding concordant results.

Discussion

We have performed an analysis of copy-number variation in the human genome by using a targeted BAC array.

Table 1

Summary of CNPs Detected by Array CGH

Ethnic Group	No. of Subjects Analyzed	Gains	Losses	No. of CNPs: Showing Both Gain and Loss	Detected in Present Study	Detected by Sebat et al. (2004)	Detected by Iafrate et al. (2004)	Novel
American Indians	7	9	22	13	44	18	9	22
Sub-Saharan Africans	16	27	31	17	75	24	14	43
Whites	12	17	22	12	51	16	13	25
Asians	12	26	27	15	68	21	14	37
Nonredundant total	47	52	50	17	119	22	21	73

NOTE.—CNPs were scored as either increased or decreased $\log_2$ ratios (i.e., gains or losses), relative to the reference DNA. In total, 46 (39%) of 119 of the CNPs we identified have been reported previously, which thus validates the ability of our array to detect known copy-number variations. In our sample population, we identified 22 (71%) of the 31 CNPs detected by Sebat et al. (2004) and 22 (39%) of the 57 CNPs detected by Iafrate et al. (2004) that were represented on the SD microarray.

Although many of the CNPs we observed were identified in previous studies—which thus validates the ability of our array to detect bona fide polymorphisms—our targeted experimental approach significantly improves the ascertainment of structural rearrangements. We grouped BACs into those that were contained within each rearrangement hotspot, those that overlapped the segmental duplications, or those that were in the flanking unique sequence (fig. 1). We observed a 4–5-fold enrichment of CNPs within regions that were flanked by or contained large, highly homologous segmental duplications, as compared with control clones. These data indicate that genomic duplication architecture is strongly associated with CNP in the human genome. Presumably, segmental duplications mediate the deletion or duplication of the intervening sequence via nonallelic homologous recombination, supporting the notion that certain regions of the genome are predisposed to rearrangement as a result of their underlying genomic architecture (Stankiewicz and Lupski 2002; Stankiewicz et al. 2003; Bailey et al. 2004). Consistent with this hypothesis, we also observed an enrichment of hotspot sequence in the more common CNPs, suggesting that the presence of flanking duplications renders these sites prone to recurrent rearrangement. In total, we detected CNPs within 51 (39%) of 130 rearrangement hotspots. It is surprising that, in most cases, CNPs were not continuous across entire hotspot regions. Several factors could account for this observation. The highly complex segmental-duplication architecture bracketing these regions means that there are multiple potential sites of rearrangement and that these configurations may differ among individuals. This provides the potential for alternate sites of rearrangement. Such an effect has been observed for the Prader-Willi and Angelman syndromes, for which atypical breakpoints have been mapped to other duplication structures (Amos-Landgraf et al. 1999; Locke et al. 2004). Other possibilities include genomic misassembly of these regions and incorrect mapping of the arrayed BAC clones. The latter possibility, however, seems less likely, because BAC end-sequence confirmation and/or FISH verification was performed for every clone on the SD microarray. Finally, if nonallelic homologous recombination is the underlying mechanism of rearrangement in these regions, then additional repair or recombination events could result in more-complex rearrangements. Nevertheless, this study demonstrates that segmental duplications play an important role in normal variation as well as in genomic disease, defining hotspots of rearrangement that are susceptible to variation among the normal population. We hypothesize that the remainder of hotspots that did not show variation in our sample population represent excellent candidate sites that may be associated with genomic disease, and this survey provides the necessary baseline to begin future studies on disease populations.

Our analysis of different ethnic groups allowed an assessment of population-specific copy-number variants. However, almost without exception, the CNPs were present in multiple populations. Of the 50 regions that were polymorphic in more than two individuals, only 2 were confined to a single ethnic group. One of these CNPs (in region 12) represents a partial deletion of two overlapping BACs at 1q31.3, observed in 6 of the 16 sub-Saharan Africans studied. The region of overlap defined by these two BACs is composed of 70 kb of sequence flanked by a pair of intrachromosomal segmental duplications with 91% identity. We suggest that this CNP likely represents a deletion of this 70-kb segment, mediated by nonallelic homologous recombination between the flanking duplications. Such ethnic predilections for copy-number variation have recently been shown to be an important determinant in disease association studies (Gonzalez et al. 2005).

The occurrence of CNPs across multiple ethnic populations suggests that these structural rearrangements either (1) are evolutionarily ancient, having occurred prior to the separation of these ethnic groups, or (2) are recurrent events that have occurred independently in multiple founders. Distinguishing between these two

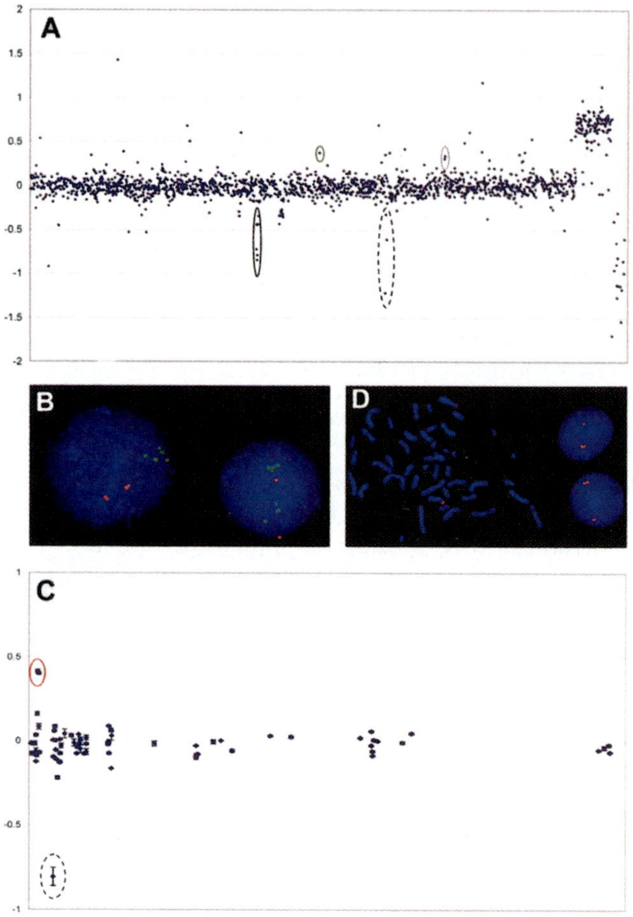

Figure 3 CNPs detected by array CGH, and verification by FISH. *A*, Genomic profile of GM10473A (a Biaka female). After quality filtering, 1,967 BAC clones were ordered sequentially from 1pter to Yqter on the basis of physical location in the July 2003 genome assembly (*X*-axis). Each data point represents the mean $\log_2$ ratio of test:reference intensity of the three replicate spots of each BAC from a single hybridization experiment (*Y*-axis). Each hybridization was repeated with reverse labeling (dye swap), and clones that yielded $\log_2$ ratios deviating >2 SDs from the mean of all autosomal clones in both experiments were classified as variant. The reference DNA is male; thus, clones located on the sex chromosomes show $\log_2$ ratios consistent with female:male hybridization. Three previously reported CNPs are circled: the β-defensin gene cluster at 8p23.1 (Hollox et al. 2003) (*solid circle*), the *IGHG1* gene cluster at 14q32.33 (Sasso et al. 1995) (*dashed circle*), and the *IGVH/SLC6A8/CDM* pseudogene cluster at 16p11.2 (Barber et al. 1999) (*dotted circle*). A novel variant locus, RP11-136P13 (chromosome 10: 81097351–81263857 [*green circle*]), yielded $\log_2$ ratios of 0.44 and 0.48 in replicate hybridizations. *B*, FISH confirmation of RP11-136P13, which is composed entirely of segmental-duplication sequence and therefore shows dual signals when used as a FISH probe (*green*). However, the presence of an additional signal in interphase nuclei shows the polymorphic nature of this locus in GM10473A. A control probe (*red*) confirms that the cells are diploid. This duplication was also observed in two other subjects. *C*, Array CGH profile of chromosome 8 in GM10493 (a Biaka). Clones are ordered by physical distance from 8pter in kb (*X*-axis), with error bars showing the SD of the $\log_2$ ratios from the three replicate spots. Two adjacent clones, RP11-159F11 and RP11-46M15 (*red circle*), yielded $\log_2$ ratios of 0.41, indicating the presence of a duplication. A BAC that yielded a $\log_2$ ratio of -0.81 in this experiment (*dashed circle*) was not confirmed in the replicate dye-swapped hybridization; thus, it was classified as nonvariant. *D*, Use of RP11-159F11 as a FISH probe, showing increased signal intensity on a chromosome 8 homologue in metaphase cells, which resolves to dual signals in interphase cells, confirming the presence of a duplication of this region. An overlapping but nonidentical duplication of 8p23.2 was also observed in GM17051.

hypotheses will require the integration of SNP haplotype and array CGH data. If CNPs play a role in phenotypic variation or susceptibility to common diseases (Buckland 2003; Gonzalez et al. 2005), the occurrence of the same CNP on multiple haplotype backgrounds as a result of recurrent rearrangement could confound conventional SNP-based association studies.

We also observed a significant enrichment of segmental duplications within regions of CNP, suggesting that these duplications themselves show marked variation in copy number. This is consistent with previous observations of polymorphic copy-number variation in segmental duplications (Fredman et al. 2004). A striking example of such polymorphism is illustrated by a series

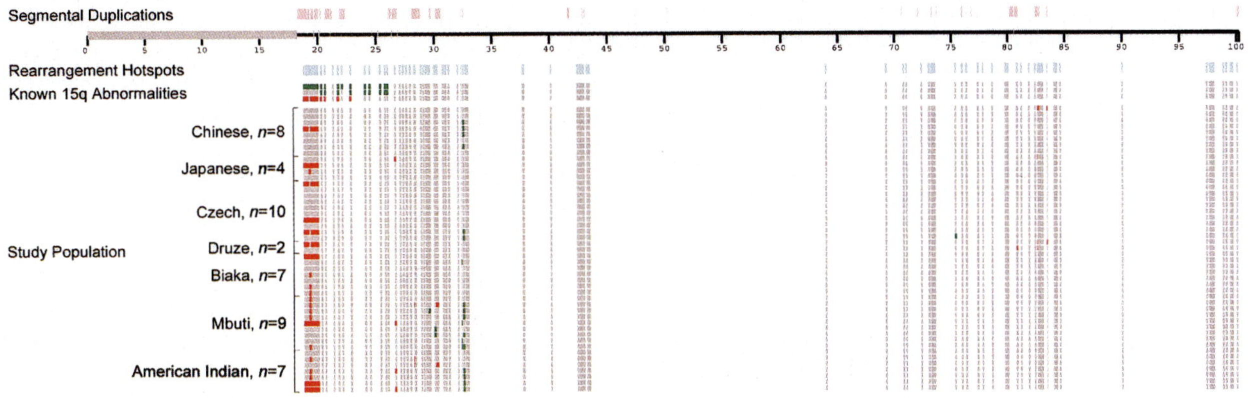

Figure 4 CNPs detected on chromosome 15. For each of the 47 individuals studied, relative duplications (*green*) and deletions (*red*) are represented, with invariant BACs shown in gray. The different sizes of the deletions and duplications in the three patients with known copy-number changes in the 15q11-q13 region (Locke et al. 2004) are clearly visible. Note that, as expected, none of the 47 normal individuals (94 chromosomes) in our population survey showed variation over these regions associated with disease. Also shown are the locations of segmental duplications >10 kb in size with >95% identity (*pink*) and of rearrangement hotspots represented on the array (*blue*), which illustrates the targeted nature of our array. Each tick mark represents 5 Mb, with gaps in the sequence assembly represented by gray bars.

of CNPs within the pericentromeric region of chromosome 9, which is composed almost exclusively of large, highly homologous (>99% identity) blocks of intrachromosomal duplication that our data suggest vary in copy number. We hypothesize that many CNPs in the human genome may be due to the presence or absence of evolutionarily recent segmental-duplication events that have not yet become fixed within the population, providing evidence that the process of duplicative transposition is ongoing within the human population. It should be noted, however, that this study likely underestimates the amount of copy-number variation that exists within regions of segmental duplication. By definition, these sequences occur at multiple genomic locations, with some present in >40 copies (Horvath et al. 2003); thus, unlike for unique portions of the genome, the gain or loss of a single duplication will often be below the resolution of array CGH, which undoubtedly biases our results. Despite the sequence complexity of these clones, they provided valuable information. We observed significantly more copy-number variation in BACs that contained segmental duplications than in unique regions of the genome. Indeed, the parallel analysis of samples on both our SD microarray and a second array with BACs spaced at an average resolution of ~1.4 Mb throughout the genome showed a >10-fold increase in the ascertainment of CNPs with the use of the duplication-targeted array. This suggests that the inclusion of BACs enriched in segmental-duplication content significantly increases the ascertainment of structurally polymorphic regions. We suggest that either the copy number or the sequence composition of these regions must differ dramatically among different individuals to produce significant differences on array CGH. However, until targeted sequencing of the variant regions from multiple individuals occurs, the true nature of the variation at these loci will not be fully ascertained.

A total of 141 genes either completely or partially overlapped variant BACs (table A3 in appendix A [online only]). However, because the majority of CNPs do not encompass complete BACs, and, because their boundaries are difficult to define accurately by use of array CGH, it is likely that only a subset of these genes vary in copy number. Because many of the genes previously confirmed as polymorphic have functions in metabolism and immunity, alterations in copy number of these genes often have profound effects on an individual's metabolic rate or resistance to environmental pathogens (Lackner et al. 1991; McLellan et al. 1997; Dalen et al. 1998; Rao et al. 2000; Sprenger et al. 2000; Townson et al. 2002; van der Burg et al. 2002; Hollox et al. 2003; Gonzalez et al. 2005) and, as such, are likely to be significant susceptibility factors for some common human diseases.

Although results yielded by array CGH only reveal copy-number changes relative to the reference sample used, deletions and duplications were observed in our sample population at approximately equal frequencies (they were observed in 50 and 52 regions, respectively). Of note, a further 17 regions showed both relative deletion and relative duplication in different individuals, which indicates that these loci have multiple variations in copy number. These may represent a variable number of tandem repeats or, alternatively, the product of reciprocal nonhomologous recombination events, as has been observed at sites of known genomic disorders (Bi

The figure is available in its entirety in the online edition of *The American Journal of Human Genetics.*

Figure 5 Genomewide map of sites of copy-number variation detected by array CGH. The legend is available in its entirety in the online edition of *The American Journal of Human Genetics.*

et al. 2003). Similarly, many other loci exhibited a wide range of hybridization ratios among different individuals, suggesting the presence of multiple alleles at these loci, such as that observed at the *AMY1A* gene cluster (Iafrate et al. 2004).

As in a previous study by Iafrate et al. [2004], we observed a significant increase in the frequency of genome assembly gaps at sites of copy-number variation. Of the 160 variant BACs, 42 (26%) were located within 100 kb of an assembly gap, compared with 130 (8%) of the 1,663 nonvariant BACs (a 3.4-fold enrichment; $\chi^2 = 58.0$; $P < .000001$), suggesting that the presence of these polymorphisms may represent a significant impediment to correct genome assembly. However, because there was also an association of segmental duplications with CNPs, which are themselves known to be correlated with gap location (Eichler et al. 2004), it is difficult to draw firm conclusions about the causality of this relationship. The coinciding of CNPs, segmental duplications, and sequence assembly gaps highlights the continued importance of resolving and studying the nature of these biologically relevant regions.

To facilitate the study of structural variation, we have compiled a Web interface, based on the UCSC Human Genome Browser, that displays all CNPs reported both here and in previous studies. Our Structural Variation Database (see Web Resources) includes an additional 297 sites of fine-scale variation (resolution ~8 kb) identified by fosmid paired-end sequence analysis (Tuzun et al. 2005), including sites of inversion not detectable by array-based approaches, as well as CNPs identified in two other studies (Iafrate et al. 2004; Sebat et al. 2004). Given the importance of this type of variation for genetic disease, a coordinated effort should be made to incorporate results and the underlying raw data into central repositories of data on human variation (such as the dbSNP and the Data Coordinating Center for the International HapMap Consortium).

In conclusion, this study demonstrates that segmental duplications define hotspots of chromosomal rearrangement in the human genome. Our data suggest not only that intrachromosomal segmental duplications frequently mediate polymorphic rearrangement of intervening sequence via nonallelic homologous recombination but also that segmental duplications themselves are often variant in copy number. Thus, the consideration of genomic architecture can significantly enrich the detection of large-scale variation. The array we have constructed includes BACs covering 25 regions associated with known pathogenic microdeletions/duplications (Stankiewicz and Lupski 2002) and includes an additional 105 regions for which the pathological relevance has not yet been determined, thus representing an excellent resource for the study of genomic disease. Although we did not detect CNPs in 79 of the 130 rearrangement hotspots in our sample population of normal individuals, we suggest that these hotspots represent excellent candidate sites of recurrent rearrangement that may be associated with novel genomic disorders (Bailey et al. 2002; Mehan et al. 2004). This survey of normal variation provides the requisite baseline for distinguishing copy-number variation associated with genomic disease.

Acknowledgments

We thank Cassy Gulden and Marla Eichler, for technical assistance. This work was supported in part by National Institutes of Health grant HD043569 (to E.E.E.).

Web Resources

The URLs for data presented herein are as follows:

Chromosome Anomaly Register, http://www.som.soton.ac.uk/research/geneticsdiv/anomaly%20register/
Structural Variation Database, http://paralogy.gs.washington.edu/structuralvariation
UCSC Human Genome Browser, http://genome.ucsc.edu/

References

Amos-Landgraf JM, Ji Y, Gottlieb W, Depinet T, Wandstrat AE, Cassidy SB, Driscoll DJ, Rogan PK, Schwartz S, Nicholls RD (1999) Chromosome breakage in the Prader-Willi and Angelman syndromes involves recombination between large, transcribed repeats at proximal and distal breakpoints. Am J Hum Genet 65:370–386

Armengol L, Pujana MA, Cheung J, Scherer SW, Estivill X (2003) Enrichment of segmental duplications in regions of breaks of synteny between the human and mouse genomes suggest their involvement in evolutionary rearrangements. Hum Mol Genet 12:2201–2208

Bailey JA, Baertsch R, Kent WJ, Haussler D, Eichler EE (2004) Hotspots of mammalian chromosomal evolution. Genome Biol 5:R23

Bailey JA, Gu Z, Clark RA, Reinert K, Samonte RV, Schwartz S, Adams MD, Myers EW, Li PW, Eichler EE (2002) Recent segmental duplications in the human genome. Science 297:1003–1007

Barber JC, Reed CJ, Dahoun SP, Joyce CA (1999) Amplification of a pseudogene cassette underlies euchromatic variation of 16p at the cytogenetic level. Hum Genet 104:211–218

Bi W, Park SS, Shaw CJ, Withers MA, Patel PI, Lupski JR (2003) Reciprocal crossovers and a positional preference for strand exchange in recombination events resulting in deletion or duplication of chromosome 17p11.2. Am J Hum Genet 73:1302–1315

Buckland PR (2003) Polymorphically duplicated genes: their relevance to phenotypic variation in humans. Ann Med 35: 308–315

Chance PF, Abbas N, Lensch MW, Pentao L, Roa BB, Patel PI, Lupski JR (1994) Two autosomal dominant neuropathies result from reciprocal DNA duplication/deletion of a region on chromosome 17. Hum Mol Genet 3:223–228

Cheung J, Estivill X, Khaja R, MacDonald JR, Lau K, Tsui LC, Scherer SW (2003) Genome-wide detection of segmental duplications and potential assembly errors in the human genome sequence. Genome Biol 4:R25

Cheung VG, Nowak N, Jang W, Kirsch IR, Zhao S, Chen XN, Furey TS, et al (2001) Integration of cytogenetic landmarks into the draft sequence of the human genome. Nature 409: 953–958

Dalen P, Dahl ML, Ruiz ML, Nordin J, Bertilsson L (1998) 10-Hydroxylation of nortriptyline in white persons with 0, 1, 2, 3, and 13 functional *CYP2D6* genes. Clin Pharmacol Ther 63:444–452

Edelmann L, Pandita RK, Morrow BE (1999) Low-copy repeats mediate the common 3-Mb deletion in patients with velo-cardio-facial syndrome. Am J Hum Genet 64:1076–1086

Eichler EE (2001) Recent duplication, domain accretion and the dynamic mutation of the human genome. Trends Genet 17:661–669

Eichler EE, Clark RA, She X (2004) An assessment of the sequence gaps: unfinished business in a finished human genome. Nat Rev Genet 5:345–354

Fantes JA, Mewborn SK, Lese CM, Hedrick J, Brown RL, Dyomin V, Chaganti RS, Christian SL, Ledbetter DH (2002) Organisation of the pericentromeric region of chromosome 15: at least four partial gene copies are amplified in patients with a proximal duplication of 15q. J Med Genet 39:170–177

Fredman D, White SJ, Potter S, Eichler EE, Den Dunnen JT, Brookes AJ (2004) Complex SNP-related sequence variation in segmental genome duplications. Nat Genet 36:861–866

Giglio S, Broman KW, Matsumoto N, Calvari V, Gimelli G, Neumann T, Ohashi H, Voullaire L, Larizza D, Giorda R, Weber JL, Ledbetter DH, Zuffardi O (2001) Olfactory receptor-gene clusters, genomic-inversion polymorphisms, and common chromosome rearrangements. Am J Hum Genet 68:874–883

Gimelli G, Pujana MA, Patricelli MG, Russo S, Giardino D, Larizza L, Cheung J, Armengol L, Schinzel A, Estivill X, Zuffardi O (2003) Genomic inversions of human chromosome 15q11-q13 in mothers of Angelman syndrome patients with class II (BP2/3) deletions. Hum Mol Genet 12:849–858

Gonzalez E, Kulkarni H, Bolivar H, Mangano A, Sanchez R, Catano G, Nibbs RJ, Freedman BI, Quinones MP, Bamshad MJ, Murthy KK, Rovin BH, Bradley W, Clark RA, Anderson SA, O'Connell RJ, Agan BK, Ahuja SS, Bologna R, Sen L, Dolan MJ, Ahuja SK (2005) The influence of *CCL3L1* gene-containing segmental duplications on HIV-1/AIDS susceptibility. Science 307:1434–1440

Hollox EJ, Armour JA, Barber JC (2003) Extensive normal copy number variation of a β-defensin antimicrobial-gene cluster. Am J Hum Genet 73:591–600

Horvath JE, Gulden CL, Bailey JA, Yohn C, McPherson JD, Prescott A, Roe BA, de Jong PJ, Ventura M, Misceo D, Archidiacono N, Zhao S, Schwartz S, Rocchi M, Eichler EE (2003) Using a pericentromeric interspersed repeat to recapitulate the phylogeny and expansion of human centromeric segmental duplications. Mol Biol Evol 20:1463–1479

Iafrate JA, Feuk L, Rivera MN, Listewnik ML, Donahoe PK, Qi Y, Scherer SW, Lee C (2004) Detection of large-scale variation in the human genome. Nat Genet 36:949–951

Ishkanian AS, Malloff CA, Watson SK, DeLeeuw RJ, Chi B, Coe BP, Snijders A, Albertson DG, Pinkel D, Marra MA, Ling V, MacAulay C, Lam WL (2004) A tiling resolution DNA microarray with complete coverage of the human genome. Nat Genet 36:299–303

Jain AN, Tokuyasu TA, Snijders AM, Segraves R, Albertson DG, Pinkel D (2002) Fully automatic quantification of microarray image data. Genome Res 12:325–332

Ji Y, Eichler EE, Schwartz S, Nicholls RD (2000) Structure of chromosomal duplicons and their role in mediating human genomic disorders. Genome Res 10:597–610

Lackner C, Boerwinkle E, Leffert CC, Rahmig T, Hobbs HH (1991) Molecular basis of apolipoprotein (a) isoform size heterogeneity as revealed by pulsed-field gel electrophoresis. J Clin Invest 87:2153–2161

Locke DP, Archidiacono N, Misceo D, Cardone MF, Deschamps S, Roe B, Rocchi M, Eichler EE (2003*a*) Refinement of a chimpanzee pericentric inversion breakpoint to a segmental duplication cluster. Genome Biol 4:R50

Locke DP, Segraves R, Carbone L, Archidiacono N, Albertson DG, Pinkel D, Eichler EE (2003*b*) Large-scale variation among human and great ape genomes determined by array comparative genomic hybridization. Genome Res 13:347–357

Locke DP, Segraves R, Nicholls RD, Schwartz S, Pinkel D, Albertson DG, Eichler EE (2004) BAC microarray analysis of 15q11-q13 rearrangements and the impact of segmental duplications. J Med Genet 41:175–182

McLellan RA, Oscarson M, Alexandrie A, Seidegård J, Price Evans DA, Rannug A, Ingelman-Sundberg M (1997) Characterization of a human glutathione S-transferase μ cluster containing a duplicated *GSTM1* gene that causes ultrarapid enzyme activity. Mol Pharmacol 52:958–965

Mehan MR, Freimer NB, Ophoff RA (2004) A genome-wide survey of segmental duplications that mediate common human genetic variation of chromosomal architecture. Hum Genomics 1:335–344

Osborne LR, Li M, Pober B, Chitayat D, Bodurtha J, Mandel A, Costa T, Grebe T, Cox S, Tsui LC, Scherer SW (2001) A 1.5 million–base pair inversion polymorphism in families with Williams-Beuren syndrome. Nat Genet 29:321–325

Pinkel D, Straume T, Gray JW (1986) Cytogenetic analysis using quantitative, high sensitivity, fluorescence hybridization. Proc Natl Acad Sci USA 83:2934–2938

Rao Y, Hoffmann E, Zia M, Bodin L, Zeman M, Sellers EM, Tyndale RF (2000) Duplications and defects in the *CYP2A6*

gene: identification, genotyping, and in vivo effects on smoking. Mol Pharmacol 58:747–755
Riley B, Williamson M, Collier D, Wilkie H, Makoff A (2002) A 3-Mb map of a large segmental duplication overlapping the α7-nicotinic acetylcholine receptor gene (*CHRNA7*) at human 15q13-q14. Genomics 79:197–209
Samonte RV, Eichler EE (2002) Segmental duplications and the evolution of the primate genome. Nat Rev Genet 3:65–72
Sasso EH, Buckner JH, Suzuki LA (1995) Ethnic differences of polymorphism of an immunoglobulin VH3 gene. J Clin Invest 96:1591–1600
Sebat J, Lakshmi B, Troge J, Alexander J, Young J, Lundin P, Maner S, Massa H, Walker M, Chi M, Navin N, Lucito R, Healy J, Hicks J, Ye K, Reiner A, Gilliam TC, Trask B, Patterson N, Zetterberg A, Wigler M (2004) Large-scale copy number polymorphism in the human genome. Science 305:525–528
Shaikh TH, Kurahashi H, Saitta SC, O'Hare AM, Hu P, Roe BA, Driscoll DA, McDonald-McGinn DM, Zackai EH, Budarf ML, Emanuel BS (2000) Chromosome 22-specific low copy repeats and the 22q11.2 deletion syndrome: genomic organization and deletion endpoint analysis. Hum Mol Genet 9:489–501
Shaw CJ, Bi W, Lupski JR (2002) Genetic proof of unequal meiotic crossovers in reciprocal deletion and duplication of 17p11.2. Am J Hum Genet 71:1072–1081
She X, Horvath JE, Jiang Z, Liu G, Furey TS, Christ L, Clark R, Graves T, Gulden CL, Alkan C, Bailey JA, Sahinalp C, Rocchi M, Haussler D, Wilson RK, Miller W, Schwartz S, Eichler EE (2004*a*) The structure and evolution of centromeric transition regions within the human genome. Nature 430:857–864
She X, Jiang Z, Clark RA, Liu G, Cheng Z, Tuzun E, Church DM, Sutton G, Halpern AL, Eichler EE (2004*b*) Shotgun sequence assembly and recent segmental duplications within the human genome. Nature 431:927–930
Siniscalco M, Robledo R, Orru S, Contu L, Yadav P, Ren Q, Lai H, Roe B (2000) A plea to search for deletion polymorphism through genome scans in populations. Trends Genet 16:435–437
Skaletsky H, Kuroda-Kawaguchi T, Minx PJ, Cordum HS, Hillier L, Brown LG, Repping S, et al (2003) The male-specific region of the human Y chromosome is a mosaic of discrete sequence classes. Nature 423:825–837
Snijders AM, Nowak N, Segraves R, Blackwood S, Brown N, Conroy J, Hamilton G, Hindle AK, Huey B, Kimura K, Law S, Myambo K, Palmer J, Ylstra B, Yue JP, Gray JW, Jain AN, Pinkel D, Albertson DG (2001) Assembly of microarrays for genome-wide measurement of DNA copy number. Nat Genet 29:263–264
Snijders AM, Segraves R, Blackwood S, Pinkel D, Albertson DG (2004) BAC microarray-based comparative genomic hybridization. Methods Mol Biol 256:39–56
Sprenger R, Schlagenhaufer R, Kerb R, Bruhn C, Brockmoller J, Roots I, Brinkmann U (2000) Characterization of the glutathione S-transferase *GSTT1* deletion: discrimination of all genotypes by polymerase chain reaction indicates a trimodular genotype-phenotype correlation. Pharmacogenetics 10:557–565
Stankiewicz P, Lupski JR (2002) Genome architecture, rearrangements and genomic disorders. Trends Genet 18:74–82
Stankiewicz P, Shaw CJ, Dapper JD, Wakui K, Shaffer LG, Withers M, Elizondo L, Park SS, Lupski JR (2003) Genome architecture catalyzes nonrecurrent chromosomal rearrangements. Am J Hum Genet 72:1101–1116
Townson JR, Barcellos LF, Nibbs RJB (2002) Gene copy number regulates the production of the human chemokine CCL3-L1. Eur J Immunol 32:3016–3026
Tuzun E, Sharp AJ, Bailey JA, Kaul R, Morrison VA, Pertz LM, Haugen E, Hayden H, Albertson D, Pinkel D, Olson MV, Eichler EE (2005) Fine-scale structural variation of the human genome. Nat Genet, published online May 15
van der Burg M, Barendregt BH, van Gastel-Mol EJ, Tümkaya T, Langerak AW, van Dongen JJM (2002) Unraveling of the polymorphic Cλ2-Cλ3 amplification and the $Ke^{+}Oz^{-}$ polymorphism in the human Iλg locus. J Immunol 169:271–276
Vissers LE, de Vries BB, Osoegawa K, Janssen IM, Feuth T, Choy CO, Straatman H, van der Vliet W, Huys EH, van Rijk A, Smeets D, van Ravenswaaij-Arts CM, Knoers NV, van der Burgt I, de Jong PJ, Brunner HG, van Kessel AG, Schoenmakers EF, Veltman JA (2003) Array-based comparative genomic hybridization for the genomewide detection of submicroscopic chromosomal abnormalities. Am J Hum Genet 73:1261–1270
Waldman AS, Liskay RM (1988) Dependence of intrachromosomal recombination in mammalian cells on uninterrupted homology. Mol Cell Biol 8:5350–5357

Am. J. Hum. Genet. 77:89–96, 2005

Identification of a Major Recombination Hotspot in Patients with Short Stature and *SHOX* Deficiency

Katja U. Schneider,[1] Nitin Sabherwal,[1] Karin Jantz,[1] Ralph Röth,[1] Nadja Muncke,[1] Werner F. Blum,[2,3] Gordon B. Cutler, Jr.,[4] and Gudrun Rappold[1]

[1]Institute of Human Genetics, University of Heidelberg, Heidelberg, Germany; [2]Lilly Research Laboratories, Eli Lilly and Company, Bad Homburg, Germany; [3]University Children's Hospital, Giessen, Germany; and [4]Lilly Research Laboratories, Eli Lilly and Company, Indianapolis

Human growth is influenced not only by environmental and internal factors but also by a large number of different genes. One of these genes, *SHOX*, is believed to play a major role in growth, since defects in this homeobox-containing gene on the sex chromosomes lead to syndromal short stature (Léri-Weill dyschondrosteosis, Langer mesomelic dysplasia, and Turner syndrome) as well as to idiopathic short stature. We have analyzed 118 unrelated patients with Léri-Weill dyschondrosteosis and >1,500 patients with idiopathic short stature for deletions encompassing *SHOX*. Deletions were detected in 34% of the patients with Léri-Weill dyschondrosteosis and in 2% of the patients with idiopathic short stature. For 27 patients with Léri-Weill dyschondrosteosis and for 6 with idiopathic short stature, detailed deletion mapping was performed. Analysis was performed by polymerase chain reaction with the use of pseudoautosomal polymorphic markers and by fluorescence in situ hybridization with the use of cosmid clones. Here, we show that, although the identified deletions vary in size, the vast majority (73%) of patients tested share a distinct proximal deletion breakpoint. We propose that the sequence present within this proximal deletion breakpoint "hotspot" region predisposes to recurrent breaks.

Introduction

Short stature has been defined as height >2 SD below the mean for age and sex. This corresponds to the shortest 2.3% of children. Although it is clear that multiple factors contribute to final height, genetic factors play a crucial role. Deletions within the distal short arm of the human X chromosome, for example, lead to multiple phenotypes, including short stature, chondrodysplasia punctata, mental retardation, steroid sulfatase deficiency, and Kallmann syndrome, and have been found as isolated entities and as part of a contiguous gene syndrome (Ballabio et al. 1989). Deletions that are normally restricted to the pseudoautosomal region (PAR1) encompassing the short-stature homeobox gene (*SHOX* [MIM 312865]) have been found in patients with Léri-Weill dyschondrosteosis (LWD [MIM 127300]) and in those with idiopathic short stature (ISS [MIM 604271]) (Ellison et al. 1997; Rao et al. 1997*b*; Belin et al. 1998; Shears et al. 1998; Cormier-Daire et al. 1999, 2001; Spranger et al. 1999; Blaschke and Rappold 2000; Grigelioniene et al. 2000; Rappold et al. 2002; Binder et al. 2003; Morizio et al. 2003). LWD is a mesomelic short-stature syndrome characterized by a skeletal forearm abnormality termed "Madelung deformity." Approximately 50%–100% of cases of LWD are due to complete deletions or intragenic mutations of the *SHOX* gene (Grigelioniene et al. 2000; Schiller et al. 2000; Cormier-Daire et al. 2001; Ross et al. 2001). Evidence suggests that roughly two-thirds of *SHOX*-deficient patients with LWD have deletions, whereas one-third of *SHOX*-deficient patients with LWD have point mutations (Cormier-Daire et al. 2001; Falcinelli et al. 2001; Grigelionience et al. 2001; Huber et al. 2001; Ross et al. 2001; Flanagan et al. 2002). In the cohort of patients with ISS, *SHOX* mutations were found in 2.4% of the patients, of which 80% (2.0% of the cohort) have been identified as carrying complete gene deletions (Rappold et al. 2002). Binder et al. (2003) confirmed these findings in a screen of individuals with ISS that revealed complete *SHOX* gene deletions in >2% of the affected individuals. On the basis of this prevalence of *SHOX* deletions in patients with ISS and under the assumption that the disorder found in most people with short stature is idiopathic, *SHOX* deletions are estimated to occur in ~1 in 2,000 individuals in the total population (Rappold et al. 2002; Binder et al. 2003). Moreover, others have found *SHOX* deletions in up to 7.1% of patients with short stature of unknown cause (Morizio et al. 2003).

Although large deletions rarely account for the majority of mutations at a given locus (Cooper et al. 1998;

Received March 18, 2005; accepted for publication May 4, 2005; electronically published June 1, 2005.

Address for correspondence and reprints: Dr. Gudrun Rappold, Institute of Human Genetics, Im Neuenheimer Feld 366, 69120 Heidelberg, Germany. E-mail: gudrun_rappold@med.uni-heidelberg.de

0002-9297/2005/7701-0009$15.00

Antonarakis et al. 2000), a high frequency of deletions has been found in several inherited disorders. For instance, large gene deletions occur in Duchenne muscular dystrophy (DMD), in which two-thirds of all affected individuals display a deletion of one or more exons of the dystrophin gene (*DMD*) (Muntoni et al. 2003), and in X-linked ichthyosis, in which the majority of the patients carry a 1.9-Mb deletion encompassing the *STS* locus (Hernandez-Martin et al. 1999).

To gain a better understanding of the mechanism underlying *SHOX* deletions, we analyzed deletion breakpoints in 27 patients with LWD and in 6 patients with ISS. We identified a high incidence of breakpoints (73%) in a 5-kb region proximal to the *SHOX* gene, suggesting that this breakpoint may represent a hotspot for deletions leading to short stature.

Material and Methods

Subjects

Peripheral blood samples were taken from 118 individuals with LWD and from >1,500 individuals with ISS after informed consent was obtained. Thirty-three patients (27 patients with LWD and 6 patients with ISS) were studied in detail for deletion sizes. Six patients with ISS and *SHOX* deletions were from a previous screen (Rappold et al. 2002 and authors' unpublished data). The patients were of both sexes (22 females and 11 males) and were of European origin (17 from Germany, 5 from the Netherlands, 5 from France, 3 from Spain, 1 from the Czech Republic, 1 from Croatia, and 1 from Poland). All individuals were unrelated and had been examined by endocrinologists. Short stature was diagnosed when height, adjusted for sex and chronological age, was below the 3rd percentile or <2 SDs of national height standards. Exclusion criteria for this study were growth hormone deficiency, growth hormone receptor defect, malignant neoplastic disease, chronic infectious disease, active rheumatoid arthritis, diabetes mellitus, renal insufficiency, hepatic disease, congestive heart failure, gonadal dysgenesis, or abnormal diet. LWD diagnosis was based on the presence of Madelung deformity, bowing of the forearms, and mesomelic short stature. For some of the patients, X-ray analysis of the forearm was performed.

PCR-Based Microsatellite Analysis

Genomic DNA was extracted from blood samples and was used for amplification with the primers DXYS201 (SHOX 5CA forward: CAT GTC ATA TAT ATA TGT GAT CC; SHOX 5CA reverse: GAC ACA GAA ATC CTT CAT AAA), DXYS233 (233 forward: TGG GAA TTC GAG GCT G; 233 reverse: TGA TTT CCA TCC TGG GGT), and CAII (CAII forward: ATA TCA GAA AAG ACT GTG TTC TAC; reverse: TAG TAG GTT GCA AAG GCA TCT G). Twenty picomoles of each primer were used with 100 ng of DNA—together with 2 U of Goldstar DNA polymerase (Eurogentec), 10 pmol dNTP (Fermentas), and 75 mmol $MgCl_2$—in the buffer provided with the enzyme. PCR was performed in a Peltier Thermal Cycler (PTC-200), starting with denaturation (95°C for 5 min), followed by 35 cycles of amplification (95°C for 30 s, 55°C for 30 s, and 72°C for 45 s) and a final elongation step (72°C for 5 min). The PCR products were loaded on a polyacrylamide gel (10%) and were stained with $AgNO_3$ solution.

FISH Analysis

Biotinylated cosmid DNA was hybridized to interphase and metaphase chromosomes of lymphocytes of patients, as described elsewhere (Lichter and Cremer 1992). FISH was performed using cosmids 11D2 (LLN0YCO3′M′11D2), 56G10 (LLN0YCO3′M′56G10), HO32 (LLNLc110HO32), 25D5 (LLN0YCO3′M′25D5), 110A7 (LLN0YCO3′M′110A7), 110E3 (LLN0YCO3′-M′110E3), 43C11 (LLN0YCO3′M′43C11), 15D10 (LLN0YCO3′M′15D10), 34F5 (LLN0YCO3′M′34F5), G0411 (ICRFc104G0411), 9E3 (LLN0YCO3′M′9E3), 29B11 (LLN0YCO3′M′29B11), P0117 (ICRFc104P0117), ANT3 (ICRFc104D0137), and 12E11 (LLN0YCO3′-M′12E11). Hybridization signals were detected via avidin-conjugated fluorescein isothiocyanate (FITC). Chromosomes were counterstained with 4′,6-diamidino-2-phenylindole (DAPI). Images of FITC- and DAPI-stained chromosomes were taken separately, using a cooled charge-coupled–device camera system (Photometrics).

SNP Analysis

SNPs that mapped to the critical breakpoint region in PAR1 were identified by searching dbSNP. Additional SNPs in this area were identified during the sequencing process and were further used for confirming heterozygosity. SNPs within the markers *DXYS86*, *DXYS59* (dbSNP accession number rs6644571), C7/SNPs (dbSNP accession numbers rs1016964 and rs3995647), C8/SNPs (dbSNP accession numbers rs2399945 and rs2399946), C9/SNPs, and C10/SNPs in the respective patients and their families were analyzed for heterozygosity by sequence analysis with the use of the following primers: P131 (forward: TCT GCC ATC CTA ATG ATG GT; reverse: AGA AGT TTC TTC TCC ACC TG), DXYS59 (forward: CAT TAA GCT GAT TAG CC AAT; reverse: AGA GCT CCA ATA TAT GCC AT), C7SNPs (forward: TAC GTG GTA GGG AGG AAG ATT GGA; reverse: ATC CAA GCA ATT GTC AGG GAT GGC), C8SNPs (forward: TCC TCC CAG TTG TCC CAG TTG TAT; reverse: GCT GCC CAT GAC AGG GGA CTA ACG), C9SNPs (forward: GCT GCT ACT AAG

TTA ACT GG; reverse: CAG ATA GAC AAT ATT TTC AG), and C10SNPs (forward: CGT CTC TTC CTT ATC ACT TG; reverse: TAA CCG CAG TGA AAC GTC CC). Sequencing was performed on a MegaBACE sequencer (Amersham Bioscience) by use of the DYEnamic ET Terminator Cycle Sequencing kit, in accordance with the manufacturer's instructions.

Secondary-Structure Prediction of the Hotspot Region by Computational Analysis

For secondary-structure prediction, a 6-kb sequence encompassing the hotspot region as well as 6-kb sequences of the direct proximal and distal adjacent regions were submitted to the Mfold server (Zuker 2003). Structures with the lowest free-energy values were selected for analysis.

Results

Deletion analysis was performed for 118 unrelated patients with LWD, by use of three polymorphic markers—*CAII, DXYS201* (CA repeat), and *DXYS233*—that reside between 520 kb and 870 kb from the telomere in PAR1 (see fig. 1). In cases of homozygosity of at least two of the three markers, deletion mapping was performed by FISH with the use of cosmids from a cosmid contig that was previously established by our group (Rao et al. 1997*a*).

In total, we found deletions encompassing *SHOX* in 40 individuals (34% of the 118 patients with LWD). For 27 patients with LWD, we were able to perform a detailed deletion mapping with the use of 15 PAR1 cosmids in total (fig. 1). The deletion sizes vary extensively, with the smallest comprising ~90 kb (patient LWD21) and the largest comprising >2.5 Mb (patients LWD25–LWD27) (table 1). However, most interestingly, 20 (74%) of 27 patients share a distinct breakpoint that is defined by the presence of a hybridization signal of cosmid P0117 and the absence of a signal of cosmid 29B11, which maps the breakpoint within the genomic sequence represented within cosmid P0117 (fig. 2).

This high incidence prompted us to investigate whether patients with ISS present similar deletion breakpoints, since 2%–3% of cases of ISS result from *SHOX* mutations (Rappold et al. 2002; Binder et al. 2003). We determined that the proximal deletion breakpoint similarly localizes within cosmid P0117 in four (67%) of the six patients with *SHOX* deletions, which indicates the clustering of the deletion breakpoint within a relatively small interval. Cosmid 29B11 harbors the probe AK1 (*DXYS163*), which detects a variable number of tandem repeats (VNTR) locus ~65 kb proximal to the *SHOX* gene (Klink et al. 1993). We used AK1 for Southern hybridization on *Taq*I-digested genomic DNAs and found that AK1 is absent in all patients carrying the deletion (data not shown). Cosmid P0117, however, was found by FISH analysis to be present in all the patients with deletions, on both alleles of the sex chromosomes.

On the basis of these findings, further mapping of the breakpoint region was achieved for seven patients (LWD1, LWD6, LWD7, LWD10, LWD15, LWD16, and ISS30) by use of SNP analysis. Cosmid P0117 contains the microsatellite marker *P117* (*DXYS417*) (Wapenaar et al. 1992), and further SNP markers were selected in the vicinity of *P117* (three distal and three proximal markers [see fig. 3]). SNP analysis mapped the breakpoints to an interval of 5 kb that is directly distal to P117 in all affected individuals. Sequence analysis of this critical region by use of the Tandem Repeat Finder of the University of California–Santa Cruz (UCSC) Genome Browser revealed a high occurrence of STRs (~85%) within the hotspot region.

Since tandem repeats can form unusual secondary structures, secondary-structure–prediction analysis was performed using the Mfold web server. Unlike the neighboring regions, the hotspot region showed (in Mfold analysis) an extensive secondary structure that is characterized by strong DNA bending and a free energy of −617.9 kcal/mol, together with hairpins and loops (fig. 4). Sequence and structure analysis of the tandem repeats revealed that they can vary in length but that they consist mostly of homologous units of 27 bp in a head-to-tail arrangement. In conclusion, the high incidence of breakpoints on cosmid P0117 is very likely due to the accumulation of STR sequences that may cause genomic instability by abnormal secondary-structure formation, including DNA bending, which, in turn, might explain the hotspot of deletions observed in the analyzed patients with short stature.

Discussion

The distal short arm of the human X chromosome is frequently subjected to deletion events that lead to genetic disorders such as short stature, chondrodysplasia punctata, mental retardation, ichthyosis, and Kallmann syndrome (Ballabio et al. 1989). We were interested in defining the deletion breakpoints in the vicinity of the *SHOX* gene, and we found that 24 (73%) of the 33 analyzed individuals share a common deletion breakpoint within a 5-kb interval. *SHOX* deletions account for 2.0%–7.1% of short stature of unknown cause (Rappold et al. 2002; Binder et al. 2003; Morizio et al. 2003), indicating that the major breakpoint that we identified contributed to the deletions in possibly >1% of patients with idiopathic short stature. Of all the tested patients with LWD and Xp deletions, the majority (73%) harbor this breakpoint on cosmid P0117. This leaves the

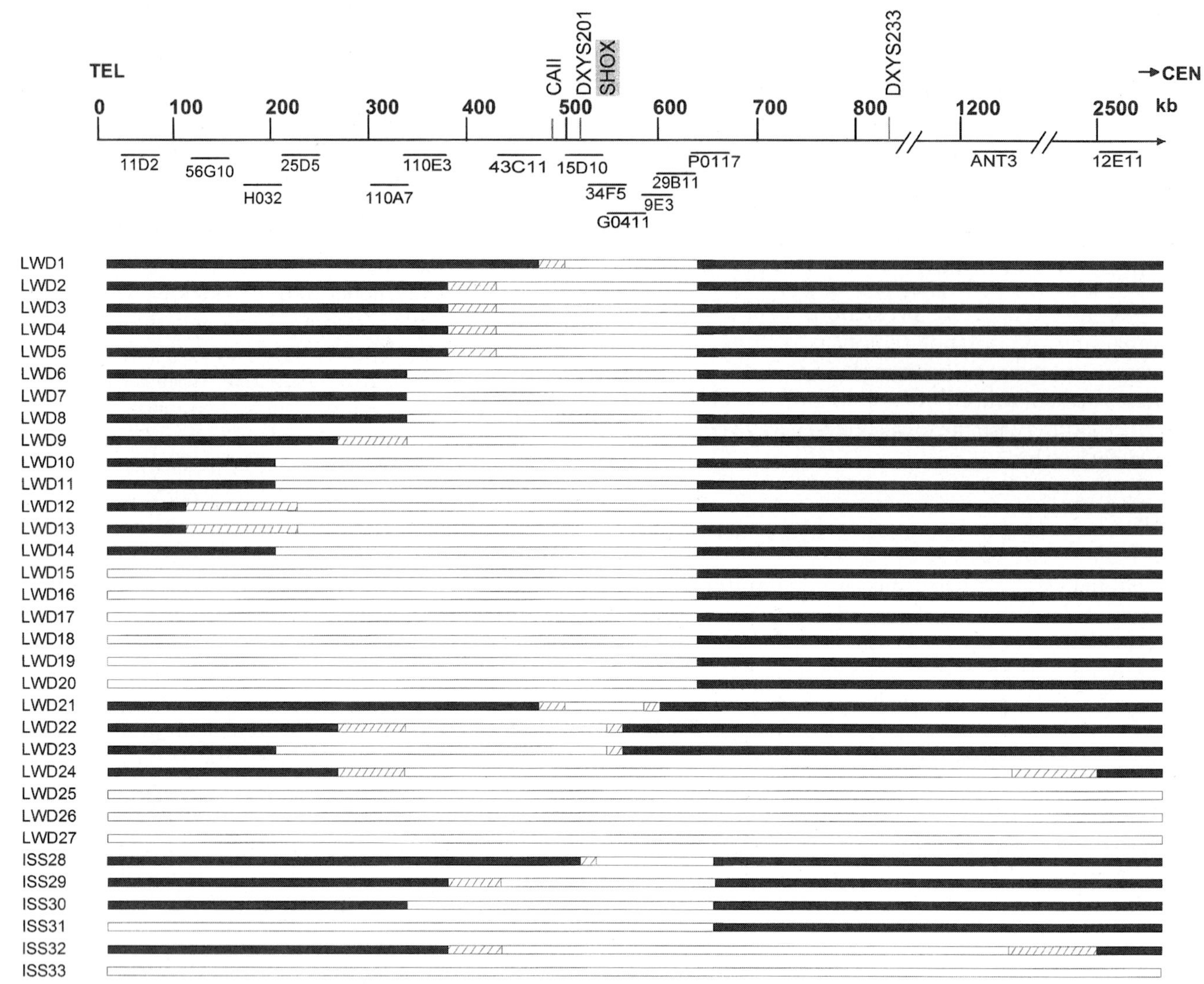

Figure 1 Deletion mapping of 27 patients with LWD (patients LWD1–LWD27) and 6 patients with ISS (patients ISS28–ISS33). Patients LWD2, LWD3, LWD4, LWD5, LWD8, LWD9, LWD19, LWD20, LWD22, and LWD28 have been described elsewhere as presenting a *SHOX* deletion (Schiller et al. 2000); however, the exact extent of the deletion sizes as well as the breakpoints were not defined. Blackened areas indicate the presence of the respective cosmid clone on both of the patient's sex chromosomes; unblackened areas indicate the absence of a cosmid clone on one sex chromosome; shaded areas indicate the breakpoint region. The map positions of the cosmid clones are indicated by horizontal lines and the clone abbreviation (see the "Material and Methods" section). The approximate distance from the telomere is given in kb. Microsatellite markers are indicated with vertical lines at their respective map position. The genomic locus of the *SHOX* gene is indicated in gray and resides ~555.1–582.3 kb from the telomere. The deletion hotspot is defined by the presence of cosmid P0117 and the absence of cosmid 29B11.

DXYS233 locus intact (fig. 1), which, in some screens, was used as an indicator of a *SHOX* deletion (e.g., Binder et al. 2003), suggesting that the true incidence of *SHOX* deletions in those studies may be considerably higher than previously estimated. A diagnostic test for *SHOX* deletions should therefore encompass markers next to the gene (e.g., CA markers *CAII* or *DXYS201*) and should not consider *DXYS233*.

The DNA instability that we observed in the overlap of cosmid clones P0117 and 29B11 is most likely due to the abundance of STRs that cause an extensive secondary-structure formation, as shown by the Mfold analysis (fig. 4). In contrast to the frequent proximal deletion breakpoint, the distal breakpoints vary considerably, with at least seven different breakpoints, as defined by FISH analysis. This variation might be due to weaker genomic instabilities at the respective positions in PAR1. PAR1 itself is a region that is highly active in recombination (Rappold et al. 1994). Crossovers are not distributed randomly but cluster in specific recom-

Table 1

Deletion Size in Patients with LWD or ISS

Patient	Presence or Absence of Hybridization Signal in Cosmid Clone															Estimated Deletion Size (kb)
	11D2 (~30 kb)	56G1 0 (~120 kb)	H032 (~180 kb)	25D5 (~240 kb)	110A7 (~300 kb)	110E3 (~320 kb)	43C11 (~440 kb)	15D10 (~490 kb)	34F5 (~530 kb)	G0411 (~560 kb)	9E3 (~580 kb)	29B11 (~600 kb)	P0117 (~650 kb)	ANT3 (~1,200 kb)	12E11 (~2,500 kb)	
LWD1							+	−	−			−	+			210
LWD2				+		+	−		−			−	+			330
LWD3				+		+	−		−			−	+			330
LWD4	+					+			−			−	+			330
LWD5				+		+	−		−			−	+			330
LWD6				+	+	−			−			−	+			350
LWD7				+	+	−	−		−			−	+			350
LWD8				+	+	−	−		−			−	+			350
LWD9				+	−	−			−			−	+			410
LWD10	+	+	+	−	−				−			−	+			470
LWD11	+	+	+	−				−	−	−		−	+			470
LWD12	+	−	−	−				−	−	−		−	+			620
LWD13	+			−			−		−	−		−	+			620
LWD14	+	+	+	−					−			−	+			470
LWD15	−			−					−			−	+			650
LWD16	−			−					−			−	+			650
LWD17	−			−				−	−	−		−	+			650
LWD18	−			−				−	−	−		−	+			650
LWD19	−								−			−	+			650
LWD20	−								−			−	+			650
LWD21						+		+/−	−	−	+	+	+			90
LWD22						+	−		−	+			+			230
LWD23	+	+	+	−		−	−	−	−	+	+	+	+			380
LWD24				+		−	−		−				−	−	+	>1,200
LWD25	−			−					−				−	−	−	>2,500
LWD26	−			−					−				−	−	−	>2,500
LWD27	−			−					−				−	−	−	>2,500
ISS28				+		+	+	−	−			−	+			210
ISS29				+		+	−		−			−	+			330
ISS30				+	+	−	−		−			−	+			350
ISS31	−			−					−			−	+			650
ISS32				+		+	−		−			−	−	−	+	>1,200
ISS33	−			−					−			−	−	−	−	>2,500

Note.—A plus sign (+) indicates the presence of a hybridization signal; a minus sign (−) indicates the absence of a signal. Cosmid clones 11D2, 25D5, 110E3, 43C11, 15D10, 34F5, G0411, 9E3, 29B11, P0117, ANT3, and 12E11 represent cosmids of PAR1, with their approximate position from the telomere (in kb). The estimated deletion size found in each patient is indicated on the right and ranges from 90 kb to >2,500 kb.

Am. J. Hum. Genet. 77:89–96, 2005

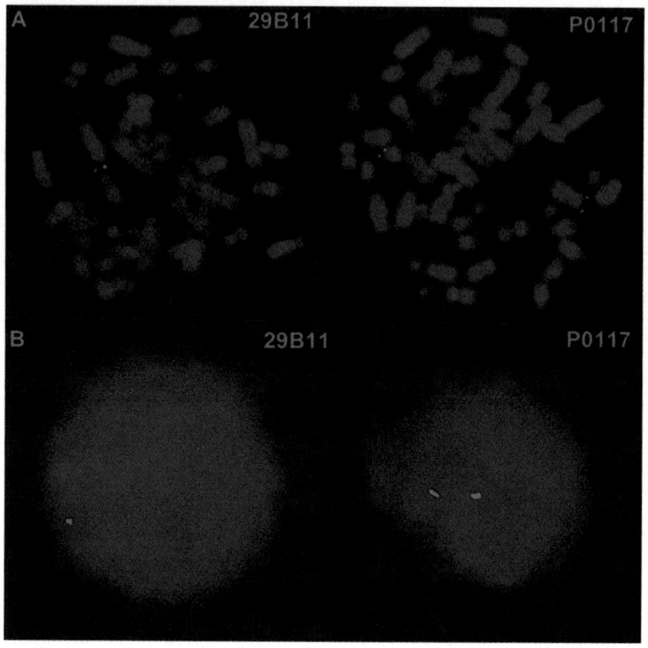

Figure 2 FISH of cosmids 29B11 and P0117 to metaphase (*A*) and interphase chromosomes (*B*) of patient LWD10. The absence of the signal of cosmid 29B11 and the presence of the signal of cosmid P0117 locates the breakpoint on cosmid P0117.

bination hotspots (May et al. 2002). Sequence comparisons of the breakpoint regions did not reveal sequence compositions that were similar to that the P0117 cosmid, suggesting that homologous recombination may not be the underlying mechanism for the deletions observed. Rather, we speculate that the unusual secondary structure of the proximal region, together, perhaps, with double-strand DNA breaks, may lead to recombination in this genomic region (Klein et al. 1996). The published sequence of the human X chromosome is 99.3% complete, and intrachromosomal duplications account for 2.6% of the X chromosome (Ross et al. 2005). Consistently, our sequence analysis and the data reported by Ross et al. (2005) exclude an intrachromosomal segmental duplication within the region of interest.

Other mechanisms underlying deletions, such as unequal crossover, have been previously described in the Xp22 region and lead to a high deletion frequency in X-linked ichthyosis (Shapiro et al. 1989; Yen et al. 1990). Interestingly, with a prevalence of 1 in 6,000 males, X-linked ichthyosis shows one of the highest incidences of deletions observed so far. Ninety percent of all patients exhibit deletion of the steroid sulfatase gene that results from homologous recombination between repetitive S232-like VNTR sequences that reside in the gene's flanking region (Yen et al. 1990; Li et al. 1992). Furthermore, approximately two-thirds of the patients suffering from DMD or Becker muscular dystrophy display deletions of one or many exons in the 2.5-Mb region encompassing the *DMD* gene (Blonden et al. 1989; Muntoni et al. 2003). Two deletion hotspots were found, one residing in the central part of the *DMD* gene and the other in the 5′ end of the gene, and screening of these two regions identified ~98% of all deletions. A detailed analysis of the more distal clustering of breakpoints in intron 44, however, has shown that the breakpoints are actually spread over a large intron of 240 kb (see the Leiden Muscular Dystrophy Pages). A real clustering at the sequence level, therefore, does not

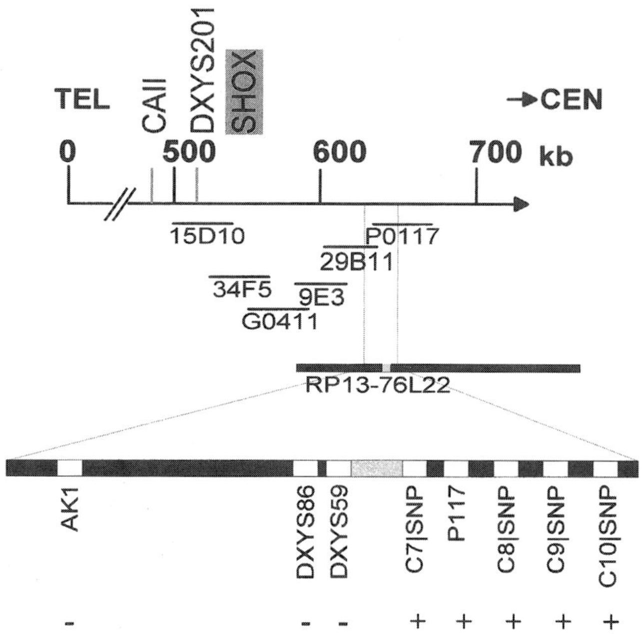

Figure 3 Results of SNP analysis of the critical breakpoint region of the overlap of cosmid clones P0117 and 29B11. This region—at ~655–678 kb from the telomere on the X chromosome and at 57–80 kb on the BAC clone RP13-76L22 (GenBank accession number AL683871.15) (on the basis of the UCSC Genome Browser human May 2004 assembly and NCBI build 35)—harbors the VNTR AK1 (655,357–656,210 bp), as well as the microsatellite marker *P117* (672,153–675,202 bp). SNPs within AK1, *DXYS86* (*P131*), *DXYS59* (dbSNP accession number rs6644571 at 666,749 bp), C7/SNP (dbSNP accession numbers rs1016964 at 671,526 bp and rs3995647 at 671,472 bp), and C8/SNP (dbSNP accession numbers rs2399945 at 676,936 bp and rs2399946 at 676,787 bp), as well as the few as-yet-unpublished SNPs within C9/SNP and C10/SNP, were checked for heterozygosity in seven families (patients LWD1, LWD6, LWD7, LWD10, LWD15, LWD16, and ISS30). The breakpoint of ~5 kb (indicated in gray) could be defined by the heterozygosity of the SNPs within C7/SNP and the absence of heterozygosity of SNPs within DXYS59. *SHOX* maps to 555,079–582,318 bp, AK1 to 655,357–656,210 bp, *DXYS86* to 665,323–665,477 bp, *DXYS59* to 666,696–666,875 bp, C7/SNP to 671,103–671,885 bp, *P117* to 672,153–675,202 bp, C8/SNP to 676,618–676,192 bp, C9/SNP to 679,663–681,329 bp, and C10/SNP to 683,363–684,552 bp (from the telomere).

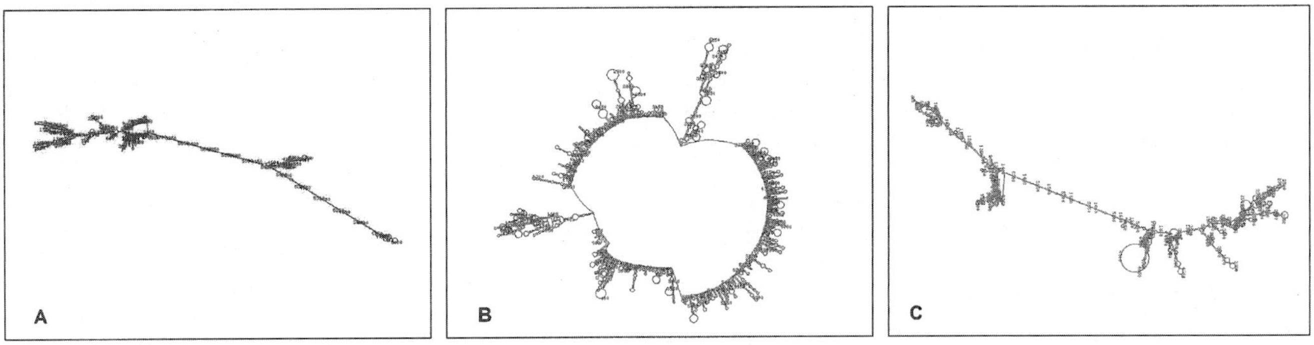

Figure 4 Secondary-structure prediction, made by use of Mfold analysis, of the sequence harboring the hotspot region (*B*) and the 6-kb sequences distal (*A*) and proximal (*C*) to it. The free-energy values for each secondary-structure prediction are −902 kcal/mol (*A*), −617.9 kcal/mol (*B*), and −677.8 kcal/mol (*C*). High DNA bending and an extensive secondary-structure formation are observed only in the hotspot region (*B*).

exist. With a prevalence of 1 in 3,500 males (i.e., 1 in 7,000 in the total population), the two deletion hotspots reach a frequency of ~1 in 11,000 individuals in the population (Bogdanovich et al. 2003).

The presence of a deletion hotspot in 73% (95% CI 56%–85%) of patients with short stature and with a *SHOX* deletion suggests a prevalence of this breakpoint of ~1:2,000 in the total population (95% CI 1:2,350–1:3,570), which is based on the assumption that the disorder found in most people with short stature is idiopathic. This implies that the recurrent deletion breakpoint identified in this study is rather frequent in the heterogeneous group of patients with short stature and, furthermore, may represent the most frequent known deletion breakpoint leading to disease.

Acknowledgments

We are indebted to all the clinicians and patients who worked closely with us. This work was performed with the support of the University of Heidelberg Medical Faculty and of Eli Lilly and Company. We thank Dr. Martijn Breuning, Beatrix Startt, and Anne Jordan for helpful comments.

Web Resources

The accession number and URLs for data presented herein are as follows:

dbSNP, http://www.ncbi.nlm.nih.gov/SNP/ (for *DXYS59* [accession number rs6644571], C7/SNPs [accession numbers rs1016964 and rs3995647], and C8/SNPs [accession numbers rs2399945 and rs2399946])

GenBank, http://www.ncbi.nih.gov/Genbank/ (for RP13-76L22 [accession number AL683871.15])

Leiden Muscular Dystrophy Pages, http://www.dmd.nl/DMD_deldup.html

Mfold, http://www.bioinfo.rpi.edu/applications/mfold/

Online Mendelian Inheritance in Man (OMIM), http://www.ncbi.nih.gov/Omim/ (for *SHOX*, LWD, and ISS)

UCSC Genome Bioinformatics, http://www.genome.ucsc.edu/

References

Antonarakis SE, Krawczak M, Cooper DN (2000) Disease-causing mutations in the human genome. Eur J Pediatr 159 Suppl 3:S173–S178

Ballabio A, Bardoni B, Carrozz R, Andria G, Bick D, Campbell L, Hame B, Ferguson-Smith MA, Gimelli G, Fraccaro M, Maraschio P, Zuffard O, Guioli S, Camerino G (1989) Contiguous gene syndromes due to deletions in the distal short arm of the human X chromosome. Proc Natl Acad Sci USA 86:10001–10005

Belin V, Cusin V, Viot G, Girlich D, Toutain A, Moncla A, Vekemans M, Le Merrer M, Munnich A, Cormier-Daire V (1998) SHOX mutations in dyschondrosteosis (Léri-Weill syndrome). Nat Genet 19:67–69

Binder G, Ranke MB, Martin DD (2003) Auxology is a valuable instrument for the clinical diagnosis of SHOX haploinsufficiency in school children with unexplained short stature. J Clin Endocrinol Metab 88:4891–4896

Blaschke RJ, Rappold GA (2000) SHOX: Growth, Léri-Weill and Turner syndromes. Trends Endocrinol Metab 11:227–230

Blonden LA, den Dunnen JT, van Paassen HM, Wapenaar MC, Grootscholten PM, Ginjaar HB, Bakker E, Pearson PL, van Ommen GJ (1989) High resolution deletion breakpoint mapping in the DMD gene by whole cosmid hybridization. Nucleic Acids Res 17:5611–5621

Bogdanovich S, Perkins K, Krag TOB, Khurana TS (2003) Therapeutics for Duchenne muscular dystrophy: current approaches and future directions. J Mol Med 82:102–115

Cooper DN, Ball EV, Krawzcak M (1998) The human mutation database. Nucleic Acids Res 26:285–287

Cormier-Daire V, Belin V, Cusin V, Viot G, Girlich D, Toutain A, Moncla A, Vekemans M, Le Merrer M, Munnich A (1999) SHOX gene mutations and deletions in dyschondrosteosis or Léri-Weill syndrome. Acta Paediatr Suppl 88:55–59

Cormier-Daire V, Huber C, Munnich A (2001) Allelic and nonallelic heterogeneity in dyschondrosteosis (Léri-Weill syndrome). Am J Med Genet 106:272–274

Ellison JW, Wardak Z, Young MF, Robey PG, Laig-Webster M, Chiong W (1997) PHOG, a candidate gene for involvement in the short stature of Turner syndrome. Hum Mol Genet 6:1341–1347

Falcinelli C, Iughetti L, Percesepe A, Calabrese G, Chiarelli F, Cisternino M, De Sanctis L, Pucarelli I, Radetti G, Wasniewska M, Weber G, Stuppia L, Bernasconi S, Forabosco A (2001) SHOX point mutations and deletions in Leri-Weill dyschondrosteosis. J Med Genet 39:E33

Flanagan SF, Munns CF, Hayes M, Williams B, Berry M, Vickers D, Rao E, Rappold GA, Batch JA, Hyland VJ, Glass IA (2002) Prevalence of mutations in the short stature homeobox containing gene (SHOX) in Madelung deformity of childhood. J Med Genet 39:758–763

Grigelioniene G, Eklof O, Ivarsson SA, Westphal O, Neumeyer L, Kedra D, Dumanski J, Hagenas L (2000) Mutations in short stature homeobox containing gene (SHOX) in dyschondrosteosis but not in hypochondroplasia. Hum Genet 107:145–149

Grigelioniene G, Schoumans J, Neumeyer L, Ivarsson A, Eklof O, Enkvist O, Tordai P, Fosdal I, Myhre AG, Westphal O, Nilsson NO, Elfving M, Ellis I, Anderlid BM, Fransson I, Tapia-Paez I, Nordenskjold M, Hagenas L, Dumanski JP (2001) Analysis of short stature homeobox-containing gene (SHOX) and auxological phenotype in dyschondrosteosis and isolated Madelung deformity. Hum Genet 109:551–558

Hernandez-Martin A, Gonzales-Sarmiento R, De Unamuno P (1999) X-linked ichthyosis: an update. Br J Dermatol 141: 617–627

Huber C, Cusin V, Le Merrer M, Mathieu M, Sulmont V, Dagoneau N, Munnich A, Cormier-Daire V (2001) SHOX point mutations in dyschondrosteosis. J Med Genet 38:323–351

Klein S, Zenvirth D, Sherman A, Ried K, Rappold GA, Simchen G (1996) Double strand breaks on YACs during yeast meiosis may reflect meiotic recombination in the human genome. Nat Genet 13:481–484

Klink A, Wapenaar M, van Ommen GJ, Rappold G (1993) AK1 detects a VNTR locus in the pseudoautosomal region. Hum Mol Genet 2:339

Li XM, Yen PH, Shapiro LJ (1992) Characterization of a low copy repetitive element S232 involved in the generation of frequent deletions of the distal short arm of the human X chromosome. Nucleic Acids Res 20:1117–1122

Lichter P, Cremer T (1992) Human cytogenetics: a practical approach. Oxford University Press, Oxford

May CA, Shone AC, Kalaydjieva L, Sajantila A, Jeffreys AJ (2002) Crossover clustering and rapid decay of linkage disequilibrium in the Xp/Yp pseudoautosomal gene SHOX. Nat Genet 31:272–275

Morizio E, Stuppia L, Gatta V, Fantasia D, Guanciali Franchi P, Rinaldi MM, Scarano G, Concolino D, Giannotti A, Verrotti A, Chiarelli F, Calabrese G, Palka G (2003) Deletion of the SHOX gene in patients with short stature of unknown cause. Am J Med Genet A 119:293–296

Muntoni F, Torelli S, Ferlini A (2003) Dystrophin and mutations: one gene, several proteins, multiple phenotypes. Lancet Neurol 2:731–740

Rao E, Weiss B, Fukami M, Mertz A, Meder J, Ogata T, Heinrich U, Garcia-Heras J, Schiebel K, Rappold GA (1997*a*) FISH-deletion mapping defines a 270-kb short stature critical interval in the pseudoautosomal region PAR1 on human sex chromosomes. Hum Genet 100:236–239

Rao E, Weiss B, Fukami M, Rump A, Niesler B, Mertz A, Muroya K, Binder G, Kirsch S, Winkelmann M, Nordsiek G, Heinrich U, Breuning MH, Ranke MB, Rosenthal A, Ogata T, Rappold GA (1997*b*) Pseudoautosomal deletions encompassing a novel homeobox gene cause growth failure in idiopathic short stature and Turner syndrome. Nat Genet 16: 54–63

Rappold GA, Fukami M, Niesler B, Schiller S, Zumkeller W, Bettendorf M, Heinrich U, Vlachopapadoupoulou E, Reinehr T, Onigata K, Ogata T (2002) Deletions of the homeobox gene SHOX (short stature homeobox) are an important cause of growth failure in children with short stature. J Clin Endocrinol Metab 87:1402–1406

Rappold GA, Klink A, Weiss B, Fischer C (1994) Double crossover in the human Xp/Yp pseudoautosomal region and its bearing on interference. Hum Mol Genet 3:1337–1340

Ross JL, Scott C Jr, Marttila P, Kowal K, Nass A, Papenhausen P, Abboudi J, Osterman L, Kushner H, Carter P, Ezaki M, Elder F, Wei F, Chen H, Zinn AR (2001) Phenotypes associated with SHOX deficiency. J Clin Endocrinol Metab 86: 5674–5680

Ross MT, Grafham DV, Coffey AJ, Scherer S, McLay K, Muzny D, Platzer M, et al (2005) The DNA sequence of the human X chromosome. Nature 434:325–337

Schiller S, Spranger S, Schechinger B, Fukami M, Merker S, Drop SL, Troger J, Knoblauch H, Kunze J, Seidel J, Rappold GA (2000) Phenotypic variation and genetic heterogeneity in Léri-Weill syndrome. Eur J Hum Genet 8:54–56

Shapiro LJ, Yen P, Pomerantz D, Martin E, Rolewic L, Mohandas T (1989) Molecular studies of deletions at the human steroid sulfatase locus. Proc Natl Acad Sci USA 86:8477–8481

Shears DJ, Vassal HJ, Goodman FR, Palmer RW, Reardon W, Superti-Furga A, Scambler PJ, Winter RM (1998) Mutation and deletion of the pseudoautosomal gene SHOX cause Léri-Weill dyschondrosteosis. Nat Genet 19:70–73

Spranger S, Schiller S, Jauch A, Wolff K, Rauterberg-Ruland I, Hager D, Tariverdian G, Troger J, Rappold, G (1999) Léri-Weill syndrome as part of a contiguous gene syndrome at Xp22.3. Am J Med Genet 83:367–371

Wapenaar MC, Petit C, Basler E, Ballabio A, Henke A, Rappold GA, van Paassen HMB, Blonden LAJ, van Ommen GJB (1992) Physical mapping of 14 new DNA markers isolated from the human distal Xp region. Genomics 13:167–175

Yen PH, Li XM, Tsai SP, Johnson C, Mohandas T, Shapiro LJ (1990) Frequent deletions of the human X chromosome distal short arm result from recombination between low copy repetitive elements. Cell 61:603–10

Zuker M (2003) Mfold web server for nucleic acid folding and hybridization prediction. Nucleic Acids Res 31:3406–3415

A Powerful and Robust Method for Mapping Quantitative Trait Loci in General Pedigrees

G. Diao and D. Y. Lin

Department of Biostatistics, University of North Carolina, Chapel Hill

The variance-components model is the method of choice for mapping quantitative trait loci in general human pedigrees. This model assumes normally distributed trait values and includes a major gene effect, random polygenic and environmental effects, and covariate effects. Violation of the normality assumption has detrimental effects on the type I error and power. One possible way of achieving normality is to transform trait values. The true transformation is unknown in practice, and different transformations may yield conflicting results. In addition, the commonly used transformations are ineffective in dealing with outlying trait values. We propose a novel extension of the variance-components model that allows the true transformation function to be completely unspecified. We present efficient likelihood-based procedures to estimate variance components and to test for genetic linkage. Simulation studies demonstrated that the new method is as powerful as the existing variance-components methods when the normality assumption holds; when the normality assumption fails, the new method still provides accurate control of type I error and is substantially more powerful than the existing methods. We performed a genomewide scan of monoamine oxidase B for the Collaborative Study on the Genetics of Alcoholism. In that study, the results that are based on the existing variance-components method changed dramatically when three outlying trait values were excluded from the analysis, whereas our method yielded essentially the same answers with or without those three outliers. The computer program that implements the new method is freely available.

Introduction

Mapping genes associated with various traits and diseases is one of the most important research areas in human genetics. A major effort in the gene-mapping process is the detection of loci that influence quantitative traits, which are referred to as "quantitative trait loci" (QTLs). Because complex diseases are associated with complex traits, many of which are quantitative, QTL analysis plays a critical role in the genetic dissection of complex human diseases. The recent explosion in genetic mapping data has placed a premium on the development of statistical methods for mapping QTLs (Pratt et al. 2000). Feingold (2001, 2002) provided excellent reviews of QTL-mapping methods, all of which are based on the principle that family members who have similar trait values should have higher-than-expected levels of identity-by-descent (IBD) allele sharing near the genes that influence those traits.

The simplest QTL-mapping method is Haseman-Elston (1972) regression, which regresses the squared differences in the trait values of sib pairs on their IBD sharing at a putative locus. Several groups (Wright 1997; Drigalenko 1998; Elston et al. 2000; Xu et al. 2000; Forrest 2001; Sham and Purcell 2001; Visscher and Hopper 2001) have attempted to improve the power of this regression by use of both the squared trait sum and the squared trait difference, whereas others (Tang and Siegmund 2001; Putter et al. 2002; Wang and Huang 2002) have proposed score statistics with similar properties. All these methods are limited to sibships or, in many cases, to sib pairs. Sham et al. (2002) offered a regression method for extended pedigrees. The idea is to reverse the Haseman-Elston paradigm by regressing the IBD sharing on an appropriate function of the trait values. This method requires specification of the correlation for each type of relative pair and does not accommodate covariate effects, gene-environment interactions, epistasis, or pleiotropy. Its type I error is inflated in some circumstances. Chiou et al. (2005) proposed to estimate the probability that a sib pair shares the same allele at the trait locus as a nonparametric function of the trait values.

An alternative approach is the variance-components model (Goldgar 1990; Schork 1993; Amos 1994; Fulker et al. 1995; Almasy and Blangero 1998; Pratt et al. 2000). This model decomposes the overall phenotypic variability among individuals within pedigrees into fixed effects due to observed covariates, random effects due to

Received February 17, 2005; accepted for publication May 6, 2005; electronically published May 25, 2005.

Address for correspondence and reprints: Dr. Danyu Lin, Department of Biostatistics, University of North Carolina, McGavran-Greenberg Hall, CB 7420, Chapel Hill, NC 27599-7420. E-mail: lin@bios.unc.edu

0002-9297/2005/7701-0010$15.00

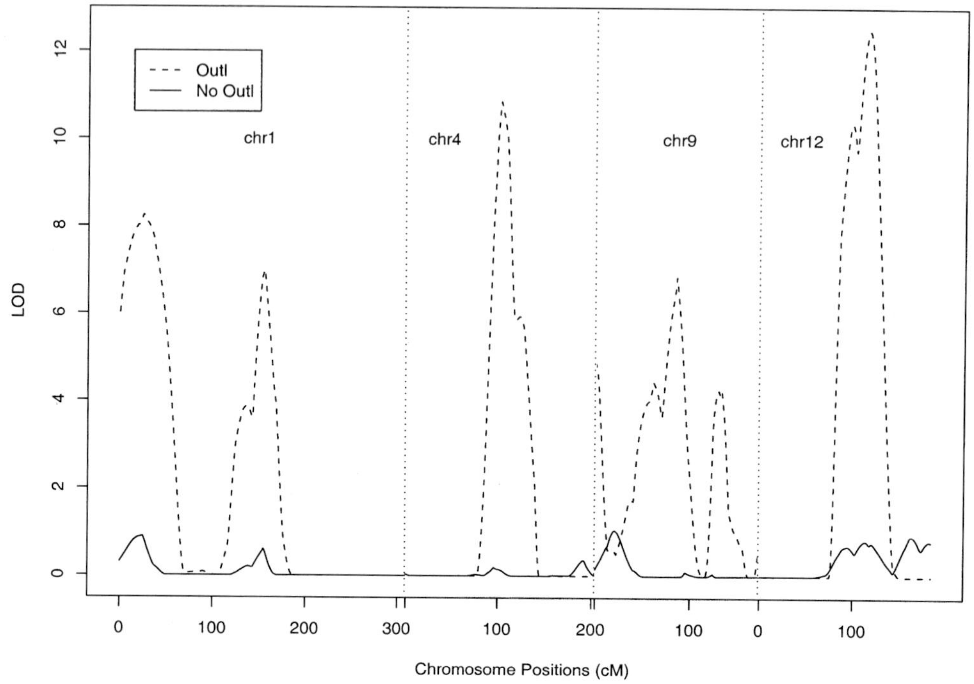

Figure 1 Multipoint LOD scores from the existing variance-components method for chromosomes 1, 4, 9, and 12 in the COGA study. Outl = outliers included; No Outl = outliers excluded.

an unobserved trait-affecting major locus, random polygenic effects, and residual nongenetic variance. The analysis is typically based on maximum-likelihood estimation. This approach is applicable to any type of pedigree and has substantially higher power than Haseman-Elston and related methods (Amos et al. 1996; Williams et al. 1997; Almasy and Blangero 1998; Pratt et al. 2000; Forrest 2001; Tang and Siegmund 2001; Feingold 2001, 2002). "It has superseded Haseman-Elston as the method of choice for most studies, particularly when large pedigrees are used" (Feingold 2002, p. 217).

The variance-components model assumes that the trait values of family members follow a multivariate normal distribution. When this assumption is violated, the parameter estimators can be severely biased, the type I error can be substantially inflated, and the power can be drastically reduced (Amos et al. 1996; Allison et al. 1999; Tang and Siegmund 2001; Feingold 2001, 2002). In this sense, the variance-components approach is less robust than Haseman-Elston regression (Allison et al. 2000). When there is nonnormality, one strategy is to perform a parametric transformation, such as the log transformation or square-root transformation on the trait values to approximate normality (Allison et al. 2000; Geller et al. 2003; Strug et al. 2003). It is often difficult to find an appropriate transformation, especially when there are negative trait values, and different transformations may yield conflicting results. Incorrect transformations will cause biased parameter estimators, inflated type I error, and loss of power. Furthermore, parametric transformations are not effective in handling outlying trait values, which can create spurious linkage signals.

Figure 1 plots the LOD scores for the variance-components analysis of monoamine oxidase B (MAOB) from the Collaborative Study on the Genetics of Alcoholism (COGA), which is a multicenter study for identification of genes that cause alcohol dependence (Begleiter et al. 1995). MAOB is a mitochondrial enzyme whose measurement is positive and can be large. The original analysis showed significant evidence of linkage on chromosomes 1, 4, 9, and 12. Three members in a family had unusually large MAOB values. When those three individuals were removed from the analysis, the evidence of linkage completely disappeared. This kind of phenomenon has deterred human geneticists from performing QTL analysis (Allison et al. 1999).

A question naturally arises as to whether there exists a method that retains the robustness of Haseman-Elston regression while approaching the greater power of the variance components model (Feingold 2001). The present article provides a positive answer to this question. We propose a novel modification of the variance-components model to allow a completely arbitrary transformation function of trait values. We then derive maximum-likelihood estimators of variance components and

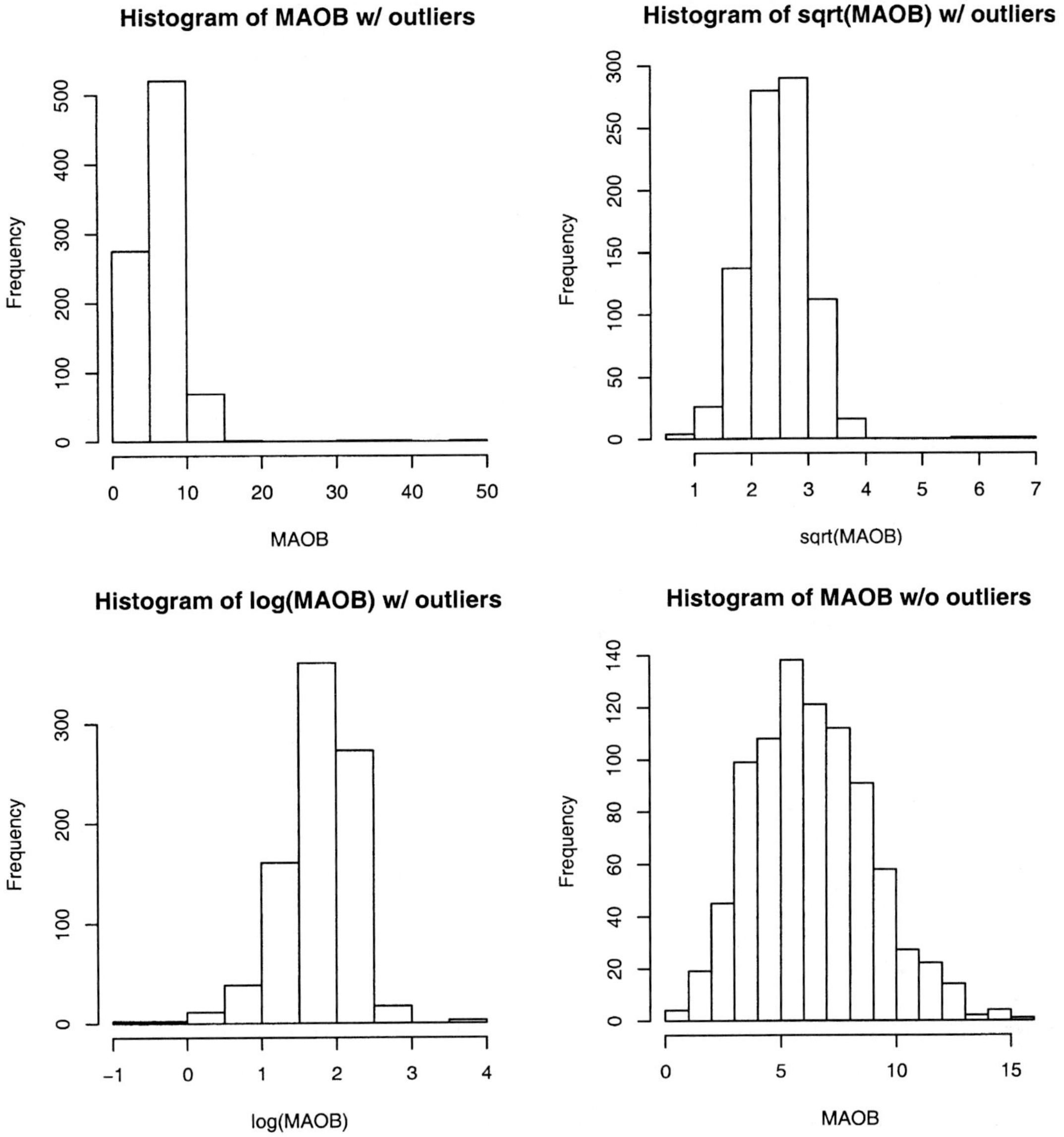

Figure 2 Histograms of MAOB activity in the COGA study

construct likelihood-ratio statistics for testing the existence of QTLs at arbitrary locations along the genome. We implement the new method in a free computer program. Extensive simulation studies demonstrate that our new method is as efficient as the existing variance-component methods when the normality assumption holds; under nonnormality, the new method continues to have proper type I error and good power, whereas the existing methods have inflated type I error and diminished power. Unlike existing methods, the new method is insensitive to outliers. The application of the new method to the aforementioned COGA data resolved the dilemma caused by the three outlying observations.

Material and Methods

Consider n general pedigrees or families and n_i relatives in the ith family, $i = 1, \ldots, n$. Let Y_{ij} denote the trait value for the jth relative of the ith family and $\mathbf{X}_{ij}$ a vector of directly observable covariates. At each genome position to be examined, we consider a variance-components model that partitions the total phenotypic variance into components that are due to a major gene at the locus, other unlinked genes, covariates, and environmental factors:

$$H(Y_{ij}) = \boldsymbol{\beta}^T\mathbf{X}_{ij} + g_{ij} + G_{ij} + e_{ij}\ , \qquad (1)$$

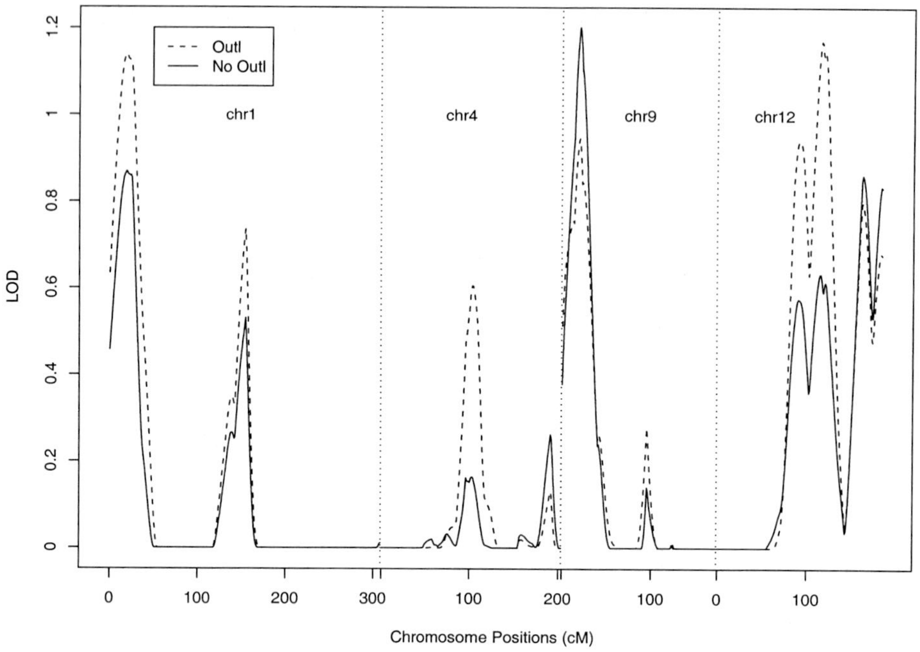

Figure 3 Multipoint LOD scores from the new method for chromosomes 1, 4, 9, and 12 in the COGA study. Outl = outliers included; No Outl = outliers excluded.

where H is an unknown increasing function, $\boldsymbol{\beta}$ is a set of fixed effects, g_{ij} is a random effect due to the major gene, G_{ij} is a random effect due to other genes at unlinked loci, and e_{ij} is an individual-specific residual environmental effect. The random effects are assumed to be normally distributed with mean 0 and variances σ_g^2, σ_G^2, and σ_e^2. Because H is an arbitrary function, we constrain the residual variance σ_e^2 to be 1, and we do not include an intercept in the model, since the intercept can be absorbed by H.

Assume that g_{ij}, G_{ij}, and e_{ij} are not correlated. Then the total trait variance Var $[H(Y_{ij})]$ is $\sigma^2 = \sigma_g^2 + \sigma_G^2 + \sigma_e^2$. The overall heritability of the trait is

$$h^2 = \frac{\sigma_g^2 + \sigma_G^2}{\sigma^2} ,$$

and the heritability attributable to the examined locus is

$$h_g^2 = \frac{\sigma_g^2}{\sigma^2} .$$

The genetic variances can be optionally decomposed into additive and dominant effects, with $\sigma_g^2 = \sigma_{ga}^2 + \sigma_{gd}^2$ and $\sigma_G^2 = \sigma_{Ga}^2 + \sigma_{Gd}^2$. We may include a household-specific random effect in the model, since the relatives in a household share the same environment. The model can also be easily extended to include interactions between different effects as well as multiple trait-affecting loci. For simplicity of description, we focus on equation (1).

We refer to equation (1) as a semiparametric linear transformation model with random effects or as semiparametric variance-components model because the true transformation function H is unspecified. By contrast, the existing variance-components model is parametric, because the transformation is assumed to be known or is implicitly incorporated in the definition of Y. Allowing an unknown transformation function is equivalent to allowing an arbitrary trait distribution, in that, for any distribution of Y, there always exists a transformation H such that $H(Y)$ has the standard normal distribution. In this sense, equation (1) generalizes the existing variance-components model to allow an arbitrary trait distribution.

The trait covariance between any two pedigree members can be expressed as a weighted sum of the variance components

$$\mathrm{Cov}\,[H(Y_{ij}),H(Y_{ik})] = \begin{cases} \sigma_{ga}^2 + \sigma_{gd}^2 + \sigma_{Ga}^2 + \sigma_{Gd}^2 + \sigma_e^2 & \text{if } j = k \\ \pi_{ijk}\sigma_{ga}^2 + \delta_{ijk}\sigma_{gd}^2 + 2\Phi_{ijk}\sigma_{Ga}^2 + \Delta_{ijk}\sigma_{Gd}^2 & \text{if } j \neq k \end{cases} , \quad (2)$$

where π_{ijk} is the proportion of alleles at the major locus that are IBD in the jth and kth relatives of the ith family, δ_{ijk} is the probability that both alleles at the locus are

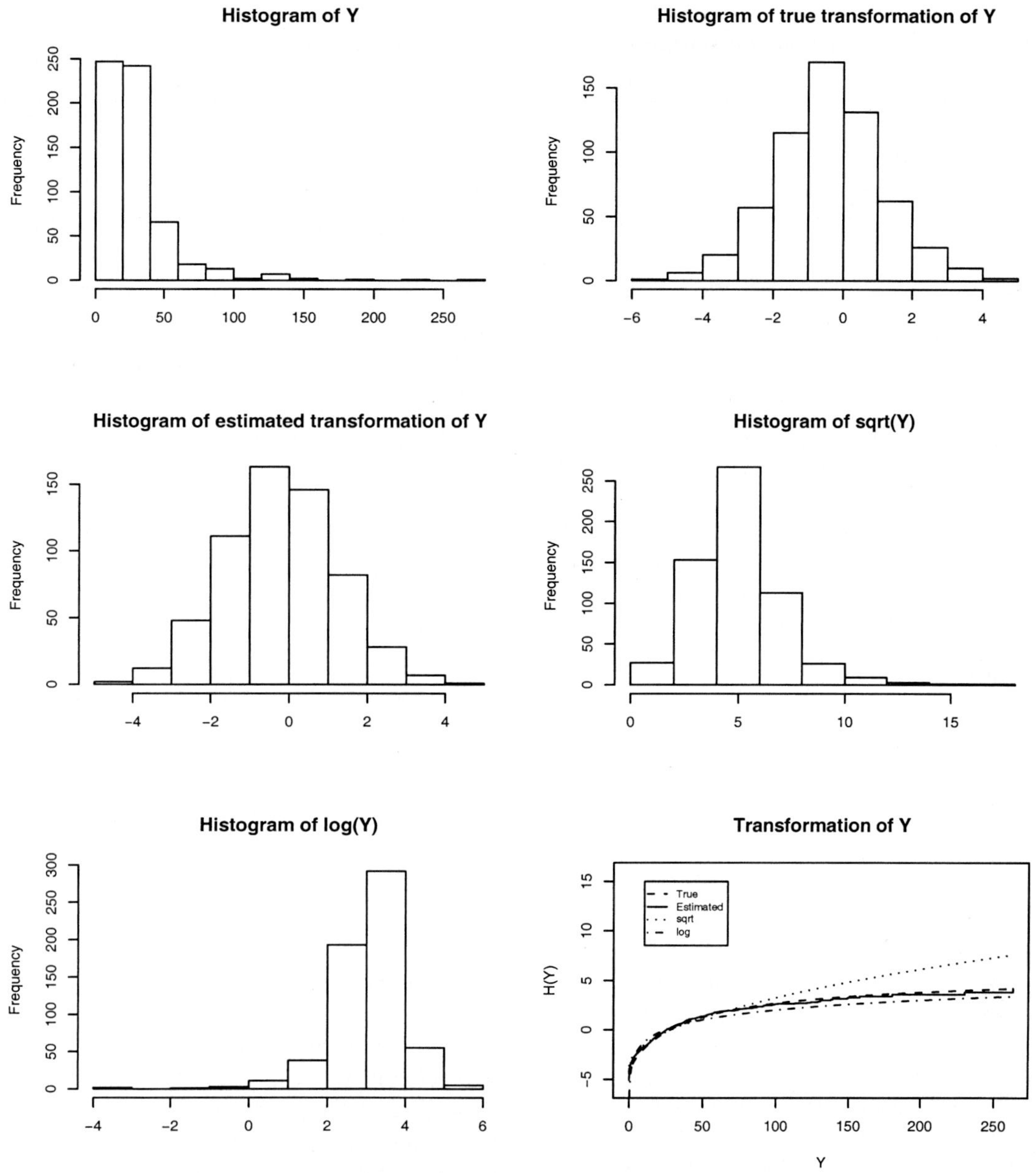

Figure 4 Histograms of trait values under various transformations and plots of the true, square-root, log, and estimated transformations for a simulated data set with 200 sib trios.

IBD, Φ_{ijk} is the kinship coefficient of relatives j and k, and Δ_{ijk} is the expected probability that the relatives share both alleles IBD. Note that π_{ijk} and δ_{ijk} are determined by the genotyping data, whereas Φ_{ijk} and Δ_{ijk} depend on only the degree of relatedness. We can infer the IBD allele–sharing probabilities at an arbitrary genome position by using the exact multipoint algorithm (Lander and Green 1987) implemented in GENEHUNTER (Kruglyak et al. 1996) or the approximation given in SOLAR (Almasy and Blangero 1998).

Write $\Lambda(y) = e^{H(y)}$. Let γ denote the variance parameters σ_{ga}^2, σ_{gd}^2, σ_{Ga}^2, σ_{Gd}^2, and σ_e^2, and let $\boldsymbol{\theta}$ denote the parameters $\boldsymbol{\beta}$, γ and $\Lambda(\cdot)$. The log likelihood for $\boldsymbol{\theta}$ is given as

$$c - \frac{1}{2}\sum_{i=1}^{n} \log|\det(\mathbf{V}_i)| - \frac{1}{2}\sum_{i=1}^{n}(\mathbf{H}_i - \mathbf{X}_i\boldsymbol{\beta})^T\mathbf{V}_i^{-1} \times(\mathbf{H}_i - \mathbf{X}_i\boldsymbol{\beta}) + \sum_{i=1}^{n}\sum_{j=1}^{n_i}\log\frac{\lambda(Y_{ij})}{\Lambda(Y_{ij})}, \quad (3)$$

where c is a constant, $\mathbf{X}_i$ is the matrix of covariates for

Table 1

Type I Error and Power (%) of Likelihood-Ratio Tests under Nonnormality, with 200 Sib Trios

	Type I Error and Power (%) for														
				Existing Methods											
	New Method			True			Square Root			Log			Untransformed		
Model	$\alpha = 5$	$\alpha = 1$	$\alpha = .1$	$\alpha = 5$	$\alpha = 1$	$\alpha = .1$	$\alpha = 5$	$\alpha = 1$	$\alpha = .1$	$\alpha = 5$	$\alpha = 1$	$\alpha = .1$	$\alpha = 5$	$\alpha = 1$	$\alpha = .1$
a	4.97	.99	.13	4.80	.92	.10	6.84	1.96	.31	6.42	1.68	.29	14.71	7.39	3.37
b	24.43	8.69	1.73	24.60	8.58	1.66	24.48	10.06	2.66	24.52	9.32	2.34	26.70	14.60	6.93
c	60.40	33.75	12.23	60.64	33.83	12.07	55.30	31.22	12.16	55.75	31.46	11.73	43.75	27.11	13.65
d	5.02	.85	.10	5.02	.85	.08	5.74	1.39	.17	5.70	1.11	.18	9.70	4.08	1.82
e	21.89	7.06	1.06	21.94	7.18	1.14	21.27	7.62	1.34	21.41	6.76	1.33	19.55	8.74	3.52
f	54.09	27.43	7.52	54.23	28.08	8.04	49.47	24.37	7.54	50.07	25.06	6.98	34.81	17.61	7.32

the ith family, $\mathbf{V}_i$ is the variance-covariance matrix of the ith family derived from equation (2), $\lambda(\cdot)$ is the derivative of $\Lambda(\cdot)$, and $\mathbf{H}_i$ is the vector of $[\log\Lambda(Y_{i1}),\ldots,\log\Lambda(Y_{in_i})]$. This is a nonparametric likelihood (Bickel et al. 1993), in that the function $H(\cdot)$ or $\Lambda(\cdot)$ is completely unspecified.

In the current variance-components literature, the transformation function H is assumed to be known, so that the log likelihood takes the form

$$c-\frac{1}{2}\sum_{i=1}^{n}\log|\det(\mathbf{V}_i)| -\frac{1}{2}\sum_{i=1}^{n}(\mathbf{H}_i-\mathbf{X}_i\boldsymbol{\beta})^T\mathbf{V}_i^{-1}(\mathbf{H}_i-\mathbf{X}_i\boldsymbol{\beta}) .$$

There are two key differences between this parametric log likelihood and the nonparametric log likelihood given in expression (3). First, the last term of expression (3) does not enter into the parametric log likelihood. Second, the values of $H(Y_{ij})$ are known in the parametric log likelihood but are unknown function of the trait values in the nonparametric log likelihood.

We wish to estimate the finite-dimensional parameters $\boldsymbol{\beta}$ and $\boldsymbol{\gamma}$, along with the infinite-dimensional parameter $\Lambda(\cdot)$, by maximizing the nonparametric log likelihood given in (3). The maximum of (3) is infinity if $\Lambda(\cdot)$ is restricted to be absolutely continuous, since we can always choose some function $\Lambda(y)$ with fixed values at the Y_{ij} while letting $\lambda(Y_{ij})$ go to infinity. Thus, we allow $\Lambda(\cdot)$ to be right-continuous and maximize the function

$$\log L(\boldsymbol{\theta}) = c-\frac{1}{2}\sum_{i=1}^{n}\log|\det(\mathbf{V}_i)| -\frac{1}{2}\sum_{i=1}^{n}(\mathbf{H}_i-\mathbf{X}_i\boldsymbol{\beta})^T\mathbf{V}_i^{-1}(\mathbf{H}_i-\mathbf{X}_i\boldsymbol{\beta}) +\sum_{i=1}^{n}\sum_{j=1}^{n_i}\log\frac{\Lambda\{Y_{ij}\}}{\Lambda(Y_{ij})} , \quad (4)$$

where $\Lambda\{Y_{ij}\}$ is the jump size of $\Lambda(y)$ at $y = Y_{ij}$; that is, the value of $\Lambda(y)$ at $y = Y_{ij}$ minus its value right before Y_{ij}. The resultant estimator, denoted by $\hat{\boldsymbol{\theta}} = (\hat{\boldsymbol{\beta}},\hat{\boldsymbol{\gamma}},\hat{\Lambda})$, is the maximum-likelihood estimator of $\boldsymbol{\theta}$ or, more precisely, the nonparametric maximum-likelihood estimator (Bickel et al. 1993).

It can be shown that $\hat{\Lambda}(\cdot)$ is a step function with jumps only at the observed values of Y_{ij}. Thus, $\hat{\boldsymbol{\theta}}$ is obtained by maximizing (4) over $\boldsymbol{\beta}$, $\boldsymbol{\gamma}$, and $\Lambda\{Y_{ij}\}$ ($i = 1,\ldots,n$; $j = 1,\ldots,n_i$). To ensure positive estimators for the jump sizes and variance parameters, we reparameterize $\Lambda\{Y_{ij}\}$ and $\boldsymbol{\gamma}$ as $\log(\Lambda\{Y_{ij}\})$ and $\log(\boldsymbol{\gamma})$ in the maximization. The maximization is realized via the quasi-Newton algorithm (Press et al. 1992). We chose the initial values of $\Lambda\{Y_{ij}\}$ in accordance with a common transformation, such as the log transformation. The first derivatives of (4) with respect to the unknown parameters are given in appendix A. In those expressions, the unknown parameters depend on the Y_{ij} only through the ranks of the Y_{ij}. This fact implies that the parameter estimators will remain the same if the trait values are replaced by their ranks. Thus, the proposed estimators are rank-based and hence robust to outliers. Note that the unknown transformation $H(y)$ is estimated by $\hat{H}(y) = \log\hat{\Lambda}(y)$.

Although it is a nonparametric maximum-likelihood estimator, $\hat{\boldsymbol{\theta}}$ possesses the familiar asymptotic properties of a parametric maximum-likelihood estimator. Specifically, $\hat{\boldsymbol{\theta}}$ is consistent, asymptotically normal, and asymptotically efficient, and its covariance matrix can be estimated by the inversed Fisher information matrix of (4). The asymptotic efficiency implies that $\hat{\boldsymbol{\theta}}$ is the most efficient estimator among all valid estimators of $\boldsymbol{\theta}$, at least in large samples. The proofs of these results involve very advanced mathematical arguments. The interested readers are referred to appendix B of Lin (2004) for an outline of arguments for this kind of problem. The detailed proofs are available from the authors on request.

We can use the familiar maximum-likelihood statis-

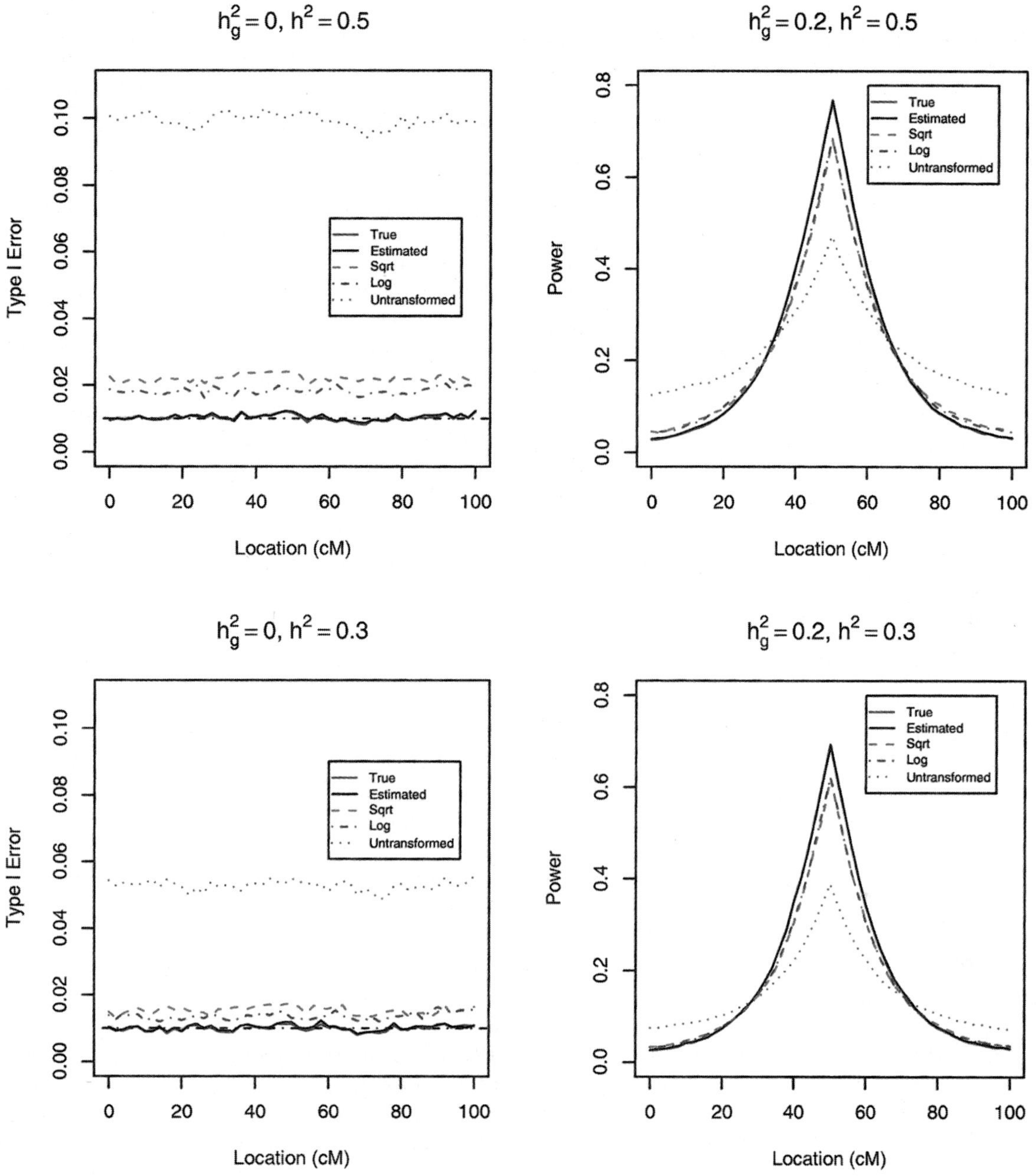

Figure 5 Type I error and power of likelihood-ratio tests with 500 sib trios at the nominal significance level of 0.01 under nonnormality. The curves for the estimated and true transformations are indistinguishable.

tics to make inferences about $\boldsymbol{\theta}$. In particular, we can perform various hypothesis tests according to the objectives of the linkage study at hand. For example, we can assess whether there is a major gene effect at the examined locus by testing the null hypothesis $H_0:\sigma^2_{ga} = \sigma^2_{gd} = 0$ against the alternative $H_A:\sigma^2_{ga} > 0$ or $\sigma^2_{gd} > 0$. We can also test the null hypothesis of no additive major-gene effect, $H_0:\sigma^2_{ga} = 0$, or the null hypothesis of no polygenic effects, $H_0:\sigma^2_{Ga} = \sigma^2_{Gd} = 0$. For each hypothesis test, we can calculate the likelihood-ratio statistic at any position along the genome with

$$LR = -2[\log L(\tilde{\boldsymbol{\theta}}) - \log L(\hat{\boldsymbol{\theta}})] \ ,$$

where $\tilde{\boldsymbol{\theta}}$ is the (restricted) maximum-likelihood estima-

Table 2

Means and SDs of Parameter Estimators under Nonnormality, with 200 Sib Pairs

	Mean (SD) of Parameter Estimator with			
	Unspecified Transformation		Known Transformation	
Model	β_1	σ_g^2	β_1	σ_g^2
a	−.486 (.115)	.080 (.120)	−.499 (.111)	.081 (.121)
b	−.486 (.115)	.212 (.178)	−.499 (.111)	.217 (.179)
c	−.486 (.114)	.388 (.205)	−.499 (.110)	.398 (.205)
d	−.493 (.118)	.086 (.129)	−.499 (.115)	.086 (.127)
e	−.494 (.117)	.210 (.181)	−.499 (.114)	.211 (.176)
f	−.497 (.117)	.368 (.202)	−.499 (.114)	.369 (.192)

tor of $\boldsymbol{\theta}$ under the null hypothesis. When we test a single variance component, the asymptotic distribution of the likelihood-ratio statistic is a half-and-half mixture of a χ_1^2 variable and a point mass at 0 (Self and Liang 1987). When multiple variance components are tested, the likelihood-ratio statistic has a more complex asymptotic distribution that continues to be a mixture of χ^2 distributions (Self and Liang 1987). The conventional LOD score is simply $LR/4.6$.

The proposed method is reminiscent of the well-known Cox (1972) regression analysis with survival data. In fact, the Cox proportional hazards model can be written as a semiparametric linear transformation model: $H(Y) = \boldsymbol{\beta}^T\mathbf{X} + \epsilon$, where H is an unknown increasing function and ϵ has the standard extreme-value distribution. The nonparametric maximum-likelihood estimators of $\boldsymbol{\beta}$ and $\Lambda(y) = e^{H(y)}$ are exactly the familiar maximum partial-likelihood estimator of the relative risk and the Breslow (1972) estimator of the cumulative hazard function. It is well known that the maximum partial likelihood estimator is rank based, the Breslow estimator is a step function, and both estimators are statistically efficient. Our estimators of $\boldsymbol{\beta}$ and Λ have the same properties.

Results

COGA Study

COGA is a six-center study aimed to detect and map susceptibility genes for alcohol dependence and related phenotypes (Begleiter et al. 1995). The study involved 105 families (typically 3 or 4 generations) with a total of 1,214 members. The largest family size was 37. A total of 992 individuals were genotyped at 285 autosomal markers on 22 chromosomes, with an average intermarker distance of 13.5 cM. We considered the quantitative trait MAOB. MAOB is a mitochondrial enzyme involved in the degradation of certain neurotransmitter amines, specifically phenylethylamine and benzylamine. Low platelet MAOB activity has been found to be associated with alcoholism (Major and Murphy 1978; Sullivan et al. 1979).

Information on MAOB activity in platelets was available for 904 of the 1,214 individuals. The mean MAOB activity was 6.48, with an SD of 3.17 and a median value of 6.17. Three outliers for MAOB activity—with values of 33.18, 38.61, and 45.44—were clustered in a single family; the values for the remaining individuals in this family were 3.53 and 6.05. Figure 2 presents the histograms of MAOB values with and without the three outliers. With the outliers, the distribution is severely right skewed and highly leptokurtic, with skewness of 4.02 and kurtosis of 40.7, as opposed to skewness of only 0.41 and kurtosis of 0.01 without outliers. Of the 904 individuals with MAOB-activity information, 432 were male, with a mean value of 5.58 and a median value of 5.36, and 472 were female, with a mean value of 7.31 and a median value of 7.20. MAOB activity tended to be lower for smokers than for nonsmokers, with mean values of 5.61 versus 7.24 and median values of 5.20 versus 7.22, respectively. MAOB activity also varied by ethnicity, with mean values of 7.72, 6.17, and 7.15 and median values of 6.98, 5.87, and 7.04 for ethnic groups "black, non-Hispanic," "white, non-Hispanic," and "white, Hispanic," respectively. We included age at interview, sex, ethnicity, and smoking status as covariates in our analysis.

We calculated the IBD allele–sharing probabilities at the 1-cM increment along the genome by using the computer package SOLAR (Almasy and Blangero 1998). We first performed the genomewide linkage scan of MAOB activity using the existing variance-components method. As shown in figure 1, significant evidence in favor of linkage with MAOB activity was observed on chromosomes 1, 4, 9, and 12, with peak LOD scores of at least 6. The peak LOD score on chromosome 12 exceeded 12. When the three outliers were deleted, the evidence of linkage completely disappeared. These results are similar to those of Barnholtz et al. (1999), who used the SAGE FSP program to break up the data set into nuclear families and then used a modified version of GENEHUNTER (Kruglyak et al. 1996; Amos et al. 1997) to calculate the multipoint IBD values. Clearly, the existing method is highly sensitive to outliers in this case.

As is evident in figure 2, parametric transformations are ineffective in handling outliers. The distributions are right skewed under the square-root transformation and left skewed under the log transformation. The kurtosis values are 6.3 and 3.0 under the square-root and log transformations, respectively. Under the square-root transformation, the peak LOD scores for chromosomes 1, 4, 9, and 12 are 2.6, 3.24, 1.67, and 3.83, respectively. Under the log transformation, the corresponding peaks are 0.88, 1.08, 1.64, and 1.18. It is disconcerting that these two transformations have conflicting results.

Table 3

Means and SDs of Estimators of h_g^2 under Nonnormality, with 200 Sib Pairs

	Mean (SD) for Estimator with				
		Specified Transformation			
Model	Unspecified Transformation	True	Square Root	Log	Identity
a	.043 (.063)	.041 (.061)	.047 (.070)	.046 (.068)	.080 (.132)
b	.113 (.093)	.109 (.090)	.110 (.097)	.109 (.097)	.126 (.150)
c	.207 (.104)	.200 (.101)	.193 (.112)	.193 (.110)	.184 (.162)
d	.044 (.065)	.043 (.064)	.046 (.069)	.046 (.067)	.064 (.108)
e	.107 (.088)	.106 (.088)	.103 (.091)	.103 (.090)	.103 (.125)
f	.184 (.093)	.185 (.094)	.175 (.099)	.176 (.098)	.149 (.133)

We also applied the new method to the COGA data and displayed the results in figure 3. No linkage signals were detected, regardless of whether the outliers were included or excluded. The two sets of LOD curves were similar to each other, and no LOD scores were >1.2. The new method is less sensitive to the outliers, so the results should be more trustworthy.

Simulation Studies

We conducted extensive simulation studies to evaluate the performance of the new method and to compare it with that of the existing methods. We generated trait values for sib trios from the model

$$H(Y_{ij}) = \beta_1 X_{1ij} + \beta_2 X_{2ij} + b_{ij} + e_{ij} , \quad (5)$$

where $\beta_1 = -0.5, \beta_2 = 0.5, X_{1ij}$ is a binary variable with 0.5 probability of being 1, X_{2ij} is an independent standard normal variable, b_{ij} consists of major gene and polygenic effects, and e_{ij} is the residual random error. The covariates X_{1ij} and X_{2ij} represent sex and standardized age, respectively. We simulated a 100-cM chromosome with 51 equally spaced markers by Markov chain under the Haldane mapping function. Each marker consisted of four equally frequent alleles. A true QTL was placed at the center of the chromosome. For simplicity, we considered only additive genetic effects. We varied the variance parameters to yield different values of overall genetic heritability h^2 and major-gene heritability h_g^2. In particular, we considered the following six scenarios.

Model	σ_g^2	σ_G^2	σ_e^2	h_g^2	h^2
a	.0	1.0	1.0	.0	.5
b	.2	.8	1.0	.1	.5
c	.4	.6	1.0	.2	.5
d	.0	.6	1.4	.0	.3
e	.2	.4	1.4	.1	.3
f	.4	.2	1.4	.2	.3

Scenarios a and d pertain to the null hypothesis, the others to alternative hypotheses. We considered 200 and 500 sib trios. For each setup, we simulated 10,000 data sets.

In the first series of studies, we generated U_{ij} from the model

$$U_{ij} = \beta_1 X_{1ij} + \beta_2 X_{2ij} + b_{ij} + e_{ij} ,$$

and set $Y_{ij} = e^{1+U_{ij}} + (5 + U_{ij})^2$. The resulting data have an average kurtosis of 44.5. After the square-root and log transformations, the average kurtosis values are 5.82 and 4.83, respectively.

We analyzed the data in five different ways: the new method and the existing methods with true transformation, log transformation, square-root transformation, and no transformation. The existing method with the true transformation pertains to the ideal situation in which the normality assumption holds (after a known transformation). Figure 4 shows the distribution of trait values for the first simulated data set. Neither the log transformation nor the square-root transformation provided a good normal approximation. The transformation estimated by the new method is almost identical to the true transformation and approximated the normal distribution very well.

We assessed the performance of the likelihood-ratio statistics for testing $H_0:\sigma_g^2 = 0$ versus $H_A:\sigma_g^2 > 0$ at the nominal significance level α of 5%, 1%, and 0.1%. Table

Table 4

Type I Error and Power (%) of Likelihood-Ratio Tests in the Presence of Outliers, with 200 Sib Trios

	Type I Error and Power (%) for					
	New Method			Existing Method		
Model	$\alpha = 5$	$\alpha = 1$	$\alpha = .1$	$\alpha = 5$	$\alpha = 1$	$\alpha = .1$
a	5.16	1.10	.08	7.95	2.85	.78
b	24.12	8.71	1.73	25.29	10.86	3.39
c	58.84	32.74	11.65	54.64	31.22	13.13
d	5.29	1.01	.10	7.62	2.33	.60
e	22.37	7.45	1.32	23.02	9.51	2.42
f	53.00	27.71	8.37	49.59	27.32	10.01

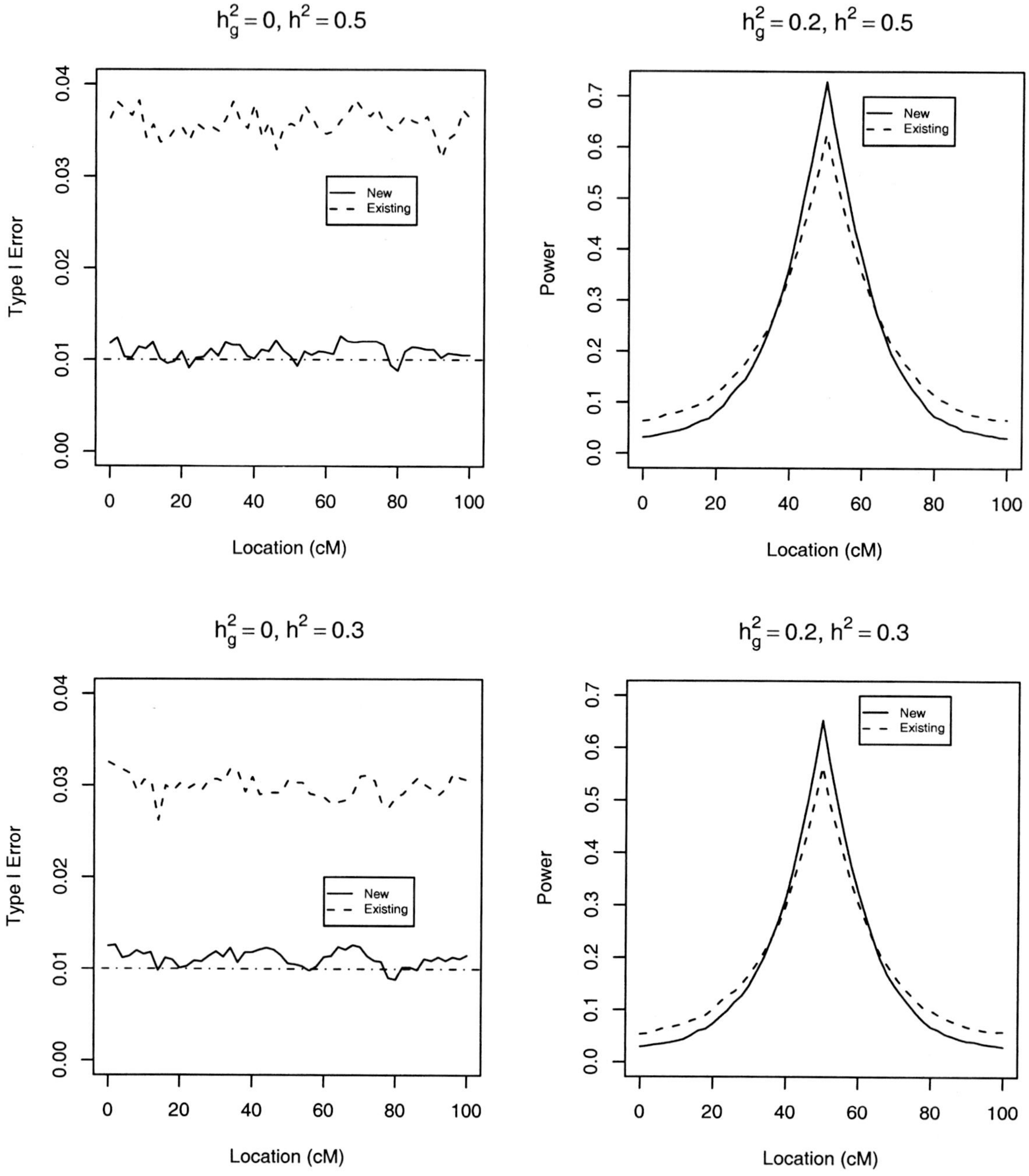

Figure 6 Type I error and power of likelihood-ratio tests with 500 sib trios at the nominal significance level of 0.01 with the presence of outliers.

1 presents the type I error and power at the true QTL with $n = 200$, whereas figure 5 displays the results of the linkage scans on the whole chromosome at the 2-cM increment with $n = 500$. The new method provides accurate control of type I error in all cases and has virtually the same power as the existing method with the true transformation. Thus, the new method performs as well as the parametric method under normality or with known transformation. Without transformation, the type I error of the existing method is very wrong. With the log or the square-root transformation, the type I error is still inflated. Although it has much smaller type I error than the existing methods, the new method tends to be more powerful than the existing methods with or without transformation, especially when there are strong genetic effects.

We also evaluated the estimators for the covariate effects, variance components, and heritability at the true

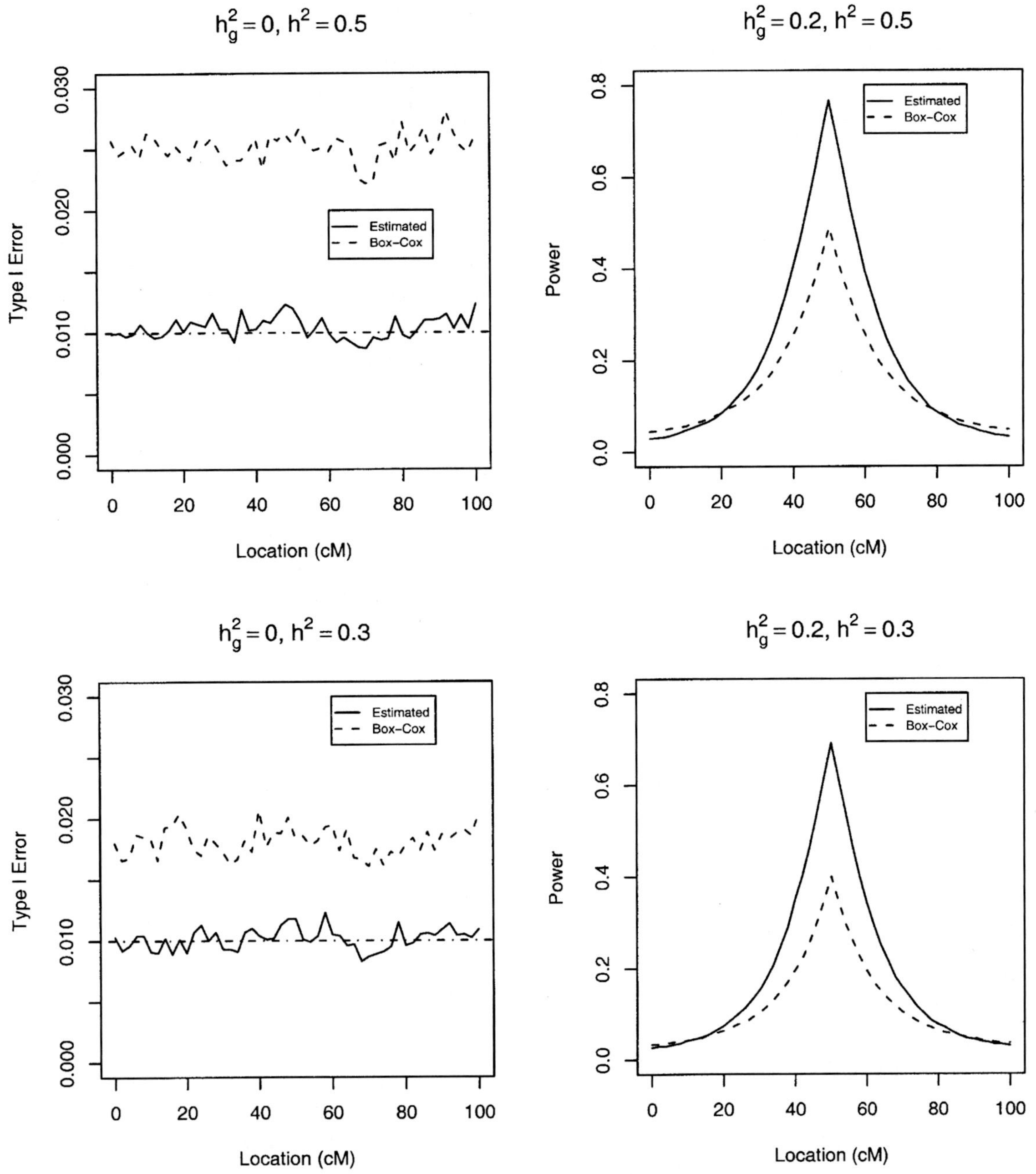

Figure 7 Type I error and power of likelihood-ratio tests with 500 sib trios at the nominal significance level of 0.01 when the true transformation is $H(y) = \log(2y - 2)/2$.

QTL. As shown in tables 2 and 3, the estimators under the new method performed as well as did the estimators with known transformation. The estimators under the existing method without transformation were quite biased, and the estimators under the existing method with the log or square-root transformation also had bias.

To mimic the COGA data, we considered model (5) with identity H but generated the residual error for 1% of the families from the exponential distribution with mean of 4. Table 4 shows the type I error and power of the new and existing methods at the true QTL, and figure 6 displays the results for the genome scans. The new method continues to provide accurate control of type I error, whereas the type I error for the existing method is vastly inflated. The former tends to be more powerful than the latter when the genetic effects are strong. In the power comparisons, we did not reset the critical values to achieve the nominal significance levels. Such compari-

Table 5

Type I Error and Power (%) of the New and Haseman-Elston Methods for Log-Normal Traits, with 500 Sib Pairs

	Type I Error and Power (%) for					
	New Method			Haseman-Elston Method		
Model	$\alpha = 5$	$\alpha = 1$	$\alpha = .1$	$\alpha = 5$	$\alpha = 1$	$\alpha = .1$
a	5.18	1.02	.10	4.38	.44	.01
b	22.45	7.80	1.42	9.59	1.51	.05
c	53.88	28.05	9.21	17.84	3.79	.32
d	5.01	.92	.02	4.61	.40	.00
e	20.16	6.26	.83	10.21	1.55	.15
f	49.23	22.76	5.71	19.18	4.41	.50

sons give unfair disadvantages to the new method, because the existing method has much higher type I error. Were the existing method adjusted to have correct type I error, its power would be drastically reduced.

For positive nonnormal trait data, one may consider the Box-Cox transformation

$$y^{(\rho)} = \begin{cases} (y^{\rho} - 1)/\rho & \text{if } \rho \neq 0 \ , \\ \log y & \text{if } \rho = 0 \ , \end{cases}$$

and include ρ as an unknown parameter in the parametric likelihood. If the true transformation belongs to the Box-Cox family or can be approximated by a member of the family, then this method will perform well. For example, the true transformation in our first series of simulation studies can be approximated very well by the Box-Cox transformation with $\rho = 0.22$. In this case, the Box-Cox transformation method performance was very similar to our proposed method (results not shown). As shown in figure 7, the Box-Cox transformation causes inflated type I error and diminished power when the true transformation cannot be approximated well by a member of the Box-Cox family. The Box-Cox transformation also performed poorly in the aforementioned simulation studies with outliers (results not shown).

We also compared the new method with the revised Haseman-Elston regression method (Elston et al. 2000). We generated trait values for sib pairs from the model $\log Y_{ij} = b_{ij} + e_{ij}$. We regressed the cross product of the sib pair's mean-centered trait values on the proportion of alleles shared IBD by the pair. The results for 500 sib pairs are shown in table 5. The new method again has proper control of type I error. The Haseman-Elston method has proper type I error at the nominal significance level of 5% but is conservative at nominal levels of 1% and 0.1%. These findings agree well with those of Allison et al. (2000). The Haseman-Elston method is substantially less powerful than the new method.

Discussion

In her invited editorial, Feingold (2002) described three criteria for evaluating QTL-mapping methods: (1) the power of the method is high when the trait is normally distributed, (2) the type I error is correct regardless of the characteristics of the data, and (3) the method is still powerful when the trait is not normally distributed. The existing variance-component methods satisfy the first criterion but perform poorly on the second and third criteria, whereas the new method meets all three criteria. If one adds a fourth criterion that the method allows arbitrary pedigrees and flexible genetic models, then the new method is the only QTL-mapping method with all these desirable properties.

The new method is independent of the estimation of multipoint IBD allele–sharing probabilities. One can choose appropriate software according to the size and complexity of the pedigrees as well as the number of markers. Software such as GENEHUNTER (Kruglyak et al. 1996) and ACT (Amos 1994) performs exact multipoint calculations that are based on a hidden Markov model (Lander and Green 1987) and can handle an arbitrary number of markers for small pedigrees, whereas the approximation method implemented in SOLAR (Almasy and Blangero 1998) can handle large pedigrees.

We have implemented an efficient and reliable algorithm for the new method in a cost-free computer program (D.Y.L.'s Web site). It is more time consuming to fit the proposed semiparametric variance-components model than the existing parametric models, but the computing time is comparable and is not a concern with current computing power. It took 1 s and 6 s on an IBM BladeCenter HS-20 machine to perform the analysis at one position for the COGA data with use of the existing and new methods, respectively. For the simulations, at one position, an analysis based on the existing and new methods took 0.75 s and 1.8 s, respectively, for 200 sib trios, and 5 and 10 s, respectively, for 500 sib trios. In the simulation studies, we generated thousands of data sets and fit millions of models. Our algorithm converged in all cases.

In some studies, families are selected on the basis of the trait values of their members. If the ascertainment criterion is known, then we can divide the likelihood by the probability that the proband falls into the specified ascertainment region. An alternative approach, which does not require knowledge of the ascertainment scheme, is to condition on the actual observed trait values. de Andrade and Amos (2000) conducted simulation studies to assess the performance of these two methods in the variance-component analysis. Their results show that (1) there is little difference between the two methods of ascertainment correction, (2) failing to correct for ascertainment affects the polygenetic and environmental components of variance but has little impact on the linked major-gene component of variance, (3) regardless of whether the data are corrected for ascertainment, the power to detect a major locus is similar, and (4) there is some inflation of type I error in the presence of a large genetic background and a rare gene. Ignoring selective sampling should have less impact on the new method, since it is robust to the induced nonnormality. Further investigation is warranted.

In the COGA data, the three outliers are so extreme that it is perhaps sensible to delete them. In general, it may not be justifiable to delete outliers unless they are known to be caused by measurement or recording error. In many studies, the distinction between outliers and nonoutliers is blurred, so that it is difficult to decide which ones to delete. Another strategy is to Winsorize the data—that is, to replace the outliers with some smaller values—but this is also a highly subjective process. The results of the variance-components analysis can change dramatically dependent on how the outliers are Winsorized, which ones are deleted, or which transformation is used. The new method avoids any manipulation of data and provides unique and reliable results.

Amos (1994) and Amos et al. (1996) considered the generalized estimating-equations approach (Prentice and Zhao 1991) for estimating variance components. This method is more robust than the parametric-likelihood method under nonnormality but is less efficient than the latter. We expect our method to perform better than the generalized estimating-equations approach, since it is robust against nonnormality and outliers and has the same efficiency as the parametric-likelihood method under normality or with known transformation. It would be worthwhile to compare the two methods by simulation.

Blangero et al. (2000) proposed robust variance-covariance estimators for the parameter estimators under the normal model. They showed that the likelihood-ratio statistics can be multiplied by a constant to yield a robust test. Finding an appropriate constant is computationally intensive and requires modeling assumptions. Although it may correct type I error, this approach may not have good power. Another strategy is to obtain P values by simulation, as recommended by Allison et al. (2000). Like the use of robust variances, this approach reduces the power. There have been some other suggestions in the literature, but they are also unsatisfactory.

In some studies, the trait values are truncated because of inability to detect values below (or above) certain thresholds. One example is the coronary artery calcification (CAC) data from the Family Heart Study (Higgins et al. 1996). The distribution of CAC exhibits a spike at the left end, since a large proportion of CAC measures are recorded as 0 because they do not exceed some threshold for detection. In addition, the positive CAC scores are highly skewed. We are currently extending our idea for analysis of such data by using a mixture model that formulates the probability of a positive CAC score with a logistic-regression model and the distribution of the positive score with model (1). The resultant procedure will be more robust than the parametric Tobit variance-component method of Epstein et al. (2003).

In many longitudinal studies, such as the Framingham Heart Study (Geller et al. 2003), quantitative traits are measured repeatedly over time. In addition to the correlation among different individuals of the same family, there is within-subject correlation among the repeated measures of the same individual. de Andrade et al. (2002) extended the parametric variance-component approach to account for the within-subject correlation. We are currently exploring the extension of our approach to this setting.

Acknowledgments

This research was supported by the National Institutes of Health (NIH). The authors are grateful to the COGA investigators, for the use of their data; and to Drs. Raymond Crowe and Jean W. MacCluer, for facilitating the transfer of the COGA data from Genetic Analysis Workshop 11, which was supported in part by NIH grant GM31575.

Appendix A

Let $\alpha_k = \Lambda\{Y_{(k)}\}$, $k = 1,\ldots,K$, where $Y_{(k)}$ is the kth order statistic of Y and K is the total number of distinct trait values. Note that α_k is the jump size of $\Lambda(y)$ at $y = Y_{(k)}$. The system of score functions—that is, the first derivatives of the log-likelihood function (4) with respect to the parameters ($\boldsymbol{\beta}$, $\boldsymbol{\gamma}$, $\alpha_1,\ldots,\alpha_K$)—are given by

$$\frac{\partial \log L}{\partial \boldsymbol{\beta}} = \sum_{i=1}^{n} \mathbf{X}_i^T \mathbf{V}_i^{-1}(\mathbf{H}_i - \mathbf{X}_i\boldsymbol{\beta}) \ ,$$

$$\frac{\partial \log L}{\partial \sigma_g^2} = -\frac{1}{2}\sum_{i=1}^{n}\left\{\mathrm{tr}\left(\mathbf{V}_i^{-T}\frac{\partial \mathbf{V}_i}{\partial \sigma_g^2}\right) - (\mathbf{H}_i - \mathbf{X}_i\boldsymbol{\beta})^T \mathbf{V}_i^{-1}\frac{\partial \mathbf{V}_i}{\partial \sigma_g^2}\mathbf{V}_i^{-1}(\mathbf{H}_i - \mathbf{X}_i\boldsymbol{\beta})\right\} \ ,$$

$$\frac{\partial \log L}{\partial \sigma_G^2} = -\frac{1}{2}\sum_{i=1}^{n}\left\{\mathrm{tr}\left(\mathbf{V}_i^{-T}\frac{\partial \mathbf{V}_i}{\partial \sigma_G^2}\right) - (\mathbf{H}_i - \mathbf{X}_i\boldsymbol{\beta})^T\mathbf{V}_i^{-1}\frac{\partial \mathbf{V}_i}{\partial \sigma_G^2}\mathbf{V}_i^{-1}(\mathbf{H}_i - \mathbf{X}_i\boldsymbol{\beta})\right\} ,$$

and

$$\frac{\partial \log L}{\partial \alpha_k} = \sum_{i=1}^{n}\sum_{j=1}^{n_i}\left\{I(Y_{ij} = Y_{(k)})\frac{1}{\alpha_k} - I(Y_{ij} \geqslant Y_{(k)})\frac{1}{\Lambda(Y_{ij})}\right\} - \sum_{i=1}^{n}(\mathbf{H}_i - \mathbf{X}_i\boldsymbol{\beta})^T\mathbf{V}_i^{-1}\frac{\partial \mathbf{H}_i}{\partial \alpha_k} ,$$

where

$$\partial \mathbf{V}_i/\partial \sigma_g^2 = \boldsymbol{\Sigma}_{gi} ,$$

$$\partial \mathbf{V}_i/\partial \sigma_G^2 = \boldsymbol{\Sigma}_{Gi} ,$$

$$\partial \mathbf{H}_i/\partial \alpha_k = [I(Y_{i1} \geqslant Y_{(k)})/\Lambda(Y_{i1}), \ldots ,I(Y_{in_i} \geqslant Y_{(k)})/\Lambda(Y_{in_i})]^T ,$$

and $I(\mathcal{A})$ is the indicator function with a value of 1 if $\mathcal{A}$ is true and of 0 otherwise. Here, $\boldsymbol{\gamma} = (\sigma_g^2,\sigma_G^2)$, and $\boldsymbol{\Sigma}_{gi}$ and $\boldsymbol{\Sigma}_{Gi}$ are the estimated IBD allele-sharing probability matrix at the major locus and the expected IBD allele-sharing probability matrix for the ith family, respectively.

By setting the system of score functions to 0, we obtain the maximum-likelihood estimators $(\hat{\boldsymbol{\beta}},\hat{\boldsymbol{\gamma}},\hat{\alpha}_1, \ldots ,\hat{\alpha}_K)$. We then estimate $\Lambda(y)$ by $\hat{\Lambda}(y) = \sum_{Y_{(k)}\leq y}\hat{\alpha}_k$ and estimate $H(y)$ by $\log \hat{\Lambda}(y)$. Note that $\hat{\Lambda}$ and $\hat{H}$ are step functions that jump at the observed trait values only. This is similar to the Breslow estimator of the cumulative hazard function and the Kaplan-Meier estimator of the survival function.

Web Resource

The URL for data presented herein is as follows:

D.Y.L.'s Web site, http://www.bios.unc.edu/~lin (for the computer program)

References

Allison DB, Fernández JR, Heo M, Beasley TM (2000) Testing the robustness of the new Haseman-Elston quantitative-trait loci–mapping procedure. Am J Hum Genet 67:249–252

Allison DB, Neale MC, Zannolli R, Schork NJ, Amos CI, Blangero J (1999) Testing the robustness of the likelihood-ratio test in a variance-component quantitative-trait loci–mapping procedure. Am J Hum Genet 65:531–544

Almasy L, Blangero J (1998) Multipoint quantitative-trait linkage analysis in general pedigrees. Am J Hum Genet 62:1198–1211

Amos CI (1994) Robust variance-components approach for assessing genetic linkage in pedigrees. Am J Hum Genet 54:535–543

Amos CI, Krushkal J, Thiel TJ, Young A, Zhu DK, Boerwinkle E, de Andrade M (1997) Comparison of model-free linkage mapping strategies for the study of a complex trait. Genet Epidemiol 14:743–748

Amos CI, Zhu DK, Boerwinkle E (1996) Assessing genetic linkage and association with robust components of variance approaches. Ann Hum Genet 60:143–160

Barnholtz JS, de Andrade M, Page GP, King TM, Peterson LE, Amos CI (1999) Assessing linkage of monoamine oxidase B in a genome-wide scan using a univariate variance components approach. Genet Epidemiol Suppl 1 17:S49–S54

Begleiter H, Reich T, Hesselbrock V, Porjesz B, Li TK, Schuckit MA, Edenberg HJ, Rice JP (1995) The Collaborative Study on the Genetics of Alcoholism. Alcohol Health Res World 19:228–236

Bickel PJ, Klassen CAJ, Ritov Y, Wellner JA (1993) Efficient and adaptive estimation in semiparametric models. Johns Hopkins University Press, Baltimore

Blangero J, Williams JT, Almasy L (2000) Robust LOD scores for variance component-based linkage analysis. Genet Epidemiol Suppl 19:S8–S14

Breslow NE (1972) Discussion of the paper by DR Cox. J R Statist Soc B 34:216–217

Chiou JM, Liang KY, Chiu YF (2005) Multipoint linkage mapping using sibpairs: non-parametric estimation of trait effects with quantitative covariates. Genet Epidemiol 28:58–69

Cox DR (1972) Regression models and life-tables (with discussion). J R Statist Soc B 34:187–220

de Andrade M, Amos CI (2000) Ascertainment issues in variance components models. Genet Epidemiol 19:333–344

de Andrade M, Gueguen R, Visvikis S, Sass C, Siest G, Amos

CI (2002) Extension of variance components approach to incorporate temporal trends and longitudinal pedigree data analysis. Genet Epidemiol 22:221–232

Drigalenko E (1998) How sib pairs reveal linkage. Am J Hum Genet 63:1242–1245

Elston RC, Buxbaum S, Jacobs KB, Olson JM (2000) Haseman and Elston revisited. Genet Epidemiol 19:1–17

Epstein MP, Lin X, Boehnke M (2003) A Tobit variance-component method for linkage analysis of censored trait data. Am J Hum Genet 72:611–620

Feingold E (2001) Methods for linkage analysis of quantitative trait loci in humans. Theor Popul Biol 60:167–180

——— (2002) Regression-based quantitative-trait–locus mapping in the 21st century. Am J Hum Genet 71:217–222

Forrest W (2001) Weighting improves the "new Haseman-Elston" method. Hum Hered 52:47–54

Fulker DW, Cherny SS, Cardon LR (1995) Multipoint interval mapping of quantitative trait loci, using sib pairs. Am J Hum Genet 56:1224–1233

Geller F, Dempfle A, Gorg T (2003) Genome scan for body mass index and height in the Framingham Heart Study. BMC Genet Suppl 4:S91

Goldgar DE (1990) Multipoint analysis of human quantitative genetic variation. Am J Hum Genet 47:957–967

Haseman JK, Elston RC (1972) The investigation of linkage between a quantitative trait and a marker locus. Behav Genet 2:3–19

Higgins M, Province M, Heiss G, Eckfeldt J, Ellison RC, Folsom AR, Rao DC, Sprafka M, Williams R (1996) NHLBI Family Heart Study: objectives and design. Am J Epidemiol 143:1219–1228

Kruglyak L, Daly M, Reeve-Daly M, Lander ES (1996) Parametric and nonparametric linkage analysis: a unified multipoint approach. Am J Hum Genet 58:1347–1363

Lander ES, Green P (1987) Construction of multilocus genetic linkage maps in humans. Proc Natl Acad Sci USA 84:2363–2367

Lin DY (2004) Haplotype-based association analysis in cohort studies of unrelated individuals. Genet Epidemiol 26:255–264

Major LF, Murphy DL (1978) Platelet and plasma amine oxidase activity in alcoholic individuals. Br J Psychiatry 132:548–554

Pratt SC, Daly MJ, Kruglyak L (2000) Exact multipoint quantitative-trait linkage analysis in pedigrees by variance components. Am J Hum Genet 66:1153–1157

Prentice RL, Zhao LP (1991) Estimating equations for parameters in means and covariances of multivariate discrete and continuous responses. Biometrics 47:825–839

Press WH, Teukolsky SA, Vetterling WT, Flannery BP (1992) Numerical recipes in C: the art of scientific computing, 2nd ed. Cambridge University Press, New York

Putter H, Sandkuijl LA, van Houwelingen JC (2002) Score test for detecting linkage to quantitative traits. Genet Epidemiol 22:345–355

Schork NJ (1993) Extended multipoint identity-by-descent analysis of human quantitative traits: efficiency, power, and modeling considerations. Am J Hum Genet 53:1306–1319

Self SG, Liang KL (1987) Asymptotic properties of maximum likelihood estimators and likelihood ratio tests under nonstandard conditions. J Am Statist Assoc 82:605–610

Sham PC, Purcell S (2001) Equivalence between Haseman-Elston and variance-components linkage analyses for sib pairs. Am J Hum Genet 68:1527–1532

Sham PC, Purcell S, Cherny SS, Abecasis GR (2002) Powerful regression-based quantitative-trait linkage analysis of general pedigrees. Am J Hum Genet 71:238–253

Strug L, Sun L, Corey M (2003) The genetics of cross-sectional and longitudinal body mass index. BMC Genet Suppl 4:S14

Sullivan JL, Cavenar JO Jr, Maltbie AA, Lister P, Zung WW (1979) Familial biochemical and clinical correlates of alcoholics with low platelet monoamine oxidase activity. Biol Psychiatry 14:385–394

Tang H-K, Siegmund D (2001) Mapping quantitative trait loci in oligogenic models. Biostatistics 2:147–162

Visscher PM, Hopper JL (2001) Power of regression and maximum likelihood methods to map QTL from sib-pair and DZ twin data. Ann Hum Genet 65:583–601

Wang K, Huang J (2002) A score-statistic approach for the mapping of quantitative-trait loci with sibships of arbitrary size. Am J Hum Genet 70:412–424

Williams JT, Duggirala R, Blangero J (1997) Statistical properties of a variance-components method for quantitative trait linkage analysis in nuclear families and extended pedigrees. Genet Epidemiol 14:1065–1070

Wright FA (1997) The phenotypic difference discards sib-pair QTL linkage information. Am J Hum Genet 60:740–742

Xu X, Weiss S, Xu X, Wei LJ (2000) A unified Haseman-Elston method for testing linkage with quantitative traits. Am J Hum Genet 67:1025–1028

Germline Susceptibility to Colorectal Cancer Due to Base-Excision Repair Gene Defects

Susan M. Farrington,[1,4,*] Albert Tenesa,[1,4,*] Rebecca Barnetson,[1,4] Alice Wiltshire,[1,4] James Prendergast,[1,4] Mary Porteous,[1,2] Harry Campbell,[1,3] and Malcolm G. Dunlop[1,2]

[1]Colon Cancer Genetics Group, School of Clinical and Molecular Medicine, [2]Clinical Genetics Department, and [3]Public Health Sciences, University of Edinburgh, and [4]Medical Research Council (MRC), Human Genetics Unit, Edinburgh

DNA repair is a key process in the maintenance of genome integrity. Here, we present a large, systematically collected population-based association study (2,239 cases; 1,845 controls) that explores the contribution to colorectal cancer incidence of inherited defects in base-excision repair (BER) genes. We show that biallelic *MUTYH* defects impart a 93-fold (95% CI 42–213) excess risk of colorectal cancer, which accounts for 0.8% of cases aged <55 years and 0.54% of the entire cohort. Penetrance for homozygous carriers was almost complete by age 60 years. Significantly more biallelic carriers had coexisting adenomatous polyps. However, notably, 36% of biallelic carriers had no polyps. Three patients with heterozygous *MUTYH* defects carried monoallelic mutations in other BER genes (*OGG1* and *MTH1*). Recessive inheritance accounted for the elevated risk for those aged <55 years. However, there was also a 1.68-fold (95% CI 1.07–2.95) excess risk for heterozygous carriers aged >55 years, with a population attributable risk in this age group of 0.93% (95% CI 0%–2.0%). These data provide the strongest evidence to date for a causative role of BER defects in colorectal cancer etiology and show, to our knowledge for the first time, that heterozygous *MUTYH* mutations predispose to colorectal cancer later in life. These findings have clinical relevance for BER gene testing for patients with colorectal cancer and for genetic counseling of their relatives.

Introduction

The role of base-excision repair (BER) in the maintenance of genome stability is primarily to counter oxidative DNA damage, which generates 8-oxoguanine products (8-oxoG). In humans, MYH (MIM 604933), OGG1 (MIM 601982), and MTH1 (MIM 600312) function in consort to identify and repair 8-oxoG incorporated into DNA, as well as to remove modified nucleoside. Recent studies have identified biallelic germline defects in *MUTYH,* in a proportion of families with multiple colorectal polyposis, that are not due to germline *APC* (MIM 175100 and 608456) mutations (Al-Tassan et al. 2002; Sieber et al. 2003). Although these studies provide indirect evidence, it is important to establish whether BER gene defects predispose to colorectal cancer (MIM 114500), to estimate the level of associated risk, and to determine the attributable contribution of such defects to overall disease incidence. Previous studies have provided some supporting evidence that biallelic mutations are associated with excess cancer risk (Croitoru et al. 2004; Fleischmann et al. 2004). Here, we present an analysis of the largest cohort study to date, thereby affording the opportunity to assess the effect of homozygous and heterozygous BER gene mutations on colorectal cancer risk. We assembled a large, systematically recruited prospective cohort of patients from across Scotland, shortly after diagnosis of colorectal cancer and irrespective of family history. We also systematically recruited healthy Scottish population control individuals through the central National Health Service (NHS). Using this population-based resource, we set out to determine, by a genetic association strategy, the role of BER genes in colorectal cancer susceptibility.

Received January 18, 2005; accepted for publication April 14, 2005; electronically published May 3, 2005.

Address for correspondence and reprints: Dr. Susan M, Farrington, Colon Cancer Genetics Group, MRC Human Genetics Unit, Western General Hospital, Edinburgh EH4 2XU, United Kingdom. E-mail: Susan.Farrington@hgu.mrc.ac.uk

* These two authors contributed equally to this work.

0002-9297/2005/7701-0011$15.00

Subjects and Methods

Assembly of the Cohort and Sample Collection

A populationwide accrual of prospective colorectal cancer cases has been in progress since 1999. Cases are ascertained through direct contact with every surgical and pathology department in Scotland. All cases had histologically confirmed adenocarcinoma of the colon or rectum. Blood DNA samples were obtained from patients after counseling and receipt of informed consent. Population-based and age- and sex-matched controls were systematically identified, and blood DNA samples were obtained from them. A questionnaire about family information and lifestyle and medical history was completed for patients and controls. Dietary risk-exposure data were also collected by use of a validated food-frequency questionnaire. For cases, tumor stage, pathology, clinical presentation, as well as the presence of synchronous polyps were documented. These studies are subject to all necessary approvals from local ethics research committee (LREC), multicenter research ethics committee (MREC), and NHS research and development management in every participating hospital.

Analysis of MUTYH *Variants Y165C and G382D*

A two-stage approach was used to efficiently identify subjects carrying heterozygous or homozygous BER gene variants. In the first step, assays were designed using Primer Express v2.0 software (Applied Biosystems [AB]) for the two commonly reported variants, Y165C and G382D, in patients with multiple polyposis. Allelic discrimination for each variant employed allele-specific *Taq*-Man MGB probes (AB), resolved on an ABI 7900 Analyzer, by use of SDS v2.1 software. Probe and primer details are available on request. Each Y165C and G382D variant identified by the *Taq*Man approach was confirmed by repeat DNA sequence analysis. In the second phase, all subjects heterozygous for Y165C and G382D underwent sequence analysis of the entire coding region of *MUTYH,* and the heterozygote cases were also screened for *OGG1* and *MTH1* gene variants. GenBank accession numbers for the genes are AF527839, NT_022517, and NT_007819, respectively. PCR products were treated with Exonuclease 1, shrimp alkaline phosphatase (Amersham Biosciences) and then were sequenced using ABI Big Dye terminator V3.0 chemistry, with precipitated products separated on an ABI 3700. Details of primer sequences are available on request. Using this approach, we identified all homozygotes or compound heterozygotes and any subjects in whom at least one allele was either Y165C or G382D. However, it should be noted that we could have missed some biallelic carriers who did not have these two common variants. Hence, if anything, our estimates may underrepresent the contribution of BER genes, but we consider this to be a marginal effect.

Assessment of Variants of BER Genes

Each variant identified by sequencing was confirmed by repeat sequence analysis. Allele frequency for each newly identified variant was then determined in at least 340 control chromosomes, to confirm that the variant was not simply a common polymorphism. Any common polymorphic variants were discarded, after which each identified variant was subjected to rigorous bioinformatic analysis. We used SIFT, which predicts deleterious coding variants on the basis of cross-species conservation; PolyPhen, which predicts the effect by use of conservation and any protein structure available in the public domain; T-Coffee, which aligns closely related Ensembl orthologues; protein domains predicted using Pfam; assessment of potential splicing effects by use of GENSCAN; ESEfinder; and Berkeley *Drosophila* Genome Project splice-site prediction.

Functional Analysis of MUTYH *nt 9639 a→g Variant*

A variant was identified that was predicted to affect splicing (*MUTYH*; nt 9639 a→g). In this case, RNA was extracted from blood leukocytes by use of Tri-reagent (Sigma) and was processed to cDNA (Boeringer Mannheim First Strand Synthesis kit). A transcript product of 475 bp was amplified using exonic primers in exons 10 and 14 (primer details available on request). The product was cloned using the Topo cloning kit (Invitrogen), and positive colonies were amplified and sequenced. Similarly, a genomic amplicon covering the nt 9639 a→g change and the G382D locus was cloned to demonstrate recessive inheritance of the two variants.

Test for Association

Association was tested using Fisher's exact test in a 3 × 2 table of genotype by colorectal cancer status, thereby making no prejudgment on potential mode of inheritance.

Estimate of Genotype Relative Risk

As an adaptation of the method of Hugot et al. (2001), the genotype relative risk (GRR) is defined as follows:

$$\mathrm{GRR}(AA) = \frac{\Pr(D|AA)}{\Pr(D|AA)} = 1 ,$$

$$\mathrm{GRR}(Aa) = \frac{\Pr(D|Aa)}{\Pr(D|AA)} = \frac{\Pr(Aa|D) \times \Pr(AA)}{\Pr(AA|D) \times \Pr(Aa)} ,$$

and

$$\mathrm{GRR}(aa) = \frac{\Pr(D|aa)}{\Pr(D|AA)} = \frac{\Pr(aa|D) \times \Pr(AA)}{\Pr(AA|D) \times \Pr(aa)} ,$$

where $\Pr(G|D)$ is the frequency of genotype G among cases and $\Pr(G)$ is the expected Hardy-Weinberg equilibrium proportion, as obtained from the allele frequency in the control population. The control population was assumed to be a representative sample of the general population. The 95% CIs for the GRRs were obtained

Table 1

Population GRR Associated with MYH Y165C

Population and Genotype	No. of Subjects with Genotype: Case	Control	GRR	95% CI
Entire cohort (P = .228):				
GG	0	0	.00	.00–.00
AG	17	8	1.76	.90–4.16
AA	2,202	1,824	1.00	1.00–1.00
U55 (P = 1.000):				
GG	0	0	.00	.00–.00
AG	7	4	1.08	.37–3.72
AA	867	535	1.00	1.00–1.00
O55 (P = .180):				
GG	0	0	.00	.00–.00
AG	10	4	2.42	.96–8.71
AA	1,335	1,289	1.00	1.00–1.00

by bootstrapping 1,000 independent samples. For each of the samples, the GRR was estimated, then the same 1,000 samples were ordered within each genotype, and the 50th and 950th estimates were taken as the lower and upper limits of the 95% CI.

Penetrance Estimates

Penetrance for colorectal cancer at a given age is defined as the probability that a randomly selected individual with genotype G will develop the disease by that age, with the assumption that that individual does not die of another cause. If A_x is the event "affected at age $x{:}x+1$, given being disease-free at x," then the probability that an individual is affected by age x, given the genotype G, is $\Pr(A_x|G)$. Similarly if $\overline{A}_x$ is the event "not affected at age $x{:}x+1$, given being disease-free at x," then the probability that an individual is not affected by age x, given genotype G, is $\Pr(\overline{A}_x|G)$. Population incidence rates, $\Pr(A_x)$, were obtained from Scottish Health Statistics, and the sex-average incidence rates were used. Then

$$\frac{\Pr(A_x|G)}{\Pr(\overline{A}_x|G)} = \frac{\Pr(G|A_x)\times\Pr(A_x)}{\Pr(G|\overline{A}_x)\times\Pr(\overline{A}_x)} ,$$

$$\frac{\Pr(A_x|G)}{1-\Pr(A_x|G)} = \frac{\Pr(G|A_x)\times\Pr(A_x)}{\Pr(G|\overline{A}_x)\times[1-\Pr(A_x)]} ,$$

and

$$\Pr(A_x|G) = \frac{\frac{\Pr(G|A_x)\times\Pr(A_x)}{\Pr(G|\overline{A}_x)\times[1-\Pr(A_x)]}}{1+\frac{\Pr(G|A_x)\times\Pr(A_x)}{\Pr(G|\overline{A}_x)\times[1-\Pr(A_x)]}} .$$

There were not enough observations for each age, so $\Pr(G|A_x)$ was estimated using logistic regression (i.e., age was used as a predictor of genotype). Similarly, $\Pr(G|\overline{A}_x)$ was estimated from controls. The penetrance for genotype G is then defined as:

$$P_G = 1-\prod_1^x[1-\Pr(A_x|G)] .$$

Estimate of CIs

The 95% CI for the estimate of the penetrance was obtained by bootstrapping (i.e., by sampling with replacement) samples of cases and controls. A total of 500 independent samples were obtained of size equal to the total number of cases and controls. Penetrance was estimated for each sample, and mean penetrance over rep-

Table 2

Population GRR Associated with MYH G382D

Population and Genotype	No. of Subjects with Genotype: Case	Control	GRR	95% CI
Entire cohort (P = .010):				
AA	8	0	121.23	44.48–325.10
GA	35	20	1.46	.93–2.43
GG	2,181	1,808	1.00	1.00–1.00
U55 (P = .402):				
AA	4	0	146.69	26.71–998.71
GA	12	6	1.24	.54–3.42
GG	864	531	1.00	1.00–1.00
O55 (P = .049):				
AA	4	0	102.19	22.09–333.10
GA	23	14	1.60	.93–2.95
GG	1,317	1,277	1.00	1.00–1.00

Table 3

Population GRR Associated with *MUTYH* Gene

Population and Genotype[a]	No. of Subjects with Genotype		GRR	95% CI
	Case	Control		
Entire cohort (P = .001):				
MM	12	0	92.65	41.60–213.20
WM	45	28	1.35	.92–2.07
WW	2,160	1794	1.00	1.00–1.00
U55 (P = .976):				
MM	7	0	91.73	22.53–293.41
WM	14	10	.87	.43–1.72
WW	851	523	1.00	1.00–1.00
O55 (P = .014):				
MM	5	0	77.26	20.51–208.98
WM	31	18	1.68	1.07–2.95
WW	1,309	1,271	1.00	1.00–1.00

[a] W = wild-type allele; M = mutant allele.

licates and standard deviation (SD) were obtained. The 95% CI was calculated using the mean ± 1.96 SD.

Results

Analysis of MUTYH *Variants Y165C and G382D*

All variants detected by *Taq*Man analysis were confirmed by genomic sequencing. Eight (0.36%) of the patients were homozygous for G382D. There were no homozygotes for Y165C, but three Y165C/G382D compound heterozygotes were identified. There were no biallelic defects in any control samples. Association was first tested, using Fisher's exact test in a 3 × 2 table of genotype by colorectal cancer status, thereby making no prejudgment on potential mode of inheritance. Next, GRR was calculated using the method of Hugot et al. (2001), because the usual method, estimated by odds ratio, is not possible because there were no homozygote controls. The frequency of Y165C and G382D alleles in cases and controls is presented in tables 1 and 2, respectively.

The data presented in table 2 establish the fact that the G382D locus is associated with colorectal cancer in the complete cohort (P = .0104; GRR 121; 95% CI 44–325 for the G382D/G382D genotype). To explore any age-specific effect, the cohort aged <55 years at diagnosis (U55) was compared with those aged >55 years at diagnosis (O55) (table 2). Because of the lower number of U55 subjects, there was no statistically significant association with G382D for the U55 cohort, whereas association for the O55 cohort remained statistically significant (P = .0494). There was no association with the Y165C locus (table 1), possibly because of the rarity of the mutant variant in the Scottish population. We consider the lack of association in the early-onset cohort to be due primarily to the low allele frequency of these individual variants and the resultant lack of statistical power, even though this study involved large case and control cohorts.

Significance of Other Variants in BER Genes

In light of prior genetic and functional evidence of an additive effect of G382D and Y165C alleles (Al-Tassan et al. 2002; Sieber et al. 2003), we next determined the overall prevalence of biallelic defects, using a pragmatic approach. To find second BER gene defects, DNA from all carriers of monoallelic Y165C or G382D mutations (n = 74) was sequenced for each exon and intron/exon boundary of *MUTYH*. BER genes *OGG1* and *MTH1* were also sequenced in cases with heterozygous Y165C or G382D MYH alleles. All identified variants were excluded as polymorphisms by confirmation of wild-type sequence in at least 340 control chromosomes and likely functional relevance assessed by bioinformatic analysis, as described in the "Subjects and Methods" section.

In addition to the eight G382D/G382D homozygotes and the three Y165C/G382D compound heterozygotes described above, we identified a further patient with a heterozygous G382D mutation who had a second genomic *MUTYH* defect (nt 9639 a→g) that we consider to be pathogenic. This variant was confirmed to reside on the wild-type allele by genomic DNA cloning and sequencing. The variant was predicted to affect splicing. This was confirmed by cDNA analysis, which showed only mutant G382D transcript and no wild-type transcript. Thus, the patient was hemizygous for G382D at the RNA level. The *Taq*Man approach used for the G382D variant identified all nt 9639 a→g variants, so we have systematically screened all samples for this variant. Thus, the genotyping strategy would have identified the *MUTYH* defect nt 9639 a→g variant with equal sensitivity in cases and controls. Hence, we have included this variant in further analyses of the effect of overall *MUTYH* genotype, for a total of 12 biallelic carriers (all cancer patients) and 73 subjects (45 patients and 28 controls) with monoallelic *MUTYH* alleles that we are confident are pathogenic (table 3).

We next considered other samples that might have a second BER gene defect. In all, there were an additional three samples with heterozygous G382D or Y165C alleles that had another BER gene defect that we consider likely to be pathogenic, but we cannot confirm or refute this. Hence, we did not include these other BER alleles in the analysis of the overall effect of putative BER gene defects (table 3). Two patients with Y165C or G382D mutations (one of each) had a second allelic variant in MTH1 (R31Q) that has been reported elsewhere in multiple polyposis (Sieber et al. 2003). Codon 31 of MTH1 is evolutionarily conserved, and bioinformatics interrogation suggests that the R31Q mutation affects protein function. Furthermore, we identified the variant in a total of 2 of 84 patient chromosomes, compared with 0 of 368 control chromosomes, which suggests that this is not a common polymorphic variant in the population (although we cannot directly compare R31Q prevalence, because these are two different groups). Taken together with previously published studies, we consider that the MTH1 R31Q variant is likely to be functionally important and consequently is likely to be a pathogenic mutation. One patient with an MTH1 R31Q variant also had a P391L variant in MYH that is at a highly conserved residue and is predicted to affect protein function. However, the significance of this variant is unclear, in light of the above discussion. A third patient with a monoallelic MYH G382D allele also had a variant in OGG1 (R197W). The variant is at a highly conserved codon, and bioinformatics analysis predicts a profound effect on protein function; again, the significance of this cannot currently be determined.

Analysis of the MUTYH *Gene and Colorectal Cancer Risk*

To assess biallelic inactivation of the entire gene, we calculated the combined risk for all significant *MUTYH* variants that had been analyzed in the complete cohort. This analysis included eight G382D/G382D homozygotes, three Y165C/G382D compound heterozygotes, and one nt 9639 a→g /G382D compound heterozygote, as discussed above. The data presented in table 3 convincingly establish the fact that the *MUTYH* gene is significantly associated with colorectal cancer ($P = .0012$). Biallelic inactivation imparts an overall 93-fold excess risk (GRR 93; 95% CI 42–213). As was the case for analysis of the G382D variant alone, the reduction in numbers for the U55 cohort resulted in loss of statistical power to detect association with the gene in that group, although the O55 group remains significant ($P = .0138$).

Separation of the cohorts by age reveals an age-specific risk effect and shows, for the first time, a significant monoallelic effect for late-onset disease when the empirical CIs produced by bootstrap analysis are used. There was a 1.68-fold excess risk (95% CI 1.07%–2.95) for heterozygous carriers aged >55 years and a population-attributable risk in this age group of 0.93% (95% CI 0%–2.0%). However, these results should be taken with some caution, because the significance was marginal, despite the fact that we have studied large case/control cohorts. Furthermore, analysis by use of standard CIs for the odd ratios in testing for association gave an almost significant result ($P = .085$; 95% CI 0.93–3) for a monoallelic effect. It was only with bootstrap analysis that this effect was significant at the 5% level. Nonetheless, these are novel observations that suggest that heterozygous *MUTYH* variants impart a modest increased risk later in life.

Estimate of Penetrance for MUTYH *Gene Defects*

We first estimated penetrance for G382D alleles at the *MUTYH* locus using the method of Satagopan et al. (2001), modified for application to a recessive trait. Figure 1 shows age-specific penetrance and 95% CIs for the G382D/G382D genotype alone. Of G382D/G382D carriers, ~55% developed colorectal cancer by age 40 years, and cancer had developed in all G382D/G382D carriers by age 65 years. Next, we estimated age-specific penetrance for all systematically determined biallelic defects identified in *MUTYH* (fig. 2). This analysis suggests that biallelic inactivation of the gene is highly penetrant, with all homozygous carriers developing cancer by age 60 years.

These findings establish the fact that there is a substantially elevated colorectal cancer risk early in life for people with biallelic MYH defects.

Synchronous Polyps in Biallelic MUTYH *Cancer Patients*

Data on polyp prevalence in cancer patients by genotype are presented in table 4. It is noteworthy that 4 (36%) of the 11 biallelic carriers with cancer for whom we had reliable polyp information had no concurrent metaplastic or adenomatous polyps. This emphasizes the fact that using polyp presence as a surrogate to enrich for *MUTYH* mutation carriers is quite insensitive. The data presented in table 4 show that there was a clear relationship between synchronous polyps and *MUTYH* genotype (all polyp types $P = .025$; adenomatous polyps $P = .007$; multiple adenomas $P < .0001$ [with use of Fisher's Exact Test]). In all, 64% of biallelic carriers had polyps; in all cases, these were multiple adenomas.

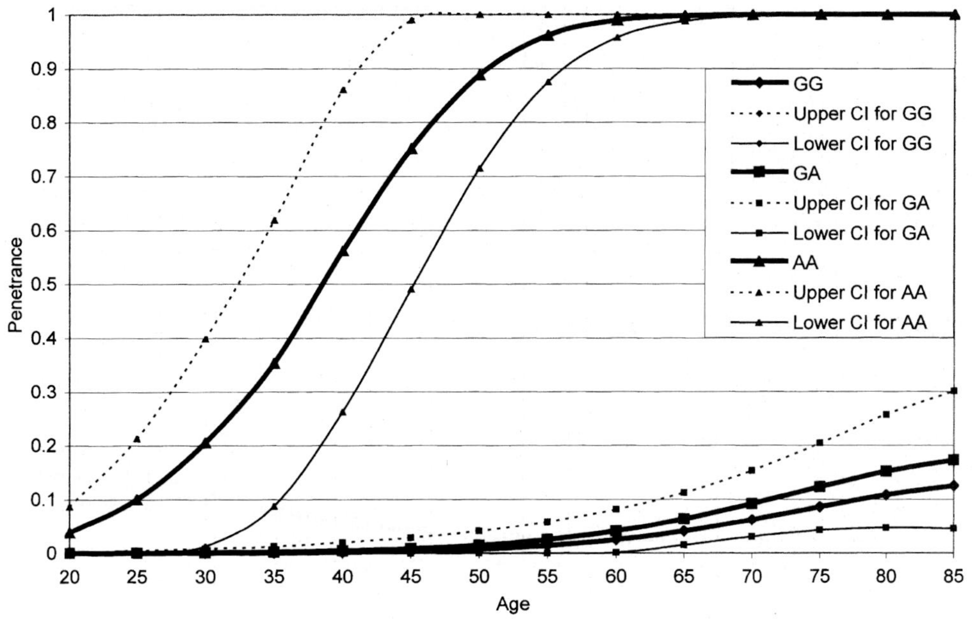

Figure 1 Penetrance curve of the MYH G382D locus. Age-related penetrance was estimated and plotted for all three genotypes, including 95% CIs.

The same analyses were performed, but with comparison of only the heterozygotes and wild-type genotypes, using 2 × 2 contingency tables; there were no significant results for presence of polyps with a heterozygote genotype ($P > .24$).

Discussion

Taken together, these data establish conclusively that defects in BER genes predispose to colorectal cancer. The findings provide robust evidence of causal involvement of biallelic BER gene defects in early-onset colorectal cancer, given the fact that there was complete penetrance by age 60 years. These findings substantially extend previous indirect evidence of involvement in colorectal cancer susceptibility through study of families with multiple polyposis (Al-Tassan et al. 2002; Sieber et al. 2003) and, combined with our findings of an excess of adenomatous polyps, suggest that polyps in such cases are premalignant. Our findings are also supported by previous suggestive evidence from smaller studies that lacked power to definitively establish whether there is an association between biallelic *MUTYH* variants and colorectal cancer (Enholm et al. 2003; Fleischmann et al. 2004; Wang et al. 2004).

There is only one previous study (Croitoru et al. 2004) that has shown an association between biallelic *MUTYH* variants and colorectal cancer. In that study, the authors proposed indirect evidence of a heterozygous effect because they observed nonrandom loss of heterozygosity of the wild-type allele in colorectal cancer. The findings presented here do, in fact, support their view and provide the first evidence of a modest colorectal cancer risk associated with heterozygous *MUTYH* mutations later in life. It is noteworthy that we found evidence of a significant excess risk associated with heterozygous *MUTYH* gene defects only when we considered the entire gene effect, and, importantly, this effect emerged only for late-onset disease. The effect was small and only just significant, and the results should be taken with some caution. Bootstrapping CIs are generally more robust than asymptotic CIs; however, it must be noted that asymptotic CIs for the odds ratio gave a slightly less significant result for the same data set. It is also possible that some of the excess risk we are detecting in heterozygotes is due to variants on the other allele that we have not detected. Data from mouse models indicates that, on an *Apc*$^{Min/+}$ background, monoallelic *Myh* inactivation does not increase tumor burden or the signature G-T transversions of the remaining *Apc* allele in the mouse tumors (Sieber et al. 2004). However, the study presented here is the largest to date, and previous studies have concentrated on early-onset disease or mixed cohorts (Fleischmann et al. 2004; Wang et al. 2004). Thus, only studies involving even larger numbers of later-onset cancer cases might be able to confirm our evidence of a monoallelic effect.

The study presented here emphasizes the requirement for very large population-based cohorts for robust assessment of the role of putative colorectal cancer sus-

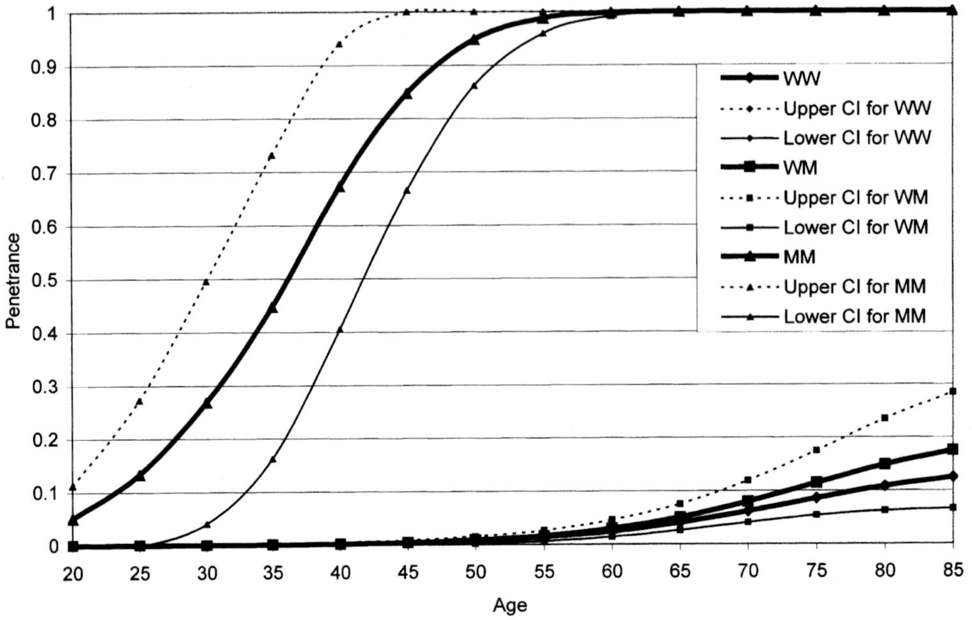

Figure 2 Penetrance curve of the *MUTYH* gene. All systematically verified and functionally deficient variants were included in the calculations, to estimate the penetrance of the entire gene. This therefore includes variants G382D, Y165C, and nt 9639 a→g. W = wild-type allele; M = mutant allele.

ceptibility alleles by genetic association strategies, even when relative risk is high. The relatively low allele frequency is likely to be a feature of many other cancer susceptibility alleles and raises some concerns for future power to detect associations where there is no prior biological hypothesis behind locus selection.

For clinical purposes, it is interesting to note that more than one-third of biallelic carriers did not have any synchronous polyps. This emphasizes the fact that use of polyps as an approach to enrich for *MUTYH* carriers with cancer is quite insensitive, in contrast with the findings of *APC*-negative multiple polyposis cases (Sampson et al. 2003; Sieber et al. 2003). Overall, there was an excess of synchronous polyps in biallelic carriers compared with others in this cohort, especially when adenomatous lesions were considered. Interestingly, monoallelic carriers did not appear to have an excess of polyps, suggesting the possibility that the excess cancer risk for heterozygotes later in life might be through a different mechanism.

Data presented here indicate that 1 of 50 patients who are diagnosed with colorectal cancer at age <40 years and 1 of 150 patients aged <55 years carry biallelic mutations in BER genes that are causally linked to cancer development. In defining the mutation carrier frequency for *MUTYH* and other BER genes, the present work informs future decisions about offering genetic testing to patients with early-onset colorectal cancer. Furthermore, the findings also have substantial clinical importance for the siblings of carriers, who have at least a 1/4 risk of colorectal cancer by age <60 years, by nature of the recessive genetic trait segregating in the family. Very large studies of late-onset disease-carrier status are required to replicate or refute the evidence

Table 4

***MUTYH* Genotype and the Presence of Synchronous Benign Polyps**

	No. (%) of Subjects with				
Genotype	No Polyps	All Polyp Types	Multiple Polyps	Adenomas	Multiple Adenomas
MM (n = 11)	4 (36)	7 (64)	7 (64)	7 (64)	7 (64)
WM (n = 44)	31 (70)	13 (30)	5 (11)	8 (18)	3 (7)
WW (n = 1,167)	859 (74)	308 (26)	100 (9)	224 (19)	54 (5)

Note.—Adenomas were either tubular or tubulovillous subtypes. Other polyps were metaplastic/hyperplastic. Three or more polyps were categorized as "multiple." Reliable concurrent polyp-prevalence data were not available for all patients with cancer, so the numbers for whom information was available are provided for each genotype.

presented here that monoallelic *MUTYH* defects contribute to colorectal cancer incidence.

Acknowledgments

We gratefully acknowledge the participation of all patients and control individuals, without whom this work would not have been possible. We thank all of the nursing and office staff employed by the Colorectal Cancer Genetic Susceptibility Study and the MRC Scottish Colorectal Cancer Study, for their tireless work in recruitment, which has been a major logistic endeavor. We also acknowledge the collaborative environment that we have enjoyed with NHS consultant surgeons and nursing teams in every Scottish hospital. We also thank the relevant departments in central Scottish NHS, including Cancer Registry, the Scottish Cancer Intelligence Unit of the Information and Statistics Division, and the Family Practitioner Committee, for invaluable help in recruiting population controls. We also thank Andrew Carothers for statistical advice. Current ethical approvals from MREC and LREC for all aspects of the study are held by M.P., H.C., and M.G.D. The work is funded by Chief Scientist Office grant CZB/4/94, Cancer Research UK grant C348/A3758, and MRC grant G0000657-53203. J.P. is funded by MRC Bioinformatics Research Studentship G74/93.

Web Resources

Accession numbers and URLs for data presented herein are as follows:

Berkeley *Drosophila* Genome Project, http://www.fruitfly.org/seq_tools/splice.html

ESEfinder, http://rulai.cshl.edu/tools/ESE/

GenBank, http://www.ncbi.nlm.nih.gov/GenBank/ (for *MUTYH* [accession number AF527839], *OGG1* [accession number NT_022517], and *MTH1* [accession number NT_007819])

GENSCAN, http://genes.mit.edu/GENSCAN.html

Online Mendelian Inheritance in Man (OMIM), http://www.ncbi.nlm.nih.gov/Omim/ (for *MYH, OGG1, MTH1, APC,* and colorectal cancer)

Pfam, http://www.sanger.ac.uk/Software/Pfam/

PolyPhen, http://www.bork.embl-heidelberg.de/PolyPhen/

SIFT, http://blocks.fhcrc.org/%7Epauline/SIFT

T-Coffee, http://www.ch.embnet.org/software/TCoffee.html

References

Al-Tassan N, Chmiel NH, Maynard J, Fleming N, Livingston AL, Williams GT, Hodges AK, Davies DR, David SS, Sampson JR, Cheadle JP (2002) Inherited variants of *MYH* associated with somatic G:C→T:A mutations in colorectal tumors. Nat Genet 30:227–232

Croitoru ME, Cleary SP, Di Nicola N, Manno M, Selander T, Aronson M, Redston M, Cotterchio M, Knight J, Gryfe R, Gallinger S (2004) Association between biallelic and monoallelic germline MYH gene mutations and colorectal cancer risk. J Natl Cancer Inst 96:1631–1634

Enholm S, Hienonen T, Suomalainen A, Lipton L, Tomlinson I, Karja V, Eskelinen M, Mecklin JP, Karhu A, Jarvinen HJ, Aaltonen LA (2003) Proportion and phenotype of *MYH*-associated colorectal neoplasia in a population-based series of Finnish colorectal cancer patients. Am J Pathol 163:827–832

Fleischmann C, Peto J, Cheadle J, Shah B, Sampson J, Houlston RS (2004) Comprehensive analysis of the contribution of germline *MYH* variation to early-onset colorectal cancer. Int J Cancer 109:554–558

Hugot JP, Chamaillard M, Zouali H, Lesage S, Cezard JP, Belaiche J, Almer S, Tysk C, O'Morain CA, Gassull M, Binder V, Finkel Y, Cortot A, Modigliani R, Laurent-Puig P, Gower-Rousseau C, Macry J, Colombel JF, Sahbatou M, Thomas G (2001) Association of NOD2 leucine-rich repeat variants with susceptibility to Crohn's disease. Nature 411:599–603

Sampson JR, Dolwani S, Jones S, Eccles D, Ellis A, Evans DG, Frayling I, Jordan S, Maher ER, Mak T, Maynard J, Pigatto F, Shaw J, Cheadle JP (2003) Autosomal recessive colorectal adenomatous polyposis due to inherited mutations of *MYH*. Lancet 362:39–41

Satagopan JM, Offit K, Foulkes W, Robson ME, Wacholder S, Eng CM, Karp SE, Begg CB (2001) The lifetime risks of breast cancer in Ashkenazi Jewish carriers of *BRCA1* and *BRCA2* mutations. Cancer Epidemiol Biomarkers Prev 10:467–473

Sieber OM, Howarth KM, Thirlwell C, Rowan A, Mandir N, Goodlad RA, Gilkar A, Spencer-Dene B, Stamp G, Johnson V, Silver A, Yang H, Miller JH, Ilyas M, Tomlinson IP (2004) *Myh* deficiency enhances intestinal tumorigenesis in multiple intestinal neoplasia ($Apc^{Min/+}$) mice. Cancer Res 64:8876–8881

Sieber OM, Lipton L, Crabtree M, Heinimann K, Fidalgo P, Phillips RK, Bisgaard ML, Orntoft TF, Aaltonen LA, Hodgson SV, Thomas HJ, Tomlinson IP (2003) Multiple colorectal adenomas, classic adenomatous polyposis, and germline mutations in *MYH*. N Engl J Med 348:791–799

Wang L, Baudhuin LM, Boardman LA, Steenblock KJ, Petersen GM, Halling KC, French AJ, Johnson RA, Burgart LJ, Rabe K, Lindor NM, Thibodeau SN (2004) *MYH* mutations in patients with attenuated and classic polyposis and with young-onset colorectal cancer without polyps. Gastroenterology 127:9–16

Am. J. Hum. Genet. 77:120–126, 2005

Report

Homozygous Nonsense Mutations in *KIAA1279* Are Associated with Malformations of the Central and Enteric Nervous Systems

Alice S. Brooks,[1] Aida M. Bertoli-Avella,[1] Grzegorz M. Burzynski,[6] Guido J. Breedveld,[1] Jan Osinga,[6] Ludolf G. Boven,[6] Jane A. Hurst,[7] Grazia M. S. Mancini,[1] Maarten H. Lequin,[2] Rene F. de Coo,[4] Ivana Matera,[6,8] Esther de Graaff,[1] Carel Meijers,[3] Patrick J. Willems,[9] Dick Tibboel,[5] Ben A. Oostra,[1] and Robert M. W. Hofstra[6]

Departments of [1]Clinical Genetics, [2]Radiology, and [3]Pathology and Departments of [4]Child Neurology and [5]Pediatric Surgery, Sophia Children's Hospital, Erasmus MC, Rotterdam; [6]Department of Medical Genetics, University of Groningen, Groningen, The Netherlands; [7]Department of Clinical Genetics, Oxford Radcliffe Hospitals, Oxford, United Kingdom; [8]Laboratorio di Genetica Molecolare, Instituto G. Gaslini, Genova; and [9]Gendia, Antwerp

We identified, by homozygosity mapping, a novel locus on 10q21.3-q22.1 for Goldberg-Shprintzen syndrome (GOSHS) in a consanguineous Moroccan family. Phenotypic features of GOSHS in this inbred family included microcephaly and mental retardation, which are both central nervous system defects, as well as Hirschsprung disease, an enteric nervous system defect. Furthermore, since bilateral generalized polymicogyria was diagnosed in all patients in this family, this feature might also be considered a key feature of the syndrome. We demonstrate that homozygous nonsense mutations in *KIAA1279* at 10q22.1, encoding a protein with two tetratrico peptide repeats, underlie this syndromic form of Hirschsprung disease and generalized polymicrogyria, establishing the importance of *KIAA1279* in both enteric and central nervous system development.

Goldberg-Shprintzen syndrome (GOSHS) (Goldberg and Shprintzen 1981) is a disorder characterized by microcephaly, mental retardation, facial dysmorphism, and Hirschsprung disease (HSCR). GOSHS shares the same accession number (MIM 235730) in the Online Mendelian Inheritance in Man (OMIM) database as the comparable disorder Mowat-Wilson syndrome (MWS) (Mowat et al. 1998). Genetically, however, they are different. MWS occurs as a de novo dominant syndrome, whereas GOSHS is most likely inherited as an autosomal recessive trait, a hypothesis based on the occurrence of the disease in consanguineous pedigrees and in affected siblings with unaffected parents (Hurst et al. 1988; Brooks et al. 1999). MWS is associated with de novo mutations in *ZFHX1B,* located at 2q22 (Amiel et al. 2001; Wakamatsu et al. 2001; Zweier et al. 2002), whereas, for GOSHS, no causative gene has yet been identified. Also, some clinical differences exist. In patients with MWS, neurological abnormalities such as epilepsy (in a high percentage of patients), agenesis of the corpus callosum (in 35% of patients), and cortical malformations (in a minority of patients) have been reported (Amiel et al. 2001; Zweier et al. 2002; Silengo et al. 2004). In the few patients with GOSHS discussed in published reports, neurological symptoms have not been studied in detail, and the cause of the microcephaly and mental retardation remains obscure (Goldberg and Shprintzen 1981; Hurst et al. 1988).

Here, we describe a family with HSCR (an anomaly of the enteric nervous system that is of neural crest origin and is histologically characterized by the absence of ganglion cells in the myenteric and submucosal plexuses) (Okamoto and Ueda 1967) as a variable feature and bilateral generalized polymicrogyria (PMG) (a developmental malformation of the cerebral cortex, characterized by an enlarged number of smaller convolutions or gyri and disruption of the normal six-layered cerebral cortical structure) (Friede 1989) as a constant feature.

Received February 22, 2005; accepted for publication April 19, 2005; electronically published May 9, 2005.

Address for correspondence and reprints: Dr. Robert M. W. Hofstra, Department of Medical Genetics, University of Groningen, Antonius Deusinglaan 4, 9713 AW Groningen, The Netherlands. E-mail: r.m.w.hofstra@medgen.umcg.nl

0002-9297/2005/7701-0012$15.00

The established diagnosis for this family was GOSHS, although bilateral generalized PMG (BGP) has not been reported as part of the syndrome before.

To unravel the genetic basis of GOSHS, we performed a complete genome scan and homozygosity mapping in a large consanguineous Moroccan family reported elsewhere (Brooks et al. 1999). The segregation of the disease in the pedigree is consistent with an autosomal recessive mode of inheritance, with several consanguineous loops (fig. 1), and the family therefore was considered suitable for homozygosity mapping (Lander and Botstein 1987). Informed consent was obtained from the parents of all subjects. In this family, five patients had the cardinal signs characterizing GOSHS (one boy lacked HSCR). One child with long-segment HSCR died in the neonatal period; his DNA was unavailable for our study. When the youngest patient was diagnosed, brain magnetic resonance imaging (MRI) revealed BGP. MRI scans of all living patients also revealed BGP (fig. 2). Gait disturbance, speech defect, excessive drooling, and

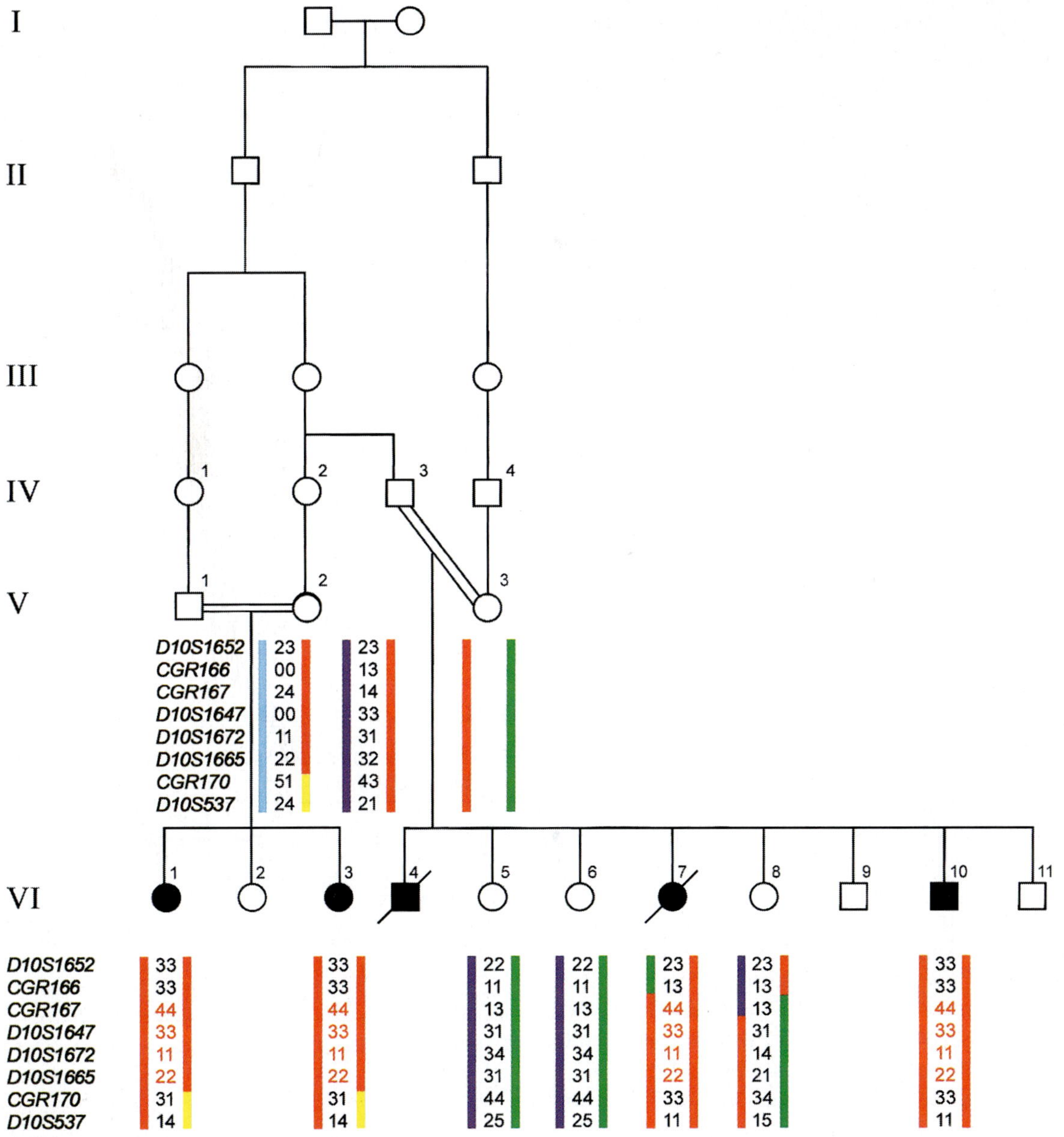

Figure 1 Pedigree structure and haplotypes of the Moroccan family with GOSHS. Patients are represented as blackened symbols. The shared region of homozygosity (*red*) in all affected cases is delimited by markers *CGR166* and *CGR170*. Six of the 11 markers typed for refining the candidate region between marker *D10S1652* and *D10S537* are shown.

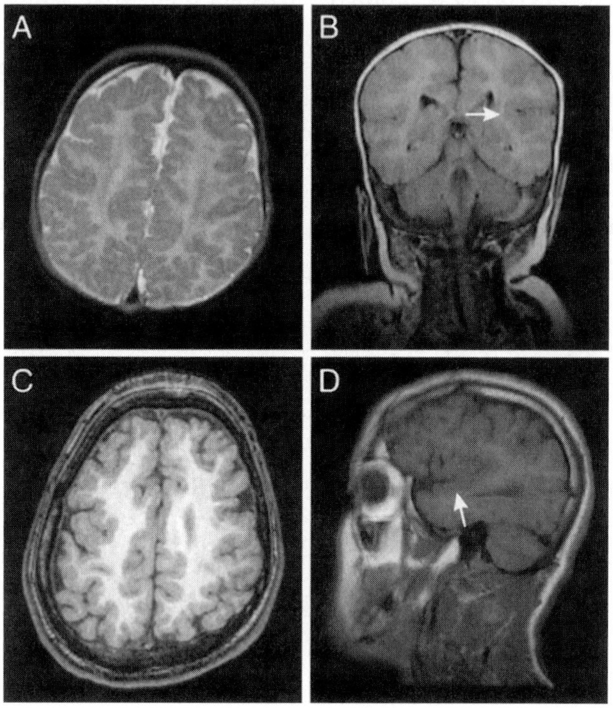

Figure 2 Representative MRIs of patient VI-1 (*panels A* and *B*) and patient VI-10 (*panels C* and *D*), showing BGP. *A*, Axial T2-weighted MRI of patient VI-1 at age 5 mo, showing frontoparietal and occipital bilateral PMG. *B*, Coronal FLAIR image of the same patient showing perisylvian PMG (*arrow*). *C*, T1-weighted axial image of patient VI-10 at age 14 years, showing BGP with distribution similar to that seen in patient VI-1. *D*, Parasagittal T1-weighted image of patient VI-10, showing PMG of the right peri-insular temporal lobe.

pseudobulbar signs indicate diffuse cortical dysfunction including the perisylvian areas.

Genomic DNA was isolated from peripheral leukocytes by use of the method described by Miller et al. (1988). By haplotyping, FISH, and sequence analyses, we excluded the *ZFHX1B* gene as a cause of GOSHS in this family (data not shown). For the systematic genome scan, 381 markers (STRPs) from the ABI Prism Linkage Mapping Set MD-10 (version 2.5), with an average spacing of 10 cM, were tested. DNA amplification was performed using 25 ng genomic DNA in 7.5-μl PCRs containing 1 × PCR Gold Buffer, 2.5 mM $MgCl_2$, 10 μM primer pair mix, and 0.4 U Ampli*Taq* Gold DNA polymerase (Applied Biosystems). Amplification conditions were 10 min at 95°C, followed by 35 cycles of 30 s at 95°C, 30 s at 55°C, and 1 min 30 s at 72°C; amplification was ended by a final extension for 5 min at 72°C. PCR products were pooled in panels and were loaded on an ABI 3100 automated sequencer. Data were analyzed using GeneMapper software (version 2.1) (Applied Biosystems).

After this initial screening, a region on 10q21.3-q22.1 was further investigated, since one of the four affected individuals was homozygous by descent for two consecutive markers, *D10S1652* and *D10S537*, whereas the other three patients were homozygous for one of these two markers. No other regions of homozygosity for consecutive markers were identified. We saturated the region between markers *D10S1652* and *D10S537* (12.3 cM) with 11 additional markers; they either were obtained from the Marshfield genetic map (Center for Medical Genetics Web site) or were newly developed. Marker order and genetic distances were obtained from the Marshfield genetic map (Center for Medical Genetics Web site) and the Celera physical map. All patients were homozygous for 7 of these 11 markers. A recombination event between loci *CGR166* and *CGR167* in patient VI-7 defined the centromeric boundary of the genetic interval. The telomeric border was defined by recombination events between markers *D10S1665* and *CGR170* in patients VI-1 and VI-3 (fig. 1). These recombination events reduced the candidate region to a minimum of 2.8 Mb and a maximum of 3.8 Mb.

Parametric two-point and multipoint linkage analyses were performed using the MLINK program from the LINKAGE (version 5.1) software package (Lathrop and Lalouel 1984) and the SimWalk2 program (version 2.9) (Sobel et al. 2002). LOD scores were calculated, under the assumption that the disease phenotype is a rare autosomal recessive disorder with 100% penetrance, with a gene frequency of 1:5,000. No phenocopies were allowed, and equal allele frequencies were used because of the limited number of available independent family members. A significant two-point LOD score was obtained (max LOD score 3.29 and $\theta = 0$ for marker *CGR167*) (table 1), which increased to a maximum mul-

Table 1

Results of Two-Point LOD Score Analysis, Performed for Markers Used in Fine Mapping

	LOD at θ =						
Marker[a]	0	.01	.05	.1	.2	.3	.4
D10S196	−13.81	−3.96	−1.52	−.65	−.08	.02	0
D10S1652	−6.96	−2.39	−1.85	−1.36	−.68	−.35	−.15
D10S1743	−4.97	1	1.39	1.31	.9	.46	.14
CGR166	−3.7	.58	1.03	1.02	.73	.4	.13
CGR167	3.29[b]	3.21	2.9	2.51	1.73	1	.4
D10S210	2.59	2.53	2.26	1.92	1.26	.67	.24
D10S1678	1.49	1.45	1.29	1.09	.72	.4	.16
D10S1647	1.84	1.79	1.58	1.33	.86	.47	.19
D10S1672	2.88	2.81	2.52	2.15	1.42	.76	.25
D10S1665	2.77	2.7	2.43	2.08	1.39	.75	.25
CGR172	1.36	1.32	1.17	.97	.62	.32	.11
CGR170	−.28	1.59	1.97	1.88	1.4	.83	.33
D10S676	−.28	1.25	1.64	1.56	1.1	.59	.18
D10S537	−.11	1.45	1.82	1.71	1.2	.65	.21

[a] Marker order follows that of the Celera physical map.
[b] Max LOD score.

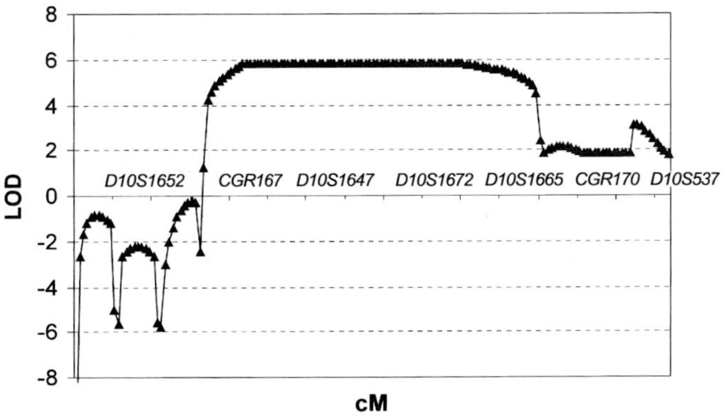

Figure 3 Multipoint LOD score analysis across and beyond the region of homozygosity, flanked by markers *D10S1652* and *CGR170*, with a peak LOD score of 5.9.

tipoint LOD score of 5.9 between markers *CGR167* and *D10S1647* (fig. 3).

The maximum 3.8-Mb linked region of shared homozygosity (defined by *CGR166* and *CGR170*) contained a total of 25 known genes and 5 genes encoding hypothetical proteins, in accordance with the National Center for Biotechnology Information (NCBI) build 34 of the human genome and the Ensembl Genome Browser (table 2). We first sequenced seven functional candidate genes on the basis of their putative involvement in neurogenesis (*CTNNA3, LRRTM3, ATOH7, DDX50, DDX21, NET-7,* and *NEUROG3*), either using cDNA obtained by RT-PCR from a lymphoblastoid cell line of patient VI-10 and from a control or using genomic DNA from both. Mutations were not identified. We then performed a systematic mutational screening of all transcripts from the candidate region. PCR products from either genomic DNA (exons including flanking intronic sequences) or reverse-transcribed products (ORFs) were amplified and purified (ExoSapIT [USB]). PCR primers, which were designed using standard software (Primer3), and conditions are available on request. Bidirectional sequencing was performed using BigDye Terminator chemistry on an ABI 3100 sequencer (Applied Biosystems). With the use of the software package SeqScape (version 2.1) (Applied Biosystems), sequences were aligned and compared with consensus sequences.

Analysis of 98% of all coding sequences from the region revealed one likely disease-causing homozygous nucleotide substitution, 303C→T, in exon 1 of the *KIAA1279* gene (fig. 4*A*). This transversion leads, at the amino acid level, to the replacement of an arginine with a stop codon (R90X), resulting in a shortened protein of 89 aa. The 303C→T mutation showed complete segregation with the disease in the family. One hundred ethnically matched control chromosomes (of North African origin) were screened for the R90X mutation, and none of the controls carried this mutation. Subsequently, one additional family of British Pakistani ancestry, with a phenotype similar to that found in the Moroccan family, was screened for mutations in this gene. This family had four affected individuals with multiple inbreeding loops. Clinical characteristics were consistent with GOSHS, and CT brain scans of this family were described in a previous study (Hurst et al. 1988) and were thought to represent an abnormality of neuronal migration. In the affected individuals, a homozygous G→T transversion was identified at nt 285, resulting, at the amino acid level, in the replacement of a glutamic acid with a stop codon (E84X) (fig. 4*B*). Two different homozygous nonsense mutations in *KIAA1279* in two independent families with GOSHS strongly indicate that *KIAA1279* is the gene responsible for GOSHS.

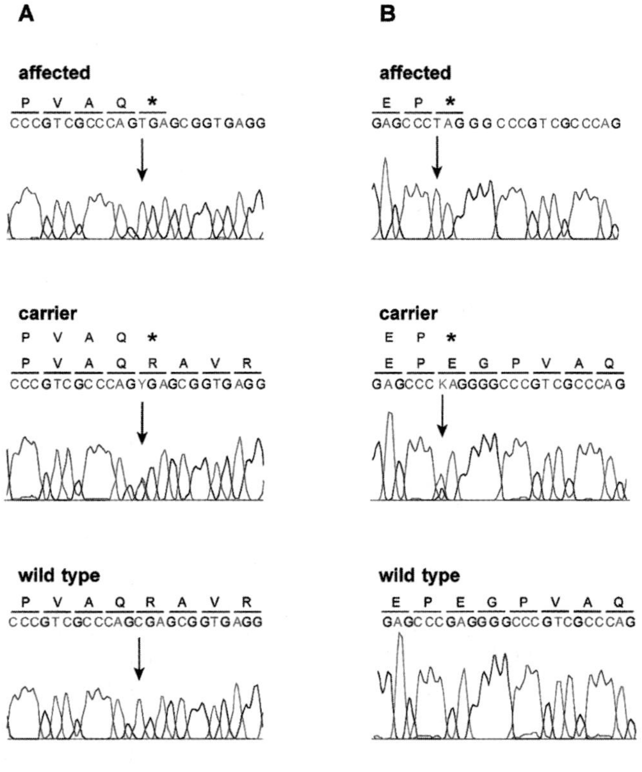

Figure 4 Mutations of *KIAA1279* associated with GOSHS. *A*, Electropherogram of the mutation identified in the Moroccan family. The 303C→T mutation causes the replacement of an arginine with a stop codon (R90X) in exon 1. *B*, Electropherogram of the mutation identified in the Pakistani family. A homozygous G→T transversion at nt 285 results in the replacement of a glutamic acid with a stop codon (E84X) in the patients.

Table 2

Gene and Marker Positions and Details

The table is available in its entirety in the online edition of *The American Journal of Human Genetics*.

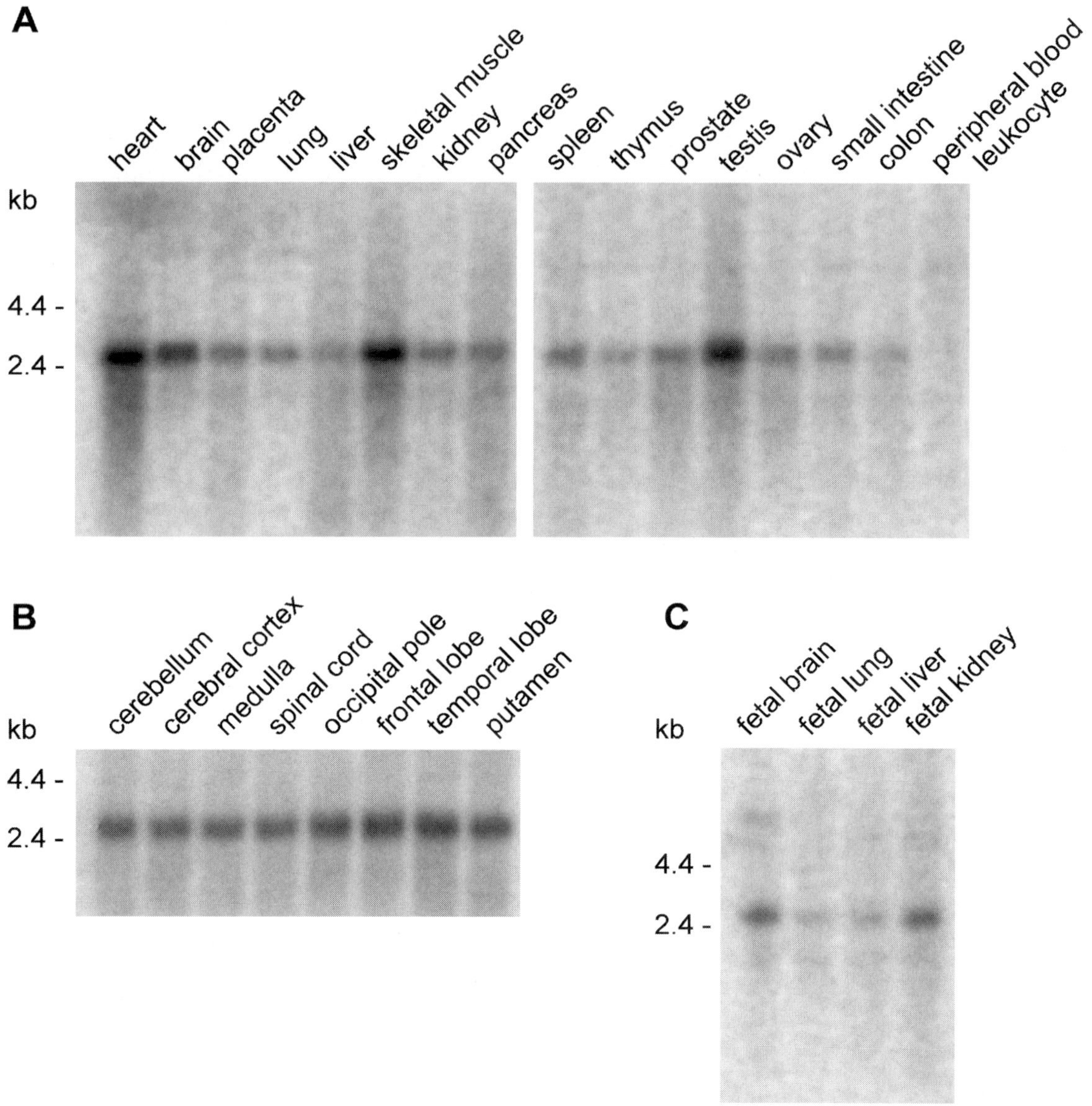

Figure 5 Expression of *KIAA1279* in human adult and fetal tissues. *A*, Multitissue northern blots, incubated with a *KIAA1279* probe, showing ubiquitous expression without a specific pattern (note the lack of expression in blood leukocytes). *B*, Northern blots from adult brain tissues, incubated with a *KIAA1279* probe. *C*, Human fetal multitissue northern blot, showing widespread expression.

KIAA1279 consists of seven exons spanning 28 kb of genomic DNA. The transcript encodes a protein of 621 aa. We identified orthologs of human KIAA1279 in fruit fly, frog, rat, mouse, bee, chicken, and Japanese puffer fish, using BLAST comparison (NCBI Web site). There is strong sequence conservation during evolution; the protein sequence of human KIAA1279 shares 89% amino acid identity with mouse product, 88% with rat product, and 29% with fruit fly product. Multitissue northern blots (both adult and fetal) (fig. 5) showed ubiquitous expression of the 2.4-kb *KIAA1279* mRNA without a specific pattern, with expression lacking only in blood leukocytes (fig. 5*A*). In addition, northern blot hybridization identified *KIAA1279* mRNA molecules in different parts of the adult CNS—namely, cerebellum, cortex, medulla, spinal cord, occipital lobe, frontal lobe, temporal lobe, and putamen (fig. 5*B*). This widespread *KIAA1279* expression is consistent with data available in gene expression databases such as the Gene Expression Omnibus, the Human Unidentified Gene-Encoded (HUGE) Protein Database, and the University of California–Santa Cruz (UCSC) Genome Browser. The function of KIAA1279 is unknown. Neither the gene nor its derived protein shows any significant sequence similarity to known human cDNA or protein sequences. Possible aspects of the molecular function of KIAA1279 may be gleaned from its primary sequence. We predicted protein motifs and domains using the program SMART (Simple Modular Architecture Research Tool). The predicted protein contains two tetratrico peptide repeats (TPRs), which are structural motifs consisting of 34 amino acid residues, in exon 1/2 and exon 4, respectively. Because of these repeats, KIAA1279 may be considered a member of the TPR protein family (D'Andrea and Regan 2003). The most basic function of TPR motifs is to mediate protein-protein interactions. Proteins with TPR motifs are involved in a variety of biological processes, such as cell-cycle regulation, transcriptional control, mitochondrial and peroxisomal protein transport, neurogenesis, and protein folding. Several diseases have been described as being caused by mutations in genes encoding proteins containing TPR domains—for example, Leber congenital amaurosis (*AIPL1*) (Sohocki et al. 2000) and Charcot-Marie-Tooth type 4C neuropathy (*KIAA1985*) (Senderek et al. 2003).

Since mutations in *KIAA1279* are associated with HSCR and PMG, its protein product may play a pivotal role in both peripheral and central nervous system development. PMG is traditionally classified as a result of a disruption such as fetal hypoxic ischemic damage, infection, or exposure to toxic drugs in the second trimester (13–21 wk) (Barth and van der Harten 1985; Barth 2003). However, the identification of *KIAA1279* as the GOSHS gene underlines the importance of genetic factors in the etiology of this neuronal migration disorder of the cortex, as was already proven (Mitchell et al. 2003; Piao et al. 2004) or suggested (Ciardo et al. 2001; Chang et al. 2004) for other forms of PMG. Under the assumption that the main function of KIAA1279 is to bind other proteins, these target peptides might be (known) HSCR- or PMG-associated susceptibility factors. More likely, however, these targets might play a more general role in neuronal development, since a malformation of cortical organization is a constant feature found in the Moroccan family, whereas HSCR is a variable feature. Elucidation of KIAA1279 function and, more important, studies of *KIAA1279* expression and protein interactions may provide new insight into the molecular basis of PMG and HSCR.

Acknowledgments

We thank the patients and their families, for their support and their willingness to donate samples; Jeannette Hoogeboom and Martijn Breuning, for patient care; Jim Barkovich, for help with classification of PMG; Martinus Niermeijer, for his guidance; Elisabeth Lodder and Peter van der Spek, for bioinformatics support; Herma van der Linde and Erik Simons, for technical assistance; and Tom de Vries Lentsch, for help with preparation of the figures. This work was funded, in part, by Nederlandse organisatie voor Wetenschappelijk Onderzoek grants 901-04-210 and 901-04-225 (to R.M.W.H.).

Web Resources

Accession numbers and URLs for data presented herein are as follows:

Celera, http://www.celeradiscoverysystem.com/
Center for Medical Genetics, Marshfield Clinic Research Foundation, http://research.marshfieldclinic.org/genetics/
Ensembl Genome Browser, http://www.ensembl.org/
GenBank, http://www.ncbi.nlm.nih.gov/Genbank/ (for *CGR170* [accession number BV212295], *CGR167* [accession number BV212296], *CGR166* [accession number BV212297], *D10S196* [accession number Z16598], *D10S1652* [accession number Z52339], *D10S1743* [accession number Z53951], *D10S210* [accession number Z16813], *D10S1678* [accession number Z52660], and *D10S1647* [accession number Z52188])
Gene Expression Omnibus, http://www.ncbi.nlm.nih.gov/geo/
Human Unidentified Gene–Encoded (HUGE) Protein Database, http://www.kazusa.or.jp/huge/
NCBI, http://www.ncbi.nlm.nih.gov/
Online Mendelian Inheritance in Man (OMIM), http://www.ncbi.nlm.nih.gov/Omim/ (for GOSHS and MWS)
Primer3, http://frodo.wi.mit.edu/cgi-bin/primer3/primer3_www.cgi
SMART, http://smart.embl-heidelberg.de/
UCSC Genome Browser, http://genome.ucsc.edu/

References

Amiel J, Espinosa-Parrilla Y, Steffann J, Gosset P, Pelet A, Prieur M, Boute O, Choiset A, Lacombe D, Philip N, Le Merrer M, Tanaka H, Till M, Touraine R, Toutain A, Vekemans M, Munnich A, Lyonnet S (2001) Large-scale deletions and *SMADIP1* truncating mutations in syndromic Hirschsprung disease with involvement of midline structures. Am J Hum Genet 69:1370–1377

Barth PG (2003) Fetal disruption as a cause of neuronal migration defects. In: Barth PG (ed) Disorders of neuronal migration. MacKeith Press, London, pp 182–194

Barth PG, van der Harten JJ (1985) Parabiotic twin syndrome with topical isocortical disruption and gastroschisis. Acta Neuropathol 67:345–349

Brooks AS, Breuning MH, Osinga J, vd Smagt JJ, Catsman CE, Buys CH, Meijers C, Hofstra RM (1999) A consanguineous family with Hirschsprung disease, microcephaly, and mental retardation (Goldberg-Shprintzen syndrome). J Med Genet 36:485–489

Chang BS, Piao X, Giannini C, Cascino GD, Scheffer I, Woods CG, Topcu M, Tezcan K, Bodell A, Leventer RJ, Barkovich AJ, Grant PE, Walsh CA (2004) Bilateral generalized polymicrogyria (BGP): a distinct syndrome of cortical malformation. Neurology 62:1722–1728

Ciardo F, Zamponi N, Specchio N, Parmeggiani R, Guerrini R (2001) Autosomal recessive polymicrogyria with infantile spasms and limb deformities. Neuropediatrics 32:325–329

D'Andrea LD, Regan L (2003) TPR proteins: the versatile helix. Trends Biochem Sci 28:655–662

Friede RL (ed) (1989) Developmental neuropathology, 2nd ed. Springer Verlag, Berlin

Goldberg RB, Shprintzen RJ (1981) Hirschsprung megacolon and cleft palate in two sibs. J Craniofac Genet Dev Biol 1: 185–189

Hurst JA, Markiewicz M, Kumar D, Brett, EM (1988) Unknown syndrome: Hirschsprung's disease, microcephaly, and iris coloboma: a new syndrome of defective neuronal migration. J Med Genet 25:494–497

Lander E, Botstein D (1987) Homozygosity mapping: a way to map human recessive traits with the DNA of inbred children. Science 236:1567–1570

Lathrop GM, Lalouel JM (1984) Easy calculations of LOD scores and genetic risks on small computers. Am J Hum Genet 36:460–465

Miller SA, Dykes DD, Polesky HF (1988) A simple salting out procedure for extracting DNA from human nucleated cells. Nucleic Acids Res 16:1215

Mitchell TN, Free SL, Williamson KA, Stevens JM, Churchill AJ, Hanson IM, Shorvon SD, Moore AT, van Heyningen V, Sisodiya SM, Mitchell TN (2003) Polymicrogyria and absence of pineal gland due to *PAX6* mutation. Ann Neurol 53:658–663

Mowat DR, Croaker GD, Cass DT, Kerr BA, Chaitow J, Ades LC, Chia NL, Wilson MJ (1998) Hirschsprung disease, microcephaly, mental retardation, and characteristic facial features: delineation of a new syndrome and identification of a locus at chromosome 2q22-q23. J Med Genet 35:617–623

Okamoto E, Ueda T (1967) Embryogenesis of intramural ganglia of the gut and its relation to Hirschsprung's disease. J Pediatr Surg 2:437–443

Piao X, Hill RS, Bodell A, Chang BS, Basel-Vanagaite L, Straussberg R, Dobyns WB, Qasrawi B, Winter RM, Innes AM, Voit T, Ross ME, Michaud JL, Descarie JC, Barkovich AJ, Walsh CA (2004) G protein-coupled receptor-dependent development of human frontal cortex. Science 303:2033–2036

Senderek J, Bergmann C, Stendel C, Kirfel J, Verpoorten N, De Jonghe P, Timmerman V, et al (2003) Mutations in a gene encoding a novel SH3/TPR domain protein cause autosomal recessive Charcot-Marie-Tooth type 4C neuropathy. Am J Hum Genet 73:1106–1119

Silengo M, Ferrero GB, Wakamatsu N (2004) Pachygyria and cerebellar hypoplasia in a patient with a 2q22-q23 deletion that includes the *ZFHX1B* gene. Am J Med Genet A 127: 109

Sobel E, Papp JC, Lange K (2002) Detection and integration of genotyping errors in statistical genetics. Am J Hum Genet 70:496–508

Sohocki MM, Bowne SJ, Sullivan LS, Blackshaw S, Cepko CL, Payne AM, Bhattacharya SS, Khaliq S, Qasim Mehdi S, Birch DG, Harrison WR, Elder FF, Heckenlively JR, Daiger SP (2000) Mutations in a new photoreceptor-pineal gene on 17p cause Leber congenital amaurosis. Nat Genet 24:79–83

Wakamatsu N, Yamada Y, Yamada K, Ono T, Nomura N, Taniguchi H, Kitoh H, Mutoh N, Yamanaka T, Mushiake K, Kato K, Sonta S, Nagaya M (2001) Mutations in *SIP1*, encoding Smad interacting protein-1, cause a form of Hirschsprung disease. Nat Genet 27:369–370

Zweier C, Albrecht B, Mitulla B, Behrens R, Beese M, Gillessen-Kaesbach G, Rott HD, Rauch A (2002) "Mowat-Wilson" syndrome with and without Hirschsprung disease is a distinct, recognizable multiple congenital anomalies-mental retardation syndrome caused by mutations in the zinc finger homeo box 1B gene. Am J Med Genet 108:177–181

Report

Disentangling Fetal and Maternal Susceptibility for Pre-Eclampsia: A British Multicenter Candidate-Gene Study

The GOPEC Consortium

The Genetics of Pre-Eclampsia (GOPEC) collaboration aims to identify genetic factors in U.K. families affected by pre-eclampsia. A number of genetic studies have reported associations with pre-eclampsia, but attempts to replicate these findings have yielded inconsistent results. We describe the results of extensive genotyping of seven candidate genes previously reported as conferring susceptibility to pre-eclampsia. Six hundred fifty-seven women affected by pre-eclampsia and their families were genotyped at 28 single-nucleotide polymorphisms in the genes encoding angiotensinogen, the angiotensin receptors, factor V Leiden variant, methylene tetrahydrofolate reductase, nitric oxide synthase, and TNFα. Genotypes were analyzed by the transmission/disequilibrium test. Genotype risk ratios (GRRs) associated with maternal genotypes had a range of 0.70–1.16; GRRs associated with fetal genotypes had a range of 0.72–1.11. No GRR achieved the prespecified criteria for statistical significance (posterior probability >.05). We conclude that none of the genetic variants tested in this large study of strictly defined pre-eclamptic pregnancies confers a high risk of disease. The results emphasize the importance of conducting rigorously designed studies of adequate size to provide precise genetic risks with narrow confidence intervals, if overreporting of false-positive results is to be avoided.

Pre-eclampsia (MIM 189800), identified clinically by maternal hypertension and proteinuria occurring after the 20th wk of gestation, affects ~3% of pregnancies in Western populations (Lie et al. 1998). Both maternal and fetal genes appear to play an etiological role; a recent analysis of 700,000 pregnancies from the Swedish Birth Registry estimated the heritability conferred by maternal genes as 0.35 (95% CI 0.33–0.36) and that due to fetal genes as 0.20 (95% CI 0.11–0.24) (Pawitan et al. 2004).

Genes that have been implicated in pre-eclampsia include angiotensinogen (*AGT*) (Ward et al. 1993), the type 1 and type 2 angiotensin receptors (*AGTR1* and *AGTR2*) (Morgan et al. 1998; Plummer et al. 2004), tumor necrosis factor α (*TNF*) (Chen et al. 1996), endothelial nitric oxide synthase (*NOS3*) (Yoshimura et al. 2000), methylene tetrahydrofolate reductase (*MTHFR*) (Sohda et al. 1997), and the Leiden variant of coagulation factor V (*F5*) (Dizon-Townson et al. 1996). Results have not been consistently reproducible, and few studies have addressed the role of the fetal genotype. It is therefore important to establish the contribution of maternal and fetal genes in a large study with adequate statistical power to detect modest genotype relative risks with narrow CIs.

The Genetics of Pre-Eclampsia (GOPEC) study, a consortium of researchers from 10 U.K. universities, recruited women affected by pre-eclampsia and their families from 2000 to 2003. We used transmission/disequilibrium testing (TDT) to distinguish between maternal- and fetal-gene effects (Mitchell 1997) and to eliminate confounding due to population stratification (admixture). All volunteers gave informed consent for the study, which was approved by the Trent Multicentre Research Ethics Committee. White western European women with pre-eclampsia, recruited at the time of diagnosis, were eligible for participation in the study if, after the 20th wk of pregnancy, their systolic blood pressure rose to ⩾140 mm Hg and their diastolic blood pressure rose to ⩾90 mm Hg on two occasions measured within 24 h and if they had proteinuria >500 mg per 24 h or 2+ (1 g/liter) on dipstick testing of urine. Women who were hypertensive or had proteinuria prior to the 20th wk of pregnancy were excluded, as were those with essential hypertension, diabetes, renal or cardiac disease, or a cur-

Received March 8, 2005; accepted for publication April 19, 2005; electronically published May 11, 2005.

Address for correspondence and reprints: Dr. Linda Morgan, Institute of Genetics, Clinical Chemistry Division, Queen's Medical Centre, Nottingham, NG14 7GZ, United Kingdom. E-mail: linda.morgan@nottingham.ac.uk

0002-9297/2005/7701-0013$15.00

Table 1

Clinical Features of 627 Index Pregnancies

Feature	5th Percentile	Median	95th Percentile
Maternal age (years)	19.9	29.7	38.4
Maternal BMI (kg/m^2)	20.37	27.01	38.60
Highest SBP[a] (mm Hg)	140	161	199
Highest DBP[b] (mm Hg)	98	110	126
Highest proteinuria (g/24 h)[c]	.50	1.67	9.59
Gestation at delivery (wk)	28	37	41
Infant birth weight (kg)	.90	2.56	3.89
Birth weight percentile[d]	0	11	89

[a] SBP = systolic blood pressure.
[b] DBP = diastolic blood pressure.
[c] 24-h protein results were available for 364 women.
[d] Calculated using GROW freeware (West Midlands Perinatal Institute Web site).

rent multiple pregnancy. Pre-eclampsia was defined as unresolved if hypertension or proteinuria persisted 13 wk after delivery. Details of recruitment protocols are available at the GOPEC Web site.

DNA was extracted from venous blood from adult participants by use of Promega Wizard DNA extraction kits. Fetal DNA was extracted from umbilical cord tissue by use of Nucleon HT kits (Amersham Biosciences). Haplotype tagSNPs with minor-allele frequencies (MAF) >0.05 were selected from bins in linkage disequilibrium ($r^2 > 0.64$) with data from the SeattleSNPs database or published data (Nakajima et al. 2002; Plummer et al. 2004). tagSNP maps generated by complete-gene resequencing were available for *AGT, TNF,* and *NOS3*; this strategy for tagSNP selection is expected to capture >80% of common haplotype diversity in these genes (Carlson et al. 2004). tagSNP maps for *AGTR1* and *AGTR2* were less complete and included flanking and exonic regions only. Two SNPs in *MTHFR* and one SNP in *F5* were selected on the basis of their functional effects (Bertina et al. 1994; Frosst et al. 1995; van der Put et al. 1998). Genotyping was undertaken using *Taq*Man 5′ exonuclease probes; assay details are available on request. Nineteen percent of samples were genotyped in duplicate, and genotyping was confirmed by DNA sequencing of a random selection of samples. The genotyping failure rate was 0.8%, and the genotyping replication rate was 99.4%.

An affected woman and her parents, or one parent and one or more siblings, formed a maternal triad for TDT of maternal genes. An affected woman, her partner, and baby formed a fetal triad for testing of fetal genes. Mendelian segregation inconsistencies, identified using PedCheck (O'Connell and Weeks 1998), may be due to either miscalling of marker alleles or incorrect information about family structure (e.g., nonpaternity or unreported ovum donation); incorrect information about family structure will reduce the power of detecting true genetic effects (Gordon et al. 1999). The information from the 28 segregating markers was used to exclude relationships on the basis of two or more discrepant genotypes (Chakraborty and Stivers 1996). Under the assumption that the probability of detecting a relationship inconsistency with one typically informative biallelic marker is .15 (Jamieson and Taylor 1997) and that the prior probability of nonpaternity/nonmaternity is ≤10%, then the posterior probability of failing to detect these inconsistent relationships using this "two strikes and you are out" rule is ≤0.7%. Maternal or fetal triads with a single SNP showing inconsistencies with Mendelian inheritance were not included in the statistical analysis of this specific marker; we assume that isolated segregation inconsistencies can be attributed to occasional genotype miscalls. From 657 families, 14 maternal and 26 fetal triads, which had more than one SNP genotyping result that was inconsistent with Mendelian inheritance, were excluded from further statistical analysis. Six hundred twenty-seven families remained, comprising 2,504 individuals, including 398 maternal triads and 536 fetal triads. Clinical features are shown in tables 1 and 2.

No deviations from Hardy-Weinberg equilibrium in founder individuals were detected using PedStats software (Center for Statistical Genetics Web site). To analyze phase-uncertain data and to study single markers or extended marker haplotypes for linkage in the presence of gene association, the TRANSMIT program was used (Clayton 1999), which implements a score test statistic that omits terms that are sensitive to population stratification. The bootstrap option was used to empirically evaluate the significance of the test statistics. Haplotypes with an estimated frequency of ≤1% were pooled for statistical analysis. Estimates of the genetic-effect size, expressed as genotype risk ratios (GRRs), (and standard errors of these estimates) were calculated from the proportion of transmitted risk alleles (Kazeem and Farrall 2005).

The results of genotyping are shown in table 3. In

Table 2

Comparison of 627 Index Pregnancies

Feature	No. (%) of Index Pregnancies
Maternal parity:	
Nulliparous	496 (79.1%)
Parous	131 (20.9%)
Sex of infant:	
Male	320 (51.0%)
Female	307 (49.0%)
Resolution[a]:	
Resolved	558 (89.0%)
Unresolved	69 (11.0%)

[a] Resolution = diastolic blood pressure <90 mm Hg and no proteinuria 13 wk postpartum.

Table 3

Results of Analysis of Maternal and Fetal SNP Genotypes by TDT

Gene, GenBank Reference Sequence, and HGVS[a] Name	Alternative Name	Location	Maternal Genotype				Fetal Genotype			
			MAF	GRR	95% CI	*P*	MAF	GRR	95% CI	*P*
AGT:										
AY436323:										
g.1718G→T	−1074G→T	5′ flanking	.11	.97	.74–1.27	.815	.11	1.04	.79–1.37	.785
g.2963C→T	172C→T	Intron 1	.08	1.16	.83–1.63	.392	.08	.82	.60–1.11	.197
g.3467G→A	676G→A	Intron 2	.37	.99	.82–1.19	.913	.36	.90	.75–1.08	.261
g.3826G→A	1035G→A	Intron 2	.25	1.00	.81–1.23	.997	.24	.91	.75–1.12	.375
g.6679C→T	174Thr→Met	Exon 2	.12	.84	.64–1.09	.185	.12	.92	.71–1.19	.519
g.6862T→C	235Met→Thr	Exon 2	.40	.94	.78–1.13	.505	.40	.92	.77–1.10	.349
g.8854C→A	6066C→A	Intron 3	.20	1.06	.84–1.33	.625	.19	.95	.77–1.18	.649
g.14321C→A	11535C→A	3′ UTR	.31	.95	.78–1.15	.583	.32	.99	.82–1.18	.882
AGTR1:										
AF245699.1:										
g.4955T→A	−810T→A	5′ flanking	.20	1.10	.88–1.38	.410	.19	1.08	.87–1.35	.495
g.5245C→T	−521C→T	5′ flanking	.35	.91	.75–1.09	.309	.32	.88	.73–1.05	.144
g.49465C→T	573C→T	Exon 5	.45	.98	.82–1.18	.848	.46	.95	.80–1.13	.569
g.50058A→C	1166A→C	3′ UTR	.31	1.01	.83–1.22	.957	.31	1.01	.85–1.21	.883
AGTR2:										
AY324607.1:										
g.2184A→T	333A→T	Intron 2	.28	***.72***	***.52–.98***	***.039***	.26	1.05	.79–1.40	.720
g.4673G→T	2812G→T	3′ UTR	.22	***.70***	***.48–1.00***	***.054***	.22	***.72***	***.52–.98***	***.038***
g.4679G→A	2818G→A	3′ UTR	.46	1.09	.80–1.47	.590	.44	1.06	.82–1.37	.655
F5:										
NM_000130:										
c.1691G→A	Leiden	Exon 10	.02	1.09	.59–2.07	.779	.02	.85	.47–1.48	.561
MTHFR:										
AY338232:										
g.8747C→T	677C→T	Exon 4	.33	1.04	.85–1.26	.723	.34	1.05	.88–1.25	.609
g.10649A→C	1298A→C	Exon 7	.30	.92	.76–1.12	.419	.29	.87	.72–1.05	.141
NOS3:										
AF519768:										
g.450T→A	−1474T→A	5′ flanking	.39	1.12	.93–1.35	.248	.38	.98	.82–1.17	.824
g.3497G→A	...	Intron 2	.14	1.13	.87–1.48	.355	.15	1.11	.86–1.43	.431
g.7164G→T	298Glu→Asp	Exon 7	.35	.93	.77–1.12	.455	.35	1.06	.88–1.28	.529
g.9932G→A	...	Intron 11	.46	1.03	.86–1.23	.724	.43	.87	.73–1.03	.116
g.13834C→A	...	Intron 13	.36	.96	.80–1.16	.676	.37	1.05	.88–1.26	.557
g.17971A→G	...	Intron 19	.24	.88	.71–1.08	.220	.23	.88	.72–1.08	.215
TNF:										
AY066019:										
g.282G→A	−308G→A	5′ flanking	.20	1.01	.81–1.26	.954	.18	.92	.73–1.14	.437
g.1893A→G	...	Intron 3	.08	.86	.62–1.19	.362	.08	***.73***	***.53–.99***	***.044***
g.4101G→A	...	3′ flanking	.15	.98	.76–1.25	.860	.12	.85	.66–1.10	.220
g.4765G→T	...	3′ flanking	.08	1.16	.82–1.65	.402	.08	1.04	.75–1.43	.833

NOTE.—Results with statistical probability ⩽.05 are shown in bold italics.

[a] HGVS = Human Genome Variation Society.

maternal triads, two SNPs in *AGTR2,* g.2184A→T and g.4673G→T, demonstrated marginally decreased transmission of the minor allele ($P = .039$ and $P = .054$, respectively). Maternal GRRs associated with minor variants at the remaining 26 SNPs fell within the range of 0.84–1.16. Analysis of fetal triads demonstrated weak evidence of transmission disequilibrium at g.4673G→T in *AGTR2* ($P = .038$) and at g.1893A→G in *TNF* ($P = .044$). GRRs associated with fetal genotype at the remaining 26 SNPs were in the range of 0.82–1.11.

The results of haplotype analysis are shown in table 4. There was weak support for transmission disequilibrium in fetal triads with *TNF* haplotypes ($P = .026$) and with the *AGT* haplotypes defined by g.6862T→C (235Met→Thr) and g.3467G→A, with the common 235Met-g.3467G allele being overtransmitted ($P = .027$).

We have analyzed our gene-association results within a Bayesian framework (Colhoun et al. 2003; Wacholder et al. 2004), which interprets the statistical significance of the results in the context of the prior probability that a candidate gene encodes disease susceptibility. The study was designed to detect moderately sized gene associations; the cohorts of 398 maternal trios and 536 fetal

Table 4

Results of Analysis of Maternal and Fetal Haplotypes

	Haplotype Analysis					
	Maternal			Fetal		
Gene	χ^2	df	*P*	χ^2	df	*P*
AGT[a]	3.56	3	.217	9.41	3	***.027***
AGTR1	6.78	9	.773	11.11	9	.305
AGTR2	6.12	3	.106	4.77	3	.189
MTHFR	2.30	3	.280	3.22	3	.173
NOS3	13.95	11	.232	19.86	11	.237
TNF	1.64	5	.898	10.49	5	***.026***

Note.—*P* values are empirical values generated using the bootstrap option of the TRANSMIT software. Results with statistical probability ⩽.05 are shown in bold italics.

[a] The computational complexities of estimating 8-marker haplotypes precluded the use of all markers for *AGT* in a single analysis. All possible pairs of markers for this gene were examined, and the most significant associations are shown. Markers are g.2963C→T and g.8854C→A (maternal haplotypes) and g.6862T→C (235Met→Thr) and g.3467G→A (fetal haplotypes). Addition of a third marker did not increase statistical significance.

trios have 85% power to detect common (MAF = 0.5) susceptibility genes with GRRs of 1.6 and 1.5, respectively, with the assumption of a type 1 error rate of 0.0005. This nominal level of significance is sufficiently stringent for detection at the 5% level of noteworthy effects of candidate genes with modest prior probabilities (⩾.01). The power of the study will inevitably be reduced for smaller GRRs, rarer SNPs, low levels of linkage disequilibrium between markers and susceptibility allele(s), or reduced prior probabilities (<.01) of gene association.

None of the examined individual SNPs or haplotypes achieved statistical significance by use of these criteria (posterior probability >.05). Genotypes and haplotypes were examined in the subgroup of nulliparous pregnancies in which hypertension and proteinuria had resolved by 13 wk postpartum, comprising 296 maternal triads and 383 fetal triads. GRRs were similar to those in the full data set, and none achieved statistical significance (posterior probability >.05).

This study of a large and very precisely phenotyped group of pregnancies excludes major risks associated with a number of SNPs in candidate genes that have dominated studies of the genetics of pre-eclampsia. The challenge remains to identify susceptibility genes that will provide greater understanding of the pathogenesis of pre-eclampsia. It is essential to study large numbers of affected women and their babies if misleading results are to be avoided. The formation of national or international consortia is one way forward. In addition, the adoption of clear definitions of phenotype and inclusion and exclusion criteria will facilitate meta-analysis of replicated studies.

Acknowledgments

We thank patients and their families, midwives, and doctors, whose support made the study possible. We are grateful to the British Heart Foundation for their generous funding. L. Morgan (Institute of Genetics, University of Nottingham) and M. Farrall (Wellcome Trust Centre for Human Genetics, Oxford) wrote the article, which was approved by all collaborators: P. N. Baker (University of Manchester); F. Broughton Pipkin, N. Kalsheker, S. O'Malley, M. Henfrey, S. Arulkumaran, and I. Symonds (University of Nottingham); A. Cameron, A. Dominiczak, M. McDade, W. Kwong Lee, and J. McCulloch (University of Glasgow); M. Caulfield (Bart's and the London, Queen Mary's School of Medicine and Dentistry); M. Habiba and C. Dodd (University of Leicester); M. Kilby and L. Davies (University of Birmingham); S. Macphail (University of Newcastle); P. M. S. O'Brien (University of Keele); K. O'Shaughnessy, B. Newcombe, and P. de la Salle (University of Cambridge); C. Redman and P. Jarrett (University of Oxford); M. de Swiet, C. Williamson, E. Byford, and F. Cheng (Imperial College London); J. J. Walker and L. Samwiil (University of Leeds); G. Chapman (University Hospital of North Staffordshire); E. Dennehy (Derby Hospitals Trust); R. Keys and S. Bjornsson (Glasgow Princess Royal Hospital); C. Mercer and M. Mohajer (Royal Shrewsbury Hospital); G. Thompson (Newcastle Royal Victoria Hospital); M. N. Fitzgibbon (Wordsley Hospital); G. Hackett (Cambridge Rosie Maternity Hospital); K. Hinshaw (Sunderland Royal Hospital); B. Lim (Hinchingbrooke Hospital); D. T. Y. Liu (Nottingham City Hospital); W. Mackenzie (Birmingham Heartlands Hospital); M. Selinger (Royal Berkshire Hospital); I. Scudamore (Leicester General Hospital); C. Sparey (Leeds General Infirmary); D. Tuffnell (Bradford Royal Infirmary); S. Ward (Kings Mill Hospital); J. Waugh (Leicester Royal Infirmary); and D. Williams (Chelsea and Westminster Hospital).

Web Resources

The URLs for data presented herein are as follows:

Center for Statistical Genetics, http://www.sph.umich.edu/csg/abecasis/PedStats/ (for PedStats)
GenBank, http://www.ncbi.nlm.nih.gov/Genbank/ (for the reference sequence numbers included in table 3)
GOPEC, http://www.gopec.org/
Online Mendelian Inheritance in Man (OMIM), http://www.ncbi.nlm.nih.gov/Omim/ (for pre-eclampsia)
SeattleSNPs, http://pga.gs.washington.edu/
West Midlands Perinatal Institute, http://www.perinatal.nhs.uk/ (for GROW freeware)

References

Bertina RM, Koeleman BP, Koster T, Rosendaal FR, Dirven RJ, de Ronde H, van der Velden PA, Reitsma PH (1994) Mutation in blood coagulation factor V associated with resistance to activated protein C. Nature 369:64–67
Carlson CS, Eberle MA, Rieder MJ, Yi Q, Kruglyak L, Nickerson DA (2004) Selecting a maximally informative set of single-

nucleotide polymorphisms for association analyses using linkage disequilibrium. Am J Hum Genet 74:106–120
Chakraborty R, Stivers DN (1996) Paternity exclusion by DNA markers: effects of paternal mutations. J Forensic Sci 41:671–677
Chen G, Wilson R, Wang SH, Zheng HZ, Walker JJ, McKillop JH (1996) Tumour necrosis factor-alpha (TNF-α) gene polymorphism and expression in pre-eclampsia. Clin Exp Immunol 104:154–159
Clayton D (1999) A generalization of the transmission/disequilibrium test for uncertain-haplotype transmission. Am J Hum Genet 65:1170–1177
Colhoun HM, McKeigue PM, Davey Smith G (2003) Problems of reporting genetic associations with complex outcomes. Lancet 361:865–872
Dizon-Townson DS, Nelson LM, Easton K, Ward K (1996) The factor V Leiden mutation may predispose women to severe pre-eclampsia. Am J Obstet Gynecol 175:902–905
Frosst P, Blom HJ, Milos R, Goyette P, Sheppard CA, Matthews RG, Boers GJ, den Heijer M, Kluijtmans LAJ, van den Heuvel LP, Rozen R (1995) A candidate genetic risk factor for vascular disease: a common mutation in methylenetetrahydrofolate reductase. Nat Genet 10:111–113
Gordon D, Matise TC, Heath SC, Ott J (1999) Power loss for multiallelic transmission/disequilibrium test when errors introduced: GAW11 simulated data. Genet Epidemiol Suppl 17:S587–S592
Jamieson A, Taylor SS (1997) Comparisons of three probability formulae for parentage exclusion. Anim Genet 28:397–400
Kazeem G, Farrall M (2005) Integrating case-control and TDT studies. Ann Hum Genet 69:329–335
Lie RT, Rasmussen S, Brunborg H, Gjessing HK, Lie-Nielsen E, Irgens LM (1998) Fetal and maternal contributions to the risk of pre-eclampsia: population based study. BMJ 316:1343–1347
Mitchell LE (1997) Differentiating between fetal and maternal genotypic effects, using the transmission test for linkage disequilibrium. Am J Hum Genet 60:1006–1007
Morgan L, Crawshaw S, Baker PN, Brookfield JFY, Broughton-Pipkin F, Kalsheker N (1998) Distortion of maternal-fetal angiotensin II type 1 receptor transmission in pre-eclampsia. J Med Genet 35:632–636
Nakajima T, Jorde LB, Ishigami T, Umemura S, Emi M, Lalouel J-M, Inoue I (2002) Nucleotide diversity and haplotype structure of the human angiotensinogen gene in two populations. Am J Hum Genet 70:108–123
O'Connell JR, Weeks DE (1998) PedCheck: a program for identification of genotype incompatibilities in linkage analysis. Am J Hum Genet 63:259–266
Pawitan Y, Reilly M, Nilsson E, Cnattingius S, Lichtenstein P (2004) Estimation of genetic and environmental factors for binary traits using family data. Stat Med 23:449–465
Plummer S, Tower C, Morgan L, Alonso P, Baker P, Broughton-Pipkin F, Kalsheker N (2004) Haplotypes of the angiotensin II receptor genes in women with normotensive pregnancy and women with pre-eclampsia. Hum Mutat 24:14–20
Sohda S, Arinami T, Hamada H, Yamada N, Hamaguchi H, Kubo T (1997) Methylenetetrahydrofolate reductase polymorphism and pre-eclampsia. J Med Genet 34:525–526
van der Put NMJ, Gabreëls F, Stevens EMB, Smeitink JAM, Trijbels FJM, Eskes TKAB, van den Heuvel LP, Blom HJ (1998) A second common mutation in the methylenetetrahydrofolate reductase gene: an additional risk factor for neural-tube defects? Am J Hum Genet 62:1044–1051
Wacholder S, Chanock S, Garcia-Closas M, El Ghormli L, Rothman N (2004) Assessing the probability that a positive report is false: an approach for molecular epidemiology studies. J Natl Cancer Inst 96:434–442
Ward K, Hata A, Jeunemaitre X, Helin C, Nelson L, Namikawa C, Farrington PF, Ogasawara M, Suzumori K, Tomoda S, Berrebi S, Sasaki M, Corvol P, Lifton RP, Lalouel J-M (1993) A molecular variant of angiotensinogen associated with preeclampsia. Nat Genet 4:59–61
Yoshimura T, Yoshimura M, Tabata A, Shimasaki Y, Nakayama M, Miyamoto Y, Saito Y, Nakao K, Yasue H, Okamura H (2000) Association of the missense Glu298Asp variant of the endothelial nitric oxide synthase gene with severe preeclampsia. J Soc Gynecol Investig 7:238–241

Am. J. Hum. Genet. 77:132–139, 2005

Report

Mapping of a Single Locus Capable of Complementing the Defective Heterochromatin Phenotype of Roberts Syndrome Cells

Lisa D. McDaniel,[1] Darrell J. Tomkins,[2,3,4] Eric J. Stanbridge,[5] Martin J. Somerville,[2,3] Errol C. Friedberg,[1] and Roger A. Schultz[1]

[1]Department of Pathology, University of Texas Southwestern Medical Center at Dallas, Dallas; Departments of [2]Medical Genetics and [3]Pediatrics, University of Alberta, and [4]Darrell J. Tomkins Genetics Consulting, Edmonton, Alberta; and [5]Department of Microbiology and Molecular Genetics, School of Medicine, University of California–Irvine, Irvine

Roberts syndrome (RS) is a developmental disorder characterized by tetraphocomelia and a broad spectrum of additional clinical features. Most patients with RS exhibit characteristic cytogenetic phenotypes, which include an abnormal appearance of pericentromeric heterochromatin on metaphase chromosomes, referred to as "heterochromatic repulsion." In the present study, we use complementation of this abnormal cytogenetic phenotype as a means to identify a specific region of the normal human genome capable of rendering phenotypic correction. We screened the entire human genome, using a transient chromosome-transfer assay, and demonstrated complementation exclusively after the transfer of proximal chromosome 8p, a result subsequently confirmed by stable microcell-mediated chromosome transfer. Additionally, homozygosity mapping was used to refine the interval of this complementing locus to 8p21. The results are consistent with the notion that the single gene defect responsible for heterochromatic splaying and developmental abnormalities maps to chromosome 8p21.

In 1919, John Roberts described a rare developmental disorder, Roberts syndrome (RS [MIM 268300]) (Roberts 1919), that is characterized by tetraphocomelia (symmetrical limb reduction) and a broad spectrum of additional variably apparent characteristics that include prenatal and postnatal growth retardation, craniofacial abnormalities, cleft lip and palate, corneal clouding, prominent phallus, and cardiac and renal abnormalities (for a review, see the work of Van Den Berg and Francke [1993*a*]). This disorder has also been referred to as "pseudothalidomide syndrome," since infants born to women who took thalidomide during pregnancy had similar limb malformations (Jurenka 1976). Although RS and the SC phocomelia syndrome (MIM #269000) were originally described as distinct entities, they are now considered to be a single disorder with significant clinical heterogeneity (Waldenmaier et al. 1978; Tomkins et al. 1979; Fryns et al. 1980; Zergollern and Hitrec 1982).

RS appears to be represented by two genetic complementation groups, designated "RS+" and "RS−." Patients are classified into the two groups on the basis of their cytogenetic and cellular phenotypes. Cells and cell lines derived from patients with RS+ manifest a phenomenon evident in mitotic chromosomes that has been previously referred to as heterochromatic repulsion (HR), heterochromatic splaying (HS), or premature centromere separation (herein referred to as "HR") (Freeman et al. 1974; Louie and German 1981). Additionally, RS+ cells exhibit mild hypersensitivity to mitomycin C, cisplatin, γ radiation, and other DNA-damaging agents (Burns and Tomkins 1989; Van Den Berg and Francke 1993*b*), as well as cell-cycle abnormalities. Importantly, RS cell lines propagated in culture, including nontransformed fibroblasts, also exhibit random chromosome loss and gain, presumably the consequence of improper chromosome segregation (Jabs et al. 1989). Hereafter, the RS+ complementation group is designated as "RS."

Microcell-mediated chromosome transfer (MMCT) (McDaniel and Schultz 1992) is a technique whereby normal human chromosomes are transferred from donor to recipient cells via a microcell intermediate. Chromo-

Received April 1, 2005; accepted for publication April 22, 2005; electronically published May 10, 2005.

Address for correspondence and reprints: Dr. Lisa D. McDaniel, Department of Pathology, University of Texas Southwestern Medical Center at Dallas, 5323 Harry Hines Boulevard, Dallas, TX 75390-9072. E-mail: lisa.mcdaniel@utsouthwestern.edu

0002-9297/2005/7701-0014$15.00

some-recipient clones are identified by selection for dominant markers and are analyzed for complementation of mutant recessive phenotypes (such as the HR associated with RS cells). However, an exhaustive analysis of all chromosomes for the identification of complementing loci by use of this approach would be very labor intensive. It would require the transfer of each tagged normal human chromosome, selection and long-term propagation of clonal isolates, and characterization of each of these clones for retention of the transferred chromosome and complementation of the relevant phenotype. Additionally, this strategy necessitates the use of immortalized cell lines representing the syndrome and maintenance of the cellular phenotype(s) of interest. Finally, with regard to the present study, initial experiments demonstrated that SV40 transformation of a fibroblast cell line (GM03913 [National Institute of General Medical Sciences Human Genetic Cell Repository]) of a patient with RS resulted in clones with an inconsistent HR phenotype, which compromised their utility in a complementation strategy (R.A.S. and L.D.M., unpublished observations).

To circumvent the aforementioned limitations, a transient whole-cell–fusion complementation assay was devised and was employed to introduce a limited number of human chromosomes from normal cells into RS cells, for rapid scoring for complementation of HR. The cell lines used were RS lymphoblastoid cell lines R20 and LB1 (Tomkins et al. 1979), Srsym1 (McDaniel et al. 2000), and Srsym2. The control donor cell line that was used, SV40-transformed VA-13 (American Type Culture Collection), was valuable because it contained both normal and rearranged copies of most chromosomes and was female in origin. Microcells were obtained from the donor cell line by treating cells in flasks with 25 μg/ml colcemid solution (Invitrogen) for 48 h, followed by centrifuging the flasks at 12,000 g for 1 h in the presence of 4 μg/ml cytochalasin B (Sigma). Microcells were collected and size selected by filtration and were fused with RS lymphoblastoid cells from patient cell lines, in the presence of 50% PEG 1500 (Roche), for 90 s. Ultimately, R20 proved to be the most efficient recipient, and all data reported are from fusions to that cell line. Complementation of a male cell line (R20) with a female donor afforded the opportunity to assess complemented metaphase cells for the presence of the Y chromosome as evidence that the metaphase originated from the R20 background. Fusion products were then grown for 48 h to allow complementation to occur in recipients that had received the complementing chromosome. Cells were grown for an additional 72 h, in the presence of hygromycin B, at a dose that did not significantly reduce the number of control metaphase cells but that lowered the overall number of R20 metaphase cells by 80%. This reduced the number of uncomplemented RS cells in the population. Surviving metaphase cells were then harvested. Chromosome-specific paints were used for FISH, to independently identify the copy number of each particular chromosome as well as to identify newly introduced rearrangements in both complemented and uncomplemented metaphase cells on the same slide. HR in RS cells is traditionally visualized by examination of fixed metaphase chromosomes stained by conventional C-banding techniques to highlight constitutive heterochromatin (Rooney and Czepulkowski 1986). In the present study, distamycin A (DA) with 4′-6-diamidino-2-phenylindole (DAPI) staining (Verma 1995) was employed to facilitate analysis of the HR effect in a fluorescence-based assay. DA/DAPI staining employed 50 μg/ml DA in PBS for 20 min. Slides were washed in PBS, stained with 0.5 μg/ml DA/DAPI for 15 min, mounted with Vectashield (Vector Laboratories). When DA and DAPI are used together, AT-rich areas of constitutive heterochromatin fluoresce in regions of chromosomes 1, 9, 15, 16, and distal Yq, which allows evaluation of HR with the simultaneous use of FISH to identify the chromosomes transferred.

Given that RS cells exhibit ongoing random chromosome loss and gain (Jabs et al. 1989), a numerical profile for each chromosome was generated for R20 parental cells by use of the same type of FISH studies employed to characterize the fusion products. Large numbers of complemented and uncomplemented metaphases were generated and analyzed on single FISH slides. Despite the aneuploid nature of the R20 cell line, our approach provided sufficient data to assess whether overrepresentation of a certain chromosome correlated with complementation. For nearly all chromosomes examined, the distribution of copy number for a given chromosome did not significantly vary among R20 parental, uncomplemented, and complemented metaphase cells (fig. 1*A*–1*C*). With use of this chromosome-painting approach, it was possible to rule out all autosomes, except chromosome 8 (fig. 1*D*). None of the other chromosomes displayed the increase in chromosome number in the complemented cells that was observed in chromosome 8. Consistent with this assignment, it was also observed that none of the complemented metaphases contained only one chromosome 8.

In addition to association of complementation with an increase in the numerical representation for a given normal chromosome, the SV40-transformed VA-13 cell line, used as the MMCT donor, offered structural rearrangements and deletions that could be identified in fusion products for correlation with complementation. BAC and YAC probes were localized to regions on the p and q arms of chromosome 8. These probes and chromosome 8 paints were then used to identify recurrent rearrangements in VA-13 metaphases. With use of these probes, it was noted that VA-13–derived 8p deletions

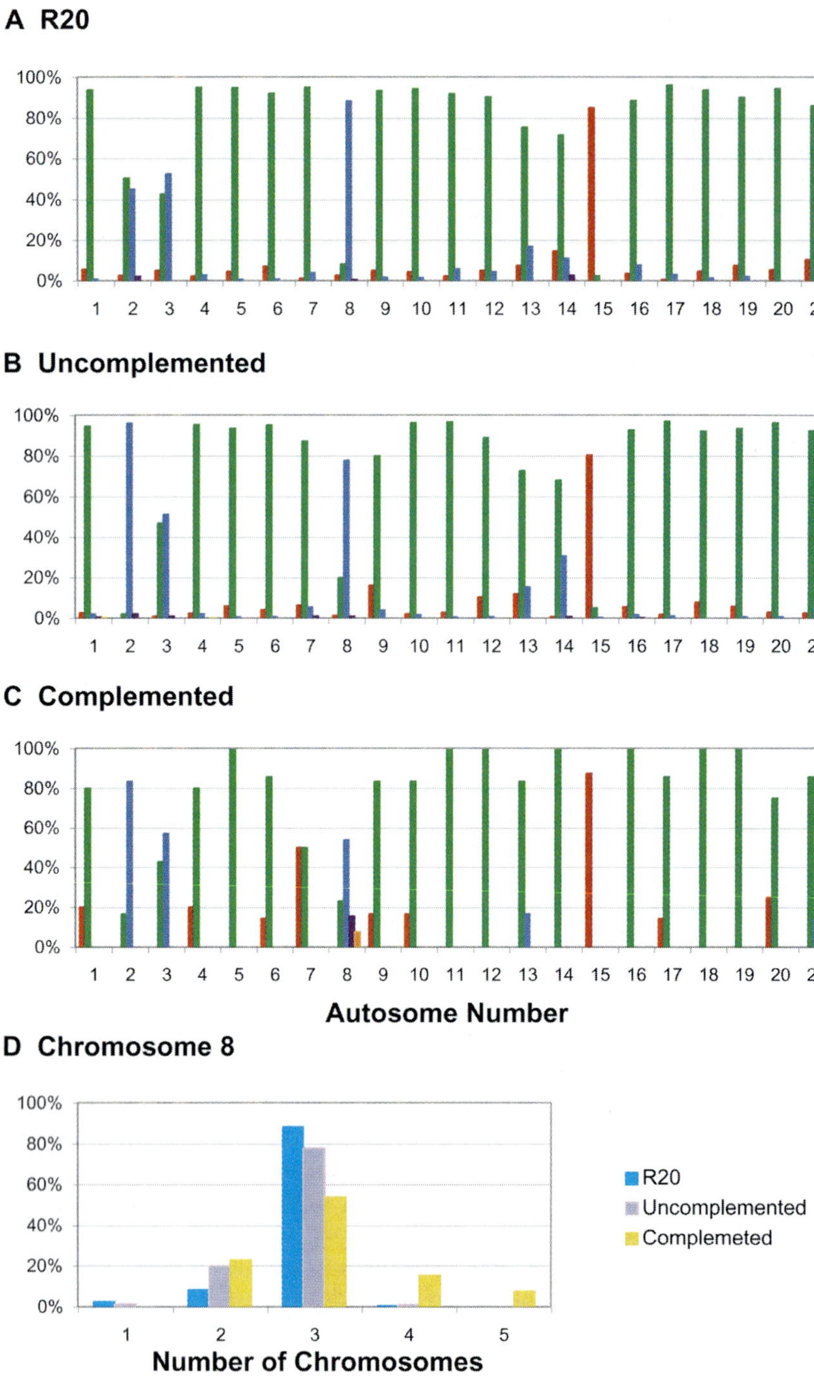

Figure 1 Profile of chromosome number in R20 parental cells, complemented cells, and uncomplemented cells after transient MMCT and FISH. *A*, R20 parental cells. With the use of one chromosome paint on each slide, 100–150 cells were characterized for chromosome number. *B*, Chromosome profile of uncomplemented metaphases after MMCT (150–500 metaphases scored). *C*, Chromosome profile of complemented metaphases on the same slide as the metaphases shown in panel B (10–30 metaphases scored). *A–C*, Bar colors indicate the percentage of metaphases with one (*red*), two (*green*), three (*blue*), four (*purple*), or five (*orange*) copies of each of the autosomes. *D*, Number of chromosome 8 sequences per metaphase in R20 parental, uncomplemented, and complemented metaphase cells in the same experiment. Chromosome 8 is the only chromosome that displayed an increased number in complemented cells.

failed to render correction (fig. 2*B*). Conversely, with retention of the p arm of chromosome 8, specifically with those metaphase cells that retained 8p12 sequences corresponding to YAC 847b12 and some distal material, results exhibited a 100% correlation with complementation. It was noted that the smallest complementing chromosome was positive for hybridization with YAC 847b12 but retained little additional distal material on the p arm of chromosome 8 (fig. 2*C*).

Collectively, the results of the transient complementation experiments are consistent with a map location of the complementing gene for RS in or near 8p12. These results predict that the stable transfer of chromosome 8 should correct the HR phenotype. To test this prediction, a mouse A9 monochromosomal hybrid bearing a human chromosome 8 that was "tagged" with a neomycin-resistance gene (neo^r) was used as a donor for MMCT to RS cells. GM03913 fibroblast cells were derived from the same patient as the R20 lymphoblastoid cells. As mentioned above, SV40-transformed GM03913 RS fibroblasts exhibited an unstable HR phenotype (R.A.S. and L.D.M., unpublished results). However, we established telomerase-immortalized GM03913 cells (reported elsewhere and herein as "TERT-RBS") (Ouellette et al. 2000) with a stable RS cellular phenotype, including HR, hygromycin B sensitivity, and random chromosome loss and gain. These cells were used as recipients for stable MMCT. Stable clones were recovered, and it was observed that one of eight clones was phenotypically complemented for HR (fig. 3*A*). In contrast, no complementation was seen after a neo-tagged chromosome 15 was introduced. These results confirm that chromosome 8 carries the complementing gene for RS. These complemented cells also exhibited resistance to hygromycin B, similar to that observed in control cells (data not shown).

Automated genotyping was used to evaluate sequences transferred from the chromosome 8 mouse/human hybrid MCH904.11 into recipient TERT-RBS cells. The seven uncomplemented clones and the single complemented clone were tested with 29 polymorphic markers spanning chromosome 8. Table 1 summarizes the allele sizes represented by the chromosome 8 sequences that are endogenous to the recipient cells and the one chromosome 8 that was provided by the donor hybrid. In this experiment, 27 of 29 markers were informative for the newly introduced chromosome 8 sequences. Analysis of the recovered clones revealed that the one complemented clone (clone 17) retained all the markers for the donated chromosome 8. Of the remaining clones, five of seven shared a common breakpoint in 8p11.2, and

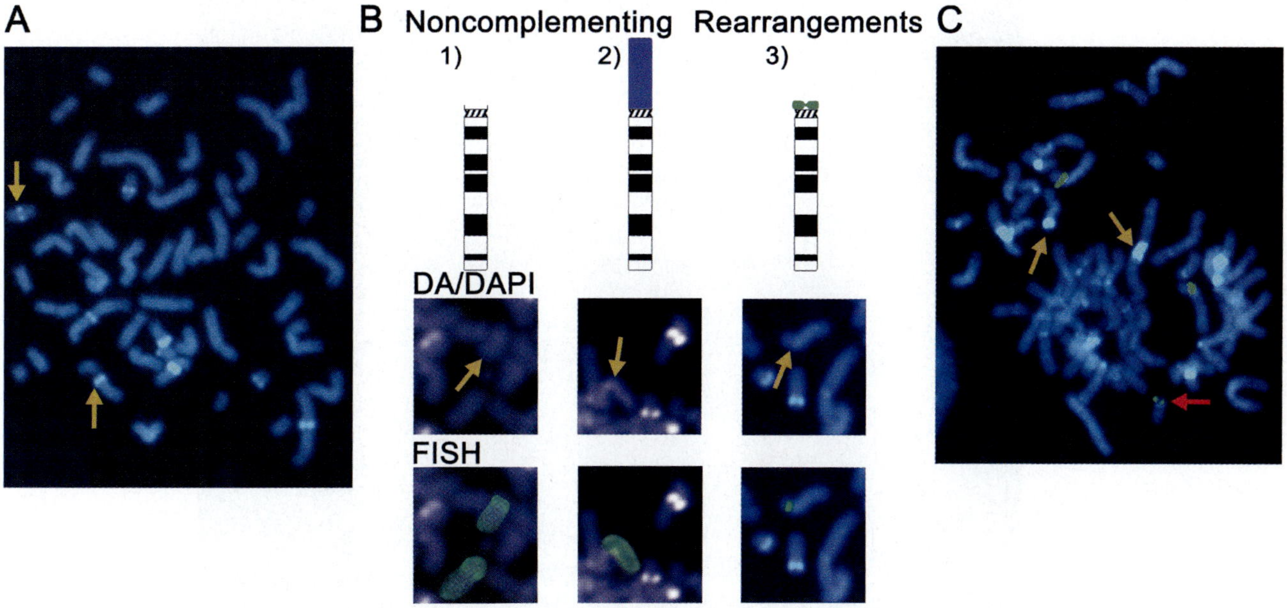

Figure 2 Characterization of metaphases observed by transient complementation. *A*, R20 metaphase, stained by DA/DAPI, displaying the HR phenotype in the constitutive heterochromatic regions of the autosomes. Yellow arrows indicate the HR phenotype in the heterochromatin of the chromosomes. *B*, Summary of the results for rearrangements that did not yield complementation of the HR phenotype, displayed by ideograms, DA/DAPI partial metaphases, and FISH. Yellow arrows indicate the uncomplementing transferred chromosome. Panels 1 and 2 show results with biotin-labeled chromosome 8 paint. Panel 3 shows results with biotin-labeled YAC 815d7 (8p11.21). All were detected with avidin–fluorescein isothiocyanate (FITC). *C*, Complemented metaphase, with the smallest fragment of chromosome 8 (indicated by the red arrow) detected by transient complementation assay probed with YAC 847b12 (8p12). Yellow arrows indicate the HR phenotype in the heterochromatin of the chromosomes.

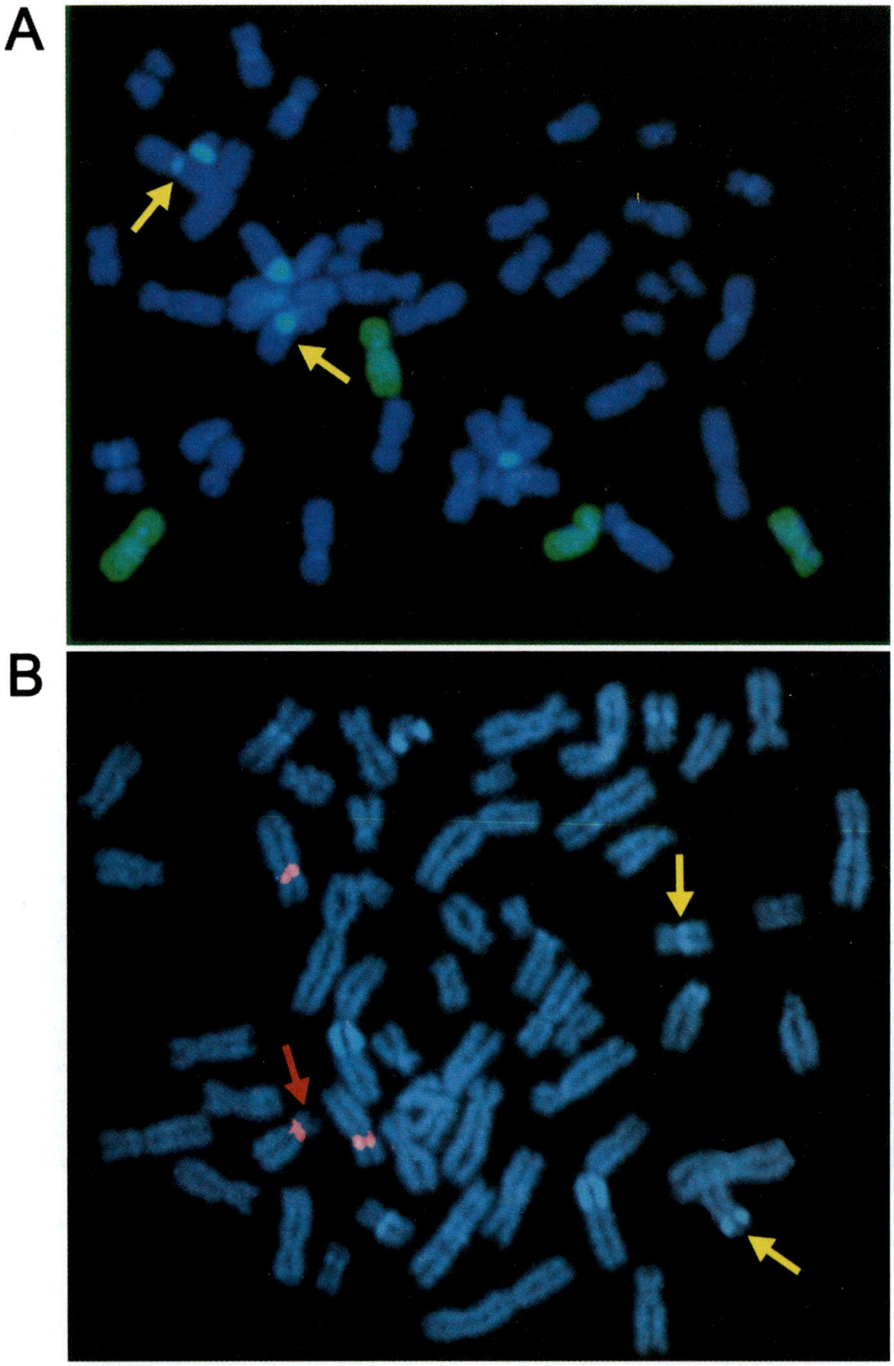

Figure 3 Stable introduction of chromosome 8 into TERT-RBS cells. Yellow arrows indicate the HR phenotype in the heterochromatin of the chromosomes in the DA/DAPI-stained metaphases. *A,* Metaphase exhibiting complementation of the HR phenotype in clone 17. Chromosome 8 paint, labeled with biotin and detected with avidin-FITC, reveals tetrasomy for chromosome 8 in the complemented metaphase, a result consistent with the fact that most of the TERT-RBS cells were trisomic for chromosome 8 prior to MMCT. *B,* The uncomplemented clone 18, probed using an chromosome 8 centromere probe directly labeled with Spectrum Orange. The red arrow indicates the contributed chromosome 8, with a significant portion of the p arm deleted.

Table 1

Allele Sizes in Parental Cell Lines and Clones from MMCT

	Allele Size(s) (bp) in										
			Clone								
Marker	MCH904.11	TERT-RBS	1	2	3	4	17	18	19	20
D8S264	155	151, 153	151, 153	151, 153	151, 153	151, 153	***151, 153, 155***	151, 153	151, 153	151, 153
D8S550	208	192, 194	192, 194	192, 194	192, 194	192, 194	***192, 194, 208***	192, 194	192, 194	192, 194
D8S1106	125	143	143	143	143	143	***134, 125***	143	143	143
D8S549	84	82	82	82	82	82	***82, 84***	82	82	82
D8S1145	270	273, 281	273, 281	273, 281	273, 281	273, 281	***270, 273, 281***	273, 281	273, 281	273, 281
D8S258	152	154, 156	154, 156	154, 156	154, 156	154, 156	***152, 154, 156***	154, 156	154, 156	154, 156
D8S282	265	267	267	267	267	267	***265, 267***	266	266	266
D8S1786	211	215	215	215	215	215	***215, 211***	215	215	215
D8S1752	156	145	145	145	145	145	***145, 156***	145	145	145
D8S1734	120	114	114	114	114	114	***114, 118***	114	114	114
D8S1725	266	268	268	268	268	268	***266, 268***	268	268	268
D8S1771	356	354	354	354	354	354	***354, 356***	354	354	354
D8S382	317	309	309	309	309	309	***309, 317***	309	309	309
D8S1048	204	204	204	204	204	204	204	204	204	204
D8S1839	175	175	175	175	175	175	175	175	175	175
D8S131	134	140	140	140	140	140	***134, 140***	140	140	140
D8S585	174	186	186	186	186	186	***174, 186***	186	186	186
D8S1820	111	119	119	119	119	119	***119, 117***	119	119	119
D8S1477	166	154	***154, 166***	***154, 166***	***154, 166***	***154, 166***	***154, 166***	***154, 166***	154	154
D8D505	115	113	***113, 115***	***113, 115***	***113, 115***	***113, 115***	***113, 115***	***113, 115***	113	113
D8S1121	118	115	***115, 118***	***115, 118***	***115, 118***	***115, 118***	***115, 118***	***115, 118***	115	115
D8S1821	142	165	***142, 165***	***142, 165***	***142, 165***	***142, 165***	***142, 165***	***142, 165***	142	142
D8S532	247	245	***245, 247***	***245, 247***	***245, 247***	***245, 247***	***245, 247***	***245, 247***	245	245
D8S1104	129	141	***129, 141***	***129, 141***	***129, 141***	***129, 141***	***129, 141***	***129, 141***	141	141
D8S1747	211	219	***219, 211***	***219, 211***	***219, 211***	***219, 211***	***219, 211***	***219, 211***	219	219
D8S1745	127	133	***127, 133***	***127, 133***	***127, 133***	***127, 133***	***127, 133***	***127, 133***	133	133
D8S1133	193	189	***189, 192***	***189, 192***	***189, 192***	***189, 192***	***189, 192***	***189, 192***	189	189
D8S1136	260	249	249	***249, 260***	249	249	***249, 260***	249	249	249
D8S1119	182	174	***174, 182***	***174, 182***	***174, 182***	***174, 182***	***174, 182***	***174, 182***	174	174

Note.—Numbers in bold italics represent cases in which the alleles from both R20 and the chromosome hybrid MCH904.11 were present in the clone. Markers that were uninformative are underlined.

two of seven had none of the alleles of the donated chromosome. FISH analysis confirmed the loss of distal 8p (fig. 3*B*). Note that the recovery of neo^r clones bearing this structure is consistent with a more proximal 8p location of the neo-tag in the chromosome 8 present in MCH904.11 hybrid cells (results documented by FISH [data not shown]). The loss of the p arm of chromosome 8 during the process of MMCT may be due to the clastogenic effects of cytochalasin B (Kolber et al. 1990) or to an event that may be stimulated by the amplification of the neo^r gene during selection.

We performed a genomewide scan for homozygosity. DNA from five unrelated patients with RS, patient S4134 and four previously mentioned patients (Tomkins et al. 1979), was amplified and analyzed for microsatellite markers. Chromosomes 1–11 were completed, and no loci were found to be homozygous in all patients, except on chromosome 8. On the basis of the above evidence for an RS complementing locus on 8p, we focused on this chromosomal arm to further refine the location of the complementing gene. In addition to known microsatellites, some SNPs and predicted variable repeats (Fondon et al. 1998) were used. The results presented in table 2 identify an interval of homozygosity, in all five patients with RS, mapping to 8p21, with no evidence of an alternative locus. Most patients exhibit homozygosity over a common 8.9-Mb interval; one patient, S4134, was homozygous for markers covering a 2.3-Mb region.

In summary, the results presented identify a single genomic interval on proximal chromosome 8p that is capable of complementing the HR phenotype and hygromycin sensitivity of RS+ cells. The results of homozygosity mapping confirmed the existence of an interval at 8p21 that is homozygous for all markers tested in five patients with RS. The results are consistent with the notion that the complementing locus for HR and the gene defect in patients with RS are one and the same and that it maps to chromosome 8p21.

Addendum.—While this manuscript was under review, *Nature Genetics* published "Roberts Syndrome Is Caused by Mutations in *ESCO2*, a Human Homolog of Yeast *ECO1* That Is Essential for the Establishment of

Table 2

Homozygosity Mapping of Patients

		Results of Mapping for Affected Patients Who Were					
		Unrelated			From an Isolated Community		
Marker	Location[a] (Mb)	R20	Srsym1	Srsym2	R23/LB1	S4134	Band
D8S264	2.1	HT	HT	HT	HT	HT	8p23.3
D8S1099	6.1	HT	HM	HT	HT	HM	8p23.2
D8S277	6.5	HT	HM	HM	HM	HM	8p23.1
D8S1469	9.1	HT	HT	HT	HT	HT	8p23.1
D8S550	10.9	HT	HM	HM	HT	HT	8p23.1
D8S1130	11.9	HT	HT	HT	HT	HT	8p23.1
D8S1106	12.9	HM	HT	HM	HT	HT	8p22
D8S511	14.7	HM	HT	HT	HM	HT	8p22
D8S549	15.7	HM	HM	HT	HM	HM	8p22
D8S1145	18.4	HT	HM	HT	HT	HT	8p22
D8S258	20.4	HT	HM	HT	HT	HM	8p21.3
D8S282	21.4	HM	HM	HM	HT	HT	8p21.3
D8S1116	21.4	HM	HM	HT	HT	HT	8p21.3
D8S136	22.5	HM	HM	HT	HT	HT	8p21.3
D8S1786	22.5	HM	HM	HM	HT	HT	8p21.3
D8S1733	22.6	HM	HM	HM	HT	HM	8p21.3
D8S1752	22.7	HM	HM	HT	HM	HT	8p21.3
D8S1734	22.9	HM	HM	HT	HT	HT	8p21.3
AF279339[b]	23.3	HM	HM	HT	HM	Not done	8p21.3
AC044891[b]	24.2	HM	HM	HM	HM	Not done	8p21.2
AC024958[b]	24.4	HM	HM	HM	HM	Not done	8p21.2
D8S1989	24.7	HM	HM	HM	HM	HT	8p21.2
D8S1725	25.1	HM	HM	HM	HM	HT	8p21.2
D8S1771	25.5	HM	HM	HM	HM	HM	8p21.2
DOCK5ca10[b]	25.5	HM	HM	HM	HM	Not done	8p21.2
D8S382	26.3	HM	HM	HM	HM	HM	8p21.2
PPP2R2A[c]	26.3	HM	HM	HM	HM	Not done	8p21.2
D8S1048	26.0	HM	HM	HM	HM	HM	8p21.2
PTK2B[d]	27.3	HM	HM	HM	HM	HM	8p21.2
Exon 26[e]	27.4	HM	HM	HM	HM	HM	8p21.2
D8S131[f]	27.4	HM	HM	HM	HM	HM	8p21.2
D8S1839	27.4	HM	HM	HM	HM	HT	8p21.1
SCARA3-F1[b]	27.5	HM	HM	HM	HM	Not done	8p21.1
D8S585	27.6	HM	HM	HM	HM	HT	8p21.1
SCARA3-F2[b]	28.0	HM	HM	HM	HM	HM	8p21.1
D8S1820	28.0	HM	HM	HM	HM	HT	8p21.1
D8S1477	32.2	HM	HM	HT	HT	HT	8p12
D8S505	34.6	HM	HM	HT	HT	HT	8p12
D8S1121	35.9	HM	HM	HT	HT	HT	8p12
D8S1747	37.1	HM	HM	HM	HT	HT	8p12
D8S1821	38.5	HT	HT	HT	HM	HT	8p12
D8S255	40.0	HM	HM	HT	HT	HT	8p11.21
D8S1104	40.7	HM	HM	HT	HT	HM	8p11.21
D8S532	40.9	HM	HM	HT	HT	HT	8p11.21

NOTE.—HM = homozygous; HT = heterozygous.

[a] Map locations are based on the University of California–Santa Cruz Genome Browser.

[b] Variable-repeat regions were predicted from the sequence by POPPOUS (Fondon et al. 1998).

[c] SNP *rs3824232*: 51 bp before exon 10 splice site (allele frequency unknown).

[d] SNP *rs1045512*: exon 2, p.Lys54Lys, Srsym1, Srsym2, and LB1 = A (allele frequency 0.775), R20 = G (allele frequency 0.225).

[e] SNP *rs751019*: p.Thr838Lys, R20, and LB1 = C (allele frequency 0.453); Srsym1 and Srsym2 = A (allele frequency 0.547).

[f] *D8S131*: all patients are homozygous for the most common allele (allele frequency 0.791).

Sister Chromatid Cohesion" (Vega et al. 2005). That publication describes homozygosity mapping and identification of the *RBS1* gene called "*ESCO2.*" *ESCO2* resides within the 8.9-Mb interval on chromosome 8p21, as defined in the present study, which confirms that the disease-causing gene and the locus that can complement the HR phenotype are one and the same.

Acknowledgments

This work was supported, in part, by National Institutes of Health grant HD32522 (to R.A.S.).

Web Resources

The URLs for data presented herein are as follows:

Online Mendelian Inheritance in Man (OMIM), http://www.ncbi.nlm.nih.gov/Omim/ (RS and SC phocomelia syndrome)
University of California–Santa Cruz Genome Bioinformatics, http://genome.cse.ucsc.edu/

References

Burns MA, Tomkins DJ (1989) Hypersensitivity to mitomycin C cell-killing in Roberts syndrome fibroblasts with, but not without, the heterochromatin abnormality. Mutat Res 216: 243–249

Fondon JW 3rd, Mele GM, Brezinschek RI, Cummings D, Pande A, Wren J, O'Brien KM, Kupfer KC, Wei MH, Lerman M, Minna JD, Garner HR (1998) Computerized polymorphic marker identification: experimental validation and a predicted human polymorphism catalog. Proc Natl Acad Sci USA 95: 7514–7519

Freeman MV, Williams DW, Schimke RN, Temtamy SA, Vachier E, German J (1974) The Roberts syndrome. Clin Genet 5:1–16

Fryns H, Goddeeris P, Moerman F, Herman F, van der Berghe H (1980) The tetraphocomelia-cleft palate syndrome in identical twins. Hum Genet 53:279–281

Jabs EW, Tuck-Muller CM, Cusano R, Rattner JB (1989) Centromere separation and aneuploidy in human mitotic mutants: Roberts syndrome. Prog Clin Biol Res 318:111–118

Jurenka SB (1976) Variations in IQ of two patients with pseudothalidomide syndrome. Dev Med Child Neurol 18:525–527

Kolber MA, Broschat KO, Landa-Gonzalez B (1990) Cytochalasin B induces cellular DNA fragmentation. FASEB J 4: 3021–3027

Louie E, German J (1981) Roberts's syndrome. II. Aberrant Y-chromosome behavior. Clin Genet 19:71–74

McDaniel LD, Prueitt R, Probst LC, Wilson KS, Tomkins D, Wilson GN, Schultz RA (2000) Novel assay for Roberts syndrome assigns variable phenotypes to one complementation group. Am J Med Genet 93:223–229

McDaniel LD, Schultz RA (1992) Elevated sister chromatid exchange phenotype of Bloom syndrome cells is complemented by human chromosome 15. Proc Natl Acad Sci USA 89:7968–7972

Ouellette MM, McDaniel LD, Wright WE, Shay JW, Schultz RA (2000) The establishment of telomerase-immortalized cell lines representing human chromosome instability syndromes. Hum Mol Genet 9:403–411

Roberts JB (1919) A child with double cleft of lip and palate, protrusion of the intermaxillary portion of the upper jaw and imperfect development of the bones of the four extremities. Ann Surg 70:252–254

Rooney DE, Czepulkowski BH (1986) Human cytogenetics: a practical approach. Constitutional analysis. IRL Press, Oxford and New York

Tomkins D, Hunter A, Roberts M (1979) Cytogenetic findings in Roberts-SC phocomelia syndrome(s). Am J Med Genet 4: 17–26

Van Den Berg DJ, Francke U (1993*a*) Roberts syndrome: a review of 100 cases and a new rating system for severity. Am J Med Genet 47:1104–1123

Van Den Berg DJ, Francke U (1993*b*) Sensitivity of Roberts syndrome cells to gamma radiation, mitomycin C, and protein synthesis inhibitors. Somat Cell Mol Genet 19:377–392

Vega H, Waisfisz Q, Gordillo M, Sakai N, Yanagihara I, Yamada M, van Gosliga D, Kayserili H, Xu C, Ozono K, Wang Jabs E, Inui K, Joenje H (2005) Roberts syndrome is caused by mutations in *ESCO2*, a human homolog of yeast *ECO1* that is essential for the establishment of sister chromatid cohesion. Nat Genet 37:468–470

Verma RS (1995) Human chromosomes: principles and techniques. McGraw-Hill, New York

Waldenmaier C, Aldenhoff P, Klemm T (1978) The Roberts' syndrome. Hum Genet 40:345–349

Zergollern L, Hitrec V (1982) Four siblings with Robert's syndrome. Clin Genet 21:1–6

Report

Genetic Variation in the Human Androgen Receptor Gene Is the Major Determinant of Common Early-Onset Androgenetic Alopecia

Axel M. Hillmer,[1,2] Sandra Hanneken,[4] Sibylle Ritzmann,[4] Tim Becker,[3] Jan Freudenberg,[2] Felix F. Brockschmidt,[2] Antonia Flaquer,[3] Yun Freudenberg-Hua,[2] Rami Abou Jamra,[2] Christine Metzen,[4] Uwe Heyn,[2] Nadine Schweiger,[4] Regina C. Betz,[2,5] Bettina Blaumeiser,[5] Jochen Hampe,[6] Stefan Schreiber,[6] Thomas G. Schulze,[7] Hans Christian Hennies,[8] Johannes Schumacher,[2] Peter Propping,[2] Thomas Ruzicka,[4] Sven Cichon,[1,5] Thomas F. Wienker,[3] Roland Kruse,[4] and Markus M. Nöthen[1,5]

[1]Department of Genomics, Life & Brain Center, and [2]Institute of Human Genetics, and [3]Institute for Medical Biometry, Informatics and Epidemiology, University of Bonn, Bonn; [4]Department of Dermatology, University of Düsseldorf, Düsseldorf; [5]Department of Medical Genetics, University of Antwerp, Antwerp; [6]Institute for Clinical Molecular Biology, Christian-Albrechts-Universität zu Kiel, Kiel, Germany; [7]Division of Genetic Epidemiology in Psychiatry, Central Institute of Mental Health, Mannheim; and [8]Department of Molecular Genetics and Gene Mapping Center, Max Delbrück Center for Molecular Medicine, Berlin

Androgenetic alopecia (AGA), or male-pattern baldness, is the most common form of hair loss. Its pathogenesis is androgen dependent, and genetic predisposition is the major requirement for the phenotype. We demonstrate that genetic variability in the androgen receptor gene (*AR*) is the cardinal prerequisite for the development of early-onset AGA, with an etiological fraction of 0.46. The investigation of a large number of genetic variants covering the *AR* locus suggests that a polyglycine-encoding GGN repeat in exon 1 is a plausible candidate for conferring the functional effect. The X-chromosomal location of *AR* stresses the importance of the maternal line in the inheritance of AGA.

Androgenetic alopecia (AGA [MIM 109200]), or male-pattern baldness, is characterized by a defined pattern of hair loss from the scalp (Hamilton 1951). In whites, the proportion of affected males increases steadily with age, so that a male in his 50s has a 50% chance of having some degree of AGA (Hamilton 1951). Association of AGA with a variety of clinical phenotypes has been suggested, including coronary heart disease (Lotufo et al. 2000), benign prostatic hyperplasia (Hawk et al. 2000), prostate cancer (Oh et al. 1998), and disorders associated with insulin resistance (Matilainen et al. 2000). Androgen dependence is an important characteristic of AGA, and genetic disposition, which is assumed to be polygenic, plays the most substantial role in the development of AGA (Küster and Happle 1984; Ellis et al. 1998; Nyholt et al. 2003). Although the only factor known to influence onset age in patients with AGA is genetic predisposition, no systematic approach has hitherto been undertaken, to our knowledge, to identify the contributing genes.

As part of a genomewide linkage study of AGA, we investigated linkage to markers covering the X chromosome. The sample consisted of 95 families in which at least two brothers had early-onset AGA (391 genotyped individuals, including 201 affected men). We obtained evidence of linkage in chromosomal region Xq12-22 (nonparametric linkage [NPL] score of 2.70 [fig. 1]) (for X-chromosomal marker information, see table 1). This region contains the *AR* gene (MIM 313700), which is an obvious candidate for explaining the development of AGA, and an association with this region has been suggested elsewhere (Ellis et al. 2001), on the basis of results from the investigation of three polymorphic sites. In the present study, we have systematically explored the contribution of the *AR* gene to the development of early-onset AGA.

Received March 21, 2005; accepted for publication April 27, 2005; electronically published May 18, 2005.

Address for correspondence and reprints: Dr. Markus M. Nöthen, Department of Genomics, Life & Brain Center, University of Bonn, Sigmund-Freud-Straße 25, 53127 Bonn, Germany. E-mail: markus.noethen@uni-bonn.de

0002-9297/2005/7701-0015$15.00

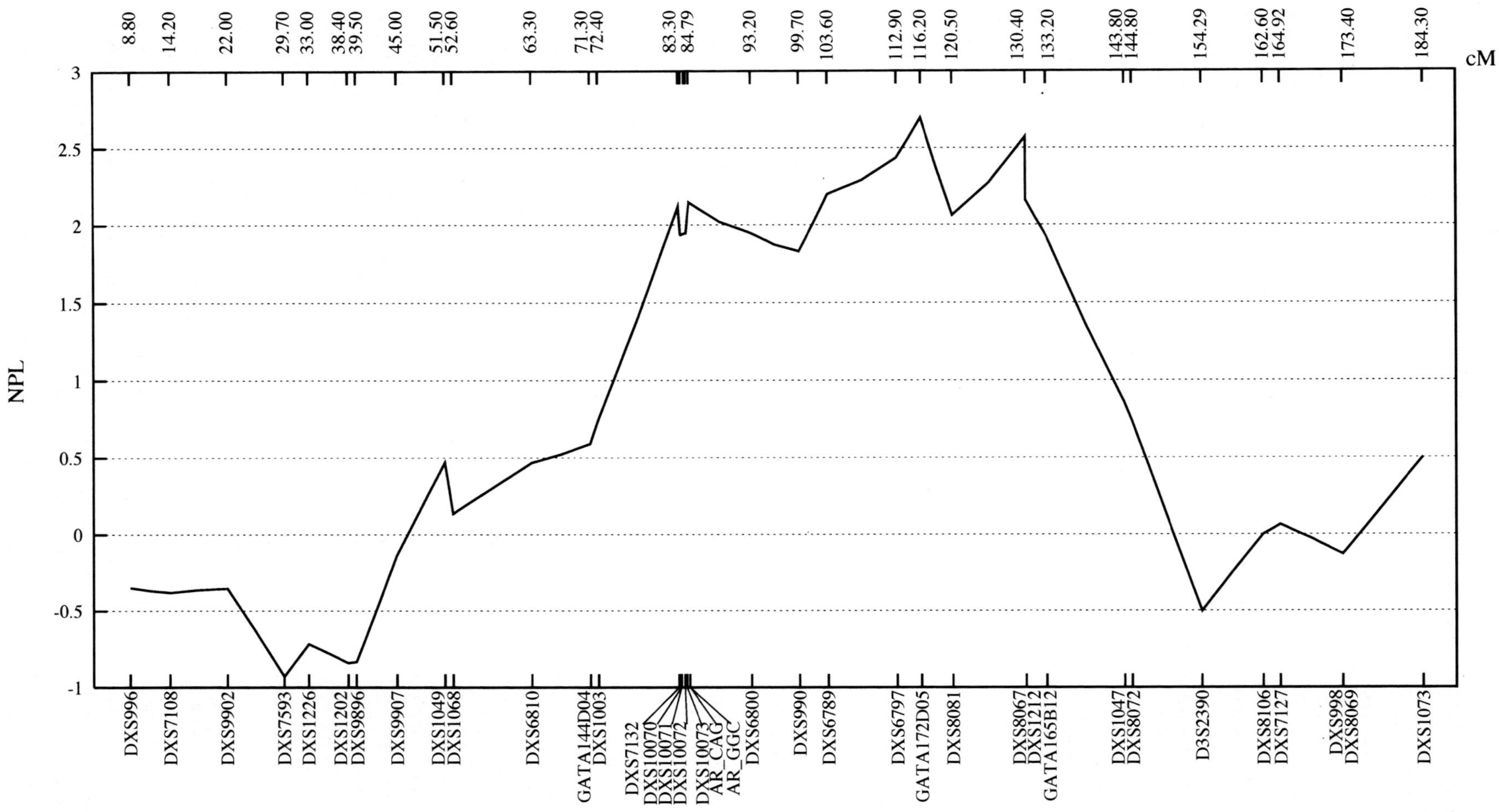

Figure 1 Multipoint NPL analysis of chromosome X, calculated by the Allegro v1.2 software (Gudbjartsson et al. 2000). The *X*-axis is the chromosome location (*top*, cM; *bottom*, STR marker), and the *Y*-axis is the LOD score.

Am. J. Hum. Genet. 77:140–148, 2005

Table 1

STR Markers Used for Linkage Analysis of Chromosome X

The table is available in its entirety in the online edition of *The American Journal of Human Genetics.*

We tested 39 SNPs, two STRs (a polyglutamine-encoding CAG repeat and a polyglycine-encoding GGN repeat in exon 1 of *AR*), and one biallelic insertion polymorphism (*XARx8insA*), in a range of 4.4 Mb at the *AR* locus, for association with AGA (fig. 2). Our analysis included the three previously studied variants (Ellis et al. 2001): the CAG and GGN repeats and *Stu*I RFLP (*rs6152*). *Taq*Man assays for genotyping of SNPs, listed in table 2, were designed by Applied Biosystems. PCRs were performed using 2.5 ng genomic DNA, Ampli*Taq* Gold DNA polymerase (Applied Biosystems), and an annealing temperature of 60°C for 45 cycles on Biometra T1 (Biometra) or Perkin Elmer GeneAmp 9700 (Applied Biosystems) thermocyclers. Fluorescence was measured with an ABI Prism 7900HT sequence detection system (Applied Biosystems). The fragment lengths of the CAG repeat, the GGN repeat, and *XARx8insA* were determined using the following fluorescence-labeled primers for PCR: CAG-F 5′-TCCAGAATCTGTTCCAGAGCGTGC-3′ and CAG-R 5′-GCTGTGAAGGTTGCTGTTCCTCAT-3′ (La Spada et al. 1991), GGN-F 5′-CCTGGCACACTCTCTTCACA-3′ and GGN-R 5′-GGATAGGGCACTCTGCTCAC-3′, and *XARx8insA*-F 5′-CACGGGAAGTTTAGAGAGCT-3′ and *XARx8insA*-R 5′-TCACCTTCTCGTCACTATTG-3′. Forty nanograms of genomic DNA was used in PCRs with Ampli*Taq* DNA polymerase (Applied Biosystems) in 38 cycles on a PTC-200 (MJ Research). The annealing temperatures were 62°C–60°C (touchdown PCR) for the CAG repeat, 58°C for the GGN repeat, and 63°C–55°C (touchdown PCR) for *XARx8insA*. MasterAmp PCR PreMix G (Epicentre) was used to amplify GGN fragments. Fragment lengths of the amplified products were analyzed on an ABI Prism 377 DNA sequencer (Applied Biosystems). Double-strand sequencing of genomic regions was performed with the ABI Prism BigDye Terminator Cycle Sequencing kit, version 2.0 (Applied Biosystems), and the ABI Prism 3730 DNA analyzer (Applied Biosystems).

For case-control analysis, we compared allele frequencies in 198 males with early-onset AGA (including 95 unrelated and randomly chosen affected individuals from the linkage-analysis families), 188 control individuals, and 157 unaffected individuals. For family-based association analysis, we studied 179 families containing at least one affected male in the youngest generation. The family-based association sample included the 95 families from the linkage analysis and overlapped with the case sample, for 179 individuals. All affected males were aged <40 years (mean [± SD] 32.0 ± 5.2) and had AGA that was representative of the most severely affected 10% of the distribution for the respective age class, on the basis of the classification of Hamilton (1951) (modified by Norwood [1975]). AGA classification, age, and ethnicity were the exclusive criteria used to select individuals for inclusion in the case sample. Unaffected males were aged >60 years (mean 67.9 ± 6.2) and without AGA, representing the least-affected 20% of the distribution for this age class. Families and unrelated individuals both with and without AGA were recruited through various sources, including press reports and advertisements in magazines, newspapers, and placards. Control individuals were male blood donors from the blood transfusion center of the University Hospital Bonn, from whom information was available only on sex, age in years (mean 29.4 ± 8.6), and ethnicity. EDTA anticoagulated venous blood samples were collected from all individuals, and lymphocyte DNA was isolated by salting out with saturated NaCl solution (Miller et al. 1988). All participants were of German descent. The study was approved by the ethics committee of the University of Bonn, and informed consent was obtained from all participants.

Association analysis was conducted using a modification of the FAMHAP software (Becker and Knapp 2004*a*, 2004*b*) for X-chromosomal data. Case-control SNP single-marker analysis was performed using the χ^2 distribution of the 2 × 2 contingency table, and multiallelic markers were evaluated with the permutational version of the χ^2 test. For case-control haplotype analysis, P values were calculated from the χ^2 distribution with $n-1$ df of the respective likelihood-ratio test (n = number of different haplotypes). The family data were analyzed with the permutation-based association test for nuclear families (Zhao et al. 2000; Knapp and Becker 2003). For each marker (single-locus analysis) and each marker combination (haplotype analysis), we used 10^{10} permutation replicates.

Pairwise distances between haplotypes were calculated as allele mismatches. By resampling markers randomly with replacement, 100 bootstrapped data sets were generated as input for the program neighbor contained in the PHYLIP package.

A region of 1 Mb showed strong association with the lowest P value of 2.1×10^{-12} for *rs10521339* in the case-control analysis of affected and unaffected individuals (table 3). As expected, the association is stronger for comparisons between individuals with AGA and individuals without AGA than between individuals with AGA and an unselected control sample (table 3). We also performed a separate analysis of the 103 cases that were not included in the linkage analysis and found that the association was also present in this sample (data not shown). The association is further supported by family-based analysis, for which SNP *rs938059* shows the lowest *P* value (4.03×10^{-6}) (table 3). *AR* is the only known gene in the strongly associated 1-Mb–spanning region (fig. 2 and table 3). The X-linked ectodysplasin-A2 receptor (*XEDAR*), which is located 900 kb 5′ of *AR*, is outside this region (fig. 2 and table 3). The significance of the association decreases within the 3′ part of the 180-kb–spanning *AR* gene, and oligophrenin 1 (*OPHN1*), which is located 320 kb 3′ of *AR*, is not within the block of strongest association (fig. 2 and table 3). *rs6152* ($P = 6.66 \times 10^{-10}$ [table 3]) in exon 1 of *AR* corresponds to the *Stu*I RFLP, for which an association has been described by Ellis et al. (2001).

The long range of the associated SNPs implies the presence of a large haplotype block, visible in fig. 2*B*. In principle, this is not unexpected in a location close to the centromere, where recombination events occur at a relatively low frequency (Nagaraja et al. 1997). To test whether the size of the haplotype block stands out even in comparison with X-chromosomal loci with similar low recombination frequencies, we analyzed average pairwise linkage disequilibrium (LD) (measured by |D′|) between SNPs retrieved from the HapMap Project database in 1-cM–sized windows. Average pairwise LD was found to be inversely correlated with recombination rate (Spearman's $\rho = -0.598$; $P < .001$). An average LD higher than that at the *AR* locus was displayed by only the six windows covering the centromere; these windows showed distinctively smaller recombination rates (fig. 3*A*). This result might suggest that the predominant *AR* haplotypes are evolutionarily more recent, perhaps indicating positive selective pressure acting at this locus (Bamshad and Wooding 2003). Since androgens mediate a wide range of developmental and physiological responses through the androgen receptor (AR) and are especially important in the male reproductive system (Lee and Chang 2003), it is conceivable that variability in *AR* can have an impact on selection. In accordance with this hypothesis, the haplotype with the highest frequency (0.45 [fig. 3*B*]) (which also confers risk of AGA) in the German population seems to be evolutionarily recent, as indicated by the low sequence identity with the ancestral haplotype (fig. 3*B*).

Table 2

Oligonucleotides for *Taq*Man Assays

The table is available in its entirety in the online edition of *The American Journal of Human Genetics.*

Sequencing of the transcribed region and of 3.4 kb of conserved sequences in the 5′ region and intron 1 of *AR* in 12 individuals revealed only two additional variants of the associated haplotype (*XARx7_01* and *XARx8insA* [table 3]). The additional variants were noncoding and did not show a stronger association than other tested markers. Of the two repeat polymorphisms in the coding region, the CAG repeat was not associated with AGA (affected/unaffected global *P* value of .1), whereas the GGN repeat was highly associated (affected/

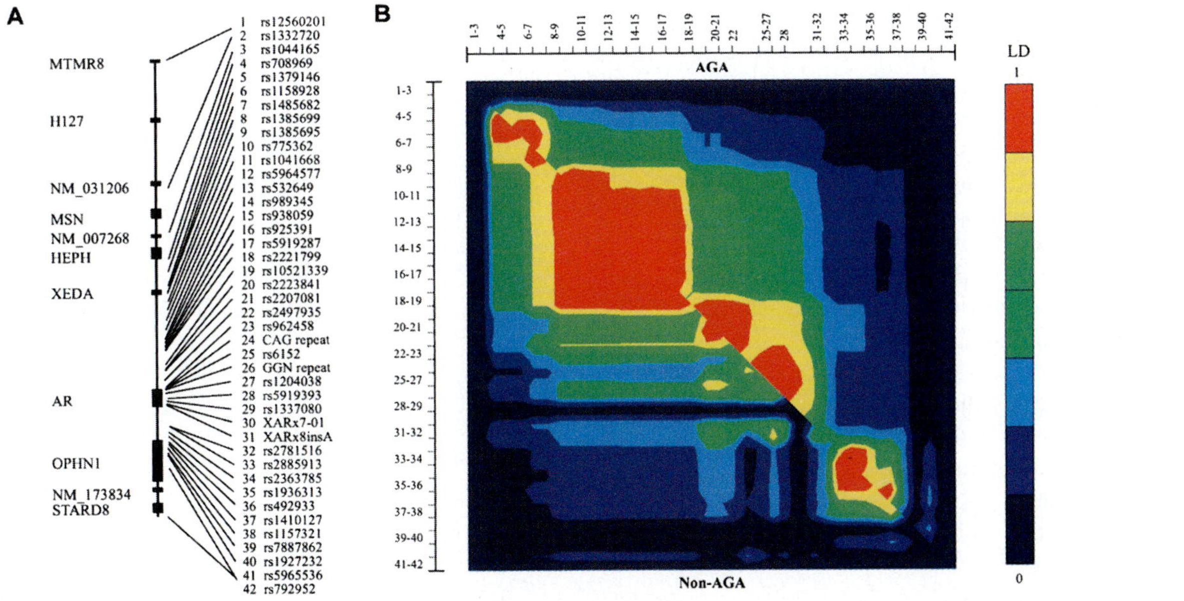

Figure 2 Gene and LD structure of the *AR* locus. *A*, Distribution of known genes (*left*) and typed SNPs and STRs (*right*) at the *AR* locus. The shown genomic region spans 4.4 Mb. Gene content information is based on Ensembl. *B*, LD in 198 individuals with AGA (*upper right diagonal*) and in 157 individuals without AGA (*lower left diagonal*) was measured with χ^2 and was visualized using the GOLD program (Abecasis and Cookson 2000).

Table 3

Association of AGA with Markers at the *AR* Locus

SNP and Allele	Frequency: Affected	Frequency: Control	Frequency: Unaffected	TDT[a]: Transmitted	TDT[a]: Nontransmitted	P^c	Affected/Control Analysis: P	Affected/Control Analysis: OR[d]	Affected/Control Analysis: CI	Affected/Unaffected Analysis: P	Affected/Unaffected Analysis: OR[d]	Affected/Unaffected Analysis: CI	Position[b]
rs12560201:						6.68×10^{-1}	8.99×10^{-1}	1.04	.55–1.82	9.38×10^{-1}	.97	.5–1.87	63,335,397
G	.112	.108	.115	23	27								
A	.888	.892	.885										
rs1332720:						1.00	1.00	ND	ND	1.00	ND	ND	64,598,557
C	.995	1.000	1.000	0	1								
T	.005	.000	.000										
rs1044165:						1.00	9.50×10^{-1}	.98	.55–1.89	1.58×10^{-1}	1.53	.85–2.76	65,024,747
A	.124	.122	.178	22	23								
G	.876	.878	.822										
rs708969:						5.35×10^{-1}	1.21×10^{-2}	2.02	1.16–3.53	3.90×10^{-3}	2.27	1.29–4	65,252,916
A	.875	.776	.755	36	29								
T	.125	.224	.245										
rs1379146:						3.25×10^{-1}	2.68×10^{-4}	2.61	1.55–4.45	4.72×10^{-4}	2.60	1.51–4.5	65,389,382
T	.872	.723	.724	39	29								
A	.128	.277	.276										
rs1158928:						1.30×10^{-1}	1.04×10^{-5}	3.23	1.89–5.56	2.08×10^{-5}	3.22	1.85–5.61	65,532,217
A	.883	.700	.701	42	27								
G	.117	.300	.299										
rs1485682:						1.30×10^{-1}	1.97×10^{-5}	3.13	1.82–5.35	3.08×10^{-5}	3.16	1.81–5.48	65,598,612
C	.883	.707	.705	42	27								
T	.117	.293	.295										
rs1385699:						1.22×10^{-1}	1.60×10^{-5}	3.23	1.86–5.59	9.41×10^{-5}	3.00	1.71–5.32	65,608,007
A	.887	.708	.722	44	28								
G	.113	.292	.278										
rs1385695:						2.97×10^{-3}	1.03×10^{-5}	4.68	2.24–9.78	2.40×10^{-8}	6.57	3.17–13.63	65,687,533
A	.949	.799	.739	38	13								
G	.051	.201	.261										
rs775362:						4.10×10^{-3}	2.09×10^{-5}	4.39	2.13–9.21	3.73×10^{-8}	6.40	3.11–13.39	65,762,194
G	.949	.809	.744	37	13								
A	.051	.191	.256										
rs1041668:						1.49×10^{-4}	1.80×10^{-6}	6.42	2.74–15.03	1.58×10^{-9}	9.29	4.03–21.44	65,868,977
G	.036	.194	.258	9	39								
A	.964	.806	.742										
rs5964577:						2.50×10^{-3}	4.24×10^{-6}	4.99	2.32–10.68	1.20×10^{-8}	7.02	3.29–15.08	65,954,512
A	.954	.806	.747	36	12								
T	.046	.194	.253										
rs532649:						5.96×10^{-6}	5.42×10^{-7}	6.38	2.75–14.71	2.33×10^{-10}	9.62	4.17–22.13	66,050,269
A	.960	.807	.735	37	7								
G	.036	.193	.265										
rs989345:						4.65×10^{-6}	1.60×10^{-6}	6.24	2.74–14.66	6.13×10^{-10}	9.56	4.2–22.29	66,084,055
A	.964	.811	.737	36	6								
G	.036	.189	.263										
rs938059:						4.03×10^{-6}	1.10×10^{-6}	6.55	2.82–15.25	9.20×10^{-10}	9.63	4.18–22.17	66,119,748
C	.036	.195	.263	7	40								
A	.964	.805	.737										
rs925391:						4.76×10^{-6}	5.97×10^{-7}	7.28	3.03–18.03	1.98×10^{-10}	11.15	4.65–27.42	66,123,458
G	.969	.811	.737	38	6								
A	.031	.189	.263										
rs5919287:						4.62×10^{-6}	2.57×10^{-7}	6.61	2.87–12.82	1.76×10^{-10}	9.70	4.22–22.45	66,143,635
C	.964	.802	.734	39	7								
T	.036	.198	.266										
rs2221799:						4.62×10^{-6}	3.37×10^{-7}	6.53	2.84–15.18	1.39×10^{-9}	9.21	4.04–21.47	66,159,637
A	.964	.804	.744	39	7								
G	.036	.196	.256										
rs10521339:						4.00×10^{-4}	1.95×10^{-7}	5.65	2.65–12.04	2.10×10^{-12}	9.89	4.62–20.7	66,291,407
A	.954	.778	.677	11	41								
T	.046	.212	.323										
rs2223841:						9.40×10^{-6}	1.20×10^{-6}	5.59	2.62–11.94	1.72×10^{-11}	9.48	4.48–20.05	66,353,192
A	.954	.789	.688	44	11								
G	.046	.211	.312										
rs2207081:						4.33×10^{-6}	7.00×10^{-7}	6.21	2.8–13.78	5.04×10^{-12}	10.72	4.89–23.75	66,356,719
A	.959	.792	.688	44	10								
G	.041	.208	.312										
rs2497935:						1.79×10^{-5}	3.10×10^{-6}	5.00	2.41–10.36	3.17×10^{-11}	8.69	4.23–17.87	66,447,287
A	.949	.790	.684	45	12								
G	.041	.208	.316										
rs962458:						2.89×10^{-3}	2.87×10^{-4}	7.32	2.12–25.3	2.56×10^{-6}	11.10	3.27–37.74	66,528,985
G	.015	.102	.146	2	17								
A	.985	.898	.854										
CAG[e]:						2.71×10^{-1} [f]							66,548,181
18	.042	.085	.110	13	12		NS	ND	ND	NS	ND	ND	
19	.110	.106	.110	30	39		NS	ND	ND	NS	ND	ND	
20	.194	.112	.103	50	19		2.66×10^{-2}	1.91	1.07–3.41	2.20×10^{-2}	2.10	1.10–3.99	

(*continued*)

Table 3 (continued)

SNP and Allele	Frequency: Affected	Frequency: Control	Frequency: Unaffected	TDT[a]: Transmitted	TDT[a]: Nontransmitted	P^c	Affected/Control Analysis: P	Affected/Control Analysis: OR[d]	Affected/Control Analysis: CI	Affected/Unaffected Analysis: P	Affected/Unaffected Analysis: OR[d]	Affected/Unaffected Analysis: CI	Position[b]
21	.147	.191	.205	32	31		NS	ND	ND	NS	ND	ND	
22	.136	.122	.096	32	28		NS	ND	ND	NS	ND	ND	
23	.126	.090	.068	26	30		NS	ND	ND	NS	ND	ND	
24	.084	.080	.096	19	36		NS	ND	ND	NS	ND	ND	
25	.047	.064	.075	12	14		NS	ND	ND	NS	ND	ND	
rs6152:						5.88×10^{-5}	3.80×10^{-6}	5.26	2.45–11.3	6.66×10^{-10}	8.21	3.86–17.45	66,548,648
T	.046	.201	.282	11	40								
C	.954	.799	.718										
GGN[e]:						7.79×10^{-5} [f]							66,549,360
23	.651	.495	.421	76	43		2.06×10^{-3}	1.91	1.26–2.88	2.07×10^{-5}	2.57	1.656–3.98	
24	.182	.367	.461	21	68		5.39×10^{-5}	.38	.24–.62	2.62×10^{-8}	.26	.161–.42	
rs1204038:						9.79×10^{-5}	1.90×10^{-6}	5.45	2.55–11.67	2.83×10^{-9}	7.72	3.62–16.46	66,571,246
A	.046	.208	.271	11	39								
G	.954	.792	.729										
rs5919393:						1.58×10^{-5}	6.00×10^{-7}	5.82	2.73–12.41	1.69×10^{-8}	7.88	3.7–16.77	66,608,378
C	.046	.218	.274	11	38								
T	.954	.782	.726										
rs1337080:						5.73×10^{-3}	6.71×10^{-4}	6.73	1.92–23.14	4.75×10^{-6}	10.78	3.12–36.19	66,661,940
A	.985	.907	.859	15	2								
G	.015	.093	.141										
XARx7_001[g]:						1.00	6.79×10^{-2}	3.95	.81–19.25	1.45×10^{-1}	3.21	.61–16.76	66,725,646
A	.010	.039	.032	3	3								
G	.990	.961	.968										
XARx8insA[h]:						3.29×10^{-3}	5.09×10^{-5}	4.11	1.99–8.47	6.62×10^{-8}	5.94	2.94–12.02	66,727,141
delA	.944	.804	.739	34	13								
A	.056	.196	.261										
rs2781516:						3.28×10^{-2}	1.00×10^{-2}	2.02	1.18–3.48	2.86×10^{-4}	2.69	1.56–4.64	66,885,052
A	.128	.228	.282	21	38								
G	.872	.772	.718										
rs2885913:						4.46×10^{-2}	1.49×10^{-4}	2.31	1.49–3.57	4.29×10^{-5}	2.53	1.62–3.97	66,898,824
G	.255	.441	.465	40	64								
A	.745	.559	.535										
rs2363785:						1.73×10^{-2}	1.82×10^{-4}	2.28	1.47–3.53	2.04×10^{-4}	2.34	1.49–3.68	66,954,319
G	.745	.562	.555	65	37								
T	.255	.438	.445										
rs1936313:						2.48×10^{-2}	7.91×10^{-5}	2.37	1.54–3.64	9.15×10^{-4}	2.15	1.36–3.37	66,983,669
T	.744	.551	.575	65	39								
C	.256	.449	.425										
rs492933:						2.44×10^{-2}	1.15×10^{-2}	1.76	1.13–2.72	2.39×10^{-2}	1.69	1.07–2.65	67,046,865
C	.736	.614	.623	67	40								
T	.264	.386	.377										
rs1410127:						2.83×10^{-2}	8.02×10^{-3}	1.79	1.16–2.76	2.13×10^{-2}	1.71	1.08–2.67	67,063,402
C	.735	.608	.619	66	40								
T	.265	.392	.381										
rs1157321:						7.83×10^{-4}	1.59×10^{-5}	2.89	1.75–4.7	2.73×10^{-5}	2.93	1.75–4.87	67,104,762
G	.848	.659	.656	64	27								
T	.152	.341	.344										
rs7887862:						1.09×10^{-1}	3.31×10^{-1}	1.34	.74–2.41	1.28×10^{-1}	1.65	.86–3.2	67,148,136
C	.152	.118	.098	36	21								
T	.848	.882	.902										
rs1927232:						6.77×10^{-1}	1.77×10^{-1}	1.36	.87–2.11	8.23×10^{-1}	1.06	.66–1.69	67,165,912
C	.719	.653	.708	49	44								
T	.281	.347	.292										
rs5965536:						1.56×10^{-1}	3.57×10^{-1}	1.33	.73–2.41	9.50×10^{-1}	1.02	.57–1.84	67,300,796
C	.154	.121	.151	35	24								
G	.846	.879	.849										
rs792952:						1.39×10^{-1}	8.45×10^{-1}	1.05	.65–1.69	8.56×10^{-1}	1.05	.64–1.71	67,766,144
C	.249	.240	.240	53	36								
G	.751	.760	.760										

NOTE.—ND = not determined; NS = not significant.

[a] Family transmission/disequilibrium test (Knapp and Becker 2003).

[b] UCSC Genome Bioinformatics Plus Strand Build 35.

[c] Permutation-based value for association.

[d] Odds ratio.

[e] Only alleles with frequencies ⩾0.05 in controls.

[f] Global *P* value.

[g] GCTTTGTCTAATGCTCCTTC[G/A]TGGGCATGCTTCCCCTCCCC (intron 6 of *AR*).

[h] ACAAGCAAACAAAAAAAAAA[A/delA]GCAAAAACAAAACAAAAAAT (exon 8 of *AR*).

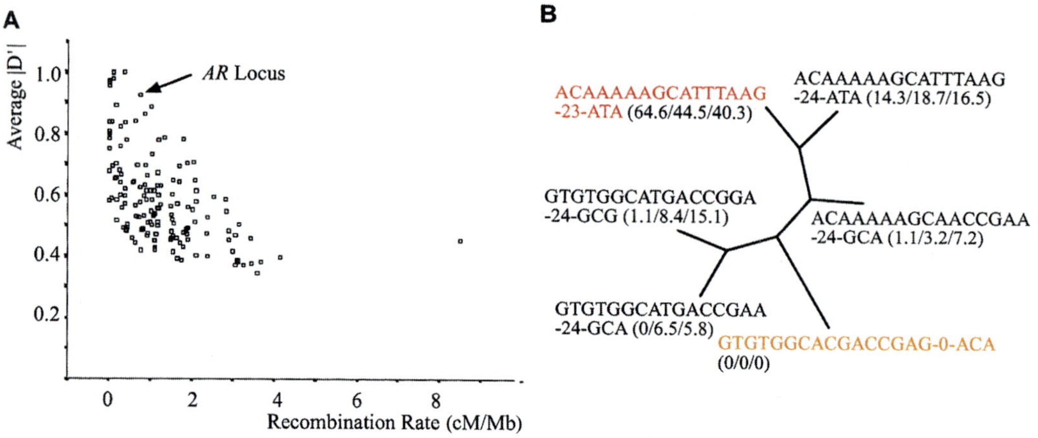

Figure 3 The *AR* locus: LD relative to the X-chromosome and haplotype structure. *A*, Average pairwise LD (measured by |D′|) between SNPs retrieved from the HapMap Project database, plotted over X-chromosomal recombination rates in 1-cM–sized windows. An average LD higher than that at the *AR* locus was displayed by only the six windows covering the centromere and showed distinctively smaller recombination rates. *B*, Neighbor-joining tree of frequent haplotype sequences (>5% in the samples from the individuals with AGA, controls, and individuals without AGA) within the most strongly associated haplotype block (genetic markers *rs1385695–XARx8insA*). The CAG repeat, *XARx7_01*, and *XARx8insA* were omitted from tree construction, because the corresponding *Pan troglodytes* allele could not be retrieved from the chimpanzee genomic sequence. The AGA haplotype is shown in red, and the chimpanzee haplotype is shown in orange. The AGA haplotype shows low sequence identity to the ancestral (chimpanzee) haplotype. Haplotype frequencies of the respective samples are indicated in parentheses (affected/control/unaffected [in %]). GGN-23 is indicated as "23"; GGN-24 is indicated as "24."

unaffected global *P* value of .0001). The study by Ellis et al. (2001) also showed a larger effect for the GGN repeat than the CAG repeat. However, the pooling of alleles in their study renders an exact comparison of results difficult. The GGN allele of 23 repeats showed a difference of affected versus unaffected allele frequencies of 0.23, which was in the range of the strongest-associated SNPs (*rs1385695–XARx8insA* [table 3]) but with a lower frequency in controls. This suggests that GGN-23 either is closer to the AGA mutation or is itself the AGA-susceptibility allele. Previously obtained functional data, in which shorter repeat alleles of the GGN repeat were associated with higher protein levels and thereby higher *AR* activity (Ding et al. 2005), support the possibility of a causal role for the repeat, and this would be compatible with current understanding of the involvement of androgens in AGA. Several studies have also suggested an effect of CAG repeat lengths on AR transactivating activity (Mhatre et al. 1993; Chamberlain et al. 1994; Kazemi-Esfarjani et al. 1995; Choong et al. 1996; Nakajima et al. 1996; Beilin et al. 2000; Ding et al. 2004). Since both repeats modulate AR activity and since we observe an association only between the GGN repeat and AGA, it may be that cells of the hair follicle lack cofactors that interact with the CAG-encoded domain.

Interestingly, shorter alleles for the GGN repeat have also been associated with prostate cancer (Hsing et al. 2000; Chang et al. 2002), whereas longer alleles have been associated with endometrial cancer (Sasaki et al. 2005), which would be in accordance with the differing effects of androgens on the endometrium and the prostate (androgens exert an inhibitory effect on endometrial cell proliferation, whereas they have a mitogenic effect in the prostate). However, the association findings with prostate cancer remain controversial, and no effect was shown in a large meta-analysis (Zeegers et al. 2004). The association with endometrial cancer has yet to be confirmed.

It remains possible that an as-yet-undetected variant in either a regulatory region affecting the expression level or an intronic variant affecting the splicing pattern of *AR* might be responsible for AGA susceptibility. The latter seems unlikely since we did not detect alternatively spliced transcripts of *AR* in human hair follicles of seven individuals representing different haplotypes. Previous studies have identified *AR* regulatory elements up to position −737 of the *AR* transcription start site (Faber et al. 1991, 1993; Supakar et al. 1993), as well as exonic enhancers in exon 1 (Faber et al. 1993) and exons 4 and 5 (Grad et al. 2001). Our sequencing analysis of 12 individuals with the associated haplotype revealed no variability in these regulatory elements of *AR*. However, there may be additional regions with regulatory effect that have not yet been fully characterized (Lower et al. 2004). Haplotypes carrying the GGN-24 allele show clearly higher frequencies in individuals without AGA than in those with AGA (fig. 3*B*). Since this effect is strikingly weaker in the ACAAAAAGCATTTAAG-24-ATA haplotype than in the other GGN-24–carrying haplotypes (fig. 3*B*), it is likely that further functionally relevant variability exists that modifies the protective effect of GGN-24–bearing haplotypes.

It is interesting to note that genetic variation in *AR*, which is located on the X chromosome, cannot explain the resemblance of fathers and sons with respect to the development of AGA (Küster and Happle 1984; Ellis et al. 1998), since sons always inherit the X chromosome from their mothers. The fact that family studies of AGA have typically stressed the resemblance of fathers and sons is understandable, given the differences in patterns of hair loss between males and females. Our genetic data, however, stress the relative importance of the maternal line in the inheritance of AGA, since we estimate an etiological fraction of 0.46 that can be attributed to having ≤23 GGN repeats within *AR*. This suggests that the average phenotypic resemblance should be greater between affected males and their maternal grandfathers than between affected males and their fathers. It is likely that the remaining etiological fraction is due to genetic variation at autosomal loci, which could explain the similarity of the AGA pattern of fathers and sons. Some autosomal candidate genes have been investigated in the past, including the insulin gene (Ellis et al. 1999), the 5α-reductase genes (Ellis et al. 1998), and the *hairless* gene (Hillmer et al. 2001, 2002), but none of these has been associated with AGA. A systematic linkage-based approach should enable the identification of additional loci.

Acknowledgments

We thank all participants for consenting to the study and for providing blood samples. This study was supported by grants from the Deutsche Forschungsgemeinschaft (DFG) (Forschergruppen "Keratinozyten—Proliferation und differenzierte Leistung in der Epidermis" and "Genetische Epidemiologie und Medizinische Genetik komplexer Erkrankungen"), the Bundesministerium für Bildung und Forschung (German Human Genome Project, "Pharmacogenomics"), and the Alfried Krupp von Bohlen und Halbach-Stiftung. R.C.B. is a recipient of a DFG Emmy Noether fellowship. We thank Faten Dahdouh and Carola Müller, for assistance in STR genotyping, and Dr. Christine Schmäl, for help in preparing the manuscript.

Web Resources

The URLs for data presented herein are as follows:

Ensembl, http://www.ensembl.org/ (for *AR* locus information)
HapMap, http://www.hapmap.org/ (for pairwise LD on the X chromosome [genotypes queried in November 2004])
Online Mendelian Inheritance in Man (OMIM), http://www.ncbi.nlm.nih.gov/Omim/ (for AGA and *AR*)
University of California–Santa Cruz (UCSC) Genome Bioinformatics, http://genome.ucsc.edu/ (for X-chromosomal recombination rates and definition of the reference strand for SNP allele calling)

References

Abecasis GR, Cookson WO (2000) GOLD—graphical overview of linkage disequilibrium. Bioinformatics 16:182–183
Bamshad M, Wooding SP (2003) Signatures of natural selection in the human genome. Nat Rev Genet 4:99–111
Becker T, Knapp M (2004*a*) A powerful strategy to account for multiple testing in the context of haplotype analysis. Am J Hum Genet 75:561–570
——— (2004*b*) Maximum-likelihood estimation of haplotype frequencies in nuclear families. Genet Epidemiol 27:21–32
Beilin J, Ball EM, Favaloro JM, Zajac JD (2000) Effect of the androgen receptor CAG repeat polymorphism on transcriptional activity: specificity in prostate and non-prostate cell lines. J Mol Endocrinol 25:85–96
Chamberlain NL, Driver ED, Miesfeld RL (1994) The length and location of CAG trinucleotide repeats in the androgen receptor N-terminal domain affect transactivation function. Nucleic Acids Res 22:3181–3186
Chang BL, Zheng SL, Hawkins GA, Isaacs SD, Wiley KE, Turner A, Carpten JD, Bleecker ER, Walsh PC, Trent JM, Meyers DA, Isaacs WB, Xu J (2002) Polymorphic GGC repeats in the androgen receptor gene are associated with hereditary and sporadic prostate cancer risk. Hum Genet 110:122–129
Choong CS, Kemppainen JA, Zhou ZX, Wilson EM (1996) Reduced androgen receptor gene expression with first exon CAG repeat expansion. Mol Endocrinol 10:1527–1535
Ding D, Xu L, Menon M, Reddy GP, Barrack ER (2004) Effect of a short CAG (glutamine) repeat on human androgen receptor function. Prostate 58:23–32
——— (2005) Effect of GGC (glycine) repeat length polymorphism in the human androgen receptor on androgen action. Prostate 62:133–139
Ellis JA, Stebbing M, Harrap SB (1998) Genetic analysis of male pattern baldness and the 5α-reductase genes. J Invest Dermatol 110:849–853
——— (1999) Insulin gene polymorphism and premature male pattern baldness in the general population. Clin Sci (Lond) 96:659–662
——— (2001) Polymorphism of the androgen receptor gene is associated with male pattern baldness. J Invest Dermatol 116:452–455
Faber PW, van Rooij HC, Schipper HJ, Brinkmann AO, Trapman J (1993) Two different, overlapping pathways of transcription initiation are active on the TATA-less human androgen receptor promoter: the role of Sp1. J Biol Chem 268: 9296–9301
Faber PW, van Rooij HC, van der Korput HA, Baarends WM, Brinkmann AO, Grootegoed JA, Trapman J (1991) Characterization of the human androgen receptor transcription unit. J Biol Chem 266:10743–10749
Grad JM, Lyons LS, Robins DM, Burnstein KL (2001) The androgen receptor (AR) amino-terminus imposes androgen-specific regulation of AR gene expression via an exonic enhancer. Endocrinology 142:1107–1116
Gudbjartsson DF, Jonasson K, Frigge M, Kong A (2000) Al-

legro, a new computer program for multipoint linkage analysis. Nat Genet 25:12–13

Hamilton JB (1951) Patterned loss of hair in man: types and incidence. Ann N Y Acad Sci 53:708–728

Hawk E, Breslow RA, Graubard BI (2000) Male pattern baldness and clinical prostate cancer in the epidemiologic follow-up of the first National Health and Nutrition Examination Survey. Cancer Epidemiol Biomarkers Prev 9:523–527

Hillmer AM, Kruse R, Betz RC, Schumacher J, Heyn U, Propping P, Nöthen MM, Cichon S (2001) Variant 1859G→A (Arg620Gln) of the *hairless* gene: absence of association with papular atrichia or androgenetic alopecia. Am J Hum Genet 69:235–237

Hillmer AM, Kruse R, Macciardi F, Heyn U, Betz RC, Ruzicka T, Propping P, Nöthen MM, Cichon S (2002) The hairless gene in androgenetic alopecia: results of a systematic mutation screening and family-based association approach. Br J Dermatol 146:601–608

Hsing AW, Gao YT, Wu G, Wang X, Deng J, Chen YL, Sesterhenn IA, Mostofi FK, Benichou J, Chang C (2000) Polymorphic CAG and GGN repeat lengths in the androgen receptor gene and prostate cancer risk: a population-based case-control study in China. Cancer Res 60:5111–5116

Kazemi-Esfarjani P, Trifiro MA, Pinsky L (1995) Evidence for a repressive function of the long polyglutamine tract in the human androgen receptor: possible pathogenetic relevance for the (CAG)n-expanded neuronopathies. Hum Mol Genet 4:523–527

Knapp M, Becker T (2003) Family-based association analysis with tightly linked markers. Hum Hered 56:2–9

Küster W, Happle R (1984) The inheritance of common baldness: two B or not two B? J Am Acad Dermatol 11:921–926

La Spada AR, Wilson EM, Lubahn DB, Harding AE, Fischbeck KH (1991) Androgen receptor gene mutations in X-linked spinal and bulbar muscular atrophy. Nature 352:77–79

Lee HJ, Chang C (2003) Recent advances in androgen receptor action. Cell Mol Life Sci 60:1613–1622

Lotufo PA, Chae CU, Ajani UA, Hennekens CH, Manson JE (2000) Male pattern baldness and coronary heart disease: the Physicians' Health Study. Arch Intern Med 160:165–171

Lower KM, Kumar R, Woollatt E, Villard L, Gecz J, Sutherland GR, Callen DF (2004) Partial androgen insensitivity syndrome and t(X;5): are there upstream regulatory elements of the androgen receptor gene? Horm Res 62:208–214

Matilainen V, Koskela P, Keinanen-Kiukaanniemi S (2000) Early androgenetic alopecia as a marker of insulin resistance. Lancet 356:1165–1166

Mhatre AN, Trifiro MA, Kaufman M, Kazemi-Esfarjani P, Figlewicz D, Rouleau G, Pinsky L (1993) Reduced transcriptional regulatory competence of the androgen receptor in X-linked spinal and bulbar muscular atrophy. Nat Genet 5: 184–188

Miller SA, Dykes DD, Polesky HF (1988) A simple salting out procedure for extracting DNA from human nucleated cells. Nucleic Acids Res 16:1215

Nagaraja R, MacMillan S, Kere J, Jones C, Griffin S, Schmatz M, Terrell J, Shomaker M, Jermak C, Hott C, Masisi M, Mumm S, Srivastava A, Pilia G, Featherstone T, Mazzarella R, Kesterson S, McCauley B, Railey B, Burough F, Nowotny V, D'Urso M, States D, Brownstein B, Schlessinger D (1997) X chromosome map at 75-kb STS resolution, revealing extremes of recombination and GC content. Genome Res 7: 210–222

Nakajima H, Kimura F, Nakagawa T, Furutama D, Shinoda K, Shimizu A, Ohsawa N (1996) Transcriptional activation by the androgen receptor in X-linked spinal and bulbar muscular atrophy. J Neurol Sci 142:12–16

Norwood OT (1975) Male pattern baldness: classification and incidence. South Med J 68:1359–1365

Nyholt DR, Gillespie NA, Heath AC, Martin NG (2003) Genetic basis of male pattern baldness. J Invest Dermatol 121: 1561–1564

Oh BR, Kim SJ, Moon JD, Kim HN, Kwon DD, Won YH, Ryu SB, Park YI (1998) Association of benign prostatic hyperplasia with male pattern baldness. Urology 51:744–748

Sasaki M, Karube A, Karube Y, Watari M, Sakuragi N, Fujimoto S, Dahiya R (2005) GGC and *Stu*I polymorphism on the androgen receptor gene in endometrial cancer patients. Biochem Biophys Res Commun 329:100–104

Supakar PC, Song CS, Jung MH, Slomczynska MA, Kim JM, Vellanoweth RL, Chatterjee B, Roy AK (1993) A novel regulatory element associated with age-dependent expression of the rat androgen receptor gene. J Biol Chem 268:26400–26408

Zeegers MP, Kiemeney LA, Nieder AM, Ostrer H (2004) How strong is the association between CAG and GGN repeat length polymorphisms in the androgen receptor gene and prostate cancer risk? Cancer Epidemiol Biomarkers Prev 13: 1765–1771

Zhao H, Zhang S, Merikangas KR, Trixler M, Wildenauer DB, Sun F, Kidd KK (2000) Transmission/disequilibrium tests using multiple tightly linked markers. Am J Hum Genet 67:936–946

Report

Strong Association of the Y402H Variant in Complement Factor H at 1q32 with Susceptibility to Age-Related Macular Degeneration

Sepideh Zareparsi,[1] Kari E. H. Branham,[1] Mingyao Li,[2] Sapna Shah,[1] Robert J. Klein,[4] Jurg Ott,[4] Josephine Hoh,[5] Gonçalo R. Abecasis,[2] and Anand Swaroop[1,3]

Departments of [1]Ophthalmology and Visual Sciences, [2]Biostatistics, [3]Human Genetics, University of Michigan, Ann Arbor; [4]Laboratory of Statistical Genetics, Rockefeller University, New York; and [5]Department of Epidemiology and Public Health, Yale University School of Medicine, New Haven

Using a large sample of cases and controls from a single center, we show that a T→C substitution in exon 9 (Y402H) of the complement factor H gene is strongly associated with susceptibility to age-related macular degeneration, the most common cause of blindness in the elderly. Frequency of the C allele was 0.61 in cases, versus 0.34 in age-matched controls ($P < 1 \times 10^{-24}$). Genotype frequencies also differ markedly between cases and controls ($\chi^2 =$ 112.68 [2 degrees of freedom]; $P < 1 \times 10^{-24}$). A multiplicative model fits the data well, and we estimate the population frequency of the high-risk C allele to be 0.39 (95% confidence interval 0.36–0.42) and the genotype relative risk to be 2.44 (95% confidence interval 2.08–2.83) for TC heterozygotes and 5.93 (95% confidence interval 4.33–8.02) for CC homozygotes.

Age-related macular degeneration (AMD) (*ARMD1* [MIM 603075]), the leading cause of untreatable blindness among the elderly in Western populations, is a clinically heterogeneous and genetically complex disease with multiple genetic and environmental risk factors (Age-Related Eye Disease Study Research Group 2000). Mutations in several genes (e.g., *ABCA4* [MIM 601691], *TIMP3* [MIM 188826], *RDS/peripherin* [MIM 179605], and *ELOVL4* [MIM 605512]) can cause early-onset macular diseases, but they do not appear to contribute significantly to AMD susceptibility (Stone et al. 2001). Particularly interesting are the fibulin-3 gene (MIM 601548) and related genes. Fibulin-3 mutations underlie drusen formation in Doyne honeycomb retinal dystrophy (MIM 126600), a disease that is phenotypically similar to AMD (Stone et al. 1999; Marmorstein et al. 2002). A mutation screen of five other fibulin genes detected missense mutations in fibulin-5 (MIM 604580) in 1.7% of patients with AMD (Stone et al. 2004). In addition, a fibulin-6 (MIM 608548) variant has been reported to cosegregate with the *ARMD1* locus in one large pedigree (Schultz et al. 2003). However, this change does not appear to play a significant role in AMD (Abecasis et al. 2004; Hayashi et al. 2004; Iyengar et al. 2004).

Linkage studies have suggested several chromosomal regions that may harbor AMD susceptibility genes. Klein and colleagues (1998) were the first to map a susceptibility locus (*ARMD1*) to chromosome 1q25-q31 in a large pedigree with AMD. Since then, many studies have been performed, and, overall, their results provide support for susceptibility loci on several chromosomes, including chromosomes 1q, 9q, 10q, and 22q (Weeks et al. 2000, 2004; Majewski et al. 2003; Seddon et al. 2003; Abecasis et al. 2004; Iyengar et al. 2004; Schmidt et al. 2004). Association studies have also been performed, and some of the identified loci appear to contribute to disease susceptibility. For example, an association between AMD and allelic variants of apolipoprotein E (*APOE* [MIM 107741]) has been widely documented, with the *APOE*-ε4 allele linked to lower risk of disease and the *APOE*-ε2 allele linked to higher risk (Klaver et al. 1998; Schmidt et al. 2002; Baird et al. 2004; Zareparsi et al. 2004). Recently, we reported an association between increased risk of AMD and the D299G variation in toll-like receptor 4 (TLR4 [MIM 603030]), a protein involved in innate immunity and

Received March 21, 2005; accepted for publication April 27, 2005; electronically published May 13, 2005.

Address for correspondence and reprints: Dr. Anand Swaroop, WK Kellogg Eye Center, University of Michigan, 1000 Wall Street, Ann Arbor, MI 48105. E-mail: swaroop@umich.edu

0002-9297/2005/7701-0016$15.00

phagocytosis by retinal pigment epithelium (Zareparsi et al. 2005). Despite these advances, the alleles that account for most of the genetic susceptibility to AMD remain undiscovered.

Recently, three independent studies have suggested that a polymorphism (Y402H) in the complement factor H gene (*CFH* [MIM 134370]) makes a substantial contribution to AMD susceptibility (Y402H has a T→C substitution at nucleotide 1277 in exon 9, which results in a tyrosine→histidine change). All three studies relied on linkage disequilibrium in the region and advances in SNP genotyping for gene identification (Abecasis et al. 2005). *CFH* maps to a region of chromosome 1q where several genome scans showed substantial evidence for linkage. One study (Klein et al. 2005), a genomewide association scan of 96 AMD cases and 50 controls by use of an Affymetrix 100K chip, identified two neighboring SNPs that were significantly associated with AMD. Another study (Edwards et al. 2005) examined noncoding SNPs across 14 Mb of the *ARMD1* locus on chromosome 1q in a sample of 224 cases and 134 controls; genotyping of 14 SNPs spanning *CFH* was performed in a larger sample. The third study (Haines et al. 2005) also focused on examination of SNPs distributed across the *ARMD1* locus, but it included a sample of 495 unrelated cases, 185 controls, and 182 families. In each study, initial associations were followed by additional genotyping that eventually led to the identification of a peak of association, which suggested the CFH-Y402H (C/T) variant as the susceptibility allele. These studies reported odds ratios (ORs) for AMD ranging between 2.4 and 4.6 for carriers of the C allele and between 3.3 and 7.4 for CC homozygotes (Edwards et al. 2005; Haines et al. 2005; Klein et al. 2005).

Independent replication studies are required to accurately assess the contribution of the associated alleles to disease susceptibility, because initial reports of association are vulnerable to a "winner's curse" effect, which can produce overestimates of the effect size (Goring et al. 2001; Lohmueller et al. 2003). We used a large sample of cases ($N = 616$) and controls ($N = 275$), collected at the Kellogg Eye Center in Ann Arbor, MI, to provide independent estimates of the effect of this common variant (CFH-Y402H) on AMD susceptibility. A majority of patients with AMD had late-stage AMD that presented as choroidal neovascularization (CNV [$N = 238$]), geographic atrophy (GA [$N = 143$]), or both CNV and GA ($N = 133$). The remaining patients had large macular drusen (LMD) in both eyes ($N = 102$) (Abecasis et al. 2004; Zareparsi et al. 2004). Control individuals were at least 68 years old and did not present any evidence of AMD in either eye after ophthalmic examination. All patients and controls reported their ethnicity as "white, not of Hispanic origin" and were recruited after informed consent. The human-genetics investigations described here were approved by the University of Michigan institutional review board. Genotyping was performed without knowledge of disease status. As shown in table 1, we detected a significantly higher frequency of the C allele in patients with AMD than in controls (0.61 vs. 0.34; $\chi^2 = 110.96$ [1 df]; $P < 1 \times 10^{-24}$). Genotype frequencies are also significantly different in affected and unaffected individuals ($\chi^2 = 112.68$ [2 df]; $P < 1 \times 10^{-24}$). OR calculations show that individuals carrying at least one copy of the C allele have a 4.36-fold increase in the risk of AMD (95% CI 3.13–6.08), whereas homozygous CC individuals exhibit a 5.52-fold increase in the risk of developing AMD (95% CI 3.54–8.59). Our results are within the range reported by the original studies (Edwards et al. 2005; Haines et al. 2005; Klein et al. 2005), and they validate the gene-dosage effect reported in two of the studies (Haines et al. 2005; Klein et al. 2005). Inclusion of age and sex as covariates in the logistic regression analysis did not affect the conclusions. Homozygous individuals for the putative risk allele were more common in all subtypes of AMD than in controls; specifically, those homozygous for the C allele included 38% of patients with GA, 34% of those with CNV, and 33% of those with LMD in both eyes, as compared with only 9% of control individuals. Interestingly, the homozygous genotype (CC) was more common in patients with a family history of AMD (38% of 261 cases) than in those without a family history (33% of 308 cases), a difference that was not statistically significant ($P > .05$). Finally, we note that the diagnosis of AMD occurred earlier for patients with at least one copy of the risk allele (mean in years [± SD] 70.9 ± 8.6) than for those without the risk allele (73.7 ± 9.2; $P = .01$).

To characterize the contribution of the Y402H polymorphism to AMD susceptibility, we fitted a series of genetic models to the data by maximum-likelihood estimation (results summarized in table 2). Model fitting was performed using the software and methods of Li et al. (2005). We performed our analysis with the assumption of a disease prevalence (K) of 0.20 (table 2), which

Table 1

Genotypic and Allele Frequencies for the T→C (Y402H) Variation in *CFH* Exon 9

Genotype or Allele	No. (Frequency) of Genotype or Allele in: Individuals with AMD [$N = 616$]	Controls [$N = 275$)]
TT	86 (.14)	114 (.415)
TC	311 (.50)	136 (.495)
CC	219 (.36)	25 (.09)
T allele	483 (.39)	364 (.66)
C allele	749 (.61)	186 (.34)

Table 2

Comparison of Fitted Genetic Models

Prevalence and Model (No. of Parameters)	ln(L)	*P*(C)[a]	*f*(TT)[b]	*f*(TC)[b]	*f*(CC)[b]	GRR1[c]	GRR2[d]	*K*	Attributable Fraction	λ_s
Constrained to *K* = .20:										
No effect (1)	−923.18	.52	.20	.20	.20	1	1	.20	…	…
General (3)	−864.86	.39	.08	.21	.47	2.81	6.30	.20	.62	1.21
Multiplicative[e] (2)	−865.75[f]	.39	.08	.20	.49	2.44	5.93	.20	.59	1.21
Additive[g] (2)	−869.14	.41	.07	.23	.38	3.05	5.10	.20	.63	1.14
Dominant[h] (2)	−893.28	.46	.09	.24	.24	2.62	2.62	.20	.53	1.05
Recessive[i] (2)	−897.67	.46	.16	.16	.36	1.00	2.24	.20	.21	1.07
Unconstrained:										
No effect (1)	−923.18	.52	NA	NA	NA	1	1	NA	…	…
General (4)	−864.46	.49	.30	.57	.83	1.88	2.77	.56	.46	1.06
Multiplicative[e] (3)	−865.54	.43	.15	.31	.66	2.10	4.40	.32	.53	1.14
Additive[g] (3)	−864.46	.49	.30	.57	.83	1.88	2.76	.56	.46	1.06
Dominant[h] (3)	−884.30	.52	.41	.75	.75	1.83	1.83	.68	.39	1.02
Recessive[i] (3)	−884.77	.53	.63	.63	.91	1.00	1.43	.71	.11	1.01

NOTE.—NA = not applicable.
[a] Estimated frequency of allele C.
[b] Estimated probability of disease for genotype.
[c] GRR1 = *f*(TC)/*f*(TT).
[d] GRR2 = *f*(CC)/*f*(TT).
[e] Constraint: GRR2 = $GRR1^2$.
[f] The best-fitting model, selected using the AIC.
[g] Constraint: GRR1 − 1 = GRR2 − GRR1.
[h] Constraint: GRR1 = GRR2.
[i] Contraint: GRR1 = 1.0.

is compatible with published estimates for elderly populations >70 years of age (Friedman et al. 2004), and without constraints on disease prevalence (table 2). With the use of a model with constrained prevalence (K = 0.20), the data suggest that the population frequency of the C allele is 0.39 (95% CI 0.36–0.42) and that the relative risk is 2.81 (95% CI 2.17–3.65) for TC heterozygotes and 6.30 (95% CI 4.53–8.72) for CC homozygotes. We also used the Akaike Information Criterium (AIC) to compare all models, including those with constrained and unconstrained prevalence, and to select the best-fitting genetic model. Our results suggest a multiplicative model—with K = 0.20, a disease-allele frequency of 0.39 (95% CI 0.36–0.42), and genotype relative risks of 2.44 (95% CI 2.08–2.83) for TC heterozygotes and 5.93 (95% CI 4.33–8.02) for CC homozygotes—as the most parsimonious model. The fitted log likelihood was ln(L) = −865.75 for the multiplicative model with K = 0.20 (two parameters, one for the genotype relative risk and another for the disease-allele frequency), versus ln(L) = −864.86 for an unconstrained model (four parameters, corresponding to three penetrances and one disease-allele frequency) and ln(L) = −923.18 for a model under the assumption of no contribution to disease susceptibility (one parameter, corresponding to the marker-allele frequency). Using this multiplicative model, we estimate the contribution of this allele to sibling-specific recurrence risk of AMD to be λ_s = 1.21 and the population-attributable fraction to be 0.62. This is the locus-specific λ_s, which can be calculated as a function of penetrances and disease-allele frequencies by use of the formulas of Risch (1990). The model predicts frequencies of 0.43, 0.47, and 0.10 among controls and 0.15, 0.48, 0.37 among cases for the TT, TC, and CC genotypes, respectively; the predicted values closely match the observed frequencies (see table 1) (goodness-of-fit χ^2 = 2.61 [2 df], not significant). An additive model also fits the data well, but dominant or recessive models are excluded. The agreement between our fitted model and observed genotype counts suggests that population stratification is not a major concern (Wittke-Thompson et al. 2005), a conclusion consistent with our analysis of previous genome-scan data.

CFH plays an essential role in regulation of complement activation, a major component of innate immunity against microbial infection. This regulation is achieved because CFH can bind to C3b (generated by cleavage of the α-chain of complement 3 [C3]), leading to the production of terminal C5b-9 complex (Giannakis et al. 2003). Many proteins of the complement system, including C5b-9 complex, have been detected in drusen from the eyes of patients with AMD (Mullins et al. 2000; Hageman et al. 2001; Johnson et al. 2001). CFH has three binding sites for C3b and additional binding sites for heparin and C-reactive protein (CRP). The Y402H change is expected to alter these interactions, since it is located within the cluster of positively charged amino acids implicated in the binding of CRP and heparin (Giannakis et al. 2003). Notably, associations have been reported between AMD and increased levels of CRP (Seddon et al. 2004) and between AMD and a polymorphism in *TLR4*, a key gene involved in innate immunity (Zareparsi et al. 2005). Hence, it is possible that certain microbial infections may be environmental triggers for AMD pathogenesis.

In summary, our data provide strong evidence for the Y402H variant being a common susceptibility allele for AMD. It is possible that another allele in strong disequilibrium with Y402H may cause disease susceptibility; this hypothesis can be tested only by evaluation of all polymorphisms and/or mechanistic functional evidence to explain the role of the Y402H variant. Our resequencing of CFH exon 9 (~500 bp) in all cases and controls did not identify any additional nearby coding variants. It will also be important to determine if the CFH-Y402H variant can explain the chromosome 1q linkage signal that is observed in independent genome scans (Klein et al. 1998; Majewski et al. 2003; Seddon et al. 2003; Abecasis et al. 2004; Iyengar et al. 2004; Weeks et al. 2004). Although *CFH* and *TLR4* are the first major AMD susceptibility genes to be identified, comprehensive studies of genetic variations are expected to lead to the identification of additional variants that contribute to this complex and debilitating disease.

Acknowledgments

We thank all the individuals who participated in this study, and we are grateful to numerous ophthalmologists and clinical staff for insights and assistance. This research was supported by grants from the National Institutes of Health (F32-EY014085, R01-EY015771, P30-EY007003, and K25-HG000060), the Foundation Fighting Blindness, the Macula Vision Research Foundation, the Elmer and Sylvia Sramek Foundation, Research to Prevent Blindness, and the Harold F. Falls Collegiate Professorship.

Web Resources

The URL for data presented herein is as follows:

Online Mendelian Inheritance in Man (OMIM), http://www.ncbi.nlm.nih.gov/Omim/ (for *ARMD1, ABCA4, TIMP3, RDS/peripherin, ELOVL4,* fibulin-3, Doyne honeycomb retinal dystrophy, fibulin-5, fibulin-6, *APOE, TLR4,* and *CFH*)

References

Abecasis GR, Ghosh D, Nichols TE (2005) Linkage disequilibrium: ancient history drives the new genetics. Hum Hered 59:118–124

Abecasis GR, Yashar BM, Zhao Y, Ghiasvand NM, Zareparsi S, Branham KE, Reddick AC, Trager EH, Yoshida S, Bahling J, Filippova E, Elner S, Johnson MW, Vine AK, Sieving PA, Jacobson SG, Richards JE, Swaroop A (2004) Age-related macular degeneration: a high-resolution genome scan for susceptibility loci in a population enriched for late-stage disease. Am J Hum Genet 74:482–494

Age-Related Eye Disease Study Research Group (2000) Risk factors associated with age-related macular degeneration. A case-control study in the age-related eye disease study: Age-Related Eye Disease Study Report Number 3. Ophthalmology 107:2224–2232

Baird PN, Guida E, Chu DT, Vu HT, Guymer RH (2004) The epsilon2 and epsilon4 alleles of the apolipoprotein gene are associated with age-related macular degeneration. Invest Ophthalmol Vis Sci 45:1311–1315

Edwards AO, Ritter R 3rd, Abel KJ, Manning A, Panhuysen C, Farrer LA (2005) Complement factor H polymorphism and age-related macular degeneration. Science 308:421–424

Friedman DS, O'Colmain BJ, Munoz B, Tomany SC, McCarty C, de Jong PT, Nemesure B, Mitchell P, Kempen J (2004) Prevalence of age-related macular degeneration in the United States. Arch Ophthalmol 122:564–572

Giannakis E, Jokiranta TS, Male DA, Ranganathan S, Ormsby RJ, Fischetti VA, Mold C, Gordon DL (2003) A common site within factor H SCR 7 responsible for binding heparin, C-reactive protein and streptococcal M protein. Eur J Immunol 33:962–969

Goring HH, Terwilliger JD, Blangero J (2001) Large upward bias in estimation of locus-specific effects from genomewide scans. Am J Hum Genet 69:1357–1369

Hageman GS, Luthert PJ, Victor Chong NH, Johnson LV, Anderson DH, Mullins RF (2001) An integrated hypothesis that considers drusen as biomarkers of immune-mediated processes at the RPE-Bruch's membrane interface in aging and age-related macular degeneration. Prog Retin Eye Res 20:705–732

Haines JL, Hauser MA, Schmidt S, Scott WK, Olson LM, Gallins P, Spencer KL, Kwan SY, Noureddine M, Gilbert JR, Schnetz-Boutaud N, Agarwal A, Postel EA, Pericak-Vance MA (2005) Complement factor H variant increases the risk of age-related macular degeneration. Science 308:419–421

Hayashi M, Merriam JE, Klaver CC, Zernant J, Bergen AA, Smith RT, Chang S, Merriam JC, Allikmets R (2004) Evaluation of the ARMD1 locus on 1q25-31 in patients with age-related maculopathy: genetic variation in laminin genes and in exon 104 of HEMICENTIN-1. Ophthalmic Genet 25:111–119

Iyengar SK, Song D, Klein BE, Klein R, Schick JH, Humphrey J, Millard C, Liptak R, Russo K, Jun G, Lee KE, Fijal B, Elston RC (2004) Dissection of genomewide-scan data in extended families reveals a major locus and oligogenic susceptibility for age-related macular degeneration. Am J Hum Genet 74:20–39

Johnson LV, Leitner WP, Staples MK, Anderson DH (2001) Complement activation and inflammatory processes in drusen formation and age related macular degeneration. Exp Eye Res 73:887–896

Klaver CC, Kliffen M, van Duijn CM, Hofman A, Cruts M, Grobbee DE, van Broeckhoven C, de Jong PT (1998) Genetic association of apolipoprotein E with age-related macular degeneration. Am J Hum Genet 63:200–206

Klein ML, Schultz DW, Edwards A, Matise TC, Rust K, Berselli CB, Trzupek K, Weleber RG, Ott J, Wirtz MK, Acott TS (1998) Age-related macular degeneration: clinical features in a large family and linkage to chromosome 1q. Arch Ophthalmol 116:1082–1088

Klein RJ, Zeiss C, Chew EY, Tsai JY, Sackler RS, Haynes C, Henning AK, Sangiovanni JP, Mane SM, Mayne ST, Bracken MB, Ferris FL, Ott J, Barnstable C, Hoh J (2005) Complement factor H polymorphism in age-related macular degeneration. Science 308:385–389

Li M, Boehnke M, Abecasis GR (2005) Joint modeling of linkage and association: identifying SNPs responsible for a linkage signal. Am J Hum Genet 76:934–949

Lohmueller KE, Pearce CL, Pike M, Lander ES, Hirschhorn JN (2003) Meta-analysis of genetic association studies supports a contribution of common variants to susceptibility to common disease. Nat Genet 33:177–182

Majewski J, Schultz DW, Weleber RG, Schain MB, Edwards AO, Matise TC, Acott TS, Ott J, Klein ML (2003) Age-related macular degeneration: a genome scan in extended families. Am J Hum Genet 73:540–550

Marmorstein LY, Munier FL, Arsenijevic Y, Schorderet DF, McLaughlin PJ, Chung D, Traboulsi E, Marmorstein AD (2002) Aberrant accumulation of EFEMP1 underlies drusen formation in malattia leventinese and age-related macular degeneration. Proc Natl Acad Sci USA 99:13067–13072

Mullins RF, Russell SR, Anderson DH, Hageman GS (2000) Drusen associated with aging and age-related macular degeneration contain proteins common to extracellular deposits associated with atherosclerosis, elastosis, amyloidosis, and dense deposit disease. FASEB J 14:835–846

Risch N (1990) Linkage strategies for genetically complex traits. I. Multilocus models. Am J Hum Genet 46:222–228

Schmidt S, Klaver C, Saunders A, Postel E, De La Paz M, Agarwal A, Small K, Udar N, Ong J, Chalukya M, Nesburn A, Kenney C, Domurath R, Hogan M, Mah T, Conley Y, Ferrell R, Weeks D, de Jong PT, van Duijn C, Haines J, Pericak-Vance M, Gorin M (2002) A pooled case-control study of the apolipoprotein E (APOE) gene in age-related maculopathy. Ophthalmic Genet 23:209–223

Schmidt S, Scott WK, Postel EA, Agarwal A, Hauser ER, De La Paz MA, Gilbert JR, Weeks DE, Gorin MB, Haines JL, Pericak-Vance MA (2004) Ordered subset linkage analysis supports a susceptibility locus for age-related macular degeneration on chromosome 16p12. BMC Genet 5:18

Schultz DW, Klein ML, Humpert AJ, Luzier CW, Persun V, Schain M, Mahan A, Runckel C, Cassera M, Vittal V, Doyle TM, Martin TM, Weleber RG, Francis PJ, Acott TS (2003) Analysis of the ARMD1 locus: evidence that a mutation in HEMICENTIN-1 is associated with age-related macular degeneration in a large family. Hum Mol Genet 12:3315–3323

Seddon JM, Gensler G, Milton RC, Klein ML, Rifai N (2004) Association between C-reactive protein and age-related macular degeneration. JAMA 291:704–710

Seddon JM, Santangelo SL, Book K, Chong S, Cote J (2003) A genomewide scan for age-related macular degeneration provides evidence for linkage to several chromosomal regions. Am J Hum Genet 73:780–790

Stone EM, Braun TA, Russell SR, Kuehn MH, Lotery AJ, Moore PA, Eastman CG, Casavant TL, Sheffield VC (2004) Missense variations in the fibulin 5 gene and age-related macular degeneration. N Engl J Med 351:346–353

Stone EM, Lotery AJ, Munier FL, Heon E, Piguet B, Guymer RH, Vandenburgh K, Cousin P, Nishimura D, Swiderski RE, Silvestri G, Mackey DA, Hageman GS, Bird AC, Sheffield VC, Schorderet DF (1999) A single EFEMP1 mutation associated with both Malattia Leventinese and Doyne honeycomb retinal dystrophy. Nat Genet 22:199–202

Stone EM, Sheffield VC, Hageman GS (2001) Molecular genetics of age-related macular degeneration. Hum Mol Genet 10:2285–2292

Weeks DE, Conley YP, Mah TS, Paul TO, Morse L, Ngo-Chang J, Dailey JP, Ferrell RE, Gorin MB (2000) A full genome scan for age-related maculopathy. Hum Mol Genet 9:1329–1349

Weeks DE, Conley YP, Tsai HJ, Mah TS, Schmidt S, Postel EA, Agarwal A, Haines JL, Pericak-Vance MA, Rosenfeld PJ, Paul TO, Eller AW, Morse LS, Dailey JP, Ferrell RE, Gorin MB (2004) Age-related maculopathy: a genomewide scan with continued evidence of susceptibility loci within the 1q31, 10q26, and 17q25 regions. Am J Hum Genet 75:174–189

Wittke-Thompson JK, Pluzhnikov A, Cox NJ (2005) Rational inferences about departures from Hardy-Weinberg equilibrium. Am J Hum Genet 76:967–986

Zareparsi S, Buraczynska M, Branham KE, Shah S, Eng D, Li M, Pawar H, Yashar BM, Moroi SE, Lichter PR, Petty HR, Richards JE, Abecasis GR, Elner VM, Swaroop A (2005) Toll-like receptor 4 variant D299G is associated with susceptibility to age-related macular degeneration. Hum Mol Genet (http://hmg.oupjournals.org/cgi/reprint/ddi154v1) (electronically published April 13, 2005; accessed May 9, 2005)

Zareparsi S, Reddick AC, Branham KE, Moore KB, Jessup L, Thoms S, Smith-Wheelock M, Yashar BM, Swaroop A (2004) Association of apolipoprotein E alleles with susceptibility to age-related macular degeneration in a large cohort from a single center. Invest Ophthalmol Vis Sci 45:1306–1310

Am. J. Hum. Genet. 77:154–160, 2005

Report

3q29 Microdeletion Syndrome: Clinical and Molecular Characterization of a New Syndrome

Lionel Willatt,[1] James Cox,[1] John Barber,[2] Elisabet Dachs Cabanas,[2] Amanda Collins,[3] Dian Donnai,[4] David R. FitzPatrick,[5] Eddy Maher,[6] Howard Martin,[1] Josep Parnau,[1] Lesley Pindar,[7] Jacqueline Ramsay,[5] Charles Shaw-Smith,[1] Erik A. Sistermans,[8] Michael Tettenborn,[9] Dorothy Trump,[4] Bert B. A. de Vries,[8] Kate Walker,[2] and F. Lucy Raymond[1]

[1]Department of Medical Genetics, Addenbrooke's Hospital, University of Cambridge, Cambridge, United Kingdom; [2]Wessex Regional Genetics Laboratory, Salisbury District Hospital, Salisbury, United Kingdom; [3]Wessex Clinical Genetics Service, Princess Anne Hospital, Southampton, United Kingdom; [4]Academic Unit of Medical Genetics, University of Manchester and Regional Genetics Service, St. Mary's Hospital, Manchester, United Kingdom; [5]MRC Human Genetics Unit and [6]Lothian Regional Genetics Service, Western General Hospital, Edinburgh, United Kingdom; [7]Department of Cytogenetics, Norfolk & Norwich Hospital, Norwich, United Kingdom; [8]Department of Human Genetics, Radboud University Nijmegen Medical Centre, Nijmegen, The Netherlands; and [9]Frimley Children's Centre, Frimley, United Kingdom

We report the identification of six patients with 3q29 microdeletion syndrome. The clinical phenotype is variable despite an almost identical deletion size. The phenotype includes mild-to-moderate mental retardation, with only slightly dysmorphic facial features that are similar in most patients: a long and narrow face, short philtrum, and high nasal bridge. Autism, gait ataxia, chest-wall deformity, and long and tapering fingers were noted in at least two of six patients. Additional features—including microcephaly, cleft lip and palate, horseshoe kidney and hypospadias, ligamentous laxity, recurrent middle ear infections, and abnormal pigmentation—were observed, but each feature was only found once, in a single patient. The microdeletion is ~1.5 Mb in length, with molecular boundaries mapping within the same or adjacent bacterial artificial chromosome (BAC) clones at either end of the deletion in all patients. The deletion encompasses 22 genes, including *PAK2* and *DLG1*, which are autosomal homologues of two known X-linked mental retardation genes, *PAK3* and *DLG3*. The presence of two nearly identical low-copy repeat sequences in BAC clones on each side of the deletion breakpoint suggests that nonallelic homologous recombination is the likely mechanism of disease causation in this syndrome.

The history of detecting microdeletion syndromes started with the recognition of discrete syndromic phenotypes associated with mental retardation, such as Prader-Willi, Miller-Dieker, Angelman, and Williams syndromes. Patients with similar phenotypes were then found to have similar submicroscopic deletions, in discrete genomic regions, that then defined the condition (Ledbetter et al. 1981; Schwartz et al. 1988; Knoll et al. 1989; Ewart et al. 1993).

Received February 28, 2005; accepted for publication May 4, 2005; electronically published May 25, 2005.

Address for correspondence and reprints: Dr. F. Lucy Raymond, Department of Medical Genetics, Cambridge Institute for Medical Research, University of Cambridge, Addenbrooke's Hospital, Cambridge CB2 2XY, United Kingdom. E-mail: flr24@cam.ac.uk

0002-9297/2005/7701-0017$15.00

In 1995, Flint et al. developed a strategy to screen for the abnormal inheritance of some subtelomeric DNA polymorphisms in individuals who had mental retardation alone and no associated clinical syndrome (Flint et al. 1995). Initially, 3 of 99 patients each had a single deletion at one of the telomeres. Since then, the technology has been developed to provide screening of all telomeres as a clinical service for suitably selected patients with mental retardation and dysmorphic features. The range of diagnostic yield is ~6%–11% (Knight et al. 1999; Slavotinek et al. 1999; Flint and Knight 2003; Koolen et al. 2004). The frequency of specific chromosome submicroscopic deletions or duplications reported in the literature varies from single case reports to >50 cases reported (De Vries et al. 2003). Conditions such as 1p36 or 2q37.3 microdeletions have been reported frequently, and these conditions now assume the status of recognizable syndromes, since common clinical features have emerged through the collection of patients with the same deletion (Shapira et al. 1997; Heilstedt et al. 2003; Aldred et al. 2004). However, several of the subtelomeric deletions have been reported only rarely to date, and the delineation of the associated clinical phenotype is therefore much more difficult.

We report here the identification of six patients with a 3q29 microdeletion. In five patients, the deletion arose de novo, and, for one patient, the parental origin could not be determined. The clinical phenotype is described in all six patients and is compared with that of a single case that was reported by Rossi et al. (2001). The molecular boundaries of the recurrent 1.5-Mb deletion are defined, and nonallelic homologous recombination is proposed as a mechanism of deletion formation in these patients.

Table 1 summarizes the clinical features of the six patients presented here and includes the few clinical details available on the patient analyzed in the study by Rossi et al. (2001). Figure 1 illustrates the patients' facial features and hands. To summarize, this condition is not associated with any antenatal abnormalities, and the birth history was uneventful in all patients. Birth measurements were within the normal range, although microcephaly was noted in patient 6. The level of developmental delay often was not fully recognized until after the 1st year of life, except in patient 6, in whom failure to thrive was noted at 5 mo of age. Growth parameters in all patients were at or below the 50th percentile but remained in the normal range. Speech delay was a particular feature, and all children needed special educational provision because of more general intellectual difficulties, although one child was in a mainstream school with substituted lessons in a specialist learning support unit. Autism was a feature of the behavior of two of the patients. Patient 1's behavior was obsessive and repetitive and met the ICD-10 (International Classification of Diseases, World Health Organization) diagnostic criteria for autism spectrum disorders; patient 3 presented at 3 years of age with moderate-to-severe cognitive learning difficulties with autistic traits but was not diagnosed as having a recognized form of autism. His psychological presentation was complex at that stage and remained so. The dysmorphology in the children is variable and not striking, but there are some facial similarities, and each child also has certain unique features. Generally, the face is long and narrow, especially in patients 2 and 4. The philtrum appears short in all patients, and a high nasal bridge is present in patients 1, 2, 3, and 4. The ears are generally large but well developed. The additional features found in at least two individuals were chest-wall deformity (pectus carinatum in one patient and pectus excavatum in another) and long and tapering fingers in two individuals, with fifth-finger clinodactyly in one of them. One additional child was noted to have fifth-finger brachydactyly, but X-ray assessment was not performed. An ungainly, ataxic gait was described in two patients, and, in patient 2, diagnoses of Angelman and Rett syndromes were considered and excluded. Each of the remaining features was identified only in a single patient: recurrent bilateral middle ear infections, requiring grommets, adenoidectomy, and removal of a cholesteatoma, in patient 2; ligamentous laxity in patient 3; downslanting palpebral fissures, posteriorly rotated ears, smooth philtrum, and prominent lower lip in patient 4; left-sided unilateral cleft lip and palate and nail hypoplasia in patient 5; progressive microcephaly and abnormal skin pigmentation in patient 6; and horseshoe kidney and hypospadias in the patient described by Rossi et al. (2001).

Molecular cytogenetic results are summarized in table 2 and figure 2. The samples were collected from laboratories in the United Kingdom and the Netherlands (Nijmegen), and FISH was performed on interphase or metaphase spreads, depending on the sample availability. G-banding at the 550 band or at a higher level, FISH probe preparation, and hybridization were performed using standard techniques. Parental samples were available for patients 1–5, and all deletions had arisen de novo. Patient 6 was adopted out of the birth family; thus, parental samples were unavailable for analysis. FISH analysis of patients 1 and 2 showed the presence of a terminal deletion of 3q29 by use of 3qter probe pVYS223B from the Totelvysion subtelomere screening kit (Vysis) on metaphase spreads. Deletions in patients 3 and 6 were initially suspected on high-resolution G-banding and were confirmed using the 3q subtelomeric probe CTC-196F4 from the study by the National Institutes of Health and Institute of Molecular Medicine Collaboration (1996). In patient 5, the deletion was detected using probe 3qtel106 from the Cytocell subtelomere screening kit. Probes pVYS223B, CTC-196F4, and 3qtel106 all map within BAC clone RP5-1061C18 (fig. 2*A*). In patient 4, the deletion was detected using multiplex ligation-dependent probe amplification (MLPA) (Koolen et al. 2004). The 3q29 deletion was not detectable with the older MLPA MRC (Medical Research Council) Holland telomere kit, PO19, which recognizes sequence in the nondeleted clone RP11-496H1, but is identifiable only with the new kit, PO36, which uses sequence within the *BDH* gene located within the deleted clones RP13-616I3 and RP11-535N19 as a MLPA probe. To refine the deletion, 26 overlapping BAC and PAC clones were identified using the then-available build 31 sequence (National Center for Biotechnology Information [NCBI] Map Viewer). The human genomic clones from the RPCI-5, -11, and -13 BAC and PAC libraries were obtained from the BACPAC Resources Center. Slides were analyzed using a fluorescence microscope (Leica DMRB), and images were recorded using

Table 1

Summary of the Clinical Features Found in the Six New Patients with the 3q29 Deletion and in the Patient from the Study by Rossi et al. (2001)

Clinical Feature	Patient 1	Patient 2	Patient 3	Patient 4	Patient 5	Patient 6	Patient from Rossi et al. (2001)
Pregnancy	Normal	Normal		Normal	Normal		
Birth weight (kg)	3.1	3.120		2.930	2.778	2.3	
Length of gestation	38 wk	Term		Term	41 wk	41 wk	
Feeding		Poor suckling				Failure to thrive	
Age at sitting	9 mo	7 mo					
Age at walking	18 mo	16 mo	Normal	21 mo		By 3 years	
Age at first words		28 mo		19 mo			
Age when developmental delay was noted	18 mo		3 years	18 mo	3 years	5 mo	
Age at talking	4–5 years	6–7 years			3 years	2 words and Makaton at 8 years, 10 mo	
Type of schooling	Special school	Special school	Special school	Special school (IQ = 70)	Learning support in mainstream school	Special school	Moderate mental retardation
Head circumference (percentile)	9th–25th		3rd	50th	10th	Progressive microcephaly[a]	
Height (percentile)	25th	25th–50th	25th	40th	3rd–10th	.4th	
Weight (percentile)	2nd–9th		25th		3rd–10th	.4th	
Hands and feet	Long and tapering fingers		Fifth-finger brachydactyly	Long and tapering fingers; clinodactyly of fifth finger and third, fourth, and fifth toes		Long	
Behavior	ICD-10 autistic		Autistic features				
Pectus	Excavatum			Carinatum			
Gait	Arm flapping when young	Ataxia and excited, stereotypical waving		Ungainly gait but neurologically normal			
Additional features		Chronic otitis media and cholesteatoma	Ligamentous laxity	Scaphoid skull (familial) and frontal bossing; downslanting palpebral fissures, smooth philtrum, and prominent lower lip; posteriorly rotated ears	Prominent metopic suture; left unilateral cleft lip and palate; nail hypoplasia	Increased pigmentation on dorsum of left foot; not toilet trained; frequent headaches	Horseshoe kidney and hypospadias

[a] Head circumference at birth: 32 cm (2 SD below the mean); at age 0.4 years: 37 cm (>4 SD below the mean); and at age 8.8 years: 46 cm (>5 SD below the mean).

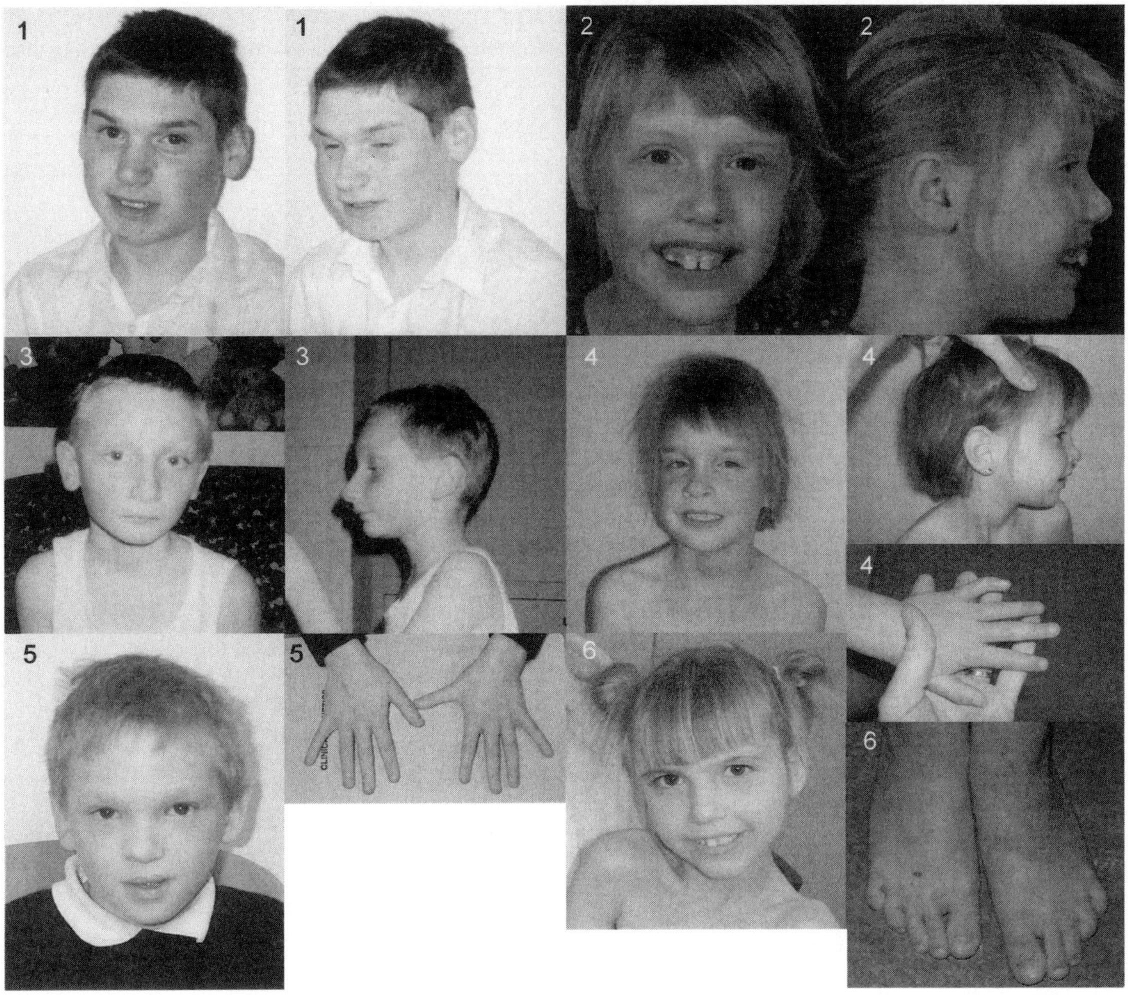

Figure 1 Photographs of patient 1, at age 9 years, 11 mo; patient 2, at age 14 years; patient 3, at age 6 years, 7 mo; patient 4, at age 6 years; patient 5, at age 7 years, 11 mo; and patient 6, at age 8 years, 10 mo. Written consent to publish these photographs was obtained from the parents of each child.

SmartCapture 2 software (Digital Scientific). Published STS primers STS-R44803, SHGC-170324, D3S4248, SHGC-34823, SHGC-149375, SHGC-10638, RH45269, SHGC-146015, RH99161, D3S2320, and RH80465 were used to check the identity of the clones (fig. 2*B*). In patients 1–4 and patient 6, the deletion endpoints were refined to within a single BAC clone. The telomeric breakpoint was within BAC clones RP11-594G13 and RP11-496H1, and the centromeric breakpoint was within BAC clones RP11-185G19 and RP11-480A16. For patient 5, there was insufficient material available to define the centromeric breakpoint, but the telomeric breakpoint was within BAC clone RP11-496H1, as for patient 2. The centromeric breakpoint lay between BAC clones RP11-171N2 and RP11-185G19 (table 2). At the telomeric breakpoint, the two BAC clones that define the deletion endpoint in the six patients overlap, and both contain STSs RH45269 and SHGC-146015. Most of clone RP11-594G13 is also contained within RP11-496H1, but clone RP11-594G13 extends ~60 kb further toward the centromere than RP11-496H1. On the basis of the resolution of FISH, the breakpoints in each of the patients are likely to be similar and to lie within 60–70 kb of each other.

The extent of the common microdeletion was determined using the finished sequence clones selected from the contigs on NCBI build 35.1 (NCBI Map Viewer). The microdeletion is estimated to be ~1.5 Mb, and it contains at least 22 transcripts, 5 of which are known genes (*PYT1A*, *PAK2* [MIM 605022], *MFI2* [MIM 155750], *DLG1* [MIM 601014], and *BDH* [MIM 603063]), 7 of which are incomplete cDNAs with two or more documented cDNA sequences, and 10 of which are hypothetical genes with no experimental evidence.

Since the deletion limits in the six patients were almost identical, the finished genomic sequence on each side of the deletion was investigated to determine whether any region-specific low-copy repeats (LCRs) were present. Nix analysis (HGMP-RC Nix Session Web site) of RP11-

496H1 (GenBank accession number AC024560) found regions of sequence homology within BAC clones RP11-480A16, RP11-352G9, and RP11-171N2. Two separate LCR sequences, designated "repeat A" and "repeat B," were identified on each side of the deletion region (fig. 2C). By use of BLAT analysis (Human BLAT Search Web site), repeat A was identified four times on chromosome 3, at positions 198832974–198852444, 197195390–197215144, and 197150598–197155588 in one orientation and at position 196868577–196884133 in the opposite orientation. Each repeat was >97.5% homologous and was ~19 kb, ~19 kb, ~5 kb, and ~15 kb long, respectively (fig. 2C). Repeat B occurred twice on chromosome 3; both repeats were in the same orientation and were located on chromosome 3 on each side of the breakpoint, at positions 198860847–198872158 and 197160541–197171848. These sequences were 98% homologous, and both were 11 kb in length (fig. 2C).

In summary, there is evidence of the presence of region-specific LCRs within the genomic sequence at each end of the microdeletion. It is likely that the formation of the similarly sized de novo microdeletions identified in the six patients was facilitated by these repeats and probably arose by nonallelic homologous recombination between LCRs on each side of the breakpoint, resulting in a single copy of the LCR and a genomic deletion between them. Alternatively, the presence of LCRs on each side of the deletion may not be directly involved in the deletion, per se, but they may act to predispose the genome to form a deletion. Both disease-causing mechanisms are now well recognized, although the presence of LCRs on each side of the deletion suggests that the former mechanism is more likely (Osborne et al. 2001; Shaw and Lupski 2004).

This analysis of six patients with an interstitial microdeletion of 3q29 is the first collation of cases to delineate 3q29 microdeletion syndrome. The clinical features of a patient from a previous report have been included for comparison, but samples from this patient were not available to establish the exact deletion breakpoints, and the family has been lost to clinical follow-up (E. Rossi, personal communication). The molecular deletion boundaries detected in the patients are strikingly similar, yet there is considerable clinical variability in the phenotype, with mild-to-moderate mental retardation being the only common and consistent feature. In addition, slightly dysmorphic facial features are similar in most patients: a long and narrow face, short philtrum, and high nasal bridge. As additional patients are screened for microdeletion syndromes on the basis of mental retardation and autism alone, it is likely that this syndrome will become increasingly well identified. Understanding the exact molecular mechanism of disease in these patients—that is, understanding how the deletion of some 22 genes in this region affects the development of an individual—is, of course, the next challenge. At this stage, it is impossible to attribute the phenotype to any one of the deleted genes, but two genes within the deleted area—*PAK2* and *DLG1*—merit further interest, since both are autosomal homologues of known X-linked mental retardation genes *PAK3* (MIM 300142) and *DLG3* (MIM 300189). Loss-of-function mutations in either *PAK3* or *DLG3* result in moderate-to-severe mental retardation (Allen et al. 1998; Tarpey et al. 2004). The *DLG1* protein SAP97, like SAP102 (*DLG3*), is a component of the postsynaptic density, and RNAi knockdown experiments of SAP97 result in reduced surface expression of GRIA1 (MIM 138248) and GRIA2 (MIM 138247) and a decrease in both AMPA (MIM 138248) and NMDA (MIM 138251) excitatory postsynaptic currents (Nakagawa et al. 2004). This sug-

Table 2

Limits of Interstitial 3q29 Microdeletion in Six Unrelated Patients

Contig and BAC/PAC Clone[a]	Accession Number	Presence or Absence of Probe in Patient[b] 1	2	3	4	5	6
NT_005612:							
513G11	AC117469	P	P	P	P	P	P
NT_005535:							
279P10	AC125362	P	P	P	P	P	P
NT_029928:							
171N2	AC069513	P	P	P	P	NT	P
352G9	AC124944	P	P	P	P	NT	P
480A16	AC024937	P	D	D	D	NT	D
185G19	AC139666	D	D	D	D	NT	D
252K11	AC026308	D	D	D	D	D	D
447L10	AC069257	D	D	D	D	NT	D
106N22	AC083822	D	D	D	D	NT	D
200I19	AC092933	D	D	D	D	NT	D
133B21	AC023797	D	D	D	D	NT	D
470E12	AC055725	D	D	D	D	NT	D
607N15	AC127904	D	D	D	D	NT	D
778E2	AC016949	D	D	D	D	D	D
432D10	AC068302	D	D	D	D	NT	D
114F20	AC092937	D	D	D	D	D	D
RP5-1061C18	AL121981	D	D	D	D	D	D
RP13-616I3	AC128709	D	D	D	D	D	D
535N19	AC126183	D	D	D	D	D	D
594G13	AC132008	P	D	P	P	D	P
496H1	AC024560	P	P	P	P	P	P
803P9	AC055764	P	P	P	P	P	P
23M2	AC022621	P	P	P	P	P	P
237O3	AC144530	P	P	P	P	NT	P
643E20	AC135893	P	P	P	P	NT	P
694O4	AC073135	P	P	P	P	NT	P

Note.—All accession numbers listed in the table are from GenBank.

[a] Unless otherwise stated, the BAC or PAC clones used were from the RP11 library.

[b] P = probe was present on both chromosome 3 homologues by FISH; D = probe was deleted on one of the chromosome 3 homologues; NT = probe was not tested, because of insufficient chromosomal material available from the patient.

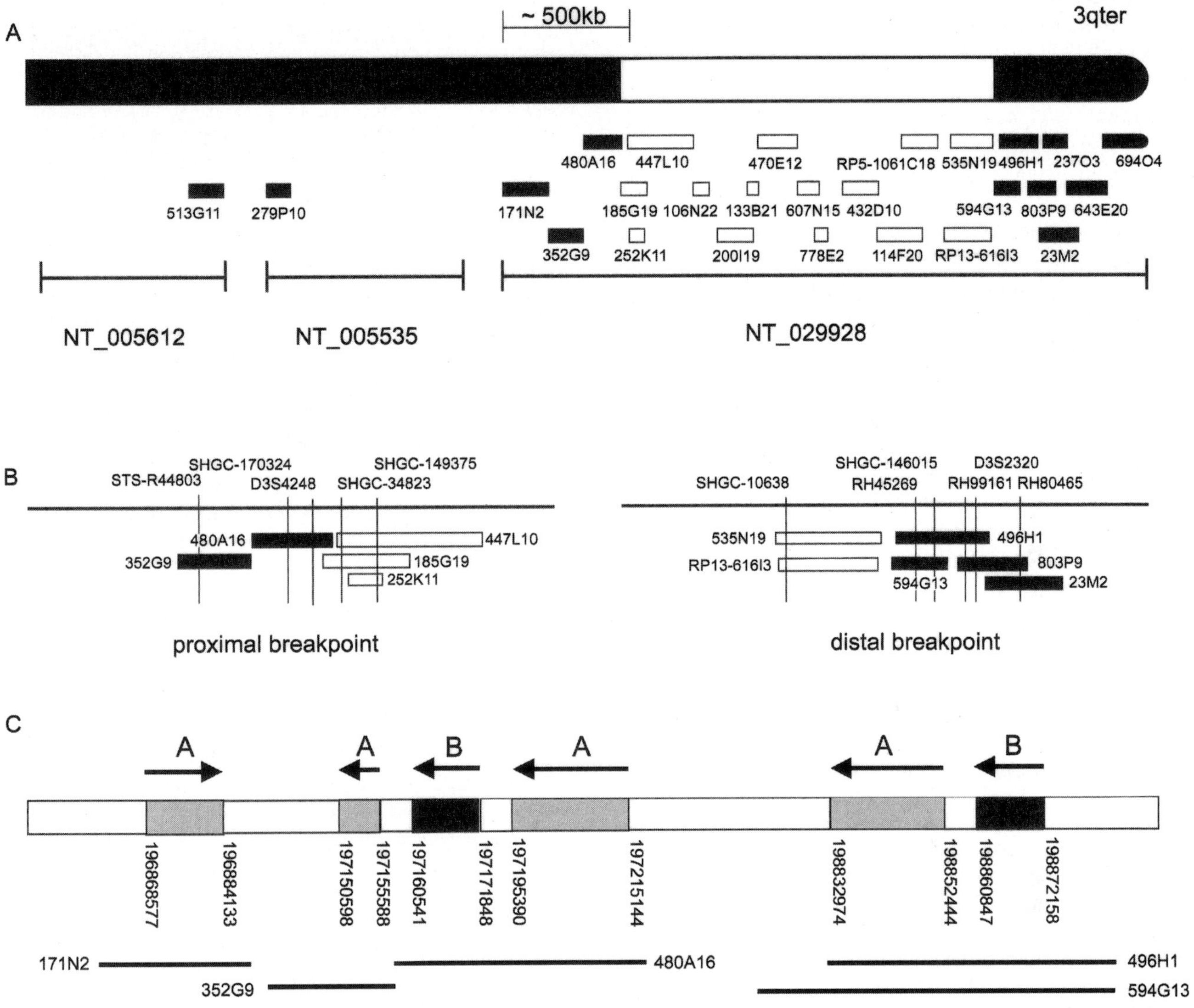

Figure 2 *A,* Genomic map of chromosome 3q, showing which clones are present (*blackened*) and which clones are deleted (*unblackened*). All six patients have deletions of BAC clones RP11-252K11–RP11-535N19 (see text). The MLPA probe, which can be used to detect the deletions in all six patients, is located within the *BDH* gene within BAC clones RP13-616I3 and RP11-535N19. The commercially available FISH probes—Vysis 3qter probe pVYS223B (D3S3560), Cytocell 3qtel106, and CTC-196F4—are all located within BAC clone RP5-1061C18. Unless otherwise stated, the BAC or PAC clones used were from the RP11 library. Contig NT_029928 and the size of the BAC clones within it are approximately to scale. The three contigs, GenBank NT_029928 (2.6 Mb), GenBank NT_005535 (1.2 Mb), and GenBank NT_005612 (100 Mb), are separated by gaps of unknown length in the sequence. *B,* The detailed positioning of BAC clones at the proximal and distal breakpoints. The relative position of each BAC clone was determined by identifying the presence or absence of known STS markers within the BAC clones and the genomic sequence around the deletion boundaries. *C,* LCR sequences in the deletion breakpoint genomic region. The region-specific LCRs designated "A" and "B" are shown (see text). The arrows above the bar show the orientation of the repeats; the position of the repeats on chromosome 3 are given below the bar. From left to right on the diagram, the repeat sizes are 15 kb, 5 kb, 11 kb, 19 kb, 19 kb, and 11 kb. The BAC clones that contain the LCRs are marked below the genomic location. The diagram is not to scale.

gests that loss of *PAK2* or *DLG1* may have a critical role in the development of mental retardation in these patients, but, clearly, this hypothesis needs further investigation.

Acknowledgments

We are grateful to the patients and families, for taking part in this study, and to the clinicians, for referring them. We thank Elizabeth Kerr for her expert technical assistance. J.C. is supported by the Medical Research Council, United Kingdom; H.M. is supported by the Department of Health, United Kingdom; B.B.A.d.V. is supported by a grant from the Netherlands Organization for Health Research and Development; and F.L.R. is supported by the Wellcome Trust.

Web Resources

Accession numbers and URLs for data presented herein are as follows:

BACPAC Resources Center, http://bacpac.chori.org/home.htm (for human genomic clones from the RPCI-5, -11, and -13 BAC and PAC libraries)
GenBank, http://www.ncbi.nlm.nih.gov/Genbank/ (for all accession numbers of BAC and PAC clones and genomic contigs listed in table 2)
HGMP-RC Nix Session, http://www.hgmp.mrc.ac.uk/Registered/Webapp/nix/ (for homology searching within BAC clone sequences)
Human BLAT Search, http://www.genome.ucsc.edu/cgi-bin/hgBlat (for homology searching within the chromosome 3 sequence)
NCBI Map Viewer, http://www.ncbi.nlm.nih.gov/mapview/ (for BLAST sequence homology search and for transcripts and genes within the 3q29 deleted region)
Online Mendelian Inheritance in Man (OMIM), http://www.ncbi.nlm.nih.gov/Omim/ (for *PAK2, MFI2, DLG1, BDH, PAK3,* and *DLG3*)

References

Aldred MA, Sanford RO, Thomas NS, Barrow MA, Wilson LC, Brueton LA, Bonaglia MC, Hennekam RC, Eng C, Dennis NR, Trembath RC (2004) Molecular analysis of 20 patients with 2q37.3 monosomy: definition of minimum deletion intervals for key phenotypes. J Med Genet 41:433–439
Allen KM, Gleeson JG, Bagrodia S, Partington MW, MacMillan JC, Cerione RA, Mulley JC, Walsh CA (1998) PAK3 mutation in nonsyndromic X-linked mental retardation. Nat Genet 20:25–30
De Vries BB, Winter R, Schinzel A, van Ravenswaaij-Arts C (2003) Telomeres: a diagnosis at the end of the chromosomes. J Med Genet 40:385–398
Ewart AK, Morris CA, Atkinson D, Jin W, Sternes K, Spallone P, Stock AD, Leppert M, Keating MT (1993) Hemizygosity at the elastin locus in a developmental disorder, Williams syndrome. Nat Genet 5:11–16
Flint J, Knight S (2003) The use of telomere probes to investigate submicroscopic rearrangements associated with mental retardation. Curr Opin Genet Dev 13:310–316
Flint J, Wilkie AO, Buckle VJ, Winter RM, Holland AJ, McDermid HE (1995) The detection of subtelomeric chromosomal rearrangements in idiopathic mental retardation. Nat Genet 9:132–140
Heilstedt HA, Ballif BC, Howard LA, Lewis RA, Stal S, Kashork CD, Bacino CA, Shapira SK, Shaffer LG (2003) Physical map of 1p36, placement of breakpoints in monosomy 1p36, and clinical characterization of the syndrome. Am J Hum Genet 72:1200–1212
Knight SJ, Regan R, Nicod A, Horsley SW, Kearney L, Homfray T, Winter RM, Bolton P, Flint J (1999) Subtle chromosomal rearrangements in children with unexplained mental retardation. Lancet 354:1676–1681
Knoll JH, Nicholls RD, Magenis RE, Graham JM Jr, Lalande M, Latt SA (1989) Angelman and Prader-Willi syndromes share a common chromosome 15 deletion but differ in parental origin of the deletion. Am J Med Genet 32:285–290
Koolen DA, Nillesen WM, Versteeg MH, Merkx GF, Knoers NV, Kets M, Vermeer S, van Ravenswaaij CM, de Kovel CG, Brunner HG, Smeets D, de Vries BB, Sistermans EA (2004) Screening for subtelomeric rearrangements in 210 patients with unexplained mental retardation using multiplex ligation dependent probe amplification (MLPA). J Med Genet 41:892–899
Ledbetter DH, Riccardi VM, Airhart SD, Strobel RJ, Keenan BS, Crawford JD (1981) Deletions of chromosome 15 as a cause of the Prader-Willi syndrome. N Engl J Med 304:325–329
Nakagawa T, Futai K, Lashuel HA, Lo I, Okamoto K, Walz T, Hayashi Y, Sheng M (2004) Quaternary structure, protein dynamics, and synaptic function of SAP97 controlled by L27 domain interactions. Neuron 44:453–467
National Institutes of Health and Institute of Molecular Medicine Collaboration (1996) A complete set of human telomeric probes and their clinical application. Nat Genet 14:86–89
Osborne LR, Li M, Pober B, Chitayat D, Bodurtha J, Mandel A, Costa T, Grebe T, Cox S, Tsui LC, Scherer SW (2001) A 1.5 million–base pair inversion polymorphism in families with Williams-Beuren syndrome. Nat Genet 29:321–325
Rossi E, Piccini F, Zollino M, Neri G, Caselli D, Tenconi R, Castellan C, Carrozzo R, Danesino C, Zuffardi O, Ragusa A, Castiglia L, Galesi O, Greco D, Romano C, Pierluigi M, Perfumo C, Di Rocco M, Faravelli F, Dagna Bricarelli F, Bonaglia M, Bedeschi M, Borgatti R (2001) Cryptic telomeric rearrangements in subjects with mental retardation associated with dysmorphism and congenital malformations. J Med Genet 38:417–420
Schwartz CE, Johnson JP, Holycross B, Mandeville TM, Sears TS, Graul EA, Carey JC, Schroer RJ, Phelan MC, Szollar J, Flannery DB, Stevenson RE (1988) Detection of submicroscopic deletions in band 17p13 in patients with the Miller-Dieker syndrome. Am J Hum Genet 43:597–604
Shapira SK, McCaskill C, Northrup H, Spikes AS, Elder FF, Sutton VR, Korenberg JR, Greenberg F, Shaffer LG (1997) Chromosome 1p36 deletions: the clinical phenotype and molecular characterization of a common newly delineated syndrome. Am J Hum Genet 61:642–650
Shaw CJ, Lupski JR (2004) Implications of human genome architecture for rearrangement-based disorders: the genomic basis of disease. Hum Mol Genet 13 Spec No 1:R57–R64
Slavotinek A, Rosenberg M, Knight S, Gaunt L, Fergusson W, Killoran C, Clayton-Smith J, Kingston H, Campbell RH, Flint J, Donnai D, Biesecker L (1999) Screening for submicroscopic chromosome rearrangements in children with idiopathic mental retardation using microsatellite markers for the chromosome telomeres. J Med Genet 36:405–411
Tarpey P, Parnau J, Blow M, Woffendin H, Bignell G, Cox C, Cox J, et al (2004) Mutations in the DLG3 gene cause nonsyndromic X-linked mental retardation. Am J Hum Genet 75:318–324

Report

Characterization of a New Syndrome That Associates Craniosynostosis, Delayed Fontanel Closure, Parietal Foramina, Imperforate Anus, and Skin Eruption: CDAGS

Roberto Mendoza-Londono,[1] Edward Lammer,[3] Rosemarie Watson,[4] John Harper,[5] Atsushi Hatamochi,[6] Saori Hatamochi-Hayashi,[7] Dobrawa Napierala,[2] Pia Hermanns,[1] Sinead Collins,[4] Benjamin B. Roa,[1] Madhuri R. Hedge,[1] Keiko Wakui,[1] Diep Nguyen,[1] David W. Stockton,[1] and Brendan Lee[1,2]

[1]Department of Human and Molecular Genetics and [2]Howard Hughes Medical Institute, Baylor College of Medicine, Houston; [3]Children's Hospital Research Institute, Oakland; [4]Our Lady's Hospital for Sick Children Crumlin, Dublin; [5]Great Ormond Street Hospital for Children, London; [6]Department of Dermatology, Dokkyo University School of Medicine, Mibu, Japan; and [7]Department of Internal Medicine, Kawasaki Medical School, Okayama, Japan

We describe the clinical characterization, molecular analyses, and genetic mapping of a distinct genetic condition characterized by craniosynostosis, delayed closure of the fontanel, cranial defects, clavicular hypoplasia, anal and genitourinary malformations, and skin eruption. We have identified seven patients with this phenotype in four families from different geographic regions and ethnic backgrounds. This is an autosomal recessive condition that brings together apparently opposing pathophysiologic and developmental processes, including accelerated suture closure and delayed ossification. Selected candidate genes—including *RUNX2, CBFB, MSX2, ALX4, TWIST1,* and *RECQL4*—were screened for mutations, by direct sequencing of their coding regions, and for microdeletions, by fluorescent in situ hybridization. No mutations or microdeletions were detected in any of the genes analyzed. A genomewide screen yielded the maximum estimated LOD score of +2.38 for markers *D22S283* and *D22S274* on chromosome 22q12-q13. We hypothesize that the gene defect in this condition causes novel context-dependent dysregulation of multiple signaling pathways, including RUNX2, during osteoblast differentiation and craniofacial morphogenesis.

In this study, we present the clinical characterization of a distinct genetic condition that associates a severe form of craniofacial dysplasia with genitourinary and skin manifestations. We have used the acronym "CDAGS" because it summarizes the most prominent features of this disorder: "C" stands for craniosynostosis and clavicular hypoplasia; "D," for delayed closure of the fontanel, cranial defects, and, in some patients, deafness; "A," for anal anomalies, including anterior placement of the anus and imperforate anus; "G," for genitourinary malformations; and "S," for skin eruption, which, in some of the patients, has been classified as porokeratosis. To date, we have identified seven patients, in four families, with the CDAGS phenotype.

The craniofacial component of CDAGS overlaps with some of the features seen in cleidocranial dysplasia (CCD [MIM 119600]), an autosomal dominant disorder characterized by hypoplastic or absent clavicles, delayed closure of the cranial sutures and fontanels, dental anomalies, and delayed skeletal development (Cooper et al. 2001). Most cases of CCD are caused by mutations in *RUNX2*, located on chromosome 6p21 (Lee et al. 1997; Mundlos et al. 1997). *RUNX2* encodes a runt domain transcriptional factor RUNX2, which is required for both osteoblast differentiation and chondrocyte maturation (Zhou et al. 1999, Zheng et al. 2003). Other conditions, such as Yunis-Varon syndrome (MIM 216340) and Crane-Heise syndrome (MIM 218090) share some phenotypic characteristics with CCD, such as cranial dysostosis and

Received March 1, 2005; accepted for publication May 4, 2005; electronically published May 27, 2005.

Address for correspondence and reprints: Dr. Brendan Lee, Department of Molecular and Human Genetics, Baylor College of Medicine, One Baylor Plaza, Room 635E, Mail Stop 225, Houston, TX 77030. E-mail: blee@bcm.tmc.edu

0002-9297/2005/7701-0018$15.00

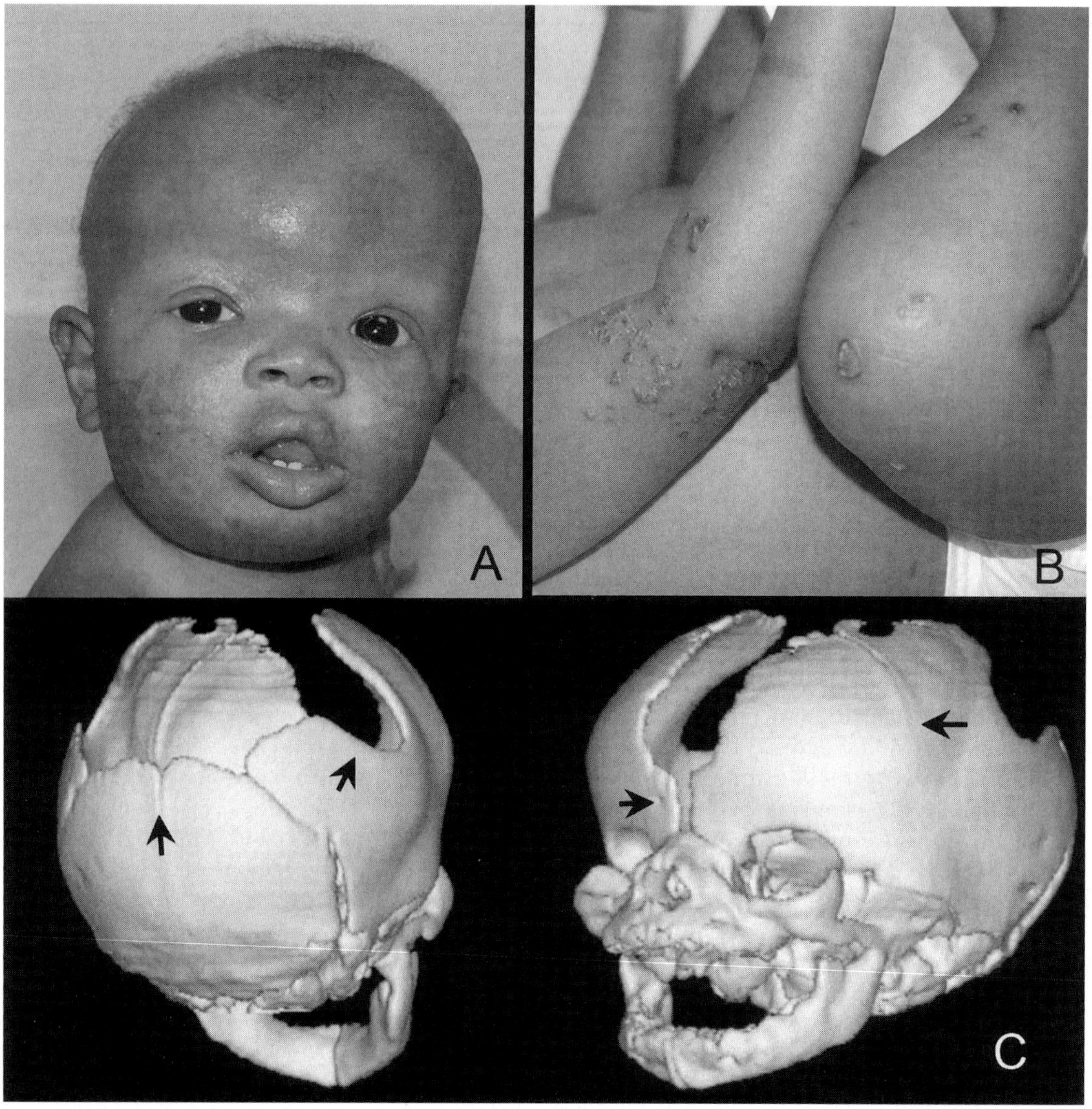

Figure 1 *A*, Craniofacial features of CDAGS syndrome in the index patient at age 8 mo. Note the brachycephaly, frontal bossing, and sparse eyelashes and eyebrows. The skin lesions on the patient's face became markedly hyperpigmented at age 2 mo. *B*, Skin lesions on arms and legs, which occur in a psoriasis-like distribution and affect the margins of the earlobes. Color pictures are included in appendix A (online only). *C*, Posterolateral and anterolateral views of the 3D reconstruction of the CT of the head of the index patient at age 1 mo. Notice the wide metopic suture extending to the nasal bridge, wide-open anterior and posterior fontanels, bilateral PF, and coronal synostosis (*arrows*).

clavicular hypoplasia; the fact that similar skeletal elements are affected in some of these conditions suggests that they may result from mutations in genes that affect the context-dependent action of RUNX2 on its downstream targets. Moreover, phenocopies of this clinical feature may help to identify in vivo regulators of the RUNX2 transcriptional network.

Our index patient is an African American female who was referred for evaluation because of imperforate anus and dysmorphic features. Initial assessment on day 1 of life demonstrated midface hypoplasia, frontal bossing, large anterior and posterior fontanels, open metopic suture extending down to the nasal bridge, and wide-open sagittal suture. Her clavicles were hypoplastic, and her shoulders could be brought together at the midline. Her genitalia appeared normal, but she had an imperforate anus with rectoperineal fistula. Skin examination revealed multiple papules over the brow and posterior hairline as well as hyperkeratotic areas on her scalp. She had very sparse hair, eyelashes, and eyebrows, which did not improve with age (fig. 1*A*). Her prenatal history was negative for complications, maternal illness, and toxic exposure. The family history is negative for consanguinity, malformations, and fetal demise.

The patient's skin lesions progressed, and, at age 4 mo, they were present on the face and extremities as papules and ruptured vesicles, with an erythematous indurated border in a psoriasis-like distribution (fig. 1*B*). A skin biopsy of a lesion on the right forearm was performed. Gross inspection revealed heavily pigmented skin with a surface plaque. Microscopic examination showed hyperkeratosis, acanthosis, and an intraepithelial pustule containing mixed inflammatory cells. There was focal disruption of the dermal-epidermal junction, and some of the keratinocytes had cytoplasmatic granules containing melanin. Skin biopsy of a lesion on the left thigh showed a lichenoid infiltrate composed of lymphocytes, neutrophils, and occasional eosinophils, with numerous colloid bodies within the epithelium.

A chest X-ray showed absence of the medial aspects of the clavicles, kyphosis of the thoracic spine, and short ribs. The scapula and vertebral bodies appeared normal. A skeletal survey also revealed poor ossification of the parietal bones and apparent hypoplasia of the sphenoid bone and of the midfacial bones involving the nasion and the maxillary bones. The remainder of the skeleton was within normal limits. A CT scan of the head showed a brachycephalic skull with bilateral coronal synostosis, wide-open metopic suture, and bilateral parietal foramina (PF) (fig. 1C). A magnetic resonance image (MRI) of the brain showed no structural abnormalities and a myelination pattern normal for age. Spinal and renal ultrasound results were normal. A hearing screen identified unilateral sensorineural hearing loss. Chromosome analysis by G-banding revealed a normal 46,XX karyotype.

We have identified and examined six additional patients from a total of four pedigrees, with similar findings. The families come from different geographic regions and ethnic backgrounds (fig. 2). Three of the families have two affected individuals, and two of those families have both male and female affected siblings. For all individuals evaluated, the family history was negative for similar defects. The pattern of transmission observed is consistent with an autosomal recessive Mendelian trait.

Family 2 is of Mexican American descent. The clinical and radiological findings for the two affected individuals in this family show striking similarities to those of the index patient, with severe skin rash, imperforate anus, and cranial defects, including bilateral PF and coronal synostosis (fig. 3). Biopsy of skin lesions on the arms showed histological findings of porokeratosis. In addition to these findings, the older affected individual in this family has profound bilateral sensorineural hearing loss and severe developmental delay. For detailed clinical information about the patients, see appendix A (online only).

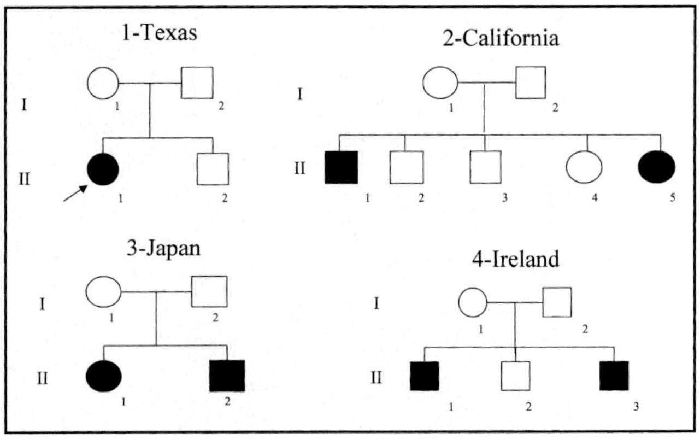

Figure 2 Pedigrees of the four families with CDAGS that have been identified to date. Three families have more than one affected individual, and two have an affected male and female. In all families, there was no history of previous affected individuals, and all families deny consanguinity.

Family 3 is of Japanese descent and comprises two affected siblings, a boy and a girl. These patients were originally described by Fukuda et al. (1981) as having an atypical form of CCD, characterized by clavicular hypoplasia, wide-open sutures and fontanel, anal atresia, and skin lesions described as erythematous plaques with erosion. Watanabe et al. (1996) published another article about these patients and described the skin lesions as a form of psoriasiform erythrokeratodermia.

Family 4 is white and is of Irish descent. Judge et al. (1990) published a study describing the older individual as having porokeratosis and craniosynostosis. Flanagan et al. (1998) described this patient and his brother as having familial craniosynostosis, anal anomalies, and porokeratosis and used the acronym "CAP" (MIM 603116) for the constellation of findings. Both individuals in this family presented with brachycephaly, wide-open anterior and posterior fontanels, and complete coronal synostosis. Flanagan et al. (1998) tested the patients of this family for mutations associated with craniosynostosis in the fibroblast growth-factor receptors 1, 2, and 3 (*FGFR1, FGFR2,* and *FGFR3*) and in the *TWIST1* genes, and no abnormalities were found (Flanagan et al. 1998).

Table 1 summarizes the clinical findings in the seven patients identified to date. The most consistent features of CDAGS syndrome are coronal synostosis, wide-open anterior and posterior fontanel with PF, underdeveloped eyebrows and eyelashes, imperforate anus, and skin lesions. In two of the families, the histological findings of the skin biopsy were compatible with a diagnosis of porokeratosis. Additional features present in some but not all of the patients include hypoplastic clavicles, sensorineural hearing loss, developmental delay, cleft palate, and hypospadias. The four patients with developmental

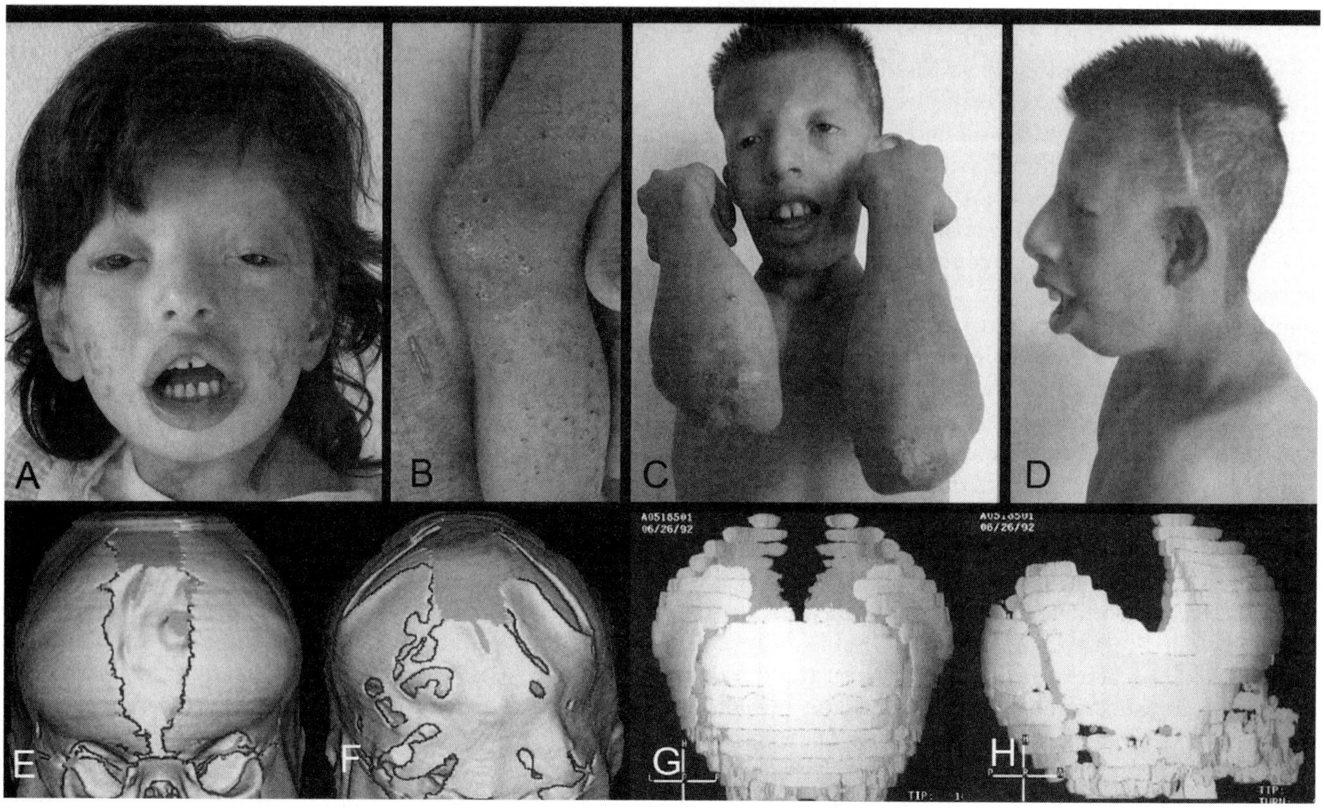

Figure 3 Clinical and radiological findings in family 2, showing striking similarities with the index patient. Notice the characteristic skin rash on the 3-year-old female's face (*A*) and extremities (*B*), whereas, in her 11-year-old brother, although there is persistence of hyperkeratotic plaques on the elbows and knees (*C*), facial skin lesions have improved significantly (*D*). Both patients have dysmorphic features and sparse eyebrows and eyelashes. Color pictures are included in appendix A (online only). Anteroposterior and lateral views of the 3D reconstruction of the CT of the head in the female (*panels E* and *F*) and male (*panels G* and *H*) at age 1 mo demonstrate the characteristic cranial defects.

delay have some degree of hearing impairment, which may account for some of the deficits. However, these patients have problems with speech and motor skills that do not improve with therapy.

To identify the molecular basis of the disorder, we initially undertook a candidate-gene approach. Figure 4 summarizes the genes that were considered on the basis of the phenotypic characteristics. Because the phenotype shares multiple characteristics with CCD, *RUNX2* and its coactivator, the core binding factor beta (*CBFB*) were attractive candidates (Kundu et al. 2002; Yoshida et al. 2002). PF are symmetric defects of parietal bone ossification that can be seen as an isolated defect or as part of different clinical syndromes. When the defects are large, they may be the main manifestation of the condition known as "parietal foramina" (PFM [MIM 168500]). PF have been described in association with CCD in two families whose affected members have hypoplastic clavicles and delayed closure of the fontanel but no additional findings (PF with CCD [MIM 168550]) (Golabi et al. 1984). Heterozygous loss-of-function mutations in *MSX2* have been described in three unrelated families with PF (Wilkie et al. 2000). Moreover, a mouse model with a targeted disruption of *Msx2* showed ossification defects in the frontal bone as well as developmental defects in three ectodermal organs, including teeth, hair follicles, and mammary glands (Satokata et al. 2000). PF are also a feature of Potocki-Shaffer syndrome (MIM 601224), which is caused by a proximal 11p deletion that includes the *ALX4* gene. Isolated mutations in *ALX4* have also been described in families segregating PF (Wuyts et al. 2000; Mavrogiannis et al. 2001). Both MSX2 and ALX4 have been shown to interact with RUNX2, and, together, these proteins participate in skull-vault differentiation (Hermanns and Lee 2001; Shirakabe et al. 2001; Antonopoulou et al. 2004).

In contrast to these developmental defects that result from loss of normal function, the premature fusion of the sutures of the cranium has been shown to result from molecular mechanisms that lead to an excess of signal. Activating mutations in *FGFR1*, *FGFR2*, and *FGFR3* cause seven different clinical syndromes that are characterized by craniosynostosis and variable degrees of skeletal abnormalities. In addition, a missense gain-of-function mutation in *MSX2* (P148H), which increases the DNA-binding ability of the protein, has been found to cause Boston-type craniosynostosis (Ma et al. 1996). Transgenic mice overexpressing wild-type *Msx2* in the skull develop craniosynostosis and ectopic bone formation, suggesting a dominant positive effect of this protein in suture closure (Liu et al. 1995). Another important player in craniofacial development and craniosynostosis is *TWIST1*. Deletions and point mutations that result in loss of function of *TWIST1* have been found in patients with Saethre-Chotzen syndrome (MIM 101400), which is characterized by craniosynostosis, delayed closure of fontanels, and hand anomalies (Johnson et al. 1998). TWIST1 has been shown to interact with RUNX2 and to repress its function (Yousfi et al. 2002; Bialek et al. 2004).

The dermatological manifestations of CDAGS syndrome are a striking and consistent finding in the families studied. The histological findings on biopsy of two families were consistent with a diagnosis of porokeratosis, a clinically heterogeneous disorder of keratinization (Hivnor et al. 2004). The genetics of this group of disorders is still poorly understood, although there are reports of multiple pedigrees that show autosomal dominant transmission, and several loci have been suggested through linkage analysis. Mutations in the gene *SSH1* (MIM 606778) on chromosome 12q24 were recently described in Chinese families with disseminated superficial actinic porokeratosis (Zhang et al. 2004). A common mechanism linking the skin findings and coronal synostosis in our patients could be the deregulation of *MSX2* expression. In addition to its expression during cranial development, *MSX2* is expressed in the matrix epithelial cells of hair follicles and the nail bed (Reginelli et al. 1995). In addition to craniosynostosis, transgenic mice overexpressing *Msx2* showed thickened skin with hyperkeratosis, desquamation, and flakiness, with fewer hairs (Jiang et al. 1999).

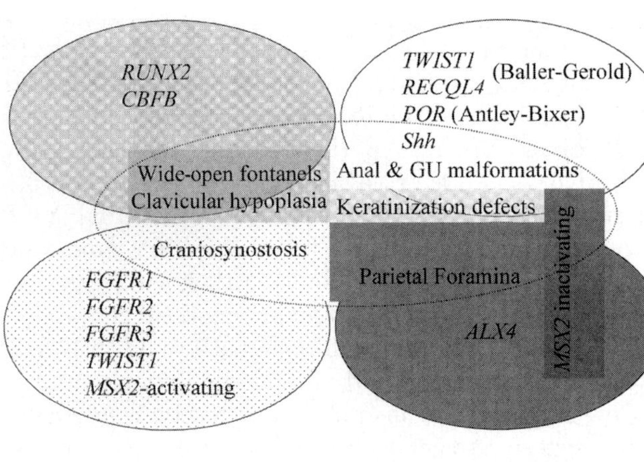

Figure 4 Venn diagram summarizing the features that characterize CDAGS syndrome and its potential molecular mechanism. GU = genitourinary.

Genitourinary and anal abnormalities are another con-

Table 1

Clinical Summary of the Most Prominent Features of CDAGS Syndrome in the Four Families Analyzed

	Finding in Patient						
Characteristic	1-II-1	2-II-1	2-II-5	3-II-1	3-II-2	4-II-1	4-II-3
Sex	F	M	F	F	M	M	M
Coronal craniosynostosis	+	+	+	ND	ND	+	+
Other craniosynostosis	−	Lambdoid[a]	Lambdoid	ND	ND	Sagittal	Sagittal
Wide-open fontanels	++	++	++	++	++	ND	+
PF	++	++	++	++	++	ND	ND
Hearing loss	Unilateral	Sensorineural	−	ND	Mixed	−[b]	−[b]
Developmental delay[c]	−	Severe	Mild	Severe	Moderate[d]	−	−
Hypoplastic clavicles	+	+	+	+	+	−	ND
Imperforate anus	+	+	+	+	+	+/−[e]	+
Hypospadias	−	+	−	−	+	+	+/−[f]
Urethrorectal fistula	−	−	+	+	+	−	−
Skin lesions[g]	+	+	+	+	+	+[h]	+[h]
Porokeratosis on biopsy	−	+	ND	−	−	+	ND

NOTE.—Plus sign (+) = present; double plus sign (++) = severe; minus sign (−) = absent; +/− = partial related finding; ND = not documented.

[a] Squamosal and lambdoid synostosis and cleft palate.

[b] Normal hearing per report, but not formally tested.

[c] The developmental delay present in some individuals is variable and affects both motor and language development.

[d] IQ < 40.

[e] Anteriorly placed anus.

[f] Bifid scrotum.

[g] The eruption is composed of hyperkeratotic papules and plaques and has a reticulate pattern on the face.

[h] Patient exhibited a Koebner phenomenon.

 Am. J. Hum. Genet. 77:161–168, 2005

sistent finding in patients with CDAGS. Imperforate anus can be found as an isolated defect or can be part of a syndrome or a sequence. Multiple genes have been studied as candidates in anorectal malformation syndromes, and there are several reports of families segregating this feature as autosomal recessive and X-linked traits (Villavicencio et al. 2000; Mo et al. 2001). The strongest evidence for genes responsible for imperforate anus is derived from animal models and points toward genes involved in the sonic hedgehog pathway (Kim et al. 2001; Mo et al. 2001). Some syndromes, such as Baller-Gerold syndrome (MIM 218600) and Antley-Bixler syndrome (MIM 207410), demonstrate an association between craniosynostosis and genitourinary/anal malformations. Although the etiology of these syndromes has not been completely elucidated, some patients with Antley-Bixler syndrome carry mutations in the P450 oxidoreductase gene (*POR* [MIM 124015]) that result in abnormal steroidogenesis (Adachi et al. 2004; Fukami et al. 2005). Patients with features of Baller-Gerold syndrome have been found to have mutations in *TWIST1* (Seto et al. 2001) as well as in the DNA helicase *RECQL4* (Van Maldergem et al. 1992, 2004). Interestingly, mutations in *RECQL4* result in a spectrum of autosomal recessive disorders that also includes Rothmund-Thomson syndrome (RTS [MIM 268400]) and RAPADILINO syndrome (MIM 266280) (Siitonen et al. 2003). RTS is characterized by short stature, cataracts, a predisposition to tumors, and a poikilodermatous rash that partly resembles the one seen in our patients (Megarbane et al. 2000; Wang et al. 2001).

All seven affected individuals and their first-degree relatives were enrolled in a research program approved by the Baylor College of Medicine institutional review board, and appropriate informed consent was obtained. We isolated genomic DNA of the two patients who were first ascertained, individuals 1-II-1 and 3-II-2, for candidate-gene studies. Sequence analysis of all eight exons and the promoter of *RUNX2* was performed as described elsewhere (Zhou et al. 1999). Similarly, the coding regions of the genes *CBFB, MSX2, TWIST1,* and *RECQL4* were amplified by PCR and were analyzed by direct sequencing. No mutations were found in the coding regions of any of these genes. Because of the possibility that this syndrome may be caused by a contiguous gene deletion, we performed FISH with probes specific for *RUNX2, CBFB,* and *ALX4.* All FISH analyses showed a normal hybridization pattern, consistent with the presence of both alleles in each case (data not shown).

On the basis of the pattern of inheritance, we assumed an autosomal recessive mode of transmission and performed simulation analysis to estimate the power to detect linkage. Assuming full penetrance, an allele frequency of 0.001, and no locus heterogeneity, we estimated the maximum LOD score to be +2.38 with a mean (±SE) of 1.66 (±0.03). We isolated DNA from all affected patients and first-degree relatives of the four families. Using Linkage Mapping Set v2.5-MD10 (Applied Biosystems), we performed a genomewide screen with 400 markers at an average resolution of 10 cM. We performed parametric two-point linkage analysis, using the Fastlink software (National Center for Biotechnology Information), to locate the genomic region harboring the gene responsible for the phenotype, and we used Allegro for multipoint analysis and fine mapping. Analysis of the genotype data showed maximum estimated LOD score of +2.38 for markers *D22S283* and *D22S274* on chromosome 22q12-q13 (fig. 5 and table B1 [online only]). Haplotype analysis allowed us to narrow the region of interest to a 34-cM interval between *D22S1163* and *D22S1170.* These results suggest that the disease gene lies in this region on 22q12-q13.

Chromosome region 22q12-q13 spans 20 Mb and contains >100 genes. There are several reports of patients with structural abnormalities involving this region, but none of them provides clues as to the possible gene responsible for CDAGS syndrome. Deletions spanning the segment 22q12-qter may result in developmental delay but only minor anomalies (Watt et al. 1985; Kirshenbaum et al. 1988). Isolated deletions of 22q13 have common features that include accelerated growth, developmental delay, hearing loss, delayed myelination, hypotonia, and minor dysmorphisms (Lindquist et al. 2005). Duplication of 22q12-qter has been associated with intrauterine growth restriction (IUGR), cleft palate, mild hearing loss, imperforate anus, and talipes (Mirza et al. 2000), and an isolated duplication of 22q13 resulted in true hermaphroditism in a patient with IUGR and am-

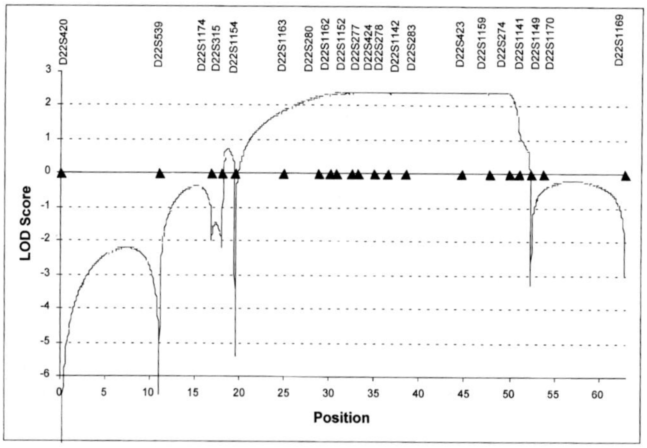

Figure 5 Multipoint linkage analysis with polymorphic markers throughout the genome demonstrated the maximum expected LOD score of +2.38 for markers *D22S283* and *D22S274* on the long arm of chromosome 22 (22q12-q13).

biguous genitalia that is due to an unbalanced translocation (Aleck et al. 1999).

In this study, we present a complete clinical characterization of CDAGS syndrome, a distinct genetic condition that associates craniofacial anomalies, clavicular hypoplasia, anal and genital abnormalities, and severe skin eruption. The clinical features of these patients point to the apparently opposing biological processes of delayed ossification and accelerated suture closure. It is well known that the function of the transcription factor RUNX2 is context dependent and is regulated by multiple coactivators and repressors. Whereas this transcription factor is essential for osteoblast cell-fate commitment, it is also a major determinant of chondrocyte maturation. Hence, it serves critical functions during both endochondral and intramembranous ossification. Interestingly, genes that have been implicated in craniosynostosis, such as *TWIST* and *MSX2,* have been reported to directly regulate *RUNX2* activity both in cell studies and in vivo. We hypothesize that the gene defect responsible for CDAGS syndrome causes novel context-dependent dysregulation of multiple signaling pathways, including RUNX2, during osteoblast differentiation and craniofacial morphogenesis. It is possible that patients with this constellation of findings have mutations in a central regulatory factor that specifies the balance of *RUNX2* activity in these diverse tissues. At the same time, this factor must also serve a function independent of *RUNX2* in tissues such as skin and in the genitourinary system, where RUNX2 is not expressed.

Acknowledgments

The authors thank all participating families, for their cooperation, and S. Carter and A. Tran, for clinical research support. This work was supported, in part, by National Institutes of Health grants ES11253 (to B.L.) and HD22657 (to D. Rimoin) and Baylor College of Medicine Mental Retardation and Developmental Disabilities Research Center grant HD24064.

Web Resources

The URLs for data presented herein are as follows:

National Center for Biotechnology Information, http://www.ncbi.nlm.nih.gov/CBBresearch/Schaffer/fastlink.html (for genetic analysis software)

Online Mendelian Inheritance in Man (OMIM), http://www.ncbi.nlm.nih.gov/Omim/ (for CCD, Yunis-Varon syndrome, Crane-Heise syndrome, CAP, PFM, PF with CCD, Potocki-Shaffer syndrome, Saethre-Chotzen syndrome, *SSH1,* Baller-Gerold syndrome, Antley-Bixler syndrome, *POR,* RTS, and RAPADILINO syndrome)

References

Adachi M, Asakura Y, Tachibana K, Shackleton C (2004) Abnormal steroidogenesis in three patients with Antley-Bixler syndrome: apparent decreased activity of 17α-hydroxylase, 17,20-lyase and 21-hydroxylase. Pediatr Int 46:583–589

Aleck KA, Argueso L, Stone J, Hackel JG, Erickson RP (1999) True hermaphroditism with partial duplication of chromosome 22 and without SRY. Am J Med Genet 85:2–4

Antonopoulou I, Mavrogiannis LA, Wilkie AO, Morriss-Kay GM (2004) Alx4 and Msx2 play phenotypically similar and additive roles in skull vault differentiation. J Anat 204:487–499

Bialek P, Kern B, Yang X, Schrock M, Sosic D, Hong N, Wu H, Yu K, Ornitz DM, Olson EN, Justice MJ, Karsenty G (2004) A twist code determines the onset of osteoblast differentiation. Dev Cell 6:423–435

Cooper SC, Flaitz CM, Johnston DA, Lee B, Hecht JT (2001) A natural history of cleidocranial dysplasia. Am J Med Genet 104:1–6

Flanagan N, Boyadjiev SA, Harper J, Kyne L, Earley M, Watson R, Jabs EW, Geraghty MT (1998) Familial craniosynostosis, anal anomalies, and porokeratosis: CAP syndrome. J Med Genet 35:763–766

Fukami M, Horikawa R, Nagai T, Tanaka T, Naiki Y, Sato N, Okuya T, Nakai H, Soneda S, Tachibana K, Matsuo N, Sato S, Hom K, Nishimura G, Hasegawa T, Ogata T (2005) POR (P450 oxidoreductase) mutations and Antley-Bixler syndrome with abnormal genitalia and/or impaired steroidogenesis: molecular and clinical studies in 10 patients. J Clin Endocrinol Metab 90:414–426

Fukuda K, Miyanomae T, Nakata E, Tanaka M, Tanaka Y, Usui T (1981) Two siblings with cleidocranial dysplasia associated with atresia ani and psoriasis-like lesions: a new syndrome? Eur J Pediatr 136:109–111

Golabi M, Carey J, Hall BD (1984) Parietal foramina clavicular hypoplasia: an autosomal dominant syndrome. Am J Dis Child 138:596–599

Hermanns P, Lee B (2001) Transcriptional dysregulation in skeletal malformation syndromes. Am J Med Genet 106:258–271

Hivnor C, Williams N, Singh F, VanVoorhees A, Dzubow L, Baldwin D, Seykora J (2004) Gene expression profiling of porokeratosis demonstrates similarities with psoriasis. J Cutan Pathol 31:657–664

Jiang TX, Liu YH, Widelitz RB, Kundu RK, Maxson RE, Chuong CM (1999) Epidermal dysplasia and abnormal hair follicles in transgenic mice overexpressing homeobox gene MSX-2. J Invest Dermatol 113:230–237

Johnson D, Horsley SW, Moloney DM, Oldridge M, Twigg SRF, Walsh S, Barrow M, Njølstad PR, Kunz J, Ashworth GJ, Wall SA, Kearney L, Wilkie AOM (1998) A comprehensive screen for *TWIST* mutations in patients with craniosynostosis identifies a new microdeletion syndrome of chromosome band 7p21.1. Am J Hum Genet 63:1282–1293

Judge MR, Michaels M, Sams VR, David TJ, Harper JI (1990) Disseminated porokeratosis in an infant with craniosynostosis. Br J Dermatol 123:249–254

Kim J, Kim P, Hui CC (2001) The VACTERL association: lessons from the sonic hedgehog pathway. Clin Genet 59:306–315

Kirshenbaum G, Chmura M, Rhone DP (1988) Long arm deletion of chromosome 22. J Med Genet 25:780

Kundu M, Javed A, Jeon JP, Horner A, Shum L, Eckhaus M, Muenke M, Lian JB, Yang Y, Nuckolls GH, Stein GS, Liu PP (2002) Cbfβ interacts with Runx2 and has a critical role in bone development. Nat Genet 32:639–644

Lee B, Thirunavukkarasu K, Zhou L, Pastore L, Baldini A, Hecht J, Geoffroy V, Ducy P, Karsenty G (1997) Missense mutations abolishing DNA binding of the osteoblast-specific transcription factor OSF2/CBFA1 in cleidocranial dysplasia. Nat Genet 16:307–310

Lindquist SG, Kirchhoff M, Lundsteen C, Pedersen W, Erichsen G, Kristensen K, Lillquist K, Smedegaard HH, Skov L, Tommerup N, Brondum-Nielsen K (2005) Further delineation of the 22q13 deletion syndrome. Clin Dysmorphol 14:55–60

Liu YH, Kundu R, Wu L, Luo W, Ignelzi MA Jr, Snead ML, Maxson RE Jr (1995) Premature suture closure and ectopic cranial bone in mice expressing Msx2 transgenes in the developing skull. Proc Natl Acad Sci USA 92:6137–6141

Ma L, Golden S, Wu L, Maxson R (1996) The molecular basis of Boston-type craniosynostosis: the Pro148→His mutation in the N-terminal arm of the MSX2 homeodomain stabilizes DNA binding without altering nucleotide sequence preferences. Hum Mol Genet 5:1915–1920

Mavrogiannis LA, Antonopoulou I, Baxova A, Kutilek S, Kim CA, Sugayama SM, Salamanca A, Wall SA, Morriss-Kay GM, Wilkie AO (2001) Haploinsufficiency of the human homeobox gene ALX4 causes skull ossification defects. Nat Genet 27:17–18

Megarbane A, Melki I, Souraty N, Gerbaka J, El Ghouzzi V, Bonaventure J, Mornand A, Loiselet J (2000) Overlap between Baller-Gerold and Rothmund-Thomson syndrome. Clin Dysmorphol 9:303–305

Mirza G, Imaizumi K, Ragoussis J (2000) Partial trisomy 22 in a liveborn resulting from a rearrangement between chromosomes 6 and 22. J Med Genet 37:E22

Mo R, Kim JH, Zhang J, Chiang C, Hui CC, Kim PC (2001) Anorectal malformations caused by defects in sonic hedgehog signaling. Am J Pathol 159:765–774

Mundlos S, Otto F, Mundlos C, Mulliken JB, Aylsworth AS, Albright S, Lindhout D, Cole WG, Henn W, Knoll JH, Owen MJ, Mertelsmann R, Zabel BU, Olsen BR (1997) Mutations involving the transcription factor CBFA1 cause cleidocranial dysplasia. Cell 89:773–779

Reginelli AD, Wang YQ, Sassoon D, Muneoka K (1995) Digit tip regeneration correlates with regions of Msx1 (Hox 7) expression in fetal and newborn mice. Development 121: 1065–1076

Satokata I, Ma L, Ohshima H, Bei M, Woo I, Nishizawa K, Maeda T, Takano Y, Uchiyama M, Heaney S, Peters H, Tang Z, Maxson R, Maas R (2000) Msx2 deficiency in mice causes pleiotropic defects in bone growth and ectodermal organ formation. Nat Genet 24:391–395

Seto ML, Lee SJ, Sze RW, Cunningham ML (2001) Another TWIST on Baller-Gerold syndrome. Am J Med Genet 104: 323–330

Shirakabe K, Terasawa K, Miyama K, Shibuya H, Nishida E (2001) Regulation of the activity of the transcription factor Runx2 by two homeobox proteins, Msx2 and Dlx5. Genes Cells 6:851–856

Siitonen HA, Kopra O, Kaariainen H, Haravuori H, Winter RM, Saamanen AM, Peltonen L, Kestila M (2003) Molecular defect of RAPADILINO syndrome expands the phenotype spectrum of RECQL diseases. Hum Mol Genet 12:2837–2844

Van Maldergem L, Megarbane A, Siitonen HA, De Roy M, Fourneau C, Jalkh N, Chouery E, Gillerot Y, Verloes A (2004) Revisiting the craniosynostosis-radial ray hypoplasia association: Baller-Gerold syndrome caused by mutations in RECQL4 helicase gene. American Society of Human Genetics, 54th Annual Meeting abstract book, p 55

Van Maldergem L, Verloes A, Lejeune L, Gillerot Y (1992) The Baller-Gerold syndrome. J Med Genet 29:266–268

Villavicencio EH, Walterhouse DO, Iannaccone PM (2000) The sonic hedgehog–patched–Gli pathway in human development and disease. Am J Hum Genet 67:1047–1054

Wang LL, Levy ML, Lewis RA, Chintagumpala MM, Lev D, Rogers M, Plon SE (2001) Clinical manifestations in a cohort of 41 Rothmund-Thomson syndrome patients. Am J Med Genet 102:11–17

Watanabe K, Hatamochi A, Arakawa M, Ueki H, Nomura S, Osawa G, Hata T (1996) Congenital psoriasiform erythrokeratodermia with cleidocranial dysplasia, urogenital anomalies and atresia ani. Dermatology 192:368–372

Watt JL, Olson IA, Johnston AW, Ross HS, Couzin DA, Stephen GS (1985) A familial pericentric inversion of chromosome 22 with a recombinant subject illustrating a "pure" partial monosomy syndrome. J Med Genet 22:283–287

Wilkie AO, Tang Z, Elanko N, Walsh S, Twigg SR, Hurst JA, Wall SA, Chrzanowska KH, Maxson RE Jr (2000) Functional haploinsufficiency of the human homeobox gene MSX2 causes defects in skull ossification. Nat Genet 24:387–390

Wuyts W, Cleiren E, Homfray T, Rasore-Quartino A, Vanhoenacker F, Van Hul W (2000) The ALX4 homeobox gene is mutated in patients with ossification defects of the skull (foramina parietalia permagna, OMIM 168500). J Med Genet 37:916–920

Yoshida CA, Furuichi T, Fujita T, Fukuyama R, Kanatani N, Kobayashi S, Satake M, Takada K, Komori T (2002) Core-binding factor β interacts with Runx2 and is required for skeletal development. Nat Genet 32:633–638

Yousfi M, Lasmoles F, Marie PJ (2002) TWIST inactivation reduces CBFA1/RUNX2 expression and DNA binding to the osteocalcin promoter in osteoblasts. Biochem Biophys Res Commun 297:641–644

Zhang Z, Niu Z, Yuan W, Liu W, Xiang L, Zhang J, Chu X, Zhao J, Jiang F, Chai B, Cui F, Wang Y, Zhang K, Wang Y, Xu S, Xia L, Gu J, Zhang S, Meng X, Wang S, Gao S, Fan M, Nie L, Zheng Z, Huang W (2004) Fine mapping and identification of a candidate gene SSH1 in disseminated superficial actinic porokeratosis. Hum Mutat 24:434–438

Zheng Q, Zhou G, Morello R, Chen Y, Garcia-Rojas X, Lee B (2003) Type X collagen gene regulation by Runx2 contributes directly to its hypertrophic chondrocyte-specific expression in vivo. J Cell Biol 162:833–842

Zhou G, Chen Y, Zhou L, Thirunavukkarasu K, Hecht J, Chitayat D, Gelb BD, Pirinen S, Berry SA, Greenberg CR, Karsenty G, Lee B (1999) CBFA1 mutation analysis and functional correlation with phenotypic variability in cleidocranial dysplasia. Hum Mol Genet 8:2311–2316

Announcements[1]

Conferences

Meeting of the Society of Craniofacial Genetics.—The forthcoming meeting of the Society of Craniofacial Genetics will take place in conjunction with the annual meeting of the American Society of Human Genetics in Salt Lake City, UT, on Tuesday, October 25, 2005. The theme of the meeting is "Craniofacial Sutures," and abstracts for presentation may be submitted to the following e-mail address: virginia.kimonis@childrens.harvard.edu. Information about the meeting can be obtained from the Society's Web site (http://craniofacial-genetics.org/).

———

Advances in Breast Cancer: Molecularly Targeted Therapies for Metastatic Disease.—A conference on Advances in Breast Cancer: Molecularly Targeted Therapies for Metastatic Disease will be held on Friday, November 11, 2005, at the Sutton Place Hotel in Toronto. Study credits are available from the American Medical Association (category 1) and the Royal College of Physicians and Surgeons of Canada. For information, please contact the Continuing Education Division of the Faculty of Medicine at the University of Toronto; telephone: (416) 978-2719 and (888) 512-8173 (North America only); fax: (416) 946-7028; e-mail: ce.med@utoronto.ca. Additional information is available on the Web site of the Continuing Education Division of the Faculty of Medicine at the University of Toronto (http://www.cme.utoronto.ca).

———

Y Chromosome and Male Germ Cell Biology in Health and Diseases in the Post Genomic Era.—An international conference on Y-chromosome and male germ cell biology will be held September 21–23, 2005, at the Asilomar Conference Center in Pacific Grove, CA. This conference is sponsored by the Laboratory of Clinical Genomics at the National Institute of Child Health and Human Development. The purpose of this conference is to bring together scientists working in various aspects of male germ cell development in health and diseases, to create an environment that is conducive to interdisciplinary collaboration in the studies of male germ cells. The conference features invited speakers in four focused sessions: "Y Chromosome and Male Reproduction," "Germ Cell Gene Expression and Regulation," "Spermatogonial Stem Cell Biology," and "Male Germ Cell Development in Health and Diseases." There will also be a poster session for other participants. A Web site (http://www.ymalegermcellconference.nichd.nih.gov/) has been set up for this conference. Please explore this Web site for further information. This conference is limited to 100 participants, and registration is on a first come, first served basis. The deadline for registration is July 10, 2005.

1. Announcements are published free of charge for members of The American Society of Human Genetics (ASHG). Please e-mail announcements to ajhg@emory.edu. Submission must be received *at least 7 weeks* before the month of issue in which publication is requested. They must be double spaced with a $1\frac{1}{2}$-inch margin on all sides. The maximum length is *250 words,* excluding the address for correspondence. Please include a cover letter indicating the name of the sponsoring ASHG member.

Information for Contributors

Postal address: **Stephen T. Warren, Ph.D., Editor, The American Journal of Human Genetics, Department of Human Genetics, Emory University School of Medicine, 615 Michael Street, Room 301, Atlanta, GA 30322-3050.** Telephone: (404) 712-9980. Fax: (404) 712-9984. E-mail: ajhg@emory.edu. Web page: http://www.ajhg.org/.

The American Journal of Human Genetics is a record of research and review relating to heredity in humans; to the applications of genetic principles in medicine, psychology, anthropology, and social services; and to areas of molecular and cell biology relevant to human genetics. It is published monthly. The *Journal* is owned and controlled by The American Society of Human Genetics and is edited, in conjunction with the publisher, by a staff appointed by the Board of Directors of the Society.

Electronic Edition

The entire content of the *Journal* is published electronically on the World Wide Web, at http://www.ajhg.org/. The full text is available to subscribers, as is material supplemental to the print version, including video and archival databases. Articles will be posted as they are ready for publication. Approximately 2 weeks before publication of the hard copy, the table of contents for that issue will be posted with final pagination, along with editorials and other material.

Editorial Policy

The *Journal* welcomes submissions of articles and reports on timely subjects concerning all aspects of human genetics, including studies of model organisms that are of direct relevance to human genetics. Letters commenting on material previously published in the *Journal* are also welcome. Review articles, editorials, and book reviews usually are solicited by the editor. The *Journal* does not publish reports of either single mutations or mutational surveys of previously identified loci unless they have unusual significance and substantial insight. Descriptions of new linkage assignments will be considered only if they are of unusual interest and significance. Reports of negative data, without substantial insight and interest, will not normally be considered. Membership in The American Society of Human Genetics is not a prerequisite for publication in the *Journal.* Papers will be considered for publication on condition that they are not currently under consideration by any other publication and that no portion of them has been published elsewhere.

• *Review process.* Manuscripts will be considered for appropriateness to the *Journal* by the editor in conjunction with the editorial board. Those considered appropriate will be reviewed by two or more external reviewers or by members of the editorial board, and those not considered appropriate will be returned to the authors. Authors are requested to suggest appropriate referees. Manuscripts will be judged on their value as original contributions to the field and on their overall presentation. Authors whose manuscripts are returned without external review may appeal by writing the editor.

• *Return of figures.* For manuscripts that are reviewed but not accepted, all figures submitted as glossy prints will be returned whenever possible.

• *Editing.* Manuscripts will be edited to conform to *Journal* style, to correct spelling and grammar where necessary, and to improve conciseness, clarity, and precision of expression. Significant editorial changes will be identified on the page proofs.

• *Publication costs.* For papers published—except for invited contributions and Letters to the Editor—authors will be charged $50.00 per printed *Journal* page or portion thereof. Each *Journal* page contains ~800 words. If authors wish, they may instead pay a single publication fee of $5,000 for an article or $2,700 for a report, to make their work freely and immediately available to all readers at publication, rather than after the usual 6-month delay for nonsubscribers. All authors will also be charged for printing of color figures (see Illustrations, below).

• *Copyright agreement.* All authors of all manuscripts accepted for publication (except U.S. government employees) must sign an agreement transferring copyright to The American Society of Human Genetics. Corresponding authors must assume responsibility for obtaining the signatures of all coauthors. Material published in the *Journal* may not be reproduced or published elsewhere without written consent of the Society and the publisher. Requests for such permission should be addressed to the publisher: Copyright, University of Chicago Press, 1427 East 60th Street, Chicago, IL 60637. Fax: (773) 702-9756.

• *Research materials.* It is assumed that authors whose research is published in the *Journal* will make cell lines, antibodies, cloned DNA sequences, and similar materials available to other investigators in noncommercial institutions, so as to permit replication of the reported work.

• *Page proofs.* Page proofs will be sent to the corresponding author for correction of typographical errors only. Corresponding authors are responsible for the return of corrected page proofs to the publisher by the designated deadline.

• *Reprints.* The corresponding author will receive an order form for reprints, along with the page proofs.

Manuscript Submission

Manuscripts should now be submitted via the *AJHG* Web Peer Review System at http://mss.uchicago.edu/AJHG. Basic instructions for submission via the WPR system can be found at the Web site (http://mss.uchicago.edu/AJHG/auth_msprep_AJHG.epl), and detailed instructions are given below.

Manuscript Preparation

Manuscripts must be written in English. MS Word, Rich Text, or LaTeX formats are acceptable. All components of the text (including references and figure legends but not tables) must

be typed double spaced in 12-point type. Tables must be single spaced. *Manuscripts that are not double spaced throughout will not be sent out for review.* Use a 1-inch margin on all four sides of each page, and do not justify the right margin. Begin each manuscript component on a separate page, and arrange components in the following order: title page, Summary (abstract), text (articles separated into Introduction, Material and Methods, Results, and Discussion), Acknowledgments, appendices (if any), Web Resources, References, tables, and figure legends. Number all pages consecutively in the upper-right-hand corner, beginning with the title page.

Cover letter. Include a letter from the author who will be responsible for correspondence regarding the manuscript as well as for communications among authors in regard to revisions, publication agreements, and approval of proofs. This letter should indicate the category of manuscript being submitted (e.g., article, report, letter, review) and highlight the significance of the manuscript in a few sentences. It should also disclose the source of funding and any affiliations with or involvement in any companies, trade associations, unions, litigants, or other groups with a direct financial interest in the subject matter or materials discussed in the manuscript by any authors and/or their immediate family within the last 5 years. Also indicate whether the first author is a student or postdoctoral fellow and a member of The American Society of Human Genetics (to be eligible for the Cotterman awards, presented at the ASHG's annual meeting).

Please indicate the category of your manuscript in the cover letter:

Articles are full-length, original research articles.

Reports are short (approximately four *Journal* pages, 800 words per page) scientific correspondence with a brief abstract but without further subdivision of the manuscript. This category is designed for timely publication of original findings that may substantially impact their field.

Letters to the Editor are brief commentaries (less than one printed page) concerning articles published in the *Journal* within the past 2 months. They may also present new data. Also included in this section are short general news items of interest to the Society. Any letter concerning a previously published article will first be sent for external review, to determine whether it meets an appropriate level of significance for publication in the *Journal.* If the letter achieves this basic level of significance, it will then be sent to the corresponding author of the pertinent article, who will be given an opportunity to submit a response. This response will be provided to the corresponding author of the letter to the editor. After considering the response, the authors may choose to withdraw their letter or to proceed with publication without further revision.

Fast-track review. If circumstances so warrant, you may request in the cover letter a fast-track review of your paper. At the editor's discretion, a 24- to 48-hour fast-track review is available to expedite manuscripts that deserve rapid review and publication.

Related manuscripts. Please submit a copy of any related papers, by any of the authors, that have been submitted but not published elsewhere or that are in press. For citation of such manuscripts, see "*Work submitted to a publication but not yet accepted, personal communications, and unpublished data,*" below.

All papers should adhere to the guidelines that follow, with two exceptions:

1) *Reports* should contain a brief summary of five sentences or fewer, but the remainder of the text should not be divided into sections.

2) *Letters to the Editor* do not contain a summary, nor should the text be divided into sections.

Otherwise, please prepare all submissions according to the following directives:

Title page. This page should contain a concise title; a running title of no more than 40 characters (including spaces); the names and institutional affiliations of all authors at the time of the study (and present affiliations, if different); and the corresponding author's name, complete current mailing address, telephone number, fax number, and e-mail address. Each paper can be assigned only one corresponding author. Joint authorship is permitted only for the first author position, with a maximum of two individuals being given this designation.

Summary (abstract). The Summary should state the purpose of the study, the basic procedures and analytical methods, the findings, and the principal conclusions. The Summary must not exceed 275 words.

Text. The text should be as concise as possible and should be organized into the following sections: Introduction, Material and Methods (or Subjects and Methods), Results, and Discussion. Some manuscripts may require different formats appropriate to their content. Brief subheadings may be used where necessary.

The Introduction should summarize the rationale for the study, without reviewing the subject extensively. Using the past tense, describe the selection of subjects and identify the methods, apparatus, and procedures in detail. Provide references for established methods and brief descriptions of those that are not well known. Describe any new or modified methods used, including reasons for their use and evaluations of their limitations.

Present results in logical sequence in the text, tables, and illustrations. Do not repeat in the text all the data that appear in the tables and illustrations. Detailed results of statistical analyses may be presented as an appendix.

Web Resources. Please provide accession numbers along with the URL of any genome or locus-specific database in which information has been deposited. (This is required for establishing links in the electronic edition of the *Journal.*) Place this information in the text and in a separate section entitled "Web Resources," following the Acknowledgments. Please do not include URLs in the text or in the References.

MIM numbers should be listed in the text after the first mention of the relevant disorder or gene. Example: adrenal hypoplasia congenita (AHC [MIM 300200]). In the Web Resources section, only the URL for the OMIM database, and not the individual MIM numbers, should be noted. Example: Online Mendelian Inheritance in Man (OMIM), http://www.ncbi.nlm.nih.gov/Omim/.

Human subjects. If the manuscript reports results of studies of either human subjects or materials obtained from human subjects, state in the Material and Methods section that the study was approved by the appropriate institutional review board and/or that appropriate informed consent was obtained from human subjects. Copies of signed consent forms from identifiable persons appearing in any photographs submitted with the manuscript must be faxed to the *AJHG* office at the time of submission: (404) 712-9984. To avoid violation of HIPAA regulations, this consent form should state that the subject understands that his or her identity (but not his or her medical records) will be divulged to the *Journal* office by the transmission of the signed consent form. Alternatively, a letter from a member of your institutional review board (IRB) can be sent to us confirming that signed consent forms have been obtained from the individuals pictured in the manuscript without naming these individuals. Your manuscript cannot be processed until we receive these consent forms or a letter from your IRB.

Acknowledgments. Acknowledge those who have made substantive contributions to the study reported, as well as the institution(s) or grant sponsor(s) that supported the research.

Reference citations. Authors must assume responsibility for the accuracy of reference citations. Reference citations in the text, tables, or figure legends should be in parentheses and include author surname(s) and year of publication. When citing a work by two authors, provide both authors' names joined by "and." When citing a work by three or more authors, provide the first author's name followed by "et al." When the author name(s) and the year of publication are identical for two or more works, distinguish between the works by appending a lowercase italic letter to the year, to match the order in which the works appear in the References section. Examples: (Charlesworth 2001), (Peters and Sandkuijl 1992), (Devriendt et al. 1997), (Stack et al. 1995*a*). List two or more works in the same citation in chronological order, separated by semicolons. When two or more works in a citation were published in the same year, arrange them alphabetically by the first author's surname. When the same author name(s) are used for two or more works in the same citation, group those works together in chronological order, with the years separated by commas. If such a group occurs in a citation that includes other works, place the group chronologically within the citation according to the first year in the group, using semicolons between the group and the other works cited. Examples: (Erdmann 1994; Braverman et al. 1997; Purdue et al. 1997), (Hellsten 1995; Redding et al. 1996*a*, 1996*b*, 2000; Kessler et al. 1997).

References section. References should be arranged alphabetically by author surname(s). References by the same author(s) should be arranged chronologically. References by the same author(s) for which the year of publication is also the same should be arranged alphabetically by title. List the names of up to 25 authors; if more than 25, list the first 7 plus "et al." Use standard abbreviations for journal titles. Do not use excess punctuation.

References examples:

Journal: Devriendt K, Matthijs G, Legius E, Schollen E, Blockmans D, van Geet C, Degreef H, Cassiman J-J, Fryns J-P (1997) Skewed X-chromosome inactivation in female carriers of dyskeratosis congenita. Am J Hum Genet 60:581–587

Chapter: Peters DJM, Sandkuijl LA (1992) Genetic heterogeneity of polycystic kidney disease in Europe. In: Breuning MH, Devoto M, Romeo G (eds) Contributions to nephrology 97: polycystic kidney disease. Karger, Basel, pp 128–139

Entire volume: Dayhoff MV (ed) (1978) Atlas of protein sequence and structure. Vol 5, suppl 3. National Biomedical Research Foundation, Washington, DC

Meeting paper: Kessler S (1997) Transcripts of genetic counseling sessions: exercises in missed opportunities. Paper presented at Talking Human Genetics: Verbal Communication, Knowledge and Genetic Makeup. Hamburg, April 24–27

Thesis/dissertation: Hellsten E (1995) Positional cloning of the infantile ceroid lipofuscinosis gene. PhD thesis, National Public Health Institute, Helsinki

Computer software: SAS Institute (1997) SAS release 6.12, Cary, NC

Work "in press": Jones TM, Peterson RW. Ethical issues in screening for genetic diseases. Am J Hum Genet (in press)

Work submitted to a publication but not yet accepted, personal communications, and unpublished data: Do not list in References. Cite in the text as "personal communication" (if none of the individuals cited are authors of the manuscript being submitted) or "unpublished data" (if at least one of the individuals cited is also an author of the manuscript being submitted). List the names (including first initials) of all individuals responsible for the unpublished data or personal communication, and include letters of authorization from the individuals named.

Tables. Each table should appear on a separate page and should be single spaced. Whenever possible, construct exceptionally large tables and pedigree diagrams in sections. Number tables consecutively and give each a brief title. Give each column a short heading. Use footnotes to explain all abbreviations that are used in each table, and denote them by letter. Titles and footnotes should be included on the same page with the tables themselves. Use the table editor of a word-processing program to create tables. Do not use tabs or spaces, and omit vertical and horizontal lines from tables. Each row of data must be in a separate row of table cells. Do not submit tables as photographs. For more detailed instructions about tables, see "Special Instructions for Tables" at the *AJHG* homepage. For further guidelines, see *Scientific Style and Format: The CBE Manual for Authors, Editors, and Publishers* and *The Chicago Manual of Style* (cited in Style Guidelines, below).

Illustrations (figures). For complete instructions on preparing figures, please refer to http://www.ajhg.org/artguide.html. Design and prepare the figures carefully; they are the visual presentation of the scientific findings and will be carefully evaluated by the reviewers and editors. Figures should be saved as Encapsulated Postscript (EPS) files or Tagged Image File Format (TIF) files. Common Web formats, such as GIF or JPEG, are not acceptable; neither are proprietary application

formats, such as PowerPoint. Most figures will be set as single column (80 mm), some as double column (175 mm), and some broadside on a page (230 mm). Prepare the figures in publication size or larger (the lettering must be large enough so that the smallest letter will be at least 2.0 mm in height when the figure is reduced to publication size).

Use patterns, such as diagonal lines, rather than shading, which does not reproduce evenly. For pedigree construction, follow the guidelines described in Bennett et al.'s "Recommendations for Standardized Human Pedigree Nomenclature" (Am J Hum Genet 56:745–752, 1995). Include the key (explanation of symbols) within the figure. For micrographs, indicate magnification either by means of a micron bar or in the legend.

Use Helvetica lettering throughout the figure. Insert uppercase letters, in a larger font size, to designate panels.

For initial submission, we require that all figures and tables be included in the main text file. The figures may be converted to the file format of the main text file, since they are being used only for evaluation purposes. External reviewers are only permitted access to the main text file, so they will see only figures and tables included in that file. Thus, it is preferable that you include supplementary materials in the main text file as well. However, if including the supplementary materials makes the main text file too large to upload on our server, they may be uploaded separately.

In submission of revised manuscripts, the figure files should be uploaded as separate files in the appropriate format (EPS or TIFF) but should also be included in the main text file, as they were in the original submission, in case your paper is sent for further external review. Hard copies of figures are required for publication, but, if you wish, you may wait to send them until acceptance of the manuscript.

Color illustrations. Authors must sign an agreement to pay the costs of production of color figures when a manuscript with color figures is accepted. Each page containing a color figure will incur a charge of $450 for the first figure or separate part of a figure, plus $200 for each additional figure.

Figure legends. These should be double spaced, beginning on a separate page. The legend should begin with a brief phrase describing the figure content. The legend should describe the illustration so that it can be understood apart from the text and should explain any labels or symbols that are not included in a key.

Supplemental material. Authors may submit additional data, at the discretion of the editor, as a supplement to the *AJHG* electronic edition.

Supplemental clinical data. For manuscripts containing clinical information, it is important that as much clinical detail as possible be provided for others to verify the conclusions drawn. Photographs, radiographs, and imaging data as well as other laboratory, historical, and clinical data outside the immediate scope of the manuscript may be included as a supplement to the *AJHG* electronic edition.

Style Guidelines

For questions of grammar, punctuation, abbreviation, and scientific style, refer to *The Chicago Manual of Style* (15th ed., University of Chicago Press, Chicago) and *Scientific Style and Format: The CBE Manual for Authors, Editors, and Publishers* (6th ed., Cambridge University Press, Cambridge, UK). The preferred or first spelling of a word in *Merriam-Webster's Collegiate Dictionary* (11th ed., Merriam-Webster, Springfield, MA) is used by the *Journal.* Mathematical equations must be typed and spaced as they should appear in print. Use metric or other internationally accepted units for all quantitative measurements.

Genetic nomenclature and notation. For human genes, use genetic notation and symbols approved by the Human Gene Mapping Workshop. Approved gene symbols may be obtained, prior to submission, from Dr. Sue Povey of the HUGO Gene Nomenclature Committee (HGNC), Department of Biology, University College London, Wolfson House, 4 Stephenson Way, London NW1 2HE, United Kingdom (telephone: 44-20-7679-7410; fax: 44-20-7387-3496; e-mail: nome@galton.ucl.ac.uk). Nomenclature guidelines are available and the Gene Name Proposal form may be completed on the HGNC Web page: http://www.gene.ucl.ac.uk/nomenclature/. See Wain et al.'s "Guidelines for Human Gene Nomenclature" (Genomics 79:464470, 2002). Use ISCN nomenclature for cytogenetic notation (see Mitelman F [ed] ISCN 1995: an international system for human cytogenetic nomenclature. S. Karger, Basel). Human gene names and loci should be written in italicized capital letters and Arabic numerals. Protein product names are not italicized. For human-mutation nomenclature, see Antonarakis et al.'s "Recommendations for a Nomenclature System for Human Gene Mutations" (Hum Mutat 11:1–3, 1998) (http://www3.interscience.wiley.com/cgi-bin/fulltext/5001291/PDFSTART).

Approved mouse nomenclature may be obtained, prior to submission, from Lois Maltais, The Jackson Laboratory, Bar Harbor, ME 04609-0800; telephone: (207) 288-6429; fax: (207) 288-6132; e-mail: nomen@informatics.jax.org; Web page: http://www.informatics.jax.org/mgihome/nomen. For other organisms, consult the appropriate authorities.

Nucleotide sequence deposition. New nucleotide data must be submitted to and deposited in the DNA Data Bank of Japan (DDBJ)/European Molecular Biology Laboratory (EMBL)/GenBank databases, and accession number(s) must be obtained before the paper can be accepted for publication. Submission to any one of the three collaborating databases is sufficient to ensure data entry in all. The accession number(s) should be included in the manuscript's Web Resources section, and the following footnote should appear on the title page: "Nucleotide sequence data reported herein are available in the DDBJ/EMBL/GenBank databases; for details, see the Web Resources section of this article." The database will withhold release of data until publication, at authors' request. The most convenient method for submission of sequence data is by World Wide Web: DDBJ, via SAKURA (http://sakura.ddbj.nig.ac.jp/); EMBL, via WEBIN (http://www.ebi.ac.uk/embl/Submission/webin.html); or GenBank, via BankIt (http://www.ncbi.nlm.nih.gov/Sequin/).

Single-nucleotide polymorphisms. Newly described single-nucleotide polymorphisms (SNPs) should be submitted to an appropriate database such as dbSNP (http://www.ncbi.nlm

.nih.gov/SNP/) prior to submission of revised manuscripts. The identification numbers should be included in the "Web Resources" section of the manuscript.

Microarray data. All newly generated microarray data referred to in the text must be submitted for publication as a supplement to the *AJHG* electronic edition. Tables of quantitated raw data and processed data are acceptable, as outlined in guidelines proposed by the Microarray Gene Expression Data Society (for full details, see http://www.mged.org/Workgroups/MIAME/miame_checklist.html). For submission, please save the tables as tab-delimited ASCII text files and submit an electronic copy (no hard copies are necessary).

Computer programs. Authors of manuscripts that describe a novel computer program must make the relevant program publicly available by the time the manuscript is published.

Manuscript-Preparation Checklist

○ Cover letter
○ Copies of signed consent forms for all identifiable photographs of patients
○ Manuscript and figures
○ All pages of text and References *fully double spaced*
○ 1-inch margin on all four sides of each page
○ Title and running title
○ Order of manuscript elements: title page, Summary, text (Introduction, Material and Methods, Results, Discussion), Acknowledgments, appendixes, Web Resources, References, tables, figure legends
○ Summary: no more than 275 words
○ Acknowledgments: all sources of support and those who have made substantive contributions to the work reported
○ References: accurate, complete, and proper style in text and reference list; up to 25 authors' names included (if more than 25, list the first 7 plus "et al.")
○ Tables: *single spaced, no vertical lines, created with the table editor of a word-processing program, not with tabs;* title and footnotes included with table
○ Figures: all guidelines followed; figure legends on a separate page, double spaced
○ A copy of related manuscripts submitted or in press

Additional Components Required at Revision

○ Permission to reproduce previously published material
○ Letters of authorization from sources of personal communications and unpublished data

Submission via the Web Peer Review System

Formatting Electronic Files

Please follow the manuscript preparation requirements above to submit a new or revised manuscript via this system. The system relies on automated processing to create an Adobe Acrobat (PDF) file from your submission. If you do not follow these instructions, your submission cannot be processed automatically and will not be received by the journal office.

The following file formats are acceptable:

- Microsoft Word (.doc; any version that can be read by Word 2000 for Windows)
- Rich Text Format (.rtf)
- Adobe Acrobat (.pdf)
- LaTeX (see special instructions below)

File contents. For initial submission, manuscripts should be submitted as single files, in one of the formats listed above, with all figures, tables, and images embedded (inserted) directly into the document. We also request that supplementary materials be included in the same file, if possible. The figures may be converted to the file format of the main text file, since they are being used only for evaluation purposes. Only materials included in the main text file (and separate supplementary files, if necessary) will be examined by external reviewers.

If we request a revision, in addition to the main text file containing all figures and tables, each figure should be uploaded separately in EPS or TIFF format. Consult your word processing program's "Help" documentation for instructions on how to embed tables and figures. You must also submit in a second file, in one of the acceptable formats, a cover letter that includes your responses to reviewer comments.

Filename requirements. All filenames must be lowercase. (All file processing by the Web Peer Review system is done on Unix machines, where filenames are case-sensitive.)

File compression and archives. Although your manuscript itself must be provided in one file that includes the tables and figures, you will have at least two files to upload into our system (i.e. the cover letter, manuscript file, and any related manuscripts). Therefore, we strongly recommend that you combine these files into an archive so that you can upload a single file for submission. Applications for Mac OS (such as StuffIt) and Windows (such as WinZip) can create this archive.

The following archive formats may be used:

- Windows or Unix zip (e.g., "archiv.zip")
- Unix tar (e.g., "archive.tar" or compressed with gzip as "archive.tar.gz" or "archive.tgz")

If you cannot create archives in these formats, you may still compress individual files to shorten upload time:

- Unix compress (e.g., "ms.tex.Z")

Electronic File Specifications

Program	Main Text File	Cover Letter	Figures	Tables
Word	ms.doc	cover_letter.doc or cover_letter.txt	[embedded in main file]	[embedded in main file]
RTF	ms.rtf	cover_letter.rtf or cover_letter.txt	[embedded in main file]	[embedded in main file]
Acrobat	ms.pdf	cover_letter.pdf or cover_letter.txt	[embedded in main file]	[embedded in main file]
LaTeX	ms.tex	cover_letter.txt	f1.eps, f2.eps, etc.	tb1.tex, tb2.tex, etc.

- Unix gzip (e.g., "ms.tex.gz")

Revisions. If you are submitting a revised manuscript and have a response to the reviewers' comments, include your response as part of the cover letter file. When submitting a revised manuscript with figures, include all the figures even if they have not changed since the previous version.

Online Submission Instructions

Preparing the manuscript file. The preferred format for submitting manuscripts online is Microsoft Word (.doc files). If you are unable to submit a Microsoft Word file, the Web Peer Review system will also accept manuscripts in Acrobat (.pdf), Rich Text Format (.rtf) or LaTeX (.tex). We have provided a drop box in the "File format" area in which to indicate the document type.

As mentioned above, manuscripts should be submitted as single files with all figures, tables, and images embedded (inserted) directly into the document. Embedded figures must be in EPS or TIF format, as these formats result in the best overall outcome when manuscripts are converted to PDF. Please note that authors whose manuscripts are accepted for publication may be required by the publisher to submit high-resolution hard copies (e.g., glossy prints) after the review process is complete and press production is about to begin.

Special instructions for LaTeX. LaTeX files prepared with the AASTeX macro package are preferred. This package uses the "natbib" style for references. If you submit a LaTeX file, figures and tables may be kept in external files, as long as they are referenced within the main "ms.tex" file.

Submission Checklist

Please have the following items readily available before beginning the online submission process:

- Your manuscript as a MS Word, Acrobat (pdf), Rich Text, or LaTeX file including all tables, figures and images embedded in the document
- Cover letter
- Information from your title page for entry into the peer review database, including the title, running title, list of contributing authors and affiliations, word count, and contact information for the corresponding author
- A list of recommended reviewers and their e-mail addresses
- Related papers, by any of the authors, that have been submitted elsewhere or that are in press.
- Copies of signed consent forms for all identifiable photographs of patients (these should be faxed to the AJHG office at [404] 712-9984 at the time of submission).

Navigating the Peer Review Web Site

Step one: describing your manuscript. Go to the *AJHG* Peer Review Web site at http://mss.uchicago.edu/AJHG/. A username and password are required to enter the site. If you already have a username and password, click on "Login/See current tasks" to view the status of your account. If you are new to the site, click on "Create account" to register. After completing your login, click on the "Begin submission" button.

Once you have logged in, fill in the fields describing your manuscript. To move from one field to the next, press the "tab" key. When all the information is complete and you are sure it is correct, click "Ready to upload files" to proceed to step two.

Step two: uploading your file(s). Click the "Browse" button to locate a file on your local system. Once a file is specified in the field, click "Upload this file" to send the file to the Web Peer Review system. You must name your manuscript file "ms," using lowercase type. (All file processing by the Web Peer Review system is done on Unix machines, where filenames are case-sensitive.) The system will assign an ID number to your manuscript during the upload.

As previously mentioned, your manuscript file must contain all figures and tables as well as the text. Remember that if you have multiple files (such as if you are providing a manuscript "in press" for the reviewers), you can compress all of them into a single archive and upload just one file. We recommend that you make an archive of all the files for your submission and then upload the single archive file.

Check your results. Only files listed in the box labeled "Files uploaded so far" have been uploaded successfully. If you need to delete a file, click the file name in the box to select it, and then click the "Delete selected file" button.

When you have uploaded all the files for your submission, click "Process uploaded files" to proceed. The system will attempt to make a PDF version of your file. The conversion to PDF reduces the size of the file and makes it easier for editors and reviewers to read. PDF files can be viewed with Adobe Acrobat Reader version 3 or higher (available free at http://www.adobe.com) or with Ghostscript 5.1 or higher compiled with PDF support turned on (available free at http://www.cs.wisc.edu/~ghost). If successful, there will be a link to the PDF on the next Web page that appears.

If you want to delete all the uploaded files and make no submission, click "Cancel submission" instead.

Step three: submitting your information. After your file has been converted to a PDF file, view the file that was generated from your submission by clicking on "ms.pdf" (a link that will be provided on the next Web page that appears). Only the manuscript file, not the cover letter or related manuscript files, will be viewable at this time. After you finish viewing the manuscript PDF file, indicate how you would like to proceed.

If you select "Approve and submit now," you assert that you have viewed the PDF file via the link provided and that the file accurately shows your manuscript as reviewers should see it. If you select "Fix and resubmit later," the files you have already uploaded will be saved (for 30 days) so that you can return later and upload new or corrected files to make a new PDF file. If you wish to return later to upload other files, please make note of the file upload ID number.

Click "Finish" to complete the final process. Click "Cancel" if you wish to abort the submission.

If your manuscript has been successfully submitted to the *AJHG* Web Peer Review system, a confirmation screen, which includes your assigned manuscript number, will appear. Please carefully note this number and use it in all future correspondence with the *AJHG* editorial office. An e-mail message confirming your submission will be sent to you.

If you do not receive either a manuscript number or confirmation e-mail message, your manuscript was not success-

fully submitted to the journal and thus cannot be sent on to peer review. Please try again or contact ajhg-help@mss.uchicago.edu for assistance.

Announcements

Announcements are posted to the electronic edition of the *Journal* as soon as they are accepted, and they are published in the earliest possible print issue. They may also be viewed at http://www.journals.uchicago.edu/AJHG/journal/announce.html. Announcements are published free of charge for members of The American Society of Human Genetics. They should be submitted via e-mail (ajhg@emory.edu). For publication in print, announcements must be received at least 7 weeks before the month of issue in which publication is desired.

2005 MEMBERSHIP APPLICATION • THE AMERICAN SOCIETY OF HUMAN GENETICS

9650 Rockville Pike • Bethesda, Maryland 20814-3998 • (301) 634-7300 • Fax: (301) 634-7079 • Toll free: (1-866) HUMGENE
E-mail: babbott@ashg.org • http://www.ashg.org/

lease keep information page for description of membership categories and discount subscriptions. Mail completed application, cluding profile form, and remittance to the above address. ***Type or print****. Use the URL above to apply online!*

ame ______________________________ Degree(s) ______________
Last First Middle

epartment ______________________________

nstitution ______________________________

treet address ______________________________

ity, state, zip, country ______________________________

Telephone ( ) ______________ Fax ( ) ______________ E-mail Address ______________
Area code Area code

Signature and membership start date: I, the undersigned, wish my membership in The American Society of Human Genetics to begin (check one): __________January 1, 2005 or__________January 1, 2006. Applications for 2006 will be accepted after September 1, 2005. I will receive all applicable subscriptions beginning in January of the calendar year indicated above.

______________________________ ______________
Applicant's signature *Date*

We will acknowledge receipt of application and send it through the process established by the Board of Directors. Notification of the Board's action is usually sent in April or November. In the interim, you will be accorded all rights and privileges of a member in good standing, except that prior to Board approval you may not vote in ASHG elections.

DUES PAYMENT (Dues include 12 monthly issues of *The American Journal of Human Genetics* and are payable on a calendar year basis.)

1. Check one box and enter dues payment on line 1 .... $ ________ 1
☐ $130 Regular ☐ $65 Trainee with Journal ☐ $70 Overseas Trainee
☐ $135 Overseas Affiliate ☐ $25 Trainee without Journal ☐ $190 Husband/Wife

2. Optional air mail postage for *AJHG* outside the United States .... $ ________ 2
☐ $40 Canada, Mexico, Central America ☐ $70 all other areas

☐ Check here if you do not want to receive commercial mailings
☐ Check here if you do not wish to receive the printed Journal.

DISCOUNT SUBSCRIPTIONS

3. $650 North America, $850 elsewhere (print only) for ***American Journal of Medical Genetics*** .... $ ________ 3
$530 North America, $690 elsewhere (print only) for ***AJMG** without **Neuropsychiatric Genetics***
4. $120 (print & online); $110 (online only) for ***BioEssays*** .... $ ________ 4
5. $115 North America, $195 elsewhere (print & online); $104 (online only) for ***Birth Defects Research: Clinical and Molecular Teratology*** .... $ ________ 5
6. $115 North America, $165 elsewhere (print & online); $104 (online only) for ***Birth Defects Research: Developmental and Reproductive Toxicology*** .... $ ________ 6
7. $799 for ***Cancer Genetics and Cytogenetics*** .... $ ________ 7
8. $159 Europe, $163 elsewhere for ***Clinical Dysmorphology*** .... $ ________ 8
9. $258 US/elsewhere not otherwise specified (online only), $271 (print & online); $276 Canada (online only), $290 (print & online); $271 Europe (online only), $285 (print & online) for ***Clinical Genetics*** .... $ ________ 9
10. $114 Europe, $117 elsewhere (print & online); $83 (online only) for ***Community Genetics*** .... $ ________ 10
11. $125 US, $134 Canada, $186 elsewhere for ***Current Biology*** .... $ ________ 11
12. $231 for ***Current Opinion in Cell Biology*** .... $ ________ 12
13. $231 for ***Current Opinion in Genetics & Development*** .... $ ________ 13
14. $623 Europe, $626 elsewhere (print & online); $557 (online only) for ***Cytogenetic and Genome Research*** .... $ ________ 14
15. $165 for ***European Journal of Human Genetics*** (includes membership in ESHG) .... $ ________ 15
$500 (print only); $550 (print & online) for ***European Journal of Human Genetics***
16. $330 North America, $390 elsewhere (print & online); $300 North America (online only) for ***Genes, Chromosomes, and Cancer*** .... $ ________ 16
17. $105 US, $189 Canada, Mexico; $225 elsewhere for ***Genes & Development*** .... $ ________ 17
18. $160 North America, $200 elsewhere (print & online); $145 (online only) for ***Genetic Epidemiology*** .... $ ________ 18
19. $316 for ***Genetics in Medicine*** .... $ ________ 19
20. $179 US, $258 elsewhere (print only); $213 US, $292 elsewhere (print & online); $179 (online only) for ***Genetic Testing*** .... $ ________ 20
21. $98 US, $154 Canada, Mexico; $178 elsewhere for ***Genome Research*** .... $ ________ 21
22. $124 for ***Genomics*** .... $ ________ 22
23. $336 US, $395 elsewhere (print only); $402 US, $462 elsewhere (print & online); $336 (online only) for ***Human Gene Therapy*** .... $ ________ 23
24. $495 for ***Human Genetics*** .... $ ________ 24
25. $394 Europe, $397 elsewhere (print & online), $356 (online only) for ***Human Heredity*** .... $ ________ 25
26. $369 US/elsewhere (print & online); $307 (online only); $394 Canada (print & online); $328 (online only) for ***Human Molecular Genetics*** (not available Europe) .... $ ________ 26
27. $280 North America, $340 elsewhere (print & online); $255 North America (online only) for ***Human Mutation*** .... $ ________ 27
28. $459 (print only) for ***Journal of Human Genetics*** .... $ ________ 28
29. $289 (print & online), $130 (online only) for ***Journal of Medical Genetics*** .... $ ________ 29
30. $113 for ***Molecular Genetics and Metabolism*** .... $ ________ 30
31. $169 US, Canada, Mexico; $215 elsewhere for ***Nature Genetics*** (not available: Japan, Korea, & China) .... $ ________ 31
32. $169 US, Canada, Mexico; $215 elsewhere for ***Nature Medicine*** (not available: Japan, Korea, & China) .... $ ________ 32
33. $169 US, Canada, Mexico; $215 elsewhere for ***Nature Reviews Genetics*** (not available: Japan, Korea, & China) .... $ ________ 33
34. $247 Europe, $254 elsewhere for ***Pharmacogenetics and Genomics*** .... $ ________ 34
35. $157 for ***Trends in Genetics*** .... $ ________ 35
36. Identify ***Annual Reviews*** by title, volume, year and price: Member price $72 per year US, $77 per year elsewhere

______________ ______ ______ $ ________
Title Vol. Year Price

California and Indiana residents add state sales tax for ***Annual Reviews***: $ ________
Canadian residents add 7% GST for ***Annual Reviews***: $ ________

Enter total payment for ***Annual Reviews*** .... $ ________ 36

37. Optional contribution to ASHG general fund: $25 ____ $50 ____ $75 ____ $100 ____ other ____ .... $ ________ 37

38. **TOTAL REMITTANCE ENCLOSED** .... $ ________ 38

PLEASE RETURN THIS NOTICE WITH YOUR REMITTANCE (U.S. currency only). See reverse for credit card information.

METHOD OF PAYMENT - 2005 ASHG MEMBER DUES

Payment may be made via money order; a check drawn on a U.S. bank, in U.S. currency only, and made payable to The American Society of Human Genetics; MasterCard, Visa, American Express (AMEX) or Discover credit card. Checks drawn on foreign banks cannot be accepted. Persons in countries with currency restrictions may apply to the Administrative Office for assistance.

For credit card remittance, please supply the following information:

Signature ____________________

Cardholder name ____________________
(please print)

Circle type of card: MasterCard VISA AMEX Discover
(no other cards accepted).

Credit card number ____________________ ☐

VISA only: Supply final 3 digits on reverse of card

Expiration date ____________________

Please note: ASHG is qualified as a 501(C) (3) organization. Dues and contributions are deductible as allowed by law. Dues payment includes $60 for a calendar year subscription to *The American Journal of Human Genetics*.

Member Profile Form

Name: ____________________
Please type or print.

PRIMARY AFFILIATION *Check one:*

MEDICAL SCHOOL DEPTS.

A.___ Genetics
B.___ Pediatrics
C.___ Pathology
D.___ Psychiatry/Psychology
E.___ Medicine
F.___ Ob/Gyn
G.___ Repro. Med.
H.___ Neurology
I.___ Family Medicine
J.___ Internal Medicine

OTHER

K.___ Hospitals and Clinics
L.___ HMO
M.___ Dental Schools
N.___ Pub Hlth & Grad School
O.___ College or University
P.___ Nursing School
Q.___ Veterinary School
R.___ Priv Practice/Consultant
S.___ Commercial Company
T.___ Institutes/Foundations
U.___ Federal Government
V.___ State/Local Government
W.___ Retired
X.___ Other
Y.___ Consultant

See box at right for codes:

Earned Degrees ☐☐☐☐ **Academic Rank** ☐ **Position** ☐☐

MAJOR TYPE OF WORK *Check one that accounts for more than 50% of your time:*
A.___ Research B.___ Teaching C.___ Administration D.___ Clinical E.___ Counseling

SECONDARY TYPE OF WORK *Check one if it represents a significant portion of time and is different from your major type of work*:
A.___ Research B.___ Teaching C.___ Administration D.___ Clinical E.___ Counseling

LABORATORY SETTING *If you are primarily in a laboratory setting, indicate focus:*
A.___ private diagnostic/reference lab
B.___ univ affiliated diagnostic/reference lab
C.___ gov't affiliated research lab
D.___ private research lab
E.___ univ affiliated research lab

SPECIAL INTEREST AREAS *Do not check more than two:*
A.___ cancer genetics
B.___ cytogenetics
C.___ DNA forensics
D.___ differentiation & development
E.___ dysmorphology
F.___ ethics/social/legal/policy issues
G.___ gene structure & function
H.___ inborn errors/biochemical genetics
I.___ late onset/adult genetic disorders
J.___ linkage mapping & polymorphisms
K.___ molecular genetics
L.___ pediatric genetics
M.___ physical mapping
N.___ population genetics/epidemiology
O.___ prenatal/perinatal genetics
P.___ genomics
Q.___ model systems
R.___ informatics
S.___ neurogenetics/behavorial genetics
T.___ public health genetics

CURRENT GRANT SUPPORT *Check all that apply (US and Canadian members only):*
A.___ NSF (NSERC in Canada)
B.___ NIH (CIHR) training grant
C.___ private industry
D.___ NIH (CIHR in Canada)
E.___ postdoc fellowship
F.___ private foundation or charity
G.___ state
H.___ province
I.___ institutional
J.___ other national agencies
K.___ HHMI

DESIGNATIONS(S) FOR YOUR RESEARCH
You may check more than one:
A.___ Applied clinical research
B.___ Applied lab research
C.___ Applied mathematical research
D.___ Basic clinical research
E.___ Basic lab research
F.___ Basic mathematical research
G.___ Other

Degree Code
A. MD
B. PhD
C. MSW
D. DVM
E. SCD
F. DDS/DMD
G. EDD
H. MS
I. MA
J. MSN
K. JD
L. MPH
M. RN
N. BSN
O. BS/BA
P. Other

Academic Rank Code
A. Professor
B. Associate Professor
C. Assistant Professor
D. Instructor
E. Nonfaculty

Position Code
A. Dean
B. Department Chair
C. Division Chief
D. Institute Center Director
E. Laboratory Director
F. Training Program Director
G. Research Program Director
H. Program Coordinator/Administrator
I. Senior Research Associate
J. Research Associate
K. Research Assistant
L. Genetic Counselor
M. Postdoctoral Research Fellow
N. Postdoctoral Clinical Fellow
O. Resident
P. Graduate Student
Q. Private Practice
R. Corporate Executive
S. Consultant
T. Other
U. Principal Investigator/Professor

OPTIONAL:
Year of Birth: _____
Gender: F ☐ M ☐

Check Box(es):
A. ☐ American Indian, Eskimo and Aleut
B. ☐ Asian, Pacific Islander
C. ☐ Black
D. ☐ White
E. ☐ Other
F. ☐ Mixed
Hispanic (Yes ☐ No ☐)

2005 ASHG MEMBERSHIP AND SUBSCRIPTIONS INFORMATION
Please keep this page for your reference.

Line 1. MEMBERSHIP CATEGORIES

Regular Membership is open to any resident of the Americas (U.S., Canada, Mexico, Caribbean, Central and South America) who is interested in research in human genetics or in issues pertaining to human genetics.

Overseas Affiliate Status is open to individuals residing outside the Americas (U.S., Canada, Mexico, Caribbean, Central and South America).

Husband/Wife Membership is open to couples who are both Regular members, but who receive only one Journal subscription. Please fill out one membership application for each person.

Trainee Membership is open to postdoctoral fellows and bona fide students enrolled in degree-granting programs at institutions in the Americas (U.S., Canada, Mexico, Caribbean, Central and South America).

Overseas Trainee Membership is open to postdoctoral fellows and bona fide students enrolled in degree-granting programs at institutions outside the Americas.

Please note: ASHG is qualified as a 501(C) (3) organization. Dues and contributions are deductible as allowed by law. Dues payment includes $60 for a calendar year subscription to *The American Journal of Human Genetics.*

Line 2. OPTIONAL AIR MAIL POSTAGE OUTSIDE THE U.S.

For those who would like to receive *The American Journal of Human Genetics* via airmail, note additional postage on line 2.

DISCOUNT SUBSCRIPTIONS

To obtain these discounts, orders must be placed through the ASHG Administrative Office. It is understood that these orders are intended for personal use only. Standing orders are not available through ASHG. Typically, the publisher will begin mailing issues one or two months after your order is received in the Administrative Office. *Annual Reviews* will be mailed at the book rate in the month of issue.

Line 3. ***American Journal of Medical Genetics,*** 40 issues, list price $685, **member price $650 North America,** list price $855, **$850 elsewhere** (print only)
AJMG without Neuropsychiatric Genetics, 32 issues, list price $565, **member price $530 North America,** list price $707, **$690 elsewhere** (print only)

Line 4. ***BioEssays, Volume 27,*** 12 issues, list price $170, **member price $120** (print & online); **$110** (online only)

Line 5. ***Birth Defects Research: Clinical & Molecular Teratology,*** 16 issues, **member price $115 North America, $195 elsewhere** (print & online); **$104** (online only)

Line 6. ***Birth Defects Research: Developmental & Reproductive Toxicology,*** 10 issues, **member price $115 North America, $165 elsewhere** (print & online); **$104** (online only)

Line 7. ***Cancer Genetics and Cytogenetics,*** 16 issues, list price $3,169 US, **member price $799**

Line 8. ***Clinical Dysmorphology,*** 4 issues, **member price $159 Europe, $163 elsewhere**

Line 9. ***Clinical Genetics,*** 12 issues, list price $371 US/elsewhere not otherwise specified, **member price $258** (online only), **$271** (print & online); **$276 Canada** (online only), **$290** (print & online); **$271 Europe** (online only), **$285** (print & online)

Line 10. ***Community Genetics,*** 4 issues, list price $147 US, **member price $114 Europe, $117 elsewhere** (print & online), **$83** (online only)

Line 11. ***Current Biology,*** 24 issues, list price $165, **member price $125 US, $134 Canada,** list price $249, **$186 elsewhere**

Line 12. ***Current Opinion in Cell Biology,*** 6 issues, list price $271, **member price $231**

Line 13. ***Current Opinion in Genetics & Development,*** 6 issues, list price $271, **member price $231**

Line 14. ***Cytogenetic and Genome Research,*** 16 issues, list price $1,841, **member price $623 Europe, $626 elsewhere** (print & online)**; $557** (online only)

Line 15. ***European Journal of Human Genetics,*** 12 issues, $165 (includes membership in ESHG); **member price $500** (print only); **$550** (print & online)

Line 16. ***Genes, Chromosomes, and Cancer,*** 12 issues, list price $365, **member price $330 North America, $390 elsewhere** (print & online); **$300 North America** (online only)

Line 17. ***Genes & Development,*** 24 issues, list price $140, **member price $105 US;** list price $260, **$189 Canada, Mexico; $225 elsewhere**

Line 18. ***Genetic Epidemiology,*** 8 issues, **member price $160 North America, $200 elsewhere** (print & online); **$145** (online only)

Line 19. ***Genetics in Medicine,*** 9 issues, list price $366, **member price $316**

Line 20. ***Genetic Testing,*** 4 issues, **member price $179 US, $258 elsewhere** (print only); **$213 US, $292 elsewhere** (print & online); **$179** (online only)

Line 21. ***Genome Research,*** 12 issues, list price $123, **member price $98 US;** list price $179, **$154 Canada, Mexico,** list price $203, **$178 elsewhere**

Line 22. ***Genomics,*** 12 issues, list price $458, **member price $124**

Line 23. ***Human Gene Therapy,*** 18 issues, **member price $336 US, $395 elsewhere** (print only); **$402 US, $462 elsewhere** (print & online); **$336** (online only)

Line 24. ***Human Genetics,*** 12 issues, list price $3,799 Europe, **member price $495**

Line 25. ***Human Heredity,*** 8 issues, list price $746 US**, member price $394 Europe, $397 elsewhere** (print & online); **$356** (online only)

Line 26. ***Human Molecular Genetics,*** 26 issues, list price $391**, member price $369 US/elsewhere** (print & online); **$307 US/elsewhere** (online only); **$394 Canada** (print & online); **$328 Canada** (online only) **(not available Europe)**

Line 27. ***Human Mutation,*** 12 issues, **member price $280 North America, $340 elsewhere** (print & online); **$255 North America** (online only)

Line 28. ***Journal of Human Genetics,*** list price $544, **member price $459** (print only)

Line 29. ***Journal of Medical Genetics,*** 12 issues, list price $478, **member price $289** (print & online); **$130** (online only)

Line 30. ***Molecular Genetics and Metabolism,*** 12 issues, list price $430, **member price $113**

Line 31. ***Nature Genetics,*** 12 issues, list price $199 US, **member price $169 US, Canada, Mexico; $215 elsewhere (not available: Japan, Korea & China)**

Line 32. ***Nature Medicine,*** 12 issues, list price $199 US, **member price $169 US, Canada, Mexico; $215 elsewhere (not available: Japan, Korea & China)**

Line 33. ***Nature Reviews Genetics,*** 12 issues, list price $199 US, **member price $169 US, Canada, Mexico; $215 elsewhere (not available: Japan, Korea & China)**

Line 34. ***Pharmacogenetics and Genomics,*** 12 issues, **member price $247 Europe, $254 elsewhere**

Line 35. ***Trends in Genetics,*** 12 issues, list price $182**, member price $157**

Line 36. ***Annual Reviews,*** **member price $72* per year US, $77* per year elsewhere**

Annual Review of:	*Genetics*	*Microbiol*	*Cell & Dev Biol*	*Ecol & Sys*	*Immunology*	*Medicine*	*Public Hlth*	*Biochem*	*Genomics & HG*
2003 Volumes	Vol. 37	Vol. 57	Vol. 19	Vol. 34	Vol. 21	Vol. 54	Vol. 24	Vol. 72	Vol. 4
2004 Volumes	Vol. 38	Vol. 58	Vol. 20	Vol. 35	Vol. 22	Vol. 55	Vol. 25	Vol. 73	Vol. 5
2005 Volumes	Available late 2005, will be offered on 2006 dues notice				Vol. 23	Vol. 56	Vol. 26	Vol. 74	Vol. 6
Month of Publication	Dec.	Oct.	Nov.	Dec.	April	February	May	July	Sept.

***California and Indiana residents add applicable sales tax. Canadian residents add 7% GST on total.**

Line 37: OPTIONAL CONTRIBUTIONS Optional contributions to the general fund are welcome. Contributions received will support projects designed to attract more young people to the field of human genetics and are tax deductible to the extent permitted by law.

THE AMERICAN SOCIETY OF HUMAN GENETICS

was organized in 1948. Its purpose is to encourage and integrate research, scholarship and education in all areas of human genetics, to bring into close contact investigators in the many general fields of research that involve human genetics, and to encourage discourse on applications of human genetics to society at large.

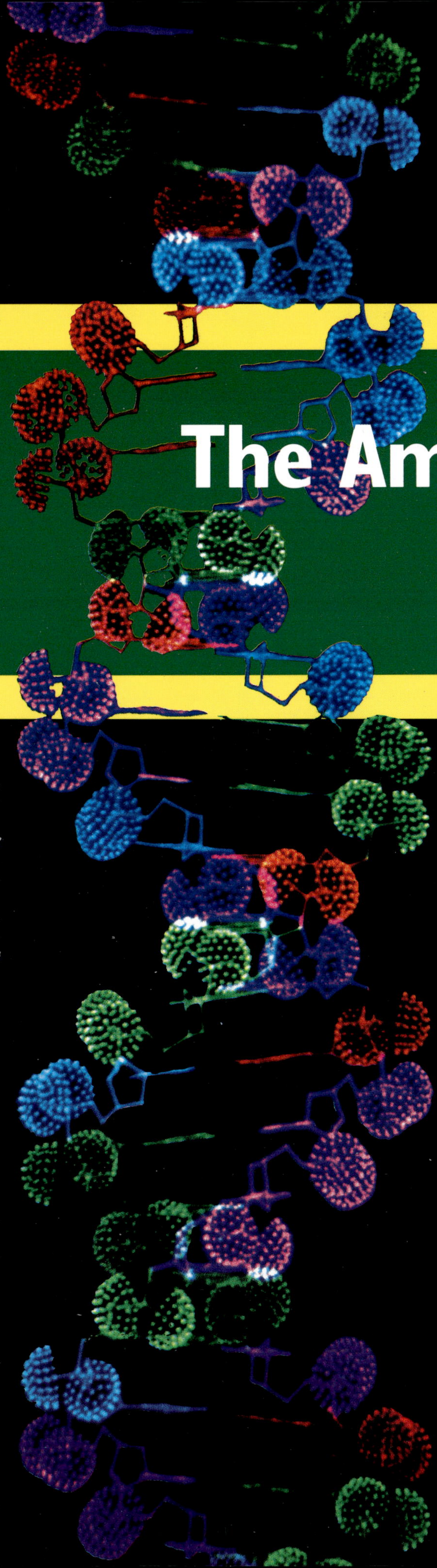

The American Journal of Human Genetics

VOLUME 77 NUMBER 2 AUGUST 2005

THE AMERICAN SOCIETY OF HUMAN GENETICS

Published for The American Society of Human Genetics
by The University of Chicago Press

DIRECT INQUIRIES AND SUBMISSIONS TO

The American Journal of Human Genetics
Department of Human Genetics
Emory University School of Medicine
615 Michael Street, Room 301
Atlanta, GA 30322-3050

Telephone: (404) 712-9980
Fax: (404) 712-9984
E-mail: ajhg@emory.edu
Web page: http://www.ajhg.org

PAST EDITORS

Subscription orders and correspondence should be addressed to the University of Chicago Press, P.O. Box 37005, Chicago, IL 60637. Checks should be made out to the University of Chicago Press. All orders must be in U.S. currency. Telephone: (8:00 A.M.–5:00 P.M. Central Standard Time, Monday–Friday) U.S. & Canada toll free, (877) 705-1878; Rest of World, (773) 753-3347. Fax: U.S. & Canada toll free, (877) 705-1879; Rest of World, (773) 753-0811. E-mail: subscriptions@press.uchicago.edu; Web site: http://www.journals.uchicago.edu. Remittance for nonmember subscription is payable to the publisher on a calendar-year basis. For domestic nonmember individuals and institutions, the single-copy rate is $88.00 and the calendar-year rate is $995.00; for foreign nonmember individuals and institutions, the single-copy rate is $88.00 (U.S. currency) and the calendar-year rate is $1050.00 (U.S. currency); the calendar-year rate for Canadian citizens, which includes GST, is $1088.65 (U.S. currency). All rates above include International Surface Airlift (ISAL) delivery to addresses outside the U.S. Subscription agent for Japan: Kinokuniya Company, Ltd. Individuals have the option to order directly from the University of Chicago Press.

Memberships.—A membership application and dues schedule appear at the back of each issue of the *Journal.*

The American Journal of Human Genetics (ISSN 0002-9297) is published monthly at 1427 East 60th Street, Chicago, IL 60637. Periodicals postage is paid at Chicago, IL, and at additional mailing offices by the American Society of Human Genetics. All rights reserved.

Postmaster: send address changes to *The American Journal of Human Genetics*, The University of Chicago Press, Journals Division, P.O. Box 37005, Chicago, IL 60637.

The American Journal of Human Genetics

Volume 77 Number 2 August 2005

i **This Month in the *Journal***
Kathryn Garber

Review Article

171 **How Malaria Has Affected the Human Genome and What Human Genetics Can Teach Us about Malaria**
Dominic P. Kwiatkowski

Articles

193 **Genotype-Phenotype Associations in Sotos Syndrome: An Analysis of 266 Individuals with *NSD1* Aberrations**
Katrina Tatton-Brown, Jenny Douglas, Kim Coleman, Geneviève Baujat, Trevor R. P. Cole, Soma Das, Denise Horn, Helen E. Hughes, I. Karen Temple, Francesca Faravelli, Darrel Waggoner, Seval Türkmen, Valérie Cormier-Daire, Alexandre Irrthum, and Nazneen Rahman, for the Childhood Overgrowth Collaboration

205 **Deletions Involving Long-Range Conserved Nongenic Sequences Upstream and Downstream of *FOXL2* as a Novel Disease-Causing Mechanism in Blepharophimosis Syndrome**
D. Beysen, J. Raes, B. P. Leroy, A. Lucassen, J. R. W. Yates, J. Clayton-Smith, H. Ilyina, S. Sklower Brooks, S. Christin-Maitre, M. Fellous, J. P. Fryns, J. R. Kim, P. Lapunzina, E. Lemyre, F. Meire, L. M. Messiaen, C. Oley, M. Splitt, J. Thomson, Y. Van de Peer, R. A. Veitia, A. De Paepe, and E. De Baere

219 **A Combined Genomewide Linkage Scan of 1,233 Families for Prostate Cancer–Susceptibility Genes Conducted by the International Consortium for Prostate Cancer Genetics**
Jianfeng Xu, Latchezar Dimitrov, Bao-Li Chang, Tamara S. Adams, Aubrey R. Turner, Deborah A. Meyers, Rosalind A. Eeles, Douglas F. Easton, William D. Foulkes, Jacques Simard, Graham G. Giles, John L. Hopper, Lovise Mahle, Pal Moller, Tim Bishop, Chris Evans, Steve Edwards, Julia Meitz, Sarah Bullock, Questa Hope, The ACTANE Consortium, Chih-lin Hsieh, Jerry Halpern, Raymond N. Balise, Ingrid Oakley-Girvan, Alice S. Whittemore, Charles M. Ewing, Marta Gielzak, Sarah D. Isaacs, Patrick C. Walsh, Kathleen E. Wiley, William B. Isaacs, Stephen N. Thibodeau, Shannon K. McDonnell, Julie M. Cunningham, Katherine E. Zarfas, Scott Hebbring, Daniel J. Schaid, Danielle M. Friedrichsen, Kerry Deutsch, Suzanne Kolb, Michael Badzioch, Gail P. Jarvik, Marta Janer, Leroy Hood, Elaine A. Ostrander, Janet L. Stanford, Ethan M. Lange, Jennifer L. Beebe-Dimmer, Caroline E. Mohai, Kathleen A. Cooney, Tarja Ikonen, Agnes Baffoe-Bonnie, Henna Fredriksson, Mika P. Matikainen, Teuvo LJ Tammela, Joan Bailey-Wilson, Johanna Schleutker, Christiane Maier, Kathleen Herkommer, Josef J. Hoegel, Walther Vogel, Thomas Paiss, Fredrik Wiklund, Monica Emanuelsson, Elisabeth Stenman, Björn-Anders Jonsson, Henrik Grönberg, Nicola J. Camp, James Farnham, Lisa A. Cannon-Albright, and Daniela Seminara

230 **Weighting Affected Sib Pairs by Marker Informativity**
Daniel Franke and Andreas Ziegler

242 **A Mutation in *SNAP29,* Coding for a SNARE Protein Involved in Intracellular Trafficking, Causes a Novel Neurocutaneous Syndrome Characterized by Cerebral Dysgenesis, Neuropathy, Ichthyosis, and Palmoplantar Keratoderma**
Eli Sprecher, Akemi Ishida-Yamamoto, Mordechai Mizrahi-Koren, Debora Rapaport, Dorit Goldsher, Margarita Indelman, Orit Topaz, Ilana Chefetz, Hanni Keren, Timothy J. O'Brien, Dani Bercovich, Stavit Shalev, Dan Geiger, Reuven Bergman, Mia Horowitz, and Hanna Mandel

252 **Identification of Risk and Age-at-Onset Genes on Chromosome 1p in Parkinson Disease**
Sofia A. Oliveira, Yi-Ju Li, Maher A. Noureddine, Stephan Züchner, Xuejun Qin, Margaret A. Pericak-Vance, and Jeffery M. Vance

265 **Allelic Heterogeneity at the Serotonin Transporter Locus (*SLC6A4*) Confers Susceptibility to Autism and Rigid-Compulsive Behaviors**
James S. Sutcliffe, Ryan J. Delahanty, Harish C. Prasad, Jacob L. McCauley, Qiao Han, Lan Jiang, Chun Li, Susan E. Folstein, and Randy D. Blakely

280 **An Autosomal Dominant Cerebellar Ataxia Linked to Chromosome 16q22.1 Is Associated with a Single-Nucleotide Substitution in the 5′ Untranslated Region of the Gene Encoding a Protein with Spectrin Repeat and Rho Guanine-Nucleotide Exchange-Factor Domains**
Kinya Ishikawa, Shuta Toru, Taiji Tsunemi, Mingshun Li, Kazuhiro Kobayashi, Takanori Yokota, Takeshi Amino, Kiyoshi Owada, Hiroto Fujigasaki, Masaki Sakamoto, Hiroyuki Tomimitsu, Minoru Takashima, Jiro Kumagai, Yoshihiro Noguchi, Yoshiyuki Kawashima, Norio Ohkoshi, Gen Ishida, Manabu Gomyoda, Mari Yoshida, Yoshio Hashizume, Yuko Saito, Shigeo Murayama, Hiroshi Yamanouchi, Toshio Mizutani, Ikuko Kondo, Tatsushi Toda, and Hidehiro Mizusawa

Reports

297 **A Mutation in the Dimerization Domain of Filamin C Causes a Novel Type of Autosomal Dominant Myofibrillar Myopathy**
Matthias Vorgerd, Peter F. M. van der Ven, Vera Bruchertseifer, Thomas Löwe, Rudolf A. Kley, Rolf Schröder, Hanns Lochmüller, Mirko Himmel, Katrin Koehler, Dieter O. Fürst, and Angela Huebner

305 **Dysregulation of Chondrogenesis in Human Cleidocranial Dysplasia**
Qiping Zheng, Eiman Sebald, Guang Zhou, Yuqing Chen, William Wilcox, Brendan Lee, and Deborah Krakow

313 **A "*Fille du Roy*" Introduced the T14484C Leber Hereditary Optic Neuropathy Mutation in French Canadians**
Anne-Marie Laberge, Michèle Jomphe, Louis Houde, Hélène Vézina, Marc Tremblay, Bertrand Desjardins, Damian Labuda, Marc St-Hilaire, Carol Macmillan, Eric A. Shoubridge, and Bernard Brais

318 **A Genomewide Scan for Intelligence Identifies Quantitative Trait Loci on 2q and 6p**
Danielle Posthuma, Michelle Luciano, Eco J. C. de Geus, Margie J. Wright, P. Eline Slagboom, Grant W. Montgomery, Dorret I. Boomsma, and Nicholas G. Martin

Letters to the Editor

327 **Use of the Term "Antley-Bixler Syndrome": Minimizing Confusion**
Deborah Cragun and Robert J. Hopkin

328 **"Antley-Bixler Syndrome"—A Reply to Cragun and Hopkin**
Walter L. Miller

330 ***LRRK2* Haplotype Analyses in European and North African Families with Parkinson Disease: A Common Founder for the G2019S Mutation Dating from the 13th Century**
Suzanne Lesage, Anne-Louise Leutenegger, Pablo Ibanez, Sabine Janin, Ebba Lohmann, Alexandra Dürr, and Alexis Brice, for the French Parkinson's Disease Genetics Study Group

Book Review

333 **Guide to Mutation Detection**
Edited by Graham R. Taylor and Ian N. Day
Reviewed by Bradford Coffee

Erratum

334 **Heterozygous Mutations of *OTX2* Cause Severe Ocular Malformations**
Ragge et al. (June 2005 [76:1008-1022])

Announcements

335 **Employment Opportunities; Cell Lines and DNA Samples**

Information for Contributors

This Month in the *Journal*

This month in the *Journal,* Dominic Kwiatkowski discusses one of the strongest selective forces that has acted on the human genome in recent times: malaria. One of the striking things about this selection is that it has resulted in several different resistance alleles that vary by location, so that a common malaria-resistance allele in Africa is rarely found in Southeast Asia, and vice versa. Not only do genetic studies of malaria resistance tell us something about humans, they also tell us about the life cycle of the malarial parasites, and they have led to novel approaches to malaria prevention.

Sotos Genotype-Phenotype Analyses, by Tatton-Brown et al. (p. 193)

Mutations in *NSD1*—and chromosome 5q35 microdeletions that include *NSD1*—cause Sotos syndrome, which is typically known as an overgrowth syndrome. It has been speculated that the phenotypes of individuals with mutations localized to *NSD1* would differ from those with microdeletions, but, since the phenotypic range for these mutations hasn't been defined, this speculation has not yet been thoroughly examined. Tatton-Brown et al. analyzed 530 individuals with a range of phenotypes and found 266 cases that had defects at *NSD1*. The mutation-positive cases were almost completely restricted to those individuals given a clinical diagnosis of typical or possible Sotos syndrome. This contrasts with previous reports that suggested some cases of Weaver and Beckwith-Wiedemann syndromes result from defects in *NSD1*. Also in contrast to previous reports is the fact that Tatton-Brown et al. ascribe the clinical features of 5q35 microdeletions to *NSD1* haploinsufficiency and not to other genes in the deleted interval. This large collection of affected individuals allowed Tatton-Brown et al. to better designate the cardinal features of Sotos syndrome, which are facial dysmorphism, learning disabilities, and childhood overgrowth. Although each is present in >90% of cases, the severity varies quite widely among individuals. Perhaps surprisingly for what has been defined an overgrowth syndrome, 10% of mutation-positive cases had growth within the normal range, so overgrowth is not a requirement for the diagnosis of Sotos syndrome.

0002-9297/2005/7702-0001$15.00

Alleles at SLC6A4/*SERT Confer Risk of Autism,* by Sutcliffe et al. (p. 265)

Linkage of autism near the serotonin transporter locus *SLC6A4* has been found in a few studies, and support for this locus seems to be stronger in families that have only affected males, which is interesting in light of the fact that the affected male:female ratio for autism is ~4:1. Although *SLC6A4* is a great candidate gene, the results of association studies of this locus have not been strong enough to explain the linkage signal in this area. Sutcliffe et al. reexamine the role of this locus in autism through studies of rare variation in this gene. In a sample in which they demonstrate highly significant linkage to this region, they report coding substitutions in *SLC6A4* that are associated with increased rigid-compulsive behaviors. In their linked families, the most common of these substitutions, Gly56Ala, is at increased frequency compared with previous reports in a control population. Gly56Ala exhibits transmission distortion, and the encoded protein has an elevated basal activity and insensitivity to certain stimuli. Sutcliffe et al. also found noncoding variations that collectively show transmission disequilibrium. They propose that multiple rare variants, rather than common variants, in *SLC6A4* confer susceptibility to autism-spectrum disorders and contribute substantially to the linkage to this region.

CCD and Growth-Plate Abnormalities, by Zheng et al. (p. 305)

Cleidocranial dysplasia (CCD) is a result of defective ossification and is characterized by a persistently open skull suture, short stature, dental anomalies, and hypo- or aplastic clavicles. CCD is caused by mutations in *RUNX2*, which encodes an osteoblast-specific transcription factor, and is thought to be due to defects in intramembranous ossification and possibly endochondral ossification. Mouse models expressing various forms and amounts of *Runx2* have provided evidence that this transcription factor is crucial for osteoblast differentiation and subsequent bone-matrix deposition by the differentiated osteoblasts, but mouse models could take researchers only so far because of phenotypic differences between *RUNX2*-deficient humans and mice. Zheng et al. characterized the effects of a *RUNX2* mutation in a rare human sample, a 20-wk fetus with CCD. This single-base insertion results in a 50% decrease in *RUNX2* mRNA in cartilage. Compared with an age-matched control, growth-plate sections in the affected fetus were disorganized and exhibited decreased chondrocyte hypertrophy as well as altered expression of collagen X. Zheng et al. also measured the expression of *RUNX2* target genes and found reduced expression of genes that are normally highly expressed in differentiated chondrocytes. This study supports the proposal that endochondral ossification defects that are the result of altered regulation of genes expressed in chondrocytes contribute to the CCD phenotype.

***French-Canadian LHON Due to* Fille du Roy,** *by Laberge et al. (p. 313)*

In contrast to many other countries, the most prevalent mutation that causes Leber hereditary optic neuropathy (LHON) in the French Canadian population is T14484C. Haplogroup analysis of this mtDNA mutation suggested that its increased prevalence is due to a founder effect, possibly from one woman. Laberge et al. investigated this idea through use of Quebec's genealogical records and found that, of the 12 genealogies they could reconstruct for LHON-affected individuals, 11 were related to the same female founder through their maternal lineage. Compared with simulations based on a sample of individuals who were geographically matched with the cases, this level of maternal relatedness was highly significant. The female founder who was identified was born in France and was sent to Nouvelle-France in the 17th century as a "*fille du roy,*" or daughter of the King. During that time, Louis XIV sent the *filles du roy* to Nouvelle-France to improve the male:female ratio in the colony. These single women, often wards of the state, were supposed to marry in the colony, thereby promoting permanent settlement. Laberge et al. traced the migration of the female descendents of this woman largely to southwest Quebec, a location that corresponds quite well with the current distribution of LHON cases due to T14484C in French Canadians.

KATHRYN GARBER
Deputy Editor

Am. J. Hum. Genet. 77:171–192, 2005

REVIEW ARTICLE
How Malaria Has Affected the Human Genome and What Human Genetics Can Teach Us about Malaria

Dominic P. Kwiatkowski

Wellcome Trust Centre for Human Genetics and University Department of Paediatrics, Oxford, United Kingdom

Malaria is a major killer of children worldwide and the strongest known force for evolutionary selection in the recent history of the human genome. The past decade has seen growing evidence of ethnic differences in susceptibility to malaria and of the diverse genetic adaptations to malaria that have arisen in different populations: epidemiological confirmation of the hypotheses that G6PD deficiency, α^{+} thalassemia, and hemoglobin C protect against malaria mortality; the application of novel haplotype-based techniques demonstrating that malaria-protective genes have been subject to recent positive selection; the first genetic linkage maps of resistance to malaria in experimental murine models; and a growing number of reported associations with resistance and susceptibility to human malaria, particularly in genes involved in immunity, inflammation, and cell adhesion. The challenge for the next decade is to build the global epidemiological infrastructure required for statistically robust genomewide association analysis, as a way of discovering novel mechanisms of protective immunity that can be used in the development of an effective malaria vaccine.

Introduction

One of the most important causes of child mortality worldwide is the malaria parasite *Plasmodium falciparum,* which annually kills >1 million children in Africa alone. This death toll is only one aspect of the global burden of malaria. *P. falciparum* is estimated to cause about half a billion episodes of disease each year (Snow et al. 2005), and there are hundreds of millions of cases due to other parasite species—*Plasmodium vivax, Plasmodium malariae,* and *Plasmodium ovale.* In regions of high malaria transmission, every member of the community might be chronically infected (Trape et al. 1994), and, in one Gambian village, it was found that about one-quarter of all children with severe complications of the disease were admitted to the hospital during the first 10 years of life (Snow et al. 1997).

When malaria's effect on child mortality is considered—and it was probably even greater before antimalarial drugs and other control measures were introduced—it is not surprising that malaria is the strongest known selective pressure in the recent history of the human genome. Malaria is the evolutionary driving force behind sickle-cell disease, thalassemia, glucose-6-phosphatase deficiency, and other erythrocyte defects that together comprise the most common Mendelian diseases of humankind. HbS, the allele that gives rise to sickle hemoglobin, is regarded as the classic paradigm of balanced polymorphisms in human populations (Feng et al. 2004; Hedrick 2004). It is a variant of the *HBB* gene (which encodes β-globin) that has arisen independently in different locations and is maintained at ~10% frequency in many malaria-endemic regions (Flint et al. 1998). HbS homozygotes suffer sickle-cell disease, but heterozygotes have a 10-fold reduced risk of severe malaria (Hill et al. 1991; Ackerman et al. 2005).

What is remarkable is the range of erythrocyte variants, apart from HbS, that have resulted from evolutionary selection by malaria. They include other variants of the *HBB* gene—namely, HbC and HbE (Agarwal et al. 2000; Modiano et al. 2001*b*; Chotivanich et al. 2002; Ohashi et al. 2004); regulatory defects of *HBA* and *HBB,* which cause α and β thalassemia (Flint et al. 1986; Williams et al. 1996; Allen et al. 1997), variation in the structural protein SLC4A1, which causes ovalocytosis (Foo et al. 1992; Genton et al. 1995; Allen et al. 1999); variation in the chemokine receptor *FY,* which causes the Duffy-negative blood group (Miller et al. 1976; Chitnis and Miller 1994; Tournamille et al. 1995; Hamblin and Di Rienzo 2000); and polymorphisms of the red-cell enzyme gene *G6PD,* which causes glucose-6-phosphate dehydrogenase deficiency (Bienzle et al. 1972; Ganczakowski et al. 1995; Ruwende and Hill 1998; Tishkoff et al. 2001; Sabeti et al. 2002*b*).

This is probably only the tip of the iceberg. Surpris-

Received June 3, 2005; accepted for publication June 3, 2005; electronically published July 6, 2005.

Address for correspondence and reprints: Dr. Dominic P. Kwiatkowski, Wellcome Trust Centre for Human Genetics, Oxford OX3 7BN, United Kingdom. E-mail: dominic@well.ox.ac.uk

0002-9297/2005/7702-0002$15.00

ingly little is currently known about the effects of malaria on the evolution of the human immune system, possibly because the phenotypic consequences are more subtle than those of the classic erythrocyte variants; for example, alteration of a splenic dendritic cell receptor is not as easy to visualize as a sickling red cell. However, the last few years have seen a rapid growth in the number of reported genetic associations with susceptibility and resistance to malaria, many of which involve immune system and inflammatory genes.

The purpose of this review is to provide an overview of what is currently known about genetic resistance to malaria and to highlight directions that are likely to see major advances in the next few years.

Evolutionary Selection by Malaria

Evolutionary selection by malaria (reviewed by Flint et al. [1998] and Tishkoff and Williams [2002]) is remarkable in two respects. First, the selective pressure is very strong; this is evident from the fact that the HbS allele has risen to high frequencies in malaria-exposed populations despite the fatal consequences for homozygotes. Second, different populations have developed independent evolutionary responses to malaria, and this is seen at both the global and the local levels. The most striking example is the *HBB* gene, in which three different coding SNPs confer protection against malaria: *Glu6Val* (HbS), *Glu6Lys* (HbC), and *Glu26Lys* (HbE). The HbS allele is common in Africa but rare in Southeast Asia, whereas the opposite is true for the HbE allele. However, a more complex picture emerges at the local level, exemplified by the Dogon people of Mali, who have a much lower frequency of the HbS allele than do most other West African groups and instead have a high frequency of the HbC allele (Agarwal et al. 2000). A further level of complexity is that, within Africa, the HbS allele is found in four distinct haplotypes (Chebloune et al. 1988; Nagel and Ranney 1990; Lapoumeroulie et al. 1992), a finding that has been generally interpreted to imply that the same mutation has arisen independently in four different Africa populations, although it has been pointed out that there may be other explanations (Flint et al. 1998). The different geographic distributions of α thalassemia, G6PD deficiency, ovalocytosis, and the Duffy-negative blood group are further examples of the general principle that different populations have evolved different genetic variants to protect against malaria.

The fact that different malaria-resistance alleles have arisen in different places suggests that a great deal of evolutionary selection by malaria has happened relatively recently in human history and certainly since humans started to migrate out of Africa. This is supported by analyses of recent positive selection in the human genome. Haplotype analysis and statistical modeling of an African malaria-resistance allele at the *G6PD* locus suggests an origin within the last 10,000 years or so (Tishkoff et al. 2001), whereas analysis of the Southeast Asian HbE allele suggests that it originated within the last 5,000 years (Ohashi et al. 2004). Studies of *G6PD* and *CD40L* malaria-resistance alleles in West Africa that made use of the long-range haplotype test are also consistent with recent positive selection (Sabeti et al. 2002*b*).

Another line of evidence comes from population-genetics analysis of malaria parasites. Malaria parasites existed long before humans—there are different *Plasmodium* species that infect birds, lizards, rodents, and other primates—but what geneticists would like to know is the timepoint at which the unusually virulent species *P. falciparum* began to expand in human populations. This has been addressed by a variety of approaches, with conflicting results (reviewed by Conway [2003] and Hartl [2004]), but the most persuasive evidence comes from a detailed analysis of 100 mtDNA sequences sampled from around the world (Joy et al. 2003). This suggests that some forms of *P. falciparum* may have existed 100,000 years ago, but that the African malaria parasite population suddenly increased ~10,000 years ago and subsequently spread to other regions. This observation, together with analysis of the speciation of human malaria vectors by polytene chromosome analysis (Coluzzi 1999; Coluzzi et al. 2002), is consistent with the hypothesis that the emergence of *P. falciparum* as a major human pathogen coincides with the beginnings of agriculture, when human populations started to form resident communities that allowed the establishment of a substantial reservoir of infection.

These findings are not just of historical interest, they may also be of practical value in the search for novel malaria-resistance loci. One of the major challenges confronting genomewide association analysis is determining how to select the most-efficient set of markers to analyze. In the case of malaria, we are particularly interested in alleles that show evidence of recent positive selection in regions where malaria is endemic. *P. falciparum* seems to have emerged as a powerful selective force subsequent to the divergence of African, Asian, and European populations, so an obvious starting point for genomewide analysis of malaria-resistance loci is to screen alleles that show large differences in frequency between major population groups.

Complex Genetic Basis of Resistance to Malaria

The genetic basis of resistance to malaria is complex at several levels. It is likely that many different genes are involved and that they interact with environmental variables and with parasite genetic factors. Here, we consider some further complexities of studying genetic resistance to malaria—namely, the range of phenotypes involved, the practical difficulties of studying families, and the remarkable geographic and ethnic heterogeneity of malaria-resistance factors.

Phenotypes

Susceptibility to and resistance to malaria can be measured in several ways. Usually, they are studied in regions with high levels of malaria transmission. When everyone is repeatedly bitten by infected mosquitoes, many children and adults are likely to have parasitemia (parasites in the blood), children may have two or three episodes of malaria fever each year, and a small minority (e.g., 1%) of malaria-fever episodes lead to severe malaria (i.e., death or life-threatening complications due to malaria). Different genetic factors may determine the risk of an exposed person for developing parasitemia, the risk of a parasitemic person for becoming ill with malaria fever, and the risk of a person with malaria fever for developing severe malaria. Parasitemia and fever can be regarded as quantitative phenotypes that are ascertained by repeated measurements within the community, whereas severe malaria is a qualitative phenotype that is typically ascertained in hospital-based studies. In principle, studies of severe malaria would be expected to detect genetic factors at each stage in the causal chain of disease progression.

Severe malaria is the phenotype that matters most to vaccine developers and to those interested in evolutionary selection. Severe malaria is composed of a number of subphenotypes that may occur alone or in combination. In African children, these are cerebral malaria, severe malarial anemia, and respiratory distress (Marsh et al. 1995). When we recruit 100 children with severe malaria who are in the hospital to a study, we are effectively identifying those, of perhaps 10,000 children who live in the hospital's catchment area, with the lowest levels of protection, and this tends to enrich the sample for strong genetic effects. For example, HbS heterozygotes have an ~2-fold reduction in the risk of malaria-fever episodes but a 10-fold reduction in the risk of severe malaria (Hill et al. 1991).

Family Studies

It is difficult to get an accurate measure of the familial component of resistance to severe malaria. Cases of severe malaria are relatively easy to identify in hospitals, but the transient nature of the illness makes it difficult to ascertain the affected status of relatives, particularly in communities that lack detailed medical records and in which there are other infectious causes of child mortality that can be confused with malaria. By careful questioning of families of affected individuals, a recent study in Mali estimated a sibling risk (λ_s) of 2.5 for cerebral malaria and 4.9 for severe malarial anemia (Ranque et al. 2005). This, of course, does not distinguish genetic effects from those of shared environment.

To do an accurate family study of malaria, it is necessary to perform detailed longitudinal analysis, which, in practice, means studying a relatively small number of individuals, such as a set of twins or a village of a few hundred people. Such studies lack power to investigate severe malaria, which is a relatively rare event, but they can evaluate quantitative traits such as the level of parasitemia or frequency of malaria-fever episodes. The fact that the level of parasitemia and the frequency of malaria fever both decline markedly with age must be factored into the analysis. A longitudinal study of Gambian twins showed that susceptibility to malaria-fever episodes is determined partly by genetic factors (Jepson et al. 1995), with linkage to the major histocompatibility complex (MHC) region on chromosome 6 (Jepson et al. 1997). A series of longitudinal family studies of parasitemia have been performed in Cameroon and Burkina Faso. An initial segregation analysis suggested the involvement of a major gene that controls blood infection levels (Abel et al. 1992), and this hypothesis seemed to be supported by a somewhat bimodal distribution of parasite density levels among pregnant women, who are particularly susceptible to malaria (Cot et al. 1993). However, subsequent studies indicate that complex genetic factors are involved (Garcia et al. 1998*a*; Rihet et al. 1998*a*) and that there is linkage to the MHC and the 5q31-33 region (Garcia et al. 1998*b*; Rihet et al. 1998*b*; Flori et al. 2003). A longitudinal family analysis in Sri Lanka concluded that there were consistent individual differences in susceptibility to clinical malaria episodes, of which about one-half appeared to have a genetic basis (Mackinnon et al. 2000).

It is also possible to estimate the genetic component of individual variation in immunological responses. A twin study in Liberia found evidence of heritability in antimalarial antibody responses that did not appear to be determined by HLA class II genes (Sjoberg et al. 1992). Familial segregation analysis of immunological responses to malaria antigens in Papua New Guinea has suggested that Mendelian effects might govern specific antigen responses, but the overall picture is complex (Stirnadel et al. 1999*a*, 2000*a*, 2000*b*).

Ethnic Differences

One of the most striking examples of differential disease susceptibility among human populations is the complete resistance of most of the population of sub-Saharan Africa to *P. vivax* infection, whereas all other human populations are vulnerable to this species of malaria parasite. This resistance is due to a SNP in the *FY* gene that results in the Duffy blood group–negative phenotype (Miller et al. 1976; Tournamille et al. 1995); the precise protective mechanism is discussed below (see the "Malaria and the Red Cell" section). Thus, whereas *P. vivax* infection is common in Asia and South America and used to be widely distributed throughout Europe, it is extremely rare in most of sub-Saharan Africa, although all the right environmental conditions exist for it to be transmitted there.

Striking differences in resistance to malaria have also been observed among ethnic groups who live in the same area. The Tharu people, who inhabit the malarious Terai region of Nepal, have a much lower prevalence of malaria than do other ethnic groups in the same region (Terrenato et al. 1988), and this may possibly be explained by the extremely high frequency of α thalassemia in the Tharu population (Modiano et al. 1991).

The Fulani people are traditionally nomadic pastoral people who are found across West Africa, often settled in close proximity to other ethnic groups. Studies in Burkina Faso (Modiano et al. 1996) and, more recently, in Mali (Dolo et al. 2005) have documented a significantly lower prevalence of malaria parasitemia and fewer clinical attacks of malaria among the Fulani than among other ethnic groups who live in neighboring villages. The Fulani have a distinctive culture, but detailed epidemiological investigations indicate that their resistance to malaria arises primarily from genetic factors. Importantly, it has also been observed that the Fulani have high levels of antimalarial antibodies (Modiano et al. 1998, 1999) and a low frequency of protective globin variants and other classic malaria-resistance factors (Modiano et al. 2001*a*). There is therefore much interest in discovering the genetic factors that determine the high antibody responses seen in the Fulani; the possible role of the *IL4* gene is discussed below (see the "Antibody Response" section) (Luoni et al. 2001; Farouk et al. 2005).

Malaria and the Red Cell

Erythrocyte Surface

Many important things happen at the erythrocyte surface in malaria (table 1). The parasite binds to erythrocyte surface molecules as the first stage in a complex and marvelous series of events—still poorly understood—that gets the parasite into the erythrocyte without destroying it (Sibley 2004). Once inside the erythrocyte, the parasite manufactures a set of proteins that it sends to the cell surface (Kyes et al. 2001). Some of these parasite-derived erythrocyte-membrane proteins bind to endothelial adhesion molecules and thereby cause parasitized erythrocytes to sequester in small blood vessels; this is thought to be a strategy for immune evasion, since it prevents the parasites from having to circulate through the spleen. But these parasite-derived molecules on the erythrocyte surface are themselves targets for immunological attack, which they counter with an extraordinary capacity for antigenic variation. We discuss in the "Cytoadherence, a Major Factor in Malaria Pathogenesis" section how human genetic variation influences endothelial cytoadherence; here, we focus on how it affects erythrocyte invasion.

The study of human genetics uncovered a key step in the molecular process of erythrocyte invasion by *P. vivax*. The Duffy antigen, encoded by the *FY* gene, is a chemokine receptor that is expressed in various cell types. The Duffy antigen is expressed in erythrocytes in most populations (but not in sub-Saharan Africa) that have a promoter SNP that disrupts a binding site for the erythroid transcription factor GATA-1 (Tournamille et al. 1995). This completely prevents *P. vivax* from invading erythrocytes, and it accounts for the remarkable absence of *P. vivax* in parts of Africa in which other species of malaria parasite are extremely common (Miller et al. 1976). It was this genetic discovery that led to the discovery of the *P. vivax* Duffy-binding protein, a parasite molecule that is critical for erythrocyte invasion by *P. vivax* (Chitnis and Miller 1994) and is now undergoing clinical trials as a candidate agent for a vaccine against this species of parasite (Yazdani et al. 2004). The African Duffy-negative allele, denoted "FY*O," has the highest F_{ST} value observed in humans and has other features that are strongly suggestive of recent positive selection (Hamblin and Di Rienzo 2000; Hamblin et al. 2002). There is further support for selective pressure at this locus, from the observation of an entirely independent *FY* polymorphism, which has emerged in Papua New Guinea, that decreases Duffy-antigen expression and acts to reduce *P. vivax* invasion efficiency (Zimmerman et al. 1999; Michon et al. 2001). The apparent strength of selection at the *FY* locus is somewhat puzzling for malariologists, since *P. vivax* infection is not generally lethal, and it has even been proposed that *P. vivax* infection may protect against the much more lethal parasite *P. falciparum* (Williams et al. 1996).

The study of human genetic polymorphisms has also been informative about how *P. falciparum* invades erythrocytes, but, in contrast to *P. vivax*, the available data suggest multiple invasion pathways with considerable redundancy (Hadley et al. 1987). A lot of attention has focused on *GYPA*, *GYPB*, and *GYPC*, the genes encoding glycophorins A, B, and C, respectively.

Various blood groups are determined by the erythrocyte-membrane sialoglycoproteins glycophorin A and B, and genetic deficiency of glycophorin A or B expression makes erythrocytes relatively resistant to invasion by *P. falciparum* (Facer 1983). Specific sialic-acid residues on the glycophorin A molecule are recognized by a Duffy-binding–like domain of *P. falciparum* erythrocyte-binding antigen 175 (Orlandi et al. 1992; Mayor et al. 2005). Sequence analysis shows evidence of strong evolutionary

Table 1

Common Erythrocyte Variants That Affect Resistance to Malaria

Gene	Protein	Function	Reported Genetic Associations with Malaria
FY	Duffy antigen	Chemokine receptor	FY*O allele completely protects against *P. vivax* infection.
G6PD	Glucose-6-phosphatase dehydogenase	Enzyme that protects against oxidative stress	G6PD deficiency protects against severe malaria.
GYPA	Glycophorin A	Sialoglycoprotein	GYPA-deficient erythrocytes are resistant to invasion by *P. falciparum.*
GYPB	Glycophorin B	Sialoglycoprotein	GYPB-deficient erythrocytes are resistant to invasion by *P. falciparum.*
GYPC	Glycophorin C	Sialoglycoprotein	GYPC-deficient erythrocytes are resistant to invasion by *P. falciparum.*
HBA	α-Globin	Component of hemoglobin	α^+ Thalassemia protects against severe malaria but appears to enhance mild malaria episodes in some environments.
HBB	β-Globin	Component of hemoglobin	HbS and HbC alleles protect against severe malaria. HbE allele reduces parasite invasion.
HP	Haptoglobin	Hemoglobin-binding protein present in plasma (not erythrocyte)	Haptoglobin 1-1 genotype is associated with susceptibility to severe malaria in Sudan and Ghana.
SCL4A1	CD233, erythrocyte band 3 protein	Chloride/bicarbonate exchanger	Deletion causes ovalocytosis but protects against cerebral malaria.

selection, not only for *GYPA* and *GYPB* in the human host (Baum et al. 2002; Wang et al. 2003), but also for EBA-175 in the *P. falciparum* parasite, which implies an ongoing evolutionary struggle between the parasite ligand and the host receptor (Wang et al. 2003).

Glycophorin C is a minor component of the erythrocyte membrane that serves as a receptor for the *P. falciparum* erythrocyte-binding antigen 140 (EBA140). The Gerbich-negative blood group, caused by a deletion of *GYPC* exon 3, is common in coastal areas of Papua New Guinea and results in reduced invasion by *P. falciparum* (Maier et al. 2003). Epidemiological studies indicate that this *GYPC* deletion does not alter the prevalence or density of asymptomatic malaria infection, but so far there has been no study of how it affects the clinical severity of infection (Patel et al. 2001, 2004).

Another erythrocyte-membrane protein that has been implicated in malaria resistance is an anion exchanger known as "band 3 protein," encoded by *SLC4A1*. A 27-bp deletion in this gene results in a form of ovalocytosis that is common in parts of Southeast Asia. It appears to be protective both against malaria infection (Cattani et al. 1987; Foo et al. 1992) and against cerebral malaria (Genton et al. 1995; Allen et al. 1999). The mechanism of protection is not yet known. It may relate to the involvement of band 3 protein in endothelial cytoadherence or to some inhibitory effect on parasite invasion or growth.

Structural Variation of Globin Genes

Erythrocytes are essentially bags filled with hemoglobin, and the malaria parasite has developed a lifestyle that is hugely dependent on its hemoglobin environment. Alterations in hemoglobin may affect the biochemical and cellular machinery of parasite development, and they may affect the ability of the spleen and other immune mechanisms to recognize parasites, by affecting the morphology, mechanical properties, or surface structure of the parasitized erythrocyte. The biological importance of these dependencies is highlighted by the huge selective pressure that malaria has exerted on the structure and regulation of α globin (encoded by the identical *HBA1* and *HBA2* genes) and β globin (encoded by *HBB*) that together comprise the tetrameric protein backbone of adult hemoglobin.

HBB has three different coding SNPs that each confer resistance against malaria and that have risen to high frequency in different populations. The HbS allele is a glutamic acid→valine substitution at codon 6 of the β globin chain, HbC is a glutamine→lysine substitution at codon 6, and HbE allele is a glutamic acid→lysine substitution at codon 26. The corresponding proteins are known as "hemoglobin S" (or "sickle hemoglobin"), "hemoglobin C," and "hemoglobin E."

The HbS allele is found across a large part of sub-Saharan African as well as parts of the Middle East. It has the distinction of being one of the first human genetic variants to be associated with a specific molecular defect (Pauling et al. 1949). Hemoglobin S tends to polymerize at low oxygen concentrations, which causes the erythrocyte to deform into a sickle-like shape (Brittenham et al. 1985). HbS homozygotes have sickle-cell disease, a debilitating and often fatal disorder caused by these red-cell deformities. The heterozygous state (denoted "HbAS") is not generally associated with any clinical abnormality and confers ~10-fold increase in protection from life-threatening forms of malaria, with a lesser degree of protection against milder forms of the disease (Allison 1954; Gilles et al. 1967; Hill et al. 1991; Allen et al. 1992; Stirnadel et al. 1999*b*; Sokhna et al. 2000; Ackerman et al. 2005). It is still not known precisely how HbAS protects against malaria. Two plausible mechanisms, which are not mutually exclusive, are suppression of parasite growth in red cells (Pasvol et al. 1978) and enhanced splenic clearance of parasitized erythrocytes (Shear et al. 1993). A study of Kenyan children found that the protective effect of HbAS against malaria increased from 20% to 56% between the ages of 2 and 10 years, which implies that it enhances or acts in synergy with the acquired immune response (Williams et al. 2005*a*). The trade-off between risks and benefits acts to maintain the HbS polymorphism at allele frequencies of ~10% in many parts of Africa, despite the lethal consequences for homozygotes, which provides the most striking known example of heterozygote advantage in human genetics.

Hemoglobin C is found in several parts of West Africa, although less commonly than is HbS. It results in a much-less-damaging clinical phenotype than sickle-cell disease: homozygotes have a relatively mild hemolytic anemia, and heterozygotes do not experience a significant reduction in hemoglobin levels (Diallo et al. 2004). Both heterozygotes and homozygotes of HbC are protected against severe malaria (Agarwal et al. 2000; Mockenhaupt et al. 2004*a*; Rihet et al. 2004), but the protective effect appears to be substantially greater in homozygotes (Modiano et al. 2001*b*). It has been proposed that the protective effect of HbC may operate by increasing immune clearance of infected erythrocytes. This is based on observations of reduced parasite cytoadherence, abnormal PfEMP1 expression, clustering of erythrocyte band 3 protein, and altered surface topography of the erythrocyte membrane in the presence of hemoglobin C (Arie et al. 2005; Fairhurst et al. 2005; Tokumasu et al. 2005).

Hemoglobin E is common in Southeast Asia, with carrier rates of 50% in some places, and analysis of haplotype structure suggests that the mutation is relatively recent and has risen rapidly in allele frequency (Ohashi et al. 2004). Homozygotes generally have symptomless anemia. Although it has not been epidemiologically proven that HbE protects against severe malaria, this is assumed to be the case, and it has been observed that erythrocytes from HbE-heterozygous individuals are relatively resistant to invasion by *P. falciparum* (Chotivanich et al. 2002).

Regulatory Variation of Globin Genes

The thalassemias are the most common Mendelian diseases of humans and constitute a major global health problem (Weatherall and Clegg 2001). They comprise a group of clinical disorders that result from defective production of α- or β-globin chains, which arise from deletions or other disruptions of the globin gene clusters on chromosomes 11 and 16. There is a broad spectrum of clinical phenotypes, reflecting the range of different genetic variants that exist and given greater complexity by the fact that α-globin is produced by two identical genes, *HBA1* and *HBA2*. Broadly speaking, homozygous thalassemia results in severe disease or is fatal, whereas heterozygotes are healthy apart from mild anemia. An exception to this general rule arises when either the *HBA1* or the *HBA2* gene, but not both, is disrupted, so that some α-globin production is possible. This condition is known as "α^+ thalassemia," and α^+ thalassemia homozygotes are only mildly anemic.

Over half a century ago, J. B. S. Haldane proposed balanced polymorphism as the explanation for why thalassemia had risen to high frequencies—approaching fixation—in certain populations (Haldane 1949). He argued that heterozygotes might be protected against some important disease, and malaria was the obvious candidate, since the global distribution of thalassemia encompasses the major malarious regions of Africa and Asia and Mediterranean regions where malaria was once common. There are many other circumstantial lines of evidence to support this concept; for example, the Tharu people have both a much higher allele frequency of α thalassemia, of ~0.8, and a much lower incidence of malarial illness than do other ethnic groups that inhabit the same region of Nepal (Modiano et al. 1991). Arguably the strongest population-genetic evidence comes from a detailed survey in Melanesia that showed that the frequency of α^+ thalassemia varied according to both altitude and latitude in a manner that was highly correlated with malaria endemicity, whereas haplotypic analysis seemed to rule out the possibility that this could have arisen because of founder effects (Flint et al. 1986).

Although the population-genetic evidence seems overwhelming, it is only relatively recently that direct evidence that thalassemia protects against malaria has emerged, and the case is still not absolutely clear-cut. A study of Kenyan children found that both heterozygous and homozygous α^+ thalassemia was protective against severe malaria (Williams et al. 2005*b*), whereas a study of Ghanaian children found that heterozygotes were protected (Mockenhaupt et al. 2004*b*). In Papua New Guinea, the risk of severe malaria was found to be reduced by 60% in children who were homozygous for α^+ thalassemia and to a lesser degree in heterozygotes, but the result did not seem to be malaria-specific, since a protective effect was also observed for other childhood infections (Allen et al. 1997).

The protective mechanism of thalassemia is unknown. Flow-cytometry studies in vitro have shown that erythrocytes with the α thalassemia phenotype show reduced parasite growth (Pattanapanyasat et al. 1999) and increased binding of antibodies from malaria-immune sera (Williams et al. 2002). Enhanced splenic clearance of malaria-infected cells is a further possibility but is difficult to test in vivo. However, much more complex explanations are also possible, as illustrated by findings of data from Vanuatu which are unusual in two respects: first, both *P. falciparum* and *P. vivax* infection are common, but severe malaria is remarkably uncommon in this population; and, second, young children with α^+ thalassemia have a significantly higher incidence of malaria than do nonthalassemic children (Williams et al. 1996). This latter result is exactly the opposite of what Williams et al. (1996) set out to prove, but they came up with a possible explanation that was based on the further observation that *P. vivax* infection, which does not cause severe disease, is acquired at an earlier age in this population than is *P. falciparum* infection. The proposal is that, in this particular epidemiological scenario, α^+ thalassemia may enhance early exposure to *P. vivax* infection, thereby in some way protecting against severe disease from later exposure to *P. falciparum*.

Oxidative Stress

Malaria parasites need to break down hemoglobin to make room to grow, quite apart from any nutritional benefit they may derive from this. This process releases by-products that are potentially toxic—particularly iron, which is a source of oxidative stress.

An important form of defense against oxidative stress within the erythrocyte is production of the electron donor nicotinamide adenine dinucleotide phosphate by the enzyme glucose-6-phosphate dehydrogenase (G6PD), encoded by *G6PD* on chromosome X. There are many different variants of *G6PD,* and those that markedly compromise enzyme activity result in hemolytic anemia. The geographical distribution of G6PD deficiency is consistent with evolutionary selection by malaria (Ganczakowski et al. 1995), and analysis of haplotypic structure at the *G6PD* locus supports the hypothesis of recent positive selection (Tishkoff et al. 2001; Sabeti et al. 2002*b*). Deficient G6PD enzyme activity has been shown to correlate with protection against severe malaria in Nigerian children (Gilles et al. 1967). A study of >2,000 Gambian and Kenyan children found that the common African form of G6PD deficiency (G6PD A^-) is associated with ~50% reduced risk of severe malaria in female heterozygotes and in male hemizygotes (Ruwende et al. 1995). Reduced parasite replication in G6PD-deficient erythrocytes is thought to be the mechanism of protection (Luzzatto et al. 1969), but the parasite appears to counter this by manufacturing G6PD itself (Usanga and Luzzatto 1985).

Haptoglobin, encoded by *HP,* is not an erythrocyte protein but is mentioned here because it is a hemoglobin-binding protein that is present in plasma. It could act to defend the malaria-infected individual in several ways: by trapping free hemoglobin, it helps to prevent hemoglobin-induced oxidative tissue damage; it has been shown to inhibit the development of malaria parasites in vitro (Imrie et al. 2004); and it appears to reduce parasite load, as determined by murine gene knockout studies (Hunt et al. 2001). The haptoglobin 1-1 genotype, characterized by protein electrophoresis, has been associated with susceptibility to severe *P. falciparum* malaria (Elagib et al. 1998; Quaye et al. 2000), although a DNA-based study of haptoglobin polymorphisms in the Gambia failed to detect such an association (Aucan et al. 2002)

Cytoadherence, a Major Factor in Malaria Pathogenesis

A critical event in the pathogenesis of severe malaria is the sequestration of *P. falciparum*–infected erythrocytes in small blood vessels (Taylor et al. 2004). A range of receptor-ligand interactions causes parasitized erythrocytes to stick to endothelium, platelets, and other erythrocytes; this is thought to be an immune-evasion strategy that allows the parasite to stay within the vascular compartment but to avoid circulating through the spleen. On the parasite side, the major ligand is *P. falciparum* erythrocyte-membrane protein-1 (PfEMP-1)—encoded by a gene family called "*var*" because each parasite contains many different copies of the gene—and, by switching expression between the copies, it is able to cause a remarkable degree of antigenic variation (Kyes et al. 2001). On the host side, a range of different adhesion molecules expressed on endothelium, platelets, macrophages, and other erythrocytes serves as binding receptors for different forms of PfEMP-1.

A number of associations have been reported between severe malaria and polymorphisms of host receptors for cytoadherence by *P. falciparum*–infected erythrocytes (table 2). When the same polymorphism has been tested in different geographical locations, the results have been variable—not simply failure to replicate but, in some cases, the association of the same polymorphism with susceptibility to severe malaria in one study and with resistance in another. As with all genetic association studies, it is possible that these results are statistical artifacts that will ultimately be resolved by larger sample sizes and by finer-scale genetic mapping of these loci. However, in this particular area of genetic analysis, it is not out of the question that the functional consequences of a single polymorphism could vary between locations and might even vary over time at a single location. As outlined above, the biological phenomenon of parasite cytoadherence to endothelium and to other cells is driven by the parasite, not by the host. The parasite varies its pattern of sequestration in different organs by constantly switching between different forms of PfEMP-1 that bind to different host receptors (and different parts of the same receptor) in a promiscuous and opportunistic manner (Roberts et al. 1992).

Many isolates of *P. falciparum* bind to endothelium via the CD36 antigen (Barnwell et al. 1989). Encoded by *CD36,* this is a receptor for a range of different molecules, including thrombospondin and long-chain fatty acids, and is expressed by platelets and dendritic cells as well as endothelium. It is a molecule of considerable interest to malaria immunologists because, as well as being a mediator of parasite sequestration, CD36 acts to bind parasitized erythrocytes to dendritic cells, an event that seems to incapacitate the dendritic cell when it comes to presenting parasite antigens (Urban et al. 1999, 2001). Several *CD36* polymorphisms have been described in malarious regions (Aitman et al. 2000; Omi et al. 2003), but the results of disease-association studies are confusing. A study of both Gambian and Kenyan case-control samples found that homozygotes for a nonsense polymorphism, the *CD36*$^+$1264G allele, were susceptible to cerebral malaria (Aitman et al. 2000), but a study of the same allele in Kenya alone found that heterozygosity was associated with protection against severe malaria (Pain et al. 2001). In Thailand, a dinucleotide repeat sequence in intron 3, implicated in alternative splicing, has been associated with protection against cerebral malaria (Omi et al. 2003).

Some isolates of *P. falciparum* bind strongly to endothelium via intercellular adhesion molecule-1 (Berendt et al. 1989). This is encoded by *ICAM1,* and its normal function is to serve as an endothelial- and immune-cell adhesion receptor for integrin-expressing leukocytes. A polymorphism in the N-terminal domain, present at high frequencies in African populations, acts to reduce binding (Fernandez-Reyes et al. 1997). A study in Gabon found that the low-binding allele was associated with reduced susceptibility to severe malaria (Kun et al. 1999), but a study in Kenya found increased susceptibility (Fernandez-Reyes et al. 1997), and another in the Gambia found no significant effect (Bellamy et al. 1998*a*).

Table 2

Host Molecules That Mediate Cytoadherence by *P. falciparum*–Infected Erythrocytes and That Have Been Reported to Show Association with Resistance or Susceptibility to Malaria

Gene	Protein	Interaction with Parasitized Erythrocyte[a]	Reported Genetic Associations with Malaria
CD36	CD36 antigen, thrombospondin receptor	PE-binding receptor on endothelium and dendritic cells	*CD36* polymorphisms show variable associations with severe malaria in the Gambia, Kenya, and Thailand.
CR1	CR1, complement receptor 1	PE-binding receptor on erythrocytes	*CR1* polymorphisms show variable associations with severe malaria in the Gambia, Thailand, and Papua New Guinea.
ICAM1	CD54, intercellular adhesion molecule-1	PE-binding receptor on endothelium	*ICAM1* polymorphisms show variable associations with severe malaria in Kenya, Gabon, and the Gambia.
PECAM1	CD31, platelet-endothelial cell–adhesion molecule	PE-binding receptor on endothelium	*PECAM1* polymorphisms show variable associations with severe malaria in Thailand, Kenya, and Papua New Guinea.

[a] PE = parasitized erythrocyte.

A survey of different ethnic groups in India found a number of novel *ICAM1* variants that merit analysis in disease-association studies (Sengupta et al. 2004).

Another endothelial-binding receptor for *P. falciparum* is the platelet–endothelial cell adhesion molecule, encoded by *PECAM1* (Treutiger et al. 1997). A common coding variant (Leu→Val at codon 125) was analyzed in case-control studies of severe malaria in Papua New Guinea and Kenya, but no significant association was identified (Casals-Pascual et al. 2001). A study from Thailand has reported a *PECAM1* haplotype that is more common in cerebral malaria than in other forms of severe malaria (Kikuchi et al. 2001).

Parasite sequestration is not due only to endothelial binding. Some *P. falciparum* isolates show a phenomenon known as rosetting, where a parasitized erythrocyte binds to other erythrocytes. One mechanism for rosetting is through PfEMP-1 binding to erythrocyte–complement receptor 1, encoded by *CR1* (Rowe et al. 1997). Up to 80% of the population of a malarious region of Papua New Guinea have erythrocyte CR1 deficiency, which has been associated both with polymorphisms in the *CR1* gene and with α^+ thalassemia, which is also common in this population (Cockburn et al. 2004). In the same study, it was found that both *CR1* polymorphisms and α thalassemia were independently associated with resistance to severe malaria. However, studies of *CR1* polymorphisms in the Gambia found no evidence of association with disease severity (Bellamy et al. 1998*a*; Zimmerman et al. 2003). In Thailand, an RFLP that is associated with reduced expression of CR1 on erythrocytes has been associated (in homozygotes) with susceptibility to severe malaria (Nagayasu et al. 2001).

Malaria and the Immune System

The genetic interaction between malaria and the immune system is potentially of huge practical interest, for two distinct reasons. First, although there is a vast literature on immunological responses to malaria in humans and in experimental model systems, there is still surprisingly little concrete evidence about precisely which immunological responses are causal mechanisms of protective immunity in naturally exposed populations, and this is a fundamental roadblock in the development of an effective malaria vaccine. One way to establish causality is to obtain clear-cut evidence that functional variation in a specific immune gene affects the clinical outcome of infection. Second, just as the selective pressure of malaria on the erythrocyte has led to common hematological disorders, such as sickle-cell disease and thalassemia, it is possible that we might learn a great deal about mechanisms of chronic immunological and inflammatory disorders if we had a better understanding of the selective pressure that malaria has exerted on the immune system.

Here, we consider a number of immune gene associations with malaria resistance and susceptibility that have emerged over the past 15 years (table 3). The same caveats, discussed above for adhesion molecules, apply here. Few of these associations have been tested in several different studies and, when this has been done, the results have been variable. Thus, much of this section should be regarded as indicative of ongoing research activity rather than definitive results. However, it is important to bear in mind that there potentially are biological reasons why the same immune gene polymorphism might have different consequences in different malarious regions. For example, HLA associations might vary according to the local prevalence of critical parasite-antigen polymorphisms. And associations with inflammatory cytokines and other immune genes may be affected by regional differences in the intensity of malaria transmission, which have complex consequences for the development of acquired immunity and the pattern of severe disease (Snow et al. 1997). These are issues that may have far-reaching implications for vaccine efficacy, and, to tackle them robustly, we need much larger sample sizes and more fine-grained genetic association maps than we have at present.

Antigen Recognition

In malaria, the opportunities for antigen presentation are limited by the fact that erythrocytes do not express MHC molecules. Liver cells, however, express MHC class I molecules and therefore provide a potential target for cytotoxic T cell (CTL) responses during the first phase of malaria infection, when parasites replicate in the liver prior to invading erythrocytes. *HLA-B* is an exceptionally polymorphic gene that encodes an MHC class I heavy chain that, together with $\beta 2$ microglobulin, makes up the *HLA-B* antigen–presentation complex. The *HLA-B53* allele is extremely common in West Africa, compared with other parts of the world, and is associated with a significantly reduced risk of severe malaria in Gambian children (Hill et al. 1991). In view of the fact that *HLA-B* is expressed by liver cells but not by erythrocytes, this genetic association implies that liver-stage parasites provide a significant target for naturally acquired protective immunity. This has boosted efforts to develop a liver-stage malaria vaccine, and it has been proposed that T cell epitope targets for malaria-vaccine development may be obtained by analyzing the peptides that bind to HLA-B53 (Hill et al. 1992).

But when a polymorphic parasite antigen interacts with a polymorphic host antigen–presenting system, there are many opportunities for complexity. For example, within a single fragment of the *P. falciparum* circumsporozoite protein (CSP), it has been observed that the Gambian parasite population has two different variants (cp26 and

Table 3

Immune Genes Reported to Be Associated with Different Malaria Phenotypes

Gene	Protein	Function	Reported Genetic Associations with Malaria
FCGR2A	CD32, low affinity receptor for Fc fragment of IgG	Clearance of antigen-antibody complexes	Association with severe malaria in the Gambia
HLA-B	HLA-B, a component of MHC class I	Antigen presentation that leads to cytotoxic T cells	HLA-B53 association with severe malaria in the Gambia
HLA-DR	HLA-DR, a component of MHC class II	Antigen presentation that leads to antibody production	HLA-DRB1 association with severe malaria in the Gambia
IFNAR1	Interferon α receptor component	Cytokine receptor	Association with severe malaria in the Gambia
IFNG	Interferon γ	Cytokine with antiparasitic and proinflammatory properties	Weak associations with severe malaria in the Gambia
IFNGR1	Interferon γ receptor component	Cytokine receptor	Association with severe malaria in Mandinka people of the Gambia
IL1A/IL1B	Interleukin-1α and -1β	Proinflammatory cytokines	Marginal associations with severe malaria in the Gambia
IL10	Interleukin-10	Anti-inflammatory cytokine	Haplotypic association with severe malaria in the Gambia
IL12B	Interleukin-12 β subunit	Promotes development of Th1 cells	Association with severe malaria in Tanzania
IL4	Interleukin-4	Promotes antibody-producing B cells	Association with antimalarial antibody levels in Fulani people of Burkina Faso
MBL2	Mannose-binding protein	Activates classic complement	Association with severe malaria in Gabon
NOS2A	Inducible NO synthase	Generates NO, a free radical	Various associations with severe malaria in Gabon, the Gambia, and Tanzania
TNF	Tumor necrosis factor	Cytokine with antiparasitic and proinflammatory properties	Various associations with severe malaria and reinfection risk in the Gambia, Kenya, Gabon, and Sri Lanka
TNFSF5	CD40 ligand	T cell–B cell interactions leading to immunoglobulin class switching	Association with severe malaria in the Gambia

cp29) that bind to *HLA-B53,* and these two variants are found together in the same individual more frequently than expected by chance. Although both cp26 and cp29 are effective targets for CTLs at the individual level, they appear to show immunological antagonism such that each acts to suppress the CTL response to the other, and it has been postulated that this is an immune-evasion strategy on the part of the parasite (Gilbert et al. 1998).

HLA-DRB1 encodes an HLA class II β chain that, together with an α chain, comprise the *HLA-DR* antigen–presenting complex. This is expressed in B lymphocytes, dendritic cells, and macrophages and is crucial for antibody production. *HLA DRB1*1302-DQB1*0501* has been associated with resistance to severe malaria in Gambian children (Hill et al. 1991), and the incidence of malaria-fever episodes in Gambian children is reported to show an overall association with distribution of MHC class II haplotypes (Bennett et al. 1993).

The Antibody Response

Interleukin-4, encoded by *IL4,* is produced by activated T cells and promotes proliferation and differentiation of antibody-producing B cells. A study of the Fulani of Burkina Faso, who have both fewer malaria attacks and higher levels of antimalarial antibodies than do neighboring ethnic groups, found that the *IL4*-524 T allele was associated with elevated antibody levels against malaria antigens, which raises the possibility that this might be a factor in increased resistance to malaria (Luoni et al. 2001).

CD40 ligand, encoded by the X chromosome gene *TNFSF5,* is expressed in T cells and binds to CD40 in B cells, which acts to regulate immunoglobulin class switching and other aspects of B cell function. In a Gambian case-control study, the *TNFSF5*-726C allele was associated with protection against severe malaria (Sabeti et al. 2002*a*), and long-range haplotype analysis of this allele suggests that it has recently undergone positive evolutionary selection (Sabeti et al. 2002*b*).

Many leukocytes express receptors for the Fc portion of IgG, which are used to engage and remove antigen-antibody complexes. A His→Arg substitution at codon 131 of *FCGR2A,* which encodes low-affinity IIa receptor for the Fc fragment of IgG, results in failure to bind to IgG2 and has been associated with protection against high levels of *P. falciparum* parasitemia in Kenya (Shi et al. 2001). Follow-up studies in Thailand and the Gambia found that homozygotes for the 131His genotype are susceptible to cerebral malaria (Omi et al. 2002; Cooke et al. 2003). In the Thai study, the *FCGR2A* association involved interaction with an *FCGR3B* gene polymorphism.

The Proinflammatory Response

Tumor necrosis factor is encoded by the *TNF* gene located in the MHC class III region, flanked by the MHC class I and II regions. It is a proinflammatory cytokine that is critical for innate immunity against malaria parasites but has also been implicated in the pathogenesis of severe malaria (reviewed by Kwiatkowski [1995] and Clark et al. [2004]). Two longitudinal family studies, in the Gambia and Burkina Faso, have identified linkage between the MHC region and susceptibility to malaria-fever episodes, and *TNF* is at the center of the linkage peaks (Jepson et al. 1997; Flori et al. 2003). Several TNF-promoter polymorphisms have been independently associated with severe malaria. Gambian children who are homozygous for the *TNF*-308A allele have been observed to have increased susceptibility to cerebral malaria (McGuire et al. 1994), and, in Gabon, it was found that those who carried this allele were more likely to encounter symptomatic reinfections with *P. falciparum* (Meyer et al. 2002). A study in Sri Lanka found that the carriers of the *TNF*-308A allele had increased risk of severe infectious diseases in general (Wattavidanage et al. 1999), whereas a study in Kenya found an increase in infant mortality and malaria morbidity (Aidoo et al. 2001). *TNF*-376A confers allele-specific binding of the transcription factor OCT-1 and has been associated with susceptibility to cerebral malaria (Knight et al. 1999), whereas the *TNF*-238A allele has been associated with susceptibility to severe malarial anemia (McGuire et al. 1999). A longitudinal study in Burkina Faso suggests that several different TNF-promoter SNPs are involved in the regulation of parasite density (Flori et al. 2005). The functional role of *TNF*-308 and other *TNF* polymorphisms remains open to question (Abraham and Kroeger 1999; Knight et al. 2003; Bayley et al. 2004), but the surrounding MHC class III region has many other interesting immunological genes and complex patterns of linkage disequilibrium (Ackerman et al. 2003). Thus, although *TNF* is unquestionably an important mediator of both immunity and pathogenesis for malaria, it remains possible that the observed genetic associations with *TNF* polymorphisms arise from functional variation in neighboring genes.

Inducible nitric oxide (NO) synthase, encoded by *NOS2A,* generates NO. This is a free radical, with antiparasitic properties, but it also has a potential immunosuppressive role and has been proposed as a factor in cerebral malaria because of its role in neurotransmission (reviewed by Clark and Rockett [1996]). The *NOS2A*-954C allele has been associated with elevated NO synthase activity in cells from Gabonese individuals, and, in that population, it has been associated with protection from severe malaria and resistance to reinfection (Kun et al. 1998, 2001), but studies in the Gambia and Tanzania failed to detect such a disease association (Levesque et al. 1999; Burgner et al. 2003). The *NOS2A*-1173T allele—which appears, on the basis of measurements in urine and plasma, to be associated with high NO production in Tanzanian children—is associated with protection from malarial illness in Tanzania and from severe malarial anemia in Kenya (Hobbs et al. 2002), but no protective effect against severe malaria was detected in the Gambia (Burgner et al. 2003). In Gambian children, an *NOS2A* microsatellite polymorphism has been associated with susceptibility to fatal malaria (Burgner et al. 1998), and a haplotype uniquely defined by the *NOS2A*-1659T allele was associated with cerebral malaria by both the transmission/disequilibrium test (TDT) and case-control analysis (Burgner et al. 2003).

Interferon-γ, encoded by *IFNG,* is a key immunological mediator that is believed to play both a protective and a pathological role in malaria (Stevenson and Riley 2004). Analysis of SNPs in the region of *IFNG* and the neighboring *IL22* gene found several weak associations with severe malaria in Gambian children but no clear-cut effect (Koch et al. 2005). A study of *IFNGR1,* which encodes the ligand-binding α chain of the interferon-γ receptor, found that in Mandinka, the major Gambian ethnic group, heterozygotes for the IFNGR1-56 polymorphism were protected against cerebral malaria (Koch et al. 2002). Reporter-gene analysis suggests that the minor allele acts to reduce levels of *IFNGR1* gene expression (Juliger et al. 2003).

IFNAR1 encodes interferon α receptor 1, a type I membrane protein that forms one of the two chains of a receptor for interferons α and β. In a murine malaria model, it has been observed that interferonα inhibits parasite development within erythrocytes (Vigario et al. 2001). A Gambian case-control study found two *IFNAR1* SNPs that were associated with protection against severe malaria, and a resistance haplotype was identified (Aucan et al. 2003).

IL12B encodes a subunit of interleukin-12, a cytokine produced by activated macrophages that is essential for the development of Th1 cells. Homozygotes for an *IL12B*-promoter polymorphism were found to have decreased NO production when measured in blood samples, and this genotype has been associated with a fatal outcome in cerebral malaria in Tanzanian but not in Kenyan children (Morahan et al. 2002)

The interleukin-1 family of cytokines, produced mainly by macrophages, are important mediators of the inflammatory response to infection and of fever. In a Gambian case-control study, a SNP in *IL1A* (encoding interleukin-1α) and another in *IL1B* (encoding interleukin-1β) showed a marginal association with susceptibility to malaria (Walley et al. 2004).

Interleukin-10, encoded by *IL10,* is a crucial anti-inflammatory cytokine. Several lines of evidence indicate that IL10 is protective against severe malaria and that IL10 production is genetically determined. An analysis of *IL10* SNPs in Gambian children found a common haplotype that was strongly associated with protection against severe malaria by case-control analysis but not by TDT analysis of the same population (Wilson et al. 2005). Since the case-control analysis was ethnically matched, this raises the question of whether *IL10* associations with severe malaria might be confounded by fetal survival rates or other sources of transmission bias, since genetic variation at the *IL10* locus has been implicated as a determinant of fertility (Westendorp et al. 2001).

Other Serum Factors

MBL2 encodes a serum mannose-binding lectin (MBL) protein that recognizes mannose and N-acetylglucosamine on bacterial pathogens and can activate the classic complement pathway. *MBL2* polymorphisms have been associated with susceptibility to various infectious diseases. A study in Gabon found that children with severe malaria had low serum MBL levels compared with those of children with mild malaria and that mutations in codons 54 and 57 of *MBL2* (which lead to low protein levels) were present at a higher frequency in those with severe malaria (Luty et al. 1998). However, a study in the Gambia failed to replicate this association with severe malaria (Bellamy et al. 1998*b*).

Differences in Resistance to Infection among Inbred Mouse Strains

Inbred strains of mice show marked and consistent differences in their response to malaria infection (Greenberg et al. 1954; Greenberg and Kendrick 1959; Rest 1982; Stevenson et al. 1982; Stevenson and Skamene 1985). Put simply, some mouse strains are more resistant to malaria than are others, but the details are somewhat more complex, since mice that are relatively resistant to one parasite strain may be relatively susceptible to a different parasite strain. For example, some strains of mice are resistant to nonlethal strains but highly susceptible to lethal strains of *Plasmodium yoelii,* whereas other mouse strains show the opposite pattern (Sayles and Wassom 1988). This confirms that both host and parasite genes—and the specific way in which they are combined—are important determinants of resistance or susceptibility to malaria.

Plasmodium chabaudi *Infection: A Model of How the Parasite Population Is Controlled*

P. chabaudi infection is controlled and cleared by some inbred strains of mice (e.g., C57BL/6J, C57L/J, DBA/2J, CBA/J, and B10.A/SgSn) much more effectively than by others (e.g., A/J, DBA/1J, BALB/c, C3H/HeJ, AKR/J, and SJL/J) (Stevenson et al. 1982). At least some of these interstrain differences show classic Mendelian patterns of segregation in crossbreeding experiments and that show resistance is generally dominant over susceptibility. When susceptible A/J and resistant C57BL mice were crossbred, it was found that the degree of splenic enlargement after infection was genetically linked to the ability to suppress parasitemia (Stevenson and Skamene 1985).

Genomewide linkage screens have been performed after crossbreeding susceptible mice (C3H, SJL, or A/J) with resistant mice (C57BL/6J). A locus on chromosome 9 (Char1) determines death or survival (Foote et al. 1997). A well-characterized locus on chromosome 8 (Char2) determines the control of parasite density (Foote et al. 1997; Fortin et al. 1997; Burt et al. 2002). A locus in the MHC region of chromosome 17 (Char3) influences parasite clearance rates at the time immediately after peak parasitemia (Burt et al. 1999).

A further resistance locus (Char4) was identified after deriving recombinant congenic strains from susceptible A/J and resistant C57BL/6J mice. The Char4 locus maps to a small congenic B6 fragment on chromosome 3 (Fortin et al. 2001). Sequencing of candidate genes across this region has identified a plausible functional mutation—namely, a loss-of-function coding variant of the pyruvate kinase gene (*Pklr*). In uninfected animals, this mutation causes hemolytic anemia that is compensated by constitutive reticulocytosis and splenomegaly (Min-Oo et al. 2003, 2004). It is possible that the malaria-protective effect is a direct consequence of impaired viability and increasing splenic clearance of host erythrocytes.

An advanced intercross line population derived from susceptible A/J and resistant C57BL/6J mice was used to identify QTLs for control of parasitemia (Hernandez-Valladares et al. 2004*a*). Of particular interest was a novel QTL (Char 8) in the chromosome 11 region that is homologous to the human 5q31-q33 region discussed above, which is rich in Th2 cytokine genes (Hernandez-Valladares et al. 2004*b*).

Plasmodium berghei *ANKA Infection: A Model of Inflammatory Pathology*

The ANKA strain of *P. berghei* causes more-severe pathology than do most other experimental murine parasites. A curious feature *of P. berghei* ANKA (PBA) infection in some inbred mouse strains (e.g., A/J and C57BL/6) is that 100% of the mice die after 5–8 d, with cerebral hemorrhages as a terminal event (Rest 1982). Cloned lines of PBA differ in their tendency to cause these cerebral changes, which indicates that pathology is determined by a specific combination of host and parasite genotype (Amani et al. 1998).

PBA-induced cerebral pathology is not a reliable model of human cerebral malaria. In particular, parasite sequestration in cerebral capillaries, a hallmark of human cerebral malaria (Taylor et al. 2004), is notable by its absence in the PBA experimental model. The pathological features of PBA in susceptible mouse strains include mononuclear cell adhesion to endothelium, which is absent in human cerebral malaria, together with hemorrhage and cerebral endothelial cell damage, with breakdown of the blood-brain barrier and cerebral edema (Thumwood et al. 1988; Neill and Hunt 1992; Neill et al. 1993). However, PBA has provided an interesting experimental system in which to study how immunopathological processes are affected by different interventions (e.g., Grau et al. [1987*a*, 1987*b*, 1989], Kremsner et al. [1991], Hunt et al. [1993], Engwerda et al. [2002], and Schofield et al. [2002]).

To search for genetic factors that determine PBA-induced cerebral pathology, one approach has been to enlarge the pool of genetic diversity by deriving new inbred mouse strains from wild-mouse populations (Bagot et al. 2002*b*). When a resistant wild-derived inbred strain (WLA) was crossed with a susceptible laboratory strain (C57BL/6J), all of the F_1 progeny and 97% of the F_2 progeny displayed resistance. A genomewide screen, performed after backcrossing the resistant wild strain onto the susceptible laboratory strain, found that resistance was linked to loci on chromosome 1 (Berr1) and chromosome 11 (Berr2) (Bagot et al. 2002*a*).

Recent analysis of the F_2 progeny of WLA and C57BL/6 strains has revealed a fascinating combinatorial effect: it seems that the WLA allele at the Berr1 locus confers resistance to early death from cerebral pathology, whereas the C57Bl/6 allele at a locus on chromosome 9 (Berr3) increases the ability of the mouse to clear the infection. Thus, the progeny have greater resistance to malaria than either of the parental strains (Campino et al. 2005).

A study that crossbred susceptible C57BL/6 mice with resistant DBA/2 mice identified a major resistance locus on chromosome 18 (Nagayasu et al. 2002). Another study that crossed susceptible CBA mice with resistant DBA/2 mice identified a susceptibility locus at the MHC region on chromosome 17 (Ohno and Nishimura 2004).

Conclusions

As geneticists brace themselves to perform genomewide association analysis of common diseases—a task that is going to require massive investment both in epidemiological infrastructure and in genotyping technology—malaria stands out as a target for which this approach is feasible and potentially of huge importance for disease prevention. In terms of feasibility, malaria is the most powerful known force for recent selection of human genetic variants, so malaria-protective polymorphisms are likely to be at high frequencies in affected populations, and, if recently selected, they may also show strong linkage disequilibrium with neighboring genetic markers.

In terms of practical importance for disease prevention, genetic studies of malaria have already yielded results: the observation that Duffy antigen–negative individuals are resistant to infection with *P. vivax* was the starting point of a chain of molecular discovery that led to a candidate vaccine against *P. vivax* that is now undergoing trials. A major impetus for researchers working in this area is the hope that large-scale genomic epidemiology will be a way of getting at basic questions that decades of immunological research have failed to resolve, such as how infected individuals clear parasites from the bloodstream or why malaria causes cerebral complications in some people but not others. The holy grail of this field is to discover novel molecular pathways for protective immunity that will provide critical insights for the development of a vaccine to reduce the massive global burden of disease due to *P. falciparum.*

Malaria research groups across the world have collected DNA samples and detailed clinical data from thousands of individuals with severe malaria, as well as from parents and population controls. Until recently, the resource has been fragmented, with different groups pursuing relatively small studies of their own samples, but there is a growing impetus to link these independent studies to form a global infrastructure for genomic epidemiology of malaria. One such initiative is Malaria Genomic Epidemiology Network (MalariaGEN), which brings together research groups in 15 different malaria-endemic countries. Large-scale epidemiological studies are needed for the sample sizes required to detect modest effects while testing perhaps a million SNP markers (Risch 2000). And once the genome-screening phase has been completed, data from different populations are needed to analyze gene-environment interactions and are needed because haplotypic diversity provides the means to dissect functional polymorphisms from nonfunctional genetic markers.

Finally, it should not be forgotten that, as recently as a century ago, malaria was found in parts of Europe and North America, in addition to its current distribution across most of Africa and large parts of Asia and South America. Sickle-cell disease and thalassemia are two classic examples of how the historical effects of malaria have left an imprint on the pattern of disease in contemporary populations. It remains an open question as to whether any of the immunological, inflammatory, and other chronic diseases that are found in modern societies are, in part, due to the evolutionary pressure that malaria exerted on our ancestors.

Acknowledgments

Funding from the Medical Research Council and the Bill and Melinda Gates Foundation is gratefully acknowledged.

Web Resource

The URL for data presented herein is as follows:

MalariaGEN, http://www.malariagen.net/

References

Abel L, Cot M, Mulder L, Carnevale P, Feingold J (1992) Segregation analysis detects a major gene controlling blood infection levels in human malaria. Am J Hum Genet 50:1308–1317

Abraham LJ, Kroeger KM (1999) Impact of the −308 TNF promoter polymorphism on the transcriptional regulation of the TNF gene: relevance to disease. J Leukoc Biol 66:562–566

Ackerman H, Usen S, Jallow M, Sisay-Joof F, Pinder M, Kwiatkowski DP (2005) A comparison of case-control and family-based association methods: the example of sickle-cell and malaria. Ann Hum Genet (http://www.blackwell-synergy.com/doi/pdf/10.1111/j.1529-8817.2005.00180.x?cookieSet=1) (electronically published April 5, 2005; accessed June 16, 2005)

Ackerman HC, Ribas G, Jallow M, Mott R, Neville M, Sisay-Joof F, Pinder M, Campbell RD, Kwiatkowski DP (2003) Complex haplotypic structure of the central MHC region flanking TNF in a West African population. Genes Immun 4:476–486

Agarwal A, Guindo A, Cissoko Y, Taylor JG, Coulibaly D, Kone A, Kayentao K, Djimde A, Plowe CV, Doumbo O, Wellems TE, Diallo D (2000) Hemoglobin C associated with protection from severe malaria in the Dogon of Mali, a West African population with a low prevalence of hemoglobin S. Blood 96:2358–2363

Aidoo M, McElroy PD, Kolczak MS, Terlouw DJ, ter Kuile FO, Nahlen B, Lal AA, Udhayakumar V (2001) Tumor necrosis factor-alpha promoter variant 2 (TNF2) is associated with pre-term delivery, infant mortality, and malaria morbidity in western Kenya: Asembo Bay Cohort Project IX. Genet Epidemiol 21:201–211

Aitman TJ, Cooper LD, Norsworthy PJ, Wahid FN, Gray JK, Curtis BR, McKeigue PM, Kwiatkowski D, Greenwood BM, Snow RW, Hill AV, Scott J (2000) Malaria susceptibility and CD36 mutation. Nature 405:1015–1016

Allen SJ, Bennett S, Riley EM, Rowe PA, Jakobsen PH, O'Donnell A, Greenwood BM (1992) Morbidity from malaria and immune responses to defined *Plasmodium falciparum* antigens in children with sickle cell trait in the Gambia. Trans R Soc Trop Med Hyg 86:494–498

Allen SJ, O'Donnell A, Alexander ND, Alpers MP, Peto TEA, Clegg JB, Weatherall DJ (1997) α^+-Thalassemia protects children against disease caused by other infections as well as malaria. Proc Natl Acad Sci USA 94:14736–14741

Allen SJ, O'Donnell A, Alexander ND, Mgone CS, Peto TE, Clegg JB, Alpers MP, Weatherall DJ (1999) Prevention of cerebral malaria in children in Papua New Guinea by Southeast Asian ovalocytosis band 3. Am J Trop Med Hyg 60: 1056–1060

Allison AC (1954) Protection afforded by sickle-cell trait against subtertian malareal infection. Br Med J 4857:290–294

Amani V, Boubou MI, Pied S, Marussig M, Walliker D, Mazier D, Renia L (1998) Cloned lines of *Plasmodium berghei* ANKA differ in their abilities to induce experimental cerebral malaria. Infect Immun 66:4093–4099

Arie T, Fairhurst RM, Brittain NJ, Wellems TE, Dvorak JA (2005) Hemoglobin C modulates the surface topography of *Plasmodium falciparum*-infected erythrocytes. J Struct Biol 150:163–169

Aucan C, Walley AJ, Greenwood BM, Hill AV (2002) Haptoglobin genotypes are not associated with resistance to severe malaria in the Gambia. Trans R Soc Trop Med Hyg 96:327–328

Aucan C, Walley AJ, Hennig BJ, Fitness J, Frodsham A, Zhang L, Kwiatkowski D, Hill AV (2003) Interferon-alpha receptor-1 (IFNAR1) variants are associated with protection against cerebral malaria in the Gambia. Genes Immun 4: 275–282

Bagot S, Campino S, Penha-Goncalves C, Pied S, Cazenave PA, Holmberg D (2002*a*) Identification of two cerebral malaria resistance loci using an inbred wild-derived mouse strain. Proc Natl Acad Sci USA 99:9919–9923

Bagot S, Idrissa Boubou M, Campino S, Behrschmidt C, Gorgette O, Guenet JL, Penha-Goncalves C, Mazier D, Pied S, Cazenave PA (2002*b*) Susceptibility to experimental cerebral malaria induced by *Plasmodium berghei* ANKA in inbred mouse strains recently derived from wild stock. Infect Immun 70:2049–2056

Barnwell JW, Asch AS, Nachman RL, Yamaya M, Aikawa M, Ingravallo P (1989) A human 88-kD membrane glycoprotein (CD36) functions in vitro as a receptor for a cytoadherence ligand on *Plasmodium falciparum*-infected erythrocytes. J Clin Invest 84:765–772

Baum J, Ward RH, Conway DJ (2002) Natural selection on the erythrocyte surface. Mol Biol Evol 19:223–229

Bayley JP, Ottenhoff TH, Verweij CL (2004) Is there a future for TNF promoter polymorphisms? Genes Immun 5:315–329

Bellamy R, Kwiatkowski D, Hill AV (1998*a*) Absence of an association between intercellular adhesion molecule 1, complement receptor 1 and interleukin 1 receptor antagonist gene polymorphisms and severe malaria in a West African population. Trans R Soc Trop Med Hyg 92:312–316

Bellamy R, Ruwende C, McAdam KP, Thursz M, Sumiya M, Summerfield J, Gilbert SC, Corrah T, Kwiatkowski D, Whittle HC, Hill AV (1998*b*) Mannose binding protein deficiency is not associated with malaria, hepatitis B carriage nor tuberculosis in Africans. QJM 91:13–18

Bennett S, Allen SJ, Olerup O, Jackson DJ, Wheeler JG, Rowe PA, Riley EM, Greenwood BM (1993) Human leucocyte antigen (HLA) and malaria morbidity in a Gambian community. Trans R Soc Trop Med Hyg 87:286–287

Berendt AR, Simmons DL, Tansey J, Newbold CI, Marsh K (1989) Intercellular adhesion molecule-1 is an endothelial cell adhesion receptor for *Plasmodium falciparum*. Nature 341:57–59

Bienzle U, Ayeni O, Lucas AO, Luzzatto L (1972) Glucose-6-phosphate dehydrogenase and malaria: greater resistance of females heterozygous for enzyme deficiency and of males with non-deficient variant. Lancet 1:107–110

Brittenham GM, Schechter AN, Noguchi CT (1985) Hemoglobin S polymerization: primary determinant of the hemolytic and clinical severity of the sickling syndromes. Blood 65:183–189

Burgner D, Usen S, Rockett K, Jallow M, Ackerman H, Cervino A, Pinder M, Kwiatkowski DP (2003) Nucleotide and haplotypic diversity of the NOS2A promoter region and its relationship to cerebral malaria. Hum Genet 112:379–386

Burgner D, Xu W, Rockett K, Gravenor M, Charles IG, Hill AV, Kwiatkowski D (1998) Inducible nitric oxide synthase polymorphism and fatal cerebral malaria. Lancet 352:1193–1194

Burt RA, Baldwin TM, Marshall VM, Foote SJ (1999) Temporal expression of an H2-linked locus in host response to mouse malaria. Immunogenetics 50:278–285

Burt RA, Marshall VM, Wagglen J, Rodda FR, Senyschen D, Baldwin TM, Buckingham LA, Foote SJ (2002) Mice that are congenic for the char2 locus are susceptible to malaria. Infect Immun 70:4750–4753

Campino S, Bagot S, Bergman ML, Almeida P, Sepulveda N, Pied S, Penha-Goncalves C, Holmberg D, Cazenave PA (2005) Genetic control of parasite clearance leads to resistance to *Plasmodium berghei* ANKA infection and confers immunity. Genes Immun (http://www.nature.com/gene/journal/vaop/ncurrent/full/6364219a.html) (electronically published June 23, 2005; accessed July 1, 2005)

Casals-Pascual C, Allen S, Allen A, Kai O, Lowe B, Pain A, Roberts DJ (2001) Short report: codon 125 polymorphism of CD31 and susceptibility to malaria. Am J Trop Med Hyg 65:736–737

Cattani JA, Gibson FD, Alpers MP, Crane GG (1987) Hereditary ovalocytosis and reduced susceptibility to malaria in Papua New Guinea. Trans R Soc Trop Med Hyg 81:705–709

Chebloune Y, Pagnier J, Trabuchet G, Faure C, Verdier G, Labie D, Nigon V (1988) Structural analysis of the 5′ flanking region of the beta-globin gene in African sickle cell anemia patients: further evidence for three origins of the sickle cell mutation in Africa. Proc Natl Acad Sci USA 85:4431–4435

Chitnis CE, Miller LH (1994) Identification of the erythrocyte binding domains of *Plasmodium vivax* and *Plasmodium knowlesi* proteins involved in erythrocyte invasion. J Exp Med 180:497–506

Chotivanich K, Udomsangpetch R, Pattanapanyasat K, Chierakul W, Simpson J, Looareesuwan S, White N (2002) Hemoglobin E: a balanced polymorphism protective against high parasitemias and thus severe *P. falciparum* malaria. Blood 100:1172–1176

Clark IA, Alleva LM, Mills AC, Cowden WB (2004) Pathogenesis of malaria and clinically similar conditions. Clin Microbiol Rev 17:509–539

Clark IA, Rockett KA (1996) Nitric oxide and parasitic disease. Adv Parasitol 37:1–56

Cockburn IA, Mackinnon MJ, O'Donnell A, Allen SJ, Moulds JM, Baisor M, Bockarie M, Reeder JC, Rowe JA (2004) A human complement receptor 1 polymorphism that reduces *Plasmodium falciparum* rosetting confers protection against severe malaria. Proc Natl Acad Sci USA 101:272–277

Coluzzi M (1999) The clay feet of the malaria giant and its African roots: hypotheses and inferences about origin, spread and control of *Plasmodium falciparum*. Parassitologia 41:277–283

Coluzzi M, Sabatini A, della Torre A, Di Deco MA, Petrarca V (2002) A polytene chromosome analysis of the *Anopheles gambiae* species complex. Science 298:1415–1418

Conway DJ (2003) Tracing the dawn of *Plasmodium falciparum* with mitochondrial genome sequences. Trends Genet 19:671–674

Cooke GS, Aucan C, Walley AJ, Segal S, Greenwood BM, Kwiatkowski DP, Hill AV (2003) Association of Fcgamma receptor IIa (CD32) polymorphism with severe malaria in West Africa. Am J Trop Med Hyg 69:565–568

Cot M, Abel L, Roisin A, Barro D, Yada A, Carnevale P, Feingold J (1993) Risk factors of malaria infection during pregnancy in Burkina Faso: suggestion of a genetic influence. Am J Trop Med Hyg 48:358–364

Diallo DA, Doumbo OK, Dicko A, Guindo A, Coulibaly D, Kayentao K, Djimde AA, Thera MA, Fairhurst RM, Plowe CV, Wellems TE (2004) A comparison of anemia in hemoglobin C and normal hemoglobin A children with *Plasmodium falciparum* malaria. Acta Trop 90:295–299

Dolo A, Modiano D, Maiga B, Daou M, Dolo G, Guindo H, Ba M, Maiga H, Coulibaly D, Perlman H, Blomberg MT, Toure YT, Coluzzi M, Doumbo O (2005) Difference in susceptibility to malaria between two sympatric ethnic groups in Mali. Am J Trop Med Hyg 72:243–248

Elagib AA, Kider AO, Akerstrom B, Elbashir MI (1998) Association of the haptoglobin phenotype (1-1) with *falciparum* malaria in Sudan. Trans R Soc Trop Med Hyg 92:309–311

Engwerda CR, Mynott TL, Sawhney S, De Souza JB, Bickle QD, Kaye PM (2002) Locally up-regulated lymphotoxin alpha, not systemic tumor necrosis factor alpha, is the principle mediator of murine cerebral malaria. J Exp Med 195: 1371–1377

Facer CA (1983) Merozoites of *P. falciparum* require glycophorin for invasion into red cells. Bull Soc Pathol Exot Filiales 76:463–469

Fairhurst RM, Baruch DI, Brittain NJ, Ostera GR, Wallach JS, Hoang HL, Hayton K, Guindo A, Makobongo MO, Schwartz OM, Tounkara A, Doumbo OK, Diallo DA, Fujioka H, Ho M, Wellems TE (2005) Abnormal display of PfEMP-1 on erythrocytes carrying haemoglobin C may protect against malaria. Nature 435:1117–1121

Farouk SE, Dolo A, Bereczky S, Kouriba B, Maiga B, Farnert A, Perlmann H, Hayano M, Montgomery SM, Doumbo OK, Troye-Blomberg M (2005) Different antibody- and cytokine-mediated responses to *Plasmodium falciparum* parasite in two sympatric ethnic tribes living in Mali. Microbes Infect 7:110–117

Feng Z, Smith DL, McKenzie FE, Levin SA (2004) Coupling ecology and evolution: malaria and the S-gene across time scales. Math Biosci 189:1–19

Fernandez-Reyes D, Craig AG, Kyes SA, Peshu N, Snow RW, Berendt AR, Marsh K, Newbold CI (1997) A high frequency African coding polymorphism in the N-terminal domain of ICAM-1 predisposing to cerebral malaria in Kenya. Hum Mol Genet 6:1357–1360

Flint J, Harding RM, Boyce AJ, Clegg JB (1998) The population genetics of the haemoglobinopathies. Baillieres Clin Haematol 11:1–51

Flint J, Hill AVS, Bowden DK, Oppenheimer SJ, Sill PR, Serjeantson SW, Bana-Koiri J, Bhatia K, Alpers MP, Boyce AJ, Weatherall DJ, Clegg JB (1986) High frequencies of alpha-thalassaemia are the result of natural selection by malaria. Nature 321:744–750

Flori L, Delahaye NF, Iraqi FA, Hernandez-Valladares M, Fumoux F, Rihet P (2005) TNF as a malaria candidate gene: polymorphism-screening and family-based association analysis of mild malaria attack and parasitemia in Burkina Faso. Genes Immun (http://www.nature.com/gene/journal/vaop/ncurrent/full/6364231a.html) (electronically published June 2, 2005; accessed June 16, 2005)

Flori L, Sawadogo S, Esnault C, Delahaye NF, Fumoux F, Rihet P (2003) Linkage of mild malaria to the major histocompatibility complex in families living in Burkina Faso. Hum Mol Genet 12:375–378

Foo LC, Rekhraj V, Chiang GL, Mak JW (1992) Ovalocytosis protects against severe malaria parasitemia in the Malayan aborigines. Am J Trop Med Hyg 47:271–275

Foote SJ, Burt RA, Baldwin TM, Presente A, Roberts AW, Laural YL, Lew AM, Marshall VM (1997) Mouse loci for malaria-induced mortality and the control of parasitaemia. Nat Genet 17:380–381

Fortin A, Belouchi A, Tam MF, Cardon L, Skamene E, Stevenson MM, Gros P (1997) Genetic control of blood parasitaemia in mouse malaria maps to chromosome 8. Nat Genet 17:382–383

Fortin A, Cardon LR, Tam M, Skamene E, Stevenson MM, Gros P (2001) Identification of a new malaria susceptibility locus (Char4) in recombinant congenic strains of mice. Proc Natl Acad Sci USA 98:10793–10798

Ganczakowski M, Town M, Bowden DK, Vulliamy TJ, Kaneko A, Clegg JB, Weatherall DJ, Luzzatto L (1995) Multiple glucose 6-phosphate dehydrogenase–deficient variants correlate with malaria endemicity in the Vanuatu archipelago (southwestern Pacific). Am J Hum Genet 56:294–301

Garcia A, Cot M, Chippaux JP, Ranque S, Feingold J, Demenais F, Abel L (1998*a*) Genetic control of blood infection levels in human malaria: evidence for a complex genetic model. Am J Trop Med Hyg 58:480–488

Garcia A, Marquet S, Bucheton B, Hillaire D, Cot M, Fievet N, Dessein AJ, Abel L (1998*b*) Linkage analysis of blood *Plasmodium falciparum* levels: interest of the 5q31-q33 chromosome region. Am J Trop Med Hyg 58:705–709

Genton B, al-Yaman F, Mgone CS, Alexander N, Paniu MM, Alpers MP, Mokela D (1995) Ovalocytosis and cerebral malaria. Nature 378:564–565

Gilbert SC, Plebanski M, Gupta S, Morris J, Cox M, Aidoo M, Kwiatkowski D, Greenwood BM, Whittle HC, Hill AV (1998) Association of malaria parasite population structure, HLA, and immunological antagonism. Science 279:1173–1177

Gilles HM, Fletcher KA, Hendrickse RG, Lindner R, Reddy S, Allan N (1967) Glucose-6-phosphate-dehydrogenase deficiency, sickling, and malaria in African children in South Western Nigeria. Lancet 1:138–140

Grau GE, Fajardo LF, Piguet PF, Allet B, Lambert PH, Vassalli

P (1987*a*) Tumor necrosis factor (cachectin) as an essential mediator in murine cerebral malaria. Science 237:1210–1212

Grau GE, Gretener D, Lambert PH (1987*b*) Prevention of murine cerebral malaria by low-dose cyclosporin A. Immunology 61:521–525

Grau GE, Heremans H, Piguet PF, Pointaire P, Lambert PH, Billiau A, Vassalli P (1989) Monoclonal antibody against interferon gamma can prevent experimental cerebral malaria and its associated overproduction of tumor necrosis factor. Proc Natl Acad Sci USA 86:5572–5574

Greenberg J, Kendrick LP (1959) Resistance to malaria in hybrids between Swiss and certain other strains of mice. J Parasitol 45:263–267

Greenberg J, Nadel EM, Coatney GR (1954) Differences in survival of several inbred strains of mice and their hybrids infected with *Plasmodium berghei.* J Infect Dis 95:114–116

Hadley TJ, Klotz FW, Pasvol G, Haynes JD, McGinniss MH, Okubo Y, Miller LH (1987) Falciparum malaria parasites invade erythrocytes that lack glycophorin A and B (MkMk): strain differences indicate receptor heterogeneity and two pathways for invasion. J Clin Invest 80:1190–1193

Haldane JBS (1949) Disease and evolution. Ricerca Sci Suppl 19:3–10

Hamblin MT, Di Rienzo A (2000) Detection of the signature of natural selection in humans: evidence from the Duffy blood group locus. Am J Hum Genet 66:1669–1679

Hamblin MT, Thompson EE, Di Rienzo A (2002) Complex signatures of natural selection at the Duffy blood group locus. Am J Hum Genet 70:369–383

Hartl DL (2004) The origin of malaria: mixed messages from genetic diversity. Nat Rev Microbiol 2:15–22

Hedrick P (2004) Estimation of relative fitnesses from relative risk data and the predicted future of haemoglobin alleles S and C. J Evol Biol 17:221–224

Hernandez-Valladares M, Naessens J, Gibson JP, Musoke AJ, Nagda S, Rihet P, ole-MoiYoi OK, Iraqi FA (2004*a*) Confirmation and dissection of QTL controlling resistance to malaria in mice. Mamm Genome 15:390–398

Hernandez-Valladares M, Rihet P, ole-MoiYoi OK, Iraqi FA (2004*b*) Mapping of a new quantitative trait locus for resistance to malaria in mice by a comparative mapping approach with human chromosome 5q31-q33. Immunogenetics 56:115–117

Hill AV, Allsopp CE, Kwiatkowski D, Anstey NM, Twumasi P, Rowe PA, Bennett S, Brewster D, McMichael AJ, Greenwood BM (1991) Common West African HLA antigens are associated with protection from severe malaria. Nature 352: 595–600

Hill AVS, Elvin J, Willis AC, Aidoo M, Allsopp CEM, Gotch FM, Gao XM, Takiguchi M, Greenwood BM, Townsend ARM, McMichael AJ, Whittle HC (1992) Molecular analysis of the association of HLA-B53 and resistance to severe malaria. Nature 360:434–439

Hobbs MR, Udhayakumar V, Levesque MC, Booth J, Roberts JM, Tkachuk AN, Pole A, Coon H, Kariuki S, Nahlen BL, Mwaikambo ED, Lal AL, Granger DL, Anstey NM, Weinberg JB (2002) A new NOS2 promoter polymorphism associated with increased nitric oxide production and protection from severe malaria in Tanzanian and Kenyan children. Lancet 360:1468–1475

Hunt NH, Driussi C, Sai-Kiang L (2001) Haptoglobin and malaria. Redox Rep 6:389–392

Hunt NH, Manduci N, Thumwood CM (1993) Amelioration of murine cerebral malaria by dietary restriction. Parasitology 107:471–476

Imrie H, Ferguson DJ, Day KP (2004) Human serum haptoglobin is toxic to *Plasmodium falciparum* in vitro. Mol Biochem Parasitol 133:93–98

Jepson A, Sisay-Joof F, Banya W, Hassan-King M, Frodsham A, Bennett S, Hill AV, Whittle H (1997) Genetic linkage of mild malaria to the major histocompatibility complex in Gambian children: study of affected sibling pairs. BMJ 315:96–97

Jepson AP, Banya WA, Sisay-Joof F, Hassan-King M, Bennett S, Whittle HC (1995) Genetic regulation of fever in *Plasmodium falciparum* malaria in Gambian twin children. J Infect Dis 172:316–319

Joy DA, Feng X, Mu J, Furuya T, Chotivanich K, Krettli AU, Ho M, Wang A, White NJ, Suh E, Beerli P, Su XZ (2003) Early origin and recent expansion of *Plasmodium falciparum.* Science 300:318–321

Juliger S, Bongartz M, Luty AJ, Kremsner PG, Kun JF (2003) Functional analysis of a promoter variant of the gene encoding the interferon-gamma receptor chain I. Immunogenetics 54:675–680

Kikuchi M, Looareesuwan S, Ubalee R, Tasanor O, Suzuki F, Wattanagoon Y, Na-Bangchang K, Kimura A, Aikawa M, Hirayama K (2001) Association of adhesion molecule PECAM-1/CD31 polymorphism with susceptibility to cerebral malaria in Thais. Parasitol Int 50:235–239

Knight JC, Keating BJ, Rockett KA, Kwiatkowski DP (2003) In vivo characterization of regulatory polymorphisms by allele-specific quantification of RNA polymerase loading. Nat Genet 33:469–475

Knight JC, Udalova I, Hill AV, Greenwood BM, Peshu N, Marsh K, Kwiatkowski D (1999) A polymorphism that affects OCT-1 binding to the TNF promoter region is associated with severe malaria. Nat Genet 22:145–150

Koch O, Awomoyi A, Usen S, Jallow M, Richardson A, Hull J, Pinder M, Newport M, Kwiatkowski D (2002) IFNGR1 gene promoter polymorphisms and susceptibility to cerebral malaria. J Infect Dis 185:1684–1687

Koch O, Rockett K, Jallow M, Pinder M, Sisay-Joof F, Kwiatkowski D (2005) Investigation of malaria susceptibility determinants in the IFNG/IL26/IL22 genomic region. Genes Immun 6:312–318

Kremsner PG, Grundmann H, Neifer S, Sliwa K, Sahlmuller G, Hegenscheid B, Bienzle U (1991) Pentoxifylline prevents murine cerebral malaria. J Infect Dis 164:605–608

Kun JF, Klabunde J, Lell B, Luckner D, Alpers M, May J, Meyer C, Kremsner PG (1999) Association of the ICAM-1^{Kilifi} mutation with protection against severe malaria in Lambarene, Gabon. Am J Trop Med Hyg 61:776–779

Kun JF, Mordmuller B, Lell B, Lehman LG, Luckner D, Kremsner PG (1998) Polymorphism in promoter region of inducible nitric oxide synthase gene and protection against malaria. Lancet 351:265–266

Kun JF, Mordmuller B, Perkins DJ, May J, Mercereau-Puijalon O, Alpers M, Weinberg JB, Kremsner PG (2001) Nitric oxide synthase 2(Lambarene) (G-954C), increased nitric oxide production, and protection against malaria. J Infect Dis 184: 330–336

Kwiatkowski D (1995) Malarial toxins and the regulation of parasite density. Parasitol Today 11:206–212

Kyes S, Horrocks P, Newbold C (2001) Antigenic variation at the infected red cell surface in malaria. Annu Rev Microbiol 55:673–707

Lapoumeroulie C, Dunda O, Ducrocq R, Trabuchet G, Mony-Lobe M, Bodo JM, Carnevale P, Labie D, Elion J, Krishnamoorthy R (1992) A novel sickle cell mutation of yet another origin in Africa: the Cameroon type. Hum Genet 89:333–337

Levesque MC, Hobbs MR, Anstey NM, Vaughn TN, Chancellor JA, Pole A, Perkins DJ, Misukonis MA, Chanock SJ, Granger DL, Weinberg JB (1999) Nitric oxide synthase type 2 promoter polymorphisms, nitric oxide production, and disease severity in Tanzanian children with malaria. J Infect Dis 180:1994–2002

Luoni G, Verra F, Arca B, Sirima BS, Troye-Blomberg M, Coluzzi M, Kwiatkowski D, Modiano D (2001) Antimalarial antibody levels and IL4 polymorphism in the Fulani of West Africa. Genes Immun 2:411–414

Luty AJ, Kun JF, Kremsner PG (1998) Mannose-binding lectin plasma levels and gene polymorphisms in *Plasmodium falciparum* malaria. J Infect Dis 178:1221–1224

Luzzatto L, Usanga FA, Reddy S (1969) Glucose-6-phosphate dehydrogenase deficient red cells: resistance to infection by malarial parasites. Science 164:839–842

Mackinnon MJ, Gunawardena DM, Rajakaruna J, Weerasingha S, Mendis KN, Carter R (2000) Quantifying genetic and nongenetic contributions to malarial infection in a Sri Lankan population. Proc Natl Acad Sci USA 97:12661–12666

Maier AG, Duraisingh MT, Reeder JC, Patel SS, Kazura JW, Zimmerman PA, Cowman AF (2003) *Plasmodium falciparum* erythrocyte invasion through glycophorin C and selection for Gerbich negativity in human populations. Nat Med 9:87–92

Marsh K, Forster D, Waruiru C, Mwangi I, Winstanley M, Marsh V, Newton C, Winstanley P, Warn P, Peshu N, Pasvol G, Snow R (1995) Indicators of life-threatening malaria in African children. N Engl J Med 332:1399–1404

Mayor A, Bir N, Sawhney R, Singh S, Pattnaik P, Singh SK, Sharma A, Chitnis CE (2005) Receptor-binding residues lie in central regions of Duffy-binding-like domains involved in red cell invasion and cytoadherence by malaria parasites. Blood 105:2557–2563

McGuire W, Hill AV, Allsopp CE, Greenwood BM, Kwiatkowski D (1994) Variation in the TNF-alpha promoter region associated with susceptibility to cerebral malaria. Nature 371:508–510

McGuire W, Knight JC, Hill AV, Allsopp CE, Greenwood BM, Kwiatkowski D (1999) Severe malarial anemia and cerebral malaria are associated with different tumor necrosis factor promoter alleles. J Infect Dis 179:287–290

Meyer CG, May J, Luty AJ, Lell B, Kremsner PG (2002) TNFalpha-308A associated with shorter intervals of *Plasmodium falciparum* reinfections. Tissue Antigens 59:287–292

Michon P, Woolley I, Wood EM, Kastens W, Zimmerman PA, Adams JH (2001) Duffy-null promoter heterozygosity reduces DARC expression and abrogates adhesion of the *P. vivax* ligand required for blood-stage infection. FEBS Lett 495:111–114

Miller LH, Mason SJ, Clyde DF, McGinniss MH (1976) The resistance factor to *Plasmodium vivax* in blacks: the Duffy-blood-group genotype, FyFy. N Engl J Med 295:302–304

Min-Oo G, Fortin A, Tam MF, Gros P, Stevenson MM (2004) Phenotypic expression of pyruvate kinase deficiency and protection against malaria in a mouse model. Genes Immun 5: 168–175

Min-Oo G, Fortin A, Tam MF, Nantel A, Stevenson MM, Gros P (2003) Pyruvate kinase deficiency in mice protects against malaria. Nat Genet 35:357–362

Mockenhaupt FP, Ehrhardt S, Cramer JP, Otchwemah RN, Anemana SD, Goltz K, Mylius F, Dietz E, Eggelte TA, Bienzle U (2004*a*) Hemoglobin C and resistance to severe malaria in Ghanaian children. J Infect Dis 190:1006–1009

Mockenhaupt FP, Ehrhardt S, Gellert S, Otchwemah RN, Dietz E, Anemana SD, Bienzle U (2004*b*) Alpha($^{+}$)-thalassemia protects African children from severe malaria. Blood 104: 2003–2006

Modiano D, Chiucchiuini A, Petrarca V, Sirima BS, Luoni G, Perlmann H, Esposito F, Coluzzi M (1998) Humoral response to *Plasmodium falciparum* Pf155/ring-infected erythrocyte surface antigen and Pf332 in three sympatric ethnic groups of Burkina Faso. Am J Trop Med Hyg 58:220–224

Modiano D, Chiucchiuini A, Petrarca V, Sirima BS, Luoni G, Roggero MA, Corradin G, Coluzzi M, Esposito F (1999) Interethnic differences in the humoral response to non-repetitive regions of the *Plasmodium falciparum* circumsporozoite protein. Am J Trop Med Hyg 61:663–667

Modiano D, Luoni G, Sirima BS, Lanfrancotti A, Petrarca V, Cruciani F, Simpore J, Ciminelli BM, Foglietta E, Grisanti P, Bianco I, Modiano G, Coluzzi M (2001*a*) The lower susceptibility to *Plasmodium falciparum* malaria of Fulani of Burkina Faso (West Africa) is associated with low frequencies of classic malaria-resistance genes. Trans R Soc Trop Med Hyg 95:149–152

Modiano D, Luoni G, Sirima BS, Simpore J, Verra F, Konate A, Rastrelli E, Olivieri A, Calissano C, Paganotti GM, D'Urbano L, Sanou I, Sawadogo A, Modiano G, Coluzzi M (2001*b*) Haemoglobin C protects against clinical *Plasmodium falciparum* malaria. Nature 414:305–308

Modiano D, Petrarca V, Sirima BS, Nebie I, Diallo D, Esposito F, Coluzzi M (1996) Different response to *Plasmodium falciparum* malaria in West African sympatric ethnic groups. Proc Natl Acad Sci USA 93:13206–13211

Modiano G, Morpurgo G, Terrenato L, Novelletto A, Di Rienzo A, Colombo B, Purpura M, Mariani M, Santachiara-Benerecetti S, Brega A, Dixit KA, Shrestha SL, Lania A, Wanachiwanawin W, Luzzatto L (1991) Protection against malaria morbidity: near-fixation of the α-thalassemia gene in a Nepalese population. Am J Hum Genet 48:390–397

Morahan G, Boutlis CS, Huang D, Pain A, Saunders JR, Hobbs MR, Granger DL, Weinberg JB, Peshu N, Mwaikambo ED, Marsh K, Roberts DJ, Anstey NM (2002) A promoter polymorphism in the gene encoding interleukin-12 p40 (IL12B) is associated with mortality from cerebral malaria and with reduced nitric oxide production. Genes Immun 3:414–418

Nagayasu E, Ito M, Akaki M, Nakano Y, Kimura M, Looareesuwan S, Aikawa M (2001) CR1 density polymorphism on erythrocytes of falciparum malaria patients in Thailand. Am J Trop Med Hyg 64:1–5

Nagayasu E, Nagakura K, Akaki M, Tamiya G, Makino S, Nakano Y, Kimura M, Aikawa M (2002) Association of a determinant on mouse chromosome 18 with experimental severe *Plasmodium berghei* malaria. Infect Immun 70:512–516

Nagel RL, Ranney HM (1990) Genetic epidemiology of structural mutations of the beta-globin gene. Semin Hematol 27: 342–359

Neill AL, Chan-Ling T, Hunt NH (1993) Comparisons between microvascular changes in cerebral and non-cerebral malaria in mice, using the retinal whole-mount technique. Parasitology 107:477–487

Neill AL, Hunt NH (1992) Pathology of fatal and resolving *Plasmodium berghei* cerebral malaria in mice. Parasitology 105:165–175

Ohashi J, Naka I, Patarapotikul J, Hananantachai H, Brittenham G, Looareesuwan S, Clark AG, Tokunaga K (2004) Extended linkage disequilibrium surrounding the hemoglobin E variant due to malarial selection. Am J Hum Genet 74:1198–1208

Ohno T, Nishimura M (2004) Detection of a new cerebral malaria susceptibility locus, using CBA mice. Immunogenetics 56:675–678

Omi K, Ohashi J, Patarapotikul J, Hananantachai H, Naka I, Looareesuwan S, Tokunaga K (2002) Fcgamma receptor IIA and IIIB polymorphisms are associated with susceptibility to cerebral malaria. Parasitol Int 51:361–366

——— (2003) CD36 polymorphism is associated with protection from cerebral malaria. Am J Hum Genet 72:364–374

Orlandi PA, Klotz FW, Haynes JD (1992) A malaria invasion receptor, the 175-kilodalton erythrocyte binding antigen of *Plasmodium falciparum* recognizes the terminal Neu5Ac (alpha 2–3)Gal- sequences of glycophorin A. J Cell Biol 116: 901–909

Pain A, Urban BC, Kai O, Casals-Pascual C, Shafi J, Marsh K, Roberts DJ (2001) A non-sense mutation in Cd36 gene is associated with protection from severe malaria. Lancet 357:1502–1503

Pasvol G, Weatherall DJ, Wilson RJ (1978) Cellular mechanism for the protective effect of haemoglobin S against *P. falciparum* malaria. Nature 274:701–703

Patel SS, King CL, Mgone CS, Kazura JW, Zimmerman PA (2004) Glycophorin C (Gerbich antigen blood group) and band 3 polymorphisms in two malaria holoendemic regions of Papua New Guinea. Am J Hematol 75:1–5

Patel SS, Mehlotra RK, Kastens W, Mgone CS, Kazura JW, Zimmerman PA (2001) The association of the glycophorin C exon 3 deletion with ovalocytosis and malaria susceptibility in the Wosera, Papua New Guinea. Blood 98:3489–3491

Pattanapanyasat K, Yongvanitchit K, Tongtawe P, Tachavanich K, Wanachiwanawin W, Fucharoen S, Walsh DS (1999) Impairment of *Plasmodium falciparum* growth in thalassemic red blood cells: further evidence by using biotin labeling and flow cytometry. Blood 93:3116–3119

Pauling L, Itano HA, Singer SJ, Wells IC (1949) Sickle cell anemia a molecular disease. Science 110:543–548

Quaye IK, Ekuban FA, Goka BQ, Adabayeri V, Kurtzhals JA, Gyan B, Ankrah NA, Hviid L, Akanmori BD (2000) Haptoglobin 1-1 is associated with susceptibility to severe *Plasmodium falciparum* malaria. Trans R Soc Trop Med Hyg 94: 216–219

Ranque S, Safeukui I, Poudiougou B, Traore A, Keita M, Traore D, Diakite M, Cisse MB, Keita MM, Doumbo OK, Dessein AJ (2005) Familial aggregation of cerebral malaria and severe malarial anemia. J Infect Dis 191:799–804

Rest JR (1982) Cerebral malaria in inbred mice. I. A new model and its pathology. Trans R Soc Trop Med Hyg 76:410–415

Rihet P, Abel L, Traore Y, Traore-Leroux T, Aucan C, Fumoux F (1998*a*) Human malaria: segregation analysis of blood infection levels in a suburban area and a rural area in Burkina Faso. Genet Epidemiol 15:435–450

Rihet P, Flori L, Tall F, Traore AS, Fumoux F (2004) Hemoglobin C is associated with reduced *Plasmodium falciparum* parasitemia and low risk of mild malaria attack. Hum Mol Genet 13:1–6

Rihet P, Traore Y, Abel L, Aucan C, Traoré-Leroux T, Fumoux F (1998*b*) Malaria in humans: *Plasmodium falciparum* blood infection levels are linked to chromosome 5q31-q33. Am J Hum Genet 63:498–505

Risch NJ (2000) Searching for genetic determinants in the new millennium. Nature 405:847–856

Roberts DJ, Craig AG, Berendt AR, Pinches R, Nash G, Marsh K, Newbold CI (1992) Rapid switching to multiple antigenic and adhesive phenotypes in malaria. Nature 357:689–692

Rowe JA, Moulds JM, Newbold CI, Miller LH (1997) *P. falciparum* rosetting mediated by a parasite-variant erythrocyte membrane protein and complement-receptor 1. Nature 388: 292–295

Ruwende C, Hill A (1998) Glucose-6-phosphate dehydrogenase deficiency and malaria. J Mol Med 76:581–588

Ruwende C, Khoo SC, Snow RW, Yates SN, Kwiatkowski D, Gupta S, Warn P, Allsopp CE, Gilbert SC, Peschu N, Newbold CI, Greenwood BM, Marsh K, Hill AVS (1995) Natural selection of hemi- and heterozygotes for G6PD deficiency in Africa by resistance to severe malaria. Nature 376:246–249

Sabeti P, Usen S, Farhadian S, Jallow M, Doherty T, Newport M, Pinder M, Ward R, Kwiatkowski D (2002*a*) CD40L association with protection from severe malaria. Genes Immun 3:286–291

Sabeti PC, Reich DE, Higgins JM, Levine HZ, Richter DJ, Schaffner SF, Gabriel SB, Platko JV, Patterson NJ, McDonald GJ, Ackerman HC, Campbell SJ, Altshuler D, Cooper R, Kwiatkowski D, Ward R, Lander ES (2002*b*) Detecting recent positive selection in the human genome from haplotype structure. Nature 419:832–837

Sayles PC, Wassom DL (1988) Immunoregulation in murine malaria: susceptibility of inbred mice to infection with *Plasmodium yoelii* depends on the dynamic interplay of host and parasite genes. J Immunol 141:241–248

Schofield L, Hewitt MC, Evans K, Siomos MA, Seeberger PH (2002) Synthetic GPI as a candidate anti-toxic vaccine in a model of malaria. Nature 418:785–789

Sengupta S, Farheen S, Mukherjee N, Dey B, Mukhopadhyay B, Sil SK, Prabhakaran N, Ramesh A, Edwin D, Usha Rani MV, Mitra M, Mahadik CT, Singh S, Sehgal SC, Majumder PP (2004) DNA sequence variation and haplotype structure of the ICAM1 and TNF genes in 12 ethnic groups of India reveal patterns of importance in designing association studies. Ann Hum Genet 68:574–587

Shear HL, Roth EF Jr, Fabry ME, Costantini FD, Pachnis A, Hood A, Nagel RL (1993) Transgenic mice expressing human sickle hemoglobin are partially resistant to rodent malaria. Blood 81:222–226

Shi YP, Nahlen BL, Kariuki S, Urdahl KB, McElroy PD, Roberts JM, Lal AA (2001) Fcgamma receptor IIa (CD32) polymorphism is associated with protection of infants against high-density *Plasmodium falciparum* infection. VII. Asembo Bay Cohort Project. J Infect Dis 184:107–111

Sibley LD (2004) Intracellular parasite invasion strategies. Science 304:248–253

Sjoberg K, Lepers JP, Raharimalala L, Larsson A, Olerup O, Marbiah NT, Troye-Blomberg M, Perlmann P (1992) Genetic regulation of human anti-malarial antibodies in twins. Proc Natl Acad Sci USA 89:2101–2104

Snow RW, Guerra CA, Noor AM, Myint HY, Hay SI (2005) The global distribution of clinical episodes of *Plasmodium falciparum* malaria. Nature 434:214–217

Snow RW, Omumbo JA, Lowe B, Molyneux CS, Obiero JO, Palmer A, Weber MW, Pinder M, Nahlen B, Obonyo C, Newbold C, Gupta S, Marsh K (1997) Relation between severe malaria morbidity in children and level of *Plasmodium falciparum* transmission in Africa. Lancet 349:1650–1654

Sokhna CS, Rogier C, Dieye A, Trape JF (2000) Host factors affecting the delay of reappearance of *Plasmodium falciparum* after radical treatment among a semi-immune population exposed to intense perennial transmission. Am J Trop Med Hyg 62:266–270

Stevenson MM, Lyanga JJ, Skamene E (1982) Murine malaria: genetic control of resistance to *Plasmodium chabaudi*. Infect Immun 38:80–88

Stevenson MM, Riley EM (2004) Innate immunity to malaria. Nat Rev Immunol 4:169–180

Stevenson MM, Skamene E (1985) Murine malaria: resistance of AXB/BXA recombinant inbred mice to *Plasmodium chabaudi*. Infect Immun 47:452–456

Stirnadel HA, Al-Yaman F, Genton B, Alpers MP, Smith TA (2000*a*) Assessment of different sources of variation in the antibody responses to specific malaria antigens in children in Papua New Guinea. Int J Epidemiol 29:579–586

Stirnadel HA, Beck HP, Alpers MP, Smith TA (1999*a*) Heritability and segregation analysis of immune responses to specific malaria antigens in Papua New Guinea. Genet Epidemiol 17:16–34

——— (2000*b*) Genetic analysis of IgG subclass responses against RESA and MSP2 of *Plasmodium falciparum* in adults in Papua New Guinea. Epidemiol Infect 124:153–162

Stirnadel HA, Stockle M, Felger I, Smith T, Tanner M, Beck HP (1999*b*) Malaria infection and morbidity in infants in relation to genetic polymorphisms in Tanzania. Trop Med Int Health 4:187–193

Taylor TE, Fu WJ, Carr RA, Whitten RO, Mueller JS, Fosiko NG, Lewallen S, Liomba NG, Molyneux ME (2004) Differentiating the pathologies of cerebral malaria by postmortem parasite counts. Nat Med 10:143–145

Terrenato L, Shrestha S, Dixit KA, Luzzatto L, Modiano G, Morpurgo G, Arese P (1988) Decreased malaria morbidity in the Tharu people compared to sympatric populations in Nepal. Ann Trop Med Parasitol 82:1–11

Thumwood CM, Hunt NH, Clark IA, Cowden WB (1988) Breakdown of the blood-brain barrier in murine cerebral malaria. Parasitology 96:579–589

Tishkoff SA, Varkonyi R, Cahinhinan N, Abbes S, Argyropoulos G, Destro-Bisol G, Drousiotou A, Dangerfield B, Lefranc G, Loiselet J, Piro A, Stoneking M, Tagarelli A, Tagarelli G, Touma EH, Williams SM, Clark AG (2001) Haplotype diversity and linkage disequilibrium at human G6PD: recent origin of alleles that confer malarial resistance. Science 293: 455–462

Tishkoff SA, Williams SM (2002) Genetic analysis of African populations: human evolution and complex disease. Nat Rev Genet 3:611–621

Tokumasu F, Fairhurst RM, Ostera GR, Brittain NJ, Hwang J, Wellems TE, Dvorak JA (2005) Band 3 modifications in *Plasmodium falciparum*-infected AA and CC erythrocytes assayed by autocorrelation analysis using quantum dots. J Cell Sci 118:1091–1098

Tournamille C, Colin Y, Cartron JP, Le Van Kim C (1995) Disruption of a GATA motif in the Duffy gene promoter abolishes erythroid gene expression in Duffy-negative individuals. Nat Genet 10:224–228

Trape JF, Rogier C, Konate L, Diagne N, Bouganali H, Canque B, Legros F, Badji A, Ndiaye G, Ndiaye P, Brahimi K, Faye O, Druilhe P, Pereira da Silva L (1994) The Dielmo project: a longitudinal study of natural malaria infection and the mechanisms of protective immunity in a community living in a holoendemic area of Senegal. Am J Trop Med Hyg 51: 123–137

Treutiger CJ, Heddini A, Fernandez V, Muller WA, Wahlgren M (1997) PECAM-1/CD31, an endothelial receptor for binding *Plasmodium falciparum*-infected erythrocytes. Nat Med 3:1405–1408

Urban BC, Ferguson DJ, Pain A, Willcox N, Plebanski M, Austyn JM, Roberts DJ (1999) *Plasmodium falciparum*-infected erythrocytes modulate the maturation of dendritic cells. Nature 400:73–77

Urban BC, Willcox N, Roberts DJ (2001) A role for CD36 in the regulation of dendritic cell function. Proc Natl Acad Sci USA 98:8750–8755

Usanga EA, Luzzatto L (1985) Adaptation of *Plasmodium falciparum* to glucose 6-phosphate dehydrogenase-deficient host red cells by production of parasite-encoded enzyme. Nature 313:793–795

Vigario AM, Belnoue E, Cumano A, Marussig M, Miltgen F, Landau I, Mazier D, Gresser I, Renia L (2001) Inhibition of *Plasmodium yoelii* blood-stage malaria by interferon alpha through the inhibition of the production of its target cell, the reticulocyte. Blood 97:3966–3971

Walley AJ, Aucan C, Kwiatkowski D, Hill AV (2004) Interleukin-1 gene cluster polymorphisms and susceptibility to clinical malaria in a Gambian case-control study. Eur J Hum Genet 12:132–138

Wang HY, Tang H, Shen CK, Wu CI (2003) Rapidly evolving genes in human. I. The glycophorins and their possible role in evading malaria parasites. Mol Biol Evol 20:1795–1804

Wattavidanage J, Carter R, Perera KL, Munasingha A, Bandara S, McGuinness D, Wickramasinghe AR, Alles HK, Mendis KN, Premawansa S (1999) TNFalpha*2 marks high risk of severe disease during *Plasmodium falciparum* malaria and other infections in Sri Lankans. Clin Exp Immunol 115:350–355

Weatherall DJ, Clegg JB (2001) Inherited haemoglobin disorders: an increasing global health problem. Bull World Health Organ 79:704–712

Westendorp RG, van Dunne FM, Kirkwood TB, Helmerhorst FM, Huizinga TW (2001) Optimizing human fertility and survival. Nat Med 7:873

Williams TN, Maitland K, Bennett S, Ganczakowski M, Peto TE, Newbold CI, Bowden DK, Weatherall DJ, Clegg JB (1996) High incidence of malaria in alpha-thalassaemic children. Nature 383:522–525

Williams TN, Mwangi TW, Roberts DJ, Alexander ND, Weatherall DJ, Wambua S, Kortok M, Snow RW, Marsh K (2005*a*) An immune basis for malaria protection by the sickle cell trait. PLoS Med 2:e128

Williams TN, Wambua S, Uyoga S, Macharia A, Mwacharo JK, Newton CR, Maitland K (2005*b*) Both heterozygous and homozygous α^+thalassemia protect against severe and fatal *Plasmodium falciparum* malaria on the coast of Kenya. Blood 106:368–371

Williams TN, Weatherall DJ, Newbold CI (2002) The membrane characteristics of *Plasmodium falciparum*-infected and -uninfected heterozygous alpha$^{(0)}$thalassaemic erythrocytes. Br J Haematol 118:663–670

Wilson J, Rockett K, Jallow M, Pinder M, Sisay-Joof F, Newport M, Newton J, Kwiatkowski D (2005) Analysis of IL10 haplotypic associations with severe malaria. Genes Immun (http://www.nature.com/gene/journal/vaop/ncurrent/full/6364227a.html) (electronically published June 3, 2005; accessed June 16, 2005)

Yazdani SS, Shakri AR, Mukherjee P, Baniwal SK, Chitnis CE (2004) Evaluation of immune responses elicited in mice against a recombinant malaria vaccine based on *Plasmodium vivax* Duffy binding protein. Vaccine 22:3727–3737

Zimmerman PA, Fitness J, Moulds JM, McNamara DT, Kasehagen LJ, Rowe JA, Hill AV (2003) CR1 Knops blood group alleles are not associated with severe malaria in the Gambia. Genes Immun 4:368–373

Zimmerman PA, Woolley I, Masinde GL, Miller SM, McNamara DT, Hazlett F, Mgone CS, Alpers MP, Genton B, Boatin BA, Kazura JW (1999) Emergence of FY*A(null) in a *Plasmodium vivax*-endemic region of Papua New Guinea. Proc Natl Acad Sci USA 96:13973–13977

Genotype-Phenotype Associations in Sotos Syndrome: An Analysis of 266 Individuals with *NSD1* Aberrations

Katrina Tatton-Brown,[1] Jenny Douglas,[1] Kim Coleman,[1] Geneviève Baujat,[2] Trevor R. P. Cole,[3] Soma Das,[4] Denise Horn,[5] Helen E. Hughes,[6] I. Karen Temple,[7] Francesca Faravelli,[8] Darrel Waggoner,[4] Seval Türkmen,[5] Valérie Cormier-Daire,[2] Alexandre Irrthum,[1] and Nazneen Rahman,[1] for the Childhood Overgrowth Collaboration*

[1]Section of Cancer Genetics, Institute of Cancer Research, Sutton, United Kingdom; [2]Department of Medical Genetics, Hopital Necker Enfants Malades, Paris; [3]Clinical Genetics Unit, Birmingham Women's Hospital, Birmingham, United Kingdom; [4]Department of Human Genetics, University of Chicago, Chicago; [5]Institut für Medizinische Genetik, Humboldt-Universität, Charité, Berlin; [6]Institute of Medical Genetics, University Hospital of Wales, Cardiff; [7]Department of Human Genetics, Southampton University Hospital, Southampton, United Kingdom; and [8]Laboratorio di Genetica Umana, Ospedali Galliera de Genova, Genova, Italy

We identified 266 individuals with intragenic *NSD1* mutations or 5q35 microdeletions encompassing *NSD1* (referred to as "*NSD1*-positive individuals"), through analyses of 530 subjects with diverse phenotypes. Truncating *NSD1* mutations occurred throughout the gene, but pathogenic missense mutations occurred only in functional domains ($P < 2 \times 10^{-16}$). Sotos syndrome was clinically diagnosed in 99% of *NSD1*-positive individuals, independent of the molecular analyses, indicating that *NSD1* aberrations are essentially specific to this condition. Furthermore, our data suggest that 93% of patients who have been clinically diagnosed with Sotos syndrome have identifiable *NSD1* abnormalities, of which 83% are intragenic mutations and 10% are 5q35 microdeletions. We reviewed the clinical phenotypes of 239 *NSD1*-positive individuals. Facial dysmorphism, learning disability, and childhood overgrowth were present in 90% of the individuals. However, both the height and head circumference of 10% of the individuals were within the normal range, indicating that overgrowth is not obligatory for the diagnosis of Sotos syndrome. A broad spectrum of associated clinical features was also present, the occurrence of which was largely independent of genotype, since individuals with identical mutations had different phenotypes. We compared the phenotypes of patients with intragenic *NSD1* mutations with those of patients with 5q35 microdeletions. Patients with microdeletions had less-prominent overgrowth ($P = .0003$) and more-severe learning disability ($P = 3 \times 10^{-9}$) than patients with mutations. However, all features present in patients with microdeletions were also observed in patients with mutations, and there was no correlation between deletion size and the clinical phenotype, suggesting that the deletion of additional genes in patients with 5q35 microdeletions has little specific effect on phenotype. We identified only 13 familial cases. The reasons for the low vertical transmission rate are unclear, although familial cases were more likely than nonfamilial cases ($P = .005$) to carry missense mutations, suggesting that the underlying *NSD1* mutational mechanism in Sotos syndrome may influence reproductive fitness.

Introduction

The nuclear receptor SET domain–containing protein 1 (*NSD1*) gene encodes a histone methyltransferase and is located at chromosome 5q35. NSD1 was initially isolated in a search for proteins that interact with the ligand-binding domain of retinoic acid receptor α and subsequently was shown to be the fusion partner of NUP98 in some cases of childhood acute myeloid leukemia (Huang et al. 1998; Jaju et al. 2001). NSD1 contains multiple functional domains, including SU(VAR)3-9,E(Z),trithorax (SET) and SET-associated (SAC) domains that together mediate the histone methyltransferase activity of NSD1; a C5HCH and five plant homeodomains (PHDs), which are implicated in chromatin regulation and are zinc finger–like motifs characterized by cysteine and histidine residues; and two proline-tryptophan-tryptophan-proline (PWWP) domains that may mediate protein-protein interactions and that are often found in proteins that act at the chromatin level (Aasland et al. 1995; Stec et al. 2000; Rayasam et al. 2003). NSD1 also contains two nuclear-receptor interaction domains, NID^{-L} and NID^{+L}, which are typical of those found in nuclear-receptor corepressors and coactivators, respectively (Huang et al. 1998).

Received April 12, 2005; accepted for publication May 19, 2005; electronically published June 7, 2005.

Address for correspondence and reprints: Dr. Nazneen Rahman, Section of Cancer Genetics, Institute of Cancer Research, 15, Cotswold Road, Sutton, Surrey, SM2 5NG, United Kingdom. E-mail: nazneen.rahman@icr.ac.uk

* The contributors to the Childhood Overgrowth Collaboration are listed in the Acknowledgments.

0002-9297/2005/7702-0003$15.00

The functions of NSD1 are not known, but it has been shown to methylate both H4 K20 and H3 K36, modifications that are individually associated with transcriptional repression (Rayasam et al. 2003). The presence of two distinct nuclear-receptor interaction domains (NIDs) has given rise to the hypothesis that differential ligand binding to NID^{-L} and NID^{+L} allows NSD1 to both negatively and positively regulate transcription (Huang et al. 1998).

In 2002, NSD1 haploinsufficiency was reported in patients with Sotos syndrome (MIM 117550), a condition characterized by facial dysmorphism, learning disability, and childhood overgrowth (Kurotaki et al. 2002). Subsequently, >100 individuals with *NSD1* abnormalities were reported in the literature (Douglas et al. 2003; Kurotaki et al. 2003; Rio et al. 2003; Türkmen et al. 2003; de Boer et al. 2004; Cecconi et al. 2005). The range and relative contributions of *NSD1* abnormalities and the spectrum of clinical phenotypes associated with *NSD1* have been unclear. In particular, the prevalence of 5q35 microdeletions in Japanese and non-Japanese individuals has been controversial. In Japan, 5q35 microdeletions are the most common cause of Sotos syndrome and are predominantly mediated by nonallelic homologous recombination between flanking low-copy repeats (Visser et al. 2005). Outside Japan, 5q35 microdeletions are uncommon, accounting for only 10% of affected individuals, and multiple mechanisms are implicated in their generation (Tatton-Brown et al. 2005). It was postulated that this difference in microdeletion frequency was due to variation in patient-selection criteria for *NSD1* analyses (Kurotaki et al. 2003). However, it seems more likely that differences in sequence architecture are responsible, since an inversion polymorphism that predisposes to microdeletions appears to be common in Japan (Tatton-Brown et al. 2005; Visser et al. 2005).

The range of clinical features associated with Sotos syndrome is broad, and it has been suggested that this variability is related to the underlying mutational mechanism. Specifically, it was proposed that the phenotypes of individuals with *NSD1* mutations and of those with 5q35 microdeletions differ because some features of Sotos syndrome, such as overgrowth and learning disability, are attributable to *NSD1,* whereas other features, such as cardiac and renal anomalies, occur only in individuals with microdeletions and are due to deletion of other genes (Nagai et al. 2003; Niikawa 2004). It has also been suggested that *NSD1* mutations can cause other overgrowth conditions such as Weaver syndrome (MIM 277590) and Beckwith-Wiedemann syndrome (BWS [MIM 130650]) (Douglas et al. 2003; Rio et al. 2003; Baujat et al. 2004).

In the present study, we screened a large series of subjects with diverse phenotypes for mutations and deletions of *NSD1,* to clarify the range and contribution of different *NSD1* abnormalities and the spectrum of associated clinical features. We compared the clinical features of individuals with mutations and microdeletions, as well as the clinical features of individuals with different-sized microdeletions, to investigate whether the deletion of other genes contributes to the phenotype of patients with 5q35 microdeletions. Additionally, we investigated the heritability and phenotypic variability of *NSD1* abnormalities, to provide information for counseling on recurrence and offspring risks and to evaluate whether prognostic information can be provided by identification of the underlying mutational mechanism in individuals with *NSD1* abnormalities.

Subjects and Methods

Patients

The research was approved by the London Multicentre Research Ethics Committee, and consent was obtained from participating subjects and/or their parents. Through analyses of 530 individuals, 266 patients with *NSD1* aberrations (referred to as "*NSD1*-positive individuals") were identified. This included 179 *NSD1*-positive individuals identified through analyses of 443 subjects in the Childhood Overgrowth Study. Patients recruited into this study have a broad range of phenotypes, including a clinical diagnosis of Sotos syndrome, overgrowth and/or macrocephaly (but without the typical facial features of Sotos syndrome), and facial features similar to Sotos syndrome (but no overgrowth). Of 179 subjects, 132 *NSD1*-positive individuals ascertained through these analyses were from the United Kingdom, and the remainder had diverse origins. NSD1 analyses of 73 of these individuals have been published elsewhere (Douglas et al. 2003, in press; Tatton-Brown et al. 2005). The remaining 87 *NSD1*-positive individuals were identified in collaborating centers in France, Germany, Italy, and the United States, and descriptions of 54 have been published elsewhere (Rio et al. 2003; Türkmen et al. 2003; Cecconi et al. 2005; Waggoner et al., in press). A standard clinical questionnaire was requested from all *NSD1*-positive individuals and was obtained from 239 of the individuals. Facial photographs of 290 of the 530 patients were evaluated independently by three clinical geneticists (T.R.P.C., H.E.H., and I.K.T.), who were unaware of the *NSD1* status, as described elsewhere (Douglas et al. 2003). The patients were categorized into four phenotypic groups: (1) "typical Sotos syndrome," (2) "possible Sotos syndrome," (3) "Weaver syndrome," and (4) "definitely not Sotos or Weaver syndrome." If another diagnosis, such as BWS, was thought possible, this was noted.

Table 1

Summary of the Number of Patients with Different *NSD1* Abnormalities

Category and Type of *NSD1* Aberration	No. of Patients
Intragenic mutations:	233
Frameshift	91
Nonsense	59
Missense	64
Splice site	11
Partial-gene deletions	8
5q35 microdeletions	33
Total	266

NSD1 *Analyses*

The 443 subjects collected through the Childhood Overgrowth Study were screened for intragenic mutations by use of conformational sensitive gel electrophoresis and sequencing, as described elsewhere (Douglas et al. 2003). To identify 5q35 microdeletions, all subjects were initially analyzed at the highly polymorphic intragenic microsatellite marker SOT3 (Douglas et al. 2003). Individuals who were homozygous at SOT3 were further analyzed by multiplex ligation-dependent probe amplification (MLPA) with the use of the SALSA P026B *NSD1* kit to identify 5q35 microdeletions, which were confirmed by quantitative fluorescent PCR and/or microsatellite analyses, as described elsewhere (Douglas et al. 2003; Tatton-Brown et al. 2005). Individuals with the classic facial features of Sotos syndrome whose mutation screening was negative were also analyzed by MLPA, even if they were heterozygous at SOT3, to identify partial-gene deletions/duplications. This revealed eight partial-gene deletions involving one or more exons (Douglas et al., in press). *NSD1* mutations in patients identified in collaborating centers were detected by sequencing and/or denaturing high-performance liquid chromatography, and 5q35 microdeletions were identified by FISH, as described elsewhere (Rio et al. 2003; Türkmen et al. 2003; Cecconi et al. 2005; Waggoner et al., in press).

Statistical Analyses

Statistical analyses were performed with the program R 2.0.1 (R Project for Statistical Computing). The statistical significance of the clustering of pathogenic mutations in the functional domains of NSD1, comprising 23% of the whole protein, was evaluated with the exact binomial test. Comparisons of proportions in two-way contingency tables were performed with the Fisher's exact test. Height, head circumference, and learning disability were compared among groups with the Wilcoxon rank-sum test. The co-occurrence of dichotomous clinical features—cardiac anomalies, renal anomalies, seizures, and scoliosis—was tested with Pearson's correlation and the Bonferroni correction. All reported P values are two-sided.

Results

Spectrum of NSD1 *Abnormalities*

We identified *NSD1* abnormalities in 266 of the 530 subjects, of whom 122 were girls and 144 were boys. The mean parental ages for 46 U.K. *NSD1*-positive individuals born between the years 1997 and 2003 were 30.2 years for mothers and 33.2 years for fathers. National averages for a comparable time period are 29.1 years for mothers and 32.3 years for fathers.

Of the 266 *NSD1*-positive individuals, 233 had 180 different intragenic *NSD1* mutations, and the remaining 33 individuals had 5q35 microdeletions encompassing *NSD1* (fig. 1*A* and tables 1 and 2). We identified 117 different truncating *NSD1* mutations, including 50 deletions of 1–10 bp, 23 insertions of 1–17 bp, 6 in/del mutations, and 37 nonsense mutations generating stop codons (table 2). One mutation was an insertion of ~190 bp from an *Alu*-Y element into exon 11, which likely results in premature protein truncation (Douglas et al., in press). We detected 10 different mutations affecting consensus splice-site residues. The precise effect of these is not known, but they likely result in premature protein truncation or exon skipping. The truncating and splice-site mutations were positioned evenly through the gene (fig. 1*B*).

To investigate the pathogenicity of missense alterations, we compared 34 de novo mutations, which we assumed were disease causing, with 24 sequence variants detected in unaffected individuals, which we assumed were nonpathogenic polymorphisms (table 2). The de novo missense mutations all occurred within functional domains that comprise 622 of the 2,696 amino acids of the protein, and this distribution was significantly different from that expected by chance (exact binomial test, $P < 2 \times 10^{-16}$) (fig. 1*B*). Furthermore, the pathogenic base substitutions were all nonsynonymous, whereas only 14 of 24 polymorphisms were nonsynonymous (Fisher's exact test, $P = 4 \times 10^{-5}$), and none of these was in a functional domain (Fisher's exact test, $P = 2 \times 10^{-12}$). Eleven de novo mutations targeted critical cysteine/histidine residues implicated in chromatin regulation (fig. 1*C*).

On the basis of these results, we considered 30 other individuals to have pathogenic missense mutations. These included 4 individuals with known mutations (i.e., mu-

Table 2

Intragenic Mutations and Exonic Polymorphisms in *NSD1*

The table is available in its entirety in the online edition of *The American Journal of Human Genetics.*

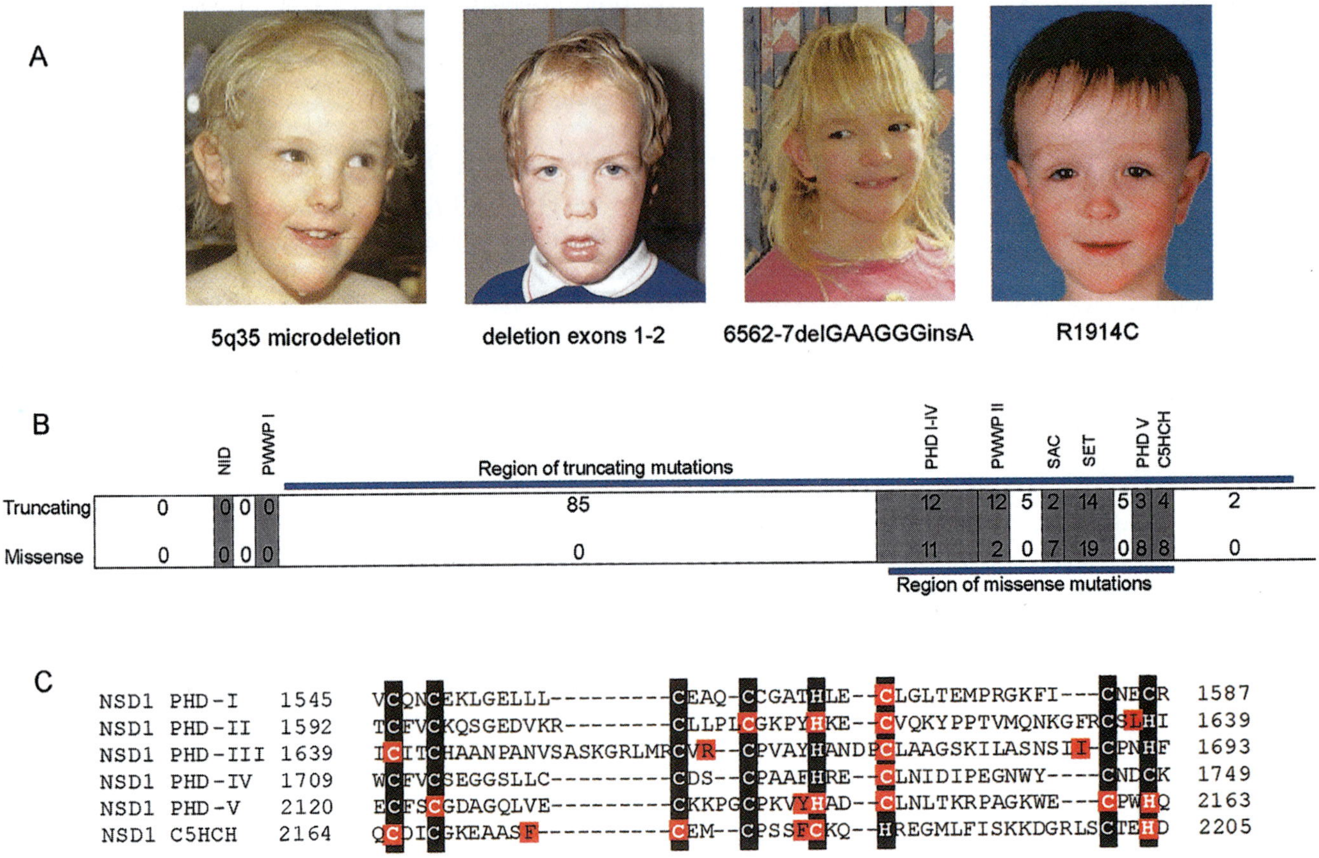

Figure 1 Facial features and *NSD1* mutations in patients with Sotos syndrome. *A*, Typical facial features of patients with different *NSD1* abnormalities: 5q35 microdeletion, partial *NSD1* deletion, truncating mutation, and missense mutation. *B*, Number of truncating and missense mutations identified in different NSD1 domains, demonstrating that missense mutations occur only within functional domains. The number of truncating mutations is at the top of each section of *NSD1*, and the number of missense mutations is shown at the bottom. Functional domains are shown as shaded boxes.*C*, Position of missense mutations (*red*) in PHD and C5HCH domains, showing bias toward mutations at consensus cysteine and histidine residues (*black*).

tations that had occurred de novo in other unrelated individuals), 10 with mutations that targeted consensus cysteine/histidine residues in functional domains, and 1 with an in-frame 3-bp deletion within PHD-V; in addition, six families (15 patients) were identified in which nonsynonymous mutations of conserved residues in functional domains segregated with Sotos syndrome in the family. Three mutations (F1177del-2, V1595A, and Y2058C) that were present in patients with classic Sotos syndrome were classified as variants of unknown significance and were excluded from further analyses. We strongly suspect that Y2058C, which alters a conserved residue in the SET domain, and F1177del-2, which results in the in-frame deletion of two amino acids, are pathogenic, but we did not have parental DNA to confirm that they arose de novo. V1595A is located in a PHD finger but does not affect a highly conserved residue. Moreover, it was present in both the affected individual and his unaffected mother and therefore may not be pathogenic.

We identified eight individuals with distinct exonic deletions of exons 1 and 2 (four individuals), exons 3–5, exons 9–13, exons 19–21, and exon 22 (Douglas et al., in press). Additionally, we identified 33 individuals with 5q35 microdeletions encompassing *NSD1* (Tatton-Brown et al. 2005). The deletion size in these individuals was very variable and ranged from 482 kb, in which only *NSD1* was deleted, to 5 Mb, in which at least 54 genes were deleted. In 18 individuals, microdeletions may have been mediated by nonallelic homologous recombination between flanking low-copy repeats. However, in 15 individuals, microdeletions cannot be mediated by recombination between these repetitive elements, and at least seven different deletion sizes were present among the 33 individuals (Tatton-Brown et al. 2005).

Familial and Recurrent NSD1 *Abnormalities*

Thirteen *NSD1*-positive individuals had affected relatives, and, in 12 families, we were able to demonstrate

Table 3

Clinical Features of Patients with Recurrent *NSD1* Mutations

Mutation and Patient ID	Clinical Feature(s)[a]
2386-9delGAAA:	
COG300	Severe LD, seizures, scoliosis, scaphocephaly
COG514	Moderate LD, seizures, ASD, VSD, PDA
COG523	Moderate LD, scoliosis
3549-50insT:	
COG073	Severe LD, seizures, complex cardiac anomaly, duplex kidney, hypercalcemia
COG095	Moderate LD, seizures, scoliosis
5279-82delTCTG:	
COG252	LD[b], ASD, scoliosis
COG288	Mild LD, conductive hearing loss
COG455	Mild LD
6596delG:	
COG265	Moderate LD, scoliosis, constipation, fixed flexion deformity of knees
COG272	Mild LD, seizures
R440X:	
COG196	No LD, bicuspid aortic valve, left pyelectasia
COG494	Moderate LD, strabismus, hyperlaxity, pectus excavatum
R604X:	
COG022	Mild LD, seizures, ASD
COG054	Mild LD, cardiac anomaly, scoliosis, strabismus
COG154	Severe LD, VSD, VUR, GOR, laryngomalacia
R611X:	
COG088	Mild LD, seizures, VSD
COG223	Moderate LD, scoliosis
R1031X:	
COG469	Moderate LD
COG502	Mild LD, scoliosis, cataracts, nystagmus
R1072X:	
COG133	Severe LD, seizures
COG497	Moderate LD
S1269X:	
COG365	Moderate LD, strabismus
COG394	Mild LD
R1322X:	
COG538	Mild LD
COG630	Moderate LD
R1811X:	
COG103	Mild LD, strabismus
COG251	Moderate LD, seizures
COG321	Mild LD, seizures, ASD, heart conduction defect, scoliosis
COG465	Moderate LD
COG495	Moderate LD, PUJ obstruction, neonatal glaucoma
R1984X:	
COG190	Mild LD, ASD, hypoplastic thyroid
COG311	Mild LD
COG458	LD[b], ASD, VUR
R2005X:	
COG323	LD[b], sacrococcygeal teratoma
COG482	Moderate LD
R1914C:	
COG131	Moderate LD
COG389	Mild LD
C1925R:	
COG034	Moderate LD, scoliosis
COG144	Mild LD, scoliosis, pectus carinatum, strabismus
R1952W:	
COG371	Mild LD, hemihypertrophy, hepatomegaly
COG434	Severe LD, TGA, scoliosis, cutis laxa
R1984Q:	
COG463	Mild LD, seizures, cardiac anomaly, chiari malformation
COG464	Moderate LD, ASD
COG490	Moderate LD, seizures, scoliosis
COG628	LD[b], cryptorchidism, phimosis
Y1997C:	
COG233	Moderate LD, scoliosis, pectus excavatum, hypospadias
COG491	Severe LD
R2017W:	
COG308	Mild LD, scoliosis, strabismus
COG500	Moderate LD, scoliosis, VUR
IVS9+3-6delGAGT:	
COG134	Moderate LD, VUR
COG227	Moderate LD, seizures, scoliosis, inguinal hernia, scaphocephaly

NOTE.—ASD = atrial septal defect; GOR = gastroesophageal reflux; PDA = patent ductus arteriosus; PUJ = pelviureteric junction; TGA = transposition of the great arteries; VSD = ventricular septal defect; VUR = vesicoureteral reflux.

[a] In addition to dysmorphism and overgrowth. LD = learning disability.

[b] Degree of LD not specified.

that the mutation segregated with the disorder (table 2). Only one of the families, with affected MZ twin boys, had a 5q35 microdeletion. Of the 12 families with inherited mutations, 7 harbored missense alterations, and this was significantly greater than the proportion of missense mutations in nonfamilial cases (48/240; Fisher's exact test, $P = .005$). The mutation was transmitted from the mother in nine individuals and from the father in three individuals. We analyzed 303 unaffected parents of *NSD1*-positive individuals, none of whom carried the mutation/deletion that was present in their children. For 141 nonfamilial cases, samples were available from both unaffected parents, and analyses confirmed that all cases had arisen de novo.

Twenty-eight mutations occurred independently in at least two unrelated individuals and are referred to as "recurrent" mutations (tables 2 and 3). Twenty-one of the recurrent mutations were base substitutions, and 18 occurred at CpG dinucleotides.

Clinical Features Associated with NSD1 *Abnormalities*

Facial dysmorphism, learning disability, and childhood overgrowth were each present in at least 90% of

NSD1-positive individuals and were designated as cardinal features.

Cardinal Features (present in ⩾90% of patients)
- Characteristic facial appearance
- Learning disability
- Overgrowth: height and/or head circumference ⩾98th percentile

Major Features (present in ⩾15% of patients)
- Advanced bone age
- Cardiac anomalies
- Cranial magnetic resonance imaging or CT abnormalities
- Hyperlaxity/pes planus
- Maternal pre-eclampsia
- Neonatal hypotonia
- Neonatal jaundice
- Neonatal poor feeding
- Renal anomalies
- Scoliosis
- Seizures

Other Features
- Astigmatism
- Behavioral problems
- Cataract
- Cholesteatoma
- Conductive hearing loss
- Constipation
- Contractures
- Craniosynostosis
- Cryptorchidism
- Gastroesophageal reflux
- Genu valgum
- Hemangioma
- Hemihypertrophy
- Hydrocele
- Hypercalcemia
- Hypermetropia
- Hyperpigmentation
- Hypopigmentation
- Hypoplastic nails
- Hypospadias
- Hypothyroid
- Inguinal hernia
- Myopia
- Neonatal hypoglycemia
- Nystagmus
- Pectus excavatum
- Phimosis
- Strabismus
- Talipes
- 2-3 toe syndactyly
- Tumors
- Umbilical hernia
- Vertebral anomalies

The strongest phenotypic feature associated with *NSD1* abnormalities was dysmorphism (fig. 1*A*). All *NSD1*-positive individuals were dysmorphic, although this was often mild. Only 2 of 166 *NSD1*-positive individuals from whom photographs were available were phenotypically scored as "definitely not Sotos or Weaver syndrome," both of whom had truncating *NSD1* mutations. Even after reviewing the subjects together with the *NSD1* results, we did not consider the facial features of these two individuals to be consistent with Sotos syndrome. The remaining 164 *NSD1*-positive individuals had been phenotypically scored as either "typical Sotos syndrome" or "possible Sotos syndrome." Only 2 of 66 individuals who were phenotypically scored as "definitely not Sotos or Weaver syndrome" had *NSD1* mutations.

Learning disability was very common (present in 97% of affected individuals). However, the degree of cognitive impairment was variable, with 21% of affected individuals considered to have "severe" impairment, 46% with "moderate" impairment, and 30% with "mild" impairment. Only seven individuals had normal intellectual development, but there is likely to be a bias toward referral of children with learning disability and, as a result, *NSD1*-positive individuals with normal development may be underrepresented in our analyses. Childhood overgrowth was also common, with 90% of affected individuals having height and/or head circumference at least 2 SDs above the mean (table 4). For these analyses, we included only individuals with height measurements taken between the ages of 1 and 10 years, to limit potential bias resulting from inaccuracies of measurement in neonates and/or the effects of puberty. In 60% of affected individuals, the height and head circumference were both above the 99.6th percentile. However, many individuals had growth

Table 4

Number of Patients with Height and Head Circumference within Each Growth Percentile, for Individuals with *NSD1* Mutations and 5q35 Microdeletions

	No. of Patients, by Measure and Mutation Type			
	Height[a]		Head Circumference[b]	
Growth Percentile	Intragenic Mutations	5q35 Microdeletions	Intragenic Mutations	5q35 Microdeletions
<.4	0	0	0	0
⩾.4	1	1	0	0
⩾2	0	0	1	0
⩾9	0	0	0	0
⩾25	2	0	2	0
⩾50	5	1	6	1
⩾75	6	6	14	0
⩾91	12	4	33	6
⩾98	27	3	31	10
⩾99.6	98	9	105	13
Total	151	24	192	30

[a] At age 1–10 years.
[b] At all ages.

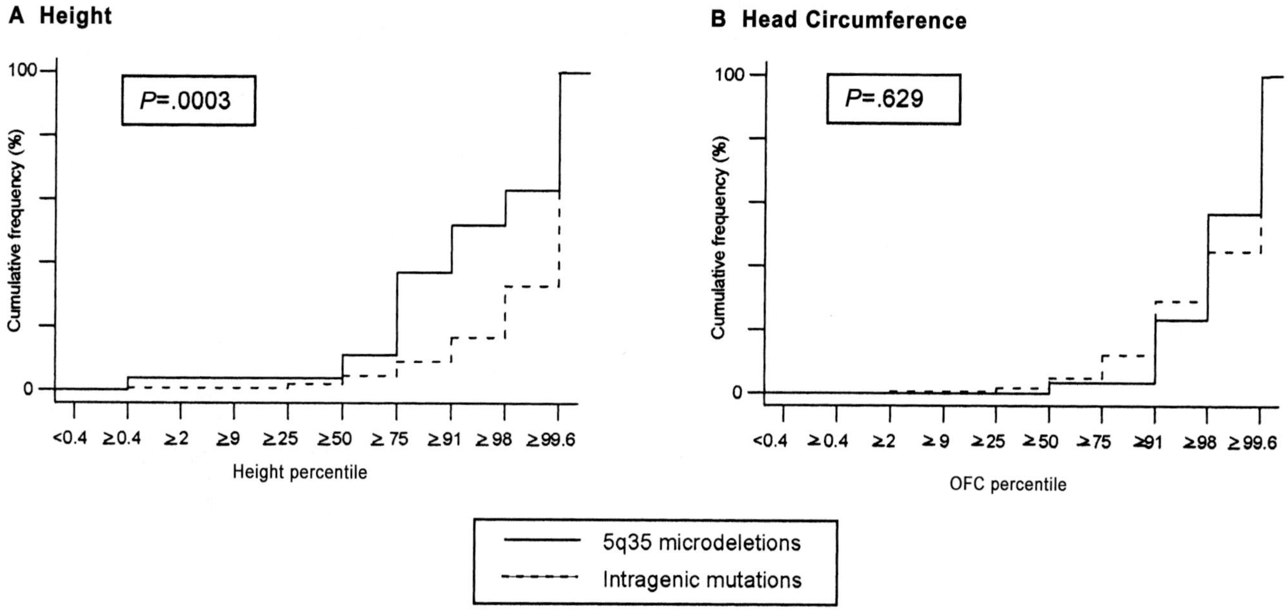

Figure 2 Cumulative frequency distribution graphs for patients with *NSD1* mutations or 5q35 microdeletions. *A*, Height distribution. *B*, Head circumference distribution. The distributions are significantly different for height (Wilcoxon rank-sum test) but not for head circumference.

parameters within the normal range, and, in four individuals, the height was below the median (table 4). We have limited data on adult growth parameters. However, the height of only 8 of 32 *NSD1*-positive adult individuals was at or above the 99.6th percentile, and 10 adults had height at or below the 50th percentile.

Eleven clinical features were present in ⩾15% of affected individuals and were designated major features of Sotos syndrome (see list above). Advanced bone age was the most common major feature and was present in 76% of affected individuals in whom it was measured. However, bone age was not advanced in nearly one-quarter of patients, and, therefore, advanced bone age should not be considered to be an essential feature of Sotos syndrome. Abnormalities on cranial imaging were also common, although these were generally nonspecific, such as dilated ventricles, prominence of the trigone and occipital horns, and/or hypoplasia of the corpus collosum. Neonatal problems, such as hypotonia, poor feeding, and jaundice, were all common (present in ~70% of patients). Scoliosis occurred in one-third of patients and was very variable in severity. Similarly, a broad spectrum of cardiac anomalies and different seizure types was present in 21% and 25% of patients, respectively. Maternal preeclampsia was reported in 17% of patients, although it was not previously known to be associated with Sotos syndrome. Renal anomalies, particularly vesicoureteral reflux, were reported for 15% of patients, but this is likely an underestimate, since relatively few patients had undergone renal investigations. More information about the clinical spectrum of associated clinical features of *NSD1*-positive individuals with Sotos syndrome is given in the study by Tatton-Brown and Rahman (2004).

Several other features were reported in at least two individuals (see list above). Apart from tumors, information about these additional features was not specifically requested on the clinical questionnaire, and their true frequency in individuals with Sotos syndrome is therefore uncertain. It is likely that some features, such as constipation or self-limiting conductive hearing loss in early childhood, occur in ⩾15% of patients and could be considered major features of Sotos syndrome. We requested information from all subjects on whether benign or malignant tumors had occurred. Only eight patients developed tumors, including one neuroblastoma, three sacrococcygeal teratomas, one presacral ganglioneuroma, two acute lymphocytic leukemias, and one small-cell lung cancer. There were many additional features that were reported in only one case, and it is unclear whether these were coincidental or related to functional NSD1 abrogation (data not shown).

Genotype-Phenotype Analyses

We compared the clinical features of individuals with intragenic *NSD1* mutations with those of individuals with 5q35 microdeletions. We compared seven features: height distribution, head circumference distribution, learning disability (scored as "none," "mild," "moderate," or "severe"), cardiac anomalies, renal anomalies, seizures, and scoliosis (all scored as either present or absent). There were highly significant differences in the height distribution and severity of learning disability. Patients with *NSD1* intragenic mutations were significantly taller than patients with 5q35 microdeletions (Wilcoxon rank-sum test, $P = .0003$) (table 4 and fig. 2*A*). By contrast, there was no difference in the head circumference distribution between patients with mutations and those with deletions (table 4 and fig. 2*B*). The individuals with 5q35 microdeletions had more-severe learning disability (Wilcoxon rank-sum test, $P = 3 \times 10^{-9}$ (fig. 3), and there was also a trend toward more cardiac anomalies (Fisher's exact test, $P = .01$) in individuals with microdeletions. However, there was no difference in the frequency of renal anomalies, scoliosis, or seizures between individuals with mutations and those with microdeletions. There were also no differences in the severity of learning disability or the frequency of associated features in patients with truncating mutations compared with patients with missense mutations. Pairwise comparisons of combinations of major features demonstrated that the occurrence of cardiac anomalies, renal anomalies, seizures, and scoliosis were all mutually independent.

All of the clinical features shown in the list above were present in at least two of the patients with mutations, but some were not seen in the patients with microdeletions, probably because only 31 individuals with microdeletions were included in these analyses, compared with 208 individuals with mutations. Conversely, nephrocalcinosis was the only feature present in individuals with microdeletions that was not reported in the individuals with mutations. Two individuals with 5q35 microdeletions, with different-sized deletions, had nephrocalcinosis. However, relatively few patients with mutations had undergone renal investigations, and it is probable that nephrocalcinosis can also occur in patients with mutations but that it has yet to be reported. The microdeletions varied in size from 482 kb to 5 Mb and included a minimum of seven different-sized deletions. There was no correlation between the clinical phenotype and the size of deletion. Additional details about the clinical features of the individuals with microdeletions are given in the study by Tatton-Brown et al. (2005).

We compared the clinical phenotypes of patients with identical mutations that had arisen independently. This revealed considerable variability in the degree of learning disability and associated clinical features in patients with recurrent mutations (table 3).

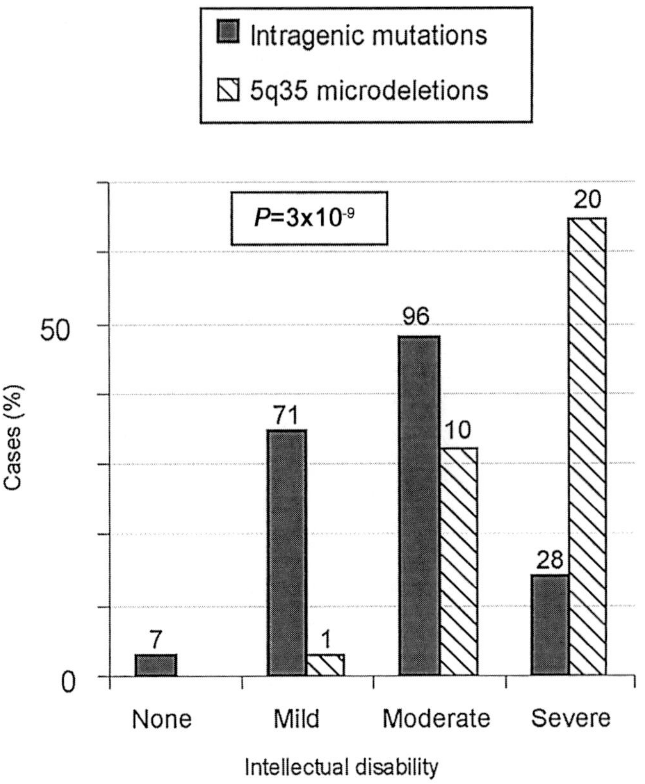

Figure 3 Bar graph showing the frequency and severity of learning disability in patients with *NSD1* mutations (*blackened*) and in those with 5q35 microdeletions (*hatched*). The actual number of patients is given above each bar. The distributions are significantly different (Wilcoxon rank-sum test).

Discussion

Multiple Mutational Mechanisms Abrogate NSD1 *Function*

Multiple mutational mechanisms—including small intragenic insertions and deletions, nonsense mutations, splicing defects, missense mutations, partial-gene deletions, and whole-gene deletions—can abrogate NSD1 function and can result in human disease. Intragenic truncating mutations occur throughout the gene, and most are unique. Sequence architecture influences both the partial- and whole-gene deletions, with several partial-gene deletions arising through nonallelic homologous recombination between *Alu* repeats (Douglas et al., in press). Similarly, a proportion of whole-gene deletions are 2-Mb 5q35 microdeletions that are mediated by nonallelic homologous recombination between low-copy repeats flanking *NSD1*. This recurrent microdeletion is particularly common in Japan, where a prevalent inversion polymorphism predisposes to the microdeletion (Tatton-Brown et al. 2005; Visser et al. 2005).

Missense *NSD1* mutations are pathogenic only if they occur within functional domains implicated in chromatin regulation. Within the PHD, SAC, and C5HCH domains, mutations predominantly occurred at the consensus cysteine and histidine residues that define these domains. Nineteen of the missense mutations were within the SET domain and may therefore result in altered methylation of K20 on H4 and/or K36 on H3. We did not identify missense mutations in the two NIDs at the 5′ end of the gene. It is uncertain whether this was because they are not pathogenic or because the NIDs together consist of only 34 amino acids. We did not have sufficient mutations to formally evaluate whether the phenotype differed in accordance with the domain affected. However, the phenotypes appeared broadly similar, suggesting that missense alterations in different domains may have comparable effects on NSD1 function. Nonsynonymous base substitutions in the central portion of *NSD1*, which is devoid of recognized functional domains, do not appear to be deleterious. The function of this part of the gene is unknown, but it is noteworthy that exon 5, which is 2.56 kb in length, is not present in the NSD1 paralogs, NSD2, or NSD3, although the functional domains are all present (Douglas et al. 2005).

NSD1 *Abnormalities Are Specific to Sotos Syndrome*

We identified 266 individuals with *NSD1* abnormalities. Of the 166 individuals for whom we had photographs, 164 were given a clinical diagnosis of "typical Sotos syndrome" or "possible Sotos syndrome," independent of the molecular analyses. Conversely, only 2 of 66 individuals given a clinical diagnosis of "definitely not Sotos or Weaver syndrome" had *NSD1* abnormalities. We analyzed >500 subjects with a broad range of phenotypes, and it is unlikely that there exists a major unidentified group of cases attributable to *NSD1* that was not included in these analyses. These data therefore indicate that *NSD1* abnormalities are essentially specific to Sotos syndrome.

It has been proposed that *NSD1* may cause other overgrowth phenotypes, such as Weaver syndrome and BWS. In a previous study, we reported three individuals with atypical Weaver syndrome and with *NSD1* mutations and proposed that *NSD1* may cause Weaver syndrome in some patients (Douglas et al. 2003). In the current analysis, these three individuals were included in the phenotypic review of 290 subjects, but instead of a single photograph in infancy, multiple pictures at different ages were available. This resulted in two of the individuals being classified as having "typical Sotos syndrome" and one as having "possible Sotos syndrome." Moreover, none of the patients with classic Weaver syndrome had *NSD1* mutations. These data suggest there is considerable clinical overlap between Sotos and Weaver syndromes, particularly at young ages, but that classic Weaver syndrome is not due to *NSD1* abnormalities. We therefore believe a diagnosis of Weaver syndrome should be given only if the presence of *NSD1* abnormalities has been excluded. Our practice is to perform *NSD1* testing for all individuals for whom a diagnosis of Weaver syndrome is being considered. If this reveals a mutation, the child is managed as for other *NSD1*-positive individuals and a diagnosis of Sotos syndrome is given.

One of the two *NSD1*-positive individuals whose facial features were not consistent with Sotos syndrome was reported elsewhere as having BWS (patient BA [Baujat et al. 2004]). The child is not typical of patients with BWS since he has learning disability and no macroglossia. The diagnosis of BWS was based on the presence of neonatal hypoglycemia, umbilical hernia, and persistent vesicoureteral reflux. However, our data demonstrate that these features are all associated with Sotos syndrome and that vesicoureteral reflux is more commonly associated with Sotos syndrome than with BWS. Since overgrowth is a cardinal feature of both conditions, they will both be included in the differential diagnosis of many children. Macroglossia is a common feature of BWS that has never been seen in an *NSD1*-positive individual, whereas characteristic facial dysmorphism and learning disability are almost universal in Sotos syndrome but are rare in BWS. For most children, these conditions should therefore be distinguishable by use of clinical criteria. For rare instances of children with overlapping phenotypes, investigations of 11p15 and *NSD1* may be required. The clinical management of such children should be in accordance with the underlying molecular cause.

The Clinical Features of Individuals with 5q35 Microdeletions Are Explicable by NSD1 *Haploinsufficiency*

It was proposed, on the basis of a comparison of only 5 individuals with mutations and 21 individuals with microdeletions (Nagai et al. 2003), that the clinical features of Sotos syndrome should be classified into two categories: those caused by *NSD1* haploinsufficiency (overgrowth and learning disability) and those ascribed to other genes in the deleted interval (such as cardiovascular and renal anomalies). Our findings, which are based on 208 individuals with mutations and 31 individuals with microdeletions, are not consistent with this model. The cardinal and major features of Sotos syndrome were identified in similar proportions of individuals with microdeletions and intragenic mutations, strongly suggesting that these features are due to functional abrogation of NSD1. Overall, individuals with microdeletions had more-severe learning disability and less-pronounced overgrowth. Although it is possible that these differences are attributable to specific genes within the deleted interval, it is more likely to be a nonspecific result of the larger chromosomal insult in patients with microdeletions, since learning disability and growth retardation are very common nonspecific features of microdeletions throughout the genome (Devriendt and Vermeesch 2004). Moreover, despite the large variability in deletion size (0.4–5 Mb), there was no correlation between deletion size and clinical phenotype. Indeed, no additional clinical features were present in the three largest deletions that were not present in at least one of the three smallest deletions (Tatton-Brown et al. 2005). Overall, our data suggest the clinical phenotype of individuals with 5q35 microdeletions is primarily attributable to haploinsufficiency of NSD1 and that the deletion of other genes exerts little phenotypic effect.

The Phenotypic Variability of Sotos Syndrome Is Largely Independent of Genotype

The phenotype of *NSD1*-positive individuals was extremely variable. The three cardinal features—characteristic facial dysmorphism, learning disability, and childhood overgrowth—were present in 90% of affected individuals, but many other features were also variably present. The presence of these additional features was not correlated with and did not appear to be strongly influenced by the underlying mutational mechanism. This was most clearly demonstrated by the differing phenotypes of individuals with identical mutations. It is currently unclear what determines the clinical variability of Sotos syndrome. Stochastic factors, intrauterine environment, functional polymorphisms in genes that interact with *NSD1,* and intrinsic variability in the regulation of downstream targets of NSD1 may all be implicated.

It is often assumed that Sotos syndrome with severe learning disability and/or multiple additional features is due to 5q35 microdeletions (Nagai et al. 2003). Although the phenotypes of individuals with microdeletions tend to be at the severe end of the spectrum, Sotos syndrome in most-severely affected individuals is attributable to intragenic mutations, which are a much more common cause of Sotos syndrome, accounting for the disorder in >80% of patients. Our data also suggest that missense and truncating *NSD1* mutations are similar with respect to degree of overgrowth, spectrum of learning disability, and nature and frequency of additional features.

Sotos Syndrome Is a Fully Penetrant Disorder That Is Usually Nonfamilial

We screened >300 parents of *NSD1*-positive individuals but identified mutations in only 11, all of whom were clinically diagnosed with familial Sotos syndrome before the molecular analyses. Thus, we have not seen a case of nonpenetrance for a confirmed pathogenic *NSD1* mutation. Neither have we seen a family with affected siblings of unaffected parents that would suggest germinal mosaicism. These data indicate that the recurrence risk for unaffected parents of a child with Sotos syndrome is extremely low and that such cases are almost always the result of de novo mutations. Familial cases had a markedly increased proportion of missense mutations, compared with nonfamilial cases, and it is interesting that all familial missense mutations occurred outside the SET domain. This suggests that certain types of mutations may be more likely to be heritable. However, affected families with truncating mutations were also identified.

The reasons for the low vertical transmission rate are currently unclear. One-third of patients with Sotos syndrome have only mild learning disability, and many of these patients are likely to consider having children in the future. Our very small series of adult patients with Sotos syndrome who have been trying to have children has not revealed any obvious problems during puberty, conception, pregnancy, or childbirth. Moreover, the outcomes have been consistent with the expected 50% offspring risk of an autosomal dominant disorder. Long-term prospective follow-up of patients with Sotos syndrome will likely be required to clarify these apparently paradoxical observations.

To date, we have undertaken all *NSD1* testing in the United Kingdom. This includes 124 U.K. subjects who were clinically judged to have Sotos syndrome by three clinical geneticists who were unaware of the molecular results. Of these 124 individuals, 96 have intragenic *NSD1* mutations, 12 have 5q35 microdeletions, 7 have partial-gene deletions, and 9 have no identified cause. These data suggest that, in at least 93% of patients, Sotos syndrome is attributable to *NSD1*—with 77% of patients having small intragenic mutations, 6% with partial-gene deletions, and 10% with whole-gene deletions. Only 7% of patients did not have an identifiable abnormality in *NSD1.* Such patients are clinically very similar to *NSD1*-positive patients with Sotos syndrome, and we suspect they also have abrogated NSD1 function. It is likely such patients harbor either mutations that were not detected by our heteroduplex analyses or aberrations that were not identifiable by our screening methods, such as regulatory abnormalities. Although we cannot exclude genetic heterogeneity as the cause of Sotos syndrome in a small proportion of patients, our analyses demonstrate that Sotos syndrome is attributable to *NSD1* in the great majority of affected individuals.

Acknowledgments

We are grateful to all the families with childhood overgrowth conditions who participated in this research and to the many clinicians who recruited them into the study. J.D. is supported by the Medical Research Council, K.T.-B. is supported by the Birth Defects Foundation, and A.I. is supported by Tenovus the Cancer Charity. This research was supported by the Institute of Cancer Research (United Kingdom) and the Medical Research Council (United Kingdom). The Childhood Overgrowth Collaboration includes the following contributors: M. Addor, A. Al Swaid, J. Amiel, S. Andries, H. Archer, A. Barnicoat, M. Barrow, J. Barwell, G.B., K. Becker, J. Berg, B. Bernhard, M. Bhat, M. Bitner, E. Blair, A. Brady, L. Brueton, S. Cavani, M. Cecconi, K. Chandler, C. Christensen, A. Clarke, J. Clayton-Smith, T.R.P.C., L. Colleaux, A. Colley, A. Collins, V.C.-D., S. Danda, S. Davies, R. Day, M. de Roy, N. Dennis,

A. Dobbie, P. Edery, F. Elmslie, F.F., H. Firth, R. Fischetto, D. FitzPatrick, F. Forzano, N. Foulds, J. Franklin, A. Fryer, S. Garcia, C. Gardiner, C. Garrett, B. Gener, R. Gibbons, Y. Gillerot, G. Gillessen-Kaesbach, D. Goudie, M. Grasso, A. Henderson, J. Hirst, S. Hodgson, S. Holder, T. Homfrey, H.E.H., B. Kerr, A. Kumar, D. Kumar, D. Lacombe, W. Lam, M. Le Merrer, N. Leonard, J. Liebelt, P. Lunt, S. Lynch, S. Lyonnet, A. Magee, M. Malacarne, S. Mansour, M. McEntagart, S. Majore, S. McKee, C. McKeown, P. Meinecke, K. Metcalfe, D. Milani, S. Mohammad, A. Munnich, A. Murray, A. Nemeth, G. Neri, S. Odent, S. Park, M. Patton, E. Penny, D. Pilz, B. Plecko, C. Pollitt, S. Price, O. Quarrell, A. Raas-Rothschild, N.R., W. Raith, J. Rankin, L. Raymond, W. Reardon, E. Reid, E. Rosser, D. Ruddy, A. Saggar-Malik, H. Santos, G. Scarano, G. B. Schaeffer, A. Schulze, A. Selicorni, A. Shaw, M. Silengo, S. Smithson, M. Splitt, F. Stewart, H. Stewart, M. Suri, E. Sweeney, K.T.-B., I.K.T., E. Thompson, M. Tischowitz, J. Tolmie, S.T., P. Turnpenny, L. Van Maldergem, P. Vasudevan, I. Vaz, D.W., C. Verellen, G. Viot, E. Wakeling, D. Weaver, K. White, L. Wilson, R. Winter, P. Zack, G. Zampino, and A. Zankl.

Web Resources

The URLs for data presented herein are as follows:

Online Mendelian Inheritance in Man (OMIM), http://www.ncbi.nlm.nih.gov/Omim/ (for Sotos syndrome, Weaver syndrome, and BWS)

R Project for Statistical Computing, http://www.R-project.org (for statistical analyses)

References

Aasland R, Gibson TJ, Stewart AF (1995) The PHD finger: implications for chromatin-mediated transcriptional regulation. Trends Biochem Sci 20:56–59

Baujat G, Rio M, Rossignol S, Sanlaville D, Lyonnet S, Le Merrer M, Munnich A, Gicquel C, Cormier-Daire V, Colleaux L (2004) Paradoxical NSD1 mutations in Beckwith-Wiedemann syndrome and 11p15 anomalies in Sotos syndrome. Am J Hum Genet 74:715–720

Cecconi M, Forzano F, Milani D, Cavani S, Baldo C, Selicorni A, Pantaleoni C, Silengo M, Ferrero GB, Scarano G, Della Monica M, Fischetto R, Grammatico P, Majore S, Zampino G, Memo L, Cordisco EL, Neri G, Pierluigi M, Bricarelli FD, Grasso M, Faravelli F (2005) Mutation analysis of the *NSD1* gene in a group of 59 patients with congenital overgrowth. Am J Med Genet A 134:247–253

de Boer L, Van Duyvenvoorde HA, Willemstein-Van Hove EC, Hoogerbrugge CM, Van Doorn J, Maassen JA, Karperien M, Wit JM (2004) Mutations in the NSD1 gene in patients with Sotos syndrome associate with endocrine and paracrine alterations in the IGF system. Eur J Endocrinol 151:333–341

Devriendt K, Vermeesch JR (2004) Chromosomal phenotypes and submicroscopic abnormalities. Hum Genomics 1:126–133

Douglas J, Coleman K, Tatton-Brown K, Hughes HE, Temple K, Cole TRP, The Childhood Overgrowth Collaboration, Rahman N (2005) Evaluation of *NSD2* and *NSD3* in overgrowth syndromes. Eur J Hum Genet 13:150–153

Douglas J, Hanks S, Temple IK, Davies S, Murray A, Upadhyaya M, Tomkins S, Hughes HE, Cole TR, Rahman N (2003) *NSD1* mutations are the major cause of Sotos syndrome and occur in some cases of Weaver syndrome but are rare in other overgrowth phenotypes. Am J Hum Genet 72: 132–143

Douglas J, Tatton-Brown K, Coleman K, Guerrero S, Berg J, Cole TRP, FitzPatrick D, Gillerot Y, Hughes HE, Pilz D, Raymond FL, Temple IK, Irrthum A, Schouten JP, Rahman N. Partial *NSD1* deletions cause 5% of Sotos syndrome and are readily identifiable by multiplex ligation-dependent probe amplification. J Med Genet (in press)

Huang N, vom BE, Garnier JM, Lerouge T, Vonesch JL, Lutz Y, Chambon P, Losson R (1998) Two distinct nuclear receptor interaction domains in NSD1, a novel SET protein that exhibits characteristics of both corepressors and coactivators. EMBO J 17:3398–3412

Jaju RJ, Fidler C, Haas OA, Strickson AJ, Watkins F, Clark K, Cross NC, Cheng JF, Aplan PD, Kearney L, Boultwood J, Wainscoat JS (2001) A novel gene, NSD1, is fused to NUP98 in the t(5;11)(q35;p15.5) in de novo childhood acute myeloid leukemia. Blood 98:1264–1267

Kurotaki N, Harada N, Shimokawa O, Miyake N, Kawame H, Uetake K, Makita Y, et al (2003) Fifty microdeletions among 112 cases of Sotos syndrome: low copy repeats possibly mediate the common deletion. Hum Mutat 22:378–387

Kurotaki N, Imaizumi K, Harada N, Masuno M, Kondoh T, Nagai T, Ohashi H, Naritomi K, Tsukahara M, Makita Y, Sugimoto T, Sonoda T, Hasegawa T, Chinen Y, Tomita Ha HA, Kinoshita A, Mizuguchi T, Yoshiura KK, Ohta T, Kishino T, Fukushima Y, Niikawa N, Matsumoto N (2002) Haploinsufficiency of *NSD1* causes Sotos syndrome. Nat Genet 30:365–366

Nagai T, Matsumoto N, Kurotaki N, Harada N, Niikawa N, Ogata T, Imaizumi K, Kurosawa K, Kondoh T, Ohashi H, Tsukahara M, Makita Y, Sugimoto T, Sonoda T, Yokoyama T, Uetake K, Sakazume S, Fukushima Y, Naritomi K (2003) Sotos syndrome and haploinsufficiency of *NSD1*: clinical features of intragenic mutations and submicroscopic deletions. J Med Genet 40:285–289

Niikawa N (2004) Molecular basis of Sotos syndrome. Horm Res 62 Suppl 3:60–65

Rayasam GV, Wendling O, Angrand PO, Mark M, Niederreither K, Song L, Lerouge T, Hager GL, Chambon P, Losson R (2003) NSD1 is essential for early post-implantation development and has a catalytically active SET domain. EMBO J 22:3153–3163

Rio M, Clech L, Amiel J, Faivre L, Lyonnet S, Le Merrer M, Odent S, Lacombe D, Edery P, Brauner R, Raoul O, Gosset P, Prieur M, Vekemans M, Munnich A, Colleaux L, Cormier-Daire V (2003) Spectrum of *NSD1* mutations in Sotos and Weaver syndromes. J Med Genet 40:436–440

Stec I, Nagl SB, van Ommen GJB, den Dunnen JT (2000) The PWWP domain: a potential protein-protein interaction domain in nuclear proteins influencing differentiation? FEBS Lett 473:1–5

Tatton-Brown K, Douglas J, Coleman K, Baujat G, Chandler

K, Clarke A, Collins A, Davies S, Faravelli F, Firth H, Garrett C, Hughes HE, Kerr B, Liebelt J, Reardon W, Schaeffer GB, Splitt M, Temple IK, Waggoner D, Weaver DD, Wilson L, Cole T, Cormier-Daire V, Irrthum A, Rahman N (2005) Multiple mechanisms are implicated in the generation of 5q35 microdeletions in Sotos syndrome. J Med Genet 42:307–313

Tatton-Brown K, Rahman N (2004) Clinical features of NSD1-positive Sotos syndrome. Clin Dysmorphol 13:199–204

Türkmen S, Gillessen-Kaesbach G, Meinecke P, Albrecht B, Neumann LM, Hesse V, Palanduz S, Balg S, Majewski F, Fuchs S, Zschieschang P, Greiwe M, Mennicke K, Kreuz FR, Dehmel HJ, Rodeck B, Kunze J, Tinschert S, Mundlos S, Horn D (2003) Mutations in *NSD1* are responsible for Sotos syndrome, but are not a frequent finding in other overgrowth phenotypes. Eur J Hum Genet 11:858–865

Visser R, Shimokawa O, Harada N, Kinoshita A, Ohta T, Niikawa N, Matsumoto N (2005) Identification of a 3.0-kb major recombination hotspot in patients with Sotos syndrome who carry a common 1.9-Mb microdeletion. Am J Hum Genet 76:52–67

Waggoner G, Raca G, Welch K, Dempsey M, Anderes E, Ostrovnaya I, Alkhateeb A, Kamimura J, Matsumoto N, Schaeffer GB, Martin CL, Das S. *NSD1* analysis for Sotos syndrome: insights and perspectives from the clinical laboratory. Genet Med (in press)

Deletions Involving Long-Range Conserved Nongenic Sequences Upstream and Downstream of *FOXL2* as a Novel Disease-Causing Mechanism in Blepharophimosis Syndrome

D. Beysen,[1] J. Raes,[3] B. P. Leroy,[1,2] A. Lucassen,[4] J. R. W. Yates,[5] J. Clayton-Smith,[6] H. Ilyina,[7] S. Sklower Brooks,[8] S. Christin-Maitre,[9] M. Fellous,[10] J. P. Fryns,[11] J. R. Kim,[12] P. Lapunzina,[13] E. Lemyre,[14] F. Meire,[3] L. M. Messiaen,[15] C. Oley,[16] M. Splitt,[17] J. Thomson,[18] Y. Van de Peer,[3] R. A. Veitia,[10] A. De Paepe,[1] and E. De Baere[1]

[1]Center for Medical Genetics and [2]Department of Ophthalmology, Ghent University Hospital, and [3]Research Group of Bioinformatics and Evolutionary Genomics, Department of Plant Systems Biology, Ghent University–Flemish Institute for Biotechnology, Ghent, Belgium; [4]Wessex Clinical Genetics Service, University of Southampton, Southampton, United Kingdom; [5]Department of Medical Genetics, University of Cambridge and Addenbrooke's Hospital, Cambridge, United Kingdom; [6]Academic Department of Medical Genetics, St. Mary's Hospital, Manchester, United Kingdom; [7]Belorussian Institute for Hereditary Disorders, Minsk, Belarus; [8]New York State Institute for Basic Research in Developmental Disabilities, New York; [9]Service d'Endocrinologie, Hôpital Saint-Antoine, and [10]INSERM U361 Reproduction et Physiopathologie Obstétricale Hôpital Cochin, Paris; [11]Center for Human Genetics, Leuven, Belgium; [12]Department of Biochemistry and Molecular Biology, Yeungnam University, Daegu, Republic of Korea; [13]Servicio de Genética, Hospital Universitario La Paz, Madrid; [14]Medical Genetics Service, Department of Pediatrics, Hôpital Sainte-Justine, Université de Montréal, Montreal; [15]University of Alabama, Birmingham; [16]Birmingham Women's Hospital, Birmingham, United Kingdom; [17]Department of Clinical Genetics, Guy's and St Thomas' Hospital National Health Service Trust, London; and [18]Clinical Genetics, St. James's University Hospital, Leeds, United Kingdom

The expression of a gene requires not only a normal coding sequence but also intact regulatory regions, which can be located at large distances from the target genes, as demonstrated for an increasing number of developmental genes. In previous mutation studies of the role of *FOXL2* in blepharophimosis syndrome (BPES), we identified intragenic mutations in 70% of our patients. Three translocation breakpoints upstream of *FOXL2* in patients with BPES suggested a position effect. Here, we identified novel microdeletions outside of *FOXL2* in cases of sporadic and familial BPES. Specifically, four rearrangements, with an overlap of 126 kb, are located 230 kb upstream of *FOXL2*, telomeric to the reported translocation breakpoints. Moreover, the shortest region of deletion overlap (SRO) contains several conserved nongenic sequences (CNGs) harboring putative transcription-factor binding sites and representing potential long-range *cis*-regulatory elements. Interestingly, the human region orthologous to the 12-kb sequence deleted in the polled intersex syndrome in goat, which is an animal model for BPES, is contained in this SRO, providing evidence of human-goat conservation of *FOXL2* expression and of the mutational mechanism. Surprisingly, in a fifth family with BPES, one rearrangement was found downstream of *FOXL2*. In addition, we report nine novel rearrangements encompassing *FOXL2* that range from partial gene deletions to submicroscopic deletions. Overall, genomic rearrangements encompassing or outside of *FOXL2* account for 16% of all molecular defects found in our families with BPES. In summary, this is the first report of extragenic deletions in BPES, providing further evidence of potential long-range *cis*-regulatory elements regulating *FOXL2* expression. It contributes to the enlarging group of developmental diseases caused by defective distant regulation of gene expression. Finally, we demonstrate that CNGs are candidate regions for genomic rearrangements in developmental genes.

Introduction

The expression pattern of many developmental genes is regulated at different levels. Usually, basal gene expression is controlled by the core promoter, located immediately upstream of the ORF. However, spatiotemporally and quantitatively correct gene expression is often controlled by long-range *cis*-acting regulatory elements as distant as 1.1 Mb (Velagaleti et al. 2005). These elements (enhancers, insulators, and locus-control regions) can be located upstream or downstream of the transcription unit of a gene. Interspecies comparative studies show a strong evolutionary conservation of these elements, which may reside in unrelated neighboring genes or intergenic regions. Genomic rearrangements involving such elements outside of a transcription unit can give rise to human disease by a dissociation of the transcrip-

Received April 22, 2005; accepted for publication May 19, 2005; electronically published June 16, 2005.

Address for correspondence and reprints: Dr. Elfride De Baere, Center for Medical Genetics, Ghent University Hospital, De Pintelaan 185, B-9000 Ghent, Belgium. E-mail: Elfride.DeBaere@UGent.be

0002-9297/2005/7702-0004$15.00

tion unit and its *cis*-acting regulatory elements, by an alteration of the chromatin structure, or by both mechanisms (reviewed by Kleinjan and van Heyningen [2005]).

Recently, it was shown that heterozygous mutations of the *FOXL2* gene (MIM 605597), which encodes a forkhead transcription factor, cause both types of blepharophimosis-ptosis-epicanthus inversus syndrome (BPES [MIM 110100]). BPES is a rare, autosomal dominant developmental disorder characterized by an eyelid malformation. Two subtypes have been identified; type I is associated with premature ovarian failure (POF), whereas type II is not (Zlotogora et al. 1983). It was shown that haploinsufficiency of *FOXL2* was caused by intragenic mutations, in most cases, and by submicroscopic deletions encompassing *FOXL2* and neighboring genes, in two cases (De Baere et al. 2001, 2003). A genotype-phenotype correlation was proposed mainly on the basis of intragenic mutations distinguishing the two BPES types at the molecular level (De Baere et al. 2003). Despite the ovarian phenotype in BPES, several studies have indicated that mutations in *FOXL2* do not play a major role in causing idiopathic POF (De Baere et al. 2001, 2002; Harris et al. 2002; Bodega et al. 2004).

A spatiotemporally restricted expression pattern of the *FOXL2* transcript and protein was demonstrated in several species (human, mouse, and goat). It was shown to be expressed in developing eyelids and in granulosa cells of fetal and adult ovaries (Crisponi et al. 2001; Cocquet et al. 2002, 2003). Recently, two studies presenting homozygous knockout mice showed that granulosa cell function is crucial not only for oocyte growth but also for ovarian maintenance, thus providing a molecular mechanism for POF in BPES in vivo (Schmidt et al. 2004; Uda et al. 2004).

During the positional cloning of *FOXL2,* three balanced translocations were characterized in patients with a classic BPES phenotype. It was shown that the breakpoints of these translocations disrupt two other genes (*BPESC1* and *MRPS22*), both devoid of pathogenic mutations in other patients with BPES, suggesting a position effect (De Baere et al. 2000; Praphanphoj et al. 2000; Crisponi et al. 2001, 2004).

Sequencing of the *FOXL2* ORF, in combination with FISH analysis with a probe encompassing the *FOXL2* gene, revealed mutations in <70% of patients with BPES (De Baere et al. 2001, 2003). Here, we applied a novel mutation-detection strategy consisting of multiplex ligation-dependent probe amplification (MLPA), genotyping with >60 microsatellites and SNPs, and comprehensive FISH analysis. This approach led to the identification of nine novel deletions encompassing *FOXL2,* which ranged from partial and total gene deletions to microdeletions and submicroscopic deletions. Notably, five novel deletions were found either upstream or downstream of the transcription unit of *FOXL2*. These genic and extragenic (micro)deletions account for 11% and 5%, respectively, of all molecular defects found in our cohort with BPES. Finally, we report the first case of germline mosaicism in a family with BPES that is confirmed at the molecular level.

Material and Methods

Patients and Diagnostic Criteria

The 37 consenting probands with BPES who were included in this study presented with blepharophimosis, ptosis, epicanthus inversus, and telecanthus. The clinical diagnosis was given by a clinical geneticist or an ophthalmologist. When possible, karyotyping was performed in the referring laboratory. The karyotype was not confirmed by us. In each proband, intragenic mutations were excluded by sequencing of the *FOXL2* ORF, as described by De Baere et al. (2001).

Custom-Made MLPA

MLPA permits relative quantification of changes in copy number of specific chromosomal sequences (Schouten et al. 2002). A custom-made deletion-detection kit for *FOXL2* was developed by MRC-Holland (P054 *FOXL2*) and contains three different probes for *FOXL2* (FOXL2-D01, FOXL2-D02, and FOXL2-D03), four probes for the *ATR* gene (located at 3q22-24), and probes for other genes (*TWIST, FOXC1, PITX2, FOXC2,* and *OA1*). Probe FOXL2-D01 is located in the forkhead domain (c.252–351; g.489–588), probe FOXL2-D02 is between the forkhead domain and the polyalanine tract (c.575–641; g.812–878), and probe FOXL2-D03 is downstream of the polyalanine tract (c.1053–1113; g.1290–1350). MLPA was performed in accordance with the manufacturer's instructions.

FISH

A genomic BAC contig of region 3q23 was obtained from the National Center for Biotechnology Information (NCBI) database. BACs were obtained from The Wellcome Trust Sanger Institute and BACPAC Resources Center. PACs and cosmids had been previously obtained from the UK–Medical Research Council and were mapped by FISH (De Baere et al. 1999). BAC, PAC, and cosmid DNA was prepared and labeled with the use of standard conditions. FISH analysis was performed as described by De Baere et al. (1999).

Microsatellite Analysis

Fifteen polymorphic microsatellites (with prefix "D3S") were selected from the NCBI on the basis of location and heterozygosity. Primer sequences of markers with

Table 1

Primer Sequences of Novel Microsatellites and SNaPshot Analysis

The table is available in its entirety in the online edition of *The American Journal of Human Genetics.*

prefixes "VY" and "NU" were obtained from Udar et al. (2003). A third series of microsatellites (Tel2 and markers with prefix "EDB") was developed by a manual search for repeats in the BAC sequences derived from NCBI. For a fourth series (with prefix "DB"), the different BAC sequences were analyzed using the Find Simple Repeats software, which selects repetitive sequences that are expected to have a very high degree of polymorphism. The search was confined to sequences presenting repetitions with a maximum of 4 nt and having a total length of at least 12 nt. Sequences with a score ⩾30 were selected for primer design. Primer sequences are given in table 1. Characterization of the polymorphic nature of the known and novel microsatellites was performed in a white population by use of an M13-system described by Schuelke (2000). For allele sizing, aliquots of PCR reaction were mixed with ROX-500 or ROX-1000 size standard (Applied Biosystems) and formamide and were separated on an ABI PRISM 3100 Genetic Analyzer (Applied Biosystems). Fragment sizing was performed automatically using GeneScan version 3.7. The different microsatellite alleles were numbered consecutively, in order of increasing size. The numbering is different for each family.

SNaPshot Analysis

Twenty-seven SNP loci were selected from the International HapMap Project database, and amplification primers were designed so that PCR products of ∼300 bp were obtained. Typing primers were designed to anneal to the target DNA flanking the 3′ end of the SNP. A standard PCR reaction was performed, followed by exonuclease I and shrimp alkaline phosphatase (SAP) treatment (Amersham). A single-nucleotide primer extension reaction was performed using an ABI PRISM SNaPshot Multiplex kit (Applied Biosystems), in accordance with the manufacturer's instructions. After SAP treatment, products were separated on an ABI PRISM 3100 Genetic Analyzer (Applied Biosystems) and were analyzed with GeneScan version 3.7. Numbers were assigned to alleles as follows: A = 1, C = 2, G = 3, and T = 4.

To assess the degree of germline mosaicism in an unaffected male, quantitative SNaPshot analysis was performed as described by Mátyás et al. (2002). For normalization, genomic samples from four unrelated individuals who have an identical SNP haplotype as that of the test sample were used as controls.

Long-Range PCR

For long-range PCR, the Expand Long Template PCR System (Roche) was used. A master mix of 50 μl contained 300 ng of genomic DNA, 0.5 μM of each primer, 5 μl of Expand Long Template PCR buffer 3 (containing 10 × PCR buffer and 27.5 mM $MgCl_2$), 3.75 U of Expand Long Template enzyme mix (containing *Taq* DNA polymerase and *Tgo* DNA polymerase), 500 μM of each dNTP, and 3 mM additional $MgCl_2$. Cycling conditions included an initial denaturation cycle at 94°C for 2 min, followed by 10 cycles at 94°C for 20 s, 65°C for 30 s, and 68°C for 12 min; 25 cycles at 94°C for 30 s and 65°C for 30 s and elongation for 12 min plus 20 s for each successive cycle; and a final extension at 72°C for 7 min.

Construction of a High-Resolution Physical Map Covering Microdeletions

First, we generated a sequence contig of 16 overlapping RPCI-11 BAC clones that span ∼1.8 Mb surrounding *FOXL2* by a search of GenBank (NCBI). The polymorphic microsatellites selected from NCBI were positioned on this BAC contig by use of the reference numbering of build 34, version 3 ("the golden path"), and by use of BLAST (NCBI). The localization of the anonymous microsatellites and SNPs was verified by BLAST searches against the BAC sequences. The exact PAC and cosmid localization was determined by BLAST after PAC and cosmid end sequencing, in accordance with standard protocol. Finally, the different known and unassigned genes that are located in this region were added to the map according to NCBI data.

Comparative Sequence Analysis

To identify conserved nongenic sequences (CNGs), comparative sequence analysis of the regions of interest was performed using the University of California–Santa Cruz (UCSC) Genome Browser. The UCSC Multiz Alignments and Conservation track contains a measure of evolutionary conservation in human, chimp, mouse, rat, dog, chicken, pufferfish, and zebrafish based on a phylogenetic hidden Markov model (phastCons). The overall conservation score across all species, as well as pairwise alignments of each species aligned to the human genome, were retrieved, and gapped alignments were included. The length of the alignment is based on the lengths of gaps in the human sequence at those alignment positions, relative to the longest nonhuman sequence. Alignments are based on the following genome assemblies: human, May 2004 (hg17); chimp, November 2003 (panTro1); mouse, May 2004 (mm5); rat, June 2003 (rn3); dog, July 2004 (canFam1); chicken, February 2004 (galGal2); *Fugu,* August 2002 (fr1); and zebrafish,

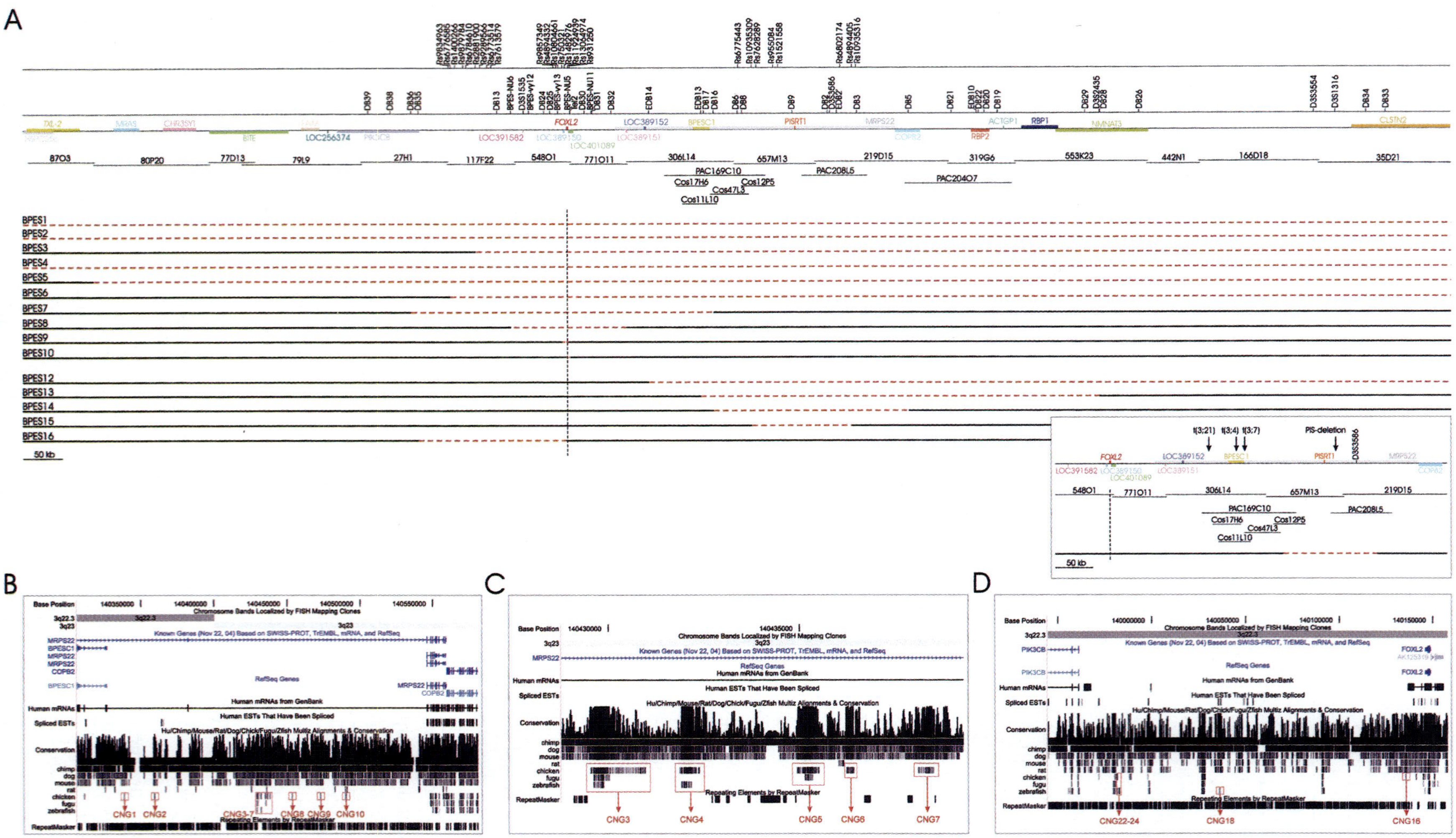
A
TXL-2
MRAS
CHR3SY1
BITE
LOC256374
PIK3CB
27H1
LOC391582
FOXL2
LOC389150
LOC401089
LOC389152
LOC389151
BPESC1
PISRT1
MRPS22
COPB2
RBP2
ACTGP1
RBP1
NMNAT3
CLSTN2
87O3
80P20
77D13
79L9
117F22
548O1
771O11
306L14
657M13
219D15
319G6
553K23
442N1
166D18
35D21
PAC169C10
Cos17H6
Cos12P5
Cos47L3
Cos11L10
PAC208L5
PAC204O7
BPES1
BPES2
BPES3
BPES4
BPES5
BPES6
BPES7
BPES8
BPES9
BPES10
BPES12
BPES13
BPES14
BPES15
BPES16
50 kb
t(3;21)
t(3;4)
t(3;7)
PIS-deletion
D3S3586
B
Base Position
Chromosome Bands Localized by FISH Mapping Clones
Known Genes (Nov 22, 04) Based on SWISS-PROT, TrEMBL, mRNA, and RefSeq
RefSeq Genes
Human mRNAs from GenBank
Human ESTs That Have Been Spliced
Hu/Chimp/Mouse/Rat/Dog/Chick/Fugu/Zfish Multiz Alignments & Conservation
Repeating Elements by RepeatMasker
CNG1
CNG2
CNG3-7
CNG8
CNG9
CNG10
C
CNG3
CNG4
CNG5
CNG6
CNG7
D
CNG22-24
CNG18
CNG16

November 2003 (danRer1). Our selection criteria included conservation at least up to chicken, pufferfish, and/or zebrafish, independent of alignment length, percentage of conservation, and presence of gaps.

The respective sequences of the selected elements and their corresponding mouse sequences were retrieved through the UCSC Genome Browser. Apart from these sequences, an available 48-kb goat sequence from the polled intersex syndrome (PIS) locus (GenBank accession number AF404302) was retrieved for human-goat comparison with the use of mVista. A pairwise alignment was performed between human and mouse, human and goat, human and chicken, human and pufferfish, and human and zebrafish by use of ClustalW. To exclude the coding potential of all putative CNGs, the human sequence of the conserved region was compared with all available EST and protein sequences in GenBank, as well as with all gene predictions for the selected region available from the UCSC Genome Browser and the Biomax Human Genome Database (blastn, blastx, tblastx, and nrprot). In addition, sequences were scanned for repetitive elements using RepeatMasker. Sequences that did not show significant similarity to known proteins, genes and/or transcripts, or transposable elements were selected as CNGs. These were searched against the Transfac database (version 8.3) of known vertebrate *cis*-acting regulatory DNA elements and *trans*-acting factors by use of the Match tool included in that database (Matys et al. 2003). Only highly significant matches with transcription-factor binding sites were considered, by use of the built-in "minimize false positive matches" setting.

Results and Discussion

The mutation detection rate of <70% in previous mutation studies of *FOXL2* in BPES could be explained by clinical misdiagnosis; the sensitivity of the strategy used, which might not allow detection of changes in gene copy number or in distant sequences outside of the transcription unit of *FOXL2* (De Baere et al. 2001, 2003); or the presence of a second BPES locus, although there is no evidence to support the existence of a second locus. Here, we developed a novel combined approach consisting of (1) custom-made MLPA for detection of changes in gene copy number of *FOXL2* and other genes; (2) a genotyping panel, comprising 15 known and 32 anonymous microsatellites and 26 SNPs; and (3) comprehensive FISH analysis whenever possible.

Genomic Rearrangements Encompassing FOXL2

A clue to subtle *FOXL2* deletions was found in similar observations for *FOXC1*, which encodes a forkhead transcription factor associated with ocular anterior segment dysgenesis (IRID1 [MIM 601631]). Irrespective of whether the gene is duplicated or deleted, a nearly identical ocular phenotype is observed, showing that exact gene dosage of *FOXC1* is critical for normal eye development (Lehmann et al. 2003).

Our approach allowed identification of 11 deletions encompassing *FOXL2*, of which 9 are novel. These deletions contribute to 11% (11/100) of all molecular defects found in our series of patients with BPES and are found in 30% (11/37) of mutation-negative patients. They occur in sporadic cases and familial cases and are absent in all unaffected family members analyzed. A graphical overview of these deletions is given in figure 1*A*. Clinical data for the 11 families and molecular details on the deletions are summarized in table 2.

The rearrangements include one partial *FOXL2* deletion (in BPES10), an 8-kb deletion removing the whole *FOXL2* ORF (in BPES9), two microdeletions of up to 420 kb, encompassing *FOXL2* and neighboring genes (in BPES7 and BPES8), four submicroscopic deletions (in BPES2, BPES4, BPES5, and BPES6), and two micro-

Figure 1 *A*, Physical map of a 1.8-Mb region flanking *FOXL2* that shows the position of the BACs, PACs, cosmids, microsatellites, and SNPs that were used for identification and delineation of the deletions. The map is drawn to scale; the size equivalent to 50 kb is given at the bottom left corner. The location of *FOXL2* is indicated by a vertical black line. The top line represents the localization of SNPs, and the second line contains the known and anonymous microsatellites used in this study. In the third line, the location of the genes in this region is shown, whereas the BACs, PACs, and cosmids used for FISH are shown below the line. The lower part of *A* is an overview of all deletions identified in this study, except one. Every line represents a patient or family in whom a deletion was found. The dashed red line shows the maximal extent of the deletion. The first 10 lines represent the deletions that encompass *FOXL2*. The deletion identified in BPES11 is not shown, since the extent of the deletion could not be determined because of a lack of material for FISH and microsatellite analysis. The second group represents the five extragenic deletions (four upstream and one downstream). Clinical details and molecular data on the patients with deletions are shown in table 2. In a box at the bottom right, a detailed view of the SRO of the four upstream extragenic deletions is shown. The position of *FOXL2* is marked by a vertical dashed black line, and the SRO is shown by the dashed red line. The positions of the known three translocation breakpoints at 3q23 in BPES and of the orthologue of the PIS locus are indicated by vertical arrows. *B* and *C*, UCSC Genome Browser map of the SRO of the four upstream extragenic rearrangements in families BPES12, BPES13, BPES14, and BPES15. CNGs are highlighted at the bottom with red boxes. Their names, based on our arbitrary numbering, are given below the boxes. Details on all CNGs can be found in table 4. The CNGs shown in *B* are evolutionarily conserved up to chicken. *C* represents a more detailed view of CNG3–CNG7. CNG3–CNG5 are conserved up to zebrafish and/or pufferfish. They all represent potential *cis*-regulatory elements of the *FOXL2* region. *D*, UCSC Genome Browser map of the sequence contained in the downstream extragenic rearrangement in family BPES16. Five CNGs are indicated in this 3′ SRO, of which several are conserved up to zebrafish and/or pufferfish (CNG14, CNG18, and CNG22–CNG24).

Table 2

Summary of Clinical and Molecular Findings in Patients with BPES Who Have Deletions Encompassing *FOXL2* or Outside of the Transcription Unit of *FOXL2*

Type of Genomic Rearrangement and Family	Type of BPES[a]	Origin[b]	Clinical Data[c]	Type of Deletion[d]	Karyotype	MLPA Finding[d]	Extent of Deletion[d]	Delineation of Centromeric Breakpoint[e]	Delineation of Telomeric Breakpoint[e]	Confirmed by FISH	Parental Origin
Encompassing *FOXL2*:											
BPES1	F2	KR	6-y-old male with psychomotor retardation and VSD (Cha et al. 2003)	Microscopic del incl. *FOXL2* in II:2	…	Total *FOXL2* and *ATR* del	>6.1 Mb in II:2 (137606245–143780323)	*D3S1238–D3S3528* (2.20 Mb)	Telomeric to *ATR*	No	Maternal
BPES2	S	NO	11-y-old male with psychomotor retardation, widely spaced nipples, scoliosis, high arched palate, and umbilical hernia (De Baere et al. 2003)	Submicroscopic del incl. *FOXL2*	Normal	Total *FOXL2* and *ATR* del	>3.8 Mb (139895393–143780323)	*D3S3617–DB39* (1.81 Mb)	Telomeric to *ATR*	Yes	Maternal
BPES3	S	GB	4-y-old female with postnatal growth retardation and microcephaly	Microscopic del incl. *FOXL2*	46,XX,del(3)(q22q23)	Total *FOXL2* del (3 probes); *ATR* normal	Max. 3.6 Mb (140031707–143650777)	*rs2881900–DB13* (26.99 kb)	*D3S1309–ATR* (1.44 Mb)	No	Maternal
BPES4	S	CA	3-y-old female with normal psychomotor development and no intrauterine and postnatal growth retardation; ultrasound of uterus and ovaries was normal at age 13 mo	Submicroscopic del incl. *FOXL2*	Normal	Total *FOXL2* del (3 probes); partial *ATR* del (1 probe)	>3.5 Mb (140058657–143651142)	*D3S3617–DB13* (1.97 Mb)	*ATR* gene	Yes	Maternal
BPES5	F	DK	II:1 had psychomotor and growth retardation and high arched palate; I:1 had growth retardation, with no clinical data about psychomotor development (De Baere et al. 2001)	Submicroscopic del incl. *FOXL2*	Normal	Total *FOXL2* del (3 probes)	Max. 3.2 Mb (139548627–142750847)	In BAC RP11-80P20 (147 kb)	*D3S3554–D3S3711* (1.66 Mb)	Yes	Unknown
BPES6	S	ES	1.5-y-old female with abnormal nose, normal psychomotor development, and no growth retardation; ultrasound of uterus and ovaries was normal	Submicroscopic del incl. *FOXL2*	Normal	Total *FOXL2* del (3 probes); *ATR* normal	Max. 2.7 Mb (140036995–142750847)	*rs9289566–rs6776585* (36.77 kb)	*D3S1309–D3S3711* (541.72 kb)	No	Paternal
BPES7	F	ES	Father and son with normal psychomotor development	Microdel incl. *FOXL2*	Normal	Total *FOXL2* del (3 probes)	Max. 412 kb (139949789–140359539)	*DB36–DB35* (9.4 kb)	*DB16–DB6* (28.21 kb)	Yes	Paternal?
BPES8	S	CD-BE	3-y-old female with normal psychomotor development	Microdel incl. *FOXL2*	…	Total *FOXL2* del (3 probes)	Max. 243 kb (140075997–140319005)	*NU6–D3S1535* (15.8 kb)	*DB 31–DB17* (45.11 kb)	Yes	Paternal
BPES9	F1	FR	II:1 had secondary amenorrhea; III:2 had heart malformation (mild interauricular communication)	Total *FOXL2* del	…	Total *FOXL2* del (3 probes)	8,226 nt (140141021–140149217)	In BAC RP11-548O1, nt 60868	BAC RP11-548O1, nt 69094	No	Unknown
BPES10	S	GB	4-y-old female with normal psychomotor development	Partial *FOXL2* del	Normal	Partial *FOXL2* del (2/3 probes)	Max. 6 kb (140147210–140150682)	In *FOXL2*, between MLPA probes 2 and 3 (416 nt)	*FOXL2*–Tel2 (2,440 nt)	No	Unknown
BPES11	S1	AU	36-y-old female with normal psychomotor development, menarche at age 18 y, only two periods, and very high FSH levels; IVF failed	(Micro)del incl. *FOXL2*	Normal	Total *FOXL2* del (3 probes)	…	…	…	No	Unknown

Outside transcription unit of *FOXL2*:										
BPES12	S	BY	15-y-old male with normal psychomotor development, intrauterine and postnatal growth retardation, microcephaly, ventricular septum defect, small mouth, contracture of interphalangeal joints, and right iris heterochromia	Microdel upstream of *FOXL2* (at 101 kb)	Normal	Two copies of *FOXL2* and *ATR* (*D3S1309* is heterozygous)	Max. 1.9 Mb (140249840–142209012)	*EDB14–DB17* (69.40 kb)	*DB33–D3S1309* (1.03 Mb)	No	Paternal
BPES13	S	PL	2-y-old female with stenosis of lacrimal duct, normal psychomotor development, microcephaly, and renal reflux	Microdel upstream of *FOXL2* (at 101 kb)	Normal	Two copies of *FOXL2*	Max. 567 kb (140249840–140816803)	*EDB14–DB16* (81.64 kb)	*DB19–D3S2435* (129.11 kb)	No	Maternal
BPES14	F2	GB	2-generation family. I:2 had astigmatism, three pregnancies, oligomenorrhea at age 40 y, and amenorrhea at age 47 y. II:1 had strabismus, normal menarche at age 12 y, and oligomenorrhea with elevated FSH and LH at age 38 y. Both I:2 and II:1 had normal growth and psychomotor development.	Microdel upstream of *FOXL2* (at 183 kb)	...	Two copies of *FOXL2* and *ATR*	Max. 244 kb (140331480–140575742)	*DB16–D3S3586* (144.53 kb)	*rs4894405–DB5* (71.90 kb)	Yes	Unknown
BPES15	F2	BE	5-generation family with typical BEPS. Affected members, normal psychomotor development	Microdel upstream of *FOXL2* (at 231 kb)	Normal	Two copies of *FOXL2*	Max. 126 kb (140377649–140503837)	*rs10935309–rs955084* (27.14 kb)	*rs6802174–rs4894405* (14.47 kb)	Yes	Unknown
BPES16	F	GB	Half-sisters II:1 and II:3 were affected; father I:2 was not affected, suggestive of germline mosaicism. II:1 had a premature birth (32 wk) with respiratory distress syndrome, intrauterine and postnatal growth retardation, microcephaly, moderate learning difficulties apparent from age 7 y, and strabismus; II:3 had normal psychomotor development	Microdel downstream of *FOXL2* (at 28.7 kb)	Normal	Two copies of *FOXL2*	Max. 188 kb (139959089–140147132)	*DB35–rs9834963* (38.27 kb)	*rs7627822–FOXL2* (28.7 kb)	Yes	Paternal

[a] F1 = familial, type I; F2 = familial, type II; F = familial, type undetermined; S = sporadic; S1 = sporadic, type I.
[b] AU = Australia; BE = Belgium; BY = Belarus; CA = Canada; CD = Congo; DK = Denmark; ES = Spain; FR = France; GB = Great Britain; KR = South Korea; NO = Norway; PL = Poland.
[c] FSH = follicle-stimulating hormone; IVF = in vitro fertilization; LH = luteinizing hormone; VSD = ventricle septum defect; y = year.
[d] del = deletion; incl. = including; Max. = at maximum.
[e] In parentheses is the length of the interval in which the centromeric and the telomeric breakpoints are located.

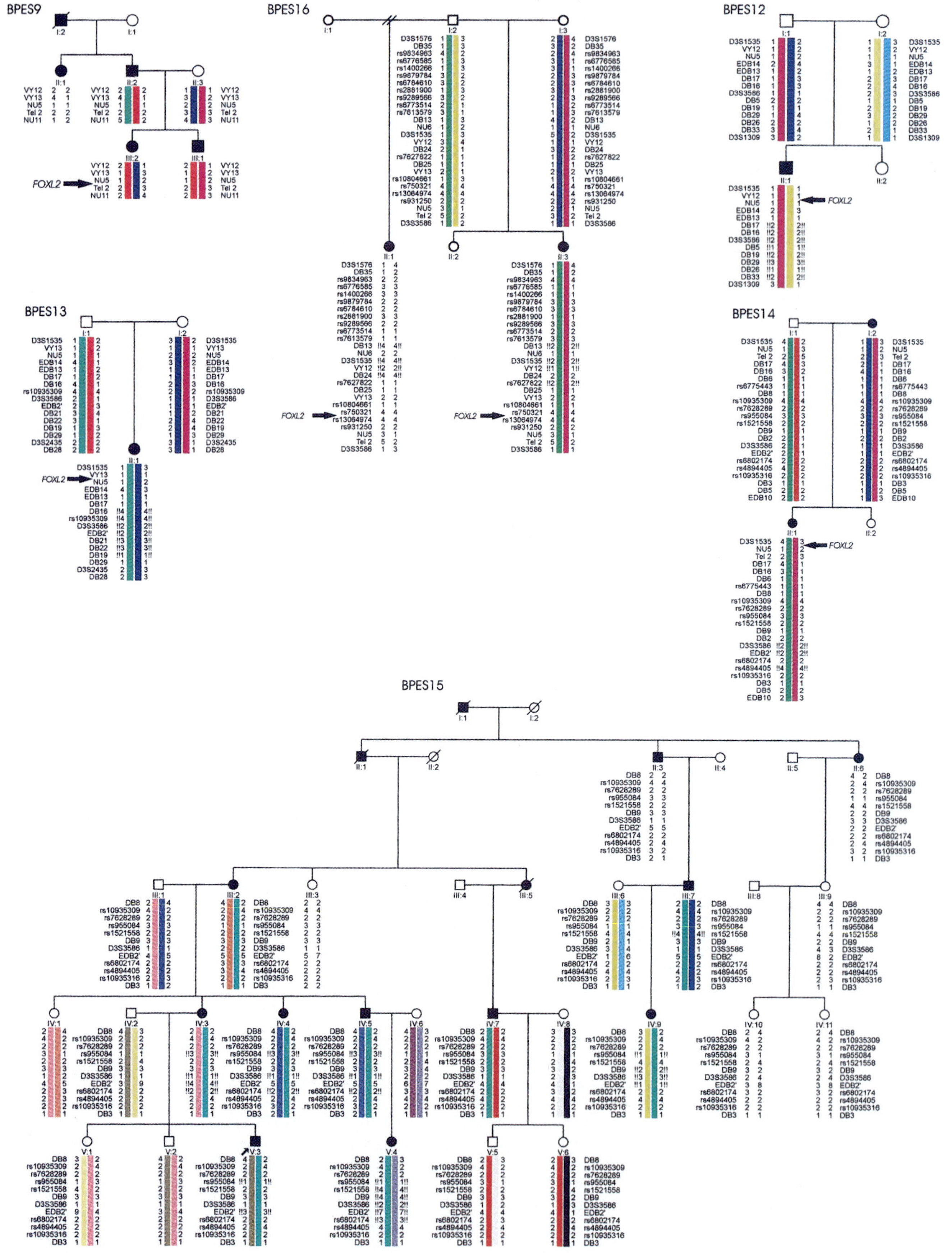
BPES9
BPES16
BPES12
BPES13
BPES14
BPES15
FOXL2

scopic deletions (in BPES1 and BPES3) (fig. 1*A* and table 2). In patient BPES11, MLPA analysis revealed a total *FOXL2* deletion; however, the extent could not be determined because of the lack of appropriate patient and parental material. The deletion breakpoints are scattered, suggesting lack of a deletion-prone region and nonhomologous end joining as the common causal mechanism (Shaw and Lupski 2004), which is supported by characterization of the junction fragment of an 8-kb deletion in family BPES9 with BPES type I (fig. 2 and fig. 3*C* and 3*D*). Attempts to characterize the junction fragments by long-range PCR failed for the other subtle deletions presented in this study.

In the three families with BPES in which several affected members are heterozygous for a total gene deletion (BPES9), a microdeletion (BPES7), or a submicroscopic deletion (BPES5), microsatellite analysis showed similar extents of the deletion in the affected family members of different generations, suggesting stability during meiosis (fig. 2 and fig. 4).

Previously, two submicroscopic deletions of >3.8 Mb and 3.2 Mb were found in patient BPES2 and the proband of BPES5, respectively, both of whom had psychomotor retardation and microcephaly as associated features. These findings led to a preliminary genotype-phenotype correlation (De Baere et al. 2001, 2003). Here, we identified a submicroscopic deletion of >3.5 Mb in a young woman with sporadic BPES (BPES4) who has microcephaly but apparently normal psychomotor development, suggesting that the extent of the deletion is not necessarily in linear correlation with the occurrence of developmental delay (table 2 and fig. 1*A*). In a recent study, it was postulated that mental retardation is associated with a heterozygous deletion of the Seckel-associated *ATR* gene located 3.6 Mb telomeric to *FOXL2* (Gille et al. 2003). In our series of patients, however, there was no consistent correlation between *ATR* haploinsufficiency and developmental delay, as seen in patient BPES4 and family BPES5 (table 2).

In addition, in 9 of 11 patients, the BPES type could not be determined (for prepubertal females or males with sporadic BPES). However, in the two families for which it was possible to assess the BPES type (BPES9 and BPES11), the deletion was found to lead to BPES and POF (type I), which is in agreement with previous genotype-phenotype correlations between heterozygous in-

The figure is available in its entirety in the online edition of *The American Journal of Human Genetics.*

Figure 3 Schematic diagram of *FOXL2* gene and protein, electropherogram of MLPA products, sequence electropherogram of the deletion junction fragment, and nucleotide sequence of the breakpoint junctions. The legend is available in its entirety in the online edition of *The American Journal of Human Genetics.*

Figure 2 Pedigrees with BPES and a rearrangement encompassing *FOXL2* or located outside of the transcription unit. Intragenic *FOXL2* mutations were excluded by sequencing of the ORF in all patients. MLPA was performed to assess changes in gene copy number, and haplotypes are based on microsatellite or SNP analysis. An exclamation mark (!) indicates hemizygosity of an allele. *BPES9,* Microsatellite analysis in two generations of this French family showed apparent linkage to *FOXL2*. However, no intragenic *FOXL2* mutation was found in affected members. MLPA analysis revealed a total gene deletion of *FOXL2*. Long-range PCR revealed the breakpoints of an 8-kb deletion (fig. 3). The occurrence of secondary amenorrhea in II:1 suggests this family has type I BPES. In addition, III:2 has a heart malformation in association with BPES. *BPES16,* In this family, two affected half-sisters (II:1 and II:3) have BPES, whereas their father (I:2) is clinically unaffected, suggesting germline mosaicism. FISH and microsatellite analysis revealed an extragenic deletion of 188 kb located 3′ of *FOXL2* in the half-sisters. Microsatellite analysis showed an apparent absence of this deletion in their father. However, quantitative studies revealed somatic mosaicism for this deletion in 5% of DNA from his leucocytes and 10% of DNA from his sperm cells, confirming germline mosaicism at the molecular level (table 3). *BPES12,* Upstream microdeletion in a 14-year-old male with sporadic BPES and additional features. MLPA showed normal *FOXL2* and *ATR* gene copy numbers, whereas several microsatellites at a distance from *FOXL2* were hemizygous, indicating a deletion outside of the transcription unit. The centromeric breakpoint of the deletion is located in a 69-kb interval between microsatellites *EDB14* and *DB17*; at the telomeric side, the deletion extends beyond the borders of the physical map in figure 1*A*, but does not contain *D3S1309*. The deletion encompasses at least several known and unknown genes (*LOC389152, BPESC1, MRPS22, COPB2, RBP2, ACTGP1, RBP1, NMNAT3,* and *CLSTN2*) and extends beyond 1.9 Mb. The contribution of each gene to the psychomotor retardation and other associated features in this patient is unclear. *BPES13,* Upstream microdeletion of maternal origin in a 2-year-old female with sporadic BPES who had normal psychomotor development and microcephaly. The deletion spans 567 kb at the most; the centromeric breakpoint is located between microsatellites *EDB14* and *DB16,* and the telomeric breakpoint is between markers *DB19* and *D3S2435*. The deletion covers part of *BPESC1, MRPS22, COPB2, RBP2, ACTGP1, RBP1,* and *NMNAT3. BPES14,* Microdeletion of ∼200 kb 5′ of *FOXL2* in two affected females, I:2 and II:1, of a two-generation family with type II BPES. FISH analysis with probes RP11-548O1, RP11-306L14, RP11-319G6, Pac204O7, and Cos11L10 showed normal hybridization signals on both chromosomes 3, whereas RP11-657M13, Cos12P5, and Pac208L5 were deleted. One normal and one lighter signal were seen with RP11-219D15 and PAC169C10, confirming that the deletion breakpoints are located in these probes. The centromeric breakpoint of the deletion is located between *DB16* and *D3S3586,* and the telomeric breakpoint is between *EDB2′* and *DB5. BPES15,* Extragenic microdeletion found in a five-generation Belgian family with BPES type II, previously linked to 3q23 (Messiaen et al. 1996). This 126-kb microdeletion is the smallest one upstream of *FOXL2* and delineates the SRO of the different microdeletions located at this side of *FOXL2* (detailed view in fig. 1*A*). FISH probes RP11-657M13 and PAC208L5 showed one lighter and one normal hybridization signal, thus indicating the borders of the deletion. Analysis with adjacent probes showed two normal signals. The hemizygous microsatellites indicate that the centromeric breakpoint is located between *rs10935309* and *rs955084* and the telomeric breakpoint is between *rs6802174* and *rs4894405* (fig. 1*A*).

The figure is available in its entirety in the online edition of *The American Journal of Human Genetics.*

Figure 4 Haplotypes of families BPES5 and BPES7, in which affected members carry a deletion encompassing *FOXL2*, illustrating the stability of deletions in the different generations. The legend is available in its entirety in the online edition of *The American Journal of Human Genetics.*

tragenic mutations leading to a *FOXL2* null allele and BPES type I (De Baere et al. 2003). Because of the small sample size, this hypothesis needs to be evaluated in additional studies of patients carrying (micro)deletions. To allow reliable genotype-phenotype correlations for psychomotor development and POF risk, an accurate delineation of deletions is a prerequisite.

In some informative families, it was possible to determine the parental origin of the deletion, but no parent-of-origin effect was observed (maternal:paternal deletion ratio was 4:3) (table 2). Thus, BPES does not belong to the group of conditions in which sex-dependent mechanisms may play a role in the origin of the underlying genomic rearrangement (e.g., Charcot-Marie Tooth 1A and hereditary neuropathy with liability to pressure palsies) (Lopes et al. 1997).

Genomic Rearrangements Outside of the Transcription Unit of FOXL2

A complex regulation of gene expression has been suggested for several forkhead transcription factors by the occurrence of chromosomal rearrangements (translocations) upstream (*FOXC1*) and downstream (*FOXC2*) of their respective transcription units (Davies et al. 1999; Fang et al. 2000). For the *FOXL2* locus, specifically, three translocation breakpoints located 170 kb upstream of the disease gene cause exactly the same phenotype as loss-of-function mutations (De Baere et al. 2000; Praphanphoj et al. 2000; Crisponi et al. 2001, 2004).

Here, we report five novel deletions mapping upstream and downstream of the transcription unit of *FOXL2* in patients with BPES with a phenotype identical to that caused by intragenic mutations. The presence of an intact transcription unit (coding sequence and copy number) was confirmed by sequencing and MLPA in all affected patients. The extragenic genomic rearrangements contribute to 5% (5/100) of all the molecular defects identified in our series of patients with BPES and are found in 14% (5/37) of our mutation-negative patients with BPES. They are found in patients with sporadic BPES and patients with familial BPES and are absent in unaffected individuals. An overview of the location and extent of these rearrangements is given in figure 1*A*, and relevant clinical data for the patients are given in table 2.

First, we identified a genomic rearrangement—presumed to be a microdeletion of ~188 kb—downstream of *FOXL2* in family BPES16, in which two affected half-sisters have typical BPES, whereas their father is clinically unaffected, which is suggestive of germline mosaicism (fig. 2 and table 2). To confirm paternal germline mosaicism at a molecular level, quantitative SNaPshot analysis was performed for three informative SNPs located in the deletion (*rs9879784*, *rs9289566*, and *rs6773514*) (table 3). We estimated that ~10% of the paternal germ cells and 5% of somatic peripheral blood lymphocytes carry the deletion (table 3). The estimated recurrence risk in this family is 10%, being significantly higher than the risk of a de novo event (<1%). This is the first case of germline mosaicism in BPES that is documented at the molecular level. This study indicates that this is an important issue to be considered in genetic counseling.

Second, we identified four overlapping microdeletions, which ranged from 126 kb to 1.9 Mb, upstream of the transcription unit of *FOXL2*. These extragenic deletions were found in two patients with a sporadic form of BPES (BPES12 and BPES13) and in two families (BPES14 and BPES15) (fig. 1*A* and fig. 2). In two of these families, assessment of the BPES type was possible; the absence of female infertility or overt POF in affected females of families BPES14 and BPES15 suggests that these 5′-located microdeletions do not significantly perturb ovarian expression of *FOXL2* and thus lead to BPES type II.

Of the two affected half-sisters in family BPES16 with the downstream microdeletion, II:3 has typical BPES with apparently normal psychomotor development at age 4 years, whereas II:1 has BPES and also presents moderate learning difficulties that were apparent from age 6 years, intrauterine and postnatal growth retardation, and microcephaly (fig. 2 and table 2). She was born at a gestational age of 32 weeks because of preeclampsia. There is no indication of a different extent of the deletion in the two patients. Another patient (BPES12), heterozygous for a 1.9-Mb upstream deletion, has BPES and presents additional features, including microcephaly, intrauterine and postnatal growth retardation, and a ventricular septum defect (fig. 2 and table 2). These additional features might represent a contiguous gene syndrome that can be explained by the extent

Table 3

Results of Quantitative SNaPshot Analysis with SNPs *rs6773514, rs9289566,* and *rs9879784*

The table is available in its entirety in the online edition of *The American Journal of Human Genetics.*

Table 4

Details of CNGs Found in the Respective SROs of the Upstream and Downstream Genomic Rearrangements

The table is available in its entirety in the online edition of *The American Journal of Human Genetics.*

of the deletion. In the other three families (BPES13, BPES14, and BPES15), no associated features were present. For the extragenic rearrangements, we can conclude that there is no association with psychomotor retardation and that there are as yet no arguments for a correlation with POF risk.

In familial cases BPES14, BPES15, and BPES16, microsatellite and FISH analysis indicated that the extent of the respective extragenic deletion is equal in each generation, suggesting stability during meiosis in these families (fig. 2). These clinical and molecular observations underscore the value of using complementary tools to delineate the extent of microdeletions together with assessment of the gene copy number of *FOXL2*.

The shortest region of deletion overlap (SRO) of the 5′ microdeletions involves a 126-kb region. Interestingly, it contains the human orthologue of the PIS locus in the goat. PIS, characterized by polledness (absence of horns) and XX intersexuality, is an animal model for BPES. Pailhoux et al. (2001) showed that it was caused by a 12-kb deletion located 280 kb upstream of *FOXL2*. This deletion does not contain any coding sequences and affects transcription of at least two genes in the PIS goat: the noncoding *PISRT1* and *FOXL2*, located at 20 kb and 280 kb from the deletion, respectively. It was suggested that the PIS locus contains elements involved in long-range *cis*-regulation of goat *FOXL2* (Pailhoux et al. 2001). Our current study lends further support to this hypothesis.

Moreover, this SRO is located telomeric to three known translocation breakpoints in BPES (fig. 1*A*). Crisponi et al. (2004) noted that these breakpoints are all located in intron 6 of the *MRPS22* gene. Using human-mouse comparative sequence analysis, they showed the presence of three highly conserved sequence blocks upstream of the most distal breakpoint, in introns 6, 11, and 12 of *MRPS22*. The PIS locus was shown to be located in the conserved sequence block in intron 11 of *MRPS22*. It was postulated that these conserved sequence blocks are candidate regions that might function as distant enhancers or have an influence on higher-order chromatin structure, both of which affect long-range *cis*-regulation of *FOXL2* expression.

CNGs in the SRO of Extragenic Rearrangements

Recent experimental approaches demonstrated that a fraction of CNGs in the genome act as *cis*-transcriptional regulators, although little is known about their function (Dermitzakis et al. 2002, 2003). Furthermore, it has been shown that conserved sequences are clustered around developmental genes and function as regulatory elements that affect embryonic development (Bejerano et al. 2004; Plessy et al. 2005). In addition, genomic variation in CNGs is presumed to be associated with phenotypic variability and even with human monogenic conditions (reviewed by Dermitzakis et al. [2005]). To identify potential CNGs, a comparative sequence analysis was undertaken in the SRO of the extragenic deletions. We made use of publicly available, gapped and ungapped alignments of the UCSC Genome Browser. Although a human-mouse alignment is generally used, we made a selection of conserved sequences across more distant species to enhance the functional significance of the selected CNGs. We performed human-chicken, human-pufferfish, human-zebrafish, and human-goat comparisons (the latter only for an available 48-kb goat sequence [GenBank accession number AF404302]). In the two regions of interest, we identified 25 putative CNGs common to human and chicken, pufferfish, and/or zebrafish and 1 common to human and goat. Seventeen of those were eventually selected as CNGs, after we filtered for coding and transposable elements (table 4). Some of them (CNG3–CNG5) are conserved up to pufferfish or zebrafish, strongly suggesting that they function as a regulatory element (table 4). CNG3–CNG7 are all contained in the human orthologue of the PIS locus. These CNGs were found to be located in the 9-kb conserved sequence block previously described by Crisponi et al. (2004).

Analysis of these sequences with a Transfac database revealed several interesting putative transcription-factor binding sites for FOXP3 in CNG5 and CNG9; for HNF-1 in CNG3, CNG9, CNG22, and CNG24; for HNF-4 in CNG1 and CNG2; and for embryonic gonadal regulator SOX9 in CNG3. Interestingly, a regulatory link between SOX9 and the PIS locus has already been suggested by Nikic and Vaiman (2004). We found that a binding site for FOXL1 (ATTCAATAAAGAAGTA), previously identified by Crisponi et al. (2004) in the 9-kb conserved sequence block, was situated in CNG3. The conserved nature of the elements located in the human orthologue of the PIS locus, together with the prediction of potentially relevant binding sites, provide arguments that they are *cis*-acting elements (e.g., an enhancer) regulating correct spatiotemporal *FOXL2* expression during embryonic development.

It is nearly impossible to obtain human samples that would allow meaningful analysis of regulation of *FOXL2* expression in developing eyelids and ovary. Such analysis currently relies on genotype-phenotype correlations of genomic rearrangements and BPES, comparative sequence analysis, and experimental validation—for instance, in animal models. In the two families in which the BPES type could be assessed, BPES14 and BPES15, we found that the 5′ extragenic rearrangements led to BPES type II. This "mild" phenotype can be explained either (1) by a selective regulation of craniofacial *FOXL2* expression by the 5′ distant elements or (2) by regulation of both craniofacial and ovarian expression but with the absence of an ovarian phenotype in the case of a heterozygous deletion. The latter situation would be identical to the regulation of *FOXL2* expression in the goat, in which both the craniofacial and ovarian expression appear to be regulated by the PIS locus, but in which phenotypic expression of polledness and XX intersexuality depend on the heterozygous and homozygous states of the deletion, respectively.

There are other diseases known to be caused by genomic rearrangements lying at considerable distances from the disease gene and leading to phenotypes identical to those resulting from intragenic mutations. However, the majority is caused by chromosomal rearrangements (translocations), and only a minority results from deletions presumably affecting a regulatory element. The first reported example was that of the locus of control region (LCR) of the β-globin gene cluster. Translocation breakpoints and deletions in this conserved element cause autosomal recessive β-thalassemia due to silencing of the β-globin gene, which maps 50 kb downstream of the LCR (Driscoll et al. 1989). A hotspot for microdeletions has been identified, in patients with X-linked deafness type 3, that is 900 kb proximal to the *POU3F4* disease gene. The 8-kb SRO of these deletions contains a 2-kb sequence that is 80% conserved between human and mouse (de Kok et al. 1996). More recently, the autosomal recessive van Buchem disease was found to be caused by a homozygous deletion that is 52 kb downstream of the disease gene *SOST* and contains two CNGs (Balemans et al. 2002). Similarly, the upstream and downstream genomic rearrangements described here dissociate putative regulatory CNGs from their target gene *FOXL2* and lead to BPES, one of the first autosomal dominant conditions for which this mechanism has been demonstrated.

Our approach led to the identification of a molecular defect in 16 (43%) of 37 mutation-negative patients with BPES analyzed in this study. The lack of a sequence variation or a rearrangement in 21 patients, representing 17% (21/121) of the total patient group, might be explained by the fact that assessment of the four diagnostic criteria of BPES was done by different clinicians. In addition, the current strategy does not allow for detection of inversions and subtle extragenic rearrangements, such as deletions, duplications, and point mutations in regulatory elements. The latter mutational mechanism was demonstrated in autosomal dominant preaxial polydactyly syndrome in humans, for which four different pathogenic point mutations were found in a regulatory element of 750 bp named "ZRS," apparently regulating expression of *SHH* that maps 1 Mb away (Lettice et al. 2003).

General Conclusions

In summary, this is the first study, to our knowledge, to show that deletions mapping downstream and upstream of the *FOXL2* transcription unit cause BPES. Several potential upstream and downstream *cis*-acting regulatory elements were identified by delineation of these genomic rearrangements and by comparative genomics. The identification of the upstream deletions containing the human orthologue of the PIS locus in four patients with BPES provides evidence of human-goat conservation of the regulation of *FOXL2* expression and of the mutational mechanism. This study provides insight into the regulation of expression of *FOXL2*, one of the earliest markers of ovarian development. More generally, it contributes to the enlarging group of human developmental diseases caused by defective long-range regulation of gene expression. It further demonstrates one of the functions of conserved noncoding regions—that is, to act as a *cis*-regulatory element. Finally, our results emphasize that CNGs may be candidate regions for harboring genomic rearrangements in monogenic developmental disorders.

Acknowledgments

We thank the families with BPES for their cooperation. We acknowledge Sarah De Jaegere, Alicia Borderé, and Evelien Vanoverschelde, for their technical assistance. This study was supported by Bijzonder Onderzoeksfonds grant BOF2002/DRMAN/047 from Ghent University (to D.B.) and by the Fund for Scientific Research-Flanders grant 1.5.244.05 (to E.D.B.).

Web Resources

Accession numbers and URLs for data presented herein are as follows:

BACPAC Resources Center, http://bacpac.chori.org/
Biomax Human Genome Database, http://www.biomax.de/products/bhgdb/bhgdb.htm
ClustalW, http://www.ebi.ac.uk/clustalw/
Find Simple Repeats software, http://zeon.well.ox.ac.uk/git-bin/microsatellite.cgi
GenBank, http://www.ncbi.nlm.nih.gov/Genbank/ (for PIS locus [accession number AF404302] and 48-kb goat sequence [accession number AF404302])
International HapMap Project, http://www.hapmap.org/index.html.en
MRC-Holland, http://www.mrc-holland.com
mVista, http://genome.lbl.gov/vista/index.shtml
NCBI, http://www.ncbi.nlm.nih.gov/
Online Mendelian Inheritance in Man (OMIM), http://www.ncbi.nlm.nih.gov/Omim/ (for *FOXL2*, BPES, and IRID1)

RepeatMasker, http://www.repeatmasker.org/
UCSC Genome Browser, http://www.genome.ucsc.edu
The Wellcome Trust Sanger Institute, http://www.sanger.ac.uk/

References

Balemans W, Patel N, Ebeling M, Van Hul E, Wuyts W, Lacza C, Dioszegi M, Dikkers FG, Hildering P, Willems PJ, Verheij JB, Lindpaintner K, Vickery B, Foernzler D, Van Hul W (2002) Identification of a 52 kb deletion downstream of the *SOST* gene in patients with van Buchem disease. J Med Genet 39:91–97

Bejerano G, Pheasant M, Makunin I, Stephen S, Kent WJ, Mattick JS, Haussler D (2004) Ultraconserved elements in the human genome. Science 304:1321–1325

Bodega B, Porta C, Crosignani PG, Ginelli E, Marozzi A (2004) Mutations in the coding region of the *FOXL2* gene are not a major cause of idiopathic premature ovarian failure. Mol Hum Reprod 10:555–557

Cha SC, Jang YS, Lee JH, Kim HK, Kim SC, Kim S, Baek SH, Jung WS, Kim JR (2003) Mutational analysis of forkhead transcriptional factor 2 (*FOXL2*) in Korean patients with blepharophimosis-ptosis-epicanthus inversus syndrome. Clin Genet 64:485–490

Cocquet J, De Baere E, Gareil M, Pannetier M, Xia X, Fellous M, Veitia RA (2003) Structure, evolution and expression of the *FOXL2* transcription unit. Cytogenet Genome Res 101: 206–211

Cocquet J, Pailhoux E, Jaubert F, Servel N, Xia X, Pannetier M, De Baere E, Messiaen L, Cotinot C, Fellous M, Veitia RA (2002) Evolution and expression of *FOXL2*. J Med Genet 39:916–921

Crisponi L, Deiana M, Loi A, Chiappe F, Uda M, Amati P, Bisceglia L, Zelante L, Nagaraja R, Porcu S, Ristaldi MS, Marzella R, Rocchi M, Nicolino M, Lienhardt-Roussie A, Nivelon A, Verloes A, Schlessinger D, Gasparini P, Bonneau D, Cao A, Pilia G (2001) The putative forkhead transcription factor *FOXL2* is mutated in blepharophimosis/ptosis/epicanthus inversus syndrome. Nat Genet 27:159–166

Crisponi L, Uda M, Deiana M, Loi A, Nagaraja R, Chiappe F, Schlessinger D, Cao A, Pilia G (2004) *FOXL2* inactivation by a translocation 171 kb away: analysis of 500 kb of chromosome 3 for candidate long-range regulatory sequences. Genomics 83:757–764

Davies AF, Mirza G, Flinter F, Ragoussis J (1999) An interstitial deletion of 6p24-p25 proximal to the *FKHL7* locus and including *AP-2*α that affects anterior eye chamber development. J Med Genet 36:708–710

De Baere E, Beysen D, Oley C, Lorenz B, Cocquet J, De Sutter P, Devriendt K, Dixon M, Fellous M, Fryns JP, Garza A, Jonsrud C, Koivisto PA, Krause A, Leroy BP, Meire F, Plomp A, Van Maldergem L, De Paepe A, Veitia R, Messiaen L (2003) *FOXL2* and BPES: mutational hotspots, phenotypic variability, and revision of the genotype-phenotype correlation. Am J Hum Genet 72:478–487

De Baere E, Dixon MJ, Small KW, Jabs EW, Leroy BP, Devriendt K, Gillerot Y, et al (2001) Spectrum of *FOXL2* gene mutations in blepharophimosis-ptosis-epicanthus inversus (BPES) families demonstrates a genotype-phenotype correlation. Hum Mol Genet 10:1591–1600

De Baere E, Fukushima Y, Small K, Udar N, Van Camp G, Verhoeven K, Palotie A, De Paepe A, Messiaen L (2000) Identification of BPESC1, a novel gene disrupted by a balanced chromosomal translocation, t(3;4)(q23;p15.2), in a patient with BPES. Genomics 68:296–304

De Baere E, Lemercier B, Christin-Maitre S, Durval D, Messiaen L, Fellous M, Veitia R (2002) *FOXL2* mutation screening in a large panel of POF patients and XX males. J Med Genet 39:e43

De Baere E, Van Roy N, Speleman F, Fukushima Y, De Paepe A, Messiaen L (1999) Closing in on the BPES gene on 3q23: mapping of a de novo reciprocal translocation t(3;4)(q23;p15.2) breakpoint within a 45-kb cosmid and mapping of three candidate genes, *RBP1*, *RBP2*, and *β′-COP*, distal to the breakpoint. Genomics 57:70–78

de Kok YJ, Vossenaar ER, Cremers CW, Dahl N, Laporte J, Hu LJ, Lacombe D, Fischel-Ghodsian N, Friedman RA, Parnes LS, Thorpe P, Bitner-Glindzicz M, Pander HJ, Heilbronner H, Graveline J, den Dunnen JT, Brunner HG, Ropers HH, Cremers FP (1996) Identification of a hot spot for microdeletions in patients with X-linked deafness type 3 (DFN3) 900 kb proximal to the DFN3 gene *POU3F4*. Hum Mol Genet 5:1229–1235

Dermitzakis ET, Reymond A, Antonarakis SE (2005) Conserved non-genic sequences—an unexpected feature of mammalian genomes. Nat Rev Genet 6:151–157

Dermitzakis ET, Reymond A, Lyle R, Scamuffa N, Ucla C, Deutsch S, Stevenson BJ, Flegel V, Bucher P, Jongeneel CV, Antonarakis SE (2002) Numerous potentially functional but non-genic conserved sequences on human chromosome 21. Nature 420:578–582

Dermitzakis ET, Reymond A, Scamuffa N, Ucla C, Kirkness E, Rossier C, Antonarakis SE (2003) Evolutionary discrimination of mammalian conserved non-genic sequences (CNGs). Science 302:1033–1035

Driscoll MC, Dobkin CS, Alter BP (1989) $\gamma\delta\beta$-Thalassemia due to a *de novo* mutation deleting the 5′ β-globin gene activation-region hypersensitive sites. Proc Natl Acad Sci USA 86:7470–7474

Fang J, Dagenais SL, Erickson RP, Arlt MF, Glynn MW, Gorski JL, Seaver LH, Glover TW (2000) Mutations in *FOXC2* (MFH-1), a forkhead family transcription factor, are responsible for the hereditary lymphedema-distichiasis syndrome. Am J Hum Genet 67:1382–1388

Gille JJP, de Ru MH, Nieuwint AWM, van Hagen JM (2003) A patient with a genomic deletion encompassing *FOXL2* and *ATR*. Am J Hum Genet Suppl 73:287

Harris SE, Chand AL, Winship IM, Gersak K, Aittomaki K, Shelling AN (2002) Identification of novel mutations in *FOXL2* associated with premature ovarian failure. Mol Hum Reprod 8:729–733

Kleinjan DA, van Heyningen V (2005) Long-range control of gene expression: emerging mechanisms and disruption in disease. Am J Hum Genet 76:8–32

Lehmann OJ, Sowden JC, Carlsson P, Jordan T, Bhattacharya SS (2003) Fox's in development and disease. Trends Genet 19:339–344

Lettice LA, Heaney SJ, Purdie LA, Li L, de Beer P, Oostra BA,

Goode D, Elgar G, Hill RE, de Graaff E (2003) A long-range *Shh* enhancer regulates expression in the developing limb and fin and is associated with preaxial polydactyly. Hum Mol Genet 12:1725–1735

Lopes J, Vandenberghe A, Tardieu S, Ionasescu V, Levy N, Wood N, Tachi N, Bouche P, Latour P, Brice A, LeGuern E (1997) Sex-dependent rearrangements resulting in CMT1A and HNPP. Nat Genet 17:136–137

Mátyás G, Giunta C, Steinmann B, Hossle JP, Hellwig R (2002) Quantification of single nucleotide polymorphisms: a novel method that combines primer extension assay and capillary electrophoresis. Hum Mutat 19:58–68

Matys V, Fricke E, Geffers R, Gossling E, Haubrock M, Hehl R, Hornischer K, Karas D, Kel AE, Kel-Margoulis OV, Kloos DU, Land S, Lewicki-Potapov B, Michael H, Munch R, Reuter I, Rotert S, Saxel H, Scheer M, Thiele S, Wingender E (2003) TRANSFAC: transcriptional regulation, from patterns to profiles. Nucleic Acids Res 31:374–378

Messiaen L, Leroy BP, De Bie S, De Pauw K, Van Roy N, Speleman F, Van Camp G, De Paepe A (1996) Refined genetic and physical mapping of BPES type II. Eur J Hum Genet 4:34–38

Nikic S, Vaiman D (2004) Conserved patterns of gene expression in mice and goats in the vicinity of the polled intersex syndrome (PIS) locus. Chromosome Res 12:465–474

Pailhoux E, Vigier B, Chaffaux S, Servel N, Taourit S, Furet JP, Fellous M, Grosclaude F, Cribiu EP, Cotinot C, Vaiman D (2001) A 11.7-kb deletion triggers intersexuality and polledness in goats. Nat Genet 29:453–458

Plessy C, Dickmeis T, Chalmel F, Strahle U (2005) Enhancer sequence conservation between vertebrates is favoured in developmental regulator genes. Trends Genet 21:207–210

Praphanphoj V, Goodman BK, Thomas GH, Niel KM, Toomes C, Dixon MJ, Geraghty MT (2000) Molecular cytogenetic evaluation in a patient with a translocation (3;21) associated with blepharophimosis, ptosis, epicanthus inversus syndrome (BPES). Genomics 65:67–69

Schmidt D, Ovitt CE, Anlag K, Fehsenfeld S, Gredsted L, Treier AC, Treier M (2004) The murine winged-helix transcription factor *Foxl2* is required for granulosa cell differentiation and ovary maintenance. Development 131:933–942

Schouten JP, McElgunn CJ, Waaijer R, Zwijnenburg D, Diepvens F, Pals G (2002) Relative quantification of 40 nucleic acid sequences by multiplex ligation-dependent probe amplification. Nucleic Acids Res 30:e57

Schuelke M (2000) An economic method for the fluorescent labeling of PCR fragments. Nat Biotechnol 18:233–234

Shaw CJ, Lupski JR (2004) Implications of human genome architecture for rearrangement-based disorders: the genomic basis of disease. Hum Mol Genet Suppl 13:R57–R64

Uda M, Ottolenghi C, Crisponi L, Garcia JE, Deiana M, Kimber W, Forabosco A, Cao A, Schlessinger D, Pilia G (2004) *Foxl2* disruption causes mouse ovarian failure by pervasive blockage of follicle development. Hum Mol Genet 13:1171–1181

Udar N, Yellore V, Chalukya M, Yelchits S, Silva-Garcia R, Small K (2003) Comparative analysis of the *FOXL2* gene and characterization of mutations in BPES patients. Hum Mutat 22:222–228

Velagaleti GV, Bien-Willner GA, Northup JK, Lockhart LH, Hawkins JC, Jalal SM, Withers M, Lupski JR, Stankiewicz P (2005) Position effects due to chromosome breakpoints that map ~900 kb upstream and ~1.3 Mb downstream of *SOX9* in two patients with campomelic dysplasia. Am J Hum Genet 76:652–662

Zlotogora J, Sagi M, Cohen T (1983) The blepharophimosis, ptosis, and epicanthus inversus syndrome: delineation of two types. Am J Hum Genet 35:1020–1027

Am. J. Hum. Genet. 77:219–229, 2005

A Combined Genomewide Linkage Scan of 1,233 Families for Prostate Cancer–Susceptibility Genes Conducted by the International Consortium for Prostate Cancer Genetics

Jianfeng Xu,[1] Latchezar Dimitrov,[1] Bao-Li Chang,[1] Tamara S. Adams,[1] Aubrey R. Turner,[1] Deborah A. Meyers,[1] Rosalind A. Eeles,[2] Douglas F. Easton,[2] William D. Foulkes,[2] Jacques Simard,[2] Graham G. Giles,[2] John L. Hopper,[2] Lovise Mahle,[2] Pal Moller,[2] Tim Bishop,[2] Chris Evans,[2] Steve Edwards,[2] Julia Meitz,[2] Sarah Bullock,[2] Questa Hope,[2] The ACTANE Consortium,[2] Chih-lin Hsieh,[3] Jerry Halpern,[3] Raymond N. Balise,[3] Ingrid Oakley-Girvan,[3] Alice S. Whittemore,[3] Charles M. Ewing,[4] Marta Gielzak,[4] Sarah D. Isaacs,[4] Patrick C. Walsh,[4] Kathleen E. Wiley,[4] William B. Isaacs,[4] Stephen N. Thibodeau,[5] Shannon K. McDonnell,[5] Julie M. Cunningham,[5] Katherine E. Zarfas,[5] Scott Hebbring,[5] Daniel J. Schaid,[5] Danielle M. Friedrichsen,[6] Kerry Deutsch,[6] Suzanne Kolb,[6] Michael Badzioch,[2,6] Gail P. Jarvik,[6] Marta Janer,[6] Leroy Hood,[6] Elaine A. Ostrander,[6] Janet L. Stanford,[6] Ethan M. Lange,[7] Jennifer L. Beebe-Dimmer,[7] Caroline E. Mohai,[7] Kathleen A. Cooney,[7] Tarja Ikonen,[8] Agnes Baffoe-Bonnie,[8] Henna Fredriksson,[8] Mika P. Matikainen,[8] Teuvo LJ Tammela,[8] Joan Bailey-Wilson,[8] Johanna Schleutker,[8] Christiane Maier,[9] Kathleen Herkommer,[9] Josef J. Hoegel,[9] Walther Vogel,[9] Thomas Paiss,[9] Fredrik Wiklund,[10] Monica Emanuelsson,[10] Elisabeth Stenman,[10] Björn-Anders Jonsson,[10] Henrik Grönberg,[10] Nicola J. Camp,[11] James Farnham,[11] Lisa A. Cannon-Albright,[11] and Daniela Seminara[12,*]

[1]Data Coordinating Center, [2]ACTANE, [3]BC/CA/HI, [4]Johns Hopkins University, [5]Mayo Clinic, [6]PROGRESS, [7]University of Michigan, [8]University of Tampere and Tampere University Hospital, [9]University of Ulm, [10]University of Umeå, [11]University of Utah, and [12]National Cancer Institute

Evidence of the existence of major prostate cancer (PC)–susceptibility genes has been provided by multiple segregation analyses. Although genomewide screens have been performed in over a dozen independent studies, few chromosomal regions have been consistently identified as regions of interest. One of the major difficulties is genetic heterogeneity, possibly due to multiple, incompletely penetrant PC-susceptibility genes. In this study, we explored two approaches to overcome this difficulty, in an analysis of a large number of families with PC in the International Consortium for Prostate Cancer Genetics (ICPCG). One approach was to combine linkage data from a total of 1,233 families to increase the statistical power for detecting linkage. Using parametric (dominant and recessive) and nonparametric analyses, we identified five regions with "suggestive" linkage (LOD score >1.86): 5q12, 8p21, 15q11, 17q21, and 22q12. The second approach was to focus on subsets of families that are more likely to segregate highly penetrant mutations, including families with large numbers of affected individuals or early age at diagnosis. Stronger evidence of linkage in several regions was identified, including a "significant" linkage at 22q12, with a LOD score of 3.57, and five suggestive linkages (1q25, 8q13, 13q14, 16p13, and 17q21) in 269 families with at least five affected members. In addition, four additional suggestive linkages (3p24, 5q35, 11q22, and Xq12) were found in 606 families with mean age at diagnosis of ≤65 years. Although it is difficult to determine the true statistical significance of these findings, a conservative interpretation of these results would be that if major PC-susceptibility genes do exist, they are most likely located in the regions generating suggestive or significant linkage signals in this large study.

Received March 22, 2005; accepted for publication May 27, 2005; electronically published June 29, 2005.

Address for correspondence and reprints: Dr. William B. Isaacs, Marburg 115, Johns Hopkins Hospital, 600 North Wolfe Street, Baltimore, MD 21287. E-mail: wisaacs@jhmi.edu

* The authors' affiliations can be found in the Acknowledgments.

0002-9297/2005/7702-0005$15.00

Introduction

Familial clustering of prostate cancer (PC [MIM 176807]) has been consistently recognized for many years (reviewed by Isaacs and Xu [2002]). Segregation analyses and twin studies strongly suggest that genetic factors explain at least some of the familial aggregation of PC (reviewed by Schaid [2004]). Research groups worldwide have recruited families with multiple members with PC and have performed linkage analyses to search for PC-susceptibility genes. More than a dozen genomewide screens have been performed (Easton et al. 2003), and numerous regions have been suggested as harboring hereditary PC (HPC) genes. Furthermore, several genes in regions linked to PC have been proposed as candidate HPC genes, notably *ELAC2* (MIM 605367), *RNASEL* (MIM 180435), and *MSR1* (MIM 153622) (Tavtigian et al. 2001; Carpten et al. 2002; Xu et al. 2002).

Despite these extensive efforts, linkage findings suggested by individual groups and proposed associations with variants in candidate genes have not been reproducibly replicated by other groups. The difficulties in mapping PC genes have been widely discussed (Isaacs and Xu 2002; Edwards and Eeles 2004; Ostrander et al. 2004; Schaid 2004). Briefly, it is likely that multiple genes predispose to PC and that no single gene is sufficiently important to provide a reliable linkage signal when a small number of families are analyzed. PC linkage may be further complicated by phenocopies, particularly given the high prevalence of the disease and widespread use of prostate-specific antigen screening. These difficulties are inherent to PC-linkage studies, and, although they cannot be completely overcome, several approaches can be used to reduce their impact. One approach is to study a much larger number of families, which should improve the statistical power to detect regions containing genes that are mutated in a small proportion of families. Another approach is to study subsets of families with PC that are more likely both to segregate mutations in genes conferring a strong PC risk and to have a reduced number of phenocopies, such as those with a large number of affected members and/or affected members with early ages at diagnosis.

The International Consortium for Prostate Cancer Genetics (ICPCG) was formed to facilitate the task of PC–susceptibility gene identification through the combined analyses of linkage data from families with PC. In the present study, we describe the results from a combined genomewide screen for PC-susceptibility genes among 1,233 PC-affected families within the ICPCG, the largest study of its kind to date.

Methods

Ascertainment of Families

The overall ICPCG study population was described in detail elsewhere (Schaid et al. 2005). All members of the ICPCG recruited their study population, supported through their own research funding. Ten ICPCG groups participated in this combined genomewide screen, ACTANE (Anglo/Canadian/Texan/Australian/Norwegian/European Union Biomed), BC/CA/HI (British Columbia, California, and Hawaii), Johns Hopkins University (JHU), Mayo Clinic, University of Michigan, PROGRESS (Prostate Cancer Genetic Research Study, Fred Hutchinson Cancer Research Center), University of Tampere in Finland, University of Ulm in Germany, University of Umeå in Sweden, and University of Utah. There were 1,233 PC pedigrees in this combined analysis. The research protocols and informed consent procedures were approved by each group's institutional review board.

Definition of Affection Status and Classification of Pedigrees

Affected individuals were defined as "those men affected with PC who had been confirmed by either medical records or death certificates." Affected individuals without either medical records or death-certificate confirmation were considered as having unknown affection status (hence, instances of self-reported PC and of PC status that was based solely on family-history interviews were considered of unknown status). Because of this restricted definition, some pedigrees had fewer affected men than were previously reported in publications by the respective groups. All men without a diagnosis of PC were coded as having unknown affection status, regardless of whether they had undergone screening for PC. Hence, all analyses were based on the sharing of marker genotypes among affected individuals, with no consideration of the phenotype for the remaining subjects. Although such an approach may result in some loss of power, it provided a uniform approach across all participating groups.

Genotyping and Consensus Genetic Map

Various methods were used by different groups to genotype microsatellite markers in their respective genomewide screen, as described in detail elsewhere (Hsieh et al. 2001; Cunningham et al. 2003; International ACTANE Consortium 2003; Janer et al. 2003; Lange et al. 2003; Schleutker et al. 2003; Wiklund et al. 2003, Xu et al. 2003; Maier et al. 2005; Camp et al., in press). Different sets of genomewide-screen markers were used by these 10 groups (see individual references for complete description of markers), with a range of information contents of 0.38–0.57 across the various groups and a total of 1,322 markers. To facilitate a combined linkage analysis, we generated a consensus map by aligning all these markers to the draft human reference sequence (physical position) on the basis of the Human hg13 assembly (released November 14, 2002). Ten of these markers could not be uniquely located in the human reference sequence and were dropped from the combined analysis. The genetic position of the aligned markers was primarily determined on the basis of the deCode map (Kong et al. 2002). Among the 1,312 mapped markers, we were able to find the deCode genetic position for 964 markers. For the remaining 348 markers, for which only physical position was available, we estimated their genetic positions by interpolation based on the flanking markers for which both physical positions and deCode positions are available.

Linkage-Analysis Methods

The combined linkage analysis was performed in two stages. In the first stage, the linkage analyses were performed by each of the 10 groups, by use of the same definition of affection status and parametric model and the same linkage programs and options. All linkage results were based on multipoint calculations implemented in the Genehunter-Plus software (Kruglyak et al. 1996; Kong and Cox 1997). Because of their large size, the Utah pedigrees were selected from the larger set of all Utah pedigrees with at least four subjects with PC with no more than two meioses separating them (Camp et al. 2005); these pedigrees were then further trimmed to allow analysis by Genehunter-Plus. The analysis performed by each group was implemented by scripts provided by the ICPCG Data Coordinating Center (DCC), to facilitate consistency and automation. Although different genomewide screen markers were used among groups, the marker position was determined on the basis of the consensus map described above; therefore, the length of each chromosome was the same across all the groups. The linkage was evaluated at a resolution of 1 cM for each chromosome. The output files containing pedigree-specific linkage information at every cM across the genome were sent to the DCC. In the second stage, a combined analysis was performed at the DCC. For nonparametric linkage analysis, the combined allele-sharing LOD score was evaluated for each chromosome on the basis of the family-specific allele sharing at each centimorgan by use of the computer program ASM (Kong and Cox 1997). For the parametric linkage analysis, the combined LOD score with the assumption of heterogeneity (HLOD) was evaluated for each chromosome, on the basis of the family-specific LOD score at each centimorgan, by use of the computer program HOMOG (Ott 1999). Throughout the present study, we used LOD scores to describe HLODs for the results of parametric analyses and allele sharing LODs for nonparametric analyses.

The allele frequencies used were population specific; that is, for each marker, allele frequencies were estimated by counting alleles across all families within each individual group, without consideration of genetic relationships. Although not fully efficient, this provides straightforward, unbiased allele-frequency estimates. Because few families within any participating group had a known nonwhite racial background, allele frequencies were estimated from the pool of all data within a group, without consideration of race. Both nonparametric and parametric linkage analyses were performed. Allele-sharing nonparametric linkage analysis was performed, because that did not require specification of a model and would be expected to have good power against a wide range of alternative models. The linear allele-sharing model was implemented using ASM (Kong and Cox 1997). Families were weighted equally, and the score function "all" was used, which provides more evidence of linkage than does the "pairs" option whenever most affected individuals in a pedigree share the same allele that is identical by descent. For the parametric linkage analyses, a dominant model and a recessive model were used. The dominant

Table 1

Characteristics of Families

	Mean Age at Diagnosis[a] (years)		No. of Affected Members				Race[b]		Total No. of Families
ICPCG Member	≤65	>65	2	3	4	≥5	White	Black	
ACTANE	41	21	18	32	11	3	64	0	64
BC/CA/HI	41	57	24	54	16	4	83	7	98
JHU	95	93	2	26	47	113	169	17	188
Mayo Clinic	72	87	70	58	21	10	158	0	159
PROGRESS	141	113	38	107	66	43	240	8	254
University of Michigan	103	73	55	76	29	16	158	16	176
University of Tampere	3	7	0	2	5	3	10	0	10
University of Ulm	84	55	60	42	29	8	139	0	139
University of Umeå	10	40	0	13	17	20	50	0	50
University of Utah	16	79	18	14	14	49	95	0	95
Total	606	625	285	424	255	269	1,166	48	1,233

[a] Information about family mean age at diagnosis was not available for two families.

[b] Nineteen families are from other ethnic groups, such as Asian, Hispanic, or Native American.

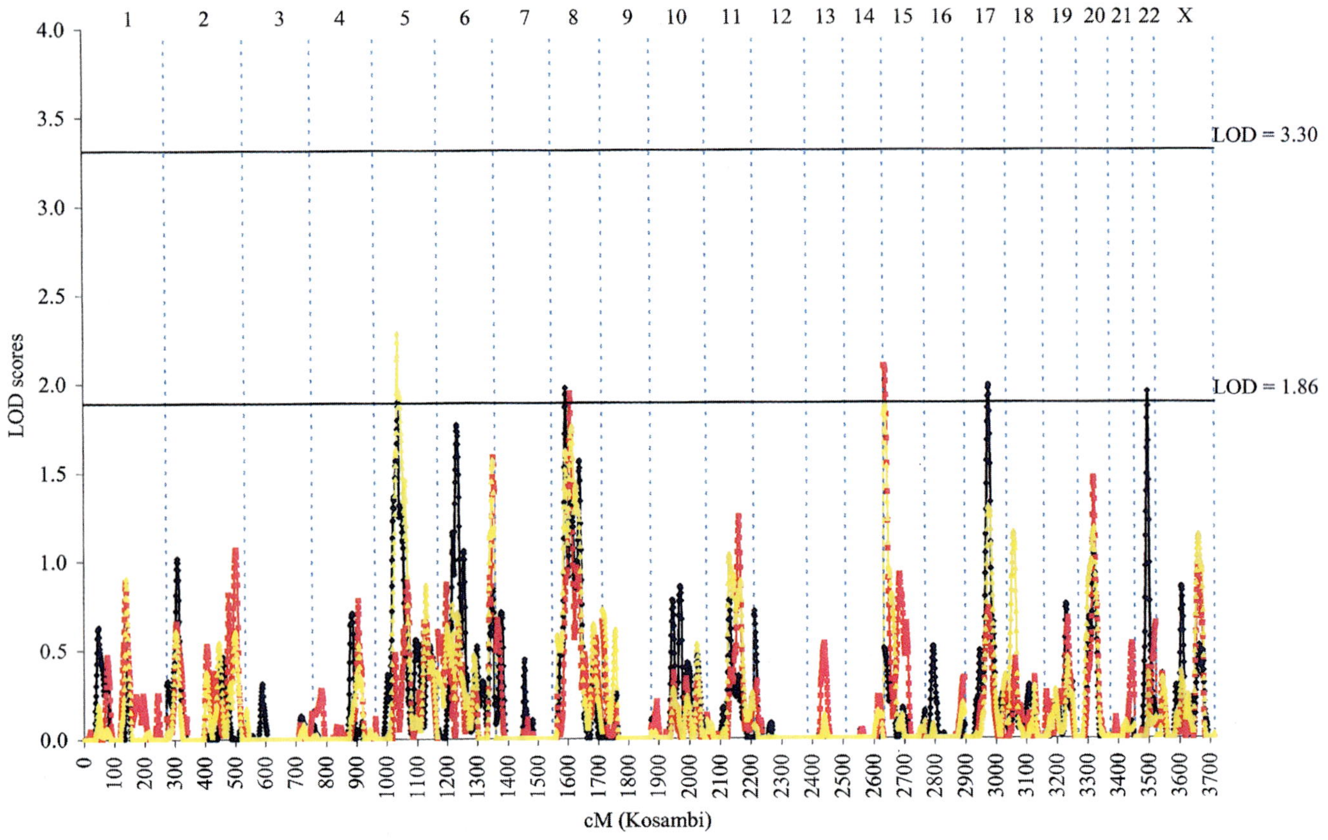

Figure 1 Combined genomewide screen for PC-susceptibility genes with use of nonparametric and parametric multipoint linkage analyses among the entire set of 1,233 PC-affected families recruited from 10 ICPCG members. LOD scores obtained from parametric analysis with use of a dominant model (*blue line*), a recessive model (*red line*), and nonparametric analysis (*yellow line*) are plotted by individual chromosome for the whole genome.

model was similar to the one used to map *HPC1* (MIM 601518) (Smith et al. 1996). The frequency of the susceptibility allele was assumed to be 0.003, with a penetrance of 0.001 for noncarriers and 1.0 for carriers. Unaffected subjects were coded as having noninformative phenotypes. The recessive model was similar to the dominant model, except that the susceptibility-allele frequency was set to 0.15 and the penetrance for heterozygous carriers was set equal to the penetrance for homozygous noncarriers. Stratified linkage analyses were also performed in two predetermined subsets of families: 269 families with at least five affected members, and 606 families with family mean age at diagnosis of ≤65 years. The planned analyses were developed and approved by members of the ICPCG.

We summarized our linkage results on the basis of the proposed guidelines for reporting linkage results of a genomewide screen: a cutoff LOD score of 3.30 as "significant" evidence of linkage and a cutoff LOD score of 1.86 as "suggestive" evidence of linkage (Lander and Kruglyak 1995). On the basis of asymptotic arguments, a LOD score of 3.30 is expected to occur 0.05 times in a genome screen that makes use of a fully informative marker set, and a LOD score of 1.86 is expected to occur once by chance.

Results

Analyses of All Families

Table 1 summarizes the characteristics of the 1,233 PC-affected families from 10 different ICPCG groups that were included in the analysis. Fifty-one percent of families had a mean age at onset of <65 years; 22% had five or more affected family members.

We first performed a combined genomewide linkage analysis of the complete set of 1,233 PC-affected families, using parametric and nonparametric approaches. Although no significant evidence of linkage was observed in the genome, evidence of suggestive PC linkage wasobserved at five chromosomal regions, 5q12, 8p21, 15q11, 17q21, and 22q12 (fig. 1 and table 2). The highest overall LOD score in the genome was 2.28 from the nonparametric analysis, found near marker *D5S2858* on

Table 2

Chromosomal Regions with Suggestive Evidence of Linkage

Population and Region	Distance from pter cM	Nearest Marker	Analysis Type	LOD	1-LOD Drop Interval Genetic (cM)	Physical (Mb)
Primary analysis: entire set of families ($N = 1,233$):						
5q12	77	*D5S2858*	Nonparametric	2.28	66–96	43–78
8p21	46	*D8S1048*	Dominant	1.97	39–52	22–32
15q11	1	*D15S817*	Recessive	2.10	0–14	0–25
17q21	77	*D17S1820*	Dominant	1.99	66–85	35–54
22q12	42	*D22S283*	Dominant	1.95	35–47	29–37
Secondary analysis: subset of families with at least five affected family members ($n = 269$):						
1q25	184	*D1S2818*	Nonparametric	2.62	170–198	165–196
8q13	81	*D8S543*	Recessive	2.41	75–90	66–75
13q14	56	*D13S1807*	Recessive	2.27	42–67	39–71
16p13	34	*D16S764*	Nonparametric	1.88	19–46	9–23
17q21	77	*D17S1820*	Dominant	2.04	66–83	39–53
22q12	42	*D22S283*	Dominant	3.57	32–50	27–42
Secondary analysis: subset of families with mean age at diagnosis of ⩽65 years ($n = 606$):						
3p24	57	*D3S2432*	Dominant	2.37	47–69	28–49
5q35	179	*D5S1456*	Dominant	2.05	166–193	162–174
11q22	102	*D11S898*	Recessive	2.20	89–112	81–111
Xq12	80	*DXS7132*	Dominant	2.30	62–90	40–85

5q12 (77 cM from pter). The linkage results for each individual family collection for each of these five chromosomal regions are shown in table 3. As seen in table 3, with the exception of 17q21, the LOD scores for each of the highlighted regions are higher in the combined analysis than those observed in any individual group, reaching a suggestive level of evidence only in the combined family data.

Analyses of Subsets of Families

We also performed linkage analyses in subsets of families that might be more likely to segregate genes conferring strong PC risk: families with at least five affected members or with family mean age at diagnosis of ⩽65 years. As hypothesized, we found stronger evidence of linkage among 269 families with at least five affected members—one region with significant evidence of linkage and four additional regions with suggestive evidence of linkage (fig. 2 and table 2). The strongest evidence of linkage in the genome was found at 22q12 with use of the dominant model, with LOD score of 3.57 at 42 cM (near marker *D22S283*). This LOD score exceeded the criterion of significant evidence of linkage in the genomewide screen. Evidence of linkage at this region was provided by multiple ICPCG groups (fig. 3). Of the 10 groups, 4 had a LOD score >1.0 at this region, including a LOD score of 2.05 from the Mayo group, a LOD score of 1.57 from the Michigan group, a LOD score of 1.31 from the Utah group, and a LOD score of 1.22 from the JHU group. It is noted that linkage evidence at this region was observed in the complete set of 1,233 families (LOD score of 1.95 at 42 cM) and was strengthened

Table 3

Support for Linkage from Each Group at Chromosomal Regions with Suggestive Linkage

Population	LOD Score by Chromosomal Region and Model: 5q12 (77 cM) Nonparametric	8p21 (46 cM) Dominant	15q11 (1 cM) Recessive	17q21 (77 cM) Dominant	22q12 (42 cM) Dominant
All groups ($N = 1,233$)	2.28	1.97	2.10	1.99	1.95
ACTANE ($n = 64$)	.00	.00	.00	.00	.00
BC/CA/HI ($n = 98$)	1.17	.00	.26	.76	.00
JHU ($n = 188$)	.29	.16	.95	.72	1.28
Mayo Clinic ($n = 159$)	.32	.09	.00	.00	1.10
PROGRESS ($n = 254$)	.25	1.64	.64	.01	.00
University of Michigan ($n = 176$)	.01	.28	1.06	3.07	.13
University of Tampere ($n = 10$)	.00	.19	.00	.42	.02
University of Ulm ($n = 139$)	.38	.77	.04	.00	.00
University of Umeå ($n = 50$)	1.62	.00	.87	.00	.00
University of Utah ($n = 95$)	.27	.17	.00	.03	1.47

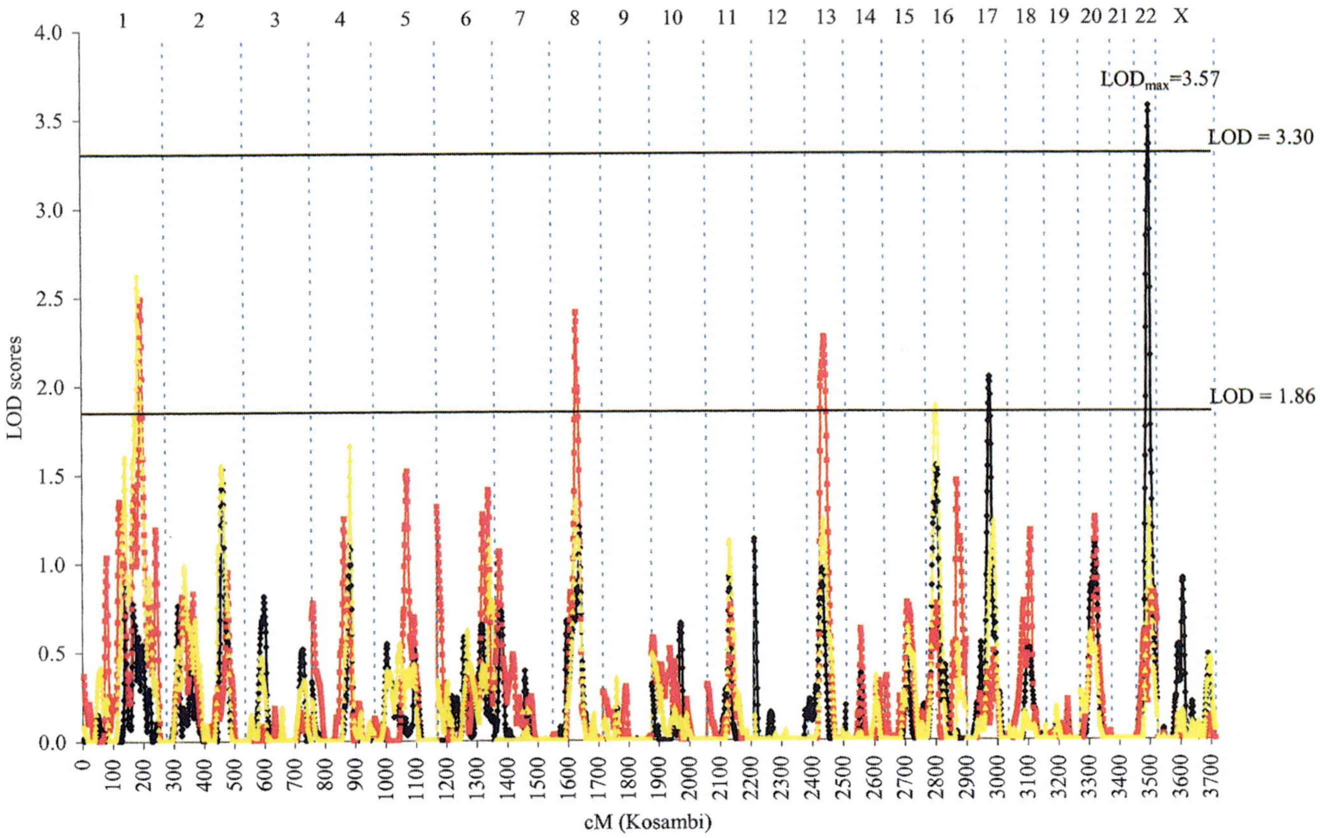

Figure 2 Combined genomewide screen for PC-susceptibility genes with use of nonparametric and parametric multipoint linkage analyses among 269 families with at least five affected members recruited from 10 ICPCG members. LOD scores obtained from parametric analysis with use of a dominant model (*blue line*), a recessive model (*red line*), and nonparametric analysis (*yellow line*) are plotted by individual chromosome for the whole genome.

in this subset. When families with at least five affected family members were removed from the analysis, no evidence of linkage at this region was found in the remaining 964 families. In addition to the 22q12 region, five additional regions reached suggestive evidence of PC linkage in this subset of families with at least five affected family members (fig. 2 and table 2).

For 606 families with family mean age at diagnosis of ≤65 years, suggestive evidence of PC linkage was found at four chromosomal regions (fig. 4 and table 2), with the highest LOD score of 2.37 near marker *D3S2432* at 3p24 (57 cM). The four PC linkages identified in this subset of families were unique to the early-age-at-diagnosis subset. No evidence of linkage at these four regions was observed in the complete set of 1,233 families.

Discussion

We have described results from the largest PC genomewide screen reported to date, with combined linkage data from 1,233 PC-affected families collected by 10 different groups in the ICPCG. From the primary analysis of the entire set of the families, we identified five chromosomal regions (5q12, 8p21, 15q11, 17q21, and 22q12) with suggestive evidence of linkage. With one exception (i.e., 17q21), the threshold for suggestive evidence of linkage was reached only in the combined analysis, which emphasizes the advantage of this combined approach.

Importantly, we found significant evidence of linkage at the 22q12 region in 269 families with at least five affected members, a subset of PC-affected families that is more likely to segregate mutations in genes conferring a strong PC risk. Suggestive evidence of linkage at five other regions (1q25, 8q13, 13q14, 16p13, and 17q21) was also observed in this subset of families. In addition, four additional regions (3p24, 5q35, 11q22, and Xq12) were found to have suggestive evidence of PC linkage in 606 families with family mean age at diagnosis of ≤65 years.

We recognize that many of the regions identified in this study may represent false positive findings due to multiple tests in a genomewide screen and that it is difficult to dissect true linkages from false signals. On the basis of the assumption of a fully informative marker

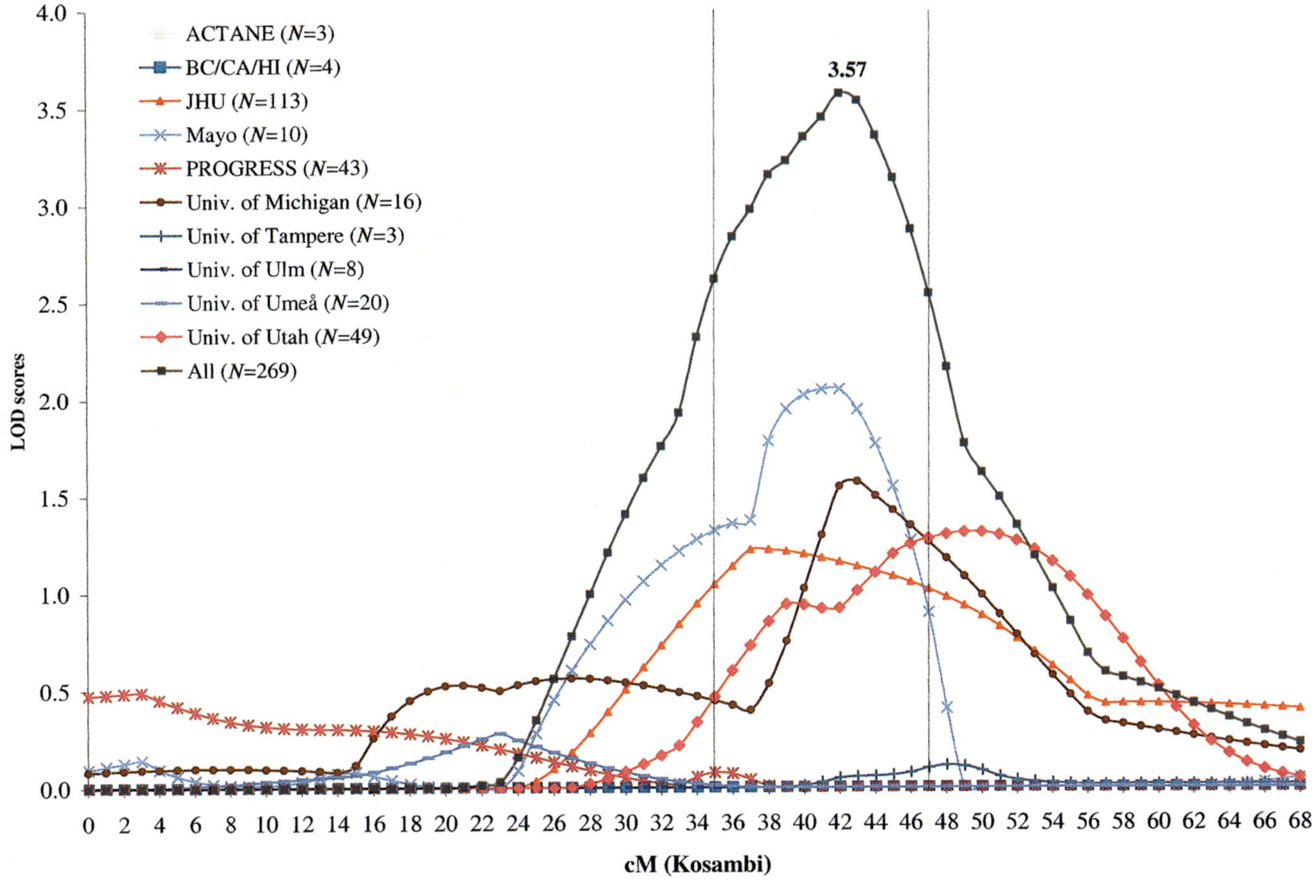

Figure 3 Parametric linkage analysis of chromosome 22 among families with at least five affected members with use of the dominant model. LOD scores are plotted for each of the 10 ICPCG groups.

map, LOD scores >3.30 or 1.86 would have been expected to occur 0.05 times and 1 time, respectively, in a single genomewide screen. Here, we performed nine genomewide screens (three in the primary analyses and six in the subgroup analyses); this needs to be considered when interpreting the results. However, these nine analyses are not independent. Using the method of Camp and Farnham (2001), we determined that the nine nonindependent analyses performed were equivalent to ~5.2 independent genomewide screens. We therefore estimate that, after correcting for multiple testing, regions with a LOD score of >3.30 (significant evidence) in at least one analysis would be expected 0.25 times in 5.2 independent screens and regions with a LOD score of >1.86 (suggestive evidence), 5.2 times. Our empirical results (one observed LOD score of 3.57 and 13 regions with LOD scores ⩾1.86) therefore exceeded the expectation under the null hypothesis of no linkage. Furthermore, these thresholds may be unduly conservative for the less-than-informative real data used in these genomewide screens. Although it is difficult to determine the true statistical significance of these findings, a conservative interpretation of these results would be that if major PC-susceptibility genes do exist, they are most likely to be located in the regions generating suggestive or significant linkage signals. Therefore, results from this analysis are likely to be helpful in prioritizing any efforts to identify PC-susceptibility genes.

Lack of reproducibility among PC-linkage studies in recent years demonstrates the difficulties faced in the effort to identify PC-susceptibility genes with the linkage approach (Isaacs and Xu 2002; Edwards and Eeles 2004; Ostrander et al. 2004; Schaid 2004). One of the major difficulties is genetic heterogeneity due to multiple but incompletely penetrant PC-susceptibility genes. Each of these genes may be responsible for a small fraction of PC-affected families. In this study, we planned two approaches to address the impact that these difficulties have on identification of PC linkage. One approach was to perform linkage analysis in a large number of PC-affected families, to increase the statistical power to detect linkage. This approach led to the identification of five regions with evidence suggestive of linkage in the complete set of 1,233 families. However, the failure to

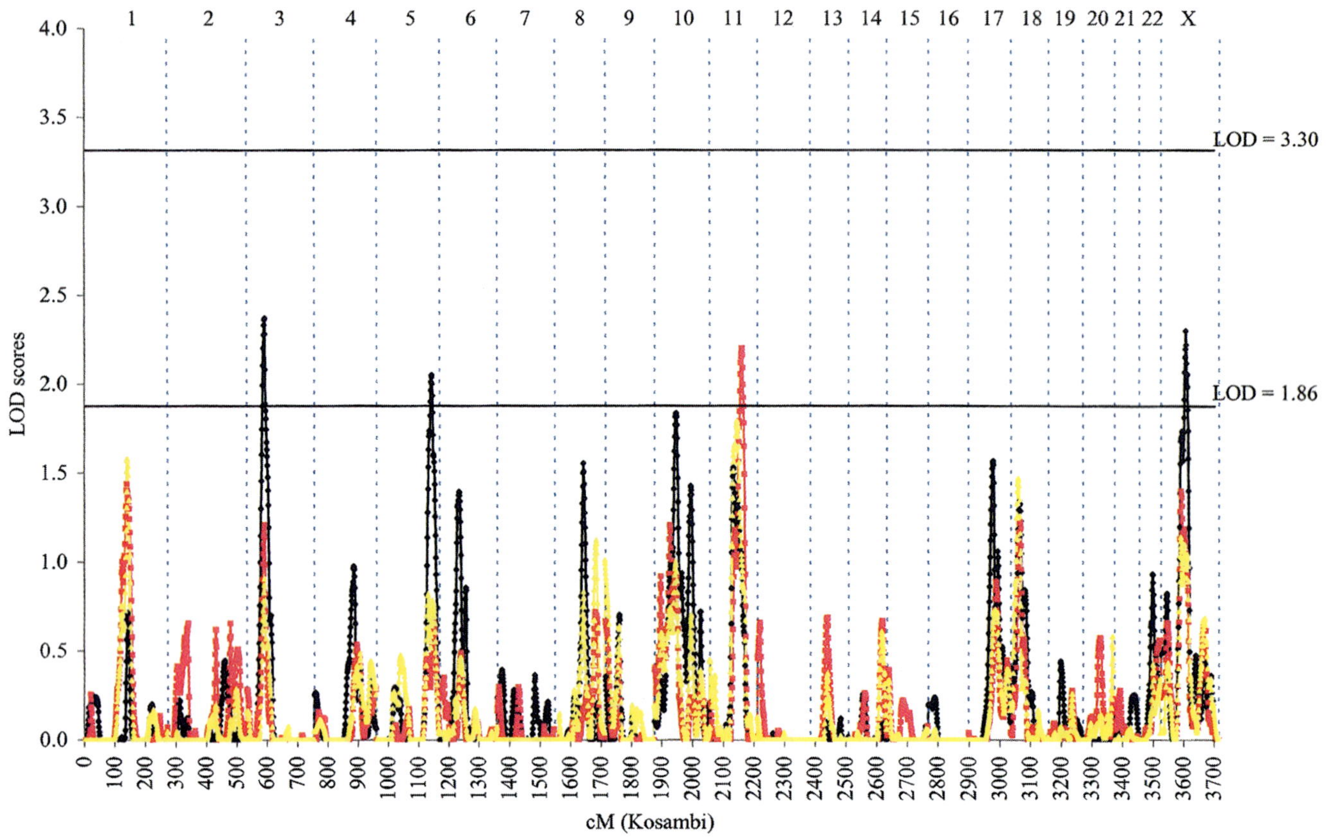

Figure 4 Combined genomewide screen for PC-susceptibility genes with use of nonparametric and parametric multipoint linkage analyses among 606 families with family mean age at diagnosis ⩽65 years recruited from 10 ICPCG members. LOD scores obtained from parametric analysis with use of a dominant model (*blue line*), a recessive model (*red line*), and nonparametric analysis (*yellow line*) are plotted by individual chromosome for the whole genome.

identify significant linkage in the genome, even with this large number of families, indicates a substantial degree of genetic heterogeneity and suggests that this approach alone is insufficient to uncover a significant signal if it is present. Our second approach was to focus on subsets of families that are more likely to segregate highly penetrant mutations, including families with large numbers of affected individuals and/or early age at diagnosis. This latter approach appeared to be more effective; stronger evidence of linkage was found in several regions among these subsets of families than from the complete set of families. The most noteworthy finding was the considerable increase in evidence of linkage at 22q12—from a LOD score of 1.95 (suggestive linkage) in the complete set of families to a LOD score of 3.57 (significant linkage) in 269 families with at least five affected members. It is important to note that the large number of families in our combined study makes it possible to analyze sufficient numbers in each subset of families. Linkage studies in families with large numbers of affected individuals and/or early ages at diagnosis have proved to be effective in identifying breast cancer–susceptibility genes (Hall et al. 1990; Easton et al. 1993).

Three pieces of evidence from our study increase our confidence that the linkage at 22q12 is due to PC-susceptibility gene(s) at this region. First, the LOD score at this region reached the criterion of significant linkage. The chance of observing this magnitude of LOD score in the genome under a null hypothesis of no linkage is <0.25 times in our study. Second, this linkage was identified in the families with at least five affected members, a subset of families that is more likely to segregate mutations in genes conferring strong PC risk. Third, the evidence of linkage at this region was supported by multiple individual groups; of six groups with ⩾10 such large families, four had LOD scores >1 in this interval. The relatively good reproducibility of this linkage finding is an unusual observation in PC-linkage studies (Easton et al. 2003). More than 129 known genes are in the 1-LOD drop interval (29–37 Mb). An important candidate gene, *CHEK2* (MIM 604373), is outside the interval, at ~27 Mb.

Because the mode of inheritance for PC is uncertain, we performed linkage analysis using both parametric (dominant or recessive) and nonparametric methods. In general, evidence of PC linkage was consistently provided by both parametric and nonparametric methods, although with different strengths at different regions. Parametric analysis will have better power to detect linkage when an assumed genetic model approximates the underlying mode of inheritance of a disease susceptibility gene (Clerget-Darpoux et al. 1986*a*, 1986*b*; Lio and Morton 1997). Nonparametric analysis, by assessment of allele sharing among affected individuals within a pedigree, may have better power when the underlying genetic model cannot be specified with any confidence (Whittemore and Halpern 1994).

Most of the linkage regions identified in the present study are broad. The information content of the marker sets used in these analyses is generally low, particularly since most of our families are small and often do not include genotypes of all parents. Further genotyping at a higher density, with use of either microsatellite markers or SNPs, should improve informativeness. An additional approach currently under way by the ICPCG incorporates clinical and pathological tumor variables in the assignment of affected status, to emphasize clinically aggressive disease in this large data set. Hopefully, these approaches should help to confirm or refute the evidence of linkage and narrow the regions of interest.

During the last decade, tremendous effort has been put forth to identify major susceptibility genes for PC. Linkage studies with smaller numbers of PC-affected families have identified and implicated many chromosomal regions that might harbor PC-susceptibility genes. The large number of different regions that have been implicated—and the general lack of reproducibility among these studies—has provided a tenuous foundation for subsequent PC-gene identification. In this context, results from the current study, with a very large number of families in the overall analysis, provides a strong basis for prioritizing regions for PC-gene identification.

Acknowledgments

We express our gratitude to the many families who participated in this study and to the many urologists who kindly assisted us by providing information and access to their patients. The ICPCG is supported by U.S. Public Health Service (USPHS) National Institutes of Health (NIH) grant CA89600. Additional support to participating groups or members within groups is as follows. **ACTANE Group**: Genotyping and statistical analysis for this study and recruitment of U.K. families was supported by Cancer Research U.K. Additional support was provided by the Prostate Cancer Charitable Trust (now Prostate Cancer Research Foundation), The Times Christmas Appeal, and the Institute of Cancer Research. Genotyping was conducted in the Jean Rook Gene Cloning Laboratory, which is supported by BREAKTHROUGH Breast Cancer–Charity 328323. The funds for the ABI 377 used in this study were generously provided by the legacy of the late Marion Silcock. We thank Mrs. Sheila Seal and Mrs. Anita Hall for kindly storing and logging the samples that were provided. D.F.E. is a principal research fellow of Cancer Research U.K. Recruitment of Australian PC-affected families was funded by National Health and Medical Research Council grant 940934 and was further supported by Tattersall's and the Whitten Foundation; infrastructure was provided by the Cancer Council Victoria. We acknowledge the work of study coordinator Margaret Staples; the research team of Bernadette McCudden, John Connal, Richard Thorowgood, Chris Costa, Melodie Kevan, and Sue Palmer; and Jolanta Karpowicz, for DNA extractions. The Texas study of familial PC was initiated by the Department of Epidemiology, M. D. Anderson Cancer Center. M.B. was supported by NCI post-doctoral fellowship in Cancer Prevention R25. **BC/CA/HI Group**: USPHS grant CA67044. **JHU Group**: USPHS grants CA58236 (to W.B.I.), CA95052-01 (to J.X.), and CA106523-01A1 (to J.X.). **Mayo Clinic Group**: USPHS grant CA72818. **Michigan Group**: USPHS grant CA079596. **PROGRESS Group**: USPHS grants CA78835 (to E.A.O.) and CA080122 (to J.L.S.) and support from the Prostate Cancer Foundation and the Fred Hutchinson Cancer Research Center (University of Washington Markey Center). **Tampere Group**: Medical Research Fund of Tampere University Hospital, Reino Lahtikari Foundation, Finnish Cancer Organizations, Sigrid Juselius Foundation, and Academy of Finland grant 201480. **Ulm Group**: Deutsche Krebshilfe grant 70–3111-V03. **Umeå Group**: Grants from the Swedish Cancer Society (Cancerfonden) and Stiftelsen för Strategisk Forskning. **Utah Group**: NIH NCI grant R01 CA90752 (to L.C.A.), a subcontract from JHU with funds provided by NIH NCI grant R01 CA89600 (to L.C.A.), and NIH grant K07 CA98364 (to N.C.). Data collection for this publication was assisted by the Utah Cancer Registry, supported by NIH Contract NO1-PC-35141 and Surveillance, Epidemiology and End Results Program, with additional support from the Utah Department of Health, the University of Utah, and Public Health Services research grant M01-RR00064 from the National Center for Research Resources. Partial support for all data sets within the Utah Population Database was provided by the University of Utah Huntsman Cancer Institute. Genotyping services were provided by the Center for Inherited Disease Research (CIDR). CIDR is fully funded through federal NIH contract N01-HG-65403 (to J.H.U.). Genotyping for the JHU, Michigan, Tampere, and Umeå groups was performed by Elizabeth Gillanders, MaryPat Jones, Derk Gildea, Erica Riedesel, Julie Albertus, Diana Freas-Lutz, Carol Markey, John Carpten, and Jeff Trent at the National Human Genome Research Institute, NIH. **Other investigators who contributed to this work: ACTANE:** *United Kingdom (Sutton)*: Rifat Hamoudi, Audrey Ardern-Jones, Christine Southgate, Anna Dowe, Kim Coleman, David Dearnaley, The Cancer Research U.K./British Prostate Group U.K. Familial Prostate Cancer Study Collaborators, British Association of Urological Surgeons' Section of Oncology, Translational Cancer Genetics Team, Molecular Genetics Team, Section of Cancer Genetics; Institute of Cancer Research, Royal Marsden NHS

Trust Foundation Hospital. *United Kingdom (Cambridge)*: M. Dawn Teare, Cancer Research U.K. Genetic Epidemiology Unit, Strangeways Research Labs. *Australia*: Dallas English, Gianluca Severi, Melissa Southey, Cancer Epidemiology Centre, The Cancer Council Victoria; University of Melbourne, Centre for Genetic Epidemiology. *Canada*: Nancy Hamel, Division of Medical Genetics, Research Institute of the McGill University Health Centre, Montreal; Steven Narod, Centre for Research in Women's Health, University of Toronto, Toronto. *Texas*: Chris Amos, M. D. Anderson Cancer Centre, Houston. *Norway (Oslo)*: Ketil Heimdal Unit of Medical Genetics, Norwegian Radium Hospital, Oslo. *Norway (Ullevaal)*: Nicolai Wessel, Tone Andersen, Department of Oncology, Ullevaal University Hospital, Oslo. *EU Biomed*: The EU Biomed Prostate Cancer Linkage Consortium, Cancer Research U.K. Genetic Epidemiology Laboratory, St. James' University Hospital, Leeds. *JHU*: Piroska Bujnovszky, Tanya Ray, Vivian Bailey, Mary Buedel, and Dawn Steinberg. *Utah*: Alan Thomas, Lewis Ershler, and Kim Nguyen.

Author affiliations.—Center for Human Genomics, Wake Forest University School of Medicine, Winston-Salem, NC (J.X., L.D., B.-L.C., T.S.A., A.R.T., and D.A.M.); Institute of Cancer Research and Royal Marsden National Health Service Trust Foundation Hospital, Sutton, United Kingdom (R.A.E., S.E., J.M., S.B., and Q.H.); Cancer Research U.K. Genetic Epidemiology Unit, Strangeways Research Labs, Cambridge, United Kingdom (D.F.E. and C.E.); Program in Cancer Genetics, Departments of Oncology and Human Genetics, McGill University, Montreal (W.D.F.); Cancer Genomics Laboratory, Centre hospitalier de l'Universite Laval Research Centre, Sainte-Foy, Quebec (J. Simard); University of Washington Medical Center (M.B. and G.P.J.) and Department of Medical Genetics, School of Public Health and Community Medicine, University of Washington (M.B. and G.P.J.), Divisions of Human Biology (D.M.F. and E.A.O.) and Public Health Sciences, Fred Hutchinson Cancer Center (S.K. and J.L.S.), and Institute for System Biology (K.D., M.J., and L.H.), Seattle; Cancer Epidemiology Centre, Cancer Council Victoria (G.G.G.), and Centre for Genetic Epidemiology, University of Melbourne (J.L.H.), Carlton, Australia; Unit of Medical Genetics, Norwegian Radium Hospital, Oslo (L.M. and P.M.); Cancer Research U.K. Genetic Epidemiology Laboratory, St. James' University Hospital, Leeds (T.B.); University of Southern California, Los Angeles (C.-l.H.); Stanford University School of Medicine, Stanford (J.H., R.N.B., and A.S.W.); Northern California Cancer Center, Union City and Stanford (I.O.-G.); Department of Urology, Johns Hopkins Medical Institutions (C.M.E., M.G., S.D.I. P.C.W., K.E.W., and W.B.I), and Inherited Disease Research Branch, National Human Genome Research Institute, NIH (J.B.-W.), Baltimore; Mayo Clinic, Rochester, MN (S.N.T., S.K.M., J.M.C., K.E.Z., S.H., and D.J.S.); Cancer Genetics Branch, National Human Genome Research Institute, (E.A.O.), and National Cancer Institute (NCI) (D.S.), NIH, Bethesda; Department of Genetics, University of North Carolina, Chapel Hill (E.M.L.); University of Michigan, Ann Arbor (J.L.B.-D., C.E.M., and K.A.C.); University of Tampere and Tampere University Hospital, Tampere, Finland (T.I., H.F., M.P.M. T.L.T., and J. Schleutker); Fox Chase Cancer Center, Division of Population Science, Philadelphia (A.B.-B.); Abteilung Humangenetik, Universität Ulm (C.M., J.J.H., and W.V.), and Urologische Universitätsklinik und Poliklinik, Abteilung für Urologie und Kinderurologie (K.H. and T.P.), Ulm, Germany; Department of Radiation Sciences, Oncology, University of Umeå, Umeå, Sweden (F.W., M.E., E.S., B.-A.J., and H.G.); Division of Genetic Epidemiology, University of Utah, Salt Lake City (N.J.C., J.F., and L.C.A).

Web Resource

The URL for data presented herein is as follows:

Online Mendelian Inheritance in Man (OMIM), http://www.ncbi.nlm.nih.gov/Omim/ (for PC, *ELAC2*, *RNASEL*, *MSR1*, *HPC1*, and *CHEK2*)

References

Camp NJ, Farnham JM (2001) Correcting for multiple analyses in genomewide linkage studies. Ann Hum Genet 65:577–582

Camp NJ, Farnham JM, Cannon-Albright LA. Genome search for prostate cancer predisposition loci in Utah pedigrees. Prostate (in press)

Carpten J, Nupponen N, Isaacs S, Sood R, Robbins C, Xu J, Faruque M, et al (2002) Germline mutations in the ribonuclease L gene in families showing linkage with HPC1. Nat Genet 30:181–184

Clerget-Darpoux F, Bonaiti-Pellie C, Hochez J (1986*a*) Effects of misspecifying genetic parameters in lod score analysis. Biometrics 42:393–399

Clerget-Darpoux F, Dizier MH, Bonaiti-Pellie C, Babron MC, Hochez J, Martinez M (1986*b*) Discrimination between genetic models for insulin dependent diabetes mellitus. Genet Epidemiol Suppl 1:313–318

Cunningham JM, McDonnell SK, Marks A, Hebbring S, Anderson SA, Peterson BJ, Slager S, French A, Blute ML, Schaid DJ, Thibodeau SN (2003) Genome linkage screen for prostate cancer susceptibility loci: results from the Mayo Clinic Familial Prostate Cancer Study. Prostate 57:335–346

Easton DF, Bishop DT, Ford D, Crockford GP (1993) Breast Cancer Linkage Consortium: genetic linkage analysis in familial breast and ovarian cancer: results from 214 families. Am J Hum Genet 52:678–701

Easton DF, Schaid DJ, Whittemore AS, Isaacs WJ (2003) Where are the prostate cancer genes? A summary of eight genome wide searches. Prostate 57:261–269

Edwards SM, Eeles RA (2004) Unravelling the genetics of prostate cancer. Am J Med Genet C Semin Med Genet 129:65–73

Hall JM, Lee MK, Newman B, Morrow JE, Anderson LA, Huey B, King MC (1990) Linkage of early-onset familial breast cancer to chromosome 17q21. Science 250:1684–1689

Hsieh C-l, Oakley-Girvan I, Balise RR, Halpern J, Gallagher RP, Wu AH, Kolonel LN, O'Brien LE, Lin IG, Van Den Berg DJ, Teh C-Z, West DW, Whittemore AS (2001) A genome screen of families with multiple cases of prostate cancer: evidence of genetic heterogeneity. Am J Hum Genet 69:148–158

Isaacs WB, Xu J (2002) Prostate cancer. In: King RA, Totter JI, Motulsky AG (eds) The genetic basis of common diseases. Oxford University Press, New York

International ACTANE Consortium (2003) Results of a genome-wide linkage analysis in prostate cancer families ascertained through the ACTANE consortium. Prostate 57:270–279

Janer M, Friedrichsen DM, Stanford JL, Badzioch MD, Kolb S, Deutsch K, Peters MA, Goode EL, Welti R, DeFrance HB, Iwasaki L, Li S, Hood L, Ostrander EA, Jarvik GP (2003) Genomic scan of 254 hereditary prostate cancer families. Prostate 57:309–319

Kong A, Cox NJ (1997) Allele-sharing models: LOD scores and accurate linkage tests. Am J Hum Genet 61:1179–1188

Kong A, Gudbjartsson D, Sainz J, Jonsdottir G, Gudjonsson S, Richardsson B, Sigurdardottir S, Barnard B, Hallbeck B, Masson M, Shlien A, Palsson S, Frigge M, Thorgeirsson T, Gulcher J, Stefansson K (2002) A high-resolution recombination map of the human genome. Nat Genet 31:241–247

Kruglyak L, Daly MJ, Reeve-Daly MP, Lander ES (1996) Parametric and nonparametric linkage analysis: a unified multipoint approach. Am J Hum Genet 58:1347–1363

Lander E, Kruglyak L (1995) Genetic dissection of complex traits: guidelines for interpreting and reporting linkage results. Nat Genet 11:241–247

Lange EM, Gillanders EM, Davis CC, Brown WM, Campbell JK, Jones M, Gildea D, Riedesel E, Albertus J, Freas-Lutz D, Markey C, Giri V, Dimmer JB, Montie JE, Trent JM, Cooney KA (2003) Genome-wide scan for prostate cancer susceptibility genes using families from the University of Michigan prostate cancer genetics project finds evidence for linkage on chromosome 17 near BRCA1. Prostate 57:326–334

Lio P, Morton NE (1997) Comparison of parametric and nonparametric methods to map oligogenes by linkage. Proc Natl Acad Sci USA 94:5344–5348

Maier C, Herkommer K, Hoegel J, Vogel W, Paiss T (2005) A genomewide linkage analysis for prostate cancer susceptibility genes in families from Germany. Eur J Hum Genet 13:352–360

Ostrander EA, Markianos K, Stanford JL (2004) Finding prostate cancer susceptibility genes. Annu Rev Genomics Hum Genet 5:151–175

Ott J (1999) Analysis of human genetic linkage. The Johns Hopkins University Press, Baltimore

Schaid D (2004) The complex genetic epidemiology of prostate cancer. Hum Mol Genet 13:R103–R121

Schaid DJ, Chang BL, International Consortium for Prostate Cancer Genetics (2005) Description of the international consortium for prostate cancer genetics, and failure to replicate linkage of hereditary prostate cancer to 20q13. Prostate 63:276–290

Schleutker J, Baffoe-Bonnie AB, Gillanders E, Kainu T, Jones MP, Freas-Lutz D, Markey C, Gildea D, Riedesel E, Albertus J, Gibbs KD Jr, Matikainen M, Koivisto PA, Tammela T, Bailey-Wilson JE, Trent JM, Kallioniemi OP (2003) Genome-wide scan for linkage in Finnish hereditary prostate cancer (HPC) families identifies novel susceptibility loci at 11q14 and 3p25-26. Prostate 57:280–289

Smith JR, Freije D, Carpten JD, Grönberg H, Xu J, Isaacs SD, Brownstein MJ, Bova GS, Guo H, Bujinovszky P, Nusskern DR, Damber JE, Bergh A, Emanuelsson M, Kallioniemi OP, Walker-Daniels J, Bailey-Wilson JE, Beaty TH, Meyers DA, Walsh PC, Collins FS, Trent JM, Isaacs WB (1996) Major susceptibility locus for prostate cancer on chromosome 1 suggested by a genome-wide search. Science 274:1371–1374

Tavtigian S, Simard J, Teng D, Abtin V, Baumgard M, Beck A, Camp N, et al (2001) A strong candidate prostate cancer susceptibility gene at chromosome 17p. Nat Genet 27:172–180

Whittemore AS, Halpern J (1994) A class of tests for linkage using affected pedigree members. Biometrics 50:118–127

Wiklund F, Gillanders EM, Albertus JA, Bergh A, Damber JE, Emanuelsson M, Freas-Lutz DL, Gildea DE, Goransson I, Jones MS, Jonsson BA, Lindmark F, Markey CJ, Riedesel EL, Stenman E, Trent JM, Grönberg H (2003) Genome-wide scan of Swedish families with hereditary prostate cancer: suggestive evidence of linkage at 5q11.2 and 19p13.3. Prostate 57:290–297

Xu J, Gillanders EM, Isaacs SD, Chang BL, Wiley KE, Zheng SL, Jones M, Gildea D, Riedesel E, Albertus J, Freas-Lutz D, Markey C, Meyers DA, Walsh PC, Trent JM, Isaacs WB (2003) Genome-wide scan for prostate cancer susceptibility genes in the Johns Hopkins hereditary prostate cancer families. Prostate 57:320–325

Xu J, Zheng SL, Komiya A, Mychaleckyj JC, Isaacs SD, Hu JJ, Sterling D, et al (2002) Germline mutations and sequence variants of the macrophage scavenger receptor 1 gene are associated with prostate cancer risk. Nat Genet 32:321–325

Am. J. Hum. Genet. 77:230–241, 2005

Weighting Affected Sib Pairs by Marker Informativity

Daniel Franke and Andreas Ziegler

Institute of Medical Biometry and Statistics, University at Lübeck, Lübeck, Germany

For the analysis of affected sib pairs (ASPs), a variety of test statistics is applied in genomewide scans with microsatellite markers. Even in multipoint analyses, these statistics might not fully exploit the power of a given sample, because they do not account for incomplete informativity of an ASP. For meta-analyses of linkage and association studies, it has been shown recently that weighting by informativity increases statistical power. With this idea in mind, the first aim of this article was to introduce a new class of tests for ASPs that are based on the mean test. To take into account how much informativity an ASP contributes, we weighted families inversely proportional to their marker informativity. The weighting scheme is obtained by use of the de Finetti representation of the distribution of identity-by-descent values. We derive the limiting distribution of the weighted mean test and demonstrate the validity of the proposed test. We show that it can be much more powerful than the classical mean test in the case of low marker informativity. In the second part of the article, we propose a Monte Carlo simulation approach for evaluating significance among ASPs. We demonstrate the validity of the simulation approach for both the classical and the weighted mean test. Finally, we illustrate the use of the weighted mean test by reanalyzing two published data sets. In both applications, the maximum LOD score of the weighted mean test is 0.6 higher than that of the classical mean test.

Introduction

A standard approach to mapping complex genetic diseases is the ascertainment of several affected sib pairs (ASPs). A variety of test statistics has been proposed for this study design, and most of the test are based on the identity-by-descent (IBD) value of an ASP. For some genetic markers, the IBD value can be determined uniquely for a given family. However, other markers may not be completely informative, so that the IBD distribution is ambiguous and has to be estimated from the observed marker data. Still, the ASP statistics can be applied by use of this estimated IBD distribution. One example of this application is the mean test statistic, which is often employed because of its elegance, simplicity, and optimality (Knapp et al. 1994; Whittemore and Tu 1998). The question of whether incomplete marker informativity affects the power of the utilized statistic remains.

The following example illustrates that incomplete informativity may lead to a decrease in the LOD score. Consider a small sample of 20 ASPs, all with an IBD value of 2. The mean test statistic gives a LOD score of 8.69. However, if the total sample comprises an additional 20 noninformative ASPs, the mean test LOD score drops to 4.34. Thus, the 20 noninformative ASPs do not increase the available information but, instead, lead to an extreme power loss. In most software packages, those completely noninformative ASPs would have been omitted from the analysis. If they are only slightly informative, sib pairs remain in the statistical calculation, although this does not alter the substantial LOD score drop.

The reason for this rather obscure observation is simple: all sib pairs receive the same weight in the linkage analysis, although their information content varies substantially. This defies basic statistical ideas summarized under the term "Horvitz-Thompson estimation" (Horvitz and Thompson 1952). On the basis of those ideas, observations should be weighted according to their informativity: the greater the degree of informativity, the greater the weight of an observation.

Weighting by informativity has already been proposed in the context of linkage studies for quantitative traits. For example, Amos et al. (1989) extended the classic Haseman-Elston method (Haseman and Elston 1972) by introducing a generalized least-squares approach in which the squared phenotypic difference of a sib pair is weighted proportional to its Fisher information. Sham and Purcell (2001) also weighted sib pairs by phenotypes. They linearly combined squared differences and squared sums, and the weights were determined by the overall trait correlation between the sibs in a population. Both statistics may lead to a substantial gain in power.

Received April 4, 2005; accepted for publication May 27, 2005; electronically published June 28, 2005.

Address for correspondence and reprints: Dr. Andreas Ziegler, Institute of Medical Biometry and Statistics, Ratzeburger Allee 160, House 4, 23538 Lübeck, Germany. E-mail: ziegler@imbs.uni-luebeck.de

0002-9297/2005/7702-0006$15.00

Unlike in studies that use quantitative phenotypes, in ASP studies, sib pairs cannot be weighted according to their phenotypic informativity, because both sibs are affected. An alternative method might be to increase power by weighting families according to marker informativity, which has already been proposed for quantitative traits. The recent regression method introduced by Sham et al. (2002) takes into account ambiguous IBD sharing by an appropriate specification of the variance-covariance matrix of IBD sharing between pairs of relatives. Sham et al. (2002) have derived the limiting distribution of the proposed test statistic and have validated their results by Monte Carlo simulations. Jacobs et al. (2003) weighted individual sib pair families for Haseman-Elston linkage analyses according to marker informativity, as measured by the difference between the allele sharing at the marker and the allele sharing at a noninformative marker. We have recently demonstrated, however, that this results in increased type I error fractions (Franke et al., in press). This led us to the conclusion that Haseman-Elston analysis with marker informativity weights should be used only in conjunction with empirical P values until the valid limiting distribution has been derived.

Weighting by informativity has been proven to be successful in the context of meta-analyses in which studies, not individual families, have been weighted (Loesgen et al. 2001; Dempfle and Loesgen 2004). The effect estimates from the single studies in the meta-analytic approach approximately follow a normal distribution by the central limit theorem, so the limiting distribution of the combined estimator can be derived easily.

In this contribution, we introduce a novel weighted mean test statistic that weights individual sib pairs according to marker informativity. Weights are based on the Euclidian distance between the IBD distribution of the marker under study and the IBD distribution of a noninformative marker. We derive the limiting distribution of the novel test statistic. We discuss the applicability of existing Monte Carlo permutation or simulation approaches, argue that previously published methods cannot be applied to the weighted test statistic, and introduce a novel method for simulating P values in ASP studies. We validate our new test statistic and the proposed simulation method in a Monte Carlo simulation study. Finally, we illustrate the application of the novel weighted mean test by reanalyzing two published data sets.

The Classical Mean Test

For the classical mean test, consider a sample of n independent ASPs, and let $\hat{f}_{1i}$ and $\hat{f}_{2i}$ denote the estimated probability that sib pair i shares 1 or 2 alleles IBD, respectively. Further, let $\hat{\tau}_i = \hat{f}_{2i} + \hat{f}_{1i}/2$ be the observed proportion of alleles shared IBD for sib pair i. Under the null hypothesis of no linkage between the marker and trait loci, the expected mean proportion of alleles shared IBD by an ASP is 1/2. In other words, if we let

$$\bar{\hat{\tau}} = \frac{1}{n}\sum_{i=1}^{n}\hat{\tau}_i$$

be the observed mean proportion of alleles shared IBD, then $E(\bar{\hat{\tau}}) = 1/2$ under the null hypothesis. The mean test statistic is given by

$$T_{\mathrm{m}} = \frac{\bar{\hat{\tau}} - \frac{1}{2}}{\sqrt{\widehat{\mathrm{Var}}(\bar{\hat{\tau}})}}$$

(see, e.g., Olson 2002), where the denominator may be replaced by $\sqrt{1/(8n)}$ under the null hypothesis of no linkage. In this case, T_{m} asymptotically follows a standard normal distribution, and its mean is >0 for ASPs under linkage.

Greater power of the mean test statistic and a better approximation to the normal distribution can be achieved by replacing the denominator with an empirical variance estimate. For example, in the software package S.A.G.E. (2004, p. 221, eq. [10.1]), $\widehat{\mathrm{Var}}(\bar{\hat{\tau}})$ is replaced by $[\sum_{i=1}^{n}(\hat{\tau}_i - \bar{\hat{\tau}})^2]/[n(n-1)]$, and we denote the resulting test statistic by T_{mev}.

Figure 1 illustrates the fundamental shortcoming that underlies the standard mean test for ASPs. It displays marker data of a notional locus for three nuclear ASP families. The IBD value of ASP (a) can be uniquely determined, whereas uncertainty remains for the other two pedigrees, (b) and (c). Although these families have markedly different degrees of informativity for linkage analysis, they share the same proportion of alleles IBD—namely, $\hat{\tau}_i = 1/2$. They thus contribute equally to T_{m},

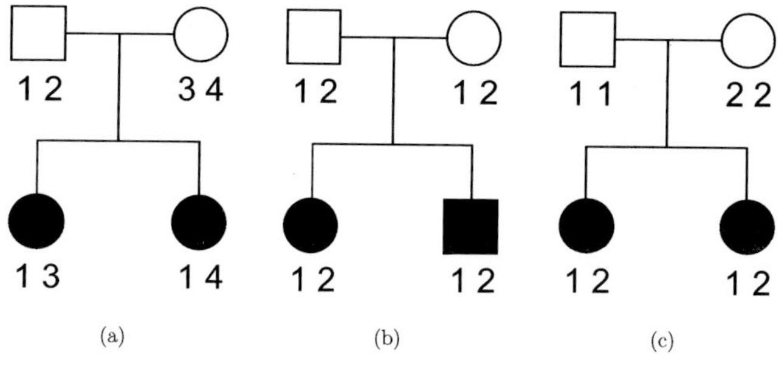

Figure 1 Three ASP families with varying degrees of informativity. Sib pair (a) shares 1 allele IBD; sib pair (b) shares either 0 or 2 alleles IBD, with equal probabilities; and sib pair (c) is completely uninformative for linkage. For all three sib pairs, the proportion of alleles shared IBD is 0.5.

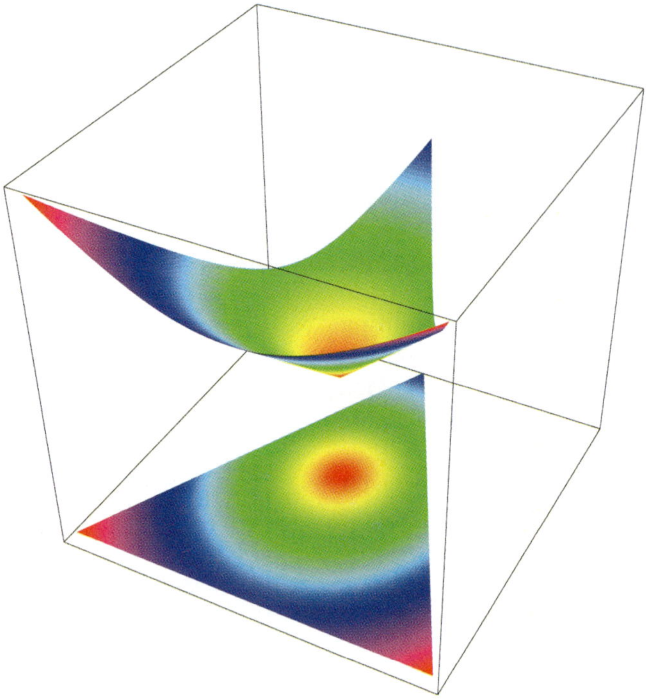

Figure 2 Euclidian distances in the space of IBD distributions. The curved plane shows the relation between the informativity of a specific IBD distribution and the weight assigned to this distribution. Weights increase with increasing distance from (1/4,1/2,1/4), which is the center of the displayed circles. The triangle below the plane is an orthogonal projection of the contours of the plane above.

since $\bar{\hat{\tau}}$ is an unweighted mean. Our alternative suggestion is to take marker informativity of a sib pair into account, and a measure for marker informativity is delineated in the next section.

Simplex Weighting Scheme

Let us begin by considering the space of IBD distributions that can be represented by an equilateral triangle of height 1, termed the "de Finetti triangle" (Franke et al., in press). If an ASP is completely noninformative at a genetic marker, its IBD distribution is (1/4, 1/2, 1/4). A natural approach to measure distance is Euclidian distance, and we (Franke et al., in press) have shown that the Euclidian distance between an uninformative marker and the actual IBD distribution $f = (f_0, f_1, f_2)$ is given by

$$d(f) = \sqrt{\frac{1}{3}(f_2 - f_0)^2 + \frac{1}{4}(1 - 2f_1)^2} \; . \qquad (1)$$

Therefore, $d = 0$ for a sib pair that is completely noninformative at a marker locus. In contrast, d equals $\sqrt{7/12}$ for sib pairs sharing 2 or 0 alleles IBD and equals 1/2 for sib pairs sharing 1 allele IBD. These different distances for sib pairs sharing 2 or 0 alleles versus 1 allele IBD naturally reflect the variability in informativity of sib pairs sharing 1 allele IBD, depending on the underlying genetic model. Thus, one expects a sharing of 2 alleles IBD under a recessive model of inheritance, whereas 1 or 2 alleles shared IBD are reasonably expected for a simple dominant genetic model.

By use of equation (1), Euclidian distance weights w_i are defined as the normalized Euclidian distance between the noninformative marker situation and the estimated IBD sharing information for ASP i, with $w_i = d(f_i)/[\sum_{j=1}^{n} d(f_j)]$ such that $\sum_{i=1}^{n} w_i = 1$. Figure 2 illustrates the Euclidian distances in both a three-dimensional representation of d_i, plotted over the triangular space of IBD distributions, and a two-dimensional representation. Points with identical colors have identical weights.

The Weighted Mean Test

As a test for linkage, we propose to replace the original unweighted mean from the classical mean test with the weighted mean

$$\bar{\hat{\tau}}_w = \sum_{i=1}^{n} w_i \hat{\tau}_i \; ,$$

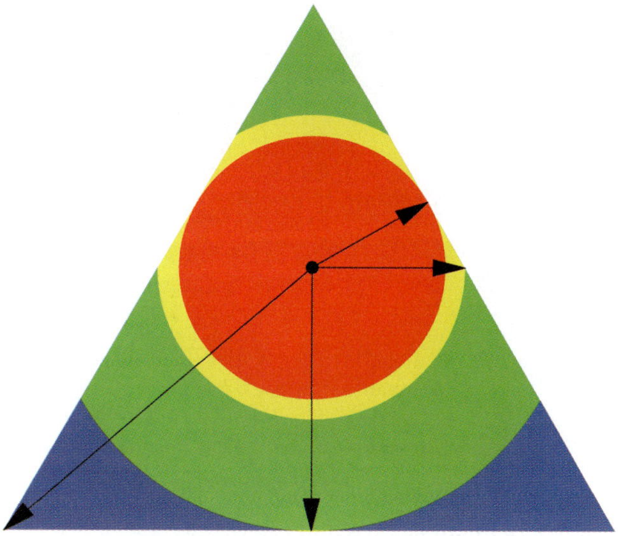

Figure 3 Space of IBD distributions and resampling restrictions. The figure visualizes the regions defined in table 1. The red area is obtained by a circular expansion from the point of noninformativity—that is, (1/4,1/2,1/4). The intersection of the circle with the side of the triangle is obtained by an orthogonal projection along the side of the triangle. The yellow circle segments are bounded by the triangle parallel to the *X*-axis. The green area is obtained by an expansion of the circle segments to the bottom line of the triangle. The blue area represents the remaining part of the triangle and is limited by the corners of the triangle.

where w_i are the Euclidian distance weights. $\bar{\hat{\tau}}_w$ has variance $\sum_{i=1}^{n} w_i^2(\tau_i - \bar{\hat{\tau}}_w)^2$, so that a weighted mean test statistic is given by

$$T_w = \frac{\bar{\hat{\tau}}_w - \frac{1}{2}}{\sqrt{\frac{n'}{n'-1}\sum_{i=1}^{n} w_i^2(\hat{\tau}_i - \bar{\hat{\tau}}_w)^2}} , \quad (2)$$

since its mean is 1/2 under the null hypothesis of no linkage for both ASPs. Here, n' denotes the number of ASPs that are not completely uninformative—that is, for which $w_i > 0$. The weighted mean test statistic reduces to the classical mean test with the empirical variance estimate if $w_i = 1/n$ for all i and $n' = n$.

In equation (2), we treat the weights as fixed, although they are estimated from the present sample. Therefore, the asymptotic properties are not obvious at first glance. However, T_w can also be derived from a generalized estimating equations (GEE) model with independence working covariance matrix (Ziegler et al. 1998). For this purpose, we assume that we can additively decompose τ_i into $\tau + \varepsilon_i$ for all n independent sib pairs. Furthermore, $E(\tau_i) = \tau$, and $\mathrm{Var}(\tau_i) = w_i$. If a generalized least squares estimator is used with weight matrix diag(w_i) for estimating τ, then the Wald statistic of equation (2) is obtained if the robust estimator of variance (Ziegler et al. 1998) is employed for this model. Therefore, T_w asymptotically follows a standard normal distribution under the null hypothesis of no linkage. To avoid slightly increased type I error, especially for small sample sizes, we recommend the use of the central t distribution, with $n - 1$ df, in applications.

Monte Carlo Simulation of *P* Values

At the beginning of this project, it was not certain whether we would discover the limiting distribution of our novel weighted mean test statistic, because weights are estimated from the current sample, thus introducing an extra random element. We therefore investigated the applicability of existing Monte Carlo permutation or simulation approaches, which can be grouped into three basic procedures, as follows.

1. For linkage analysis of quantitative traits in sib pairs and for case-control association studies, one may permute phenotypes or genotypes to disperse the dependency of genotypes and phenotypes (Wan et al. 1997; Zhao et al. 2000). In ASP studies, however, all sib pairs have identical phenotypic values, and this approach is not applicable.
2. One may generate new marker genotypes under the null hypothesis of no linkage with a prespecified heterozygosity (see, e.g., Zinn-Justin et al. 2001). This, in turn, alters the weights, and thus the degree of informativity is not adequately reflected.

Table 1

Mapping Rules

Case	Distance d	Range of t
1	$0 \leq d \leq \frac{1}{4}$	$0 \leq t < 2\pi$
2	$\frac{1}{4} < d < \frac{1}{2\sqrt{3}}$	$0 < t \leq 2\arctan\left(3^{-1/2} - a - A\right)$ $2\arctan\left(3^{-1/2} - a + A\right) \leq t \leq 2\arctan\left(-3^{-1/2} + b - B\right)$ $-2\arctan\left(3^{-1/2} - b - B\right) \leq t < \pi$ $\pi \leq t \leq 2\pi$
3	$d = \frac{1}{2\sqrt{3}}$	$\frac{\pi}{3} \leq t \leq \frac{2\pi}{3}$ $\pi \leq t \leq 2\pi$
4	$\frac{1}{2\sqrt{3}} < d \leq \frac{1}{2}$	$2\arctan\left(3^{-1/2} - a + A\right) \leq t \leq 2\arctan\left(-3^{-1/2} + b + B\right)$ $2\pi - 2\arctan\left(3^{-1/2} - b + B\right) \leq t \leq 2\pi - 2\arctan\left(-3^{-1/2} + a + A\right)$
5	$\frac{1}{2} < d \leq \sqrt{\frac{7}{12}}$	$2\pi - 2\arctan\left(3^{-1/2} - b + B\right) \leq t \leq 2\pi - 2\arctan\left(2r + \sqrt{4r^2 - 1}\right)$ $2\pi - 2\arctan\left(2r - \sqrt{4r^2 - 1}\right) \leq t \leq 2\pi - 2\arctan\left(-3^{-1/2} + a + A\right)$

NOTE.—Valid IBD distributions are calculated in terms of polar coordinates (d,t) with origin in $(f_0,f_1,f_2) = (1/4,1/2,1/4)$. These rules specify, for any d, the valid angles t (in radians), so that the pair (d,t) maps back to a valid IBD sharing value. Except for the first area, which describes a whole circle, distances d correspond to the union of different circle segments. In addition, $a = \left(\sqrt{3} + 6d\right)^{-1}$, $A = \sqrt{a^2 3(16d^2 - 1)}$, $b = \left(\sqrt{3} - 6d\right)^{-1}$, and $B = \sqrt{b^2 3(16d^2 - 1)}$.

3. Zhao et al. (1999) proposed a randomization procedure for the inheritance vectors obtained from the Lander-Green algorithm (Idury and Elston 1997; Kruglyak and Lander 1998). Again, this approach does not hold the weights w_i constant and therefore does not adequately reflect the informativity of the individual sib pairs.

To conclude, all existing approaches do not keep the weight constant for an individual sib pair. They are therefore not suitable for the proposed weighted mean test, and we suggest instead the use of the following approach. If we consider lines tracking the circles around the IBD distribution of an uninformative marker, we see that these represent ASPs with identical informativity and, thus, equal weights. Although the weights are constant, their specific IBD distribution may vary, as shown by a specific position on the circle. For a given weight w_i, we therefore simulate new ASPs on the line describing the circle belonging to weight w_i, as shown in figure 3.

With increasing weights, circles around (1/4, 1/2, 1/4) do not completely fit into the triangle of IBD distributions in figure 3. In this situation, one could first simulate a point on the corresponding circle, as before, and, second, check whether the point corresponds to a valid IBD distribution by lying within the triangle. This may, however, be quite inefficient. For example, in the most extreme case (i.e., a sib pair with either 2 or 0 alleles shared IBD), the circle intersects the triangle at only those two points. Consequently, the probability that a point on the circle exactly corresponds to one of the two possible IBD distributions is 0. For this reason, we mathematically derived the circles and circle segments, given a specific weight. Four areas have to be distinguished, as shown in figure 3. The first area is the red circle, which is obtained by moving from (1/4, 1/2, 1/4) in all directions toward the sides of the triangle. The first intersection is obtained orthogonal to f_0 and f_2. The second area, marked in yellow, is bounded by the intersection orthogonal to the Y-axis. The third area, displayed in green, is limited by the intersection orthogonal to the X-axis. The remaining area is shown in blue.

Areas according to Euclidian distances and corresponding valid IBD distributions are calculated using polar coordinates (d,t). These specify the valid angles t (in radians) for any distance d (table 1). With the angles t, given the distance d, the following simulation algorithm for ASPs may be employed.

1. Compute the weighted mean test statistic T_w, using the original n sib pairs. Keep the Euclidian distances d_i and weights w_i.
2. For sib pairs i, from 1 to n,
   a. Draw t_i from a continuous uniform distribution in accordance with table 1.
   b. Calculate the simulated IBD sharing values

$$f_{0i} = \frac{1}{4} + \frac{d_i}{2}\left[\sqrt{3}\cos(t_i) - \sin(t_i)\right] ,$$

$$f_{1i} = \frac{1}{2} + d_i \sin(t_i), \text{ and}$$

$$f_{2i} = 1 - f_{0i} - f_{1i} .$$

Table 2

Possible IBD Distributions (f_0,f_1,f_2) and Their Probabilities at a Marker Locus with r Equifrequent Alleles

IBD Distribution	Probability: No Linkage[a]	Probability: Dominant Model[b]	Probability: Recessive Model[b]
(1,0,0)	$\frac{r^3-r^2+1}{4r^3}$	$\frac{r-1}{8r^3}[(3r^2-3r-4)p^4-(4r^2-4r-6)p^3+(3r^2-3r-4)p^2]$	$\frac{1}{4r^3}(r^3-2r^2+1)p^4$
(0,1,0)	$\frac{r-1}{2r^2}$	$\frac{(r-1)^2}{8r^2}(5p^4-5p^3+3p^2+p)$	$\frac{(r-1)^2}{8r^2}(3p^4+p^3)$
(0,0,1)	$\frac{r^3-r^2+1}{4r^3}$	$\frac{1}{16r^3}[(5r^3-10r^2-r+6)p^4-(4r^3-8r^2-2r+6)p^3+(r^3-2r^2-r+2)p^2+(2r^3-4r^2+2)p]$	$\frac{r-1}{16r^3}[(3r^2-3r-2)p^4-p^3+(r^2-r)p^2]$
$\left(\frac{1}{2},\frac{1}{2},0\right)$	$\frac{r-1}{r^2}$	$\frac{r-1}{4r^2}(5p^4-5p^3+3p^2+p)$	$\frac{r-1}{r^2}p^4$
$\left(\frac{1}{2},0,\frac{1}{2}\right)$	$\frac{r-1}{2r^3}$	$\frac{r-1}{8r^3}(7p^4-9p^3+5p^2+p)$	$\frac{r-1}{8r^3}(3p^4+p^3)$
$\left(0,\frac{1}{2},\frac{1}{2}\right)$	$\frac{r-1}{r^2}$	$\frac{r-1}{8r^2}(11p^4-12p^3+7p^2+2p)$	$\frac{r-1}{8r^2}(5p^4+p^3+p^2)$
$\left(\frac{1}{2},\frac{1}{4},\frac{1}{2}\right)$	$\frac{1}{r^2}$	$\frac{1}{16r^2}(21p^4-22p^3+13p^2+4p)$	$\frac{1}{16r^2}(13p^4+2p^3+p^2)$

[a] Displays the probability of an ASP for a specific IBD distribution at an unlinked autosomal genetic marker—that is, $\theta = 0.5$.

[b] The probability of an ASP for a specific IBD distribution at a linked genetic marker with $\theta = 0$ for an autosomal dominant disease (dominant model) or a recessive disease (recessive model) with complete penetrance and a diallelic trait locus with minor-allele frequency p. Both loci are in Hardy-Weinberg equilibrium, and there is no linkage disequilibrium between the loci.

3. Compute the simulated test statistic, T_{sim}, of the resampled pairs, using weights w_i.
4. Repeat steps 2 and 3, say, M times.
5. Compute the empirical P value, P_{emp}, by $\#\{T_{\text{sim}} \geqslant T_w\}/M$. Here, # denotes the number operator.

To explain step 2a of the algorithm in greater detail, we consider the following example. If the estimated IBD distribution is $f = (1/2, 1/4, 1/4)$, then one obtains $d = \sqrt{13}/12$, corresponding to case 4 in table 1. This distance d falls within the interval $[1/(2\sqrt{3}); 1/2]$. With $a = 1/(\sqrt{3} + \sqrt{13}/2) \approx 0.282899$, $b = 1/(\sqrt{3} - \sqrt{13}/2) \approx -14.1393$, $A = (4/3)(-6 + \sqrt{39}) \approx 0.326664$, and $B = (4/3)(6 + \sqrt{39}) \approx 16.3267$, t is drawn from a continuous uniform distribution, with values that fall within the interval

$$\left[2\arctan\left(\frac{4+\sqrt{13}}{6+\sqrt{39}}\right); -2\arctan\left(\frac{-4+\sqrt{13}}{-6+\sqrt{39}}\right)\right]$$
$$\cup\left[2\pi\arctan\left(\frac{4+\sqrt{13}}{6-\sqrt{39}}\right); 2\pi\arctan\left(\frac{-4+\sqrt{13}}{6+\sqrt{39}}\right)\right]$$
$$\approx [1.1116; 2.0300] \cup [3.2060; 6.2188] .$$

Simulation Studies

In this section, we demonstrate the validity of the proposed weighted mean test and the Monte Carlo simulation approach. Furthermore, we show the gain in power that can be achieved by the weighted mean test, in comparison with the classical mean test.

In the simulation study, we wanted to avoid computer time–consuming simulation of parental alleles, segregation of alleles to offspring, disease assignment, and subsequent calculation of IBD values in a two-point setting. We therefore derived the probabilities for the seven possible IBD distributions for ASPs at an unlinked marker locus with r equifrequent alleles (table 2). A similar distribution has been presented by Risch (1990) for identity-by-state values. We also deduced the probabilities of the seven possible IBD distributions for ASPs, assuming an autosomal dominant and recessive disease with complete penetrance, no phenocopies, a diallelic trait locus with minor-allele frequency p, $\theta = 0$, and a marker locus with r equifrequent alleles. Both loci are assumed to be in Hardy-Weinberg equilibrium, and there is no linkage disequilibrium between the loci.

Parameters subject to variation were the probability of the disease allele ($p = 1/100{,}000$), the number of families ($n = 50$ and $n = 200$), and the number of equally frequent alleles at the marker locus (r). The scenario $r = 2$ corresponds to a heterozygosity of 0.5, which is comparable to the usual two-point situation. The scenario $r = 4$ (i.e., heterozygosity of 0.75) is similar to the informativity in a microsatellite genome scan, and $r = 100$ corresponds to an almost completely informative chromosomal position, which can be achieved in genomewide scans with SNP chips.

The number of replications was set to 100,000 under

Table 3

Asymptotic and Empirical Type I Error Fractions for the Classical Mean Test with Empirical Variance (Classic) and the Weighted Mean Test with Euclidian Distance Weights (Euclid)

	Type I Error											
	$n = 50; r = 2$		$n = 50; r = 4$		$n = 50; r = 100$		$n = 200; r = 2$		$n = 200; r = 4$		$n = 200; r = 100$	
Nominal α	Classic	Euclid	Classic	Euclid	Classic	Euclid	Classic	Euclid	Classic	Euclid	Classic	Euclid
Asymptotic:												
.001	.00113	.00146	.00098	.00195	.00098	.00183	.00091	.00132	.00077	.00089	.00097	.00104
.01	.00986	.01377	.01025	.01357	.00965	.01195	.00952	.01024	.00960	.01011	.01010	.01023
.02	.02049	.02598	.01972	.02398	.02115	.02197	.01973	.02049	.01940	.01952	.02040	.02026
.03	.03058	.03764	.02999	.03406	.03127	.03204	.02967	.03062	.02918	.02977	.03092	.03024
.04	.04085	.04869	.04033	.04426	.04013	.04251	.03991	.04117	.03908	.03974	.04084	.04008
.05	.05034	.05989	.04907	.05462	.04979	.05315	.05019	.05141	.04908	.05002	.05109	.05062
Empirical:												
.001	.00117	.00051	.00083	.00078	.00099	.00130	.00121	.00096	.00100	.00072	.00092	.00097
.01	.01071	.00819	.01026	.01000	.00957	.01042	.01060	.00892	.01009	.00955	.01032	.01011
.02	.02025	.01756	.01982	.01991	.01995	.02044	.02119	.01853	.02033	.01891	.02061	.02027
.03	.03037	.02808	.02953	.02978	.02971	.03033	.03133	.02845	.03021	.02880	.03094	.02999
.04	.04040	.03812	.03992	.03970	.04007	.04029	.04149	.03879	.04006	.03910	.04128	.03956
.05	.05029	.04855	.04918	.05000	.05002	.05075	.05167	.04929	.05058	.04907	.05153	.05010

Note.—Error values were calculated for n ASPs and r equifrequent alleles. Asymptotic type I errors are obtained from the t distribution with $n - 1$ df. Empirical type I error fractions are estimated from the novel Monte Carlo simulation approach.

the null hypothesis, H_0, for the unlinked marker and to 1,000 for a completely linked marker locus. Asymptotic P values were obtained from the t distribution, with $n - 1$ df, for the standard mean tests and the weighted mean test. The number of simulations was set to $M = 10{,}000$ for the computation of empirical P values for both T_{mev} and T_w. For the empirical determination of P values, data were simulated on circles or circle segments. Distances, however, were ignored in the computation of T_{mev} by setting weights to $1/n$. Power at type I error level α was determined by using the upper α fractile from both the asymptotic and the empirical distribution of P values simulated under the null hypothesis of no linkage. All Monte Carlo simulations were performed by a fast and flexible simulation utility in C++, which is available upon request.

Simulation results for type I error fractions and power for the dominant genetic model are summarized in tables 3 and 4, respectively. As displayed in figure 4, asymptotic type I error levels based on the t distribution agree well with the nominal levels, if the sample size is at least $n = 100$, and the approximation improves with sample size, regardless of the underlying marker informativity. Asymptotic normality begins to take effect later for the novel weighted mean test (dashed line in fig. 4) than for the classical mean test with empirically estimated variance (solid line in fig. 4) because of the extra random element introduced by the weight w_i. However, differences are negligible when the sample size exceeds 150 (fig. 4). No such pattern can be observed for empirically determined type I errors. Here, the nominal level coincides well with the simulated level for both mean tests, regardless of the sample size and marker informativity (table 3), except for $n = 50$ and $r = 2$, for which the weighted mean test appeared to be slightly conservative.

Because the weighted mean test with the use of the asymptotic distribution is liberal for $n = 50$, power for this test is presented only for a sample size of $n = 200$ (table 4). As expected, power increases with the number of ASPs and the number of alleles at the linked marker locus. Power varies only slightly between asymptotically and empirically determined type I error levels. There is, however, a remarkable gain in power between the classical mean test with empirically estimated variances and the weighted mean test, for many configurations. For instance, for a significance level of 0.001, with $n = 200$ ASPs and a low heterozygosity of 50%, corresponding to $r = 2$, the power increases from 28% to 70%. Furthermore, there is no configuration in our simulations for which the classical mean test has greater power than the weighted mean test.

Application to Sample Data

As a first example, we reanalyzed the ASP sample data given by Risch (1990, table 1), which are displayed in table 5. Only 32 of the 74 ASPs have definite information about IBD. The mean test statistic T_m, with variance fixed to $1/(8n)$, gives a LOD score of 1.95 (table 6) when T_m statistics are converted to LOD scores via $T_m^2/(2 \ln 10)$. As expected, the mean test statistic with empirical variance T_{mev} has a higher LOD score of 2.63. The weighted mean test statistic outperforms both mean

Table 4

Asymptotic and Empirical Power of the Classical Mean Test with Empirical Variance (Classic) and the Weighted Mean Test with Euclidian Distance Weights (Euclid)

	Power											
	n = 50; r = 2		n = 50; r = 4		n = 50; r = 100		n = 200; r = 2		n = 200; r = 4		n = 200; r = 100	
Nominal α	Classic	Euclid	Classic	Euclid	Classic	Euclid	Classic	Euclid	Classic	Euclid	Classic	Euclid
Asymptotic:												
.001	.01734	...	.78372	...	1.00000	...	.27522	.69777	.99991	1.00000	1.00000	1.00000
.01	.06973	...	.86694	...	1.00000	...	.39528	.88785	.99999	1.00000	1.00000	1.00000
.02	.13617	...	.91924	...	1.00000	...	.53396	.93070	.99999	1.00000	1.00000	1.00000
.03	.17692	...	.93668	...	1.00000	...	.59950	.94601	.99999	1.00000	1.00000	1.00000
.04	.20631	...	.95779	...	1.00000	...	.62774	.95875	.99999	1.00000	1.00000	1.00000
.05	.24086	...	.96311	...	1.00000	...	.65765	.96887	.99999	1.00000	1.00000	1.00000
Empirical:												
.001	.02291	.05394	.78853	.90693	.99901	.99870	.28467	.69713	.99900	1.00000	1.00000	1.00000
.01	.07334	.23344	.86252	.98124	1.00000	1.00000	.39984	.88308	1.00000	1.00000	1.00000	1.00000
.02	.14210	.34297	.91689	.98798	1.00000	1.00000	.54142	.92321	1.00000	1.00000	1.00000	1.00000
.03	.18063	.41545	.93584	.99095	1.00000	1.00000	.60576	.94377	1.00000	1.00000	1.00000	1.00000
.04	.21263	.49261	.95330	.99401	1.00000	1.00000	.63758	.95470	1.00000	1.00000	1.00000	1.00000
.05	.24729	.56199	.96008	.99606	1.00000	1.00000	.65720	.96530	1.00000	1.00000	1.00000	1.00000

Note.—Power was calculated for n ASPs under an autosomal dominant genetic model with complete penetrance, no phenocopies, and $\theta = 0$ in a two-locus setting. The linked marker was assumed to have $r = 2$, $r = 4$, and $r = 100$ equally frequent alleles. Empirical P values are based on 100,000 simulations. The asymptotic weighted mean is liberal for a sample size of $n = 50$; therefore, we present asymptotic power of the weighted mean test only for $n = 200$.

test statistics T_m and T_{mev}, with a LOD of 3.09, because the ASPs with IBD values equal to 2 receive greater weight than the ASPs with IBD values equal to 1.

The IBD distribution estimated from the completely informative ASP sample is $\hat{f}_2 = 0.44$, $\hat{f}_1 = 0.44$, and $\hat{f}_0 = 0.06$, and it therefore lies in the possible triangle (Holmans 1993). Subsequently, the maximum LOD score (MLS) and the triangle test statistic (TTS) have identical LOD scores of 2.20. Nevertheless, the asymptotic distributions of these test statistics are different (for details, see Holmans 1993).

When the incompletely informative families are added to the sample, the LOD scores of both classical mean tests decrease. In contrast, the weighted mean test shows an increase in the LOD score to 3.20. A higher LOD score of 2.79 can also be observed for the MLS and TTS. The IBD distribution estimated for the complete sample is an inner point of the possible triangle, so that the LOD scores are identical. Nonetheless, the LOD score of the weighted mean test statistic T_w is higher than the LOD score of the MLS and TTS.

As a second example, we consider the data of Mein et al. (1998). On the basis of a genomewide scan that included a total of 356 ASP families collected in the United Kingdom, they reported a susceptibility locus on chromosome 16q22-q24 (*D16S515–D16S520*) for type 1 diabetes (see fig. 1*b* in Mein et al. 1998). Seventeen of the ASPs were drawn from families with three affected offspring, from which a single ASP was selected that comprised the proband and the next diagnosed individual; thus, a sample of independent ASPs was assembled. Details on subjects, genotyping, and map construction can be found in the work of Mein et al. (1998). The information content varied between 65% and 90% for chromosome 16 (for details, see fig. 1*a* in Mein et al. 1998), and it was ~80% at the peak position.

Mein et al. (1998) used the TTS under the assumption of dominance variance, as implemented in Genehunter (Kruglyak and Lander 1998) for multipoint linkage analysis. We reanalyzed the published data with use of the TTS, the classical mean test with variance evaluated under H_0, the mean test with empirical variance, and the weighted mean test (fig. 5). While the maximum LOD for T_m is 2.8, both T_{mev} and TTS have maximum LOD scores of ~3.4. They are outperformed by the T_w, which shows a LOD of 3.9 at *D16S3098*. It is important to note that the general shapes of the LOD score curves look similar for all displayed test statistics.

Discussion

Informativity of families for linkage analysis is an important issue in human genetics, and, consequently, it has been studied by several investigators using different concepts. Teng and Siegmund (1998), for example, analytically compared differences between two-point and multipoint analyses. They showed that multipoint analyses exploit available information better than two-point analyses. However, even in multipoint situations, the IBD value cannot be determined unambiguously for ev-

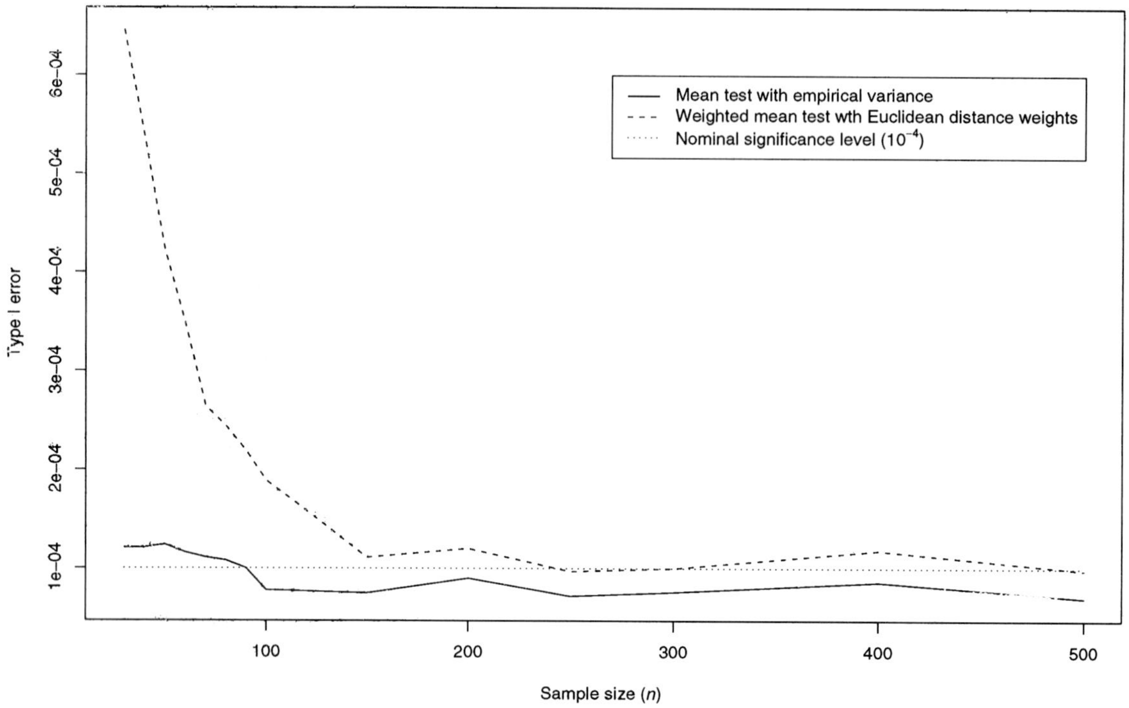

Figure 4 Asymptotic type I error of the classical mean test with empirical variance and of the weighted mean test with an increasing number of sib pairs (n). Under H_0, 1,000,000 samples of size n were simulated. P values were obtained by use of Student's t distribution, with $n-1$ df and at a nominal significance level of $\alpha = 10^{-4}$.

ery chromosomal position, since markers are not placed at any genomic location and the number of distinct alleles at each marker locus is restricted. Therefore, weighting by marker informativity, as proposed here, can still increase power to detect linkage.

Another focus in the consideration of informativity is the family size, since families of different sizes also have different degrees of informativity. This has been studied by Hodge (1984) for linkage analysis with ASPs. Hodge examined the Shannon information contained in sibships of size s and showed that a complete sibship contains $(2s-3+0.5^{s-1})/1.5$ pair-equivalents of information. Thus, a sibship of size 4 has the informativity of ~3.4 independent ASPs, although 6 different pairs can be constructed. Hodge therefore proposed to down-weight multiple sibships accordingly. For the more general case of affected relative pairs, weighting on the basis of pedigree structure has also been discussed in the context of the nonparametric linkage (NPL) statistic (see, e.g., Whittemore 1996; Kong and Cox 1997; Teng and Siegmund 1997).

A third interpretation for informativity has been employed successfully in meta-analyses in which studies have been weighted according to their information content (Loesgen et al. 2001; Dempfle and Loesgen 2004). Weighting families by marker informativity has already

Table 5

Sample Data for Comparison of Test Statistics in Table 6

No. of Sib Pairs	f_2	f_1	f_0
14	1	0	0
16	0	1	0
2	0	0	1
22	2/3	1/3	0
13	0	1/3	2/3
7	1/2	0	1/2

Table 6

Comparison of MLS, Holman's TTS, and the Mean Test Statistics for the Sample Data in Table 5

	LOD Score for	
Test Statistic[a]	Informative Families	All Families
MLS and TTS	2.20	2.79
T_m	1.95	1.90
T_{mev}	2.63	2.55
T_w	3.09	3.20

[a] T_m is the classical mean test statistic with variance evaluated under the null hypothesis, H_0. T_{mev} is the classical mean test statistic with empirical variance. T_w is the weighted mean test statistic.

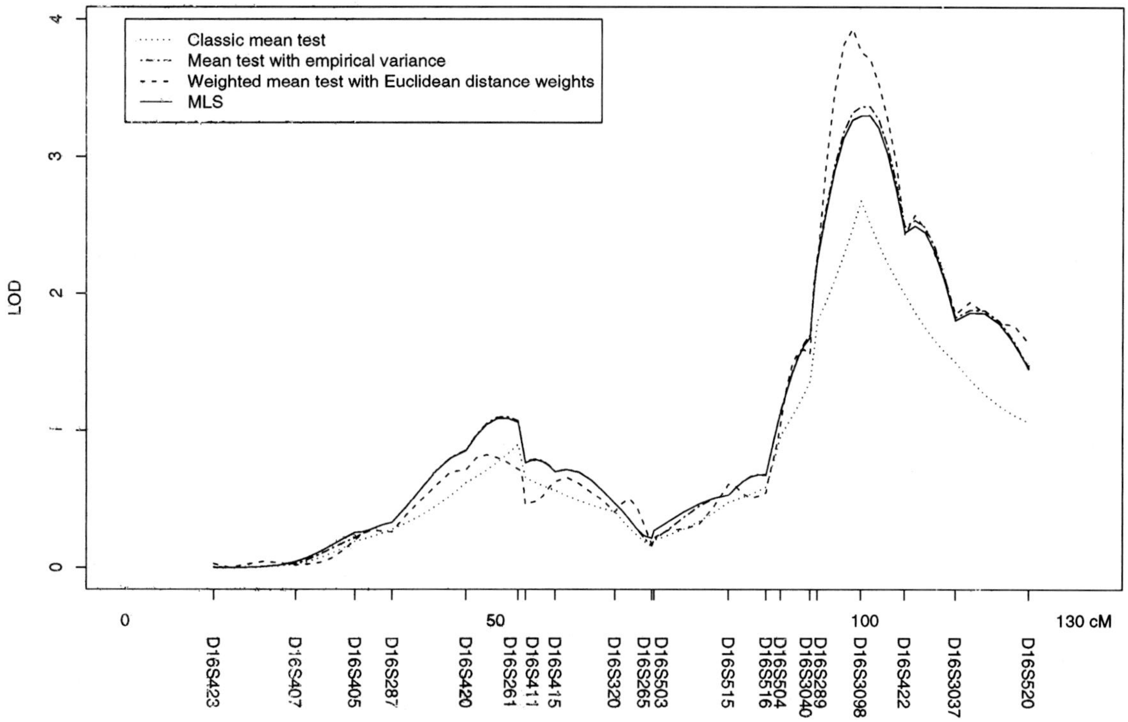

Figure 5 Multipoint linkage analysis of chromosome 16 with use of the data from Mein et al. (1998). Multipoint TTS statistic was calculated under the assumption of dominance variance. The classical mean test with variance was evaluated under H_0, and the weighted mean test with Euclidian distance weights was computed from the same individual ASP IBD estimates.

been incorporated in the analysis by Sham et al. (2002), who specified and estimated the covariance matrix of IBD sharing between relative pairs in the framework of a new regression-based method for linkage analysis of quantitative traits.

If marker informativeness is neglected in the analyses, a severe loss of power can occur, as recently discussed (Abecasis et al. 2004; Cordell 2004; Mukhopadhyay et al. 2004; Schork and Greenwood 2004*a*, 2004*b*; Sieberts et al. 2004; Visscher and Wray 2004). A simple solution to the problem is to remove uninformative relative pairs from the analysis. This corresponds to a discrete weighting scheme with all-or-nothing weights, which is already implemented in some software packages. However, Schork and Greenwood (2004*b*) also pointed out that, in practice, it will be difficult to decide which pairs should be discarded from the analyses. They have, therefore, also proposed to consider the use of more complicated test statistics that downweight partially informative relative pairs in some way.

In this article, we have taken up this idea and have weighted ASP families by marker informativity: the greater the degree of informativity of an ASP, the greater its weight in linkage analysis. We thus extended the classical mean test, proposed a weighted mean test, and derived its limiting distribution. Because weights are estimated from current data, asymptotic normality begins to take effect later for the novel weighted mean test than for the classical mean test. Although significance levels of 10^{-4}, which correspond to a LOD score of 3, can be maintained for ~50 ASPs with the classical mean test, between 100 and 150 ASPs are required for the weighted mean test. However, for most applications, this should not be a relevant restriction. In cases in which the number of ASPs is low, our new method for simulation of P values may be employed instead. This keeps Euclidian distance weights fixed, and new ASPs are generated using a continuous uniform distribution on the corresponding circle or circle segment. Our simulation method clearly shows that the weighted mean test is, in principle, able to detect any deviation from the null hypothesis. This is in contrast to the TTS, for which IBD estimates for the whole sample are restricted to the so-called possible triangle.

Weighting as discussed here may be employed in some other tests as well. Whittemore and Tu (1998), for example, derived a set of constraints for the IBD probabilities of affected sib triples and used common features of the shapes of the two constraint sets to introduce the minmax tests. For other test statistics, weighting by marker informativity seems to be impossible. For instance, in likelihood-ratio statistics like the MLS, the weights cancel out in both the numerator and the denominator. Here, an all-or-none weighting scheme seems to be the only possibility to exclude partially informative families from the analysis. Uninformative families are already discarded. For a sample consisting of ASPs only, the standard NPL statistic is equivalent to the classical mean test with theoretical variance (see, e.g., Cordell 2004). Though weighting is meaningful for the standard NPL statistic, different degrees of marker informativity are adequately considered in the further development by Kong and Cox (1997).

For validation of results, it may be worthwhile to investigate the effect of additionally recruited discordant sib pairs (DSPs), in which one offspring is affected and the other is unaffected (Guo and Elston 2000; Elston et al. 2005). Because the classical mean test has been used for the analysis of DSPs (Risch and Zhang 1996; Guo and Elston 2000), the weighted mean test is adopted easily for this situation—instead of a higher sharing under linkage, it should be <1/2 for DSPs. The weighted mean test for ASPs and DSPs will soon be available in the software package S.A.G.E., which can be obtained for free by nonprofit organizations.

In two applications, we have illustrated the use of the weighted mean test in two-point and multipoint analyses. However, our new approach is currently restricted to independent ASPs. Two approaches to overcome this restriction are possible. First, large sibships can be treated as independent ASPs, as shown by Blackwelder and Elston (1985). This result is based on asymptotic arguments with identical weights; thus, P values are possibly too liberal in small samples. In addition, the generalization of the argument used by Blackwelder and Elston (1985) for the classical mean test to the weighted mean test needs to be demonstrated in a Monte Carlo simulation study. Second, the same GEE technique that has been used for deriving the asymptotic normality of the proposed weighted mean test may be employed here, with a correction for large sibships. Similarly, our approach for simulation of P values requires extension to large sibships.

Another area of possible improvement is our use of Euclidian distance weights for the novel weighted mean test. We validated the asymptotic distribution of the proposed test statistic with Euclidian distance weights in a Monte Carlo simulation study and demonstrated that the power of the weighted mean test can be substantially higher than the power of the classical mean test. However, our simulations were based on simple Mendelian traits—that is, fully penetrant without phenocopies. Furthermore, we did not study the effect of missing parental genotypes and of misspecified allele frequencies. Use of the diabetes data in our example yielded results consistent with findings from our simple simulation studies. However, we recognize that diabetes is a more complex genetic disease, and we therefore presume that our weighted mean test is also powerful in more complex models.

Since we did not show the optimality of the proposed weights, other weighting schemes based on different distance or informativity measures, such as Shannon's entropy or the Fisher information, may be even more powerful. We cannot exclude the notion that the classical mean test with empirical variance might be more powerful in some configurations. Although the numerical derivation of optimal weights is possible in principle, a theoretical result most likely cannot be derived, since weights appear in both the numerator and the denominator of the weighted mean test statistic. Further research is required to extend the weighted mean test to large sibships, or even to affected relative pairs.

Acknowledgments

We are grateful to Inke R. König for helpful discussions on a previous version of the manuscript. We gratefully acknowledge the Juvenile Diabetes Research Foundation/Wellcome Trust Diabetes and Inflammation Laboratory for providing genotype data (from Mein et al. [1998], data version 1.0) for independent analysis by our group. This work was supported by Deutsche Forschungsgemeinschaft grant ZI 591/12-1.

Web Resources

The URL for data presented herein is as follows:

S.A.G.E. software, http://darwin.cwru.edu/ (Note: the weighted mean test will be available soon from S.A.G.E. Nonprofit organizations can obtain S.A.G.E. for free.)

References

Abecasis G, Cox N, Daly MJ, Kruglyak L, Laird N, Markianos K, Patterson N (2004) No bias in linkage analysis. Am J Hum Genet 75:722–723

Amos CI, Elston RC, Wilson AF, Bailey-Wilson JE (1989) A more powerful robust sib-pair test of linkage for quantitative traits. Genet Epidemiol 6:435–449

Blackwelder WC, Elston RC (1985) A comparison of sib-pair linkage tests for disease susceptibility loci. Genet Epidemiol 2:85–97

Cordell HJ (2004) Bias toward the null hypothesis in model-free linkage analysis is highly dependent on the test statistic used. Am J Hum Genet 74:1294–1302

Dempfle A, Loesgen S (2004) Meta-analysis of linkage studies for complex diseases: an overview of methods and a simulation study. Ann Hum Genet 68:69–83

Elston RC, Song D, Iyengar SK (2005) Mathematical assumptions versus biological reality: myths in affected sib pair linkage analysis. Am J Hum Genet 76:152–156

Franke D, Kleensang A, Elston RC, Ziegler A. Haseman-Elston weighted by marker informativity. BMC Genet (in press)

Guo X, Elston RC (2000) Two-stage global search designs for

linkage analysis. II. Including discordant relative pairs in the study. Genet Epidemiol 18:111–127
Haseman JK, Elston RC (1972) The investigation of linkage between a quantitative trait and a marker locus. Behav Genet 2:3–19
Hodge SE (1984) The information contained in multiple sibling pairs. Genet Epidemiol 1:109–122
Holmans P (1993) Asymptotic properties of affected–sib-pair linkage analysis. Am J Hum Genet 52:362–374
Horvitz DG, Thompson DJ (1952) A generalization of sampling without replacement from a finite universe. J Am Stat Assoc 47:663–685
Idury RM, Elston RC (1997) A faster and more general hidden Markov model algorithm for multipoint likelihood calculations. Hum Hered 47:197–202
Jacobs KB, Gray-McGuire C, Cartier KC, Elston RC (2003) Genome-wide linkage scan for genes affecting longitudinal trends in systolic blood pressure. BMC Genet Suppl 4:82
Knapp M, Seuchter SA, Baur MP (1994) Linkage analysis in nuclear families. I. Optimality criteria for affected sib-pair tests. Hum Hered 44:37–43
Kong A, Cox NJ (1997) Allele-sharing models: LOD scores and accurate linkage tests. Am J Hum Genet 61:1179–1188
Kruglyak L, Lander ES (1998) Faster multipoint linkage analysis using Fourier transforms. J Comput Biol 5:1–7
Loesgen S, Dempfle A, Golla A, Bickeböller H (2001) Weighting schemes in pooled linkage analysis. Genet Epidemiol Suppl 21:142–147
Mein CA, Esposito L, Dunn MG, Johnson GC, Timms AE, Goy JV, Smith AN, et al (1998) A search for type 1 diabetes susceptibility genes in families from the United Kingdom. Nat Genet 19:297–300
Mukhopadhyay I, Feingold E, Weeks DE (2004) No "bias" toward the null hypothesis in most conventional multipoint nonparametric linkage analyses. Am J Hum Genet 75:716–718
Olson JM (2002) Linkage analysis, model free. In Elston RC, Olson JM, Palmer L (eds) Biostatistical genetics and genetic epidemiology. John Wiley & Sons, New York, pp 460–472
Risch N (1990) Linkage strategies for genetically complex traits. III. The effect of marker polymorphism on analysis of affected relative pairs. Am J Hum Genet 46:242–253 (erratum 51:673–675)
Risch NJ, Zhang H (1996) Mapping quantitative trait loci with extreme discordant sib pairs: sampling considerations. Am J Hum Genet 58:836–843
S.A.G.E. (2004) Statistical analysis for genetic epidemiology. Statistical Solutions, Cork, Ireland
Schork NJ, Greenwood TA (2004*a*) Got bias? The authors reply. Am J Hum Genet 75:723–727
——— (2004*b*) Inherent bias toward the null hypothesis in conventional multipoint nonparametric linkage analysis. Am J Hum Genet 74:306–316
Sham PC, Purcell S (2001) Equivalence between Haseman-Elston and variance-components linkage analyses for sib pairs. Am J Hum Genet 68:1527–1532
Sham PC, Purcell S, Cherny SS, Abecasis GR (2002) Powerful regression-based quantitative-trait linkage analysis of general pedigrees. Am J Hum Genet 71:238–253
Sieberts SK, Broman KW, Gudbjartsson DF (2004) Conventional multipoint nonparametric linkage analysis is not necessarily inherently biased. Am J Hum Genet 75:720–722
Teng J, Siegmund D (1997) Combining information within and between pedigrees for mapping complex traits. Am J Hum Genet 60:979–992
——— (1998) Multipoint linkage analysis using affected relative pairs and partially informative markers. Biometrics 54: 1247–1265
Visscher PM, Wray NR (2004) Conventional multipoint nonparametric linkage analysis is not necessarily inherently biased. Am J Hum Genet 75:718–720
Wan Y, Cohen J, Guerra R (1997) A permutation test for the robust sib-pair linkage method. Ann Hum Genet 61:79–87
Whittemore AS (1996) Genome scanning for linkage: an overview. Am J Hum Genet 59:704–716
Whittemore AS, Tu IP (1998) Simple, robust linkage tests for affected sibs. Am J Hum Genet 62:1228–1242
Zhao H, Merikangas KR, Kidd KK (1999) On a randomization procedure in linkage analysis. Am J Hum Genet 65: 1449–1456
Zhao JH, Curtis D, Sham PC (2000) Model-free analysis and permutation tests for allelic associations. Hum Hered 50: 133–139
Ziegler A, Kastner C, Blettner M (1998) The generalised estimating equations: an annotated bibliography. Biom J 40: 115–139
Zinn-Justin A, Ziegler A, Abel L (2001) Multipoint development of the weighted pairwise correlation (WPC) linkage method for pedigrees of arbitrary size and application to the analysis of breast cancer and alcoholism familial data. Genet Epidemiol 21:40–52

Am. J. Hum. Genet. 77:242–251, 2005

A Mutation in *SNAP29,* Coding for a SNARE Protein Involved in Intracellular Trafficking, Causes a Novel Neurocutaneous Syndrome Characterized by Cerebral Dysgenesis, Neuropathy, Ichthyosis, and Palmoplantar Keratoderma

Eli Sprecher,[1,4] Akemi Ishida-Yamamoto,[7] Mordechai Mizrahi-Koren,[1,5] Debora Rapaport,[8] Dorit Goldsher,[2,4] Margarita Indelman,[1] Orit Topaz,[1,4] Ilana Chefetz,[1,4] Hanni Keren,[1] Timothy J. O'Brien,[9] Dani Bercovich,[10] Stavit Shalev,[11] Dan Geiger,[6] Reuven Bergman,[1,4] Mia Horowitz,[8] and Hanna Mandel[3,4]

[1]Department of Dermatology and Laboratory of Molecular Dermatology, [2]MRI Institute, [3]Metabolic Disease Unit and Department of Pediatrics B, Rambam Medical Center; [4]Rappaport Faculty of Medicine, [5]Biotechnology Interdisciplinary Unit, and [6]Computer Science Department, Technion-Israel Institute of Technology, Haifa, Israel; [7]Department of Dermatology, Asahikawa Medical College, Asahikawa, Japan; [8]Department of Cell Research and Immunology, Tel Aviv University, Ramat Aviv, Israel; [9]Department of Obstetrics and Gynecology, University of Arkansas for Medical Sciences, Little Rock; [10]Human Molecular Genetics & Pharmacogenetics, Migal-Galilee Technology Center, Kiryat-Shmona, Israel; [11]Genetic Institute, Ha'emek Medical Center, Afula, Israel

Neurocutaneous syndromes represent a vast, largely heterogeneous group of disorders characterized by neurological and dermatological manifestations, reflecting the common embryonic origin of epidermal and neural tissues. In the present report, we describe a novel neurocutaneous syndrome characterized by cerebral dysgenesis, neuropathy, ichthyosis, and keratoderma (CEDNIK syndrome). Using homozygosity mapping in two large families, we localized the disease gene to 22q11.2 and identified, in all patients, a 1-bp deletion in *SNAP29,* which codes for a SNARE protein involved in vesicle fusion. SNAP29 expression was decreased in the skin of the patients, resulting in abnormal maturation of lamellar granules and, as a consequence, in mislocation of epidermal lipids and proteases. These data underscore the importance of vesicle trafficking regulatory mechanisms for proper neuroectodermal differentiation.

Introduction

Endocytosis and exocytosis, which are a hallmark of eukaryotic cells, involve tightly orchestrated mechanisms ensuring trafficking of numerous molecules and particles through the formation of membrane carriers, often vesicles (Deitcher 2002). Membrane fusion between vesicles and target membranes, a critical step in these processes, is mediated by a large number of the so-called soluble n-ethylmaleimide sensitive factor attachment protein (SNAP) receptor (SNARE) proteins (Bonifacino and Glick 2004). Two classes of SNAREs can be distinguished: v-SNAREs, located on vesicular membranes, and t-SNAREs, located on target membranes. SNAREs self-assemble into extremely stable four-helix bundles, composed of two cognate parts, which mediate fusion between vesicle and target membrane (Ungar and Hughson 2003). SNAP proteins are ubiquitous t-SNARE proteins that have been shown to promote membrane fusion in numerous physiological systems (Ungar and Hughson 2003).

To date, very few genetic diseases associated with mutations in genes coding for modulators of vesicle trafficking have been described (Chediak Higashi syndrome [MIM 214500]; Griscelli syndrome [MIM 214450, MIM 607624]; Hermansky-Pudlak syndrome [MIM 203300]; chylomicron retention disease [MIM 246700]; familial hemophagocytic lymphohistiocytosis type 4 [MIM 267700]) (Barbosa et al. 1996; Pastural et al. 1997; Menasche et al. 2000; Huizing and Gahl 2002; Jones et al. 2003; Gissen et al. 2004; zur Stadt et al. 2005), and none caused by mutations in genes coding for SNAP molecules have been reported, possibly owing to a large degree of functional redundancy among SNARE proteins or to early lethality associated with mutations in these genes. The present report describes the severe clinical consequences of abnormal expression of a SNAP protein in humans.

Material and Methods

Patients and Biological Materials

All participants or their legal guardians provided written and informed consent according to a protocol ap-

Received April 22, 2005; accepted for publication June 6, 2005; electronically published June 20, 2005.

Address for correspondence and reprints: Dr. Eli Sprecher, Laboratory of Molecular Dermatology, Department of Dermatology, Rambam Medical Center, Haifa, Israel. E-mail: e_sprecher@rambam.health.gov.il

0002-9297/2005/7702-0007$15.00

Table 1

***SNAP29* Oligonucleotide Sequences**

Process and Exon	Oligonucleotide Sequence: Forward	Oligonucleotide Sequence: Reverse	Annealing Temperature (°C)
Genomic DNA amplification:			
1	F-GGAGTTCGCGCGACGACCGC	R-CAAGAATCTATGCTAGGCAAC	60
2	F-GATGACAGTACCCGTCTCCAG	R-GCACTGACGTGGACTGAAAGTC	60
3	F-GAGTTTGGCACAGAGGAGGC	R-CTTTGGCTAGCATGGGTGATGC	60
4	F-CATGAGCCTGCGCTGTGCTC	R-GACAGTGGCTTACAGAAGCTG	60
5	F-GACAGTGGCTTACAGAAGCTG	R-CATCACAATAGAGTGGAAATC	60
dHPLC screening:			
1	F-GCGGACAGGCAGCAGTACTTG	R-CAAGAATCTATGCTAGGCAAC	60
RT-PCR:			
1–5	F-GAGTCCTGGAGCGCACAGAGAAGATG	R-CAGCTCATCTAGGTTGCTGTCGATC	60
Quantitative real-time PCR:			
3–4	F-GAAGCTATAAGTACAAGTAAAG	R-CATCAGTACTCATGGCAGAAC	55

proved by the local Helsinki Committee and by the Committee for Genetic Studies of the Israeli Ministry of Health. Blood samples were drawn from all family members, and DNA was extracted according to standard procedures. Skin-biopsy samples were fixed either in formaldehyde for subsequent immunohistochemistry, in Karnowski's fixative for transmission electron microscopy, or in paraformaldehyde for immunoelectron microscopy. Fibroblast cell cultures were obtained from punch biopsies from patients or healthy controls after written informed consent was obtained, and they were maintained in DMEM supplemented with fetal calf serum 10%.

Transformation of Fibroblasts by SV40 Large T-Antigen Transfection

Fibroblasts, grown in 10-cm plates, were stably transfected with 10 μg of a plasmid containing the SV40 large T-antigen coupled to the SV40 early promoter (a gift from Dr. Danny Canaani, Tel Aviv University, Israel) (Canaani et al. 1986), by use of 20 μl Lipofectamine 2000 transfection reagent (Invitrogen), according to the manufacturer's instructions. Twelve days later, all colonies in each plate were trypsinized and split. Transformation was confirmed by indirect immunofluorescence. Cells, grown on cover slips, were fixed with 4% paraformaldehyde and were incubated first with a monoclonal anti-SV40 large T-antigen antibody (Gurney et al. 1980) and then with Cy3-conjugated goat anti-mouse secondary antibodies (Jackson Immunoresearch Laboratories).

Genotyping

Genomic DNA was PCR amplified using either fluorescently labeled primer pairs (PE Applied Biosystems) or, for fine mapping, nonlabeled primer pairs. PCR conditions were: 95°C for 4 min, followed by 35 cycles of 95°C for 30 s, 55°C for 30 s, and 72°C for 30 s, with a final extension step of 72°C for 5 min. For semiautomated genotyping, PCR products were separated by PAGE on an ABI 310 sequencer system, and allele sizes were determined with Genescan 3.1 and Genotyper 2.0 software. For manual genotyping, amplicons were electrophoresed on 6% acrylamide gels, followed by silver staining. Multipoint LOD score analysis was performed with the SuperLink software (Fishelson and Geiger 2002), under the assumptions of autosomal recessive inheritance and a mutation frequency of 0.001. Allele frequencies were calculated from analysis of a pool of population-matched DNA samples.

Sequencing

Genomic DNA was PCR amplified using primer pairs encompassing all exons and exon-intron boundaries of the *SNAP29* gene (MIM 604202) (table 1). Gel-purified (QIAquick gel extraction kit, Qiagen) amplicons were subjected to bidirectional DNA sequencing using the BigDye terminator system on an ABI Prism 3100 sequencer (PE Applied Biosystems).

To confirm and screen for the 220delG mutation, we used WAVE analysis (Transgenomic). PCR products were denatured at 95°C for 5 min and were cooled to 65°C down a temperature gradient of 1°C/min. Five μl of each sample were applied to a preheated C18 reversed phase column based on nonporous polystyrene-divinyl-benzene particles (DNA-Sep Cartridge, Transgenomic). DNA was eluted within a linear acetonitrile gradient consisting of buffer A (0.1 M triethylammonium acetate (TEAA)/ buffer B (0.1 M TEAA, 25% acetonitrile) (Transgenomic). The melting profile of the DNA fragment was determined using Wavemaker 4.2 software and the Stanford DHPLC Melt program (Bercovich and Beaudet 2003).

RT-PCR

For semiquantitative RT-PCR, total RNA was extracted from cultured fibroblasts harvested from skin-

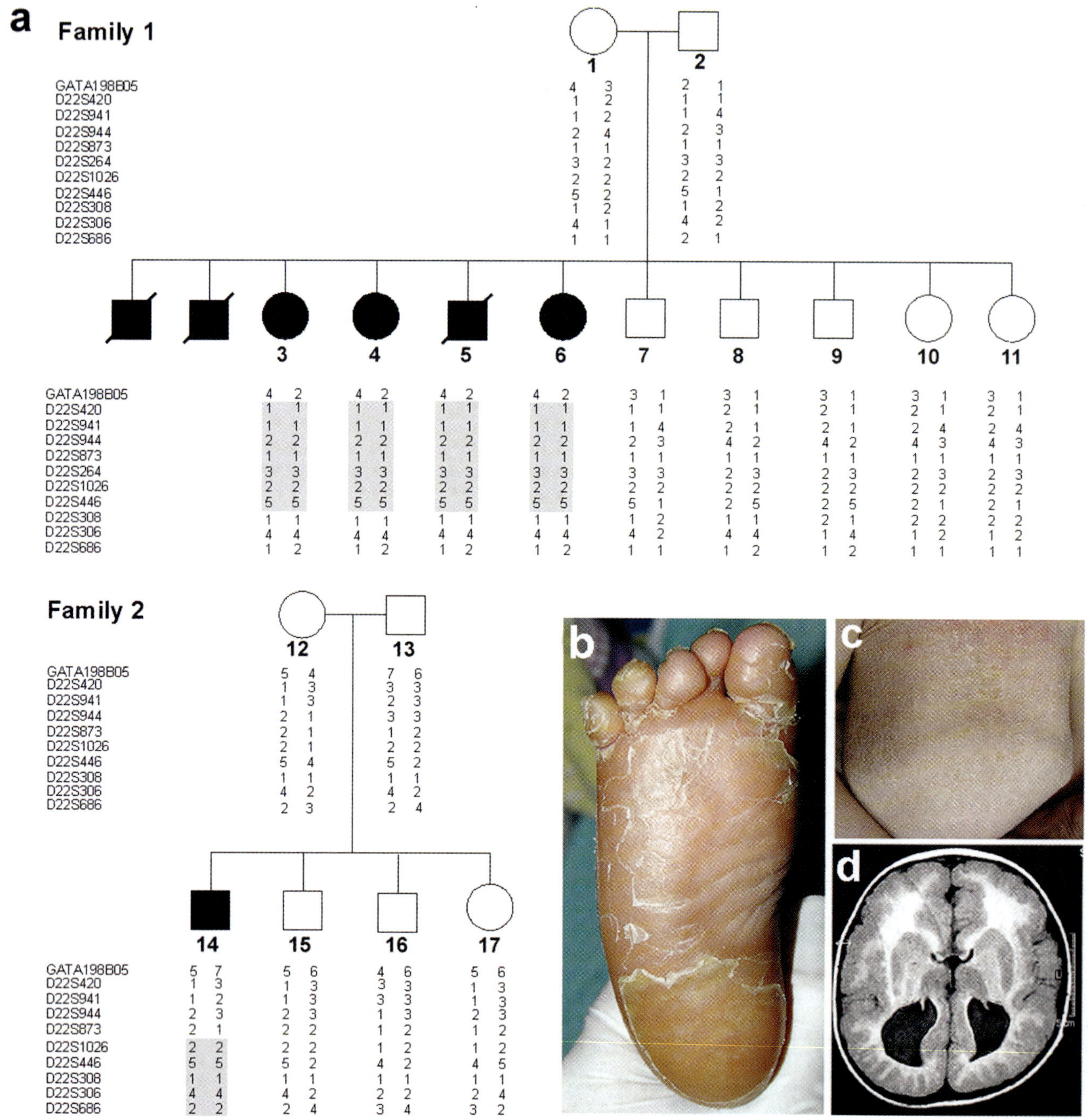

Figure 1 Family trees, genotyping, and clinical spectrum of CEDNIK syndrome. *a,* Haplotype analysis in two families affected with CEDNIK syndrome, performed using polymorphic microsatellite markers on 22q11.2. Homozygous disease-associated haplotypes for each family are marked in gray. *b,* Severe thickening (keratoderma) of the plantar skin in patient 3. *c,* Lamellar ichthyosis over the abdominal surface in patient 14. *d,* Axial T1 (SE) weighted MR image demonstrating cortical dysplasia and pachygyria with polymicrogyria, as well as typical absence of corpus callosum, in patient 5.

biopsy samples (RNeasy extraction kit, Qiagen) and was amplified using the TITAN One Tube RT-PCR kit (Roche Molecular Biochemicals) and intron-crossing primer pairs specific for *SNAP29* (table 1) or *ACTB* (MIM 102630), encoding β-actin (forward, F-CCAAGGCCAACCGCG-AGAAGATGAC; reverse, R-AGGGTACATGGTGGT-GCCGCCAGAC). PCR conditions were: 50°C for 30 min; 94°C for 2 min; 10 cycles of 94°C for 30 s, 60°C for 30 s, and 68°C for 90 s; 25 cycles of 94°C for 30 s, 60°C for 30 s, and 68°C for 90 s + 5 additional s at each cycle; and a final extension step at 68°C for 7 min.

For quantitative real-time PCR, cDNA was synthesized from 1 μg of total RNA extracted from cultured fibroblasts using the Reverse-iT first strand synthesis kit (ABgene) and random hexamers. cDNA PCR amplification was performed using the Absolute QPCR SYBR Green Mix (ABgene) on a Rotor-Gene 3000 multifilter system (Corbett Research) with primer pairs specific for *SNAP29* (table 1) or *ACTB* (F-TTGCCGACAGGATGCAGAAGGA and R-AGGTGGACAGCGAGGCCAGGAT). To ensure the specificity of the reaction conditions, at the end of the individual runs, the melting temperature (T_m) of the amplified products was measured to confirm its homogeneity. Cycling conditions were as follows: 95°C for 15 min; 95°C for 1 s, 55°C for 5 s, and 72°C for 5 s for a total of 40 cycles. Each sample was analyzed in triplicate. For quantification, standard curves were obtained using serially diluted cDNA amplified in the same real-time PCR run. Results were normalized to β-actin mRNA levels. After the quantification procedure, the products were resolved by 2.5% agarose gel electrophoresis to confirm that the reaction had amplified the correct DNA fragments of known size.

Western Blotting

Cells were homogenized in lysis buffer (10 mM Hepes, 100 mM NaCl, 1 mM $MgCl_2$, 0.5% NP-40, and a protease-inhibitors mix including 1 mM PMSF and 1 μg/ml aprotinin and leupeptin [Sigma]). After centrifugation at 10,000 g for 15 min at 4°C, proteins were electrophoresed through a 10% SDS-PAGE and transferred onto a nitrocellulose membrane (Schleicher Schuell). After 1 h blocking with PBS containing 5% skim milk, blots were interacted with rabbit anti-SNAP29 antibodies (Rotem-Yehudar et al. 2001). The blots were washed three times with TBS-Tween (20 mM Tris HCl, 4 mM Tris base, 140 mM NaCl, 1 mM EDTA, 0.1% Tween-20). After incubation with secondary HRP-conjugated goat anti-rabbit IgG antibodies (Jackson ImmunoResearch) and subsequent washings, proteins were detected using the western blotting Luminol Reagent (Santa Cruz Biotechnology). To compare the amount of protein in the different samples, the blots were reprobed with anti-Erk antibodies (Santa Cruz Biotechnology).

Immunohistochemistry

Formaldehyde-fixed 5-μm paraffin-embedded sections were treated with 3% H_2O_2 in methanol for 15 min at room temperature, were warmed in a microwave oven in citrate buffer for 15 min at 90°C, and were stained with polyclonal anti-SNAP29 antibodies (Abnova Corporation), anti-keratin 14 antibodies (BioGenex), or preimmune rabbit antiserum for 1 h at room temperature. After extensive washings in phosphate-buffered saline, the antibodies were revealed using the ABC technique (Zymed), and the slides were counterstained using hematoxylin.

Electron Microscopy

Transmission electron microscopy (TEM) and immunoelectron microscopy (IEM) analyses were performed as described elsewhere (Ishida-Yamamoto et al. 2005). For IEM, ultrathin cryosections were incubated with antibodies against glucosylceramides (Glycobiotech), kalikrein 5 (KLK5) (Santa Cruz Biotechnology), and KLK7 (Tanimoto et al. 1999).

Results

Clinical Features of CEDNIK Syndrome

We identified two unrelated, consanguineous Arab Muslim families from northern Israel (fig. 1*a*), comprising seven affected individuals (four boys and three girls) displaying a unique constellation of clinical signs. All patients were born at term after an uneventful gestation, with normal APGAR scores and birth weight. Roving eye movements, poor head and trunk control, and failure to thrive were the presenting symptoms during the first 4 mo of life. All patients had progressive microcephaly and facial dysmorphism including elongated faces, antimongolian eye slant, slight hypertelorism, and flat broad nasal root. Palmoplantar keratoderma (fig. 1*b*) and ichthyosis (fig. 1*c*) appeared between 5 and 11 mo of age, with progressive worsening during the 2nd year of life. By the age of 8–15 mo, psychomotor retardation became apparent as major developmental milestones, like unaided sitting and walking, were not attained. Tendon reflexes could not be elicited, and peripheral nerve conduction studies performed in three patients demonstrated low-amplitude responses. Muscle biopsies performed in two patients disclosed neurogenic atrophy and normal activity of the mitochondrial respiratory chain complexes. Ophthalmologic evaluation revealed hypoplastic optic disk; electrophysiological studies were suggestive of reduced conductance from peripheral retina and macular atrophy. Mild sensorineural deafness was demonstrated in three patients studied. Brain MRI performed on four patients showed various degrees of corpus callosum abnormalities and cortical dysplasia, with pachygyria and polimicrogyria (fig. 1*d*). Three male patients died of aspiration pneumonia between 5 and 12 years of age. To date, four patients, aged 5–13 years, are alive, with features including severe psychomotor retardation, ichthyosis, and palmoplantar keratoderma.

The results of routine laboratory studies, plasma and urinary amino acids, urinary organic acids, serum lac-

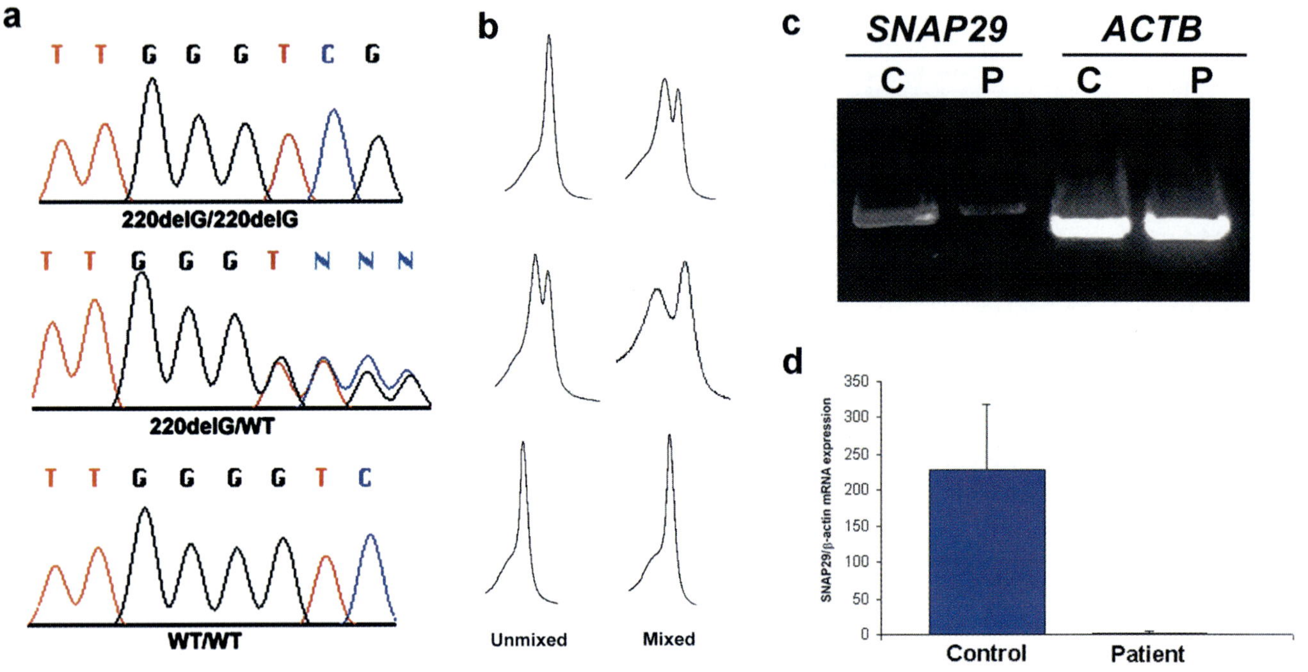

Figure 2 Mutation analysis and gene expression. *a*, Sequence analysis revealed a homozygous G deletion at *SNAP29* cDNA position 220 in all affected individuals of both families (*upper panel*). All obligatory carriers were shown to carry the mutation in a heterozygous state (*middle panel*). The wild-type sequence is given for comparison (*lower panel*). *b*, The corresponding dHPLC tracings obtained by running PCR samples unmixed and mixed with control DNA are depicted. *c*, Expression of *SNAP29* and *ACTB*, coding for β-actin, assessed using RT-PCR in fibroblasts harvested from a patient (P) and from a healthy control individual (C). Note the lower amounts of the *SNAP29* RT-PCR products in the patient relative to the control. *d*, Quantitative real-time PCR analysis for gene expression of *SNAP29* in fibroblasts obtained from control and patient skin. Expression levels are expressed as absolute values normalized relative to β-actin RNA levels.

tate, copper, and ceruloplasmin were within normal limits. Karyotype was normal. Using a battery of enzymatic and biochemical assays, as well as lipid staining in leukocytes and hair microscopy, we excluded a large number of syndromes with closely related clinical manifestations, including Sjogren Larsson syndrome (MIM 270200), peroxisomal disorders, congenital disorders of N- and O-glycosylation, Chanarin-Dorfman disease (MIM 275630), trichothiodystrophy (MIM 601675), Gaucher disease (MIM 230900), steroid sulfatase (MIM 308100), and multiple sulfatase deficiency (MIM 272200).

Mapping of CEDNIK Syndrome

Given the apparent rarity of the syndrome and the fact that the two affected families were consanguineous and lived a few miles from one another, we assumed the existence of a single homozygous causative mutation. We therefore established the genotypes at 332 microsatellite loci of five patients from whom DNA was available and scrutinized our results for regions of homozygosity. A homozygous haplotype spanning 4 Mb on 22q11.2 was found to be shared by all affected individuals and to be absent or carried in a heterozygous state by other healthy family members (not shown). We subsequently genotyped all family members, using 13 markers saturating the putative disease interval. Multipoint LOD score analysis generated a maximum score of 4.85 at marker *D22S446*. Haplotype analysis identified a critical recombination event in individual 8 and loss of homozygosity in individual 14, at markers *D22S308* and *D22S873*, respectively, thereby establishing the telomeric and centromeric boundaries of the disease-associated interval.

SNAP29 Mutation Analysis

The CEDNIK-associated interval, spanning ~2 Mb, was found to harbor 84 genes, among which *SNAP29*, coding for a SNARE protein involved in intracellular vesicle fusion, was chosen as our prime candidate because it modulates critical physiological processes in the central and peripheral nervous system (Su et al. 2001). Sequencing of this gene revealed in all patients a G deletion at cDNA position 220 (starting from ATG) (fig. 2*a*), which was predicted to result in frameshift and in the synthesis of a significantly truncated protein due to premature termination of translation 28 amino acids

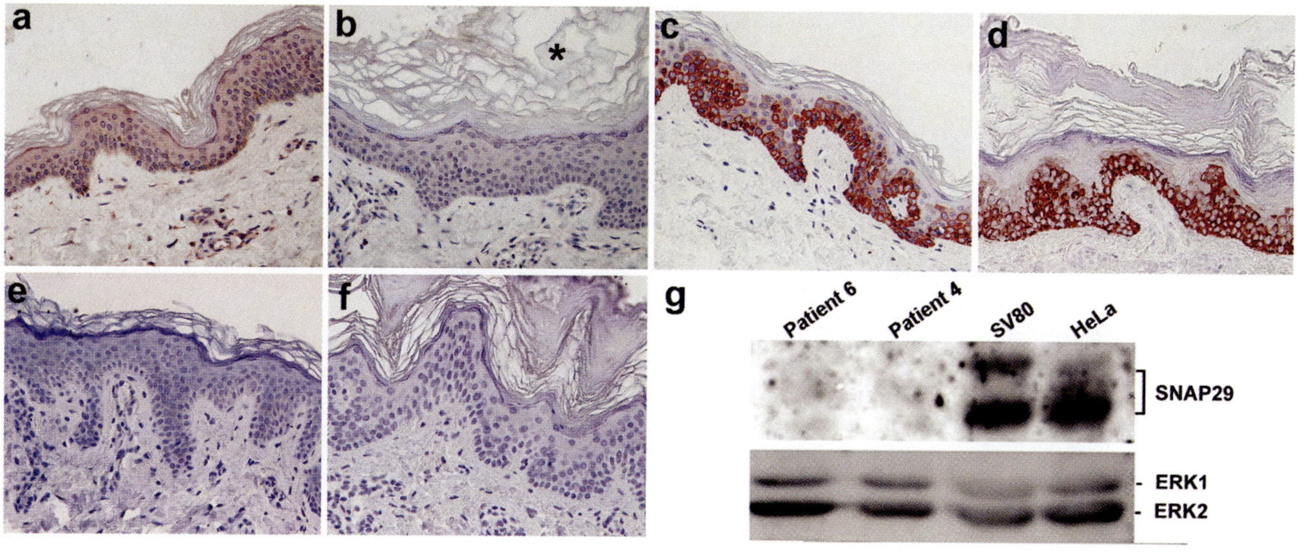

Figure 3 SNAP29 protein expression. Skin biopsy sections obtained from a control individual (*a*, *c*, and e) and a patient with CEDNIK (*b*, *d*, and *f*) were stained with antibodies directed against SNAP29 (*a* and *b*) and keratin 14 (*c* and *d*) and with preimmune rabbit antiserum (*e* and *f*). Note the very thickened stratum corneum (hyperkeratosis), marked by an asterisk (*). Cytoplasmic staining for SNAP29 shows positive results in keratinocytes as well as dermal fibroblasts in control skin, but not in the skin of the patient (original magnification ×400). *g*, To confirm the immunostaining results, protein was extracted from transformed fibroblast cell cultures established from patient skin (patients 4 and 6), from control transformed skin fibroblasts (SV80), and from HeLa cells. Cell lysates containing 80 μg of protein were electrophoresed through 10% SDS-PAGE, and the corresponding immunoblot was reacted with anti-SNAP29 antibodies. Detection was performed with HRP-conjugated goat anti-rabbit antibodies. Membranes were reblotted with anti-Erk antibodies to control for protein loading.

downstream of the mutation. Using dHPLC heteroduplex analysis, we confirmed segregation of the mutation in the two families (fig. 2*b*) and excluded the mutation from a panel of 200 population-matched control chromosomes.

SNAP29 Expression in Skin of Patients with CEDNIK Syndrome

The 220delG mutation in SNAP29 gene was found to be associated with decreased levels of *SNAP29* transcripts (fig. 2*c*), possibly reflecting nonsense-mediated mRNA decay. Using quantitative RT-PCR, we found that *SNAP29* RNA expression was decreased 99-fold in patient fibroblasts relative to control fibroblasts (fig. 2*d*). To assess the consequences of the mutation at the protein level, we stained skin-biopsy samples obtained from patients and control individuals with anti-recombinant SNAP29 antiserum. *SNAP29* was found to be expressed by virtually all cells in the normal epidermis and dermis (fig. 3*a*). In contrast, SNAP29 expression was markedly reduced in the skin of affected individuals (fig. 3*b*). This decrease in SNAP29 expression was specific, since the expression of unrelated proteins such as keratin 14 was unchanged (fig. 3*c* and 3*d*) and staining with preimmune rabbit serum showed negative results (fig. 3*e* and 3*f*). We then confirmed these results using western blot analysis of protein extracted from SV40-transformed normal fibroblasts and SV40-transformed fibroblasts grown from skin-biopsy samples obtained from two patients (fig. 3*g*). Similar results were obtained using primary fibroblast cell cultures (not shown). Thus, 220delG mutation results in SNAP29 deficiency in the skin of patients with CEDNIK syndrome.

Ultrastructural Consequences of SNAP29 Deficiency in CEDNIK Syndrome

Lamellar granules are abundant organelles typically found in the upper epidermal layers and responsible for delivering to the stratum corneum lipids, proteases, and their inhibitors during the process of epidermal barrier formation (Fartasch 2004). A large body of evidence supports the concept that lamellar granules originate from the Golgi complex (Ishida-Yamamoto et al. 2005). In parallel, a number of studies have shown that SNAP29, in contrast with other SNAP proteins (Gonelle-Gispert et al. 2000; Feng et al. 2002), is prominently found in intracellular membrane structures (Steegmaier et al. 1998; Ugur and Jones 2000; Hohenstein et al. 2001) and have suggested a specific role for SNAP29 in mediating Golgi trafficking (Wong et al. 1999). To assess the possibility that SNAP29 deficiency interferes with epidermal granule maturation, we examined skin-biopsy samples obtained from a CEDNIK patient by TEM. The most striking ultrastructural abnormality in the patient epidermis

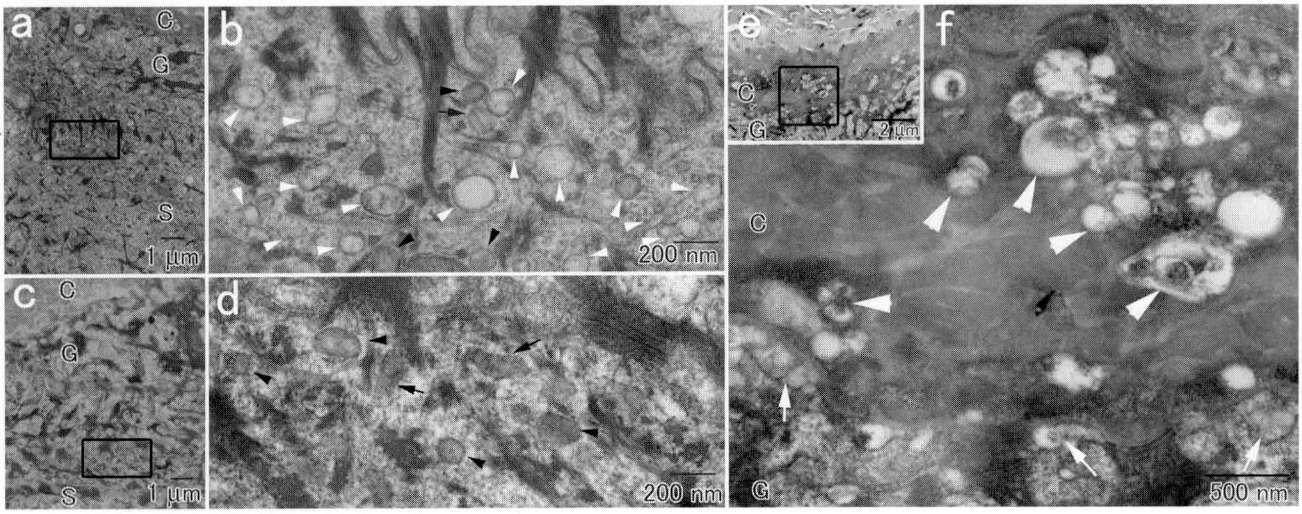

Figure 4 Transmission electron micrograph of a skin-biopsy sample obtained from a patient (*a, b, e,* and *f*) and from a healthy control individual (*c* and *d*). Panels b, d, and f show higher-magnification views of the areas marked in panels a, c, and e, respectively. In addition to normal appearing lamellar granules with (*black arrows*) or without (*black arrowheads*) lamellar internal structures, numerous empty vesicles (*white arrowheads*) are seen in the patient epidermis (*b*) but not in the control skin (*d*). *e* and *f,* The extracellular spaces between the most superficial granular cells and the cornified cells in the patient skin contain secreted lamellar granule contents (*white arrows* in panel *f*). In addition, countless abnormal vesicles are observed in the lower stratum corneum (*white arrowheads*). The letters C, G, and S identify the epidermal cornified, granular, and spinous cell layers, respectively.

was the presence of countless clear vesicles in the spinous and granular epidermal layers (fig. 4*a* and 4*b*) that were not found in control epidermis (fig. 4*c* and 4*d*). Vesicles of various sizes and contents were also present, abnormally, in the lower layers of the significantly thickened stratum corneum in patient skin (fig. 4*e* and 4*f*) but not in normal skin (not shown). It is of note that normal-looking lamellar granules, loaded with lipid molecules, were also seen (fig. 4*b*), and they were released into the extracellular space between the superficial granular and cornified layers (fig. 4*e* and 4*f*). We did not observe any additional abnormality in other epidermal structures.

Epidermal differentiation is critically dependent on proper spatial deposition of lipids and proteolytic enzymes, which contribute to the formation of the skin barrier and mediate desquamation, respectively (Ishida-Yamamoto et al. 2005). Because the transfer of these molecules to the stratum corneum is, in turn, dependent on correct formation of lamellar granules, and because lamellar granule maturation was found to be abnormal in CEDNIK syndrome (fig. 4), we assessed the distribution of glucosylceramides in patient skin, using IEM. Glucosylceramides are precursor molecules for ceramides, the most abundant intracorneal lipids, and are normally secreted between granular and cornified epidermal cells (Ishida-Yamamoto et al. 2005) (fig. 5, *left panel*). In the skin of our patients, considerable amounts of glucosylceramides were retained, abnormally, within the cells of lower stratum corneum (fig. 5, *middle panel*) and numerous vesicles with positive glucosylceramide labeling were seen in the lower cornified layer (fig. 5, *right panel*), indicating that lamellar granules are not correctly secreted in the skin of patients with CEDNIK syndrome. Abnormal vesicles in the cornified cells were also found to contain KLK5 and KLK7, two proteases of major importance for normal desquamation (Caubet et al. 2004) (not shown).

Discussion

In the present study, we describe a novel neurocutaneous disease, termed "CEDNIK syndrome," characterized by severe developmental abnormalities of the nervous system as well as aberrant differentiation of the epidermis. We show that this disorder results from decreased expression of SNAP29, a SNARE protein involved in vesicle fusion. Although neural tissues were not available for examination, ultrastructural features of the syndrome in the skin of patients, including the presence of abnormal vesicles in the granular and lower cornified cell layers of the epidermis, are consonant with deranged function of SNARE-mediated vesicle transport/fusion. Interestingly, abnormal vesicles were also observed in dermal fibroblasts (not shown), suggesting a generalized defect in vesicle trafficking in patient tissues. Although, to our knowledge, similar ultrastructural features have

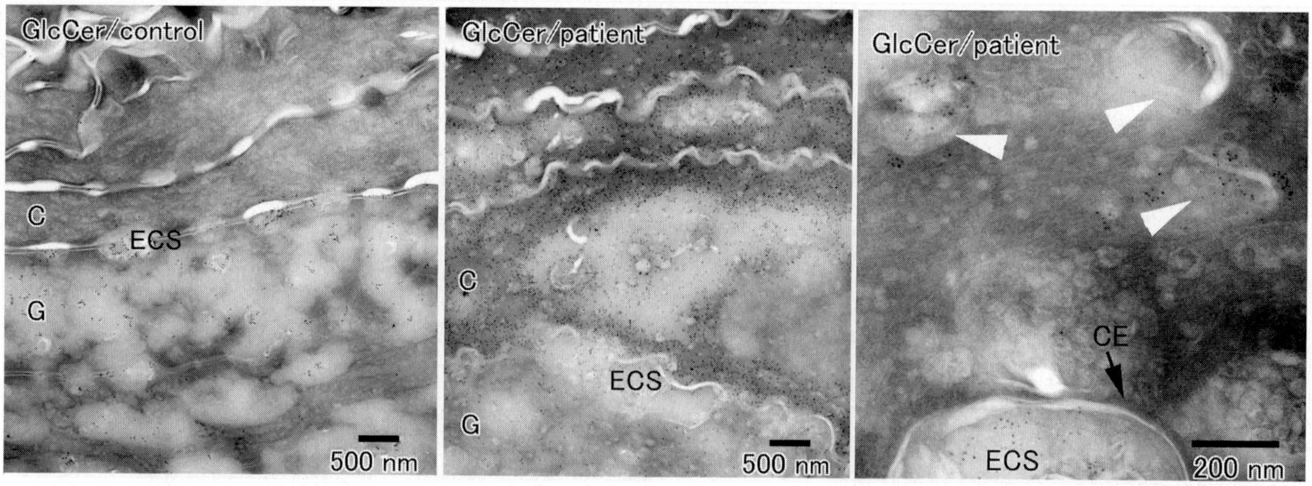

Figure 5 Immunoelectron microscopy of skin-biopsy samples obtained from two CEDNIK patients and a control individual with antibodies directed against glucosylceramides (GlcCer). Glucosylceramides appear as black dots. In the control samples, glucosylceramides are found in lamellar granules, and they are secreted between the epidermal granular cells (G) and cornified cells (C) (*left panel*). By contrast, in patient skin, only a small proportion of glucosylceramide-positive granules is secreted into the extracellular spaces (ECS) between the granular and cornified cells, a large amount of glucosylceramides is found in the lower cornified cells (*middle panel*), which are shown to retain a very large number of glucosylceramide-positive vesicles (*white arrowheads* in *right panel*). The black arrow marks the cornified cell envelope (CE).

never previously been described in a human disease, they bear striking resemblance to the phenotype observed in mutant yeasts with abnormal SNARE complex function causing defective fusion of transport vesicles with the Golgi apparatus (Bonifacino and Glick 2004). As mentioned above, SNAP29 has been shown to play an important role in Golgi trafficking (Wong et al. 1999).

Abnormal SNAP29-mediated vesicle fusion may explain the major clinical features characteristic of CEDNIK syndrome. Indeed, numerous studies have underscored the importance of the SNARE machinery during brain development, axonal growth, synaptogenesis, and neurotransmission (Hepp and Langley 2001; Chen and Olson 2005). SNARE proteins have also been shown to play an important role in the development of the retina (West-Greenlee et al. 1998). The prominent ophthalmologic signs observed in patients with CEDNIK syndrome—including roving eye movements during the first months of life (or even at birth, in one patient), early macular atrophy, and reduced conductance from peripheral retina demonstrated by electrophysiological studies—together suggest a pivotal function for SNAP29 in the development of the visual system. SNAP29 regulates neurotransmitter release by slowing the recycling of the fusion machinery and down-regulating synaptic vesicle turnover (Su et al. 2001; Pan et al., in press). The process of synaptic vesicle recycling, including SNARE complex formation and dissociation, is essential for ongoing synaptic transmission (Sudhof 2004). SNAP29 deficiency may therefore explain the development of the severe neuropathy displayed by patients with CEDNIK syndrome. Moreover, the skin findings in CEDNIK syndrome are likely to result from abnormal lamellar granule maturation and secretion (figs. 4 and 5). Although in normal skin, lamellar granules release lipids and proteases beneath the stratum corneum, reinforcing the epidermal barrier and mediating desmosome dissolution during desquamation, respectively, in CEDNIK syndrome, glucosylceramide and kallikrein-containing granules are aberrantly retained in the stratum corneum, leading to abnormal barrier formation and retention hyperkeratosis (fig. 6).

CEDNIK syndrome includes a number of features overlapping with clinical characteristics of other genetic diseases, which is suggestive of intersecting pathophysiologies. For example, lamellar body degeneration has been observed in type II pneumocytes in Hermansky-Pudlak syndrome, another autosomal recessive disorder associated with impaired vesicle trafficking (Nakatani et al. 2000). Also, the occurrence of neurocutaneous signs associated with abnormal distribution of glucosylceramides in the skin of patients with CEDNIK syndrome is reminiscent of the clinical phenotype resulting from decreased hydrolysis of glucosylceramide to ceramide in type II Gaucher disease (Holleran et al. 1994), where severe ichthyosis can be observed along with neurological deficits.

In conclusion, we have described a novel human genetic disease, caused by decreased expression of SNAP29 and resulting in abnormal vesicle maturation and se-

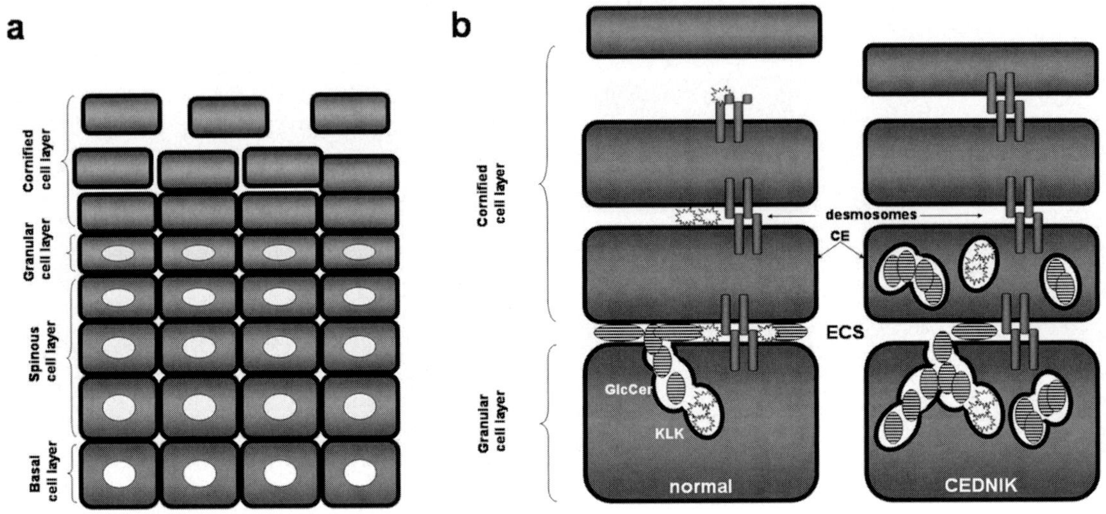

Figure 6 Pathogenesis of CEDNIK syndrome. *a,* Formation of the epidermal barrier occurs at the end of a complex differentiation process during which keratinocytes, derived from the proliferating basal cell layer, sequentially transform into spinous cells, granular cells, and cornified cells as they migrate outwards throughout the epidermis. *b,* The epidermal barrier is composed of the cornified cell envelope (CE), a protein scaffold, which replaces the plasma membrane; intracellular cross-linked and polymerized keratin filament bundles; and extracellular lipid layers. Lipids, such as glucosylceramides (GlcCer), are normally secreted from lamellar granules present in granular cells into the extracellular space (ECS) between the granular and the cornified cell layers. Lamellar granules also secrete proteases, such as KLK5 and KLK7, which dissolve desmosomal plates in the upper cornified cell layers, thereby enabling cells to separate one from the other, a process known as "desquamation." In CEDNIK syndrome, lamellar granules are retained within the cornified cell layer, and the diminished secretion of lipids and proteases in the ECS, causes impaired barrier formation and decreased desquamation, respectively, which explains the increased thickness of the outer epidermal layers in patients.

cretion. These data underscore the importance of the SNARE complex in general and of SNAP29 in particular for normal neuroectodermal differentiation.

Acknowledgments

We are grateful to the family members for their participation in our study. We thank Dr. Vered Friedman, for services in nucleic acid analysis; Ma'ayan Fishelson and Anna Tzemach, for computer assistance; and Dr. Peter Itin, Dr. Gabriele Richard, Dr. Eddie Karnieli, Dr. Tsipora Kra-Oz, Alon Hirshberg, and Dr. Gila Maor, for stimulating discussions. This study was supported in part by grants provided by the Ruth and Allen Ziegler Fund for Pediatric Research (to E.S.) and the Japanese Ministry of Education, Culture, Sports, Science and Technology (to A.I.Y.). Electron microscopy samples were observed at the Electron Microscopy Unit, Central Laboratory for Research and Education, Asahikawa Medical College.

Web Resources

The URLs for data presented herein are as follows:

DHPLC Melt program, http://insertion.stanford.edu/meltdoc.html

Online Mendelian Inheritance in Man (OMIM), http://www.ncbi.nlm.nih.gov/Omim/

Superlink, http://bioinfo.cs.technion.ac.il/pedtool/

References

Barbosa MDFS, Nguyen QA, Tchernev VT, Ashley JA, Detter JC, Blaydes SM, Brandt SJ, Chotai D, Hodgman C, Solari RCE, Lovett M, Kingsmore SF (1996) Identification of the homologous beige and Chediak-Higashi syndrome genes. Nature 382:262–265

Bercovich D, Beaudet AL (2003) Denaturing high-performance liquid chromatography for the detection of mutations and polymorphisms in UBE3A. Genet Test 7:189–194

Bonifacino JS, Glick BS (2004) The mechanisms of vesicle budding and fusion. Cell 116:153–166

Canaani D, Naiman T, Teitz T, Berg P (1986) Immortalization of xeroderma pigmentosum cells by simian virus 40 DNA having a defective origin of DNA replication. Somat Cell Mol Genet 12:13–20

Caubet C, Jonca N, Brattsand M, Guerrin M, Bernard D, Schmidt R, Egelrud T, Simon M, Serre G (2004) Degradation of corneodesmosome proteins by two serine proteases of the kallikrein family, SCTE/KLK5/hK5 and SCCE/KLK7/hK7. J Invest Dermatol 122:1235–1244

Chen EH, Olson EN (2005) Unveiling the mechanisms of cell-cell fusion. Science 308:369–373

Deitcher D (2002) Exocytosis, endocytosis, and development. Semin Cell Dev Biol 13:71–76

Fartasch M (2004) The epidermal lamellar body: a fascinating secretory organelle. J Invest Dermatol 122:XI–XII

Feng D, Crane K, Rozenvayn N, Dvorak AM, Flaumenhaft R (2002) Subcellular distribution of 3 functional platelet SNARE proteins: human cellubrevin, SNAP-23, and syntaxin 2. Blood 99:4006–4014

Fishelson M, Geiger D (2002) Exact genetic linkage computations for general pedigrees. Bioinformatics 18:S189–S198

Gissen P, Johnson CA, Morgan NV, Stapelbroek JM, Forshew T, Cooper WN, McKiernan PJ, Klomp LW, Morris AA, Wraith JE, McClean P, Lynch SA, Thompson RJ, Lo B, Quarrell OW, Di Rocco M, Trembath RC, Mandel H, Wali S, Karet FE, Knisely AS, Houwen RH, Kelly DA, Maher ER (2004) Mutations in VPS33B, encoding a regulator of SNARE-dependent membrane fusion, cause arthrogryposis-renal dysfunction-cholestasis (ARC) syndrome. Nat Genet 36:400–404

Gonelle-Gispert C, Molinete M, Halban PA, Sadoul K (2000) Membrane localization and biological activity of SNAP-25 cysteine mutants in insulin-secreting cells. J Cell Sci 113: 3197–3205

Gurney EG, Harrison RO, Fenno J (1980) Monoclonal antibodies against simian virus 40 T antigens: evidence for distinct sublcasses of large T antigen and for similarities among nonviral T antigens. J Virol 34:752–763

Hepp R, Langley K (2001) SNAREs during development. Cell Tissue Res 305:247–253

Hohenstein AC, Roche PA (2001) SNAP29 is a promiscuous syntaxin-binding SNARE. Biochem Biophys Res Commun 285:167–171

Holleran WM, Ginns EI, Menon GK, Grundmann JU, Fartasch M, McKinney CE, Elias PM, Sidransky E (1994) Consequences of beta-glucocerebrosidase deficiency in epidermis: ultrastructure and permeability barrier alterations in Gaucher disease. J Clin Invest 93:1756–1764

Huizing M, Gahl WA (2002) Disorders of vesicles of lysosomal lineage: the Hermansky-Pudlak syndromes. Curr Mol Med 2:451–467

Ishida-Yamamoto A, Deraison C, Bonnart C, Bitoun E, Robinson R, O'Brien TJ, Wakamatsu K, Ohtsubo S, Takahashi H, Hashimoto Y, Dopping-Hepenstal PJ, McGrath JA, Iizuka H, Richard G, Hovnanian A (2005) LEKTI is localized in lamellar granules, separated from KLK5 and KLK7, and is secreted in the extracellular spaces of the superficial stratum granulosum. J Invest Dermatol 124:360–366

Jones B, Jones EL, Bonney SA, Patel HN, Mensenkamp AR, Eichenbaum-Voline S, Rudling M, Myrdal U, Annesi G, Naik S, Meadows N, Quattrone A, Islam SA, Naoumova RP, Angelin B, Infante R, Levy E, Roy CC, Freemont PS, Scott J, Shoulders CC (2003) Mutations in a Sar1 GTPase of COPII vesicles are associated with lipid absorption disorders. Nat Genet 34:29–31

Menasche G, Pastural E, Feldmann J, Certain S, Ersoy F, Dupuis S, Wulffraat N, Bianchi D, Fischer A, Le Deist F, de Saint Basile G (2000) Mutations in RAB27A cause Griscelli syndrome associated with haemophagocytic syndrome. Nat Genet 25:173–176

Nakatani Y, Nakamura N, Sano J, Inayama Y, Kawano N, Yamanaka S, Miyagi Y, Nagashima Y, Ohbayashi C, Mizushima M, Manabe T, Kuroda M, Yokoi T, Matsubara O (2000) Interstitial pneumonia in Hermansky-Pudlak syndrome: significance of florid foamy swelling/degeneration (giant lamellar body degeneration) of type-2 pneumocytes. Virchows Arch 437:304–313

Pan PY, Cai Q, Lin L, Lu PH, Duan SM, Sheng ZH. SNAP-29–mediated modulation of synaptic transmission in cultured hippocampal neurons. J Biol Chem (in press) (accepted manuscript version available at http://www.jbc.org/cgi/content/abstract/M502356200v1)

Pastural E, Barrat FJ, Dufourcq-Lagelouse R, Certain S, Sanal O, Jabado N, Seger R, Griscelli C, Fischer A, de Saint Basile G (1997) Griscelli disease maps to chromosome 15q21 and is associated with mutations in the myosin-Va gene. Nat Genet 16:289–292

Rotem-Yehudar R, Galperin E, Horowitz M (2001) Association of insulin-like growth factor 1 receptor with EHD1 and SNAP29. J Biol Chem 276:33054–33060

Steegmaier M, Yang B, Yoo JS, Huang B, Shen M, Yu S, Luo Y, Scheller RH (1998) Three novel proteins of the syntaxin/SNAP-25 family. J Biol Chem 273:34171–3419

Su Q, Mochida S, Tian JH, Mehta R, Sheng ZH (2001) SNAP29: a general SNARE protein that inhibits SNARE disassembly and is implicated in synaptic transmission. Proc Natl Acad Sci USA 98:14038–14043

Sudhof TC (2004) The synaptic vesicle cycle. Annu Rev Neurosci 27:509–547

Tanimoto H, Underwood LJ, Shigemasa K, Yan Yan MS, Clarke J, Parmley TH, O'Brien TJ (1999) The stratum corneum chymotryptic enzyme that mediates shedding and desquamation of skin cells is highly overexpressed in ovarian tumor cells. Cancer 86:2074–2082

Ugur O, Jones TL (2000) A proline-rich region and nearby cysteine residues target XLalphas to the Golgi complex region. Mol Biol Cell 11:1421–1432

Ungar D, Hughson FM (2003) SNARE protein structure and function. Annu Rev Cell Dev Biol 19:493–517

West-Greenlee MH, Finley S, Wilson MC, Jacobson CD, Sakaguchi DS (1998) Transient, high levels of SNAP-25 expression in cholinergic amacrine cells during postnatal development of the mammalian retina. J Comp Neurol 394:374–385

Wong SH, Xu Y, Zhang T, Griffiths G, Lowe SL, Subramaniam VN, Seow KT, Hong W (1999) GS32, a novel Golgi SNARE of 32 kDa, interacts preferentially with syntaxin 6. Mol Biol Cell 10:119–134

zur Stadt U, Schmidt S, Kasper B, Beutel K, Diler AS, Henter JI, Kabisch H, Schneppenheim R, Nurnberg P, Janka G, Hennies HC (2005) Linkage of familial hemophagocytic lymphohistiocytosis (FHL) type-4 to chromosome 6q24 and identification of mutations in syntaxin 11. Hum Mol Genet 14:827–834

Am. J. Hum. Genet. 77:252–264, 2005

Identification of Risk and Age-at-Onset Genes on Chromosome 1p in Parkinson Disease

Sofia A. Oliveira,* Yi-Ju Li,* Maher A. Noureddine, Stephan Züchner, Xuejun Qin, Margaret A. Pericak-Vance, and Jeffery M. Vance

Department of Medicine and Center for Human Genetics, Duke University Medical Center, Durham, NC

We previously reported a linkage region on chromosome 1p (LOD = 3.41) for genes controlling age at onset (AAO) in Parkinson disease (PD). This region overlaps with the previously reported *PARK10* locus. To identify the gene(s) associated with AAO and risk of PD in this region, we first applied a genomic convergence approach that combined gene expression and linkage data. No significant results were found. Second, we performed association mapping across a 19.2-Mb region centered under the AAO linkage peak. An iterative association mapping approach was done by initially genotyping single-nucleotide polymorphisms at an average distance of 100 kb apart and then by increasing the density of markers as needed. Using the overall data set of 267 multiplex families, we identified six associated genes in the region, but further screening of a subset of 83 families linked to the chromosome 1 locus identified only two genes significantly associated with AAO in PD: the γ subunit of the translation initiation factor EIF2B gene (*EIF2B3*), which was more significant in the linked subset and the ubiquitin-specific protease 24 gene (*USP24*). Unexpectedly, the human immunodeficiency virus enhancer-binding protein 3 gene (*HIVEP3*) was found to be associated with risk for susceptibility to PD. We used several criteria to define significant results in the presence of multiple testing, including criteria derived from a novel cluster approach. The known or putative functions of these genes fit well with the current suspected pathogenic mechanisms of PD and thus show great potential as candidates for the *PARK10* locus.

Introduction

Parkinson disease (PD [MIM 168600]) is the second most common neurodegenerative disorder and is characterized clinically by rigidity, bradykinesia, and resting tremor. PD has been shown to have a genetic component contributing to the disorder, including mutations in several genes (e.g., *α-synuclein, Parkin, UCHL1, LRRK2,* and *PINK1*) that lead to rare Mendelian forms of the disease (Polymeropoulos et al. 1997; Kitada et al. 1998; Leroy et al. 1998; Paisan-Ruiz et al. 2004; Valente et al. 2004).

The age at which an individual first manifests symptoms of the disease (i.e., age at onset [AAO]) also appears to be genetically controlled (Destefano et al. 2002; Li et al. 2002), but only a few genes (e.g., *APOE, GSTO1/2,* and *IDE*) that affect AAO have been identified (Karamohamed et al. 2003; Li et al. 2003, 2004; Blomqvist et al. 2004). We previously conducted a genomic screen to identify chromosomal regions harboring genes influencing AAO in PD and found significant evidence of linkage on chromosome 1p (LOD = 3.41) (Li et al. 2002). Interestingly, this AAO linkage peak is essentially identical to a risk linkage peak for PD (at locus *PARK10*) reported by Hicks et al. (2002) in their study of an Icelandic population (fig. 1), which provides strong evidence that there is a major PD gene in this region.

Several approaches have been undertaken to identify susceptibility genes located in linkage regions. One is the candidate-gene approach. However, because of our limited understanding of the biological systems involved in PD, this approach has not provided much insight into which genes to select. We proposed a second approach, which we termed "genomic convergence," whereby genes that lie under a linkage peak and are differentially expressed between cases and controls in a relevant tissue (e.g., substantia nigra of the midbrain for PD) are tested for association (Hauser et al. 2003). This approach was successful in identifying the glutathione *S*-transferase omega-1 and -2 complex (GSTO1/2), located in the chromosome 10q linkage region for AAO, as having an influence on AAO in Alzheimer disease and PD (Li et al. 2003). The possible role of GSTO1/2 in modifying the AAO of Alzheimer disease has been recently cor-

Received March 2, 2004; accepted for publication June 7, 2004; electronically published June 28, 2005.

Address for correspondence and reprints: Dr. Jeffery M. Vance, 595 LaSalle Street, Duke University Medical Center, Box 3445, Durham, NC 27710. E-mail: jeff.vance@duke.edu

* These two authors contributed equally to this work

0002-9297/2005/7702-0008$15.00

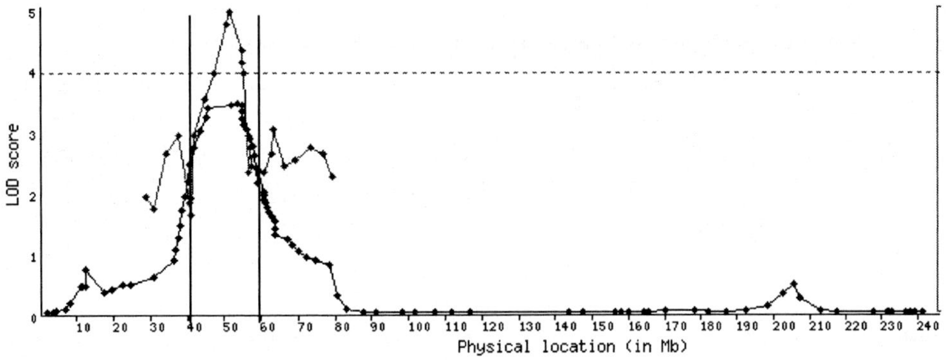

Figure 1 Linkage curves. The lower line depicts a chromosome 1 AAO linkage curve (Li et al. 2002), and the upper line shows the overlapping PD risk linkage peak derived from the Icelandic study (Hicks et al. 2002). The vertical lines indicate the 1-LOD score region screened in the iterative association map.

roborated by others (Kolsch et al. 2004). A third approach relies on genotyping a dense set of SNPs across a linkage region and subsequently testing those SNPs for association with the trait of interest. However, this process can become extremely costly for a large number of markers and samples.

In this article, we present the application of the genomic convergence approach combined with a process we term "iterative association mapping" to screen a dense map of SNPs in the region that were 1 LOD score down from the peak (hereafter, the 1-LOD score region) of the chromosome 1p linkage peak. In this region, there are 199 Ensembl genes (National Center for Biotechnology Information [NCBI] build 35) and 4,924 SNPs with a minor-allele frequency (MAF) >10% in the white population. Our proposed approach allows us to extract valuable information on the basis of reasonable genotyping efforts. Using this approach, we have identified several genes that show association with AAO and, surprisingly, one gene that shows association with risk for PD.

Material and Methods

Patients and Families

Affected individuals and family members were collected by the Morris K. Udall Parkinson Disease Research Center of Excellence (PDRCE) located within the Duke Center for Human Genetics (DCHG) and by the 13 centers of the Parkinson Disease Genetics Collaboration (Scott et al. 2001). A standard clinical evaluation involves neurological examination, including evaluation with the Unified Parkinson's Disease Rating Scale (Goetz et al. 2003). A rigorous clinical assessment was performed by all participating clinicians to provide a clear diagnosis of PD and to exclude any individuals who displayed atypical features of parkinsonism (Hubble et al. 1999; Scott et al. 2001). Individuals categorized as "affected" showed at least two of the cardinal signs of PD (resting tremor, bradykinesia, and rigidity). AAO for affected individuals was defined as the age at which an affected individual first noticed one of the cardinal signs of PD. Participants categorized as "unaffected" demonstrated no signs of the disease, and participants categorized as "unclear" showed only one cardinal sign and/or atypical features. All participants signed informed consent forms prior to blood and data collection. Institutional review boards at each participating center approved the study protocols and consent forms.

Table 1

SNPs Analyzed

The table is available in its entirety in the online edition of *The American Journal of Human Genetics.*

The data set consists of multiplex (n = 267) and singleton (n = 361) white families. We defined singleton and multiplex families on the basis of the total number of parent-child triads and discordant sib pairs (DSPs) in the family that can contribute to the association test. Singleton families have only one group (either a triad or a DSP) contributing to the association test—that is, they have one affected individual—and either the parent (affected or unaffected) or the unaffected sibling is sampled in addition to the affected individual. Multiplex families have at least two groups (triads or DSPs) contributing to the association test—that is, they have at least two affected siblings sampled in the family. Families with *Parkin* mutation carriers were excluded from this study. The multiplex data set includes 609 affected individuals (average AAO ± SD = 61.0 ± 11.6 years; range 14–90 years; 58.8% males) and 666 unaffected individuals

Table 2

Genes that Map to the Chromosome 1p AAO Linkage Peak, Differentially Expressed in Patients with PD versus Controls in Microarray and SAGE Experiments

Gene Name	Gene Symbol	UniGene ID	Fold Change in Patients with PD versus Controls	*P* Value[a]
Ubiquinol–cytochrome c reductase hinge protein	*UQCRH*	Hs. 481571	−1.4	.0244[b]
ATPase, H^+ transporting, lysosomal 21-kD, V0 subunit c	*ATP6V0B*	Hs. 7476	−1.3	.0356[b]
Ring finger protein 11	*RNF11*	Hs. 96334	−4.1	<.0001[c]
Chromosome 1 ORF 8	*C1orf8*	Hs. 416495	3.6	.0006[c]
Tetratricopeptide repeat domain 4	*TTC4*	Hs. 412482	−12.3	.0149[c]
Phosphatidic acid phosphatase type 2B	*PPAP2B*	Hs. 432840	−6.2	.0359[c]

[a] These *P* values were not corrected for multiple testing.
[b] Obtained from Hauser et al. (2005).
[c] Obtained from Noureddine et al. (2005).

(42.8% males). The singleton families include 391 affected individuals (average AAO ± SD = 55.5 ± 13.0 years; range 15–85 years; 69% males) and 356 unaffected individuals (42.7% males).

DNA Extraction and Genotyping

DNA samples were prepared and stored by the DCHG DNA bank core. Genomic DNA was extracted from whole blood by use of the PureGene system (Gentra Systems Autopure LS). A total of 284 SNPs (table 1) were genotyped with the use of Applied Biosystems (ABI) Assays-on-Demand (AoDs) or Assays-by-Design (AbDs) or with the use of primers and probes designed using ABI Primer Express 2.0 software. The SNPs were chosen first on the basis of their location (e.g., SNPs were initially chosen with an average distance of 100 kb between them) and then on the basis of frequency to capture a wide range of frequencies among all selected SNPs. The TaqMan allelic discrimination assay was used to genotype all SNPs. PCR amplification was performed in 5-μl reactions (comprising 2.6 ng of dried DNA, 1 × TaqMan universal PCR master mix [ABI], and 1 × genotyping mix for AoDs and AbDs or, for self-designed assays, 900 nM of each primer and 200 nM of each probe). PCR was performed using the GeneAmp PCR system 9700 thermocycler (ABI), with a 40-cycle program (1 cycle at 95°C for 10 min, followed by 40 cycles at 95°C for 15 s and at T_m for 1 min, where T_m is 60°C for AoDs and AbDs and ranges from 58°C to 64°C for self-designed assays). The fluorescence generated during the PCR amplification was read using the ABI Prism 7900HT sequence detection system and was analyzed with SDS software (ABI).

Stringent quality-control measures were taken to ensure data consistency. Internal controls consisted of 24 duplicated individuals per 384-well plate. In addition, two samples from CEPH were plated eight times per plate to assure plate-to-plate consistency. All genotypers were blinded to these internal controls. Quality-control samples were compared at the DCHG Data Coordinating Center. Data were stored and managed by the PEDIGENE system (Haynes et al. 1995). To pass quality control, genotyping plates must have retained a 100% match for quality-control samples and must have at least 95% overall efficiency.

Candidate Genes Derived from the Genomic Convergence Approach

Two independent gene expression studies on human midbrain tissues from patients with PD and normal controls, by use of microarray and serial analysis of gene expression (SAGE) technologies, were conducted as part of current projects of the Duke PDRCE (Hauser et al. 2003; Noureddine et al. 2005). By combining these two studies, we found six genes that were significantly differentially expressed between patients with PD and controls and that mapped to the chromosome 1p AAO linkage region (table 2). In the present study, we tested SNPs in these six genes for association with risk and AAO in PD.

Iterative Association Mapping

We developed a second approach, iterative association mapping, to identify candidate genes in a linkage region. The overall concept is to reduce the number of SNPs genotyped while maximizing the chance of discovering a significant association. SNPs are first chosen at 100-kb intervals and then tested for association with traits of interest, which, in this case, are risk and AAO in PD. If no significant association is detected, the marker-to-marker distance is decreased by one-half each time (to 50 kb, 25 kb, etc.), until a significant association result is found. When a significant association is detected, additional SNPs in the surrounding region are then tested on the basis of known linkage disequilibrium (LD) patterns or physical iteration in the surrounding region

Table 3

Pairwise Pearson Correlation Coefficient (r^2) for *ATP6V0B*

The table is available in its entirety in the online edition of *The American Journal of Human Genetics.*

of the associated SNP if no previous LD patterns are available.

Statistical Analyses

All SNPs were tested for Hardy-Weinberg equilibrium (HWE) and LD in the affected group (comprising one affected individual from each family) and the unaffected group (comprising one unaffected individual from each family). An exact test implemented in the Genetic Data Analysis program was used to test HWE, for which 3,200 permutations were performed to estimate the empirical *P* value for each marker (Zaykin et al. 1995). The Graphical Overview of Linkage Disequilibrium (GOLD) package was used to calculate LD (as measured by the Pearson correlation coefficient, r^2, and Lewontin's standardized disequilibrium coefficient, D') between pairs of SNPs (Abecasis and Cookson 2000). Both r^2 and D' range from 0 (no LD) to 1 (perfect LD). However, there is no clear definition to use for interpretation of intermediate LD values. Here, we chose an arbitrary cutoff and considered two markers to be in strong LD if $r^2 > 0.60$ or $D' > 0.90$.

AAO was treated as a quantitative trait. We used both the orthogonal model (OM) (Abecasis et al. 2000) and the Monks-Kaplan method (MKM) (Monks and Kaplan 2000) implemented in the Linkage Disequilibrium Analyses for Quantitative and Discrete Traits (QTDT) program (see Web Resources) to test the association between markers and AAO. The MKM not only provides an association signal but also detects the direction of association—that is, positive association for allele A is declared when the majority of allele A carriers have an AAO higher than the average AAO. In addition to obtaining nominal *P* values, we also performed 10,000 permutation tests to obtain an empirical *P* value for each marker on the basis of the MKM. The global significance level was derived from permutation tests.

We performed haplotype analysis for genes with significant markers. Prior to the haplotype analysis, we identified tagging SNPs (tagSNPs) for each gene by using the ldSelect program (see Web Resources) (Carlson et al. 2004). The ldSelect program generates groups of markers in LD on the basis of a given threshold for r^2. These groups are referred to as "LD bins." A tagSNP is then selected from each LD bin. To perform the haplotype association analysis for AAO on the tagSNPs, we first used the FBAT –o option (Laird et al. 2000) to estimate the optimal offset of the AAO for each tagSNP. We then performed the HBAT –e option (Horvath et al. 2004) on the adjusted AAO data (subtracting from AAO the average optimal offset estimate), to test the association between haplotypes and AAO. When the number of tagSNPs is large, the computational time is substantial and the haplotype frequencies tend to be small, which makes interpretation difficult, even if significant *P* values are found. Therefore, we limited our haplotype computations to five tagSNPs. For genes with more than five tagSNPs, we analyzed all possible combinations of five tagSNPs.

The pedigree disequilibrium test (PDT) (Martin et al. 2000, 2003) was used to determine the association between markers and PD risk. Two PDT statistics were used: the PDT-sum statistic, for allelic effects, and the GenoPDT statistic, for genotypic effects. We also performed haplotype analysis on the risk genes detected by the PDT. The approach of selecting tagSNPs was as described above. We used the HBAT –e option to test the haplotype association between a set of tagSNPs and PD.

Several criteria were used to determine the final levels of significance in the presence of multiple comparisons. First, a significance level of $P \leqslant .05$ was used for evaluating the initial set of markers with 100-kb spacing. Second, a cluster approach (described below) was used to generate a significance level for further iterations. This approach requires that two or more markers, which have an r^2 correlation <0.6, be significant within a cluster of SNPs. Finally, at least one marker in the candidate gene or region needs to meet the global significance level derived from the permutation test.

Assume a total of *N* markers with low LD ($r^2 < 0.6$) across the region of interest and *x* markers located in each cluster, which leads to *y* clusters ($y = N/x$). We hypothesized that a cluster would be significant only if two markers within the cluster are significant. We can formulate the probability (α_c) that 1 of the *y* clusters is significant as a function of the probability that a marker is significant (where α is the significance level of a marker):

$$\alpha_c = \binom{y}{1}\binom{x}{2}\alpha^2(1-\alpha)^{x-2}\left[1-\binom{x}{2}\alpha^2(1-\alpha)^{x-2}\right]^{y-1} .$$

By restricting the significance level of a cluster to be α_c, we can compute the probability that a marker is significant. In other words, the probability that two

Table 4

Pairwise Pearson Correlation Coefficient (r^2) for *UQCRH*

The table is available in its entirety in the online edition of *The American Journal of Human Genetics.*

Table 5

Pairwise Pearson Correlation Coefficient (r^2) for *RNF11*

The table is available in its entirety in the online edition of *The American Journal of Human Genetics.*

markers within a cluster are significant at the level of α will result in the probability α_c that one cluster is significant. Clearly, α decreases when the number of significant markers within a cluster decreases or when α_c, the significance level of a cluster, decreases. The calculation of the global significance level is described above.

The multiplex families used in this study include 167 families that were studied in the previous AAO linkage study (hereafter called "the linkage data set") (Li et al. 2002). We performed SOLAR (Almasy and Blangero 1998) PEDLOD analysis with our previously found chromosome 1 peak marker (*D1S2134*), to obtain family-specific LOD scores for the 167 families. We then stratified the linkage data set into positive- and negative-linkage subsets on the basis of the family-specific LOD scores. The genes significantly associated with AAO in the overall data set were also tested for association with AAO by use of the MKM in the positive- and negative-linkage subsets. We did not use the OM, because it requires a normal distribution for the quantitative trait of interest, which is a problem for these small stratified data sets.

mRNA Analysis of USP24

Total RNA was isolated from human midbrain tissue and was reverse transcribed using poly-dT primers to generate a cDNA library. Primers used to amplify fragments of the *USP24* transcript were designed using Primer3 (see Web Resources). (The sequences are available on request.) We generated several PCR products of the expected size from the cDNA library and sequenced them. The exon-intron structure of the complete *USP24* transcript was deduced from genomic alignment of the overlapping RT-PCR fragments.

Results

Identification of the Linkage Subsets of Families

The SOLAR PEDLOD analysis of *D1S2134* identified 83 families with positive LOD scores (i.e., with positive linkage) and 84 with negative LOD scores (i.e., with negative linkage) from the linkage data set (Li et al. 2002). Throughout the present study, we performed association analyses with the overall PD data set as well as with these two stratified linkage subsets.

Genomic Convergence

We identified two differentially expressed genes from a previous microarray study (Hauser et al. 2005) and four from a SAGE study (Noureddine et al. 2005) that mapped to our chromosome 1p AAO linkage region (table 2). We analyzed SNPs (table 1) in each of these six genes, using the PD multiplex data set. The LD patterns of these six genes (pairwise r^2 values) are shown in tables 3–8.

The exclusion of a gene as a candidate from an association study is not always straightforward. The degree of confidence with which one excludes a gene from association is based on the depth of the search. One measure is at the level of LD defined by the current HapMap data set. Because we began genotyping our data set prior to the availability of the HapMap data set, and because we genotyped as many SNPs with as wide a variety of frequencies as possible from what was available in public (NCBI) and private (ABI) databases, some of our markers are not in the HapMap data set. To evaluate whether we have sufficiently covered each gene, we compared our SNP coverage of each gene with that available in the current HapMap data. The number of LD bins identified on the basis of HapMap SNPs with an MAF >10% is as follows: one LD bin each for *ATP6V0B, UQCRH,* and *C1orf8*; two for *TTC4*; three for *RNF11*; and 12 for *PPAP2B*. Overall, our SNPs included the HapMap tagSNPs in all genes except *RNF11* and *PPAP2B*; we missed one HapMap tagSNP in *RNF11* and covered only two HapMap tagSNPs (of seven genotyped SNPs) in *PPAP2B*.

None of these genes show significant association with PD risk, and only SNP 193 in *C1orf8* showed significant association with AAO in PD (fig. 2). The association of SNP 193 was not verified in the positive-linkage subset.

ELAVL4

The embryonic-lethal, abnormal vision, *Drosophila*-like 4 gene (*ELAVL4*) encodes for a neuron-specific RNA-binding protein. This gene was studied as a biological candidate gene through an ongoing project of the Duke PDRCE (Antic and Keene 1997). Two polymorphisms (SNPs 136 and 143) were previously found to be significantly associated with AAO in PD (Noureddine et al. 2005). However, these markers were not found to reach significant P values in the positive-linkage subset in the present study.

Table 6

Pairwise Pearson Correlation Coefficient (r^2) for *C1orf8*

The table is available in its entirety in the online edition of *The American Journal of Human Genetics.*

Iterative Association Mapping and LD

The initial association map consisted of 200 SNPs (1 SNP genotyped, on average, every 100 kb) in the 1-LOD score region (40.4–59.2 Mb on NCBI build 34) (fig. 1). With additional genotyping in the regions of interest, the average SNP density in our final association map was 1 marker every 66 kb, with a total of 284 SNPs genotyped. The MAFs of the SNPs varied from 0.03 to 0.50 (median and average of 0.29). All but 20 (7%) of the SNPs were in HWE in both the affected and unaffected samples at a $P = .05$ level (table 1). The genotype distributions of these 20 SNPs were reexamined by a technician in the laboratory and were tested for HWE again. The results remained the same. Given a 5% random chance of obtaining markers not in HWE, the 7% frequency detected in our project is within a reasonable range. Furthermore, it is important to note that the MKM and the PDT do not require HWE.

Figure 3 depicts the overall LD structure in this region (for SNPs that did not deviate from HWE, since LD calculations assume equilibrium) in the unaffected group. A similar LD pattern was observed in the affected group. LD is mostly restricted to intragenic areas, with no extensive LD for long stretches of DNA, or across distant loci for the majority of polymorphisms. Only SNPs with a low MAF (recent SNPs) show high values of D' with most neighboring SNPs.

To obtain a P value for the cluster analysis, 210 markers were identified whose r^2 was <0.6 for LD. Using these 210 markers and assuming 7 markers within each cluster, we derived a significance level of .01 for each marker. In addition, we obtained a global significance level of .001. Figures 2 and 4 depict the nominal P values of all 284 markers in $-\log_{10}$ scale. Among the first 200 SNPs studied (from the 100-kb map), evidence for association with AAO was found by either the OM or the MKM in the genes for the eukaryotic translation initiation factor EIF2B3 (for SNP 63, $P = .009$ by the OM and .0004 by the MKM), the testis-specific protein kinase 2 (TESK2 [for SNP 76, $P = .008$ by the MKM]), hypothetical protein FLJ14442 (for SNP 117, $P = .01$ by the MKM), and the ubiquitin-specific protease 24 (USP24 [for SNP 220, $P = .004$ by the OM]) (figs. 2 and 5). All these markers have empirical P values by the permutation test that are slightly lower than the nominal P values. For example, the empirical P value for SNP 63 in *EIF2B3* was .0002. Evidence of association with risk for PD by use of the multiplex data set was found only in the HIV type 1 enhancer-binding protein 3 gene (*HIVEP3*), for SNPs 13 ($P = .008$) and 19 ($P = .004$) (fig. 4). We proceeded to increase the SNP density in these genes.

Table 7

Pairwise Pearson Correlation Coefficient (r^2) for *TTC4*

The table is available in its entirety in the online edition of *The American Journal of Human Genetics.*

TESK2 *and* FLJ14442

Additional SNPs (SNPs 72, 74, and 75 in *TESK2* and SNPs 116, 118, 120, 122, and 124 in *FLJ14442*) were genotyped, to a final average density of 1 marker per 29 kb for *TESK2* and 1 marker per 51 kb for *FLJ14442*. Although we detected two sets of cluster markers for AAO association, no markers were significant after correction for multiple testing, nor did they show evidence of association in the positive-linkage subset.

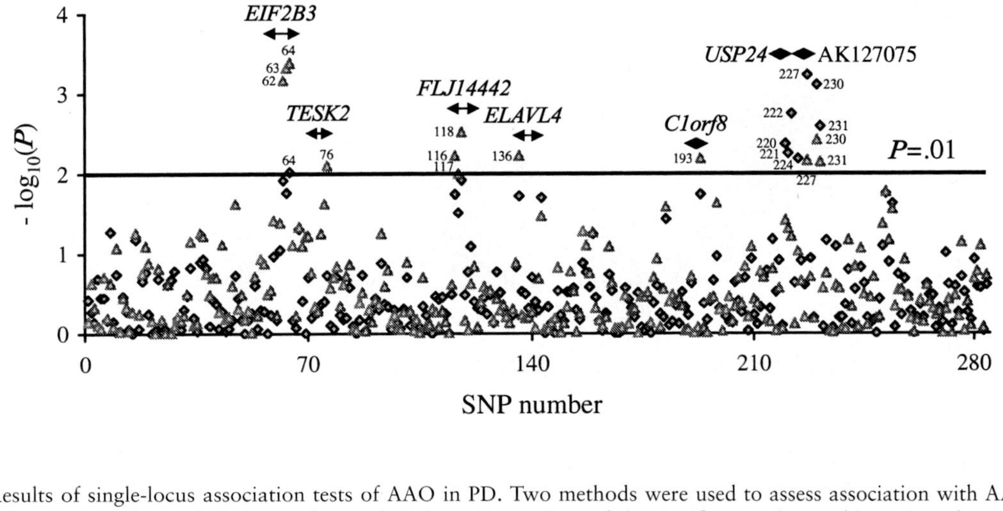

Figure 2 Results of single-locus association tests of AAO in PD. Two methods were used to assess association with AAO in the overall PD data set: the MKM (*triangles*) and the OM (*diamonds*). The SNP numbers of the significant polymorphisms (i.e., those with $P \leq .01$) are indicated. The candidate genes are *EIF2B3, TESK2, FLJ14442, ELAVL4, C1orf8, USP24,* and AK127075.

EIF2B3

Ten additional SNPs (SNPs 57–62 and 64–67) were genotyped in the *EIF2B3* gene (size 136 kb), leading to a final average density of 1 marker per 12 kb (fig. 2). Interestingly, several markers that were close to significance in the overall data set became significantly associated with AAO in the positive-linkage subset (table 9), despite the fact that the subset is only one-third (83 families) of the total sample. Therefore, at least two clusters of markers in low LD ($r^2 < 0.6$) (SNPs 59–61 and 62–64) are strongly associated with AAO in this gene. More interestingly, SNPs 62–64 are still significant after correction for multiple testing ($P < .001$).

Five tagSNPs (SNPs 59, 60, and 64–66) were found in *EIF2B3*. Haplotype analysis with these five tagSNPs and the use of the overall PD data set produced two haplotypes significantly associated with AAO: C-C-G-

Table 8

Pairwise Pearson Correlation Coefficient (r^2) for *PPAP2B*

The table is available in its entirety in the online edition of *The American Journal of Human Genetics*.

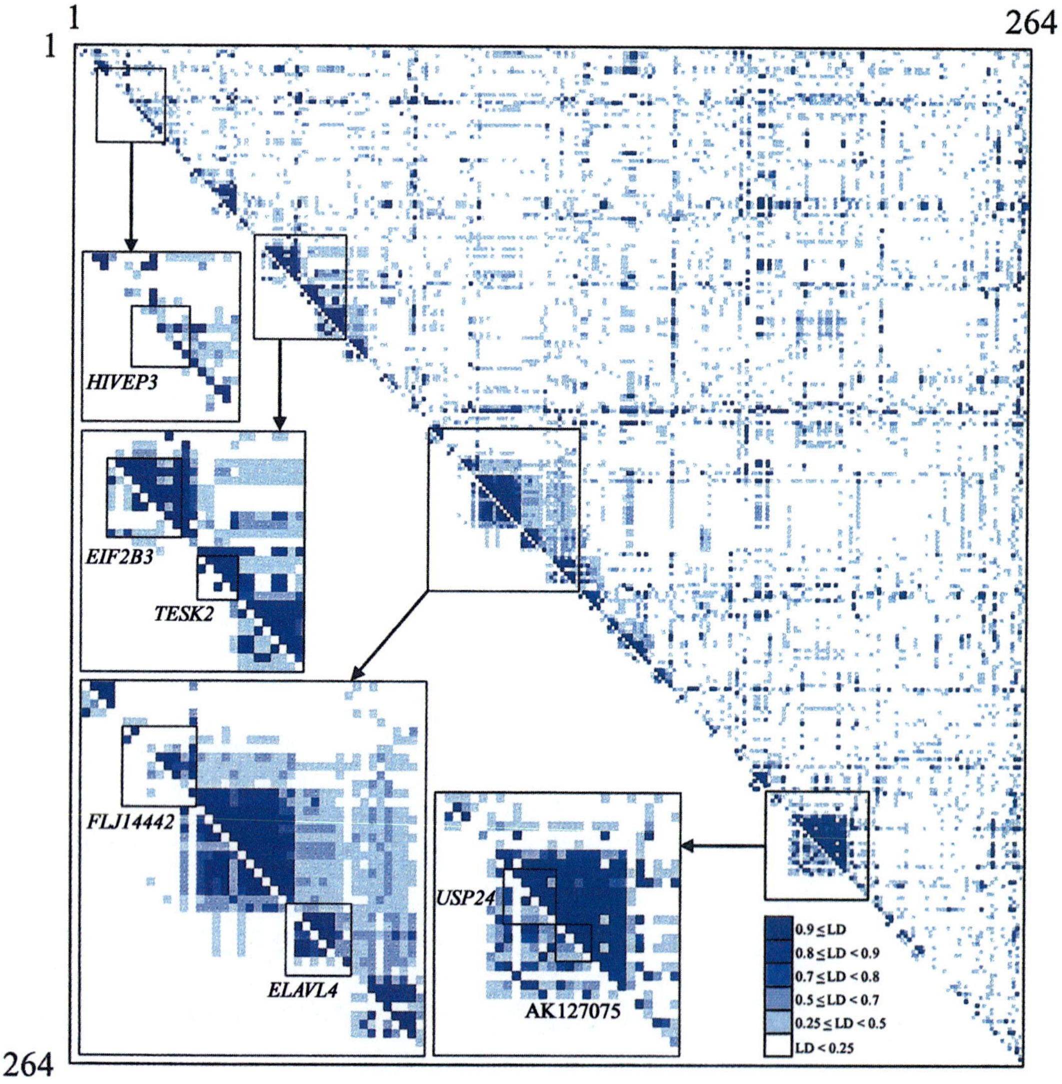

Figure 3 LD plot. The pairwise LD (as measured by the Pearson correlation coefficient, r^2, and Lewontin's standardized disequilibrium coefficient, D') in the group without PD, between all 264 markers in HWE, is depicted. The top-right triangle shows the D' coefficients, and the lower-left triangle shows the r^2 values (the stronger the LD, the darker the LD dot). The inserts in the lower left triangle constitute amplifications of the LD plots in the significantly associated genes (the boxes in these inserts indicate the SNPs inside the gene of interest).

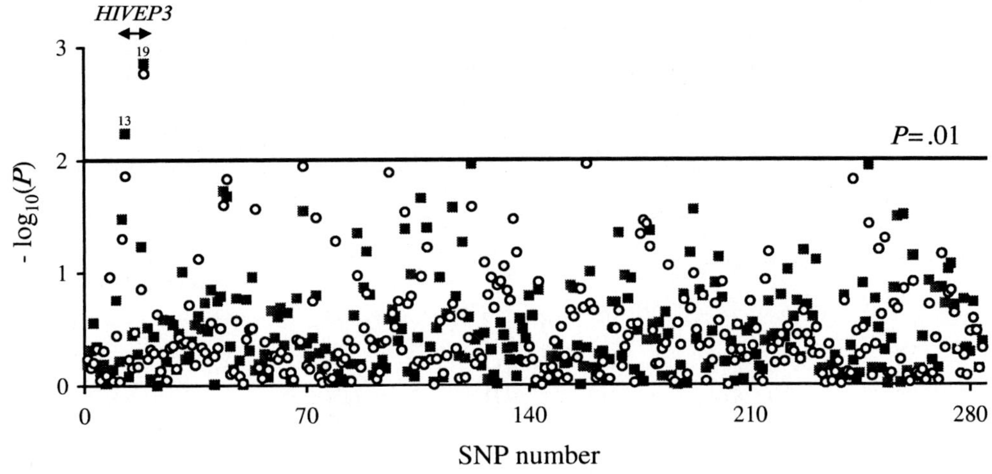

Figure 4 Results of single-locus association tests of risk for PD. The allelic association with PD was tested using the PDT (*squares*), and the genotypic association was tested using the the GenoPDT (*circles*) with the overall PD data set. The SNP numbers of the significant polymorphisms (i.e., those with $P \leqslant .01$) are indicated next to their P values.

T-G (haplotype frequency 17.2%; $P = .002$) and A-C-A-T-G (haplotype frequency 15.2%; $P = .002$) (table 10). These two haplotypes showed P values comparable to what we detected for SNP 64 alone ($P = .01$ by the OM and .0001 by the MKM).

USP24 *and AK127075*

In total, we genotyped 14 SNPs (SNPs 218–231) with ~17-kb spacing in the region from *USP24* to the cDNA *FLJ45132* clone BRAWH3037979 (GenBank accession number AK127075), a region in which seven SNPs (SNPs 220–222, 224, 227, 230, and 231) are significantly associated with AAO ($P < .01$) (fig. 2). The most significant marker was SNP 227, with $P = .0006$ by the OM and .007 by the MKM.

In silico, several lines of evidence suggested that the annotated *USP24* gene in NCBI build 34 (as defined by the mRNA for KIAA1057 protein [GenBank accession number AB028980]) may actually be a truncated version of the full-length *USP24* transcript. The 5′ end of the AB028980 transcript (exons 1–11) matches the 3′ end of the AK127075 mRNA (exons 25–35), and the human THC1877380 transcript from the TIGR Human Gene Index overlaps both genes. GenScan predicts the existence of the NT_032977.390 mRNA (composed of the AB028980 and AK127075 mRNAs and 12 additional exons at the 5′ end), and there is a cluster of human overlapping spliced ESTs (e.g., GenBank accession numbers BM458550, AW853346, and CD687922) that support the existence of a longer *USP24* transcript. Furthermore, the mouse AK045043 significantly overlaps with this cluster of ESTs but has two additional distant exons at the 5′ end. The putative first exon is supported by the FirstEF program prediction, contains an ATG start codon with sequences conforming to a Kozak consensus ([A/G]CC ATG G), has a nearby CpG island, and is close to predicted promoter sequences; all of which strongly reinforce the idea that it encodes the first exon of the larger *USP24* ORF. This gene produces a predicted mRNA of ~8 kb.

To evaluate the existence of this larger *USP24* transcript, termed "$USP24_L$," we used strategically positioned primers to amplify overlapping transcript fragments from a human midbrain cDNA library. We obtained RT-PCR products of the expected sizes, and direct sequencing of these products confirmed the existence of $USP24_L$. Using the BLAST tool implemented at the University of California–Santa Cruz Web site, we aligned the experimentally amplified composite cDNA with the genomic sequence. The sequence of our $USP24_L$ transcript carried more exons than the GenScan NT_032977.390 and XM_371254 predictions, some of which are supported by human or mouse ESTs. All splice junctions followed the canonical AG/GT rule. The composite cDNA is predicted to encode a protein of 2,590

The figure is available in its entirety in the online edition of *The American Journal of Human Genetics.*

Figure 5 Characterization of $USP24_L$, with mRNA and predicted protein sequence of the $USP24_L$ transcript. The legend is available in its entirety in the online edition of *The American Journal of Human Genetics.*

Table 9

Summary of *P* Values Obtained by the OM and MKM for SNPs in *EIF2B3* and *USP24*, in the Overall, Positive-Linkage, and Negative-Linkage Data Sets

Gene and SNP ID	Probe dbSNP Number	Overall Data Set[a] (n = 267) by OM	Overall Data Set[a] (n = 267) by MKM	Subsets by MKM[b] Positive Linkage (n = 83)	Subsets by MKM[b] Negative Linkage (n = 84)
EIF2B3:					
57	*rs12733586*	1.000	.325	.714	.460
58	*rs12139143*	.584	.288	.820	.496
59	*rs263977*	.109	.039	***.005***	.138
60	*rs263978*	.663	.590	.160	.850
61	*rs263965*	.099	.041	***.003***	.210
62	*rs1022814*	.012	***.001***	***.001***	.034
63	*rs12405721*	.018	***.0005***	***.001***	.045
64	*rs546354*	***.01***	***.0004***	***.0003***	.096
65	*rs566063*	.663	.078	.655	.250
66	*rs364482*	.842	.598	.767	.890
67	*rs489676*	.055	.046	.013	.160
USP24:					
218	*rs13312*	.122	.274	.068	.483
219	*rs1043671*	.791	.850	NA	NA
220	*rs487230*	***.004***	.039	.115	.655
221	*rs683880*	***.006***	.049	.057	.245
222	*rs667353*	***.002***	.061	.273	.811
223	*rs615652*	.232	.757	.177	.743
224	*rs594226*	***.007***	.094	.052	.889
225	*rs567734*	.124	.221	.071	.714
226	*rs625219*	.249	.626	.113	.736
227	*rs1165226*	***.001***	***.007***	.440	.662
228	*rs1024305*	.116	.196	.071	.714
229	*rs287234*	.632	.648	NA	NA
230	*rs287235*	***.001***	***.004***	.058	.166
231	*rs2047422*	***.003***	***.007***	.648	.487

NOTE.—*P* values ≤.01 are in bold italics, and *P* values ≤.05 and >.01 are underlined. NA = markers that are not informative with the MKM.

[a] In total, 167 of the 267 families were included in the previously published AAO genomic screen study (Li et al. 2002).

[b] The positive-linkage subset includes families with a positive LOD score at *D1S2134*, and the negative-linkage subset includes families with a negative LOD score at *D1S2134*.

aa (fig. 5), distributed over 69 exons and spanning 146 kb of genomic sequence (54904635–55050704 bp in chromosome 1). The LD block observed from SNP 216 through SNP 231 (fig. 3), which encompasses USP24$_L$ and flanking regulatory sequences only, also supports the predicted size of USP24$_L$.

Since the SNPs significantly associated with AAO in this region completely span USP24$_L$, and since strong LD exists throughout USP24$_L$ but not with neighboring genes, we concluded that the association originates from USP24$_L$ itself. Three LD bins were found in this region on the basis of 14 SNPs genotyped in this study (SNPs 218–231). The seven SNPs significantly associated with AAO were, in fact, originating from two LD bins. The first LD bin is formed by SNPs 220, 221, 224, and 230 (maximum P = .007), and the second is formed by SNPs 222, 227, and 231 (maximum P = .003), which implies that there are two independent polymorphisms in USP24$_L$ that have significant effect on AAO. Although none of the SNPs in USP24$_L$ were significantly associated in either the positive- or negative-linkage subsets by the MKM, SNPs 221, 224, and 230 were close to significant ($.05 < P < .06$) in the positive-linkage subset (table 9).

Three tagSNPs (SNPs 218, 219, and 227) were identified in *USP24*. Two haplotypes, C-T-T (frequency 62.6%; P = .003) and C-T-C (frequency 19.9%; P = .026), were found to be significantly associated with AAO (table 10). Overall, these haplotypes in *USP24* did not provide any more information on the association with AAO than did SNP 227 alone.

HIVEP3

A total of nine markers in this gene were genotyped, with a final average density of 1 marker every 45 kb. The new SNPs failed to reveal any further significant

Table 10

Summary of Haplotypes Showing Significant Association with AAO in the Overall PD Data Set

Haplotype							
Marker 1	Marker 2	Marker 3	Marker 4	Marker 5	Gene	Frequency (%)	*P*
SNP 192_G	SNP 193_A	SNP 194_C	...	...	*C1orf8*	66.4	.004
SNP 192_G	SNP 193_T	SNP 194_C	...	...	*C1orf8*	29	.009
SNP 72_C	SNP 75_A	SNP 76_A	...	...	*TESK2*	40.6	.012
SNP 117_T	SNP 118_A	SNP 119_C	SNP 121_A	SNP 123_A	*FLJ14442*	7.5	.037
SNP 117_G	SNP 118_C	SNP 119_C	SNP 121_A	SNP 123_A	*FLJ14442*	6.7	.018
SNP 59_C	SNP 60_C	SNP 64_G	SNP 65_T	SNP 66_G	*EIF2B3*	17.2	.002
SNP 59_A	SNP 60_C	SNP 64_A	SNP 65_T	SNP 66_G	*EIF2B3*	15.2	.002
SNP 218_C	SNP 219_T	SNP 227_T	...	...	*USP24*	62.6	.003
SNP 218_C	SNP 219_T	SNP 227_C	...	...	*USP24*	19.9	.026
SNP 13_A	SNP 15_G	SNP 17_T	SNP 19_G	SNP 21_C	*HIVEP3*	2.1	.003

NOTE.—The details on SNP numbers are listed in table 1.

association with risk for development of PD (fig. 4). However, SNP 12 was close to significant in both the allelic ($P = .058$) and the genotypic ($P = .057$) association tests, and SNP 18 ($P = .059$) was close to significant in the PDT, since it is in relatively high LD with SNP 19 ($r^2 = 0.75$ in the unaffected group). To test for association of SNPs 13 and 19 in a second independent data set, we genotyped these two markers in the PD singleton data set. We did not find evidence of association of these SNPs in the singleton data set alone. However, both markers showed stronger significant association in the combined multiplex and singleton data set ($P = .006$ for SNP 13; $P = .002$ for SNP 19) than in the multiplex data set. Clearly, some singleton families also contribute to the association of these two markers.

We identified eight tagSNPs (SNPs 13–17 and 19–21) in *HIVEP3*. Haplotype analyses based on five tagSNPs revealed the best results by use of tagSNPs 13, 15, 17, 19, and 21, in which a rare A-G-T-G-C haplotype (frequency 2.1%) was significantly associated with risk for PD ($P = .003$) (table 10). *HIVEP3* is a relatively large gene (408 kb), and very low levels of LD were observed among the SNPs genotyped (fig. 3). The lack of LD between SNPs 13 and 19 ($r^2 = 0$; $D' = 0.02$) provides two independent lines of evidence for the involvement of this gene in controlling risk for development of PD.

Discussion

The present study was motivated by the results of our previous genomic screen for AAO in PD, in which we reported a linkage region on chromosome 1p near *D1S2134* (LOD = 3.41) (Li et al. 2002). In the present study, we present a systematic approach, termed "iterative association mapping," to identify susceptibility genes and genetic modifiers in a linkage region. This methodology has the advantage of being unbiased by any preconceived ideas about the pathogenic mechanisms of a disease (as in candidate-gene studies). In addition, our analysis strategies include single-locus association tests in the overall set and in the positive- and negative-linkage subsets, as well as haplotype association analysis based on tagSNPs in the overall data set.

Because a large number of SNPs was tested in this study, we wished to correct for multiple testing while maintaining an appropriate threshold to screen for potential areas of association without eliminating any potential candidates. The Bonferroni correction is too conservative and would become exclusionary at a point when we want to avoid missing any potential associations. One can prioritize genes on the basis of the order of *P* values or use the global significance level derived from the permutation test, but either method may exclude too many potential leads; thus, these options do not fit the purpose of the first few iterations. Therefore, we added an intermediate criterion for analysis, since we considered the presence of multiple significant markers in low LD within a regional cluster to be more important than sporadic results across the region. The concept of this method is relatively straightforward: if multiple comparisons lead to significant SNPs only by chance, then these false-positive SNPs (if we assume, for the moment, that all SNPs in high LD have the same measure) should be randomly distributed across the physical region being tested. That is, there is no reason for them to be clustered together physically if they are significant only due to chance. Thus, we are seeking two SNPs with a defined level of significance that lie within a small physical region and that have a correlation that is low enough ($r^2 < 0.6$) that the significant associations of each individual marker with AAO are not likely to be the result of measuring the same chance event. This approach allows us to lower the significance level, which is more stringent than the conventional approach of using a nominal significance level, and to take into account the locations of the significant markers.

EIF2B3 ranks as the most significant AAO gene in this region. Two clusters of markers in this gene were significantly associated with AAO in the overall set and positive-linkage subsets. We also detected two clusters of markers in *USP24* that are significantly associated with AAO at both significance levels $P = .01$ and $P = .001$. However, the association evidence was not as strong as it was for *EIF2B3*, because of less significant findings in the positive-linkage subset. We therefore would consider *USP24* to be the second most significant AAO gene in the region for further follow-up. Finally, *HIVEP3* is the only gene found in this region that is associated with risk for development of PD.

The finding of multiple associated genes under the peak was somewhat unexpected. If one assumes that not all the statistically significant genes found here are biologically important in PD, is there a way to prioritize them for further study? Conceptually, since linkage analysis localized the initial peak (Li et al. 2002), the associations we identified should be "responsible" for the linkage. Thus, we identified those families contributing to the chromosome 1 linkage localization and examined that subset for association. However, by reducing the sample size to one-third (only 83 families had positive LOD scores at marker *D1S2134*), one would expect that the P values of the associated SNPs would become less significant, on the basis of power alone. But, in reducing the sample size, we also expect to render our sample more homogeneous and therefore to increase the significance for the true susceptibility polymorphisms. Interestingly, the most significant polymorphism in *EIF2B3* remained equally significant despite the sample size decrease, whereas two polymorphisms in *EIF2B3* (SNPs 59 and 61) that were close to significant in the overall data set became more significant in the positive-linkage subset. This implicates *EIF2B3* in controlling the AAO of PD. The ability to subdivide the data on the basis of linkage also demonstrates one of the additional strengths of family-based association data.

EIF2B3 is the γ subunit of the heteropentamer *EIF2B* (which includes α, β, γ, δ, and ε subunits). The translation initiation factor *EIF2B* catalyzes the exchange of guanine nucleotides on the initiation factor, *EI2F*, which itself mediates the binding of the initiator Met-tRNA to the 40S ribosomal subunit during translation initiation. *EIF2B* is important because it regulates global rates of protein synthesis, particularly when the cell is under mild cellular stress. Protein synthesis is generally decreased during periods of cellular stress, to lower the amount of detrimental unfolded and damaged proteins that can be toxic to the cell (van der Knaap et al. 2002). Interestingly, *EIF2B* causes vanishing white-matter disease (VWM [MIM 603896]), an autosomal recessive disorder characterized by cerebellar ataxia, spasticity, inconstant optic atrophy, and a relatively mild mental decline. The early onset of this disease reflects the hypothetical maximum expression levels of *EIF2B*-β, -γ, -δ, and -ε during embryonic development and the lower levels associated with aging (Inamura et al. 2003). It is well known that mild head trauma or fever is highly correlated with rapid clinical decline in these patients. van der Knapp et al. (2002) suggested that this clinical deterioration is the result of the failure of *EIF2B* in the critical role of regulating protein synthesis under mild cellular stress. Furthermore, the observed phenotypic variation in patients with identical *EIF2B* mutations suggests that genetic polymorphisms may influence the mutation's effect (van der Knaap et al. 2002). Thus, the biological activity of this gene fits well with the current ideas about cellular stress having a major role in PD.

USP24, the second most significant AAO gene, is a member of the family of the ubiquitin-specific proteases that remove polyubiquitin from target proteins, rescuing them from degradation by the proteosome. Whereas genes involved in the proteolytic pathway and aggregation of proteins (*Parkin* and *α-synuclein*) contribute to PD pathology, *USP24* appears to be an excellent biological candidate gene for controlling AAO in PD. We identified several polymorphisms in *USP24* significantly associated with AAO, one of which (SNP 220) is nonsynonymous (alanine→valine). The effect of this polymorphism on protein function is not currently known.

Unlike *EIF2B3* and *USP24*, *HIVEP3* was found to be associated with the risk for development of PD. The HIVEP3 protein is a member of the HIV enhancer-binding protein family that encodes large zinc-finger proteins and that regulates transcription via the κB enhancer motif (Allen et al. 2002). This motif is an important element controlling the transcription of viral genes and many cellular genes that are involved in immunity, cell-cycle regulation, and inflammation. As we reported elsewhere, *GSTO1* is associated with AAO in PD (Li et al. 2003) and also possibly plays a role in inflammation during the pathogenesis of PD, because of its involvement in the posttranslational modification of the inflammatory cytokine interleukin-1β (Laliberte et al. 2003). The mouse homolog of HIVEP3, the κ recognition component (KRC), participates in the signal transduction pathway leading from the tumor necrosis factor receptor to gene activation and may play a critical role in inflammatory and apoptotic responses (Oukka et al. 2002). Interestingly, patients with HIV have been reported to have decreased levels of dopamine but normal levels of other neurotransmitters, which suggests selective and profound loss of dopamine neurons (Lopez et al. 1999).

As mentioned above, our linkage peak for AAO in chromosome 1 has a surprisingly accurate overlap with the risk linkage peak from the Hicks et al. (2002) study of an Icelandic population. It is interesting to note that we did not detect linkage signals in chromosome 1 in our genomic screen (Scott et al. 2001). However, this may be because of the genetically heterogeneous nature of our study population, compared with the population of Iceland.

In summary, through the use of a genomic iterative association mapping technique, we have identified three novel and biologically pertinent genes associated with risk or AAO in PD. We also demonstrate the potential usefulness of using linked subsets to further prioritize genes when presented with multiple associated genes in the same region. We are currently examining the biological role of these genes in modifying AAO and risk in PD.

Acknowledgments

We are grateful to all of the families whose participation made this project possible. We thank the members of the PD Genetics collaboration (Martha A. Nance, Ray L. Watts, Jean P. Hubble, William C. Koller, Kelly Lyons, Rajesh Pahwa, Matthew B. Stern, Amy Colcher, Bradley C. Hiner, Joseph Jankovic, William G. Ondo, Fred H. Allen Jr., Christopher G. Goetz, Gary W. Small, Donna Masterman, Frank Mastaglia, and Jonathan L. Haines) who contributed multiplex families to the study. We also thank the core personnel at the Center for Human Genetics, Duke University Medical Center, and the members of the clinical core of the Duke PDRCE. This research was supported by National Institutes of Health/National Institute of Neurological Disorders and Stroke grants R01 NS311530-10 and P50-NS-039764. S.A.O. received funding from a postdoctoral fellowship (BPD/5733/2001) granted by the Portuguese Science and Technology Foundation.

Web Resources

Accession numbers and URLs for data presented herein are as follows:

dbSNP, http://www.ncbi.nlm.nih.gov/SNP/index.html

GenBank, http://www.ncbi.nlm.nih.gov/Genbank/ (for cDNA *FLJ45132* clone BRAWH3037979 [accession number AK127075], the mRNA for KIAA1057 protein [accession number AB028980], and ESTs [accession numbers BM458550, AW853346, and CD687922])

GenScan, http://www.ncbi.nlm.nih.gov (for accession numbers NT_032977.390 and XM_371254)

ldSelect program, http://droog.gs.washington.edu/ldSelect.html

Online Mendelian Inheritance in Man (OMIM), http://www.ncbi.nlm.nih.gov/Omim/ (for PD and VWM)

Primer3, http://frodo.wi.mit.edu/cgi-bin/primer3/primer3_www.cgi

QTDT, http://www.sph.umich.edu/csg/abecasis/QTDT/index.html

TIGR Human Gene Index, http://www.tigr.org/tdb/hgi/

References

Abecasis GR, Cardon LR, Cookson WO (2000) A general test of association for quantitative traits in nuclear families. Am J Hum Genet 66:279–292

Abecasis GR, Cookson WO (2000) GOLD—graphical overview of linkage disequilibrium. Bioinformatics 16:182–183

Allen CE, Mak CH, Wu LC (2002) The κB transcriptional enhancer motif and signal sequences of V(D)J recombination are targets for the zinc finger protein HIVEP3/KRC: a site selection amplification binding study. BMC Immunol 3:10

Almasy L, Blangero J (1998) Multipoint quantitative-trait linkage analysis in general pedigrees. Am J Hum Genet 62:1198–1211

Antic D, Keene JD (1997) Embryonic lethal abnormal visual RNA-binding proteins involved in growth, differentiation, and posttranscriptional gene expression. Am J Hum Genet 61:273–278

Blomqvist ME, Silburn PA, Buchanan DD, Andreasen N, Blennow K, Pedersen NL, Brookes AJ, Mellick GD, Prince JA (2004) Sequence variation in the proximity of IDE may impact age at onset of both Parkinson disease and Alzheimer disease. Neurogenetics 5:115–119

Carlson CS, Eberle MA, Rieder MJ, Yi Q, Kruglyak L, Nickerson DA (2004) Selecting a maximally informative set of single-nucleotide polymorphisms for association analyses using linkage disequilibrium. Am J Hum Genet 74:106–120

Destefano AL, Lew MF, Golbe LI, Mark MH, Lazzarini AM, Guttman M, Montgomery E, et al (2002) PARK3 influences age at onset in Parkinson disease: a genome scan in the *Gene*PD study. Am J Hum Genet 70:1089–1095

Goetz CG, Poewe W, Rascol O, Sampaio C, Stebbins GT, Fahn S, Lang AE, Martinez-Martin P, Tilley B, Van Hilten B, Cleczka C, Seidl L (2003) The Unified Parkinson's Disease Rating Scale (UPDRS): status and recommendations. Mov Disord 18:738–750

Hauser MA, Li YJ, Takeuchi S, Walters R, Noureddine M, Maready M, Darden T, Hulette C, Martin E, Hauser E, Xu H, Schmechel D, Stenger JE, Dietrich F, Vance J (2003) Genomic convergence: identifying candidate genes for Parkinson's disease by combining serial analysis of gene expression and genetic linkage. Hum Mol Genet 12:671–677

Hauser MA, Li YJ, Xu H, Stenger J, Noureddine M, Shao Y, Gullans S, Scherzer CR, Jensen R, McLaurin A, Scott B, Jewett RM, Hulette C, Schmechel DE, Vance JM (2005) Expression profiling of substantia nigra in Parkinson, PSP, and FTDP-17. Arch Neurol 62:917–921

Haynes C, Speer MC, Peedin M, Roses AD, Haines JL, Vance JM, Pericak-Vance MA (1995) PEDIGENE: a comprehensive data management system to facilitate efficient and rapid disease gene mapping. Am J Hum Genet Suppl 57:A193

Hicks AA, Petursson H, Jonsson T, Stefansson H, Johannsdottir HS, Sainz J, Frigge ML, Kong A, Gulcher JR, Stefansson K, Sveinbjornsdottir S (2002) A susceptibility gene for late-onset idiopathic Parkinson's disease. Ann Neurol 52:549–555

Horvath S, Xu X, Lake SL, Silverman EK, Weiss ST, Laird NM (2004) Family-based tests for associating haplotypes with general phenotype data: application to asthma genetics. Genet Epidemiol 26:61–69

Hubble JP, Weeks CC, Nance M, Watts RL, Koller WC, Stern MB, Colcher A, Ondo W, Jankovic J, Goetz C, Pappart E, Deane-Glaxo WPGC, Stajich JM, Scott BL, Vance JM, Pericak-Vance MA (1999) Parkinson's disease: clinical features in sibships. Neurology Suppl 52:A13

Inamura N, Nawa H, Takei N (2003) Developmental changes of eukaryotic initiation factor 2B subunits in rat hippocampus. Neurosci Lett 346:117–119

Karamohamed S, Destefano AL, Wilk JB, Shoemaker CM, Golbe LI, Mark MH, Lazzarini AM, et al (2003) A haplotype at the *PARK3* locus influences onset age for Parkinson's disease: the GenePD study. Neurology 61:1557–1561

Kitada T, Asakawa S, Hattori N, Matsumine H, Yamamura Y, Minoshima S, Yokochi M, Mizuno Y, Shimizu N (1998) Mutations in the *parkin* gene cause autosomal recessive juvenile parkinsonism. Nature 392:605–608

Kolsch H, Linnebank M, Lutjohann D, Jessen F, Wullner U, Harbrecht U, Thelen KM, Kreis M, Hentschel F, Schulz A, von Bergmann K, Maier W, Heun R (2004) Polymorphisms in glutathione *S*-transferase omega-1 and AD, vascular dementia, and stroke. Neurology 63:2255–2260

Laird NM, Horvath S, Xu X (2000) Implementing a unified approach to family-based tests of association. Genet Epidemiol Suppl 1 19:S36–S42

Laliberte RE, Perregaux DG, Hoth LR, Rosner PJ, Jordan CK, Peese KM, Eggler JF, Dombroski MA, Geoghegan KF, Gabel CA (2003) Glutathione *S*-transferase omega 1-1 is a target of cytokine release inhibitory drugs and may be responsible for their effect on interleukin-1β posttranslational processing. J Biol Chem 278:16567–16578

Leroy E, Anastasopoulos D, Konitsiotis S, Lavedan C, Polymeropoulos MH (1998) Deletions in the Parkin gene and genetic heterogeneity in a Greek family with early onset Parkinson's disease. Hum Genet 103:424–427

Li YJ, Hauser MA, Scott WK, Martin ER, Booze MW, Qin XJ, Walter JW, Nance MA, Hubble JP, Koller WC, Pahwa R, Stern MB, Hiner CB, Jankovic J, Goetz CG, Small GW, Mastaglia F, Haines JL, Pericak-Vance MA, Vance JA (2004) Apolipoprotein E controls the risk and age at onset of Parkinson disease. Neurology 62:2005–2009

Li YJ, Oliveira SA, Xu P, Martin ER, Stenger JE, Scherzer CR, Hauser MA, et al (2003) Glutathione *S*-transferase omega-1 modifies age-at-onset of Alzheimer disease and Parkinson disease. Hum Mol Genet 12:3259–3267

Li YJ, Scott WK, Hedges DJ, Zhang F, Gaskell PC, Nance MA, Watts RL, et al (2002) Age at onset in two common neurodegenerative diseases is genetically controlled. Am J Hum Genet 70:985–993

Lopez OL, Smith G, Meltzer CC, Becker JT (1999) Dopamine systems in human immunodeficiency virus-associated dementia. Neuropsychiatry Neuropsychol Behav Neurol 12: 184–192

Martin ER, Bass MP, Gilbert JR, Pericak-Vance MA, Hauser ER (2003) Genotype-based association test for general pedigrees: the genotype-PDT. Genet Epidemiol 25:203–213

Martin ER, Monks SA, Warren LL, Kaplan NL (2000) A test for linkage and association in general pedigrees: the pedigree disequilibrium test. Am J Hum Genet 67:146–154

Monks SA, Kaplan NL (2000) Removing the sampling restrictions from family-based tests of association for a quantitative-trait locus. Am J Hum Genet 66:576–592

Noureddine MA, Li YJ, van der Walt JM, Walters R, Jewett RM, Xu H, Wang T, Walter JW, Scott BL, Hulette C, Schmechel DE, Stenger J, Dietrich F, Vance JM, Hauser MA (2005) Genomic convergence to identify candidate genes for Parkinson disease: SAGE analysis of the substantia nigra. Mov Disord (electronically published June 17; available at: http://www3.interscience.wiley.com/cgi-bin/abstract/110541328) (accessed 22 June 2005)

Oukka M, Kim ST, Lugo G, Sun J, Wu LC, Glimcher LH (2002) A mammalian homolog of *Drosophila schnurri,* KRC, regulates TNF receptor-driven responses and interacts with TRAF2. Mol Cell 9:121–131

Paisan-Ruiz C, Jain S, Evans EW, Gilks WP, Simon J, van der BM, de Munain AL, Aparicio S, Gil AM, Khan N, Johnson J, Martinez JR, Nicholl D, Carrera IM, Pena AS, de Silva R, Lees A, Marti-Masso JF, Perez-Tur J, Wood NW, Singleton AB (2004) Cloning of the gene containing mutations that cause *PARK8*-linked Parkinson's disease. Neuron 44: 595–600

Polymeropoulos MH, Lavedan C, Leroy E, Ide SE, Dehejia A, Dutra A, Pike B, Root H, Rubenstein J, Boyer R, Stenroos ES, Chandrasekharappa S, Athanassiadou A, Papapetropoulos T, Johnson WG, Lazzarini AM, Duvoisin RC, Di Iorio G, Golbe LI, Nussbaum RL (1997) Mutation in the α-synuclein gene identified in families with Parkinson's disease. Science 276:2045–2047

Scott WK, Nance MA, Watts RL, Hubble JP, Koller WC, Lyons K, Pahwa R, et al (2001) Complete genomic screen in Parkinson disease: evidence for multiple genes. JAMA 286: 2239–2244

Valente EM, Abou-Sleiman PM, Caputo V, Muqit MM, Harvey K, Gispert S, Ali Z, Del Turco D, Bentivoglio AR, Healy DG, Albanese A, Nussbaum R, Gonzalez-Maldonado R, Deller T, Salvi S, Cortelli P, Gilks WP, Latchman DS, Harvey RJ, Dallapiccola B, Auburger G, Wood NW (2004) Hereditary early-onset Parkinson's disease caused by mutations in *PINK1*. Science 304:1158–1160

van der Knaap MS, Leegwater PA, Konst AA, Visser A, Naidu S, Oudejans CB, Schutgens RB, Pronk JC (2002) Mutations in each of the five subunits of translation initiation factor eIF2B can cause leukoencephalopathy with vanishing white matter. Ann Neurol 51:264–270

Zaykin D, Zhivotovsky L, Weir BS (1995) Exact tests for association between alleles at arbitrary numbers of loci. Genetica 96:169–178

Am. J. Hum. Genet. 77:265–279, 2005

Allelic Heterogeneity at the Serotonin Transporter Locus (*SLC6A4*) Confers Susceptibility to Autism and Rigid-Compulsive Behaviors

James S. Sutcliffe,[1,2,3,4] Ryan J. Delahanty,[2,4] Harish C. Prasad,[6] Jacob L. McCauley,[2,4] Qiao Han,[6] Lan Jiang,[2,4] Chun Li,[3,5] Susan E. Folstein,[7] and Randy D. Blakely[1,6]

Centers for [1]Molecular Neuroscience and [2]Human Genetics Research, [3]Vanderbilt Kennedy Center for Research on Human Development, and Departments of [4]Molecular Physiology and Biophysics, [5]Biostatistics, and [6]Pharmacology, Vanderbilt University, Nashville; and [7]Department of Psychiatry and Behavioral Sciences, Johns Hopkins University, Baltimore

Autism is a spectrum of neurodevelopmental disorders with a primarily genetic etiology exhibiting deficits in (1) development of language and (2) social relationships and (3) patterns of repetitive, restricted behaviors or interests and resistance to change. Elevated platelet serotonin (5-HT) in 20%–25% of cases and efficacy of selective 5-HT reuptake inhibitors (SSRIs) in treating anxiety, depression, and repetitive behaviors points to the 5-HT transporter (5-HTT; SERT) as a strong candidate gene. Association studies involving the functional insertion/deletion polymorphism in the promoter (5-HTTLPR) and a polymorphism in intron 2 are inconclusive, possibly because of phenotypic heterogeneity. Nonetheless, mounting evidence for genetic linkage of autism to the chromosome 17q11.2 region that harbors the SERT locus (*SLC6A4*) supports a genetic effect at or near this gene. We confirm recent reports of sex-biased genetic effects in 17q by showing highly significant linkage driven by families with only affected males. Association with common alleles fails to explain observed linkage; therefore, we hypothesized that preferential transmission of multiple alleles does explain it. From 120 families, most contributing to linkage at 17q11.2, we found four coding substitutions at highly conserved positions and 15 other variants in 5′ noncoding and other intronic regions transmitted in families exhibiting increased rigid-compulsive behaviors. In the aggregate, these variants show significant linkage to and association with autism. Our data provide strong support for a collection of multiple, often rare, alleles at *SLC6A4* as imposing risk of autism.

Introduction

In 1943, Leo Kanner published a series of 11 case reports of children with a condition he termed "infantile autism" or "autistic disturbances of affective contact" (Kanner 1943). Autism (MIM 209850) is now recognized as a spectrum of phenotypes that spans a range of clinical severity but fundamentally represents deficits in three domains: (1) development and use of language, (2) development of social relationships and interactions with family and peers, and (3) patterns of repetitive behaviors, restricted interests and activities, and a strong desire to maintain "sameness" in environment and daily routines (reviewed by Folstein and Rosen-Sheidley [2001]). Pharmacotherapies include antipsychotic medications for disruptive and aggressive behaviors and selective serotonin-reuptake inhibitors (SSRIs) for treatment of anxiety, depression, and repetitive behaviors (Cook and Leventhal 1996; Hollander et al. 2005). Of interest regarding the partial efficacy of SSRIs are findings of elevated levels of platelet serotonin (5-hydroxytryptamine [5-HT]) in ~20%–25% of affected individuals (Schain and Freedman 1961) and correlation with levels in first-degree relatives (Cook et al. 1993). Other findings supporting 5-HT involvement in autism are reviewed elsewhere (Cook and Leventhal 1996; Veenstra-VanderWeele et al. 2000).

Since the first twin study of autism by Folstein and Rutter in 1977 (Folstein and Rutter 1977), evidence has mounted to support a predominantly genetic etiology of autism (reviewed by Folstein and Rosen-Sheidley [2001]). The prevalence of narrowly defined autism is ~1/1,000 (Chakrabarti and Fombonne 2001), and inclusion of the broader spectrum increases this rate to ~1/300–1/500 (Fombonne 2003; Yeargin-Allsopp et al. 2003). Males are affected more often, with a male:female ratio of 4:1. Twin data show that MZ twins have an average concordance of ~60%–70% for classic autism and up to 90% when milder language and social deficits seen in the broader phenotype are considered. This contrasts with DZ twin concordance rates, shown to be 0%–10%, depending on the study. Sibling-recurrence risk in narrowly defined autism is ~6%–8% (Jones and Szatmari 1988; Ritvo et al. 1989). Modeling the above data

Received June 2, 2005; accepted for publication June 10, 2005; electronically published July 1, 2005.

Address for correspondence and reprints: Dr. James S. Sutcliffe, Department of Molecular Physiology and Biophysics, 702 Light Hall, Vanderbilt University, Nashville, TN 37232-0615. E-mail: james.s.sutcliffe@vanderbilt.edu

0002-9297/2005/7702-0009$15.00

Table 1

Autism Family Samples for Linkage and Association Studies

Sample	No. of Families						
	Multiplex			Trio			Grand Total
	MO	FC	Total	MO	FC	Total	
AGRE	156	111	267	11	5	16	283
Tufts/Vanderbilt University	46	28	74	22	5	27	101
Total	202	139	341	33	10	43	384

has led to estimates of ∼5–15 genes that contribute to genetic risk, possibly involving epistasis (Pickles et al. 1995), and locus heterogeneity (Risch et al. 1999). The data may best be explained by oligogenic inheritance, with different families possessing varying constellations of risk alleles (Folstein and Rosen-Sheidley 2001). A genetic-heterogeneity framework has important implications for the clinical variability observed in autism, in that specific risk loci, or distinct alleles at a given locus, are likely to influence the phenotype differently.

Several groups have undertaken family-based genetic studies to (1) identify regions of the genome commonly inherited by affected family members in multiplex-family samples (i.e., genomic linkage screens) and/or (2) test-specific loci for evidence of common alleles that confer genetic risk on the basis of tests of allelic association (reviewed by Folstein and Rosen-Sheidley [2001] and Veenstra-VanderWeele et al. [2004]). Chromosomal intervals identified in linkage studies with use of either a categorical diagnosis or indexing on specific traits include 7q, 2q, and 17q (International Molecular Genetic Study of Autism Consortium [IMGSAC] 1998, 2001*a*, 2001*b*; Ashley-Koch et al. 1999; Collaborative Linkage Study of Autism (CLSA) et al. 1999; Philippe et al. 1999; Risch et al. 1999; Auranen et al. 2000; Buxbaum et al. 2001, 2004; CLSA 2001; Liu et al. 2001; Shao et al. 2002*a*, 2002*b*; Yonan et al. 2003; McCauley et al. 2004, 2005; Stone et al. 2004; Cantor et al. 2005). For 17q, second-stage genomic screens with use of different samples (IMGSAC 2001*a*; Yonan et al. 2003) detected highly suggestive or significant linkage at or near the serotonin transporter (SERT) locus (*SLC6A4* [MIM 182138]) and evidence of a sex-restricted pattern of genetic effects (Stone et al. 2004). Our own reports of linkage to this region, with use of family data sets that contain partial overlap with the Autism Genetics Resource Exchange (AGRE) sample (Yonan et al. 2003), lend further support to involvement of this region (McCauley et al. 2004, 2005).

Studies of allelic association at *SLC6A4* with autism have focused primarily on a functional, insertion-deletion polymorphism in the promoter (5-HTTLPR) or a variable number tandem repeat (VNTR) marker in intron 2. Results of these studies are inconsistent, with associations shown either to the short (S) or long (L) alleles or absent association (Cook et al. 1997; Klauck et al. 1997; Maestrini et al. 1999; Persico et al. 2000; Tordjman et al. 2001; Yirmiya et al. 2001). Four studies have reported more-comprehensive analyses of common alleles and haplotypes that span the locus, including multiple SNPs (Kim et al. 2002; Conroy et al. 2004; McCauley et al. 2004; Devlin et al., in press). These studies find at least nominal association of the S allele at 5-HTTLPR and other markers or haplotypes. Our study of multiplex families (McCauley et al. 2004) also showed very suggestive linkage that cannot be explained by the modest association of HTTLPR and *rs140700* at *SLC6A4*. The two possible explanations for these results are (1) that *SLC6A4* is not the risk locus accounting for linkage or (2) that multiple different alleles at *SLC6A4* contribute to genetic risk independently. We report further investigation of chromosome 17 linkage in families with autism and an in-depth analysis of the *SLC6A4* gene, testing the hypothesis that allelic heterogeneity may account for the genetic liability to autism. Using a large sample of multiplex families, we find that *SLC6A4* exhibits strong evidence of linkage to autism, driven by allele-sharing in males. We find multiple coding and noncoding variants preferentially transmitted to affected individuals, and we identify significant correlations with increased rigid-compulsive behaviors, which indicates that *SLC6A4* is a likely susceptibility locus for autism, where allelic heterogeneity supports disease risk.

Subjects and Methods

Sample and Genetic Analyses

The sample for the present study consisted of 73 families recruited from the Tufts-Vanderbilt Consortium and 267 from the AGRE Consortium (table 1). The demographics of these populations have been reported elsewhere (Yonan et al. 2003; McCauley et al. 2005) as have diagnostic inclusion and exclusion criteria for linkage analysis (McCauley et al. 2005). Families were selected on the basis of the presence of a single proband who met full Autism Diagnostic Interview (ADI) criteria for autism and a second sibling who received the diagnosis of autism or presented on the broader spectrum. In the current report, we further examined linkage in a larger sample of 341 families with at least two affected children; for association studies and screening for known variants (e.g., Gly56Ala), we included an additional 43 trios (proband and both parents). As reported elsewhere (McCauley et al. 2005), Tufts/Vanderbilt families were genotyped at deCODE by use of the deCODE 500 marker panel with an average intermarker spacing of ~8 cM. Two-point and multipoint heterogeneity LOD (HLOD) scores for individual and combined samples, respectively, were calculated with Allegro, under both dominant and recessive models (Gudbjartsson et al. 2000). Disease-allele frequencies were estimated to be 0.01 and 0.1 for dominant and recessive models, respectively. Phenotypic status was considered only for affected individuals, and other family members were designated as having an unknown phenotypic status. Nonparametric allele-sharing LOD* values were calculated using affected relative pair data that was based on an exponential model with use of the S_{pairs} scoring function, as recommended by McPeek (1999). Nonparametric linkage (NPL) scores and corresponding *P* values were also calculated with Allegro. The position of chromosome 17 markers is based on the deCODE genetic map (Kong et al. 2002).

Association tests of 5-HTTLPR and *rs140700* were performed using the pedigree disequilibrium test (PDT) statistic (Martin et al. 2000), a variant of the transmission/disequilibrium test (TDT), developed for use with general pedigrees. Genotype analysis of these markers has been reported elsewhere (McCauley et al. 2004). Other tests of association or comparison of allele frequencies involved generation of a χ^2 statistic and corresponding *P* values with use of standard 2 × 2 contingency tables. Comparison of male:female affection for autism in the presence of Gly56Ala alleles was performed using Fisher's exact test. Comparison of ADI-derived variable cluster scores was performed using the *T* test—with incorporation of subject numbers, means, and standard deviations for the overall data set and either (1) individuals within a given family or (2) family means across multiple families—to evaluate the significance of score differences. Significance is reported as two-tailed *P* values. Approval for these studies was granted by the respective institutional review boards at Tufts University School of Medicine/New England Medical Center and Vanderbilt University Medical Center. All studies were performed with the informed consent of the families participating in the research.

Variant Discovery

Known but rare *SLC6A4* coding variants reported in previous studies (Cargill et al. 1999; Glatt et al. 2001; Hahn and Blakely 2002; Ozaki et al. 2003) were screened in 327 multiplex families and 57 parent-child trios by use of TaqMan allelic discrimination assays (table 2). When possible, variants were assayed within exons to permit inclusion of in vitro mutagenized plasmid cDNA samples either alone or mixed with wild-type cDNAs, to provide homozygous and heterozygous controls, respectively. ABI TaqMan (Holloway et al. 1999) reactions were performed in a 5-μl volume in accordance with manufacturer's recommendations (Applied Biosystems). Cycling conditions included an initial denaturation at 95°C for 10 min, followed by 50 cycles of 92°C for 15 s and 60°C for 1 min. Samples were analyzed using an ABI 7900HT Sequence Detection System.

Screening for unknown variants involved arbitrary selection of one affected individual from each of 120 families, ranked by family-specific nonparametric LOD* scores from the overall 341-family data set. Screening of PCR products for all exons was performed on the first 24 samples, with temperature-gradient capillary electrophoresis (TGCE) (Li et al. 2002), on a 96-capillary Reveal system, in accordance with manufacturer's recommendations (Spectrumedix). Putative variants detected by TGCE were confirmed by direct sequencing of PCR product by use of ABI dye terminators in the Center for Molecular Neuroscience Neurogenomics Core. The promoter for the initial 24 individuals and both exons and the promoter for samples from one proband from each of the remaining 96 (of 120) families were analyzed for variation by double-stranded direct sequencing of PCR products with use of ABI dye terminator chemistry. ABI electropherogram data obtained from Vanderbilt Cores or from Polymorphic DNA Technologies were imported and were analyzed for variation with the Phred/Phrap/Consed and PolyPhred suite of sequence analysis tools (Nickerson et al. 1997, 2001; Gordon et al. 2001). Variant confirmation and segregation of rare variants were determined by sequencing available family members and the original proband in the same manner. Location of variation within the gene was documented in table 3 with nomenclature described by den Dunnen and Antonarakis (2001).

Functional Analysis of Gly56Ala Activity and Regulation

Epstein-Barr virus (EBV)–transformed lymphocyte cell lines from AGRE or Tufts/Vanderbilt families with autism who carried either the Gly56 or 56Ala allele were obtained from the National Institute of Mental Health

Table 2

***SLC6A4* SNP Marker Information**

The table is available in its entirety in the online edition of *The American Journal of Human Genetics*.

Table 3

TD of Multiple Coding and Noncoding Alleles at *SLC6A4*

Location and dbSNP Number	Position[a]	Protein	No. of Families	No. of Transmissions to: All Affected Individuals[b]	All but Proband[c]	No. of NT	No. of Autistic: Males	Females
Exon 1b:								
ss38318598	c.147C→A	5′ UTR	2	4	2	1	3	1
Exon 2:								
rs6355	c.462G→C	Gly56Ala[d]	7	15	8	5	11	4
Exon 9:								
ss38318599	c.1568A→C	Ile425Leu	1	2	1	0	2	0
Exon 10:								
ss38318600	c.1688T→C	Phe465Leu	1	2	1	1	1	1
Exon 12:								
ss38318601	c.1943G→C	Leu550Val	1	2	1	0	2	0
Exon 13:								
rs6352	c.2110A→C	Lys605Asn	1	0	0	2	0	0
Exon 14:								
rs13306796	c.2516A→G	3′ UTR	1	2	1	0	2	0
Promoter:								
ss38318589	g.15622G→A	NA	1	1	0	1	1	0
rs2020932	g.14519A→T	NA	3	8	5	0	6	0
ss38318590	g.14289A→C	NA	1[e]	1	0	1	1	0
rs25533	g.13912T→C	NA	1	4	3	0	2	0
ss38318591	g.13754C→T	NA	(1)[f]	(1)	(0)	(1)	(1)	(0)
Intron 1a:								
ss38318592	IVS1a+20C→T	NA	1	1	0	0	1	0
ss38318593	IVS1a+133G→A	NA	1	1	0	0	1	0
hcv11414117	IVS1a−47G→C	NA	5	10	5	2	8	2
hcv11414114	IVS1a−25G→A	NA	4	9	5	0	7	2
Intron 1b:								
ss38318594	IVS1b+28G→A	Gly56Ala[g]	3	NA	NA	NA	NA	NA
Intron 6:								
ss38318595	IVS6−44G→C	NA	1	2	1	0	2	0
Intron 7:								
ss38318596	IVS7+83C→T	NA	4	9	5	0	9	2
Intron 8:								
ss38318597	IVS8−33C→T	NA	2	4	2	0	4	0
Total			31	76	40	12	63	12

NOTE.—NA = not applicable.

[a] Changes in the cDNA are indicated relative to the GenBank *SLC6A4* reference sequence (accession number NM_001045); genomic variants are designated by +1 corresponding to the initiating ATG or position within an intron.

[b] Transmissions to all affected individuals, including the proband in whom the variant was first identified (T:NT = 76:12; $\chi^2 = 26.82$; 1 df; $P = 2.2 \times 10^{-7}$).

[c] Transmissions excluding the screened proband in whom the variant was initially identified (T:NT = 39:12; $\chi^2 = 8.13$; 1 df; $P = .0042$).

[d] Four 56Ala NTs derive from two heterozygous couples transmitting only one 56Ala allele to affected children.

[e] Redundant transmissions are not counted toward total transmissions.

[f] Family does not contribute to linkage; corresponding counts are not included in the totals.

[g] IVS1b+28G→A lies on the Gly56Ala allele; therefore, to avoid redundancy, transmission was not considered.

(NIMH) Center for Collaborative Genetic Studies on Mental Disorders repository. Lymphocytes were cultured in suspension in RPMI 1640 medium (supplemented with 15% fetal bovine serum, 2 mM L-glutamine, 100 units/ml penicillin, and 100 μg/ml streptomycin) at 37°C in a humidified incubator at 5% CO_2 prior to assay. Lymphocytes were pelleted at 1,500 rpm for 5 min and were washed with Krebs-Ringers-HEPES (KRH) assay buffer. A total of 1×10^6 cells in triplicate were prewarmed (37°C) in a shaking water bath (10 min) in 12 × 75 polypropylene tubes in KRH buffer that contained 100 μM pargyline and 100 μM ascorbic acid. After a 5-min incubation with [^{3}H]5-HT (20 nM) at 37°C, uptake assays were terminated by immersion on ice, and uptake in pelleted, 1% SDS-extracted cells was quantitated by scintillation spectrometry. Specific 5-HT uptake was determined by subtracting the amount of [^{3}H]5-HT accumulated in the presence of 10 μM paroxetine (SmithKline Beecham). [^{3}H]L-glutamate transport assays were conducted as described for [^{3}H]5-HT, except with use of 100 nM substrate and definition of nonspecific uptake, with parallel accumulation acquired at 4°C.

Results

Linkage

On the basis of our initial linkage results (McCauley et al. 2004) and other reports of linkage to 17q (IMGSAC 2001*a*; Yonan et al. 2003), we substantially increased our sample of 73 Tufts/Vanderbilt and 85 AGRE families through acquisition from the NIMH repository; we reassessed evidence of linkage in the larger sample that contained 182 additional AGRE families. We found striking linkage in an overall data set of 341 multiplex families, with a peak recessive HLOD ($HLOD_{REC}$) score of 5.8 (fig. 1*A*) at two adjacent markers at ∼53 cM (*D17S1800* [∼1.4 Mb from *SLC6A4*] and *D17S1294* [∼150 kb from *SLC6A4*]). Results from all parametric and NPL analyses are detailed in table 4. Influenced by two recent reports (Stone et al. 2004; Weiss et al. 2005), we incorporated a sex-specific approach in our linkage analysis of chromosome 17. We queried for male-specific effects by splitting the data set into (1) families containing only affected males (MO) and (2) the remaining female-containing (FC) families, similar to the approach of Stone and colleagues (2004). Linkage increased substantially in the MO sample ($HLOD_{REC} = 8.0$; $n = 202$), with negligible contribution from the 138 remaining FC families. The magnitude of linkage overall and in the MO families, extraordinary for a complex behavioral disorder, encouraged us to pursue more-detailed studies to identify autism-associated alleles within *SLC6A4*.

Association

Initially, we tested for evidence of allelic association using the two markers (5-HTTLPR and the intron 5 SNP *rs140700*) that previously demonstrated modest association in a smaller sample (McCauley et al. 2004). In a sample of 384 combined multiplex and trio families, we detected evidence of allelic association with autism (i.e., transmissions [T] > nontransmissions [NT]) only at the intron 5 marker *rs140700* (minor allele T:NT = 93:124; $\chi^2 = 4.47$; $P = .03$). However, when MO and FC subsets were examined separately, modest association of the S allele of 5-HTTLPR was detected in the MO data set ($n = 235$ families; T:NT = 362:314; $\chi^2 = 4.90$; $P = .03$) as well as persistent undertransmission of the minor allele at *rs140700* (T:NT = 47:76; $\chi^2 = 6.84$; $P = .009$), whereas no association or trend toward association was seen in the 149 FC families (HTTLPR-S: T:NT = 223:231, $\chi^2 = 0.07$, $P = .79$; *rs140700*: T:NT = 46:48, $\chi^2 = 0.021$, $P = .88$). The association in MO families is consistent with previous results (McCauley et al. 2004) and the male bias in linkage (Stone et al. 2004), but it fails to explain the highly significant linkage in MO families shown above.

Allelic Heterogeneity at SLC6A4

Since *common* alleles across the *SLC6A4* locus do not explain the observed linkage, we considered the hypothesis that multiple, possibly rare, *SLC6A4* risk alleles exist and confer risk of autism. We tested our hypothesis using two parallel strategies. We first screened all families for known rare coding variants to determine if one or more is present at elevated frequency in our autism sample and, by inference, is potentially related to disease risk. Our second approach involved (1) selecting unrelated probands from the multiplex families that contribute most to linkage and, at minimum, have a positive LOD score at the linkage peak and (2) screening their *SLC6A4* exons and promoter sequences for novel variants. In our combined sample of 384 multiplex families and parent-child trios, we screened for known nonsynonymous variants using TaqMan allelic discrimination assays. We detected multiple individuals who carried one or two copies of the 56Ala-encoding allele and a single subject heterozygous for an allele encoding the nonsynonymous variant Lys605Asn.

Detailed analysis of families with the Gly56Ala substitution reveal its presence in both "linked" (positive LOD scores) and "unlinked" multiplex families and trios. Within the 120 families with the highest family-specific LOD scores, we found the 56Ala allele present on 11 (2.3%) of 480 independent chromosomes. Three homozygous 56Ala subjects were identified in these families. In contrast, Glatt et al. (2001) reported the 56Ala variant occurred on only 4 of 900 chromosomes in the only large *nonclinical* comparison sample described, with a minor-allele frequency (MAF) of 0.44% and no homozygous subjects. In our remaining families with autism, we found a lower frequency of the 56Ala allele, with 12 (1.1%) of 1,056 chromosomes harboring the variant; no homozygotes were identified for this group. An alternative comparison comes from our screening of a predominantly white population ascertained for Axis I Mood Disorders. Here, we identified 3 (1.1%) of 272 chromosomes with 56Ala alleles (J. R. Field, H.C.P., R.D.B., E. Sanders-Bush, and R. C. Shelton, unpublished findings).

A parallel strategy involved screening the promoter, exons, and flanking sequence of unrelated probands from, initially, 24 families who most contributed to linkage in this region, on the basis of ranking for family-specific LOD scores. TGCE followed by direct sequencing of PCR products comprised the initial effort, and one proband sample from each of the remaining 96 (of 120) families was subjected to direct sequencing of PCR prod-

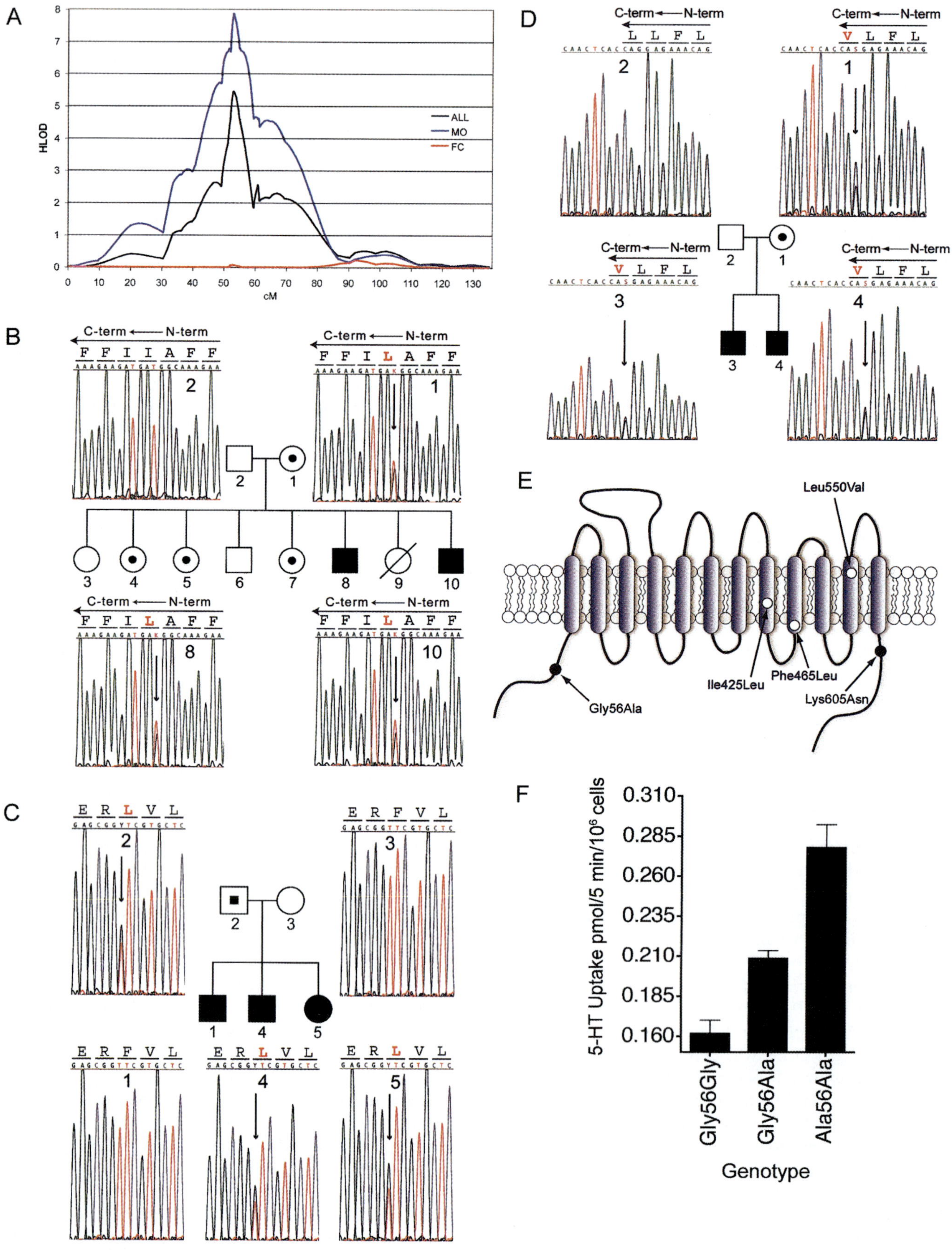

A
HLOD
cM
ALL
MO
FC
B
C-term ← N-term
F F I I A F F
F F I L A F F
C
E R L V L
E R F V L
D
L L F L
V L F L
E
Leu550Val
Ile425Leu
Phe465Leu
Gly56Ala
Lys605Asn
F
5-HT Uptake pmol/5 min/10^6 cells
Gly56Gly
Gly56Ala
Ala56Ala
Genotype

ucts. In addition to the independent identification of one 56Ala homozygote, two novel coding variants (Ile425Leu and Leu550Val) (fig. 1*B* and 1*D*) were detected in the 24 most-linked families (4/48 = 8.3% allele frequency). In the remaining 96 families, several 56Ala alleles and a Phe465Leu nonsynonymous substitution (fig. 1*C*) were detected (table 3). All three coding substitutions occur within transmembrane domains (fig. 1*E*) and are highly conserved (fig. 2). The least conserved of the novel variants corresponds to residue Ile425, which is present within all SERT proteins from human to *Drosophila*. The other two nonsynonymous variants occur at residues conserved from human to *Drosophila* in all monoamine transporters—including SERT, the norepinephrine transporter (NET), and the dopamine transporter (DAT)—for which sequence was available.

To consider the genetic relevance of the coding variants to autism risk, we asked if these variants segregated with disease in each family. Two of the three novel coding variants were transmitted to all affected individuals (5 males and 1 female) in the three families (fig. 1*B*–1*D*). One affected male did not inherit the paternally transmitted Phe465Leu variant allele. The 425Leu allele exhibited a particularly intriguing overall segregation pattern (fig. 1*B*). This variant was maternally transmitted to both affected sons. Three unaffected daughters also inherited the allele, but two other unaffected siblings, one male and one female, did not. When the clear sex bias in linkage is considered, segregation of the 425Leu allele in this family is consistent with but not proof of male-biased genetic risk or elevated penetrance associated with the allele. No unaffected siblings were present in the other two families. The 56Ala allele was detected in seven linked families, in which the T:NT was 15:5 (table 3). Of the five nontransmissions, four correspond to two distinct instances in which both parents were carriers (expected to occur in ~1 of every 2,000 couples, under the assumption of Hardy-Weinberg equilibrium [HWE]), and offspring received only one Ala56 allele. The other nontransmitted 56Ala allele was present in the mother of the family that paternally transmitted the Phe465Leu variant. Of the three homozygous individuals in the 120 linked/screened families, two were affected male offspring and one was a mother for whom medical history information was unavailable but who transmitted the allele to two affected male offspring. Analysis of the unlinked multiplex and simplex families with a 1.1% (12/1056) 56Ala frequency did not show bias in transmission (data not shown). There was a significant effect in a larger 643 multiplex/trio data set for autism in males carrying one or two 56Ala alleles compared with females (23:14 affected:unaffected males vs. 7:16 affected:unaffected females; $P = .016$).

Clinical Correlations

To explore phenotypic correlates with the coding variants, we compared scores for trait subsets of autism that were based on ADI-Revised (ADI-R)–derived variable clusters (table 5) identified elsewhere from a principal-components analysis of ADI-R items (Tadevosyan-Leyfer et al. 2003). These clusters reflect (1) language, (2) social intent, (3) developmental milestones, (4) savant skills, (5) rigid-compulsive, and (6) sensory-aversion aspects of the autism phenotype. There was a significant increase in rigid-compulsive behaviors associated with the novel variants ($P = .0003$) (table 5), and the effect was most pronounced for the Ile425Leu and Leu550Val families. The Ile425Leu substitution tracked with more-severe language deficits ($P = .0031$), although the brothers harboring the allele were generally more affected across most factor domains, with the exception of sensory aversions. The Leu550Val and Phe465Leu variants were associated with lesser impairment in language and social-intent domains, significantly so for the Phe465Leu variant ($P < .0001$ and $P = .0021$, respectively). The Gly56Ala variant (heterozygous or homozygous) in the linked families similarly demonstrated a significant as-

Figure 1 Male-biased linkage of autism and novel coding variants at the 17q11.2 *SLC6A4* locus. *A*, Male-biased linkage of autism to 17q11.2. Multipoint linkage analysis on chromosome 17 is shown for the overall 341-family data set (*black line*), 202 MO families (*blue line*), or the remaining 138 FC families (*red line*). HLOD scores were calculated under a recessive model and were plotted as a function of marker position in centimorgans (cM) along chromosome 17. *B–D*, Sequence detection of novel nonsynonymous *SLC6A4* variants in families with autism. Sequence-based detection is shown for each of the three novel coding variants, with corresponding pedigrees. *B*, Ile425Leu. *C*, Phe465Leu. *D*, Leu550Val. Blackened circles or squares reflect individuals with an autism diagnosis, unblackened circles or squares reflect individuals without autism, and allele carriers without autism are indicated by small blackened circles or squares within the larger pedigree symbol. Electropherogram data is shown in either sense (*B*) or antisense (*A* and *C*) orientations, with corresponding coding sequence. Antisense sequences (*A* and *C*) indicate the reversed orientation of amino acid codons, represented by lines across each three-base sequence. Variant amino acids are shown in red, and corresponding heterozygous sequence changes are indicated by an arrow. Individual numbers in the respective pedigrees correspond to numbers within each of the sequence frames. *E*, Schematic representation of the 5-HT transporter. Amino acid substitutions are indicated by location within transmembrane or cytoplasmic domains. *F*, Dosage-dependent elevated 5-HT transporter activity of Ala56-encoded hSERT in native lymphoblastoid cells. Lymphocytes genotype-matched at 5-HTTLPR (L/L) and the intron 2 VNTR (10/10) and bearing Gly/Gly–, Gly/Ala–, or Ala/Ala–encoding genotypes at residue 56 were assayed for [^{3}H]5-HT transport activity, as described (see the "Subjects and Methods" section). Three independent experiments were performed in triplicate for each line, and the combined basal uptake data were plotted.

sociation with more severe rigid-compulsive behaviors ($P = .0085$). When all linked families with individuals carrying a coding variant were considered together, the significance in elevated severity of rigid-compulsive behaviors increased ($P = .0002$). No consistent pattern was observed across all Gly56Ala families, regardless of sex, for other ADI clusters; however, there appeared to be a trend toward two subgroups. In one group, patients had greater severity for rigid-compulsive and sensory-aversion behaviors, with fewer impairments in language and social domains. The second group did not show the sensory-aversion finding but was more impaired in language (table 5).

Functional Properties of Gly56Ala SERT

The presence of multiple homozygous 56Ala subjects in our multiplex autism sample allowed evaluation of the functional impact of a 56Ala substitution on SERT activity and regulation by use of genotyped, EBV-transformed lymphocytes, since *SLC6A4* is natively expressed in those cells (Khan et al. 1996; Lesch et al. 1996; Faraj et al. 1997). Basal 5-HT transport activity was elevated in Ala56-expressing cells (T test, $P < .05$) compared with Gly56 homozygous, Gly56Ala heterozygous, or combined Gly56 genotypes; significance remains after normalization to L-glutamate transport activity and does not segregate with the *SLC6A4* genotype (fig. 3). To control for potential confounding effects of variation in *SLC6A4* gene expression and downstream basal 5-HT uptake associated with 5-HTTLPR and intron 2 VNTR genotypes (Lesch et al. 1996; Ogilvie et al. 1996; MacKenzie and Quinn 1999), we repeated studies with two cell lines of each Gly56Ala genotype that carried identical 5-HTTLPR (L/L) and intron 2 VNTR (10/10) genotypes. Figure 1*F* demonstrates a 56Ala dosage-dependent effect on basal 5-HT transport activity, with ~75% increase evident for the 56Ala homozygous lines as compared with lines homozygous for 56Gly. In these cells, we also demonstrated that the 56Ala allele is refractory to regulation by acute application of activators of protein kinase G (PKG) or p38 mitogen-activated protein kinase (MAPK) (Miller and Hoffman 1994; Qian et al. 1997; Ramamoorthy and Blakely 1999; Zhu et al. 2004, 2005; Samuvel et al. 2005) (fig. 4*A* and 4*B*), which suggests that intrinsic features of function unlikely to be attributable to a linked, noncoding variant are evident. We recently described a similar loss of regulation despite normal surface density for 56Ala cDNA transfected into HeLa cells (Prasad et al., in press).

The figure is available in its entirety in the online edition of *The American Journal of Human Genetics*.

Figure 2 ClustalW alignment of hSERT amino acid sequence versus other species of SERT and other biogenic amine transporters. The legend is available in its entirety in the online edition of *The American Journal of Human Genetics*.

Association of Heterogeneous Alleles with Autism

To more completely evaluate the *SLC6A4* locus for novel alleles, we expanded our screen to cover proximal promoter sequences and noncoding 5′ and 3′ exons. We subsequently analyzed 31 families for allelic segregation patterns for rare, noncoding variants discovered across the locus. Variants were identified in the promoter, exon 1b, exon 14, and intronic sequences in the linked families (table 3). Several variants are known polymorphisms with existing database identifiers, although many are novel. Other polymorphisms with modest-to-high MAF were tested elsewhere for association and are not included in table 3. Allelic segregation patterns reveal a stark pattern of transmission disequilibrium (TD) when all variants are combined for purposes of considering segregation. Redundant allelic transmissions represented by two or more SNPs were not counted more than once. TD was evident from a T:NT count of 76:12, which represents a highly significant deviation from the null hypothesis of no association ($\chi^2 = 26.82$; 1 df; $P = 2.2 \times 10^{-7}$). There is an a priori expectation of transmission (or de novo sequence change) to index cases in whom variants were originally detected. To reduce this bias, transmissions to these individuals were excluded, yet segregation remained significant (T:NT = 40:12; $\chi^2 = 8.13$; 1 df; $P = .0042$). Therefore, these multiple coding and noncoding alleles persist in demonstrating a collective link-

Table 4

Autism Linkage Data for Chromosome 17

Family Sample	Marker	Position[a] (cM)	HLOD Dominant	HLOD Recessive	LOD*	LOD* P[b]	NPL	NPL P[b]
Overall ($n = 340$)	*D17S1800*	53	4.98	5.44	5.82	1.59×10^{-7}	4.88	6.63×10^{-8}
MO ($n = 189$)	*D17S1800*	53	5.35	7.86	6.65	4.85×10^{-8}	5.18	1.64×10^{-8}
FC ($n = 138$)	*D17S1800*	53	.4	.06	.46	.085	2.21	.073

[a] Position on the deCODE chromosome 17 genetic map.

[b] P values are nominal and are not corrected.

Table 5

ADI Cluster Scores for Families with *SLC6A4* Coding Variant

ADI Cluster	No. of Subjects	Mean for Sample				All Novel Variants		No. of Subjects with	Mean for Carriers with						All G56A Carriers		Male Gly56Ala Carriers			All Coding	
		Total	Ile425Leu	Leu550Val	Phe465Leu	Mean	*P*	G56A	G56A-1	G56A-2	G56A-3	G56A-4	G56A-5	G56A-6	Mean	*P*	No. of Subjects	Mean	*P*	Mean	*P*
Language	770	***.457 ± .268***	***.838***[a]	.314	***.231***[b]	.461 ± .329	NS	13	.647	.378	.552	.207	.378	.436	.462 ± .156	NS	9	.541 ± .297	NS	.442 ± .205	NS
Social Intent	770	***.439 ± .228***	***.605***[c]	.325	***.200***[d]	.377 ± .207	NS	13	.564	.164	.314	.454	.165	.344	***.334 ± .158***	.075	9	.444 ± .203	NS	.370 ± .169	.095
Milestones	758	***.738 ± .068***	.809	.740	.763	.771 ± .035	.052	13	.723	.734	.750	.780	.757	.759	.742 ± .026	NS	9	.754 ± .056	NS	***.757 ± .026***	***.0069***
Savant Skills	730	***.124 ± .150***	.000	.083	.028	***.037 ± .042***	***.0031***	13	.088	.671	.111	.033	.671	.109	.215 ± .238	NS	9	.150 ± .157	NS	.199 ± .270	NS
Rigid Compulsive	747	***.288 ± .209***	.402	.428	.351	***.394 ± .039***	***.0003***	13	.317	.412	.210	.497	.413	.606	***.409 ± .138***	***.0085***	9	***.343 ± .138***	NS	***.404 ± .11***	***.0002***
Sensory Aversion	708	***.331 ± .269***	.060	.245	.340	.215 ± .142	.08	11	.305	.667	.319	.667	.667	NA	***.525 ± .195***	***.0005***	7	.353 ± .272	NS	.409 ± .231	NS

NOTE.—Values shown in bold italics are statistically significant ($P < .05$) in comparison with overall means. NS = not significant.

[a] Ile425Leu-Language mean = .838 ± .34; $P = .0031$.

[b] Social Intent mean = .605 ± .026; $P = .011$.

[c] Phe465Leu-Language mean = .231 ± .0035; $P < .0001$.

[d] Social Intent mean = .200 ± .06; $P = .0021$.

The figure is available in its entirety in the online edition of *The American Journal of Human Genetics.*

Figure 3 Altered basal 5-HT transport activity and regulation associated with the Gly56Ala variant. The legend is available in its entirety in the online edition of *The American Journal of Human Genetics.*

age to and allelic segregation with autism, despite failure to identify association of *common* alleles (apart from HTTLPR and *rs140700*) at *SLC6A4* in these families.

Discussion

Two recent reports are notable for leveraging the sex bias of disease affection in autism to define an analytical framework that identified significant male-biased genetic effects at 17q. The AGRE Consortium reported a genomewide analysis with use of sex (as presented here) to stratify a 257-family data set (Stone et al. 2004), and they have recently replicated evidence for male-biased linkage to 17q (Cantor et al. 2005). They compared overall linkage with that of MO families and of FO families. They found a significant effect at 17q11.2 near the *SLC6A4* locus (~53 cM), with MO families showing an empirically significant increase of linkage from a maximum LOD score (MLS) of 3.2 in the overall data set to an MLS of 4.3 in the 148-family MO data set. Our analyses, which include AGRE and Tufts/Vanderbilt families, confirm these previous observations by the AGRE Consortium yet show more-pronounced overall and male-biased genetic effects at this locus. In the second report, Weiss et al. (2005) showed significant association of marker alleles at *SLC6A4* and the 17q31 integrin $\beta 3$ (*ITGB3* [MIM 173470]) locus, with male-specific genetic influences on 5-HT levels. *ITGB3* was detected earlier by Weiss et al. (2005) as a QTL for circulating serotonin levels. Our own recently published genomic linkage screen showed two adjacent linkage peaks on proximal 17q (McCauley et al. 2005). Conditional linkage analyses revealed locus- or peak-specific effects, which supports the premise that both *SLC6A4* at 53 cM and another more telomeric locus (possibly *ITGB3*) contribute to genetic effects in this region. We speculate on the basis of published linkage patterns—including the AGRE replication study that showed linkage (MLS = 3.6) to a more distal site in 17q21 (Cantor et al. 2005)—that overall linkage in this region represents two loci, with the likely stronger effect at *SLC6A4*.

We were struck by the extraordinary evidence of linkage, given that common alleles and haplotypes fully representing LD across the locus failed to explain the linkage, as would be predicted under the "common disease-common allele" hypothesis. Given the above observations, we considered the alternative hypothesis that allelic heterogeneity explained risk at *SLC6A4*. We have discovered three novel highly conserved coding variants in families that strongly contribute to linkage in this region. Two of the three novel coding variants (Ile425Leu and Leu550Val), a 56Ala homozygous proband, and a novel intron 6 SNP (IVS6-44G→C) were identified among 24 probands (8.3% allele frequency) from families with the highest family-specific LOD scores. These two novel alleles segregate to all affected individuals in their respective families and thus are associated with disease. These findings spawned further discovery efforts that led to the identification of 13 novel SNPs, including the Phe465Leu nonsynonymous variant. The family with this latter variant is of interest because the mother carried but did not transmit the 56Ala allele. She did trans-

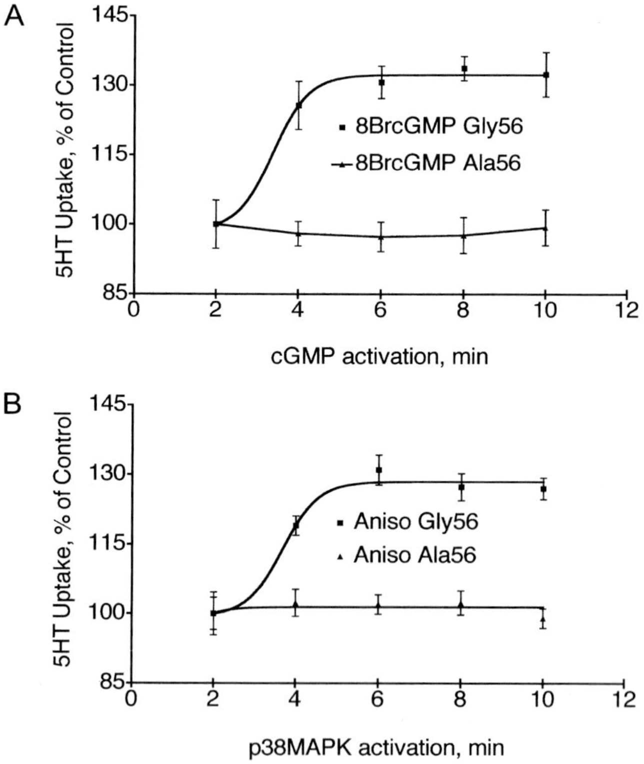

Figure 4 SERT is refractory to regulation through PKG and p38 MAP kinase signaling pathways. *A,* SERT Ala56 lacks sensitivity to 8BrcGMP. Homozygous Ala56 cells (10^6/tube) were preincubated for various lengths of time at 37°C, with 10 μM 8BrcGMP prior to [^{3}H]5-HT transport assays. *B,* SERT Ala56 lacks sensitivity to the p38 MAPK activator anisomycin; 8BrcGMP effects on Gly56 SERT are completely blocked by coincubation with the PKG inhibitor H8 (10 μM), whereas the p38 MAPK inhibitor SB203580 (1 μM) prevented anisomycin stimulation (data not shown). Data plotted represent mean data ± SD (n = 3) for a single cell line of each genotype assayed in parallel. Findings were replicated with identical results in an additional line for each genotype.

mit a rare genomic variant (hCV11414114) (table 3) to all affected children. The study by Glatt and colleagues (2001) did not detect the three novel coding alleles in the 450 individuals (900 chromosomes) sequenced; this indicates that these alleles are rare and have a frequency of <1/900, or <0.11%.

Cross-species conservation of novel coding-variant residues and their identification in linked families suggests an increased likelihood of altered functionality for the variant transporter, although future study will be required to fully elaborate this premise. All three novel substitutions occur within transmembrane domains (fig. 1*E*), and the 425Leu allele affects the identical residue and nucleotide—as does the Ile425Val mutant in the pedigrees described by Ozaki and colleagues (2003)—that segregates Asperger syndrome (MIM 608638), obsessive-compulsive disorder (OCD [MIM 164230]), and other psychiatric phenotypes. The Ile425Leu variant does, therefore, have an a priori increased likelihood of functional effect that is based on prior precedent from disease association and subsequent functional characterization of the Ile425Val substitution showing ~2-fold elevated basal activity in transfection studies (Kilic et al. 2003; Prasad et al., in press).

The Gly56Ala substitution shows a very suggestive increase of MAF to 2.3% in the 120 linked families, compared with the 1.1% seen in the remaining families. A 2.3% allele frequency represents a noticeable increase over the single *nonclinical* reference study (Glatt et al. 2001), which shows 4 of 900 (0.44%) chromosomes (and no homozygotes) carrying a 56Ala allele. HWE would dictate a frequency of homozygous individuals to be ~1/2,000 in unrelated individuals (or ~1/5,000 on the basis of a 0.44% frequency in the Glatt et al. [2001] comparison sample). Therefore, our finding of three homozygotes and two additional (unrelated) instances of dual heterozygous couples is highly unlikely by chance ($P \approx 0$). The findings of (1) an apparent fivefold increase in 56Ala allele frequency in the linked families, with a trend toward overtransmission, (2) a substantial deviation from HWE, and (3) a male-biased trend toward autism affection in the presence of this allele compared with females indicates a role for the 56Ala allele as a genetic risk factor in autism. The infrequency of the allele, however, makes this more difficult to quantitate. Larger autism population studies are indicated.

Equally important are functional data that demonstrate that the 56Ala SERT protein displays an elevated basal activity and insensitivity to regulation through PKG and p38 MAPK signaling pathways in a native cell system. Importantly, down-regulation in response to protein kinase C–activating phorbol esters was equivalent between Gly56 and Ala56 lines (data not shown). We do not believe that PKG/p38 MAPK regulatory insensitivity derives directly from altered basal activities, since we have demonstrated transport regulation through these pathways with other variants that differed up to 10-fold in activity (Prasad et al., in press), although over-expression in transfected cells can blunt regulation (C.-B. Zhu and R.D.B., unpublished findings). Elevated basal 5-HT uptake is also not due to enhanced transcription, since RealTime PCR analysis revealed equal SERT mRNA levels in the Gly56 and Ala56 lines (data not shown). Elevated basal activity of the Ala56-encoded transporter is intriguing in light of a similar effect with 425Val-encoded SERT in patients with Asperger syndrome and OCD. Although altered regulation was not seen with the Ile425Val mutation, the elevated basal transporter activity may suggest a common functional mechanism important in autism, OCD, and other phenotypes. It is possible that prolonged expression of a variant lacking regulation induces other compensatory changes that influence basal transporter activity. Regardless, these findings suggest that Gly56Ala carriers may possess an *inflexibility to regulatory stimuli* that could thereby compromise appropriate demand-dependent modulation of SERT surface expression and/or catalytic activity.

Phenotypically, the three novel variants and Gly56Ala are significantly associated with increased rigid-compulsive behaviors. These include (1) stereotyped utterances, (2) unusual preoccupations, (3) compulsions/rituals, (4) resistance to trivial changes in the environment, and (5) unusual attachment to objects (Tadevosyan-Leyfer et al. 2003). This is important for several reasons. Our previous study of linkage in a smaller sample demonstrated a significant increase in linkage at ~53 cM when the same rigid-compulsive trait was used to stratify the data set (McCauley et al. 2004). It is consistent with the finding of Asperger syndrome, OCD, and other traits in families segregating the functionally abnormal (Prasad et al., in press) Ile425Val substitution (Ozaki et al. 2003). Obsessive-compulsive–type traits and clinical OCD are seen more frequently in families with autism than in the general population (Bolton et al. 1998). Repetitive behaviors and associated anxiety in autism and OCD are often effectively treated with SSRIs, targeting the SERT protein (Hollander et al. 2005). Whereas other phenotypic findings associated with specific variants were variable across families with all four variants, increased severity for the rigid-compulsive domain was a consistent finding for these variants. Given the magnitude of the observed genetic effect, the possibility exists that our sample may be enriched by chance or selection methods for phenotypic traits (or regional alleles) that bias in favor of an effect at this locus.

The functionality of promoter and other noncoding variants is unknown; however, the segregation of these multiple variants in aggregate, in addition to the coding variants, provides additional genetic evidence of an allelic heterogeneity framework for disease risk involving *SLC6A4*. Several previously documented variants (*rs2020932*, hCV11414117, and hCV11414114) were each found in multiple families. These heterogeneous variants arose largely on independent haplotypic backgrounds, which indicates that they are rare independent events and are not the result of an effect of some common genetic background. The clustering of collectively associated rare genomic variants in the promoter and near the 5′ end of the gene raises the possibility of transcriptional effects at *SLC6A4*. Intronic or noncoding transcribed variants may, if they are risk factors with biological relevance, affect transcription, transcript stability, or RNA splicing (Pagani and Baralle 2004). An expression-based mechanism for potentially disease-related 5′ variants is consistent with association of the HTTLPR marker, since the insertion/deletion variant exhibits differential transcription. Even with a relatively conservative analysis of transmission by eliminating the subject from each family in whom the variant was discovered, association data in the presence of linkage must be interpreted cautiously. The analysis of transmissions in families with an a priori expectation of variable allele-sharing would inflate any measure of allelic association, and the TDT analysis of *multiplex* families in this unusual context would yield a measure of linkage (Spielman and Ewens 1996). Nevertheless, the context in which these observations are made supports the significance of association in the aggregate of these multiple variants. The modest association at 5-HTTLPR and the intron 5 SNP *rs140700* in the current MO sample is not only consistent with but is also supportive of this proposed risk framework. Other common alleles are not associated with autism, whereas the heterogeneous rare alleles described in this report are. Thus, the most parsimonious model involves multiple different risk alleles (including 5-HTTLPR) that act in different families to collectively account for the observed linkage.

The import of our data is summarized by the constellation of findings, including (1) three novel highly conserved coding variants, one of which affects a residue (Ile425) with known phenotypic and functional relevance; (2) the dysfunctional properties of SERT encoded with the Gly56Ala substitution; (3) the stark deviation from HWE and increased frequency in linked families; (4) a phenotypic correlation between coding variants and increased rigid-compulsive behaviors; and (5) the aggregate association shown by heterogeneous promoter 5′ and intragenic noncoding variants. These data collectively support the premise that *SLC6A4* represents a susceptibility locus for autism-spectrum disorders. Our findings must be examined in larger independent autism family populations with similar phenotypic representation to determine their ultimate significance. Given the linkage reported at *SLC6A4* by IMGSAC (as well as AGRE) and incomplete screening in the current sample (only one affected individual per family was screened for exon and promoter variants), we suspect that additional coding and noncoding variants will be discovered at this locus. As they stand now, our findings provide compelling evidence that the *SLC6A4* locus is a bona fide autism-susceptibility gene, with variants predisposing to rigid-compulsive traits.

Acknowledgments

This work was supported, in part, by National Institutes of Health (NIH) grants MH61009 (to J.S.S.), MH55135 (to S.E.F.), and DA07390 (to R.D.B.); Vanderbilt Kennedy Center Hobbs Research Awards (to J.S.S. and R.D.B.); a Family Research Award (to J.S.S.); generous support from the National Alliance for Autism Research (to J.S.S.); and a Pre-Doctoral fellowship (J.L.M.). We thank Jonathan L. Haines for helpful discussions and evaluation of the manuscript. We acknowledge the important contributions to this work by the staff at the Vanderbilt Center for Human Genetics Research, including the DNA Resources, Data Analysis, Family Ascertainment, and Bioinformatics Cores, and the Center for Molecular Neuroscience Neurogenomics Core. Some of this work was also supported by Vanderbilt General Clinical Research Center grant M01 RR-00095, NIH Center for Research Resources. We especially acknowledge the families that have participated in this research and resources provided by the NIMH Center for Collaborative Genetic Studies on Mental Disorders repository, without which this work would not have been possible.

Biomaterials and phenotypic data provided through the NIMH Autism Genetics Initiative came from three projects: (1) Data and biomaterial collection was supported by NIH grant MH55135 ("Collaborative Linkage Study of Autism") to S.E.F., and her key Clinical and Phenotypic Coordinators were Brian Winklosky and Beth Rosen-Sheidley, M.S., C.G.C. Coinvestigators included J.S.S. and Jonathan L. Haines. (2) Data and biomaterial collection was also supported by a supplement to NIH grant MH61009 ("Molecular Genetics of 15q11-q13 Defects in Autism") and by Development Funds from the Vanderbilt Centers for Human Genetics Research and the Kennedy Center for Research on Human Development (to J.S.S.). The clinical and phenotypic coordinator for this project was Genea Crocket, M.S. (3) Data and biomaterial collection from the AGRE collection was supported by NIH grant MH64547 to Daniel H. Geschwind, M.D., Ph.D. (University of California at Los Angeles [UCLA]) and the Cure Autism Now Foundation. Coprincipal investigators include Stanley F. Nelson, M.D., and Rita Cantor, Ph.D. (UCLA) and Christa Lese Martin, Ph.D., and T. Conrad Gilliam, Ph.D. (University of Chicago). Coinvestigators include Maricela Alarcón, Ph.D., Kenneth Lange, Ph.D., and Sarah J. Spence M.D., Ph.D. (UCLA), David H. Ledbetter Ph.D. (Emory), and Hank Juo, M.D., Ph.D. (Columbia). Scientific oversight of AGRE is provided by the AGRE steering committee (chair: Daniel H. Geschwind, M.D., Ph.D.; members: W. Ted Brown, M.D., Ph.D., Maja Bucan, Ph.D., Joseph Buxbaum, Ph.D., T. Conrad Gilliam, Ph.D., David Greenberg, Ph.D., David Ledbetter, Ph.D., Bruce Miller, M.D., Stanley F. Nelson, M.D., Jonathan

Pevsner, Ph.D., Carol Sprouse, Ed.D., Gerard Schellenberg, Ph.D., and Rudolph Tanzi, Ph.D.

Web Resources

Accession numbers and URLs for data presented herein are as follows:

GenBank, http://www.ncbi.nlm.nih.gov/Genbank/ (for *SLC6A4* [accession number NM_001045])
NIMH Center for Collaborative Genetic Studies on Mental Disorders, http://www.nimhgenetics.org/
Online Mendelian Inheritance in Man (OMIM), http://www.ncbi.nlm.nih.gov/Omim/ (for autism, *SLC6A4, ITGB3,* Asperger syndrome, and OCD)
Single Nucleotide Polymorphism, http://www.ncbi.nlm.nih.gov/SNP/ (for dbSNP numbers *ss38318598, ss38318599, ss38318600, ss38318601, ss38318589, ss38318590, ss38318591, ss38318592, ss38318593, ss38318594, ss38318595, ss38318596,* and *ss38318597*)

References

Ashley-Koch A, Wolpert CM, Menold MM, Zaeem L, Basu S, Donnelly SL, Ravan SA, Powell CM, Qumsiyeh MB, Aylsworth AS, Vance JM, Gilbert JR, Wright HH, Abramson RK, DeLong GR, Cuccaro ML, Pericak-Vance MA (1999) Genetic studies of autistic disorder and chromosome 7. Genomics 61:227–236
Auranen M, Nieminen T, Majuri S, Vanhala R, Peltonen L, Jarvela I (2000) Analysis of autism susceptibility gene loci on chromosomes 1p, 4p, 6q, 7q, 13q, 15q, 16p, 17q, 19q and 22q in Finnish multiplex families. Mol Psychiatry 5:320–322
Bolton PF, Pickles A, Murphy M, Rutter M (1998) Autism, affective and other psychiatric disorders: patterns of familial aggregation. Psychol Med 28:385–395
Buxbaum JD, Silverman J, Keddache M, Smith CJ, Hollander E, Ramoz N, Reichert JG (2004) Linkage analysis for autism in a subset families with obsessive-compulsive behaviors: evidence for an autism susceptibility gene on chromosome 1 and further support for susceptibility genes on chromosome 6 and 19. Mol Psychiatry 9:144–150
Buxbaum JD, Silverman JM, Smith CJ, Kilifarski M, Reichert J, Hollander E, Lawlor BA, Fitzgerald M, Greenberg DA, Davis KL (2001) Evidence for a susceptibility gene for autism on chromosome 2 and for genetic heterogeneity. Am J Hum Genet 68:1514–1520
Cantor RM, Kono N, Duvall JA, Alvarez-Retuerto A, Stone JL, Alarcón M, Nelson SF, Geschwind DH (2005) Replication of autism linkage: fine-mapping peak at 17q21. Am J Hum Genet 76:1050–1056
Cargill M, Altshuler D, Ireland J, Sklar P, Ardlie K, Patil N, Shaw N, Lane CR, Lim EP, Kalyanaraman N, Nemesh J, Ziaugra L, Friedland L, Rolfe A, Warrington J, Lipshutz R, Daley GQ, Lander ES (1999) Characterization of single-nucleotide polymorphisms in coding regions of human genes. Nat Genet 22:231–238
Chakrabarti S, Fombonne E (2001) Pervasive developmental disorders in preschool children. JAMA 285:3093–3099
Collaborative Linkage Study of Autism (2001) Incorporating language phenotypes strengthens evidence of linkage to autism. Am J Med Genet 105:539–547
Collaborative Linkage Study of Autism, Barrett S, Beck JC, Bernier R, Bisson E, Braun TA, Casavant TL, et al (1999) An autosomal genomic screen for autism. Am J Med Genet 88:609–615
Conroy J, Meally E, Kearney G, Fitzgerald M, Gill M, Gallagher L (2004) Serotonin transporter gene and autism: a haplotype analysis in an Irish autistic population. Mol Psychiatry 9:587–593
Cook EH, Leventhal BL (1996) The serotonin system in autism. Curr Opin Pediatr 8:348–354
Cook EH Jr, Arora RC, Anderson GM, Berry-Kravis EM, Yan SY, Yeoh HC, Sklena PJ, Charak DA, Leventhal BL (1993) Platelet serotonin studies in hyperserotonemic relatives of children with autistic disorder. Life Sciences 52:2005–2015
Cook EH Jr, Courchesne R, Lord C, Cox NJ, Yan S, Lincoln A, Haas R, Courchesne E, Leventhal BL (1997) Evidence of linkage between the serotonin transporter and autistic disorder. Mol Psychiatry 2:247–250
den Dunnen JT, Antonarakis SE (2001) Nomenclature for the description of human sequence variations. Hum Genet 109: 121–124
Devlin B, Cook Jr EH, Coon H, Dawson G, Grigorenko EL, McMahon W, Minshew N, Pauls D, Smith M, Spence MA, Rodier PM, Stodgell C, Network CG, Schellenberg GD. Autism and the serotonin transporter: the long and short of it. Mol Psychiatry (in press)
Faraj BA, Olkowski ZL, Jackson RT (1997) Prevalence of high serotonin uptake in lymphocytes of abstinent alcoholics. Biochem Pharmacol 53:53–57
Folstein S, Rutter M (1977) Genetic influences and infantile autism. Nature 265:726–728
Folstein SE, Rosen-Sheidley B (2001) Genetics of autism: complex aetiology for a heterogeneous disorder. Nat Rev Genet 2:943–955
Fombonne E (2003) The prevalence of autism. JAMA 289:87–89
Glatt CE, DeYoung JA, Delgado S, Service SK, Giacomini KM, Edwards RH, Risch N, Freimer NB (2001) Screening a large reference sample to identify very low frequency sequence variants: comparisons between two genes. Nat Genet 27: 435–438
Gordon D, Desmarais C, Green P (2001) Automated finishing with autofinish. Genome Res 11:614–625
Gudbjartsson DF, Jonasson K, Frigge ML, Kong A (2000) Allegro, a new computer program for multipoint linkage analysis. Nat Genet 25:12–13
Hahn MK, Blakely RD (2002) Monoamine transporter gene structure and polymorphisms in relation to psychiatric and other complex disorders. Pharmacogenomics J 2:217–235
Hollander E, Phillips A, Chaplin W, Zagursky K, Novotny S, Wasserman S, Iyengar R (2005) A placebo controlled crossover trial of liquid fluoxetine on repetitive behaviors in childhood and adolescent autism. Neuropsychopharmacology 30: 582–589
Holloway JW, Beghe B, Turner S, Hinks LJ, Day IN, Howell WM (1999) Comparison of three methods for single nucleotide polymorphism typing for DNA bank studies: sequence-specific oligonucleotide probe hybridisation, TaqMan liquid

phase hybridisation, and microplate array diagonal gel electrophoresis (MADGE). Hum Mutat 14:340–347

International Molecular Genetic Study of Autism Consortium (1998) A full genome screen for autism with evidence for linkage to a region on chromosome 7q. Hum Mol Genet 7: 571–578

——— (2001*a*) A genomewide screen for autism: strong evidence for linkage to chromosomes 2q, 7q, and 16p. Am J Hum Genet 69:570–581

——— (2001*b*) Further characterization of the autism susceptibility locus *AUTS1* on chromosome 7q. Hum Mol Genet 10:973–982

Jones MB, Szatmari P (1988) Stoppage rules and genetic studies of autism. J Autism Dev Disord 18:31–40

Kanner L (1943) Autistic disturbance of affective contact. Nervous Child 2:217–250

Khan NA, Meyneil JP, Deschaux P (1996) Ca^{2+}/calmodulin and protein kinase C regulation of serotonin transport in human K562 lymphocytes. Cell Immunol 172:269–274

Kilic F, Murphy DL, Rudnick G (2003) A human serotonin transporter mutation causes constitutive activation of transport activity. Mol Pharmacol 64:440–446

Kim SJ, Cox N, Courchesne R, Lord C, Corsello C, Akshoomoff N, Guter S, Leventhal BL, Courchesne E, Cook Jr EH (2002) Transmission disequilibrium mapping at the serotonin transporter gene (*SLC6A4*) region in autistic disorder. Mol Psychiatry 7:278–288

Klauck SM, Poustka F, Benner A, Lesch KP, Poustka A (1997) Serotonin transporter (5-HTT) gene variants associated with autism. Hum Mol Genet 6:2233–2238

Kong A, Gudbjartsson DF, Sainz J, Jonsdottir GM, Gudjonsson SA, Richardsson B, Sigurdardottir S, Barnard J, Hallbeck B, Masson G, Shlien A, Palsson ST, Frigge ML, Thorgeirsson TE, Gulcher JR, Stefansson K (2002) A high-resolution recombination map of the human genome. Nat Genet 31:241–247

Lesch KP, Bengel D, Heils A, Sabol SZ, Greenberg BD, Petri S, Benjamin J, Muller CR, Hamer DH, Murphy DL (1996) Association of anxiety-related traits with a polymorphism in the serotonin transporter gene regulatory region. Science 274:1527–1531

Li Q, Liu Z, Monroe H, Culiat CT (2002) Integrated platform for detection of DNA sequence variants using capillary array electrophoresis. Electrophoresis 23:1499–1511

Liu J, Nyholt DR, Magnussen P, Parano E, Pavone P, Geschwind D, Lord C, Iversen P, Hoh J, the Autism Genetic Resource Exchange, Ott J, Gilliam TC (2001) A genomewide screen for autism susceptibility loci. Am J Hum Genet 69: 327–340

MacKenzie A, Quinn J (1999) A serotonin transporter gene intron 2 polymorphic region, correlated with affective disorders, has allele-dependent differential enhancer-like properties in the mouse embryo. Proc Natl Acad Sci USA 96: 15251–15255

Maestrini E, Lai C, Marlow A, Matthews N, Wallace S, Bailey A, Cook EH, Weeks DE, Monaco AP, the International Molecular Genetic Study of Autism Consortium (1999) Serotonin transporter (*5-HTT*) and γ-aminobutyric acid receptor subunit $\beta 3$ (*GABRB3*) gene polymorphisms are not associated with autism in the IMGSA families. Am J Med Genet 88:492–496

Martin ER, Monks SA, Warren LL, Kaplan NL (2000) A test for linkage and association in general pedigrees: the pedigree disequilibrium test. Am J Hum Genet 67:146–154

McCauley JL, Li C, Jiang L, Olson LM, Crockett G, Gainer K, Folstein SE, Haines JL, Sutcliffe JS (2005) Genome-wide and Ordered-Subset linkage analyses provide support for autism loci on 17q and 19p with evidence of phenotypic and interlocus genetic correlates. BMC Med Genet 6:1

McCauley JL, Olson LM, Dowd M, Amin T, Steele A, Blakely RD, Folstein SE, Haines JL, Sutcliffe JS (2004) Linkage and association analysis at the serotonin transporter (*SLC6A4*) locus in a rigid-compulsive subset of autism. Am J Med Genet B Neuropsychiatr Genet 127:104–112

McPeek MS (1999) Optimal allele-sharing statistics for genetic mapping using affected relatives. Genet Epidemiol 16:225–249

Miller KJ, Hoffman BJ (1994) Adenosine A3 receptors regulate serotonin transport via nitric oxide and cGMP. J Biol Chem 269:27351–27356

Nickerson DA, Kolker N, Taylor SL, Rieder MJ (2001) Sequence-based detection of single nucleotide polymorphisms. Methods Mol Biol 175:29–35

Nickerson DA, Tobe VO, Taylor SL (1997) PolyPhred: automating the detection and genotyping of single nucleotide substitutions using fluorescence-based resequencing. Nucleic Acids Res 25:2745–2751

Ogilvie AD, Battersby S, Bubb VJ, Fink G, Harmar AJ, Goodwim GM, Smith CA (1996) Polymorphism in serotonin transporter gene associated with susceptibility to major depression. Lancet 347:731–733

Ozaki N, Goldman D, Kaye WH, Plotnicov K, Greenberg BD, Lappalainen J, Rudnick G, Murphy DL (2003) Serotonin transporter missense mutation associated with a complex neuropsychiatric phenotype. Mol Psychiatry 8:933–936

Pagani F, Baralle FE (2004) Genomic variants in exons and introns: identifying the splicing spoilers. Nat Rev Genet 5: 389–396

Persico AM, Militerni R, Bravaccio C, Schneider C, Melmed R, Conciatori M, Damiani V, Baldi A, Keller F (2000) Lack of association between serotonin transporter gene promoter variants and autistic disorder in two ethnically distinct samples. Am J Med Genet 96:123–127

Philippe A, Martinez M, Guilloud-Bataille M, Gillberg C, Rastam M, Sponheim E, Coleman M, Zappella M, Aschauer H, van Malldergerme L, Penet C, Feingold J, Brice A, Leboyer M (1999) Genome-wide scan for autism susceptibility genes. Hum Mol Genet 8:805–812

Pickles A, Bolton P, Macdonald H, Bailey A, Le Couteur A, Sim CH, Rutter M (1995) Latent-class analysis of recurrence risks for complex phenotypes with selection and measurement error: a twin and family history study of autism. Am J Hum Genet 57:717–726

Prasad HC, Zhu C-B, McCauley JL, Samuvel DJ, Ramamoorthy S, Shelton R, Hewlett WA, Sutcliffe JS, Blakely RD. Human serotonin transporter variants display selective insensitivity to protein kinase G and p38 mitogen activated protein kinase. Proc Natl Acad Sci USA (in press)

Qian Y, Galli A, Ramamoorthy S, Risso S, DeFelice LJ, Blakely RD (1997) Protein kinase C activation regulates human serotonin transporters in HEK-293 cells via altered cell surface expression. J Neurosci 17:45–57

Ramamoorthy S, Blakely RD (1999) Phosphorylation and sequestration of serotonin transporters differentially modulated by psychostimulants. Science 285:763–766

Risch N, Spiker D, Lotspeich L, Nouri N, Hinds D, Hallmayer J, Kalaydjieva L, et al (1999) A genomic screen of autism: evidence for a multilocus etiology. Am J Hum Genet 65:493–507

Ritvo ER, Freeman BJ, Pingree C, Mason-Brothers A, Jorde L, Jenson WR, McMahon WM, Petersen PB, Mo A, Ritvo A (1989) The UCLA–University of Utah epidemiologic survey of autism: prevalence. Am J Psychiatry 146:194–199

Samuvel DJ, Jayanthi LD, Bhat NR, Ramamoorthy S (2005) A role for p38 mitogen-activated protein kinase in the regulation of the serotonin transporter: evidence for distinct cellular mechanisms involved in transporter surface expression. J Neurosci 25:29–41

Schain RJ, Freedman D (1961) Studies on 5-hydroxyindole metabolism in autistic disorder and other mentally retarded children. J Pediatr 58:315–320

Shao Y, Raiford KL, Wolpert CM, Cope HA, Ravan SA, Ashley-Koch AA, Abramson RK, Wright HH, DeLong RG, Gilbert JR, Cuccaro ML, Pericak-Vance MA (2002*a*) Phenotypic homogeneity provides increased support for linkage on chromosome 2 in autistic disorder. Am J Hum Genet 70: 1058–1061

Shao Y, Wolpert CM, Raiford KL, Menold MM, Donnelly SL, Ravan SA, Bass MP, McClain C, von Wendt L, Vance JM, Abramson RH, Wright HH, Ashley-Koch A, Gilbert JR, DeLong RG, Cuccaro ML, Pericak-Vance MA, McCoy PA (2002*b*) Genomic screen and follow-up analysis for autistic disorder. Am J Med Genet 114:99–105

Spielman RS, Ewens WJ (1996) The TDT and other family-based tests for linkage disequilibrium and association. Am J Hum Genet 59:983–989

Stone JL, Merriman B, Cantor RM, Yonan AL, Gilliam TC, Geschwind DH, Nelson SF (2004) Evidence for sex-specific risk alleles in autism spectrum disorder. Am J Hum Genet 75:1117–1123

Tadevosyan-Leyfer O, Dowd M, Mankoski R, Winklosky B, Putnam S, McGrath L, Tager-Flusberg H, Folstein SE (2003) A principal components analysis of the Autism Diagnostic Interview–Revised. J Am Acad Child Adolesc Psychiatry 42: 864–872

Tordjman S, Gutknecht L, Carlier M, Spitz E, Antoine C, Slama F, Carsalade V, Cohen DJ, Ferrari P, Roubertoux PL, Anderson GM (2001) Role of the serotonin transporter gene in the behavioral expression of autism. Mol Psychiatry 6: 434–439

Veenstra-VanderWeele J, Anderson GM, Cook EH Jr (2000) Pharmacogenetics and the serotonin system: initial studies and future directions. Eur J Pharmacol 410:165–181

Veenstra-VanderWeele J, Christian SL, Cook EH Jr (2004) Autism as a paradigmatic complex genetic disorder. Annu Rev Genomics Hum Genet 5:379–405

Weiss LA, Abney M, Cook EH Jr, Ober C (2005) Sex-specific genetic architecture of whole blood serotonin levels. Am J Hum Genet 76:33–41

Yeargin-Allsopp M, Rice C, Karapurkar T, Doernberg N, Boyle C, Murphy C (2003) Prevalence of autism in a US metropolitan area. JAMA 289:49–55

Yirmiya N, Pilowsky T, Nemanov L, Arbelle S, Feinsilver T, Fried I, Ebstein RP (2001) Evidence for an association with the serotonin transporter promoter region polymorphism and autism. Am J Med Genet 105:381–386

Yonan AL, Alarcón M, Cheng R, Magnusson PKE, Spence SJ, Palmer AA, Grunn A, Hank Juo S-H, Terwilliger JD, Liu J, Cantor RM, Geschwind DH, Gilliam TC (2003) A genome-wide screen of 345 families for autism-susceptibility loci. Am J Hum Genet 73:886–897

Zhu C-B, Carneiro AM, Dostmann WR, Hewlett WA, Blakely RD (2005) p38 MAPK activation elevates serotonin transport activity via a trafficking-independent, protein phosphatase 2a-dependent process. J Biol Chem 280:15649–15658

Zhu C-B, Hewlett WA, Feoktistov I, Biaggioni I, Blakely RD (2004) Adenosine receptor, protein kinase G, and p38 mitogen-activated protein kinase-dependent up-regulation of serotonin transporters involves both transporter trafficking and activation. Mol Pharmacol 65:1462–1474

Am. J. Hum. Genet. 77:280–296, 2005

An Autosomal Dominant Cerebellar Ataxia Linked to Chromosome 16q22.1 Is Associated with a Single-Nucleotide Substitution in the 5′ Untranslated Region of the Gene Encoding a Protein with Spectrin Repeat and Rho Guanine-Nucleotide Exchange-Factor Domains

Kinya Ishikawa,[1,*] Shuta Toru,[1,*] Taiji Tsunemi,[1] Mingshun Li,[1] Kazuhiro Kobayashi,[8] Takanori Yokota,[1] Takeshi Amino,[1] Kiyoshi Owada,[1] Hiroto Fujigasaki,[1] Masaki Sakamoto,[1] Hiroyuki Tomimitsu,[1] Minoru Takashima,[1] Jiro Kumagai,[2] Yoshihiro Noguchi,[3] Yoshiyuki Kawashima,[3] Norio Ohkoshi,[9] Gen Ishida,[10] Manabu Gomyoda,[11] Mari Yoshida,[12] Yoshio Hashizume,[12] Yuko Saito,[5] Shigeo Murayama,[5] Hiroshi Yamanouchi,[6] Toshio Mizutani,[7] Ikuko Kondo,[13] Tatsushi Toda,[8] and Hidehiro Mizusawa[1,4]

Departments of [1]Neurology and Neurological Science, [2]Pathology, and [3]Audiovestibular Science, Graduate School, and [4]The 21st Century Center of Excellence Program on Brain Integration and Its Disorders, Tokyo Medical and Dental University, [5]Department of Neuropathology, Tokyo Metropolitan Institute of Gerontology, [6]Department of Neurology, Tokyo Metropolitan Geriatric Hospital, and [7]Department of Pathology, Tokyo Metropolitan Neurological Hospital, Tokyo; [8]Division of Functional Genomics, Department of Post-Genomics and Diseases, Course of Advanced Medicine, Osaka University Graduate School of Medicine, Osaka, Japan; [9]Department of Neurology, Institute of Clinical Medicine, University of Tsukuba, Tsukuba, Japan; Departments of [10]Neurology and [11]Clinical Laboratory, National Matsue Hospital, Matsue, Japan; [12]Department of Neuropathology, Institute of Medical Science of Aging, Aichi Medical University, Aichi, Japan; and [13]Department of Medical Genetics, Ehime University School of Medicine, Ehime, Japan

Autosomal dominant cerebellar ataxia (ADCA) is a group of heterogeneous neurodegenerative disorders. By positional cloning, we have identified the gene strongly associated with a form of degenerative ataxia (chromosome 16q22.1–linked ADCA) that clinically shows progressive pure cerebellar ataxia. Detailed examination by use of audiogram suggested that sensorineural hearing impairment may be associated with ataxia in our families. After restricting the candidate region in chromosome 16q22.1 by haplotype analysis, we found that all patients from 52 unrelated Japanese families harbor a heterozygous C→T single-nucleotide substitution, 16 nt upstream of the putative translation initiation site of the gene for a hypothetical protein DKFZP434I216, which we have called "puratrophin-1" (Purkinje cell atrophy associated protein-1). The full-length *puratrophin-1* mRNA had an open reading frame of 3,576 nt, predicted to contain important domains, including the spectrin repeat and the guanine-nucleotide exchange factor (GEF) for Rho GTPases, followed by the Dbl-homologous domain, which indicates the role of puratrophin-1 in intracellular signaling and actin dynamics at the Golgi apparatus. Puratrophin-1—normally expressed in a wide range of cells, including epithelial hair cells in the cochlea—was aggregated in Purkinje cells of the chromosome 16q22.1–linked ADCA brains. Consistent with the protein prediction data of puratrophin-1, the Golgi-apparatus membrane protein and spectrin also formed aggregates in Purkinje cells. The present study highlights the importance of the 5′ untranslated region (UTR) in identification of genes of human disease, suggests that a single-nucleotide substitution in the 5′ UTR could be associated with protein aggregation, and indicates that the GEF protein is associated with cerebellar degeneration in humans.

Introduction

Autosomal dominant cerebellar ataxia (ADCA) is a clinical entity of heterogeneous neurodegenerative diseases that show dominantly inherited, progressive cerebellar ataxia that can be variably associated with other neurological and systemic features (Harding 1982). Circumscribed groups of neurons in the cerebellum, brainstem, basal ganglia, or spinal cord are selectively involved in different combinations and to varying extents among diseases (Graham and Lantos 2002). ADCA is now classified by the responsible mutations or gene loci. To date, 24 subtypes have been identified: spinocerebellar ataxia type (SCA) 1, 2, 3 (or, Machado-Joseph disease [MJD]), 4–8, 10–19/22, 21, 23, 25, 26; dentatorubral and pallidoluysian atrophy (DRPLA); and ADCA with mutation in fibroblast growth factor (FGF) 14 (Stevanin et

Received March 15, 2005; accepted for publication June 3, 2005; electronically published July 6, 2005.

Address for correspondence and reprints: Dr. Hidehiro Mizusawa, Professor and Chairman, Department of Neurology and Neurological Science, Graduate School, Tokyo Medical and Dental University, 1-5-45 Yushima, Bunkyo-ku 113-8519, Tokyo, Japan. E-mail: h-mizusawa.nuro@tmd.ac.jp

* These two authors contributed equally to this work.

0002-9297/2005/7702-0010$15.00

al. 2000, 2004; Margolis 2002; van Swieten et al. 2003; Yu et al. 2005). Among these, mutations in SCA1, SCA2, SCA3/MJD, SCA6, SCA7, SCA17, and DRPLA have been identified as the expansion of a trinucleotide (CAG) repeat that encodes the polyglutamine tract, uniformly causing aggregation of polyglutamine-containing causative protein (Ross and Poirier 2004). Expansion of noncoding trinucleotide (CAG or CTG) or pentanucleotide (ATTCT) repeats are involved in SCA8, SCA10, and SCA12 (Holmes et al. 1999; Koob et al. 1999; Matsuura et al. 2000). Very few families are affected by missense mutations in the protein kinase Cγ (PKCγ) (SCA14 [see Chen et al. 2003]) and *FGF14* genes (ADCA with *FGF14* mutation [see van Swieten et al. 2003]). However, genes or even their loci remain unidentified for >20%–40% of families with ADCA (Sasaki et al. 2003).

We had previously mapped mutations in six Japanese families with ADCA to a 10-cM interval in human chromosome 16q13.1-q22.1, identifying 16q-linked ADCA type III, or spinocerebellar ataxia 4 (SCA4 [MIM 600223]) (Ishikawa et al. 2000). Clinically, our families show cerebellar ataxia without obvious evidence of extracerebellar neurological dysfunction (i.e., "pure cerebellar ataxia," or "ADCA type III") (Harding 1982; Ishikawa et al. 2000). The average age at onset of ataxia was >55 years (Ishikawa et al. 1997), which suggests that this disease shows the oldest age at onset among ADCA types with assigned loci. Another important clinical feature of this disease is that a substantial number of patients show progressive sensorineural hearing impairment (Owada et al., in press). Since the hearing impairment can be very mild and of later onset, presence of hearing impairment can be easily overlooked. However, this finding may indicate that the mutated gene could cause hearing impairment as well as ataxia. In this sense, it would be more appropriate to use the term "chromosome 16q22.1–linked ADCA" instead of "ADCA type III" to describe our families. Neuropathological examination showed peculiar degeneration of Purkinje cells that was not described in other degenerative ataxias (Owada et al., in press). Many Purkinje cells undergo shrinkage and are surrounded by amorphous materials composed of Purkinje-cell somato-dendritic sprouts and an increased number of presynaptic terminals. These findings may indicate that certain proteins involved in the cytoskeleton of Purkinje cells are disturbed in chromosome 16q22.1–linked ADCA.

Chromosome 16q22.1–linked ADCA has been assigned to the same locus as another ADCA, SCA4 (Flanigan et al. 1996; Hellenbroich et al. 2003). Although SCA4 and chromosome 16q22.1–linked ADCA may be allelic, SCA4 is clinically distinct from chromosome 16q22.1–linked ADCA, because SCA4 shows prominent sensory axonal neuropathy and pyramidal tract signs, with an age at onset earlier than that of chromosome 16q22.1–linked ADCA (Flanigan et al. 1996; Hellenbroich et al. 2003). Several groups, including ours, have refined the loci of SCA4/chromosome 16q22.1–linked ADCA and have, so far, excluded repeat expansions as mutations (Hellenbroich et al. 2003; Li et al. 2003; Hirano et al. 2004). The minimum candidate region of SCA4 and chromosome 16q22.1–linked ADCA is set at the region between markers *D16S3031* and *D16S3095*. A strong founder effect has been observed for chromosome 16q22.1–linked ADCA (Li et al. 2003), which indicates the need to recruit a large number of families to narrow the critical region.

To discover the causative gene of chromosome 16q22.1–linked ADCA, we embarked on a positional cloning study by recruiting 52 families from diverse regions of Japan. Here, we describe the identification of a strong association between a single-nucleotide change and chromosome 16q22.1–linked ADCA and show the consequence of this genetic change on mRNA and protein levels. The data presented here also suggest that a single-nucleotide change in the 5′ UTR could be associated with aggregation of the gene product.

Patients, Material, and Methods

Recruitment of Families with Chromosome 16q22.1–Linked ADCA

We attempted to include families clinically diagnosed with late-onset ADCA type III from a wide region of Japan. Fifty-two families, including 109 affected individuals and 48 at-risk individuals, were ultimately recruited. These families originated from seven of eight districts of Japan (Hokkaido, Tohoku, Kanto, Chu-bu, Kinki, Chu-goku, and Kyu-shu), which indicates that their origins are widespread. Clinical features of these patients were consistent with those of families described elsewhere (Ishikawa et al. 1997, 2000; Li et al. 2003).

Detailed neuro-otological examinations, including pure-tone audiometry, were performed on 13 families at the Departments of Neurology and Otolaryngology, Tokyo Medical and Dental University. Progressive hearing impairment was assessed when the pure-tone average calculated from thresholds at the frequencies of 0.5, 1, and 2 kHz was more severe than the mean +2 SD of age-matched normal Japanese population (Tsuiki et al. 2002). By that criterion, 6 (42.9%) of 14 families had a hearing impairment other than age-related hearing loss. When we used the recommendations for the description of genetic and audiological data composed by the GENDEAG study group (see The Hereditary Hearing Loss Homepage), all of the patients with the hearing impairment were confirmed to have bilateral sensorineural hearing loss of mild-to-moderate severity. The audiometric configurations of these patients include mid-frequency U-shaped, flat, and high-frequency sloping. These data would suggest that the hearing impairment in our families is not a coincidence.

Preparation of DNA and RNA Samples

After informed consent was obtained, genomic DNA was extracted from peripheral-blood lymphocytes or lymphoblastoid cell lines by use of methods described elsewhere (Ishikawa et al. 1997). All families were excluded for SCA1, SCA2, SCA3/MJD, SCA6, SCA7, SCA8, SCA12, SCA14, SCA17, and DRPLA by testing mutations in the disease genes. For expression analysis on an RNA level, frozen cerebellar tissues of four brains affected with Alzheimer disease (AD) (age at death, range 65–85 years; duration of the disease, range 5–10 years) were used as controls. Clinically, these patients with AD showed a moderate-to-severe degree of dementia, as measured by the Clinical Dementia Rating (Hughes et al. 1982). Neuropathology in the cerebella of these patients showed only a few senile plaques without neuronal losses. For chromosome 16q22.1–linked ADCA, two patients were studied (ages at death, 74 and 78 years). Both control and 16q22.1-linked ADCA brains were obtained at autopsy, with the families' written consents approved by each institutional ethical committee. These brains were immediately frozen and stored at −80°C until use. Total RNA was extracted from frozen cerebellar tissues as described elsewhere (Ishikawa et al. 1999). Poly-A^+ RNA was selected from total RNA by NucleoTrap (Macherey-Nagel).

Restriction of Candidate Interval by Genotyping and Haplotype Analysis

Genotypes were determined for 23 informative markers, including five new markers we identified (*GGAA10, TTCC01, TA001, GA001,* and *AAT01* [GenBank accession numbers AB13610, AB13611, AB13612, AB197662, and AB13613, respectively]) (table 1). Standard PCR was performed in a final volume of 20 μl, containing 10 ng of genomic DNA, 3.4 pmol of each primer, 2.5 mM of dNTP, and 0.75 U of *Taq* polymerase (Takara). Thermal cycling was performed at 94°C for 5 min for initial denaturing, 30 cycles of denaturation (94°C for 30 s), annealing (55°C for 30 s), and extension (72°C for 30 s), followed by a final extension at 72°C for 5 min in an ABI GeneAmp PCR system 9700 (PE Applied Biosystems). The amplified product was separated in the Automated Laser Fluorescent DNA Sequencer II (Pharmacia Biotech), and genotypes were determined with Fragment Manager (Pharmacia Biotech) (Ishikawa et al. 1997). Allele frequencies in the general population were analyzed in 500 unrelated individuals without personal or family history of ataxia or other degenerative diseases.

Table 1

Microsatellite Markers and Primer Sequences

The table is available in its entirety in the online edition of *The American Journal of Human Genetics.*

Haplotypes of 16q22.1 markers were determined for 10 families (fig. 1) that were informative for determining the phase of alleles. The remaining 42 families were not sufficiently informative for determining the phase. Paucity of informative families was mainly due to the late age at onset of this disease. For these uninformative families, only combinations of genotypes were assessed, and the region of genotypes shared with the larger 10 families was compared.

Screening for Mutation in 21 Different Candidate Genes

Within the most critical interval, 21 genes or clusters of ESTs were retrieved from the Ensembl, UniGene, National Center for Biotechnology Information (NCBI), and Celera databases. Primers were designed to amplify individual exon and intron-exon boundaries for each gene, and genomic DNA was amplified by the aforementioned standard PCR protocol (primer sequences are available on request). Amplicons from controls and patients were first separated on 2% agarose gels, to determine by screening whether any aberrant bands were amplified from patient DNA samples. Residual solutions of PCR products were then purified with QIAquick PCR purification kit (Qiagen) and were directly sequenced using Applied Biosystems Model 377 or 3100 Automated Sequencer, as described elsewhere (Li et al. 2003). The mutation was analyzed by comparing sequenced data and annotated databases, with use of the software DNASIS (Hitachi). Genomic rearrangement was screened by Southern-blot analysis by use of cosmid clones for probe synthesis as described elsewhere (Kobayashi et al. 1998). In brief, cosmid clones, tandemly covering the chromosome 16q22.1–linked ADCA critical region, were generated by subcloning from the BAC contig (Li et al. 2003). Then, the radiolabeled (^{32}P) probe was generated from each cosmid clone. Genomic DNA extracted from lymphoblastoid cell lines of control individuals and patients with chromosome 16q22.1–linked ADCA was digested with a restriction enzyme and was subjected to Southern-blot analysis. To screen gene arrangement, analysis was performed with six different restriction enzymes (*Bam*HI, *Bgl*II, *Eco*RI, *Eco*RV, *Hind*III, and *Xba*I).

Twenty-one exons and 20 introns of the *puratrophin-1* gene, partially annotated as "*Q9H7K4*," were sequenced entirely. The genomic region between the *puratrophin-1* gene and *SLC9A5* was also screened (fig. 2).

Families	P2	P4	P6	P12	P14	P15	T1	T2	T3	T4	T5	T6	T7	T8	T9	T10	T11	T12
No. of patients	7	6	4	6	3	2	5	4	6	8	2	2	2	2	2	2	2	3
No. of at-risk individuals	12	1	2	2	7	2	3	3	3	4	4	0	0	0	0	0	2	2
DNA marker																		
D16S3031	9	9	9	9	9	9	9	9	10	9	10	1	10	3/9	9	9	9	9
GGAA05	1	6	1	1	1	1	1	2	5	1	1	1	2	1/2	1/2	1/6	1	1
GGAA10	3	3	3	3	3	3	3	3	4	3/5	3	3	3	3/4	3/5	3/4	3	3
TTCC01	6	6	6	6	6	5/6	6	6	6	6/7	6	6/7	6	6	6	6	6	6/7
D16S3086	2	2	2	2	2	2	2	2	2	2	2	2	2	2	2	2	2	2/3
GATA01	2	2/3	2	2	2	1/2	2	2	2	3	3	3	2	2	2	2/3	2	2
D16S421	3	3	3	3	3	3	3	3	3	3	3	3	3	3/5	3	3	3	3
***Q9H7K4* /exon 1**	T	T	T	T	T	T/C	T	T	T	T	T	T/C	T/C	T/C	T/C	T/C	T/C	T/C
TA001	1	1	1	1	1	1	1	1	1	1	1	1	1	1/8	1	1	1	1
GA001	4	4	4	4	4	4	4	4	4	4	4	4/7	4/7	4/7	4/7	4/5	4	4
TTTA001	4	4	4	4	4	4	4	4	4	4	4	4	4	4	3/4	4	4	4
CATG003	4	4	4	4	4	4	4	4	4	4	4	4	4	4	4	4	4	4
17msm	2	2	2	2	2	2	2	2	2	2	2	2	2	2	2	2	2/3	5
D16S3107	7	7	7	7	7	7	7	7	7	7	6	7	7	6	7	4/7	7	7
D16S3085	2	2	2	2	2	2	2	2	2	2	2	2	2	2	2	2	2	2
ATT01	2	2	2	2	2	2	2	2	2	2	2/4	2	2	2/3	2	2	2	2
GGAA01	6	6	6	6	6	6	6	6	6	6	6	7	6	5/6	5	6	4/6	6
D16S3025	4	4	4	4	4	4	4	4	4	4	3/4	4	4	4	4	4	4	4
CTTT01	8	8	8	8	8	8	8	8	9/10	8	5	9	8	8/10	4/10	9/10	12	10
D16S496	5	5	5	5	5	5	5	5	5	5	5	5	5	5	5	1/5	5	5
D16S3141	3	3	3	3	3	3	3	3	3	3	3	3	3	3	3	3/6	4	3
D16S3067	5	5	5	5	5	5	5	5	5	5	5	5	5	5	5	5	5	5
GT01	6	6	6	6	6	6	1/6	6	6	6	7	6	6	3/6	2/6	4/6	5	4
D16S3095	2	3	1	1	1	1	2	2	1	1	2	3	2	1/3	1	1/2	1	1/2

Families	T13	T14	T15	T16	T17	T18	T19	T20	T21	T22	T23	T24	T25	T26	T27	T28	T29	T30
No. of patients	4	2	2	2	2	1	1	1	1	1	1	1	1	1	1	1	1	1
No. of at-risk individuals	0	0	1	0	0	0	0	0	0	0	0	0	0	0	0	0	0	0
DNA marker																		
D16S3031	8/9	9	9/10	9/10	9	9	9	9/10	9	9	9	9	9	9	9	1/9	9	9
GGAA05	1	1/4	2/4	1	1	1/5	1/3	1/4	1/5	1/5	1/2	1/5	5	1/2	1/5	1/7	1/5	1/5
GGAA10	3/5	3	3	3	3	2/3	3/6	3/6	2/3	3/5	3/4	1/3	2/4	3/7	3/6	3/5	1/3	3/8
TTCC01	6	6	5/6	6	6	6	6	6	6	6	6	6	6	6/7	6/7	6/7	6	5/6
D16S3086	2	2/3	2	2	2	2	2	2	2	2	2	2	2	2/3	2/3	2/3	2	2/3
GATA01	2	2	2	1/2	2	2	2/3	2	1/3	2	2	2/3	3/4	1/3	2	1/3	2	1
D16S421	3	3	3	3	3	3	3	3/4	3	3	3	3/4	3	3	3	3	3/4	3
***Q9H7K4* /exon 1**	T/C	T/C	T/C	T/C	T/C	T/C	T/C	T/C	T/C	T/C	T/C	T/C	T/C	T/C	T/C	T/C	T/C	T/C
TA001	1	1	1	1	1	1	1/9	1/10	1/7	1/8	1/7	1/6	2/8	1/6	1/10	1/10	1/7	1/9
GA001	4	4/7	4/5	4	4/7	4/7	1/4	4/7	4/8	4/7	4/5	4/7	4/5	4/7	4/7	4/7	4/7	4/6
TTTA001	4	4	4	4	4	4	4	4	3/4	3/4	3/4	3/4	4	4	3/4	4	4	3/4
CATG003	4/5	4	4	4	4	4	4	2/4	1/4	4	4/7	4	4/5	4	1/4	4	4/5	4
17msm	2	2/4	2/3	2	2	2	2/5	2/4	2/5	2/4	2/5	2/3	2/4	2/4	2/5	2/4	2/4	2/4
D16S3107	7	7/11	7	5	7/8	7	6	7	5/6	5/7	4/7	7	3/7	6/10	6/7	6	7	7
D16S3085	2	2	2	2	2	2	2	2	2	2	2	2	2	2	2/4	2	2/3	2
ATT01	2	2	2	2	2/3	2/6	2/3	2/3	2	2/3	2	2	2/3	2	2	2	2/4	2
GGAA01	6	6	5/6	1/6	6	4/6	3/6	6	2/6	4/6	6	4/6	2/6	4/6	5/6	6/7	6	6
D16S3025	4	4	4	4	4	4	4	4	4	4	4	4/6	4	4	4	4/5	4	4
CTTT01	8	9	8	8	8	9/10	9/10	5/10	3/9	8	9/10	10	9/10	8/10	8	8	7/8	8/11
D16S496	5	5	5	5	5	5	5	5/6	5	5/8	5/6	5	3/5	5	5	5	5	5
D16S3141	3	3/6	3	3/4	3	3/12	3	3	3/8	3/6	3/6	3/5	5	3	3/5	3/8	3	3
D16S3067	5	5	5	5	5	5	5	5	5	5	5	5	5	5	5	5	5	5
GT01	6	4/6	3/6	6	6	1/6	2/6	6	1/6	6/7	6	2/6	4/6	4/6	4/6	2/6	4/6	5/6
D16S3095	1	1/2	2	1	1/3	1	1	2	1/2	1/2	1/3	1/2	1/2	1/2	1/2	1/3	1/3	1

Families	T31	T32	T33	T34	T35	T36	T37	T38	T39	T40	T41	T42	T43	T44	T45	T46	Allele frequency (%)	Linkage disequilibrium (*P* value)
No. of patients	1	1	1	1	1	1	1	1	1	1	1	1	1	1	1	1		
No. of at-risk individuals	0	0	0	0	0	0	0	0	0	0	0	0	0	0	0	0		
DNA marker																		
D16S3031	8/9	8/9	1/9	9	9	8/9	9	9	9/10	8/9	9	9	9	9	9	9	68.1	
GGAA05	1/5	2/5	1/4	1/4	1/5	1/3	1/3	1/4	1/6	1/2	1/5	1/3	1/5	2/4	1/4	2/6	1.4	
GGAA10	3	3	3/4	3/4	3/5	3/5	4/6	3/4	3	3/5	3/6	3	3/6	3/5	3/5	3/7	13.2	
TTCC01	4/6	6	6/7	6	5/6	6/7	5/6	6	5/6	6	6/7	6	5/6	5/6	6/7	5/6	60.5	
D16S3086	2/3	2	2/4	2	2/3	2/3	2/3	2	2/5	2	2	2	2/3	2	2	2	65.7	
GATA01	1/2	2/4	2/3	2	2	2	2	2	2	2/3	2	3	1/3	2/3	2	2/3	44.1	
D16S421	3	3	3	3	3	3	3	3	3	3	3/5	3/4	3	3	3	3	75.7	<.0001*
***Q9H7K4* /exon 1**	T/C	T/C	T/C	T/C	T/C	T/C	T/C	T/C	T/C	T/C	T/C	T/C	T/C	T/C	T/C	T/C	0	<.0001*
TA001	1/9	1/8	1/16	1/9	1/7	1/5	1/9	1/10	1/9	1	1/10	1	1/9	1/9	1/6	1/5	23.8	<.0001*
GA001	4/8	4/5	4/7	4/8	4/7	4/6	4/11	4/5	4/8	4/5	4/7	4/5	4/7	4/5	4/7	4/7	0.1	<.0001*
TTTA001	4	3/4	4	4	4	1/4	4	3/4	3/4	4	1/4	4	4	4	4	3/4	65	<.0001*
CATG003	4	4	4	4	2/4	4	4	4	4	4	4/6	4	4	4	4	4	76.9	<.0001*
17msm	2	2/3	2/6	1/2	2	2/4	2/5	2/3	2/5	2/4	2/10	2/4	2/4	4/6	2/4	2/4	8.3	
D16S3107	6/7	6/7	5/7	7/11	7/10	2	5/7	3/7	5/7	4/7	5/7	3/7	6/7	4/7	5/7	6/7	13.9	
D16S3085	2/3	2	2	2/3	2/3	2	2/4	2	2	2	2	2	2	2	2	2	81.8	
ATT01	2/3	2/4	2	2/3	2/3	2/4	2/3	2/4	2/5	2	2/3	2	2	2	2	2	47.5	
GGAA01	4/6	6	5/6	3/6	2/6	3/6	6	6/7	6/9	6/7	3/6	6	6/7	6/7	5/6	5/6	18.8	
D16S3025	4/5	4/5	4	4	4	4	4	4	4/5	4	4	4/5	4	4/6	4	4	75	
CTTT01	7/9	8/9	3/9	9	5/9	4/8	6/9	8/14	8/10	7/9	8/10	8/15	9/10	1/7	7/9	3/8	28.2	
D16S496	5	5	5	5	5	5	5	5	5	5	5	5	5	5	5	5	54.2	
D16S3141	3/5	3/5	3	4/6	3/4	3	3	3/5	3/5	3/4	3	3	3	3/5	3/6	3/7	44.4	
D16S3067	5	5	5	5	5	5	5	5	5	5	5	5	5	5	5	5	41.9	
GT01	6	1/6	4/6	6	2/6	4/6	4/6	4/6	5/6	5/6	6/7	6	3/6	3/4	4/6	4/6	15.8	
D16S3095	1/2	1/2	1/2	1/3	1/2	1	1	2/3	1/3	1/3	1/4	1/2	1/3	2	1/2	1	-	

Figure 1 Haplotype analysis in the chromosome 16q22.1–linked ADCA critical locus. Ten families (P2, P4, P6, P12, P14, and T1–T5) large enough for haplotype analysis are indicated (*yellow boxes at top*). A founder haplotype "3-1-4-4-4" was seen in all patients for markers 16cen-*D16S421-TA001-GA001-TTTA001-CATG003*-16qter, between *GATA01* and *17msm.* Two alleles are shown (separated by a virgule [/]) for cases in which phase could not be determined. An asterisk (*) indicates that *P* values show significant linkage disequilibrium by Fisher's exact probability test. The specific C→T change in the *puratrophin-1* gene lies within the founder chromosomal region.

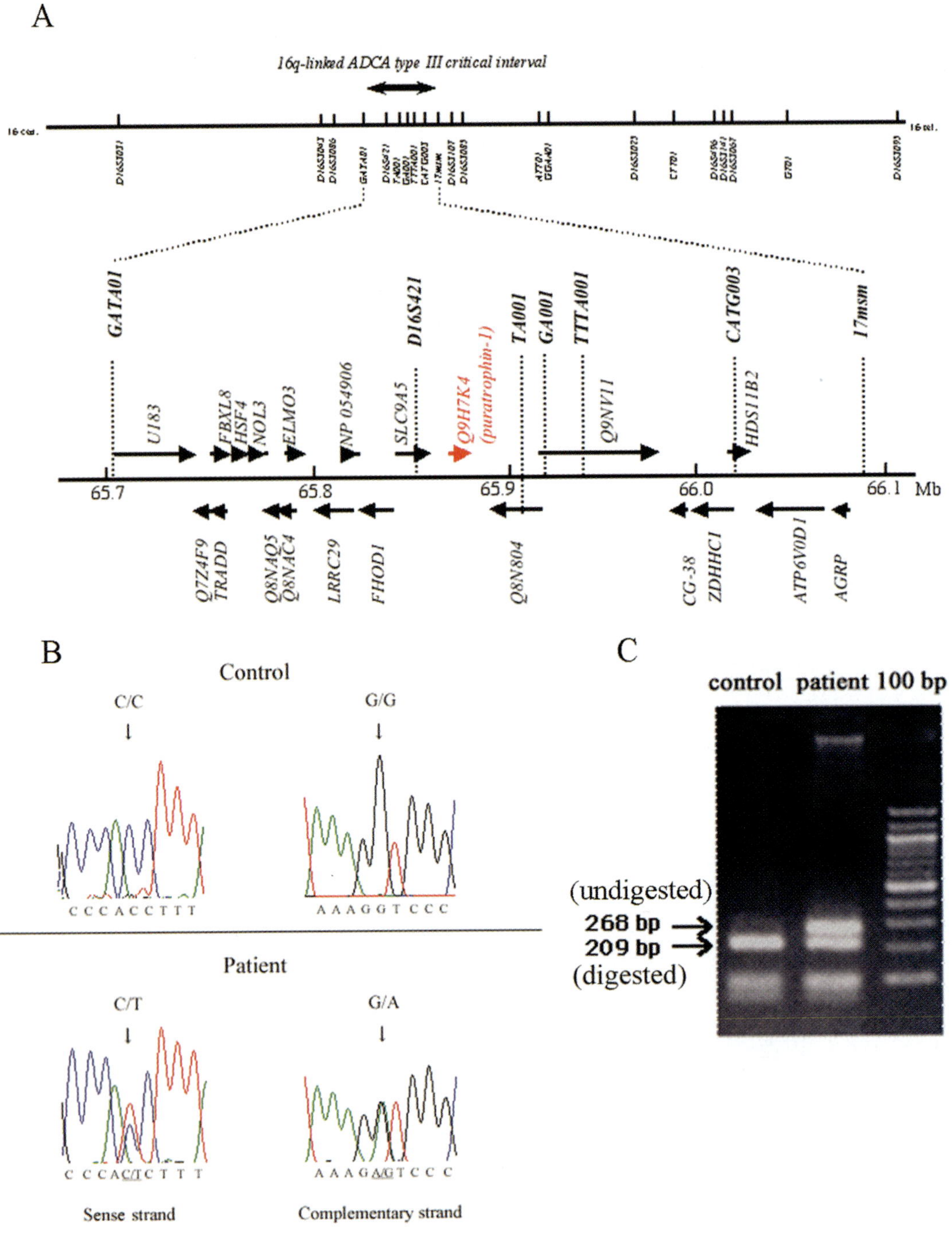

Figure 2 Positional cloning of the chromosome 16q22.1–linked ADCA gene. *A*, Genetic and physical maps of the interval in chromosome 16q22.1, showing microsatellite markers used to refine the interval. Twenty-one genes and their direction of transcription (Ensembl) are shown. *B*, Nucleotide sequences of exon 1 flanking the C→T single-nucleotide change in control and patient DNA samples. The patient harbors a heterozygous C→T substitution on the sense strand. *C*, RFLP by digestion with *Eco*NI. PCR was performed with primers UK1-E1F1 and UK1-E1R1. Whereas the normal allele produces digested fragments of 209, 92, and 59 bp, the C→T change in the mutant allele disrupts one *Eco*NI site, producing fragments of 268 and 92 bp.

The C→T change in the 5′ UTR was detected by amplifying genomic DNA with forward primer UK1-E1F1 (5′-CAGCGCGGTTCACACTGAGA-3′) and reverse primer UK1-E1R1 (5′-GGCCCTTTCTGACAGGACTGA-3′), which yielded a specific product of 360 bp. This amplicon harbors two *Eco*NI sites, one of which is destroyed by the C→T change.

Expression Analysis of Puratrophin-1 *mRNA by RT-PCR*

To characterize *puratrophin-1* mRNA in the human brain, poly-A$^+$RNA obtained from control human cerebellar tissues was reverse transcribed with SuperScript II (Stratagene), and the entire coding region was amplified with primers UKI-RT-025F (5′-TTCGCCTGCATTGCCCACTGAG-3′) and UK1-RT-005R (5′-CACACACATCAGAAAGGGTAGTCAAC-3′), which yielded a major product of 3,835 bp. To analyze alternative transcription, the PCR products were subcloned into pCR2.1-TOPO (Invitrogen), and 10 randomly selected clones from each brain mRNA (2 AD and 2 chromosome 16q22.1–linked ADCA cerebella) were sequenced and compared with partially annotated sequences (*Q9H7K4*, NCBI accession numbers BC054486 and AK024475). Rapid cloning of the 5′ and 3′ ends (5′- and 3′-RACE) was performed using Marathon-ready cDNA kit (Clontech [BD Biosciences]) as described elsewhere (Tsunemi et al. 2002). The entire 5′ UTR was amplified with primers UK1-RT-493F (5′-TGAGACAGTCTCAGTCAGGTCAC-3′) and UK1-RT-021R (5′-GTGGGCACACAGAAGCAGCACTGC-3′), was subcloned into pCR2.1-TOPO (Invitrogen), and was sequenced.

Expression of the *puratrophin-1* gene in various human tissues was studied by RT-PCR with use of primers UKI-RT-025F and UK1-RT-005R on human Multiple Tissue Panels I and II (Clontech [BD Bioscience]). Expression levels of *puratrophin-1* mRNA were compared among control and patient cerebellar cortices by RT-PCR with use of primers UK1-RT-BF001F (5′-TCACGGTTCCCCGCGGCTCG-3′) and UK1-RT-BF019R (5′-GGTTGCATGGCCCTGAGAGTCTGG-3′), which yielded PCR products of 291, 419, and 505 bp, depending on alternative transcription. To compare *puratrophin-1* mRNA levels more precisely, real-time RT-PCR analysis was performed on four control (individuals with AD) and two chromosome 16q22.1–linked ADCA cerebella by use of TaqMan technique (Applied Biosystems) on Applied Biosystems 7700 Sequence Detection System. PCR was performed for total *puratrophin-1* mRNAs (i.e., full-length and short-form mRNAs [GenBank accession numbers AB197663 and AB197664, respectively]; definitions of these two isoforms are described in the "Results" section) with primers total-taq-F (5′-TGGAGAGATGAGTGTCAAGACTTTG-3′) and total-taq-R (5′-AATGACTTGGGTCTGCCTTGG-3′). The short-form *puratrophin-1* mRNA was specifically assessed with primers short-taq-F (5′-ATGCCACCGACTGGAGATTT-3′) and short-taq-R (5′-GCTGCCCTGTAGCTCCTCAT-3′). The TaqMan probe for total *puratrophin-1* mRNA was 5′-FAM-CCAGATGCACGTTAAGGACCCAGGTC-TAMRA-3′, and that for short-form *puratrophin-1* mRNA was 5′-FAM-TCTCTGACCCTACTCAGGCTGAAGCCC-TAMRA-3′. The experiments were performed three times and were averaged. The level of *puratrophin-1* mRNA was assessed relative to the level of *G3PDH* mRNA amplified with primers supplied from the manufacturer (Applied Biosystems). Since the expression level of *G3PDH* mRNA was >1,000-fold higher than that of *puratrophin-1* mRNA, one control individual was chosen and the value of *puratrophin-1* mRNA:*G3PDH* mRNA ratio (designated "*puratrophin-1* mRNA/*G3PDH* mRNA index") was standardized as "1"; another three control individuals and two patients were compared relatively. The difference between the control and patient groups was statistically analyzed with the Mann-Whitney *U* test.

To see the effect of the C→T change in the 5′ UTR of *puratrophin-1* gene on expression in vitro, the partial 5′-UTR fragment containing the mutation site was amplified with forward primers UK1-UF10-F2 (5′-CCGGAATTCCAGGCCTGAATTGCAGTTC-3′) and UK1-UF10-R2 (5′-CCAGGCATCCCTGAAACT-3′) and was subcloned into the *Hind*III-*Nco*I sites of the luciferase assay vector, pGL3-Control Vector (Promega). The C→T mutation was then generated by site-directed mutagenesis (Stratagene). Three types of vectors (mock, empty pGL3-Control Vector; wild-type, pGL3 with normal *puratrophin-1* 5′ UTR with allele C; and mutant, pGL3 with mutant *puratrophin-1* 5′ UTR with allele T) were separately transfected with Renilla vector (Promega) into HEK293 cells to equalize the transfection efficiency. The transfection experiment was performed independently three times. Luciferase activity (F/R: fire-fly luciferase activity against Renilla activity) was assayed in accordance with the manufacturer's protocol and was statistically analyzed with the Mann-Whitney *U* test.

Generation of Rabbit Polyclonal Antibodies against Puratrophin-1

On the basis of the deduced amino acid sequence of "full-length" and "short-form" puratrophin-1, the secondary structure of each isoform was predicted, and five synthetic peptides were designed: polypeptide *FL01* (aa 1–13), N-MERPLENGDESPD-C; *FL02* (aa 421–432), N-MDKADELYDRVD-C; *FL03* (aa 570–583), N-EEGQRVLAELEQER-C; *FL04* (aa 991–1003), N-RFEIWFRRRKARD-C; and *SV01* (aa 13–26), N-REVWEGNGDAWRDE-C. The polypeptide FL01 lies at the amino terminus of the puratrophin-1 (fig. 3). Therefore, the

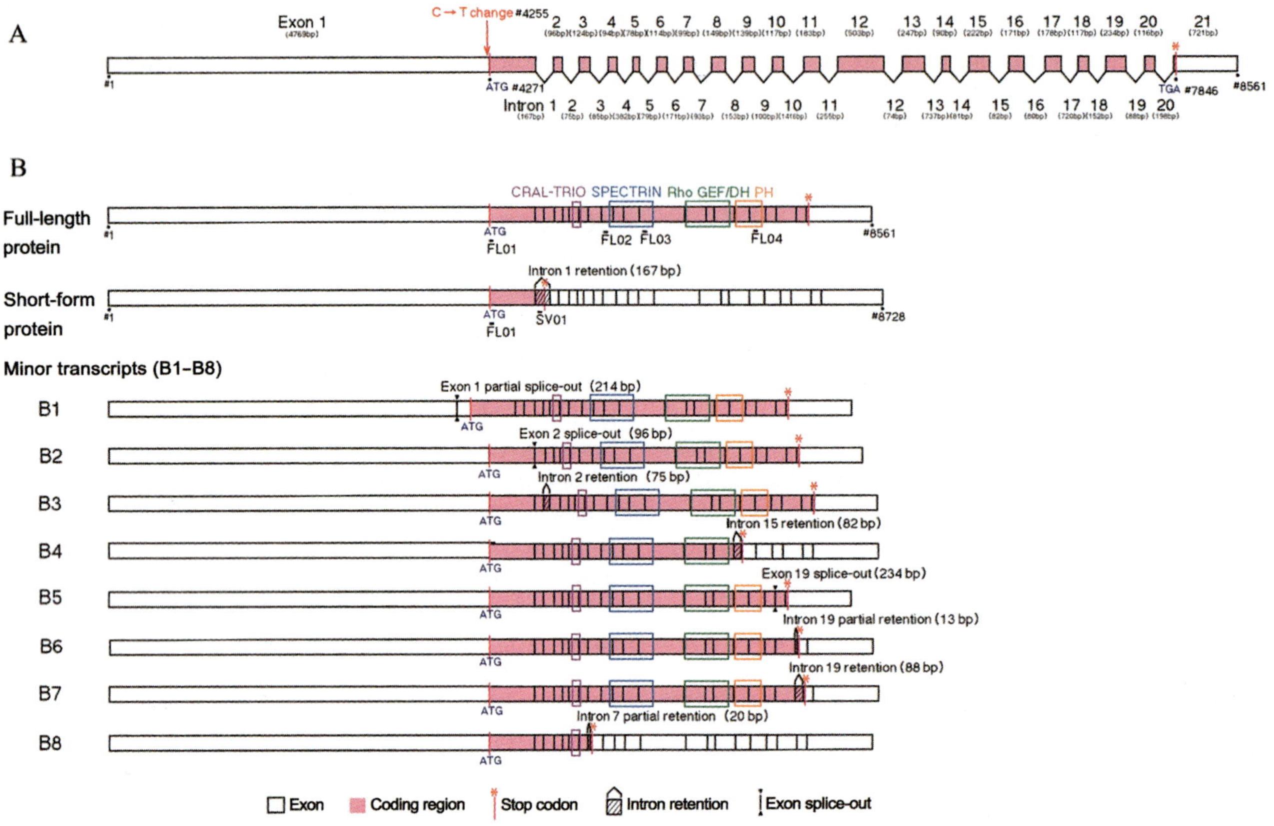

Figure 3 Genomic and mRNA structure of the *puratrophin-1* gene. *A*, Intron-exon structure of *puratrophin-1*. Exons are shown as vertical bars, and coding regions are shown in red. The C→T change at nt 4255 (or, 16 nt upstream of the translation initiation codon) is indicated. Nucleotide numbers (indicated by a number sign [#]) are counted from the 5′ end. *B*, *Puratrophin-1* mRNAs cloned from the human cerebellum. Major transcripts are full-length and short-form *puratrophin-1* mRNAs; minor transcripts (B1–B8) were also cloned. The CRL-TRIO, spectrin, Rho GEF/DH, and PH domains are indicated. Epitopes for five rabbit anti–puratrophin-1 antibodies (FL01–FL04 and SV01) are also mapped. Antibodies FL02, FL03, and FL04 are designed to specifically detect full-length puratrophin-1, the antibody SV01 specifically detects short-form puratrophin-1, and the antibody FL01 detects both full-length and short-form puratrophin-1.

antibody Prtrphn1-Ab FL01 would detect both full-length and short-form puratrophin-1. The polypeptides FL02, FL03, and FL04 are specific for the full-length puratrophin-1 (fig. 3). Notably, FL03 is at the spectrin repeat motif. The polypeptide SV01 lies at the carboxyl-terminus of the short-form puratrophin-1. Therefore, the antibody Prtrphn1-Ab SV01 would specifically recognize the short-form puratrophin-1. Each antigen was immunized into rabbit, and polyclonal antibodies were obtained as described elsewhere (Ishikawa et al. 1999).

The specificity of Prtrhn1-Abs was assessed by detection of recombinant puratrophin-1 protein. For this purpose, an antisense-strand primer was designed to encode hemagglutinin A (HA) in-frame at the carboxyl-terminus of the puratrophin-1. By PCR, full-length *puratrophin-1* cDNA with the HA-coding nucleotide sequence at its 3′ end was generated and was then cloned into pcDNA1 expression vector (Invitrogen). The puratrophin-1–HA fusion protein, transiently expressed in HEK293 cells, was first immunoprecipitated with Prtrhn1-Abs and then was detected with rat monoclonal anti-HA High Affinity antibody (3F10 [Roche Mannheim]) (fig. 4). The fusion protein immunoprecipitated with preimmune sera was not detected with anti-HA antibody.

Specificity of Prtrphn1-Abs on immunohistochemistry was assessed by immunoabsorption test. Solutions containing Prtrphn1-Ab and different concentrations of antigen (synthetic peptide) (0, 0.01, 0.1, and 1 mg/

The figure is available in its entirety in the online edition of *The American Journal of Human Genetics*.

Figure 4 Immunoprecipitation of puratrophin-1–HA fusion protein and immunoabsorption test with antiserum against puratrophin-1. The legend is available in its entirety in the online edition of *The American Journal of Human Genetics*.

liter) were made. Sections were incubated overnight with these solutions as other immunohistochemical staining. Prtrphn1-Abs were completely absorbed by peptides of higher concentrations (fig. 4).

Immunohistochemical Analyses of Puratrophin-1, Golgi-Apparatus Protein G58K, and Spectrin in Control Mouse, Human, and 16q22.1-Linked ADCA Tissues

Five polyclonal antibodies against puratrophin-1 (Prtrphn1-Ab types *FL01, FL02, FL03, FL04,* and *SV01*) were used for immunohistochemistry. Mouse monoclonal antibody against the microtubule-binding peripheral Golgi-apparatus membrane protein G58K (Sigma) and the mouse monoclonal antibody for α- and β-spectrin (MAB372 [Chemicon International]) were also used for immunohistochemistry.

Formalin-fixed paraffin-embedded tissue sections were prepared. Examined tissues were C57BL/6J wild-type mouse tissue, including cochlea (1 d postnatal), normal-control human tissues (testis, pancreas, prostate gland, lung, liver, heart, kidney, and brain from three individuals who died with nonneurological diseases), disease-control human brains (AD [$n = 3$], SCA6 [$n = 2$], multiple-system atrophy [MSA] [$n = 3$], and SCA3/MJD [$n = 3$]), and three brains with chromosome 16q22.1–linked ADCA. Immunohistochemistry was performed as described elsewhere (Ishikawa et al. 1999). In brief, sections were incubated overnight with Prtrphn1-Abs (diluted 1:200 with PBS), G58K (diluted 1:400), or MAB372 (diluted 1:200) at 4°C, after which the primary antibody was serially detected with avidin-biotinylated peroxidase complex method (Vector), was developed with 3,3′-diaminobenzidine (DAB), and was counterstained with hematoxylin.

Results

Restriction of the Critical Interval to <600 kb within Human Chromosome 16q22.1

Haplotype reconstruction of 10 informative families revealed that all affected individuals in these families were segregated with the haplotype 3-1-4-4-4 for markers *16cen-D16S421-TA001-GA001-TTTA001-CATG003-16qter* lying between *GATA01* and *17msm* (fig. 1). Genotypes of all affected individuals in the remaining 42 families that were not informative enough for haplotype reconstruction were also consistent with the common haplotype. Particularly, a dinucleotide (GA) repeat marker *GA001* showed strong linkage disequilibrium: the allele 4 of GA001 was seen in all affected individuals in all families with chromosome 16q22.1–linked ADCA, whereas that allele was seen very rarely (frequency 0.1%) in 1,000 control chromosomes (fig. 1). Whereas only one common haplotype was seen between *GATA01* and *17msm,* different alleles were seen for *GATA01* and other centromeric markers or for *17msm* and other telomeric markers (fig. 1). These results indicate that the gene for chromosome 16q22.1–linked ADCA is most likely to exist in the interval between *GATA01* and *17msm.* This region was within the previously refined intervals (Hellenbroich et al. 2003; Li et al. 2003) and was considered to be <600 kb in size in the database Ensembl.

Identification of a Single-Nucleotide Substitution in the 5′ UTR of the Gene Encoding Puratrophin-1 in the Critical Interval

Within the critical interval between *GATA01* and *17msm,* 21 different genes were identified (fig. 2*A*). We screened all 21 genes by direct sequencing of amplified genomic PCR products of all coding exons and flanking intronic sequences. Genomic Southern-blot analyses were also performed but did not detect any rearrangement (fig. 5).

We found that all patients with chromosome 16q22.1–linked ADCA harbored a heterozygous C→T single-nucleotide substitution at the position 16 nt upstream of the putative translation initiation codon of the gene *Q9H7K4,* encoding hypothetical protein DKFZP434I216 (NCBI accession number BC054486) (fig. 2*B*). All the at-risk individuals who had the founder haplotype between *GATA01* and *17msm* also harbored the C→T change. The ages of these individuals were below the maximum age at disease onset in their families, which indicates that they could be in presymptomatic stages. On the other hand, this C→T substitution was not seen in 500 healthy Japanese individuals (1,000 chromosomes), confirmed by *Eco*NI RFLP analysis (fig. 2*C*). All intronic sequences between the 21 exons and all the 8-kb sequences upstream of the *Q9H7K4* gene were also directly sequenced. Although there was a G→A SNP 44 nt upstream of the 3′ splice site of intron 9 of the *Q9H7K4* gene, the allele segregating with the disease was also seen in 75% of control chromosomes. As far as we examined, the C→T change at the position 16 nt upstream of the putative translation initiation codon of the gene *Q9H7K4* was the only specific change seen for patients with chromosome 16q22.1–linked ADCA. We renamed this protein "puratrophin-1," meaning Purkinje cell atrophy associated

The figure is available in its entirety in the online edition of *The American Journal of Human Genetics.*

Figure 5 Southern-blot analysis. The legend is available in its entirety in the online edition of *The American Journal of Human Genetics.*

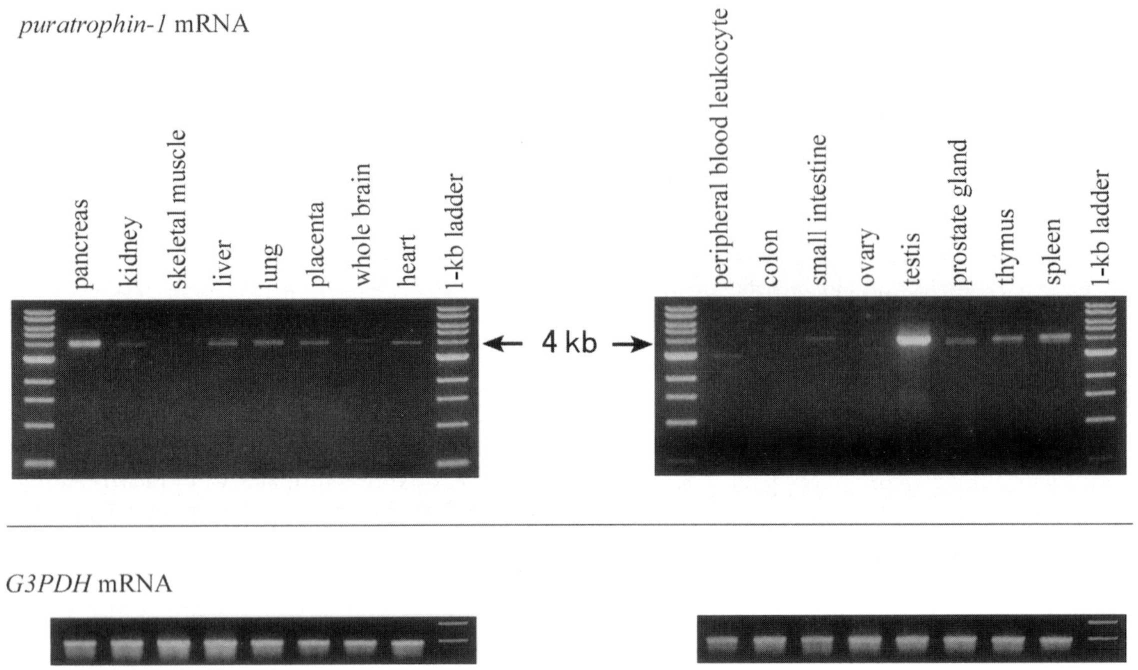

Figure 6 *Puratrophin-1* mRNA expression in various control human tissues. With this nonquantitative RT-PCR analysis, a relatively stronger expression was observed in the testis and pancreas, whereas mild or moderate expression was seen in the spleen, thymus, prostate gland, heart, placenta, lung, liver, and kidney. *Puratrophin-1* mRNA expression was low in the ovary, small intestine, colon, peripheral-blood leukocytes, whole brain, and skeletal muscle.

protein-1. (We reserved the nomenclature "ataxin-4" for families with original SCA4.)

Characterization of the Puratrophin-1 *Gene and Its Expression*

The *puratrophin-1* gene comprises 20 introns and 21 exons spanning a 13.7-kb genomic region (fig. 3*A*). RT-PCR and RACE experiments revealed that this gene is expressed in the human brain with an 8,561-nt mRNA and a single ORF of 3,576 nt (from nt 4,271 to nt 7,846) (fig. 3*B*). The first exon was 4,769 nt in length. This "full-length" transcript is predicted to encode a 134-kD protein, consisting of 1,192 aa, that contains four important domains: the cellular retinaldehyde-binding (CRAL)/triple function domain (TRIO) (at codons 304–338), the spectrin-repeat domain in the middle portion (at codons 447–601), the guanine-nucleotide exchange factor (GEF) for Rho/Rac/Cdc42-like GTPases followed by the Dbl-homologous (Rho GEF/DH) domain (at codons 733–907), and the pleckstrin-like homology (PH) domain (at codons 921–1027). The presence of these four domains suggests the role of puratrophin-1 in intracellular signaling and actin dynamics targeted to the Golgi apparatus (Godi et al. 1998; Fucini et al. 2000).

Besides the full-length *puratrophin-1* mRNA, we also found several alternative transcripts in human cerebellar cDNA (fig. 3*B*). The most common one had an unspliced intron 1 between exons 1 and 2 ("short-form" *puratrophin-1* mRNA). This intron retention produced a frameshift after exon 1 that resulted in a premature stop codon after 26 aa residues in intron 1. There were several other alternative transcripts (B1–B8 [fig. 3*B*]) in addition to full-length and short-form *puratrophin-1* mRNA. However, expression levels of these transcripts were considered lower than those of full-length or short-form *puratrophin-1* mRNA, as judged from cloning frequencies. *Puratrophin-1* mRNA was expressed in many tissues with various expression levels (fig. 6). The strongest expression was observed in the testis and pancreas, whereas its expression level was low in the "whole" brain. The expression was very weak on northern-blot analysis, even in the testis and pancreas (data available on request), which indicates that the expression of *puratrophin-1* mRNA was not abundant.

The Consequence of a C→T Change for Puratrophin-1 *mRNA Expression*

The consequence of the C→T change in the *puratrophin-1* gene was assessed by RT-PCR on frozen cerebellar tissues of two patients. No aberrant *puratrophin-1* mRNA was detected, which indicates that the mutation in the 5′ UTR does not affect alternative transcrip-

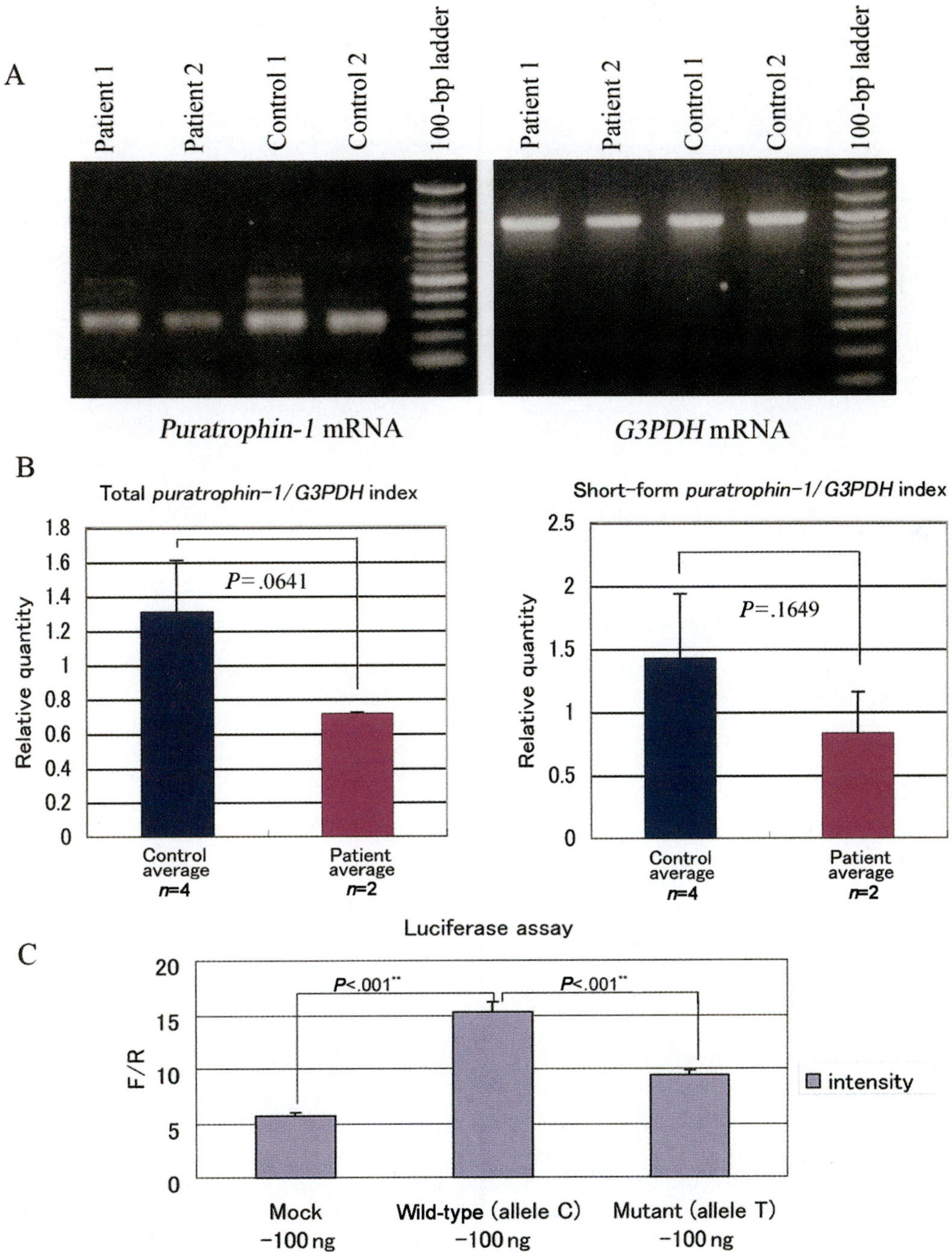

Figure 7 The consequence of a C→T change in the 5′ UTR of *puratrophin-1* mRNA. *A*, The *puratrophin-1* mRNA level assessed relative to *G3PDH* mRNA levels. The *puratrophin-1* mRNA levels in the cerebella of individuals with chromosome 16q22.1–linked ADCA appear slightly decreased compared with levels in control individuals. *B*, Quantitative analysis of *puratrophin-1* mRNA, with the use of the TaqMan technique in cerebellar mRNAs of four control individuals (with AD) and of two individuals with chromosome 16q22.1–linked ADCA. Both total *puratrophin-1* mRNA (i.e., full-length and short-form mRNAs) and short-form *puratrophin-1* mRNAs tended to be reduced in cerebella of individuals with chromosome 16q22.1–linked ADCA, although the significance was not statistically proven ($P = .0641$ for total mRNA; $P = .1649$ for short-form mRNA). *C*, Histogram of in vivo luciferase assay. "F/R" denotes fire-fly luciferase activity versus Renilla activity. The wild-type construct with allele C increases luciferase expression compared with an empty vector (Mock), whereas the mutant construct with allele T demonstrates significantly reduced luciferase activity ($P < .001$).

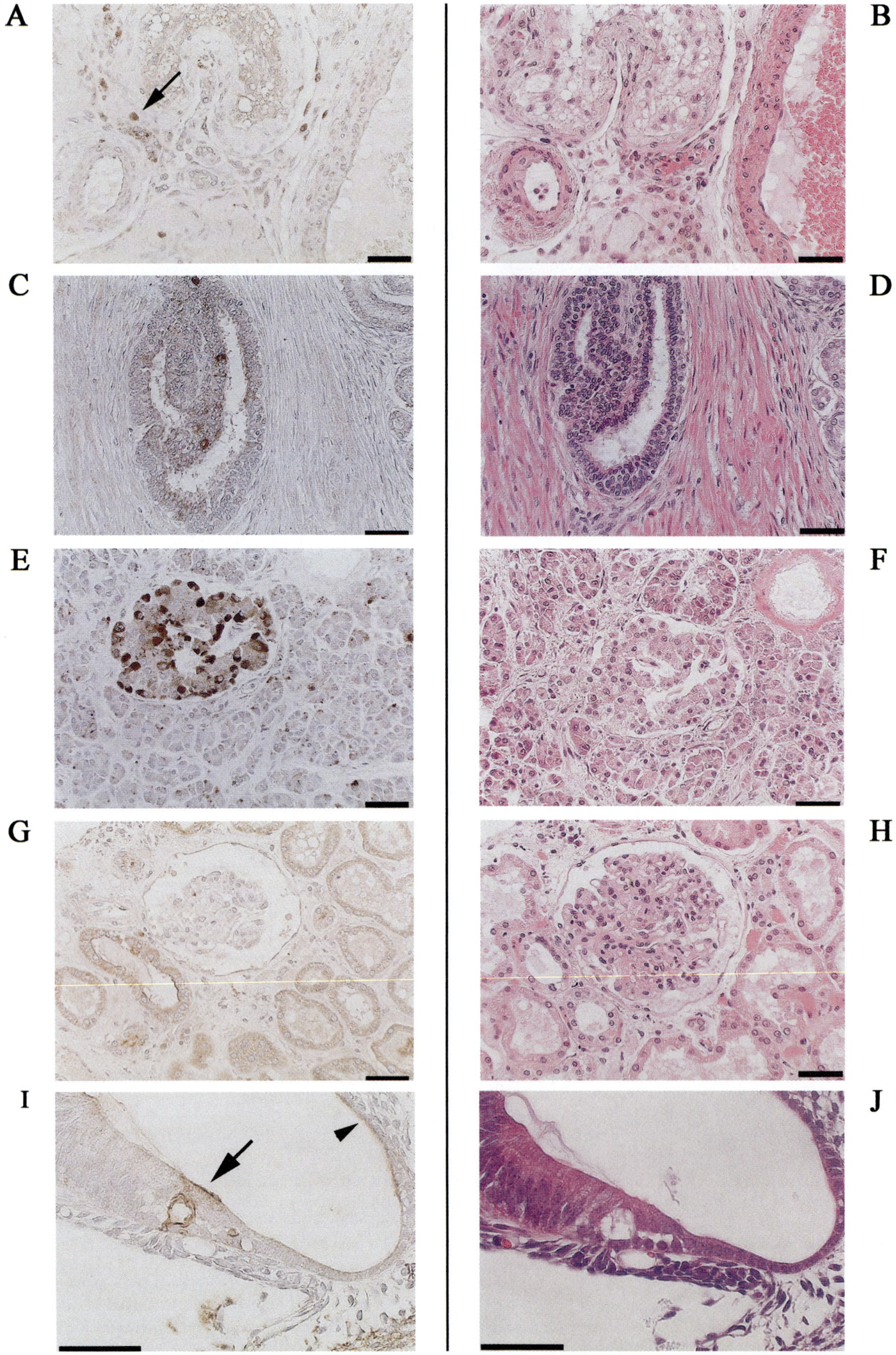
A
B
C
D
E
F
G
H
I
J

tion significantly. Instead, the expression level of *puratrophin-1* mRNA in the patient cerebella appeared slightly low compared with that in control cerebella (fig. 7*A*). On real-time RT-PCR analysis by TaqMan technique, the expression of *puratrophin-1* mRNA in the patient cerebella appeared lower than that in the control samples (fig. 7*B*). The tendency of reduction was seen for both total and short-form *puratrphin-1* mRNAs, although the significance was not proven statistically ($P = .0641$ for total *puratrophin-1* mRNA; $P = .1649$ for short-form *puratrophin-1* mRNA).

The in vitro study with *puratrophin-1* 5′-UTR sequences subcloned into luciferase expression vectors showed significantly reduced luciferase activity; the construct had mutant allele T, and the wild-type construct had allele C (fig. 7*C*). These data suggest that the C→T change in the *puratrophin-1* 5′ UTR could lead to reduced mRNA expression.

Expression of Puratrophin-1 in Control Human and Mouse Tissues and in Brains of Patients with 16q22.1–Linked ADCA

We next examined puratrophin-1 expression by immunohistochemistry using rabbit polyclonal Prtrhn1-Abs. Puratrophin-1 expression was seen in many control human tissues and mouse cochlea (fig. 8). Interestingly, puratrophin-1 expression was commonly seen in epithelial cells, such as epithelial cells in the human testis and hair cells in the mouse cochlea. As far as we examined in human tissues, the strength of immunoreactivity correlated with the mRNA expression level revealed by RT-PCR experiments (fig. 6).

In control human brains, both full-length and short-form puratrophin-1 was expressed faithfully in various neurons but most strongly in Purkinje cells (fig. 9*A*). In chromosome 16q22.1–linked ADCA brains, a striking difference was noted: the presence of microscopic aggregates of puratrophin-1 in the cytoplasm of Purkinje cells (fig. 9*B*). These aggregates were detected with all Prtrhn1-Abs, which indicates that full-length puratrophin-1 and short-form puratrophin-1 were both involved in the aggregate. On the other hand, puratrophin-1 aggregates were not obvious in neurons other than Purkinje cells. The finding of puratrophin-1 aggregates was specific to chromosome 16q22.1–linked ADCA brains, since the aggregates were not seen in other diseases showing degeneration of Purkinje cells, such as SCA6 or MSA.

We next examined the expression of G58K and of the α- and β-spectrin on control and chromosome 16q22.1–linked ADCA brains. Whereas G58K and spectrin were homogeneously stained in control brains (fig. 9*C* and 9*E*), these proteins both formed aggregation within the Purkinje cell of chromosome 16q22.1–linked ADCA brains (fig. 9*D* and 9*F*). This further suggests that formation of puratrophin-1 aggregates is abnormal and associates with disturbances of Golgi apparatus and spectrin.

Discussion

The single-nucleotide C→T substitution in the 5′ UTR of the *puratrophin-1* gene is strongly associated with chromosome 16q22.1–linked ADCA, as evidenced by the following three points. First, this single-nucleotide change was the only specific difference detected in patients, as far as we screened all exons and intron-exon boundaries of the 21 annotated genes lying within the founder chromosome. The change completely segregated with the disease in 52 unrelated families that originated in all sections of Japan, whereas such a change was not seen in 1,000 control chromosomes. We also screened for genomic rearrangement by Southern-blot analysis, but we did not observe any changes. Second, the C→T change was not a mere polymorphism present in the founder chromosome, since it resulted in reduced expression in the in vitro luciferase assay. Consistently, tendency for reduction in mRNA expression was seen in the cerebellum of chromosome 16q22.1–linked ADCA. Third, puratrophin-1 was aggregated in the major target neuron (i.e., the Purkinje cell) of chromosome 16q22.1–linked ADCA. The Golgi-apparatus membrane protein (G58K) and spectrin, both important cytoskeletal proteins, were also aggregated. Since aggregation of mutated protein is a common feature of many neurodegenerative disorders (Ross and Poirier 2004), a single-nucleotide change in the 5′ UTR in the *puratrophin-1* gene appears to be the mutation that causes chromosome 16q22.1–linked ADCA. Most mutations that cause ADCAs reside in genes encoding proteins whose functions are not well understood, except for the α1A-calcium channel ($Ca_v2.1$) for SCA6 (Zhuchenko et al. 1997), PKCγ for

Figure 8 Expression of puratrophin-1 in control human and mouse tissues. *A* and *B*, Human testis. *C* and *D*, Human prostate gland. *E* and *F*, Human pancreas. *G* and *H*, Human kidney. *I* and *J*, Mouse cochlea. *A*, *C*, *E*, *G*, and *I*, Immunohistochemical analysis with use of the polyclonal anti–puratrophin-1 antibody SV01. *B*, *D*, *F*, *H*, and *J*, Hematoxylin and eosin stain of the section adjacent to that shown in *A*, *C*, *E*, *G*, and *I*, respectively. Puratrophin-1 is expressed in many tissues, with varying strength. In particular, Leydig cells in the testis (*arrow* in *A*), epithelial cells in the prostate gland (*C*), and Langerhans islet in the pancreas (*E*) showed strong immunoreactivity. Immunoreactivity in the kidney was weak (*G*). Expression in the cochlea was particularly intense at the sensory hairlets (*arrow* in *I*). Hair cells of the stria vascularis also showed immunoreactivity (*arrowhead* in *I*). All scale bars = 50 μm.

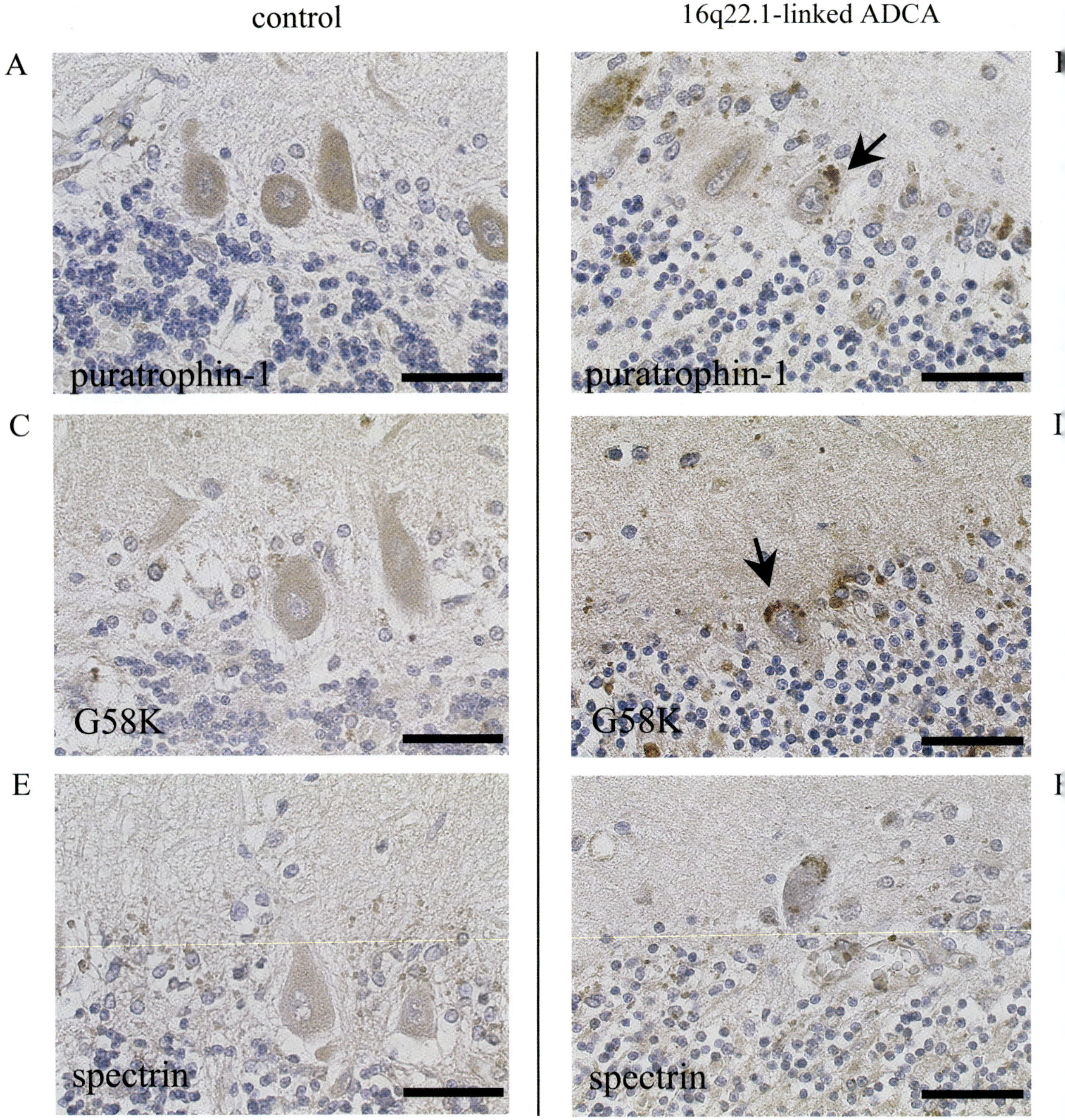

Figure 9 Immunohistochemical analysis of puratrophin-1, Golgi-apparatus membrane protein (G58K), and spectrin in control cells and samples from a patient's cerebellum. *A*, Puratrophin-1 expression in the cell body of Purkinje cells, visualized with use of rabbit polyclonal anti–puratrophin-1 antibody (FL01). *B*, With use of same antibody FL01, aggregation of puratrophin-1 (*arrow*), seen in a Purkinje cell of a brain affected with chromosome 16q22.1–linked ADCA. *C*, G58K expression, seen diffusely in the cell body of control Purkinje cells. *D*, G58K aggregation (*arrow*), morphologically quite similar to the puratrophin-1 aggregate, seen in a patient's Purkinje cell. *E*, Spectrin expression, seen in the cell body of a control Purkinje cell. *F*, Spectrin aggregation in a patient's Purkinje cell. All scale bars = 50 μm.

SCA14 (Chen et al. 2003), TATA-binding protein for SCA17 (Koide et al. 1999), and FGF14 for ADCA with FGF14 mutation (van Swieten et al. 2003). Puratrophin-1 is the first known protein related to intracellular signaling and cytoskeleton that is associated with ADCA. Our preliminary results suggest that the frequency of chromosome 16q22.1–linked ADCA is relatively high, since it was ranked the third most frequent ADCA in Japan, after MJD/SCA3 and SCA6. Since chromosome 16q22.1–linked ADCA had a strong founder effect, it will be important to clarify whether this specific C→T change is seen in other ethnic groups. Particularly, it is extremely important to clarify whether original patients with SCA4 reported from North American and German populations harbor mutation within the *puratrophin-1* gene (Flanigan et al. 1996; Hellenbroich et al. 2003).

A heterozygous, single-nucleotide substitution in the 5′ UTR that is associated with aggregation of the gene product is a unique feature as a cause of human disease. Generally, a single-nucleotide substitution in the 5′ UTR may result in expression of aberrant mRNA, abnormal trafficking of mutant transcripts due to conformational changes, or reduced transcription of mRNA, as in β thalassemia intermedia (Sgourou et al. 2004). In the present study, no aberrant transcripts were cloned from patient brains. Instead, the result from the in vitro study suggested that the transcription efficiency could be reduced significantly by the C→T substitution in the 5′ UTR of the *puratrophin-1* gene. Consistent with this in vitro finding, levels of *puratrophin-1* mRNA tended to be lower in cerebella of patients with 16q22.1-linked ADCA than in those of AD-affected controls. Further studies comprising a larger number of samples that include "neurologically normal" controls will be necessary to confirm that reduced *puratrophin-1* mRNA expression is associated with the C→T change in the 5′ UTR. Although aggregations of mutated proteins in most neurodegenerative diseases are due to conformational changes produced by amino acid alterations, reduced protein expression may also cause protein aggregation, such as the neurofilament light-chain aggregation in anterior horn cells of patients with amyotrophic lateral sclerosis (ALS) (Bergeron et al. 1994). It is currently not known how the C→T change in the *puratrophin-1* gene leads to puratrophin-1 aggregation. However, it is possible that alteration in the stoichiometry or changes in the protein stability, observed in neurofilament proteins in ALS (Ge et al. 2003), also exist for puratrophin-1 in chromosome 16q22.1–linked ADCA. In addition, it should be noted that since reduction of *puratrophin-1* mRNA levels in patient cerebella was small, that may not be a sufficient explanation of the formation of aggregation. It will be important to assess the *puratrophin-1* mRNA levels specifically in Purkinje cells, where the protein aggregates.

Puratrophin-1 is a novel protein with four important domains: the spectrin repeat, CRAL/TRIO, Rho GEF/DH, and PH domains. Therefore, the *puratrophin-1* gene would be the fifth gene that encodes Rho GEF protein to be associated with human disease, after the *FGD1GEF* gene for faciogenital dysplasia (Pasteris et al. 1994), the *ARHGEF6* gene for X-linked nonsyndromic mental retardation (Kutsche et al. 2000), the *ARHGEF10* gene for autosomal dominant neuropathy with thin myelinated fibers (Verhoeven et al. 2003), and the *ALS2* gene for the autosomal recessive juvenile motor neuron disease ALS2 (Hadano et al. 2001; Yang et al. 2001). GEFs exert diverse functions in intracellular-membrane trafficking and microtubule dynamics and ultimately regulate numerous cellular responses—such as proliferation, differentiation, and movement—by activating small G-protein GTPases (Rossman et al. 2005). Although Rho GEF/DH and PH domains are typical for Rho GEF proteins, the presence of a spectrin repeat suggests that puratrophin-1 could be targeted to the Golgi-apparatus membrane, where it may regulate certain membrane dynamics through modulating actin (Godi et al. 1998; Lemmon et al. 2002). The CRAL/TRIO domain is implicated in the nerve growth factor (NGF) pathway that leads to neurite outgrowth through activating Rho G (Estrach et al. 2002), which indicates that puratrophin-1 may also have a role in cell differentiation signaling through NGF. In the present study, we showed that the Golgi-apparatus membrane protein and spectrin both form aggregation in the Purkinje cells of patient brains, which strongly supports the hypothesis that puratrophin-1 indeed interacts with these essential cytoskeletons. Formation of these aggregations, which seems to be a new phenomenon implicated in pathogenesis of human disease, could be deleterious for cells, since Golgi-apparatus membrane proteins and spectrin are important in maintaining cellular architecture, as noted for autosomal dominant polycystic kidney diseases (Charron et al. 2000). In addition, it also seems rational to speculate that disturbance of puratrophin-1 may affect Purkinje-cell morphology and eventually cause the peculiar Purkinje-cell atrophy that characterizes chromosome 16q22.1–linked ADCA, since Rho GEFs are implicated particularly in neural morphogenesis and connectivity by regulating actin dynamics (Godi et al. 1998).

Finally, the association of progressive hearing impairment in patients with chromosome 16q22.1–linked ADCA may suggest a role of puratrophin-1 in hearing. As far as we were able to examine by auditory tests, 42.8% of study families had hearing impairment. Audiometric configurations showing mid-frequency U-shaped or flat-shaped pattern also suggested that the hearing impairment of these patients was not a simple age-related hearing loss. However, it should be noted that some families had moderate hearing impairment, whereas other families had only mild hearing impairment, which may indicate the presence of other modifying genetic factors for this phenotype. Further clinical analyses with use of detailed auditory tests are needed to ascertain how strongly hearing impairment is associated with ataxia. If hearing impairment is confirmed as being complicated by chromosome 16q22.1–linked ADCA, puratrophin-1 will be the first deafness/hearing-impairment protein related to Rho GEF. Since mutations in the γ-actin gene (*ACTG1*; DFN20/26) (Zhu et al. 2003), genes coding proteins that interact with actin (e.g., the myosins espin and harmonin), or a gene coding proteins that coordinate actin polymerization (Mburu et al. 2003) are known to cause deafness, it is possible that puratrophin-1 disruption causes hearing impairment by disturbing actin dynamics in the cochlea. In support of this hypothesis, expression of puratrophin-1 was seen in mouse cochlear hair cells, in which actin is also expressed (Mburu et al. 2003). Rho GTPases are also important regulators of actin cytoskeleton in stereocilia development, which is crucial for auditory transduction (Kollmar 2001). We hypothesize that the *puratrophin-1* gene mutation ultimately causes hearing impairment by dysregulation of actin in the cochlea. Further studies, such as targeted disruption of puratrophin-1 in mouse, will be important for clarifying whether puratrophin-1 has a role in hearing.

In summary, we have identified that a single-nucleotide C→T substitution in the 5′ UTR of the gene *puratrophin-1* is strongly associated with chromosome 16q22.1–linked ADCA. If patients with SCA4 are found to harbor mutations in this gene, it would suggest that the chromosome 16q22.1–linked ADCA in Japan is allelic with SCA4. Identification of the mechanism of puratrophin-1 expression, the upstream signaling cascade that activates puratrophin-1, and the actual Rho GTPase activated by puratrophin-1 would be the next key steps for understanding the molecular mechanisms that underlie cellular degeneration of chromosome 16q22.1–linked ADCA and hearing impairment.

Acknowledgments

We thank the doctors who participated in this work by recruiting families with chromosome 16q22.1–linked ADCA: Drs. Hidenao Sasaki, Department of Neurology, Graduate School, Hokkaido University; Masashi Aoki, Department of Neurology, Graduate School, Tohoku University; Yoshihisa Takiyama, Department of Neurology, Jichi Medical School; Kazuo Yoshizawa, National Mito Hospital; Kazuko Mitani and Yu-ichi Fumimura, Department of Neurology, Tokyo Metropolitan Geriatric Hospital; Hirohiko Murakami, Department of Neurology, Tokyo Women's Medical School; Satoshi Orimo, Department of Neurology, Kanto Central Hospital; Souichiro Mochio, Department of Neurology, Jikei Medical School, The Third Hospital; Kunihiro Yoshida, Department of Clinical Genetics, Shinshu University; Isao Sahashi, Fourth Department of Internal Medicine, Aichi Medical University; Masanori Nakagawa, Department of Neurology, Kyoto Prefectural Medical College; Akihumi Goto, Department of Neurology, Nagasaki Medical Center of Neurology; Hideki Kida, Kida Hospital; Eiichiro Uyama, Department of Neurology, Kumamoto University of Medicine; Jun Goto and Shoji Tsuji, Department of Neurology, Graduate School, University of Tokyo; and Miho Murata and Ichiro Kanazawa, National Center of Neurology and Psychiatry, Ministry of Health, Labor and Welfare. For human and mouse control specimens, we also thank Professors Morio Koike, Department of Pathology, and Ken Kitamura, Department of Audio-Vestibular Neuroscience, Graduate School, Tokyo Medical and Dental University. We thank Ms. Iku Sudo and Ms. Minori Kono for technical assistance. We deeply acknowledge Professors Ichiro Kanazawa, Director of National Center of Neurology and Psychiatry, Ministry of Health, Labor and Welfare, and Shoji Tsuji, Department of Neurology, Graduate School, University of Tokyo, for supporting this study. This study was supported by Grant-in-Aids for Scientific Research on Priority Areas—Advanced Brain Science Project—from Ministry of Education, Culture, Sports, Science and Technology, Japan (to K.I. and H.M.), as well as grants from Research on Intractable Disorders (to H.M.) and from Human Genome and Regenerative Medicine, Ministry of Health, Labor and Welfare, Japan (to K.I. and H.M.).

Web Resources

Accession numbers and URLs for data presented herein are as follows:

Celera Discovery System, http://www.celeradiscoverysystem.com/index.cfm (for candidate genes)

Ensembl, http://www.ensembl.org/ (for genetic map, genomic sequences, ESTs, and 21 candidate genes, including *Q9H7K4* and *SLC9A5*)

GenBank, http://www.ncbi.nlm.nih.gov/Genbank/ (for microsatellite DNA markers *GGAA10* [accession number AB13610], TTCC01 [accession number AB13611], *TA001* [accession number AB13612], *GA001* [accession number AB197662], and *AAT01* [accession number AB13613] and full-length and short-form *puratrophin-1* mRNAs [accession numbers AB197663 and AB197664])

NCBI, http://www.ncbi.nlm.nih.gov/ (for DKFZP434I216 [accession numbers BC054486 and AK024475])

Online Mendelian Inheritance in Man (OMIM), http://www.ncbi.nlm.nih.gov/Omim/ (for 16q-linked ADCA type III, or SCA4)

The Hereditary Hearing Loss Homepage, http://webhost.ua.ac.be/hhh/

UniGene, http://www.ncbi.nlm.nih.gov/UniGene/ (for candidate genes and ESTs)

References

Bergeron C, Beric-Maskarel K, Muntasser S, Weyer L, Somerville M, Percy ME (1994) Neurofilament light and polyaden-

ylated mRNA levels are decreased in amyotrophic lateral sclerosis motor neurons. J Neuropathol Exp Neurol 53:221–230
Charron AJ, Bacallao RL, Wandinger-Ness A (2000) ADPKD: a human disease altering Golgi function and basolateral exocytosis in renal epithelia. Traffic 1:675–686
Chen D-H, Brkanac Z, Verlinde CLMJ, Tan X-J, Bylenok L, Nochlin D, Matsushita M, Lipe H, Wolff J, Fernandez M, Cimino PJ, Bird TD, Raskind WH (2003) Missense mutations in the regulatory domain of PKCγ: a new mechanism for dominant nonepisodic cerebellar ataxia. Am J Hum Genet 72:839–849
Estrach S, Schmidt S, Diriong S, Penna A, Blangy A, Fort P, Debant A (2002) The human Rho-GEF trio and its target GTPase RhoG are involved in the NGF pathway, leading to neurite outgrowth. Curr Biol 12:307–312
Flanigan K, Gardner K, Alderson K, Galster B, Otterud B, Leppert MF, Kaplan C, Ptacek LJ (1996) Autosomal dominant spinocerebellar ataxia with sensory axonal neuropathy (SCA4): clinical description and genetic localization to chromosome 16q22.1. Am J Hum Genet 59:392–399
Fucini RV, Navarrete A, Vadakkan C, Lacomis L, Erdjument-Bromage H, Tempst P, Stamnes M (2000) Activated ADP-ribosylation factor assembles distinct pools of actin on Golgi membranes. J Biol Chem 275:18824–18829
Ge WW, Leystra-Lantz C, Wen W, Strong MJ (2003) Selective loss of trans-acting instability determinants of neurofilament mRNA in amyotrophic lateral sclerosis spinal cord. J Biol Chem 278:26558–26563
Godi A, Santone I, Pertile P, Devarajan P, Stabach PR, Morrow JS, DiTullio G, Polishchuk R, Petrucci TC, Luini A, DeMatteis MA (1998) ADP ribosylation factor regulates spectrin binding to the Golgi complex. Proc Natl Acad Sci USA 95: 8607–8612
Graham DI, Lantos PL (eds) (2002) Greenfield's neuropathology, 7th ed. Arnold, London
Hadano S, Hand CK, Osuga H, Yanagisawa Y, Otomo A, Devon RS, Miyamoto N, Showguchi-Miyata J, Okada Y, Singaraja R, Figlewicz DA, Kwiatkowski T, Hosler BA, Sagie T, Skaug J, Nasir J, Brown RH Jr, Scherer SW, Rouleau GA, Hayden MR, Ikeda JE (2001) A gene encoding a putative GTPase regulator is mutated in familial amyotrophic lateral sclerosis 2. Nat Genet 29:166–173
Harding AE (1982) The clinical features and classification of the late onset autosomal dominant cerebellar ataxias: a study of 11 families, including descendants of "Drew family of Walworth." Brain 105:1–28
Hellenbroich Y, Bubel S, Pawlack H, Opitz S, Vieregge P, Schwinger E, Zuhlke C (2003) Refinement of the spinocerebellar ataxia type 4 locus in a large German family and exclusion of CAG repeat expansion in this region. J Neurol 250:668–671
Hirano R, Takashima H, Okubo R, Tajima K, Okamoto Y, Ishida S, Tsuruta K, Arisato T, Arata H, Nakagawa M, Osame M, Arimura K (2004) Fine mapping of 16q-linked autosomal dominant cerebellar ataxia type III in Japanese families. Neurogenetics 5:215–221
Holmes SE, O'Hearn EE, McInnis MG, Gorelick-Feldman DA, Kleiderlein JJ, Callahan C, Kwak NG, Ingersoll-Ashworth RG, Sherr M, Sumner AJ, Sharp AH, Ananth U, Seltzer WK, Boss MA, Vieria-Saecker AM, Epplen JT, Riess O, Ross CA, Margolis RL (1999) Expansion of a novel CAG trinucleotide repeat in the 5′ region of PPP2R2B is associated with SCA12. Nat Genet 23:391–392
Hughes CP, Berg L, Danziger WL, Coben LA, Martin RL (1982) A new clinical scale for the staging of dementia. Br J Psychiatry 140:566–572
Ishikawa K, Fujigasaki H, Saegusa H, Ohwada K, Fujita T, Iwamoto H, Komatsuzaki Y, Toru S, Toriyama H, Watanabe M, Ohkoshi N, Shoji S, Kanazawa I, Tanabe T, Mizusawa H (1999) Abundant expression and cytoplasmic aggregation of α1A voltage-dependent calcium channel protein associated with neurodegeneration in spinocerebellar ataxia type 6. Hum Mol Genet 8:1185–1193
Ishikawa K, Nagaoka U, Takashima M, Yoshizawa K, Yoshizawa T, Ishikawa M, Yamawaki T, Shoji S, Mizusawa H (2000) A gene on SCA4 locus causes dominantly-inherited pure cerebellar ataxia. Neurology 54:1971–1975
Ishikawa K, Tanaka H, Saito M, Ohkoshi N, Fujita T, Yoshizawa K, Ikeuchi T, Watanabe M, Hayashi A, Takiyama Y, Nishizawa M, Nakano I, Matsubayashi K, Miwa M, Shoji S, Kanazawa I, Tsuji S, Mizusawa H (1997) Japanese families with autosomal dominant pure cerebellar ataxia map to chromosome 19p13.1-p13.2 and are strongly associated with mild CAG expansions in the spinocerebellar ataxia type 6 gene in chromosome 19p13.1. Am J Hum Genet 61:336–346
Kobayashi K, Nakahori Y, Miyake M, Matsumura K, Kondo-Iida E, Nomura Y, Segawa M, Yoshioka M, Saito K, Osawa M, Hamano K, Sakakihara Y, Nonaka I, Nakagome Y, Kanazawa I, Nakamura Y, Tokunaga K, Toda T (1998) An ancient retrotransposal insertion causes Fukuyama-type congenital muscular dystrophy. Nature 394:388–392
Koide R, Kobayashi S, Shimohata T, Ikeuchi T, Maruyama M, Saito M, Yamada M, Takahashi H, Tsuji S (1999) A neurological disease caused by an expanded CAG trinucleotide repeat in the TATA-binding protein gene: a new polyglutamine disease? Hum Mol Genet 8:2047–2053
Kollmar R (2001) Who does the hair cell's 'do? Rho GTPases and hair-bundle morphogenesis. Curr Opin Neurobiol 9:394–398
Koob MD, Moseley ML, Schut LJ, Benzow KA, Bird TD, Day JW, Ranum LP (1999) An untranslated CTG expansion causes a novel form of spinocerebellar ataxia (SCA8). Nat Genet 21:379–384
Kutsche K, Yntema H, Brandt A, Jantke I, Nothwang HG, Orth U, Boavida MG, David D, Chelly J, Fryns J-P, Moraine C, Ropers H-H, Hamel BCJ, van Bokhoven H, Gal A (2000) Mutations in *ARHGEF6*, encoding a guanine nucleotide exchange factor for Rho GTPases, in patients with X-linked mental retardation. Nat Genet 26:247–250
Lemmon MA, Ferguson KM, Abrams CS (2002) Pleckstrin homology domains and cytoskeleton. FEBS Lett 513:71–76
Li M, Ishikawa K, Toru S, Tomimitsu H, Takashima M, Goto J, Takiyama Y, Sasaki H, Imoto I, Inazawa J, Toda T, Kanazawa I, Mizusawa H (2003) Physical map and haplotype analysis of 16q-linked autosomal dominant cerebellar ataxia (ADCA) type III in Japan. J Hum Genet 48:111–118
Margolis RL (2002) The spinocerebellar ataxias: order emerges from chaos. Curr Neurol Neurosci Rep 2:447–456

Matsuura T, Yamagata T, Burgess DL, Rasmussen A, Grewal RP, Watase K, Khajavi M, McCall AE, Davis CF, Zu L, Achari M, Pulst SM, Alonso E, Noebels JL, Nelson DL, Zoghbi HY, Ashizawa T (2000) Large expansion of the ATTCT pentanucleotide repeat in spinocerebellar ataxia type 10. Nat Genet 26:191–194

Mburu P, Mustapha M, Varela A, Weil D, El-Amraoui A, Holme RH, Rump A, Hardisty RE, Blanchard S, Coimbra RS, Perfettini I, Parkinson N, Mallon A-M, Glenister P, Rogers MJ, Paige AJ, Moir L, Clay J, Rosenthal A, Liu XZ, Blanco G, Steel KP, Petit C, Brown SDM (2003) Defects in whirlin, a PDZ domain molecule involved in stereocilia elongation, cause deafness in the whirler mouse and families with DFNB31. Nat Genet 34:421–428

Owada K, Ishikawa K, Toru S, Ishida G, Gomyoda M, Tao O, Noguchi Y, Kitamura K, Kondo I, Noguchi E, Arinami T, Mizusawa H. A clinical, genetic and neuropathologic study in a family with 16q-linked ADCA type III. Neurology (in press)

Pasteris NG, Cadle A, Logie LJ, Porteous ME, Schwartz CE, Stevenson RE, Glover TW, Wilroy RS, Gorski JL (1994) Isolation and characterization of the faciogenital dysplasia (Aarskog-Scott syndrome) gene: a putative Rho/Rac guanine nucleotide exchange factor. Cell 79:669–678

Ross CA, Poirier MA (2004) Protein aggregation and neurodegenerative disease. Nat Med Suppl 10:S10–S17

Rossman KL, Der CJ, Sondek J (2005) GEF means go: turning on RHO GTPases with guanine nucleotide-exchange factors. Nat Rev Mol Cell Biol 6:167–180

Sasaki H, Yabe I, Tashiro K (2003) The hereditary spinocerebellar ataxias in Japan. Cytogenet Genome Res 100:198–205

Sgourou A, Routledge S, Antoniou M, Papachatzopoulou A, Psiouri L, Athanassiadou A (2004) Thalassaemia mutations within the 5′ UTR of the human β-globin gene disrupt transcription. Br J Haematol 124:828–835

Stevanin G, Bouslam N, Thobois S, Azzedine H, Ravaux L, Boland A, Schalling M, Broussole E, Durr A, Brice A (2004) Spinocerebellar ataxia with sensory neuropathy (SCA25) maps to chromosome 2p. Ann Neurol 55:97–104

Stevanin G, Durr A, Brice A (2000) Clinical and molecular advances in autosomal dominant cerebellar ataxias: from genotype to phenotype and physiopathology. Eur J Hum Genet 8:4–18

Tsuiki T, Sasamori S, Minami Y, Ichinohe T, Murai K, Murai S, Kawashima H (2002) [Age effect on hearing: a study on Japanese.] Audiol Japan 45:241–250

Tsunemi T, Saegusa H, Ishikawa K, Nagayama S, Murakoshi T, Mizusawa H, Tanabe T (2002) Novel $Ca_v2.1$ splice variants isolated from Purkinje cells do not generate P-type Ca^{2+} current. J Biol Chem 277:7214–7221

van Swieten JC, Brusse E, de Graaf BM, Krieger E, van de Graaf R, de Koning I, Maat-Kievit A, Leegwater P, Dooijes D, Oostra BA, Heutink P (2003) A mutation in the fibroblast growth factor 14 gene is associated with autosomal dominant cerebellar ataxia. Am J Hum Genet 72:191–199 (erratum 72:1078)

Verhoeven K, De Jonghe P, Van de Putte T, Nelis E, Zwijsen A, Verpoorten N, De Vriendt E, Jacobs A, Van Gerwen V, Francis A, Ceuterick C, Huylebroeck D, Timmerman V (2003) Slowed conduction and thin myelination of peripheral nerves associated with mutant Rho guanine-nucleotide exchange factor 10. Am J Hum Genet 73:926–932

Yang Y, Hentati A, Deng HX, Dabbagh O, Sasaki T, Hirano M, Hung WY, Ouahchi K, Yan J, Azim AC, Cole N, Gascon G, Yagmour A, Ben-Hamida M, Pericak-Vance M, Hentati F, Siddique T (2001) The gene encoding alsin, a protein with three guanine-nucleotide exchange factor domains, is mutated in a form of recessive amyotrophic lateral sclerosis. Nat Genet 29:160–165

Yu GY, Howell MJ, Roller MJ, Xie TD, Gomez CM (2005) Spinocerebellar ataxia type 26 maps to chromosome 19p13.3 adjacent to SCA6. Ann Neurol 57:349–354

Zhu M, Yang T, Wei S, DeWan AT, Morell RJ, Elfenbein JL, Fisher RA, Leal SM, Smith RJH, Friderici KH (2003) Mutations in the γ-actin gene (*ACTG1*) are associated with dominant progressive deafness (DFNA20/26). Am J Hum Genet 73:1082–1091

Zhuchenko O, Bailey J, Bonnen P, Ashizawa T, Stockton DW, Amos C, Dobyns WB, Subramony SH, Zoghbi HY, Lee CC (1997) Autosomal dominant cerebellar ataxia (SCA6) associated with small polyglutamine expansions in the α1A-voltage-dependent calcium channel. Nat Genet 15:62–69

Am. J. Hum. Genet. 77:297–304, 2005

Report

A Mutation in the Dimerization Domain of Filamin C Causes a Novel Type of Autosomal Dominant Myofibrillar Myopathy

Matthias Vorgerd,[1,*] Peter F. M. van der Ven,[2,4,*] Vera Bruchertseifer,[3] Thomas Löwe,[2] Rudolf A. Kley,[1] Rolf Schröder,[5,6] Hanns Lochmüller,[7] Mirko Himmel,[2] Katrin Koehler,[3] Dieter O. Fürst,[2,4] and Angela Huebner[3]

[1]Department of Neurology, Neuromuscular Center Ruhrgebiet, Ruhr-University Bochum, Bochum, Germany; [2]Department of Cell Biology, University of Potsdam, Potsdam, Germany; [3]Children's Hospital, Technical University Dresden, Dresden; Departments of [4]Molecular Cell Biology and [5]Neurology, University of Bonn, Bonn; [6]Center for Biochemistry, University of Cologne, Cologne, Germany; and [7]Department of Neurology, Friedrich-Baur-Institute, Munich

Myofibrillar myopathy (MFM) is a human disease that is characterized by focal myofibrillar destruction and pathological cytoplasmic protein aggregations. In an extended German pedigree with a novel form of MFM characterized by clinical features of a limb-girdle myopathy and morphological features of MFM, we identified a cosegregating, heterozygous nonsense mutation (8130G→A; W2710X) in the filamin c gene (*FLNC*) on chromosome 7q32.1. The mutation is the first found in *FLNC* and is localized in the dimerization domain of filamin c. Functional studies showed that, in the truncated mutant protein, this domain has a disturbed secondary structure that leads to the inability to dimerize properly. As a consequence of this malfunction, the muscle fibers of our patients display massive cytoplasmic aggregates containing filamin c and several Z-disk–associated and sarcolemmal proteins.

Myofibrillar myopathy (MFM) is a neuromuscular disorder, usually with adult onset and an autosomal dominant inheritance pattern, that results in slowly progressive weakening of limb muscles. MFM may lead to multisystem involvement (eye, peripheral nerve, and heart), and progressive cardiorespiratory complications are potentially lethal (Goldfarb et al. 1998, 2004; Selcen and Engel 2003; Bär et al. 2005). Typically, skeletal-muscle fibers of patients with MFM show Z-disk pathologies in association with cytoplasmic accumulation of several Z-disk and cytoplasmic proteins (Selcen and Engel 2004*b*). MFM is genetically heterogeneous. Thus far, four genes have been associated with MFM: the genes encoding desmin (*DES* [MIM 125660]) (Goldfarb et al. 1998), myotilin (*TTID* [MIM 604103]) (Hauser et al. 2000; Selcen and Engel 2004*a*), Z-band alternatively spliced PDZ motif-containing protein (*LDB3* [MIM 605906]) (Selcen and Engel 2005), and αB-crystallin (*CRYAB* [MIM 123590]) (Vicart et al. 1998). However, in the majority of patients with MFM, the presence of mutations in these genes was excluded (Selcen and Engel 2005), indicating that mutations in other genes are also causative of this disease.

In the present study, we have identified an extended family of German origin with MFM, and we have excluded the involvement of the *DES, TTID*, and *CRYAB* genes by haplotype analysis (data not shown). Informed consent was obtained from all subjects (with approval of the ethics committee of Ruhr-University Bochum [#2221]). A total of 17 individuals (12 females and 5 males) were clinically affected. All patients presented with slowly progressive skeletal-muscle weakness, beginning in the lower extremities, which is compatible with the clinical signs of limb-girdle muscular dystrophy (LGMD). Eight of these patients (five females and three males) had been examined clinically (table 1). Their weakness started between the ages of 37 years and 57 years and was more prominent proximally in seven patients, whereas one patient (IV:16) had distal weakness of the calf muscles only. Serum creatine kinase levels were moderately elevated, up to 8-fold higher than the normal upper limit. Four of the patients had respiratory symp-

Received March 24, 2005; accepted for publication May 13, 2005; electronically published May 31, 2005.

Address for correspondence and reprints: Dr. Angela Huebner, Children's Hospital, Technical University Dresden, Fetscherstraße 74, 01307 Dresden, Germany. E-mail: angela.huebner@mailbox.tu-dresden.de

* These two authors contributed equally to this work.

0002-9297/2005/7702-0011$15.00

toms, and, in two of them (III:14 and III:16), nocturnal ventilation was required. One affected individual (IV:3) revealed findings compatible with cardiac involvement; three of the eight patients had evidence of an additional peripheral neuropathy (table 1). Individual IV:18 carries the *FLNC* mutation but appears to be presymptomatic as a result of his young age (28 years).

In patients III:18 and IV:3, the histological findings of muscle biopsies from a clinically affected muscle were typical of MFM. Many fibers showed structural changes harboring amorphous, granular, or hyaline deposits best recognized in trichrome-stained frozen sections (fig. 1*A*), whereas some fibers showed vacuoles. Oxidative enzyme activities (nicotinamide adenine dinucleotide dehydrogenase, succinic dehydrogenase, and cytochrome oxidase) were sharply reduced in these abnormal fiber regions. In each biopsy, increased internal nuclei, fiber splitting, and isolated necrotic fibers were present. Serial transverse cryostat sections (4 μm) of skeletal-muscle biopsies from these patients were studied by immunofluorescence assays with the use of monoclonal antibodies against filamin c (clone RR90; dilution 1:2) (van der Ven et al. 2000*a*), desmin (D33; 1:500 [DAKO]), myotilin (RSO34; 1:20), dystrophin (Dy8/6C5; 1:20), α-, β-, γ-, and δ-sarcoglycan (Ad1/20A6, βSarc/SB1, 35DAG/21B5, δ-Sarc3/12C1; 1:100 [Novocastra]), and isotype-specific secondary antibodies conjugated with fluorescein isothiocyanate or Cy2 (Southern Biotech). In each patient, many abnormal fibers revealed a marked accumulation of desmin, the histopathological hallmark of MFM, as well as filamin c in massive aggregates. These aggregates also showed strong immunoreactivity for the filamin c–binding Z-disk protein myotilin, for the sarcolemma-associated protein dystrophin, and for all sarcoglycans (fig. 1*A*). Ultrastructural analysis of skeletal muscle from patient IV:3 showed myofibrillar changes, including Z-disk streaming and extensive nemaline-rod formation (data not shown). As in MFMs that are due to heterozygous desmin mutations (Schröder et al. 2003; Goldfarb et al. 2004; Selcen and Engel 2004*b*; Bär et al. 2005), multiple fibers displayed intermyofibrillar and subsarcolemmal granulofilamentous protein aggregates (fig. 1*B*).

The dramatic mislocalization of filamin c in the muscle fibers of our patients prompted us to perform haplotype analysis, by use of microsatellite markers of the *FLNC* gene region, and subsequently to screen the family with MFM for mutations within the *FLNC* gene (MIM 102565). For haplotype and mutational analyses, genomic DNA was isolated from peripheral blood lymphocytes in accordance with standard procedures. Haplotype analysis of the candidate *FLNC* gene on chromosome 7q32.1 was performed with markers included in the deCODE genetic map. Primer pairs were designed with the OLIGO software (primer sequences are available on request). The primers were labeled with one of four fluorophores: FAM, VIC, PET, or NED. PCR amplifications were performed in a T3 thermal cycler (Biometra), and amplicons were separated on an ABI 3100 Genetic Analyzer (Applied Biosystems). The pedigree was drawn with Cyrillic software, version 2.1 (Cherwell Scientific Publishing), and haplotype analysis was performed manually. Two-point LOD score calculations were

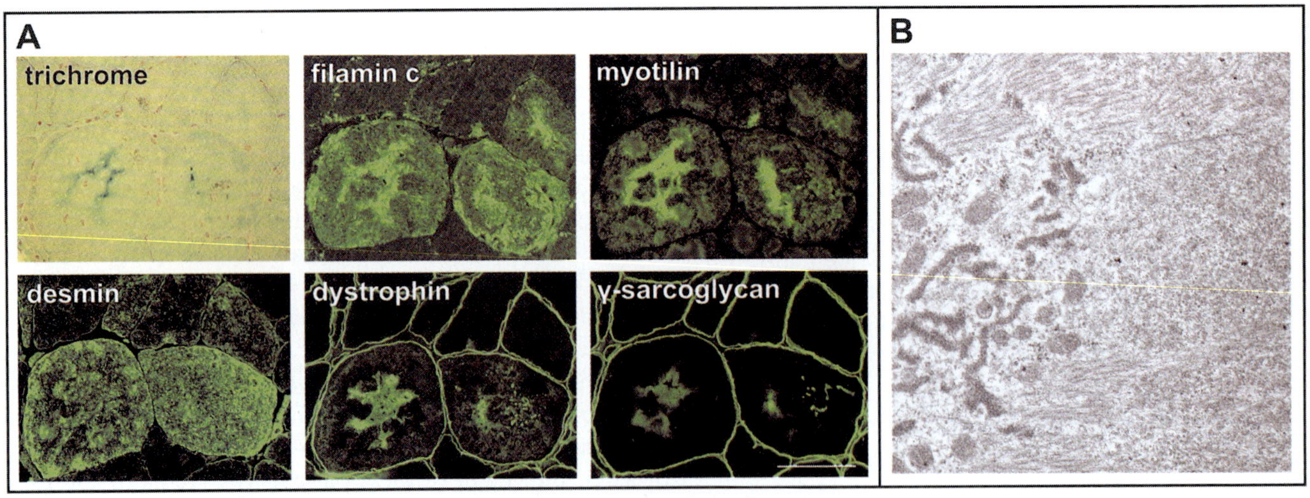

Figure 1 Immunohistochemical and ultrastructural analysis of aggregates in patient IV:3 from the pedigree with MFM. *A*, Several muscle fibers with structural changes in the trichrome-stained sections, showing intracytoplasmic accumulation of the Z-disk–associated proteins filamin c, myotilin, and desmin. Aggregates also show strong immunoreactivity for dystrophin and the sarcoglycans (as exemplified by γ-sarcoglycan), which are main components of the sarcolemmal dystrophin-glycoprotein complex (bar = 100 μm). *B*, Ultrastructural analysis of skeletal muscle, showing multiple fibers displaying intermyofibrillar granulofilamentous protein aggregates (original magnification: × 20,000).

Table 1

Clinical Data of Eight Affected Individuals in a Pedigree with a Proven *FLNC* W2710X Mutation

Patient	Sex	Age at Onset of MFM (years)	Age at Examination (years)	Initial Symptoms	Distribution of Weakness and Muscle Atrophy	Evidence of Peripheral Nerve/Eye/Cardiac Involvement	Creatine Kinase Increase
III:14	F	37	64	Weakness when climbing stairs, back pain	Proximal > distal, lower > upper extremities; respiratory insufficiency	No	2-fold
III:16	M	45	62	Weakness when climbing stairs, lower back pain	Proximal > distal, lower > upper extremities; respiratory insufficiency	No	6-fold
III:18	M	45	58	Waddling gait, chronic lumbar back pain	Proximal > distal, lower > upper extremities; respiratory insufficiency	No	8-fold
III:19	F	49	54	Waddling gait, lower back pain	Proximal in lower extremities	Peripheral nerve	3-fold
III:20	F	44	48	Weakness in legs, lower back pain	Proximal in upper extremities; proximal > distal in lower extremities	No	2-fold
IV:3	M	57	60	Weakness when climbing stairs or walking uphill	Proximal > distal, lower > upper extremities; respiratory insufficiency	Peripheral nerve/incomplete right bundle branch block, ejection fraction 66%	2-fold
IV:16	F	43	50	Unsteady gait	Distal in lower extremities	No	4-fold
IV:17	F	46	48	Waddling gait, weakness when climbing stairs, lower back pain	Proximal-dorsal and distal-anterior in lower extremities	Peripheral nerve	2-fold

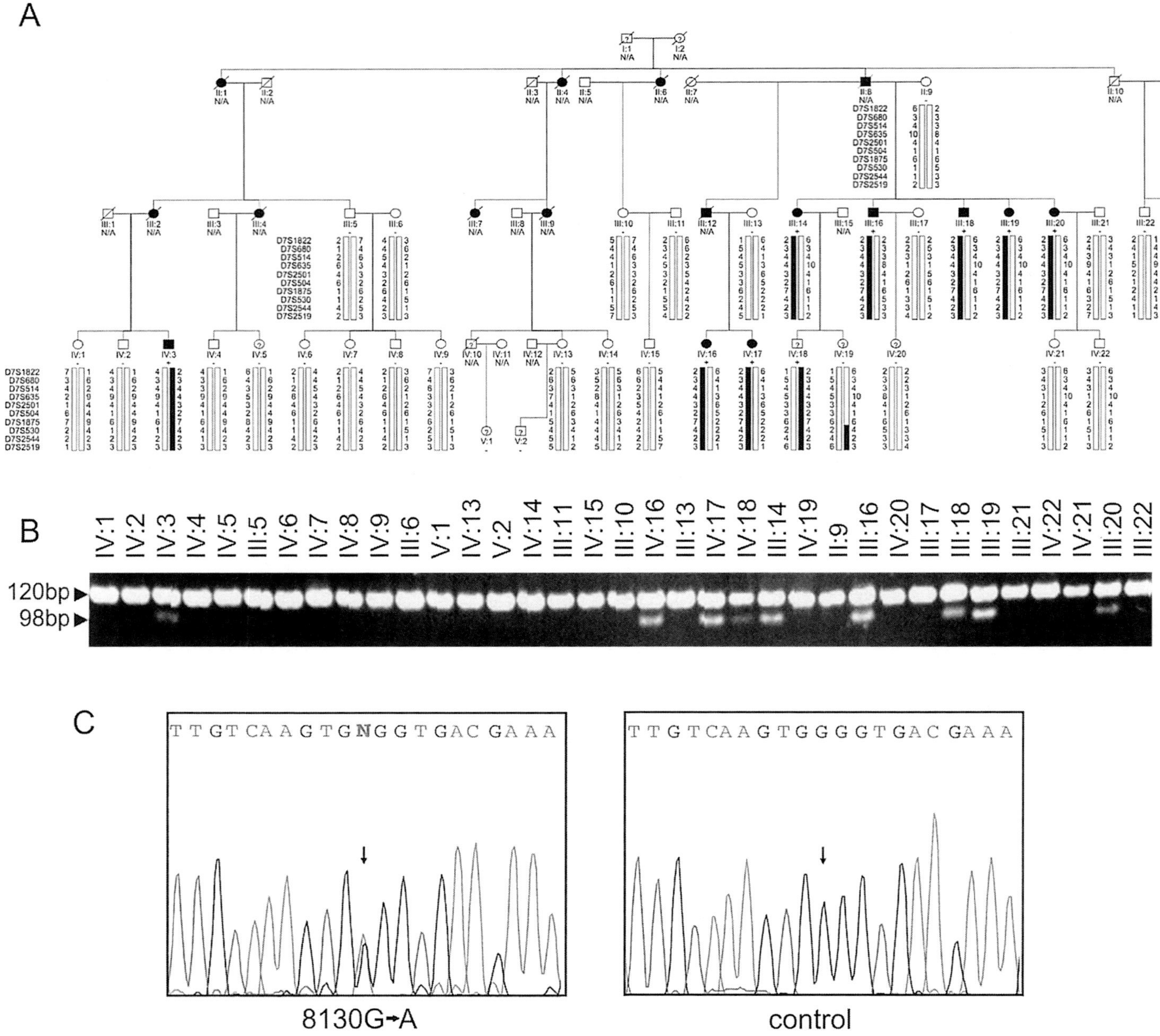
A
B
120bp
98bp
IV:1 IV:2 IV:3 IV:4 IV:5 III:5 IV:6 IV:7 IV:8 IV:9 III:6 V:1 IV:13 V:2 IV:14 III:11 IV:15 III:10 IV:16 III:13 IV:17 IV:18 III:14 IV:19 II:9 III:16 IV:20 III:17 III:18 III:19 III:21 IV:22 IV:21 III:20 III:22
C
TTGTCAAGTGNGGTGACGAAA
TTGTCAAGTGGGGTGACGAAA
8130G→A
control

Table 2

Two-Point LOD Scores between Chromosome 7 Markers and the *FLNC* Locus

	LOD AT θ =								
MARKER	.000	.001	.010	.050	.100	.150	.200	.300	.400
D7S487	2.458	2.453	2.407	2.207	1.964	1.727	1.492	1.014	.509
D7S2527	.299	.306	.355	.490	.546	.533	.479	.307	.124
D7S1873	2.310	2.306	2.274	2.117	1.894	1.655	1.410	.931	.470
D7S1822	2.417	2.415	2.393	2.262	2.050	1.807	1.548	1.020	.505
D7S680	2.871	2.865	2.808	2.549	2.218	1.885	1.553	.914	.360
D7S514	2.501	2.495	2.444	2.213	1.922	1.629	1.340	.787	.317
D7S635	4.879	4.870	4.786	4.408	3.920	3.416	2.897	1.827	.767
D7S2501	2.798	2.793	2.750	2.549	2.274	1.983	1.682	1.075	.499
D7S504	3.022	3.015	2.954	2.682	2.343	2.007	1.678	1.050	.483
D7S1875	4.286	4.278	4.203	3.865	3.434	2.994	2.547	1.640	.741
D7S530	1.822	1.817	1.771	1.575	1.352	1.143	.941	.550	.219
D7S2544	2.902	2.894	2.829	2.549	2.220	1.907	1.604	1.003	.419
D7S2519	1.460	1.458	1.437	1.338	1.202	1.057	.906	.597	.294
D7S2531	.294	.296	.312	.359	.375	.358	.315	.186	.056
D7S640	−2.090	1.047	1.988	2.417	2.366	2.178	1.926	1.317	.639

performed using the LINKAGE program package, with the help of the LINKRUN program (T. F. Wienker, personal communication), under the assumption of autosomal dominant inheritance, equal male and female recombination rates, full penetrance, and a disease-allele frequency of 0.0001. The National Center for Biotechnology Information (NCBI) Map Viewer and Ensembl Genome Browser databases were used for localization of the microsatellite marker loci and identification of transcripts in the candidate region. The GDB Human Genome Database was used for information about microsatellite markers and their primer sequences. Indeed, haplotype analyses established linkage of the disease to the *FLNC* locus (fig. 2*A*), with a maximum LOD score of 4.879 ($\theta = 0$) at marker *D7S635* (table 2).

Sequence analysis of *FLNC* included all 48 exons and was performed on genomic DNA from individuals IV:3 and IV:16 of the present family, as well as on DNA from four sporadic cases with similar clinical and morphological features pointing to LGMD or MFM. Sequencing was performed with an ABI 3100 Genetic Analyzer (Applied Biosystems) by use of the BigDye Terminator v 1.1 Cycle Sequencing kit (Applied Biosystems). Although no *FLNC* mutations were found in the sporadic cases, a single heterozygous nucleotide substitution (8130G→A), resulting in a substitution of tryptophan at position 2710 by a stop codon (W2710X) (human *FLNC* [GenBank accession number AF252549], human chromosome 7 clones containing *FLNC* [GenBank accession numbers AC025594 and AC024952], and FLNC [accession number Q14315]), was identified in exon 48 in patients IV:3 and IV:16 from the present family (fig. 2*C*).

To confirm cosegregation of the mutation with the MFM disease phenotype, all available family members and 110 control individuals were investigated for the 8130G→A mutation by RFLP analysis and/or direct sequencing. Since the mutation did not delete or introduce a restriction site, a new *Alu*I restriction site was created in the mutant PCR product by use of a lower primer with a single-nucleotide mismatch at the penultimate 3′ position (primer sequences are available on request). For restriction-enzyme digestion, the PCR product was incubated with *Alu*I, and the cleaved fragments were separated on a 2% agarose gel and were visualized by ethidium bromide staining (for details, see the legend to fig. 2*B*). The 8130G→A mutation was detected in all affected family members and was confirmed by direct sequencing (fig. 2*B*). It was not observed in 220 control chromosomes.

Recently, a large five-generation Spanish family with LGMD, with clinical features similar to those seen in the German family, was described (Gamez et al. 2001), and,

Figure 2 *A*, Pedigree and genotypic analysis of the German family with autosomal dominant MFM segregating with *FLNC*. Marker haplotypes on chromosome 7q31.33-7q32.3 that are linked to MFM are indicated by blackened bars. Blackened and unblackened symbols represent clinically affected individuals and unaffected individuals, respectively; unblackened symbols with question marks represent individuals of undetermined disease status. Presence (+) or absence (−) of the *FLNC* mutation in those individuals available for mutation analysis is indicated. N/A = not available for genetic diagnosis. *B*, RFLP analysis of the 8130G→A mutation, by digestion of a PCR product with *Alu*I. Undigested PCR product (120 bp) corresponds to the G allele, and digested PCR product (98 bp + unverifiable 22 bp) corresponds to the A allele. *C*, Sequence chromatograms demonstrating the heterozygous mutation (8130G→A; W2710X) found in affected family members (*left*) and the corresponding normal sequence (*right*).

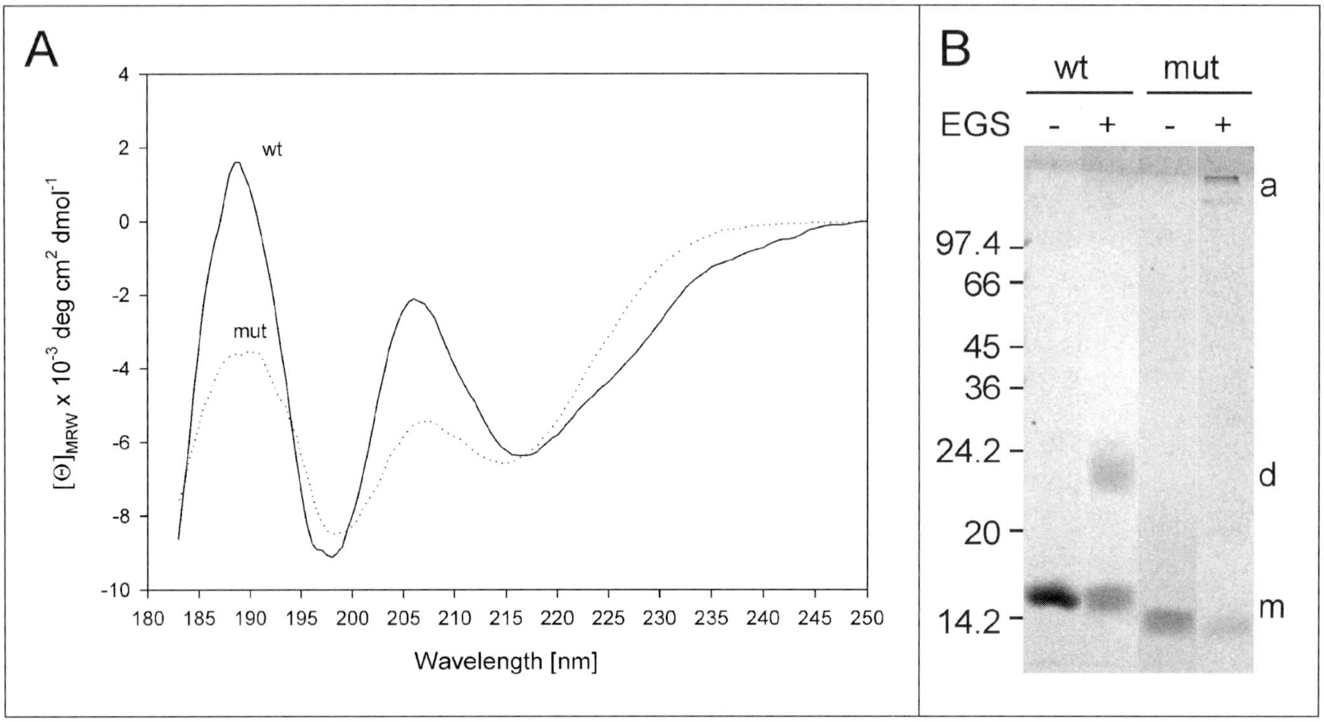

Figure 3 Functional studies of the *FLNC* W2710X mutation. *A*, Circular dichroism spectrometry of filamin c domain 24 in the far UV range, performed with purified, bacterially expressed proteins. Note that the wild-type protein (wt) shows the typical β-sheet secondary structure, whereas the mutant-protein (mut) spectrum has lower amplitudes, indicating improper folding. deg = degrees; $[\Theta]_{MRW}$ = mean residue weight ellipticity. *B*, The same recombinant polypeptides as above were cross-linked using ethylene glycol bis(succinimidylsuccinate) (EGS). Proteins were separated by SDS-PAGE, and the gel was stained with Coomassie Brilliant Blue. Without cross-linking (−), only monomers (m) of the wild type and the truncated mutant polypeptide are visible. Note that, on cross-linking (+), the wild-type protein yields dimers (d), whereas the mutant protein yields aggregates (a) of higher molecular mass.

subsequently, the disorder was referred to as "LGMD1F" (MIM 608423) and was mapped to chromosome 7q32, which includes the *FLNC* locus. However, in this family, *FLNC* was excluded as a candidate gene (Palenzuela et al. 2003). In the Spanish family, skeletal-muscle weakness, predominantly involving the pelvic and shoulder girdle, started between the ages of 1 year and 58 years, whereas, in the German family, no patient with a juvenile-onset form was observed. In the Spanish family, the histochemical and immunohistochemical findings were compatible with LGMD; desmin immunostaining was not reported. In contrast, the massive protein aggregates in the German family clearly indicated MFM. Despite substantial overlap in the clinical phenotype, patients in the German family are distinct—not only genetically but also morphologically—from patients with LGMD1F. Because of the protein defect, we suggest classification of the disease found in the German family as "autosomal dominant filaminopathy," a novel form of MFM.

Filamins are a family of actin-binding proteins involved in reshaping the actin cytoskeleton and its associated structures (Stossel et al. 2001; van der Flier and Sonnenberg 2001). Actin binding is conferred by a pair of amino-terminal CH domains. For their actin filament–bundling and cross-linking activities, the filamins depend on their C-terminal region—more specifically, the immunoglobulin-like domain 24, which is responsible for dimer formation (Himmel et al. 2003). Furthermore, filamins interact with a plethora of cellular proteins of great functional diversity, indicating that they are multifunctional signaling adapter proteins (van der Flier and Sonnenberg 2001). Although mutations in the ubiquitously expressed genes encoding filamin a (Fox et al. 1998; Robertson et al. 2003) and filamin b (Krakow et al. 2004) are causative for a strikingly wide range of human diseases (Feng and Walsh 2004), up to the present, no disease-causing mutations had been found in *FLNC*, the gene encoding the muscle-specific filamin isoform. Its up-regulation during initial stages of myocyte differentiation, its localization predominantly at the periphery of Z-disks (van der Ven et al. 2000*a*), and its direct interaction with myotilin (van der Ven et al. 2000*b*) imply an important role for this filamin isoform during myofibrillogenesis. Since filamin c also binds γ- and δ-sarcoglycan at the sarcolemma (Thompson et al. 2000), it was hypothesized that filamin c is involved in signaling pathways from the sarcolemma to the myofibril (Thompson et al. 2000; van der Ven et al. 2000*b*).

The W2710X mutation in the reported family with MFM leads to a truncation of the filamin c immunoglobulin domain that is responsible for dimerization (Himmel et al. 2003). To assess the pathogenic potential of the mutation, we examined its effects on the secondary structure of the mutant domain 24 and on its ability to dimerize. cDNA fragments encoding the wild-type and mutant domain 24 were cloned in pET23-T7 (Obermann et al. 1998), and recombinant proteins were expressed in and purified from *Escherichia coli* BL21-CodonPlus-RP cells by use of standard procedures (Himmel et al. 2003). Circular dichroism spectra were recorded from both proteins on a Jasco J-715 spectropolarimeter. Whereas analysis of the wild-type domain resulted in the typical β-sheet secondary structure that was previously reported for this domain (Himmel et al. 2003; Pudas et al. 2005), analysis of the truncated, mutated domain resulted in significantly lower signals, suggesting improper folding (fig. 3*A*).

We next examined dimerization of mutant filamin c by chemical cross-linking experiments, essentially using previously established conditions for the wild-type protein (Himmel et al. 2003), except that PBS was used instead of cross-linking buffer. Whereas the dimerization of the wild-type variant was reproduced under these conditions, cross-linking of the truncated domain 24 did not result in the detection of dimers. Instead, high–molecular mass aggregates of the mutated filamin fragment were observed on the SDS-polyacrylamide gel (fig. 3*B*) and on immunoblots (not shown). Although the precise structural changes that occur in the mutated filamin c are currently unknown, the formation of aggregates in the cross-linking assay and the tendency to precipitate in solution (not shown) imply a weaker stability of mutated filamin c in comparison with the wild-type protein and indicate a strong tendency for uncontrolled aggregation rather than defined dimerization.

We have provided evidence of an altered distribution of myotilin and the dystrophin-sarcoglycan complex in affected individuals. We hypothesize that the fine balance of filamin c and its binding partners in both the Z-disk and the cell membrane may be disturbed. Therefore, defects in this protein may weaken myofibrils and, at the same time, destabilize the muscle cell membrane. This may ultimately result in clinical and molecular features resembling both MFM and LGMD.

In summary, we describe here the first disease-related mutation within the *FLNC* gene and also the first mutation in a dimerization domain in the filamin family. The mutation results in the inability of the mutant protein to dimerize and leads to the generation of large filamin c–containing aggregates within the skeletal-muscle fibers. Biochemical experiments provide an explanation for this observation and show that dimer formation is essential for the biological function of filamin.

Acknowledgments

We thank the family members for participation in this study; A. Hartmann-Schreiner, M. Fey, P. Mitzscherling, and G. Nürnberg, for technical assistance; and A. Freiberg and R. Seckler, for help with the circular dichroism spectrometry and for helpful discussions. M.V. and R.A.K. are supported by the Scientific Committee of the Kliniken Bergmannsheil Bochum and by the FoRUM program of the Ruhr-University Bochum. A.H., V.B., and K.K. were supported by the MeDDrive program of the Medical Faculty of Technical University Dresden. M.V., H.L., D.O.F., and A.H. are members of the German Network on Muscular Dystrophies (MD-NET), which is supported by the Bundesministerium für Forschung und Bildung (01GM0302).

Web Resources

Accession numbers and URLs for data presented herein are as follows:

Ensembl Genome Browser, http://www.ensembl.org/
GDB Human Genome Database, http://www.gdb.org/
GenBank, http://www.ncbi.nih.gov/Genbank/ (for human *FLNC* [accession number AF252549], human chromosome 7 clones containing *FLNC* [accession numbers AC025594 and AC024952], and FLNC [accession number Q14315])
NCBI Map Viewer, http://www.ncbi.nlm.nih.gov/mapview/
Online Mendelian Inheritance in Man (OMIM), http://www.ncbi.nlm.nih.gov/entrez/Omim/ (for *DES, TTID, LDB3, CRYAB, FLNC*, and LGMD1F)

References

Bär H, Fischer D, Goudeau B, Kley RA, Clemen CS, Vicart P, Herrmann H, Vorgerd M, Schröder R (2005) Pathogenic effects of a novel heterozygous R350P desmin mutation on the assembly of desmin intermediate filaments in vivo and in vitro. Hum Mol Genet 14:1251–1260

Feng Y, Walsh CA (2004) The many faces of filamin: a versatile molecular scaffold for cell motility and signalling. Nat Cell Biol 6:1034–1038

Fox JW, Lamperti ED, Eksioglu YZ, Hong SE, Feng Y, Graham DA, Scheffer IE, Dobyns WB, Hirsch BA, Radtke RA, Berkovic SF, Huttenlocher PR, Walsh CA (1998) Mutations in filamin 1 prevent migration of cerebral cortical neurons in human periventricular heterotopia. Neuron 21:1315–1325

Gamez J, Navarro C, Andreu AL, Fernandez JM, Palenzuela L, Tejeira S, Fernandez-Hojas R, Schwartz S, Karadimas C, DiMauro S, Hirano M, Cervera C (2001) Autosomal dominant limb-girdle muscular dystrophy: a large kindred with evidence for anticipation. Neurology 56:450–454

Goldfarb LG, Park KY, Cervenakova L, Gorokhova S, Lee HS, Vasconcelos O, Nagle JW, Semino-Mora C, Sivakumar K, Dalakas MC (1998) Missense mutations in desmin associated with familial cardiac and skeletal myopathy. Nat Genet 19:402–403

Goldfarb LG, Vicart P, Goebel HH, Dalakas MC (2004) Desmin myopathy. Brain 127:723–734

Hauser MA, Horrigan SK, Salmikangas P, Torian UM, Viles KD, Dancel R, Tim RW, Taivainen A, Bartoloni L, Gilchrist JM, Stajich JM, Gaskell PC, Gilbert JR, Vance JM, Pericak-Vance MA, Carpen O, Westbrook CA, Speer MC (2000) Myotilin is mutated in limb girdle muscular dystrophy 1A. Hum Mol Genet 9:2141–2147

Himmel M, van der Ven PFM, Stöcklein W, Fürst DO (2003) The limits of promiscuity: isoform-specific dimerization of filamins. Biochemistry 42:430–439

Krakow D, Robertson SP, King LM, Morgan T, Sebald ET, Bertolotto C, Wachsmann-Hogiu S, Acuna D, Shapiro SS, Takafuta T, Aftimos S, Kim CA, Firth H, Steiner CE, Cormier-Daire V, Superti-Furga A, Bonafe L, Graham JM Jr, Grix A, Bacino CA, Allanson J, Bialer MG, Lachman RS, Rimoin DL, Cohn DH (2004) Mutations in the gene encoding filamin B disrupt vertebral segmentation, joint formation and skeletogenesis. Nat Genet 36:405–410

Obermann WMJ, van der Ven PFM, Steiner F, Weber K, Fürst DO (1998) Mapping of a myosin-binding domain and a regulatory phosphorylation site in M-protein, a structural protein of the sarcomeric M band. Mol Biol Cell 9:829–840

Palenzuela L, Andreu AL, Gamez J, Vila MR, Kunimatsu T, Meseguer A, Cervera C, Fernandez Cadenas I, van der Ven PFM, Nygaard TG, Bonilla E, Hirano M (2003) A novel autosomal dominant limb-girdle muscular dystrophy (LGMD 1F) maps to 7q32.1-32.2. Neurology 61:404–406

Pudas R, Kiema TR, Butler PJ, Stewart M, Ylanne J (2005) Structural basis for vertebrate filamin dimerization. Structure 13:111–119

Robertson SP, Twigg SR, Sutherland-Smith AJ, Biancalana V, Gorlin RJ, Horn D, Kenwrick SJ, Kim CA, Morava E, Newbury-Ecob R, Orstavik KH, Quarrell OW, Schwartz CE, Shears DJ, Suri M, Kendrick-Jones J, Wilkie AO (2003) Localized mutations in the gene encoding the cytoskeletal protein filamin A cause diverse malformations in humans. Nat Genet 33:487–491

Schröder R, Goudeau B, Casteras Simon M, Fischer D, Eggermann T, Clemen CS, Li Z, Reimann J, Xue Z, Rudnik-Schöneborn S, Zerres K, van der Ven PFM, Fürst DO, Kunz WS, Vicart P (2003) On noxious desmin: functional effects of a novel desmin insertion mutation on the extrasarcomeric desmin cytoskeleton and mitochondria. Hum Mol Genet 12: 657–669

Selcen D, Engel AG (2003) Myofibrillar myopathy caused by novel dominant negative α-B-crystallin mutations. Ann Neurol 54:804–810

——— (2004*a*) Mutations in myotilin cause myofibrillar myopathy. Neurology 62:1363–1371

——— (2004*b*) Myofibrillar myopathy. In: Engel AG, Franzini-Armstrong C (eds) Myology. McGraw-Hill, New York, pp 1187–1202

——— (2005) Mutations in ZASP define a novel form of muscular dystrophy in humans. Ann Neurol 57:269–276

Stossel TP, Condeelis J, Cooley L, Hartwig JH, Noegel A, Schleicher M, Shapiro SS (2001) Filamins as integrators of cell mechanics and signalling. Nat Rev Mol Cell Biol 2:138–145

Thompson TG, Chan YM, Hack AA, Brosius M, Rajala M, Lidov HG, McNally EM, Watkins S, Kunkel LM (2000) Filamin 2 (FLN2): a muscle-specific sarcoglycan interacting protein. J Cell Biol 148:115–126

van der Flier A, Sonnenberg A (2001) Structural and functional aspects of filamins. Biochim Biophys Acta 1538:99–117

van der Ven PFM, Obermann WMJ, Lemke B, Gautel M, Weber K, Fürst DO (2000*a*) Characterization of muscle filamin isoforms suggests a possible role of γ-filamin/ABP-L in sarcomeric Z-disc formation. Cell Motil Cytoskeleton 45: 149–162

van der Ven PFM, Wiesner S, Salmikangas P, Auerbach D, Himmel M, Kempa S, Hayess K, Pacholsky D, Taivainen A, Schröder R, Carpén O, Fürst DO (2000*b*) Indications for a novel muscular dystrophy pathway: γ-filamin, the muscle-specific filamin isoform, interacts with myotilin. J Cell Biol 151:235–248

Vicart P, Caron A, Guicheney P, Li Z, Prevost MC, Faure A, Chateau D, Chapon F, Tome F, Dupret JM, Paulin D, Fardeau M (1998) A missense mutation in the αB-crystallin chaperone gene causes a desmin-related myopathy. Nat Genet 20:92–95

Report

Dysregulation of Chondrogenesis in Human Cleidocranial Dysplasia

Qiping Zheng,[1] Eiman Sebald,[3] Guang Zhou,[1] Yuqing Chen,[1,2] William Wilcox,[3,4,5] Brendan Lee,[1,2] and Deborah Krakow[3,5]

[1]Department of Molecular and Human Genetics and [2]Howard Hughes Medical Institute, Baylor College of Medicine, Houston; and [3]Medical Genetics Institute, [4]Department of Pediatrics, Cedars-Sinai Medical Center, and [5]David Geffen School of Medicine at University of California–Los Angeles, Los Angeles

Cleidocranial dysplasia (CCD) is an autosomal dominant skeletal dysplasia caused by heterozygosity of mutations in human *RUNX2*. The disorder is characterized by delayed closure of the fontanel and hypoplastic clavicles that result from defective intramembranous ossification. However, additional features, such as short stature and cone epiphyses, also suggest an underlying defect in endochondral ossification. Here, we report observations of growth-plate abnormalities in a patient with a novel *RUNX2* gene mutation, a single C insertion (1228insC), which is predicted to lead to a premature termination codon and thus to haploinsufficiency of *RUNX2* and the CCD phenotype. Histological analysis of the rib and long-bone cartilages showed a markedly diminished zone of hypertrophy. Quantitative real-time reverse transcription–polymerase chain reaction analysis of limb cartilage RNA showed a 5–10-fold decrease in the hypertrophic chondrocyte molecular markers *VEGF, MMP13,* and *COL10A1.* Together, these data show that humans with CCD have altered endochondral ossification due to altered *RUNX2* regulation of hypertrophic chondrocyte–specific genes during chondrocyte maturation.

Runx2 is a well-characterized critical transcriptional regulator of osteoblast differentiation (Ducy et al. 1997; Komori et al. 1997; Otto et al. 1997). Heterozygosity for mutations in *RUNX2* causes cleidocranial dysplasia (CCD [MIM 119600]), an autosomal dominant skeletal dysplasia characterized by hypoplastic clavicles, short stature, and tooth anomalies (Lee et al. 1997; Mundlos et al. 1997; Lee and Zhou 2004). *Runx2*-deficient mice (−/−) have no bone formation, whereas the heterozygote mice (+/−) display abnormalities similar to those seen in individuals with CCD (Shapiro 1999). *Runx2* heterozygote mice have fewer osteoblasts and bone-specific proteins, and the enzyme activity of alkaline phosphatase is low (Shapiro 1999). Furthermore, molecular and mouse genetic studies demonstrate that the abnormal bone formation is mainly due to *Runx2* transcriptional regulation of its target genes during osteoblast differentiation. In osteoblasts, transcription of the bone-specific osteocalcin gene is principally regulated by the *Runx2* transcription factor and is stimulated in response to vitamin D_3 via the vitamin D_3 receptor complex (Sierra et al. 2003). Beyond the skeleton, studies suggest that *Runx2* regulates the expression of molecules in mesenchyme that act reciprocally on the dental epithelium to control its growth and differentiation, and this partly explains the dental abnormalities found in patients with CCD and in *Runx2* heterozygote mice (D'Souza et al. 1999; Zou et al. 2003).

The CCD characteristics of delayed closure of the fontanel and hypoplastic clavicles reflect defective intramembranous ossification. However, the significantly hypoplastic or absent clavicles point to an effect on both intramembranous and endochondral ossification, because the clavicle ossifies embryologically by both routes (Huang et al. 1997). Recent reports that emphasize short stature as a prominent feature in CCD provide supporting evidence for *RUNX2* effects on endochondral ossification (Cooper et al. 2001; Morava et al. 2002). In addition, mouse genetics studies have shown altered chondrocyte maturation or defective chondrocyte hypertrophy in some long bones of *Runx2* null mice (Inada et al. 1999; Enomoto et al. 2000). Growth-plate compression and decreased expression of *Col10a1* (a hy-

Received March 21, 2005; accepted for publication May 26, 2005; electronically published June 10, 2005.

Address for correspondence and reprints: Dr. Brendan Lee, Department of Molecular and Human Genetics, Baylor College of Medicine, One Baylor Plaza, Room 635E, Houston, TX 77030. E-mail: blee@bcm.tmc.edu

0002-9297/2005/7702-0012$15.00

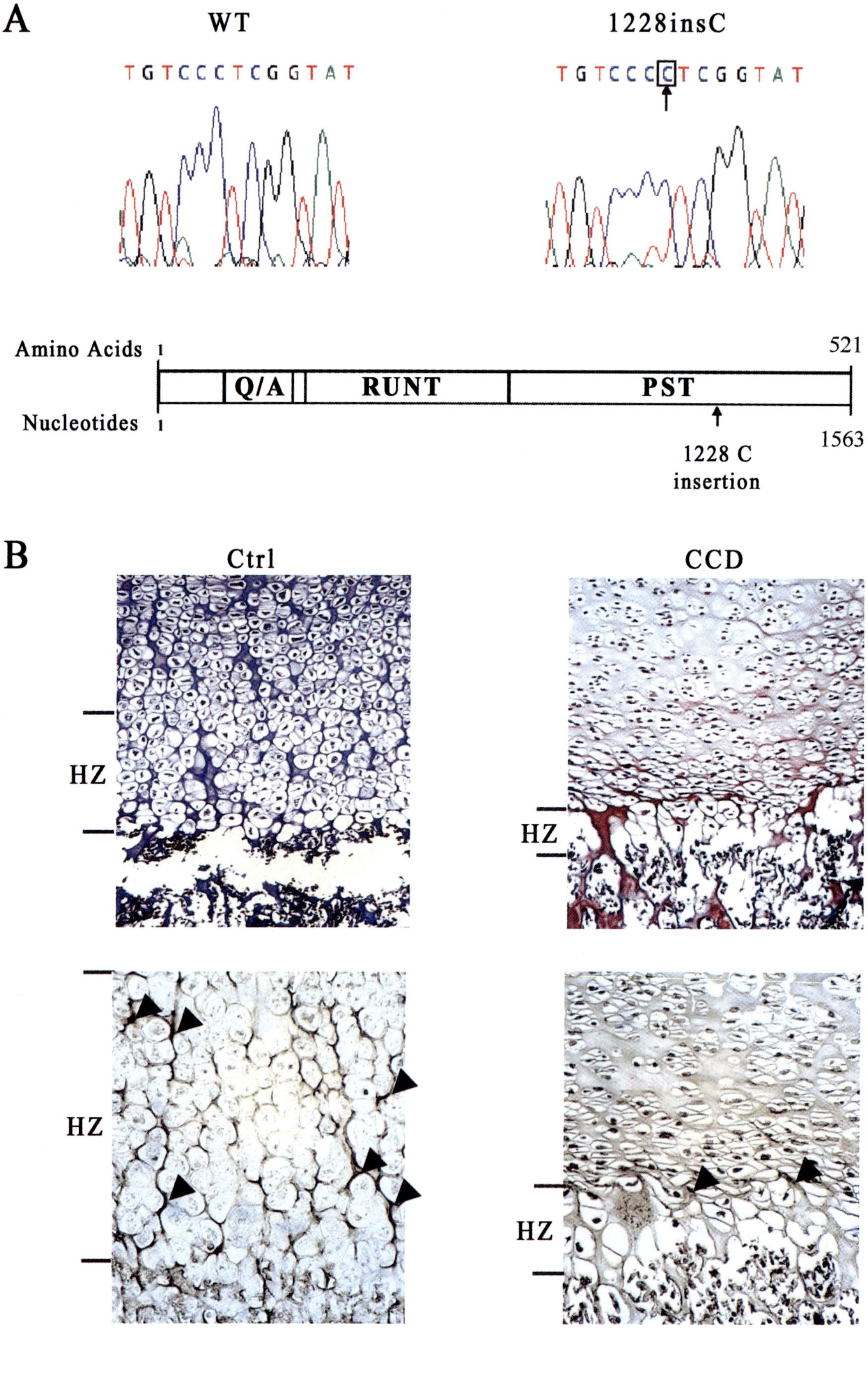
A
WT
TGTCCCTCGGTAT
1228insC
TGTCCCCTCGGTAT
Amino Acids 1
521
Q/A
RUNT
PST
Nucleotides 1
1563
1228 C
insertion
B
Ctrl
CCD
HZ
HZ
HZ
HZ

pertrophic chondrocyte–specific molecular marker) have also been reported in *Runx2* heterozygote mice (Zheng et al. 2003). However, the molecular and histological correlates in human development have only been extrapolated.

In this study, we report the molecular, immunohistochemical, and histological characterization of growth-plate abnormalities in a 20-wk fetus with CCD and a novel *RUNX2* gene mutation. Prenatal diagnosis of a de novo case of CCD was made by ultrasonography at 19 wk. On the basis of ultrasound long-bone measurements, the 20-wk fetus was smaller than normal, with limb lengths consistent with 19-wk gestation, and absent clavicles and a hypomineralized calvarium were noted. Relevant tissues, including the entire distal femoral cartilage, were harvested at autopsy. *RUNX2* exons were PCR amplified from genomic DNA by use of intron-specific primers, as described elsewhere (Lee et al. 1997). Direct sequencing of this PCR-amplified *RUNX2* gene revealed a single C insertion (1228insC) resulting in a frameshift mutation in codon 410 (fig. 1*A*). The mutation was confirmed by cloning and sequencing of each allele. This mutation is predicted to lead to a premature termination codon at amino acid 489 in the proline, serine, and threonine–rich (PST) transactivation domain and to alteration of the identity of the last 112 amino acids in the peptide (fig. 1*A*). On the basis of previous work, this mutation is predicted to cause haploinsufficiency and to produce the CCD phenotype (Lee et al. 1997; Mundlos et al. 1997; Zhou et al. 1999). Interestingly, one nearby mutation (1205insC), which leads to a frameshift in codon 402, was reported to cause a severe CCD phenotype, with osteoporosis, recurrent bone fractures, and scoliosis (Quack et al. 1999). Another adjacent R391X premature termination mutation was previously reported to be associated with classic CCD; in an in vitro transfection study, this mutated protein showed only 20% transactivation of the reporter activity, compared with wild-type Runx2 (Zhou et al. 1999).

To study the putative skeletal deficiency in this fetus with CCD, we performed histologic analysis of rib and other long-bone cartilage from the fetus and an age-matched control. The rib, tibia, and femur from the fetus with CCD and the control were formalin-fixed and embedded in paraffin. Von Kossa staining was performed on 5-μm sagittal sections (Lowe and Bancroft 1996). The rib growth-plate sections of the fetus with CCD showed a markedly diminished zone of hypertrophy and disorganized growth-plate chondrocytes, compared with those of the age-matched control (fig. 1*B*, *upper panel*). Similar findings were also found for the ulna and tibia (data not shown). Because of the significant shortened zone of hypertrophy, we performed immunohistochemical analysis with both rib and limb sections, using an antibody specific to type X collagen (from Dr. Robin Pool, Montreal), a molecular marker of chondrocyte hypertrophy during endochondral ossification. The result showed altered type X collagen expression and localization. In the control growth plate, type X collagen staining was seen primarily in the pericellular matrix. In contrast, in the CCD growth plate, the type X collagen staining was poorly visible in the extracellular matrix and was more localized to intracellular space (fig. 1*B*, *lower panel*, and figs. 2 and 3). These data together suggest an important function for *RUNX2* in human endochondral ossification, linking haploinsufficiency of *RUNX2*, decreased chondrocyte hypertrophy, and altered type X collagen expression and distribution in CCD.

Runx2 has been shown to be an important regulator of chondrocyte maturation, by in vitro cell culture and in vivo mouse genetics studies (Inada et al. 1999; Kim et al. 1999; Enomoto et al. 2000; Takeda et al. 2001; Ueta et al. 2001). In *Runx2*-deficient mice (−/−), chondrocyte differentiation was reported to be severely disturbed (Inada et al. 1999), and lack of hypertrophic chondrocytes with delayed onset of hypertrophy has also

The figure is available in its entirety in the online edition of *The American Journal of Human Genetics.*

Figure 2 Hematoxylin and eosin staining and immunohistochemical analysis of the CCD and control femur sections. The legend is available in its entirety in the online edition of *The American Journal of Human Genetics.*

Figure 1 Molecular and histological analyses of a fetus with CCD. *A*, Sequencing of exon 9 of *RUNX2* alleles shows the mutant allele with a C insertion in the PST domain (1228insC) and the wild-type allele (WT). The relative position of this mutation is shown in the schematic representation of the RUNX2 structure. Q/A = polyglutamine/polyalanine domain; RUNT = DNA-binding runt domain. *B*, Von Kossa staining and immunohistochemical analysis of the CCD rib cartilage. For an age-matched control fetal rib section (Ctrl), Von Kossa histological analysis shows a normal hypertrophic zone (*top left panel*), and type X collagen immunostaining exhibits normal extracellular staining of type X collagen in the hypertrophic zone (*arrowheads in bottom left panel*). Separation of primary spongiosa is an artifact of tissue preparation. For the rib section from the fetus with CCD, Von Kossa staining shows a much shortened hypertrophic zone (*top right panel*), and type X collagen immunostaining shows flattened hypertrophic chondrocytes, with both reduced and asymmetric type X collagen expression within the compressed hypertrophic zone (*arrowheads in bottom right panel*). HZ = hypertrophic zone of growth plate.

The figure is available in its entirety in the online edition of *The American Journal of Human Genetics.*

Figure 3 Von Kossa staining and immunohistochemical analysis of the CCD and control rib cartilage sections. The legend is available in its entirety in the online edition of *The American Journal of Human Genetics.*

been observed (Kim et al. 1999). Although type X collagen was barely detectable in *Runx2* null mice, osteopontin, bone sialoprotein, and collagenase 3 (MMP-13) were also not expressed in hypertrophic chondrocytes, indicating that they are regulated by *Runx2* in terminal hypertrophic chondrocytes (Inada et al. 1999). In recent studies, this has been shown to be the result of direct *Runx2* regulation of their respective promoters (Sato et al. 1998; Jimenez et al. 1999; Zheng et al. 2003; Wang et al. 2004). Vascular endothelial growth factor (VEGF), a critical regulator of angiogenesis during development, is another direct transcriptional target of *Runx2*. *Runx2* is required for a tissue-specific genetic program that regulates VEGF during endochondral bone formation (Zelzer et al. 2001). More recently, mouse genetics studies have pointed out the possible cooperative function of Runt gene family members—*Runx1*, *Runx2*, and *Runx3*—in skeletal development. *Runx1* mediates early events of endochondral and intramembranous bone formation, *Runx3* cooperates with *Runx2* in promoting chondrocyte maturation, and *Runx2* is a potent inducer of late stages of chondrocyte and osteoblast differentiation (Yoshida et al. 2004; Smith et al. 2005).

To further characterize the molecular mechanisms and signaling pathways that are involved in the pathogenesis of CCD in humans, we performed quantitative real-time RT-PCR analysis of growth-plate RNA, to determine the status of the *RUNX2* transcriptional network in cartilage. We performed assays for the relative expression levels of known *RUNX2* targets *VEGF*, *MMP13*, and *COL10A1*, as well as for the transcription factor genes *RUNX1*, *RUNX2*, *RUNX3*, and *SOX9*. Total RNAs from CCD and age-matched control cartilages (from bilateral distal femurs) were extracted as described elsewhere (Zheng et al. 2003). cDNA synthesis from the total RNA, real-time PCR amplification of target genes, and analysis of the real-time PCR results for fold induction of gene expression were performed in accordance with the manufacturer's protocol and as in previously reported procedures with modifications (Livak and Schmittgen 2001; Pfaffl 2001; Zheng et al. 2003). The sequences of the primers used for PCR amplification of *RUNX1*, *RUNX2*, *RUNX3*, *COL10A1*, *MMP13*, *SOX9*, *VEGF*, and *GAPDH* are listed in table 1. The *GAPDH* gene was used as an internal control for the quantity and quality of the cDNAs.

Our results showed that the level of *RUNX2* mRNA was ~50% downregulated in the CCD cartilage, as compared with the control cartilage, suggesting that haploinsufficiency of *RUNX2* results from the frameshift mutation described above (figs. 1*A* and 4*A*). This mutation, which sits in the last exon of *RUNX2*, is predicted to lead to a premature termination codon (PTC). However, nonsense-mediated mRNA decay (NMD) cannot be excluded for this mutant allele (Maquat 2004). It has been reported that a PTC mutation leading to complete NMD causes collagen X haploinsufficiency in Schmid metaphyseal chondrodysplasia cartilage (Bateman et al. 2003). However, since this mutation resides in the last exon, a potential translated mRNA that escapes NMD is possible, although the production of a truncated protein has never been demonstrated for this condition. Interestingly, sequencing of 10 independent RT-PCR cDNAs showed that 3 of 10 contain the mutant allele, which suggests the possibility that the transcript escapes NMD. We also examined the hypertrophic chondrocyte–related molecular markers *COL10A1*, *MMP-13*, and *VEGF*, and they all showed a 5–10-fold decrease in mRNA levels (fig. 4*B*, 4*C*, and 4*D*). These genes are highly expressed in terminally differentiated chondrocytes. Because of the significantly shortened zone of hypertrophy, we dissected the whole growth-plate cartilages to examine the expression level of the specific genes mentioned above, with normalization to the house-keeping gene *GAPDH*. Although the reduced expression of target genes might be partially due to the reduced number of hypertrophic chondrocytes, these data generated in human tissue correlate well with the in vitro and in vivo data for mice showing the direct regulation of the respective target promoters by *Runx2* during skeletal development (Jimenez et al. 1999; Zelzer et al. 2001; D'Alonzo et al. 2002; Zheng et al. 2003). The observation of a shortened zone of hypertrophy was previously reported for *Runx2* heterozygote mice and also correlates well with human data (Zheng et al. 2003). No change in mRNA levels was observed for *RUNX1* (fig. 4*E*). Interestingly, we also examined the *RUNX3* mRNA level by real-time RT-PCR analysis, and it showed a 4-fold upregulation in CCD cartilage, compared with control cartilage (fig. 4*F*). This raises the question of whether *RUNX3* expression may be upregulated in compensation for loss of *RUNX2*. Recent

Table 1

Sequences of Primers Used for PCR Amplification

The table is available in its entirety in the online edition of *The American Journal of Human Genetics.*

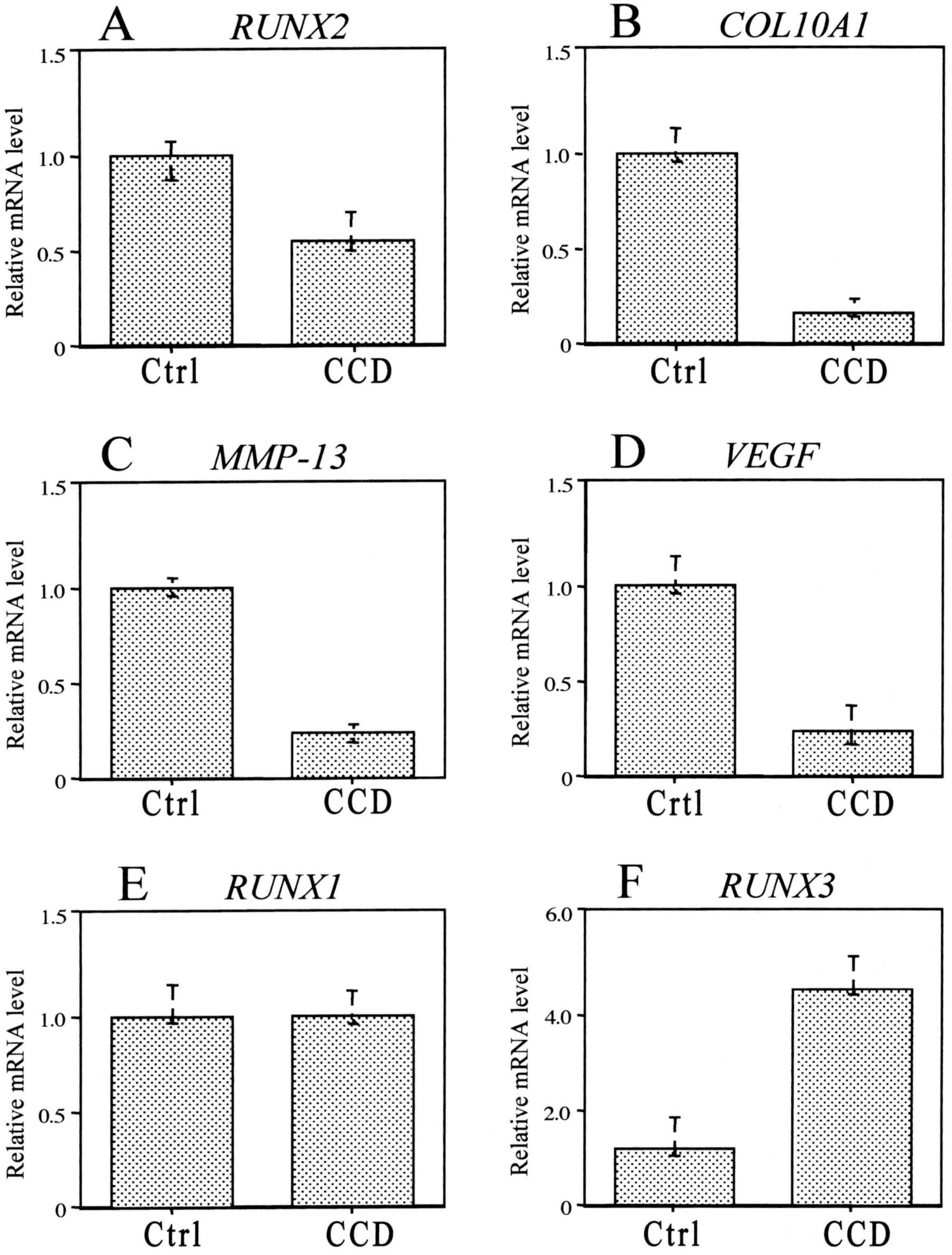

Figure 4 Real-time RT-PCR analysis of genes expressed in limb cartilage. Amplification was performed on a LightCycler (Fast Start DNA Master SYBR Green I [Roche Diagnostics]). Analysis of the results (i.e., the relative gene expression level) was achieved by normalization to *GAPDH* and by comparison with the age-matched control for fold induction. *A*, The mRNA level of *RUNX2* is decreased by 50% in the fetus with CCD, compared with the control. *B*, *C*, and *D*, The hypertrophic chondrocyte–related molecular markers *COL10A1*, *MMP-13*, and *VEGF* showed 10-, 7.6-, and 8-fold decreases in mRNA levels, respectively. *E*, No change in mRNA level was observed for *RUNX1*. *F*, *RUNX3* showed 4-fold up-regulation in fetus with CCD, compared with the age-matched control. Each real-time RT-PCR experiment was performed in triplicate, and one representative set of results is presented here, with SDs shown by error bars. Ctrl = age-matched control.

mouse genetics studies suggest that both *Runx2* and *Runx3* are essential for chondrocyte maturation and that the delayed chondrocyte maturation in *Runx2* heterozygotes on a *Runx3* null background demonstrated that *Runx3* is required for endochondral ossification when the *Runx2* gene dosage is halved (Yoshida et al. 2004; Komori 2005). No mRNA level change was observed for *SOX9*, a transcription factor required for chondrogenesis and a regulator of the type II collagen gene (Lefebvre et al. 1998). This supports the selective defect present in prehypertrophic and hypertrophic chondrocytes and not in the proliferating and resting chondrocytes of the growth plate in this fetus with CCD.

CCD is caused by haploinsufficiency of *RUNX2,* and no significant phenotypic differences have been observed between patients with deletions or frameshifts and patients with missense mutations of *RUNX2* (Quack et al. 1999). There is a correlation between phenotypic short stature and tooth anomalies in some patients with CCD (Yoshida et al. 2003). Unlike many skeletal dysplasias that primarily affect cartilage, CCD affects both cartilage and bone (Mundlos 1999; Hermanns and Lee 2001; Lee and Zhou 2004). Since *RUNX2* is required for both osteoblast differentiation and chondrocyte maturation, it links chondrocyte and osteoblast differentiation during endochondral bone formation (Mundlos 1999; de Crombrugghe et al. 2001). Many other transcription factors, such as the Sox family members, and signaling molecules, including Indian hedgehog, parathyroid hormone, and related peptide (PTH/PTHrP) and fibroblast growth factors, also link chondrocyte and osteoblast differentiation pathways during endochondral bone formation (Lanske et al. 1996; Vortkamp et al. 1996; Schipani et al. 1997; St-Jacques et al. 1999; Chung et al. 2001; de Crombrugghe et al. 2001). Not surprisingly, some of these pathways have been shown to impinge on Runx2 activity. Our studies demonstrate altered chondrocyte hypertrophy in human CCD, with decreased expression of hypertrophic chondrocyte–related markers that have been shown to be transcriptional targets of *Runx2* in mouse genetics studies (Jimenez et al. 1999; Zelzer et al. 2001; Wong et al. 2003; Zheng et al. 2003; Varghese et al. 2005). On the basis of these data and observations in mice, we can conclude that abnormal endochondral ossification in CCD results from altered *RUNX2* regulation of chondrocyte hypertrophy and is associated with downregulation of important *RUNX2* transcriptional targets, including *COL10A1, VEGF,* and *MMP13.*

Acknowledgments

This work was supported by National Institutes of Health grants ES 11253 (to B.L.) and HD22657 (to B.L., W.W., and D.K.), General Clinical Research Center grant MO1-RR00425 (to D.K.), the Arthritis Foundation (to Q.Z.), the Drown Foundation (to D.K.), and Baylor College of Medicine Mental Retardation and Developmental Disability Research Center grant HD24064 (to B.L.).

Web Resources

The URL for data presented herein is as follows:

Online Mendelian Inheritance in Man (OMIM), http://www.ncbi.nlm.nih.gov/Omim/ (for CCD)

Reference

Bateman JF, Freddi S, Nattrass G, Savarirayan R (2003) Tissue-specific RNA surveillance? Nonsense-mediated mRNA decay causes collagen X haploinsufficiency in Schmid metaphyseal chondrodysplasia cartilage. Hum Mol Genet 12: 217–225

Chung UI, Schipani E, McMahon AP, Kronenberg HM (2001) Indian hedgehog couples chondrogenesis to osteogenesis in endochondral bone development. J Clin Invest 107:295–304

Cooper SC, Flaitz CM, Johnston DA, Lee B, Hecht JT (2001) A natural history of cleidocranial dysplasia. Am J Med Genet 104:1–6

D'Alonzo RC, Selvamurugan N, Karsenty G, Partridge NC (2002) Physical interaction of the activator protein-1 factors c-Fos and c-Jun with Cbfa1 for collagenase-3 promoter activation. J Biol Chem 277:816–822

de Crombrugghe B, Lefebvre V, Nakashima K (2001) Regulatory mechanisms in the pathways of cartilage and bone formation. Curr Opin Cell Biol 13:721–727

D'Souza RN, Aberg T, Gaikwad J, Cavender A, Owen M, Karsenty G, Thesleff I (1999) Cbfa1 is required for epithelial-mesenchymal interactions regulating tooth development in mice. Development 126:2911–2920

Ducy P, Zhang R, Geoffroy V, Ridall AL, Karsenty G (1997) Osf2/Cbfa1: a transcriptional activator of osteoblast differentiation. Cell 89:747–754

Enomoto H, Enomoto-Iwamoto M, Iwamoto M, Nomura S, Himeno M, Kitamura Y, Kishimoto T, Komori T (2000) Cbfa1 is a positive regulatory factor in chondrocyte maturation. J Biol Chem 275:8695–8702

Hermanns P, Lee B (2001) Transcriptional dysregulation in skeletal malformation syndromes. Am J Med Genet 106: 258–271

Huang LF, Fukai N, Selby PB, Olsen BR, Mundlos S (1997) Mouse clavicular development: analysis of wild-type and cleidocranial dysplasia mutant mice. Dev Dyn 210:33–40

Inada M, Yasui T, Nomura S, Miyake S, Deguchi K, Himeno M, Sato M, Yamagiwa H, Kimura T, Yasui N, Ochi T, Endo N, Kitamura Y, Kishimoto T, Komori T (1999) Maturational disturbance of chondrocytes in Cbfa1-deficient mice. Dev Dyn 214:279–290

Jimenez MJ, Balbin M, Lopez JM, Alvarez J, Komori T, Lopez-Otin C (1999) Collagenase 3 is a target of Cbfa1, a transcription factor of the runt gene family involved in bone formation. Mol Cell Biol 19:4431–4442

Kim IS, Otto F, Zabel B, Mundlos S (1999) Regulation of

chondrocyte differentiation by Cbfa1. Mech Dev 80:159–170

Komori T (2005) Regulation of skeletal development by the Runx family of transcription factors. J Cell Biochem 95: 445–453

Komori T, Yagi H, Nomura S, Yamaguchi A, Sasaki K, Deguchi K, Shimizu Y, Bronson RT, Gao YH, Inada M, Sato M, Okamato R, Kitamura Y, Yoshiki S, Kishimoto T (1997) Targeted disruption of *Cbfa1* results in a complete lack of bone formation owing to maturational arrest of osteoblasts. Cell 89:755–764

Lanske B, Karaplis AC, Lee K, Luz A, Vortkamp A, Pirro A, Karperien M, Defize LH, Ho C, Mulligan RC, Abou-Samra AB, Juppner H, Segre GV, Kronenberg HM (1996) PTH/PTHrP receptor in early development and Indian hedgehog-regulated bone growth. Science 273:663–666

Lee B, Thirunavukkarasu K, Zhou L, Pastore L, Baldini A, Hecht J, Geoffroy V, Ducy P, Karsenty G (1997) Missense mutations abolishing DNA binding of the osteoblast-specific transcription factor OSF2/CBFA1 in cleidocranial dysplasia. Nat Genet 16:307–310

Lee B, Zhou G (2004) RUNX2 and cleidocranial dysplasia. In: Epstein CJ, Erickson RP, Wynshaw-Boris A (eds) Inborn errors of development. Oxford; New York, pp 331–339

Lefebvre V, Li P, de Crombrugghe B (1998) A new long form of *Sox5* (*L-Sox5*), *Sox6* and *Sox9* are coexpressed in chondrogenesis and cooperatively activate the type II collagen gene. EMBO J 17:5718–5733

Livak KJ, Schmittgen TD (2001) Analysis of relative gene expression data using real-time quantitative PCR and the $2^{-\Delta\Delta C_T}$ method. Methods 25:402–408

Lowe J, Bancroft JD (1996) Bone. In: Bancroft JD, Stevens A (eds) Theory and practice of histological techniques, fourth edition. Churchill Livingstone, New York, pp 309–339

Maquat LE (2004) Nonsense-mediated mRNA decay: splicing, translation and mRNA dynamics. Nat Rev Mol Cell Biol 5: 89–99

Morava E, Karteszi J, Weisenbach J, Caliebe A, Mundlos S, Mehes K (2002) Cleidocranial dysplasia with decreased bone density and biochemical findings of hypophosphatasia. Eur J Pediatr 161:619–622

Mundlos S (1999) Cleidocranial dysplasia: clinical and molecular genetics. J Med Genet 36:177–182

Mundlos S, Otto F, Mundlos C, Mulliken JB, Aylsworth AS, Albright S, Lindhout D, Cole WG, Henn W, Knoll JHM, Owen MJ, Mertelsmann R, Zabel BU, Olsen BR (1997) Mutations involving the transcription factor CBFA1 cause cleidocranial dysplasia. Cell 89:773–779

Otto F, Thornell AP, Crompton T, Denzel A, Gilmour KC, Rosewell IR, Stamp GWH, Beddington RSP, Mundlos S, Olsen BR, Selby PB, Owen MJ (1997) *Cbfa1*, a candidate gene for cleidocranial dysplasia syndrome, is essential for osteoblast differentiation and bone development. Cell 89: 765–771

Pfaffl MW (2001) A new mathematical model for relative quantification in real-time RT-PCR. Nucleic Acids Res 29: e45

Quack I, Vonderstrass B, Stock M, Aylsworth AS, Becker A, Brueton L, Lee PJ, Majewski F, Mulliken JB, Suri M, Zenker M, Mundlos S, Otto F (1999) Mutation analysis of core binding factor A1 in patients with cleidocranial dysplasia. Am J Hum Genet 65:1268–1278

Sato M, Morii E, Komori T, Kawahata H, Sugimoto M, Terai K, Shimizu H, Yasui T, Ogihara H, Yasui N, Ochi T, Kitamura Y, Ito Y, Nomura S (1998) Transcriptional regulation of osteopontin gene in vivo by PEBP2αA/CBFA1 and ETS1 in the skeletal tissues. Oncogene 17:1517–1525

Schipani E, Lanske B, Hunzelman J, Luz A, Kovacs CS, Lee K, Pirro A, Kronenberg HM, Juppner H (1997) Targeted expression of constitutively active receptors for parathyroid hormone and parathyroid hormone-related peptide delays endochondral bone formation and rescues mice that lack parathyroid hormone-related peptide. Proc Natl Acad Sci USA 94:13689–13694

Shapiro IM (1999) Discovery: *Osf2/Cbfa1*, a master gene of bone formation. Clin Orthod Res 2:42–46

Sierra J, Villagra A, Paredes R, Cruzat F, Gutierrez S, Javed A, Arriagada G, Olate J, Imschenetzky M, Van Wijnen AJ, Lian JB, Stein GS, Stein JL, Montecino M (2003) Regulation of the bone-specific osteocalcin gene by p300 requires Runx2/Cbfa1 and the vitamin D3 receptor but not p300 intrinsic histone acetyltransferase activity. Mol Cell Biol 23: 3339–3351

Smith N, Dong Y, Lian JB, Pratap J, Kingsley PD, van Wijnen AJ, Stein JL, Schwarz EM, O'Keefe RJ, Stein GS, Drissi MH (2005) Overlapping expression of Runx1(Cbfa2) and Runx2(Cbfa1) transcription factors supports cooperative induction of skeletal development. J Cell Physiol 203: 133–143

St-Jacques B, Hammerschmidt M, McMahon AP (1999) Indian hedgehog signaling regulates proliferation and differentiation of chondrocytes and is essential for bone formation. Genes Dev 13:2072–2086

Takeda S, Bonnamy JP, Owen MJ, Ducy P, Karsenty G (2001) Continuous expression of Cbfa1 in nonhypertrophic chondrocytes uncovers its ability to induce hypertrophic chondrocyte differentiation and partially rescues Cbfa1-deficient mice. Genes Dev 15:467–481

Ueta C, Iwamoto M, Kanatani N, Yoshida C, Liu Y, Enomoto-Iwamoto M, Ohmori T, Enomoto H, Nakata K, Takada K, Kurisu K, Komori T (2001) Skeletal malformations caused by overexpression of Cbfa1 or its dominant negative form in chondrocytes. J Cell Biol 153:87–100

Varghese S, Rydziel S, Canalis E (2005) Bone morphogenetic protein-2 suppresses collagenase-3 promoter activity in osteoblasts through a runt domain factor 2 binding site. J Cell Physiol 202:391–399

Vortkamp A, Lee K, Lanske B, Segre GV, Kronenberg HM, Tabin CJ (1996) Regulation of rate of cartilage differentiation by Indian hedgehog and PTH-related protein. Science 273:613–622

Wang X, Manner PA, Horner A, Shum L, Tuan RS, Nuckolls GH (2004) Regulation of MMP-13 expression by RUNX2 and FGF2 in osteoarthritic cartilage. Osteoarthritis Cartilage 12:963–973

Wong M, Siegrist M, Goodwin K (2003) Cyclic tensile strain and cyclic hydrostatic pressure differentially regulate expression of hypertrophic markers in primary chondrocytes. Bone 33:685–693

Yoshida CA, Yamamoto H, Fujita T, Furuichi T, Ito K, Inoue

K, Yamana K, Zanma A, Takada K, Ito Y, Komori T (2004) Runx2 and Runx3 are essential for chondrocyte maturation, and Runx2 regulates limb growth through induction of *Indian hedgehog*. Genes Dev 18:952–963

Yoshida T, Kanegane H, Osato M, Yanagida M, Miyawaki T, Ito Y, Shigesada K (2003) Functional analysis of *RUNX2* mutations in cleidocranial dysplasia: novel insights into genotype-phenotype correlations. Blood Cells Mol Dis 30: 184–193

Zelzer E, Glotzer DJ, Hartmann C, Thomas D, Fukai N, Soker S, Olsen BR (2001) Tissue specific regulation of VEGF expression during bone development requires Cbfa1/Runx2. Mech Dev 106:97–106

Zheng Q, Zhou G, Morello R, Chen Y, Garcia-Rojas X, Lee B (2003) Type X collagen gene regulation by Runx2 contributes directly to its hypertrophic chondrocyte-specific expression in vivo. J Cell Biol 162:833–842

Zhou G, Chen Y, Zhou L, Thirunavukkarasu K, Hecht J, Chitayat D, Gelb BD, Pirinen S, Berry SA, Greenberg CR, Karsenty G, Lee B (1999) *CBFA1* mutation analysis and functional correlation with phenotypic variability in cleidocranial dysplasia. Hum Mol Genet 8:2311–2316

Zou SJ, D'Souza RN, Ahlberg T, Bronckers AL (2003) Tooth eruption and cementum formation in the Runx2/Cbfa1 heterozygous mouse. Arch Oral Biol 48:673–677

Report

A *"Fille du Roy"* Introduced the T14484C Leber Hereditary Optic Neuropathy Mutation in French Canadians

Anne-Marie Laberge,[1,5] Michèle Jomphe,[6] Louis Houde,[7] Hélène Vézina,[7] Marc Tremblay,[7] Bertrand Desjardins,[2] Damian Labuda,[3] Marc St-Hilaire,[8] Carol Macmillan,[9] Eric A. Shoubridge,[4] and Bernard Brais[1]

[1]Laboratoire de Neurogénétique, Centre Hospitalier de l'Université de Montréal, [2]Department of Demography, Faculty of Arts and Sciences, and [3]Department of Pediatrics, Faculty of Medicine, Université de Montréal, and [4]Montreal Neurological Institute and Departments of Human Genetics and Neurology and Neurosurgery, McGill University, Montreal; [5]Institute for Public Health Genetics, Department of Epidemiology, School of Public Health and Community Medicine, University of Washington, Seattle; [6]Projet BALSAC and [7]Groupe de Recherche Interdisciplinaire en Démographie et en Épidémiologie Génétique, Université du Québec à Chicoutimi, Saguenay; [8]Department of Geography, Université Laval, Quebec City; and [9]Departments of Neurology and Pediatrics, University of Illinois at Chicago, Chicago

The predominance of the T14484C mutation in French Canadians with Leber hereditary optic neuropathy is due to a founder effect. By use of genealogical reconstructions of maternal lineages, a woman married in Quebec City in 1669 is identified as the shared female ancestor for 11 of 13 affected individuals, who were previously not known to be related. These individuals carry identical mitochondrial haplogroups. The current geographic distribution of French Canadian cases overlaps with that of the founder's female descendants in 1800. This is the first example of genealogical reconstruction to identify the introduction of a mitochondrial mutation by a woman in a founder population.

Leber hereditary optic neuropathy (LHON [MIM 535000]) presents as acute or subacute loss of central vision in an individual with previously normal vision (Man et al. 2002). In most cases, both eyes are affected, either simultaneously or sequentially. In some cases, vision eventually improves. LHON is maternally transmitted and affects primarily young adult males. In >95% of cases, LHON is caused by one of three mutations—G3640A, G11778A, or T14484C—located in the mitochondrial genes encoding respiratory chain complex I subunits. G11778A is the most prevalent mutation worldwide (52%–92% of cases), T14484C is usually the second most prevalent (3%–19% of cases), and G3640A is the least prevalent (1%–33% of cases) (Rosenberg et al. 1995; Yen et al. 2002; Howell et al. 2003; Kim et al. 2003; Man et al. 2003). In contrast, the most frequently found mutation in French Canadian patients is T14484C, which accounts for 86% of French Canadians cases, whereas G11778A and G3640A account for 12% and 2%, respectively (Macmillan et al. 1998). Haplogroup analysis suggested that the predominance of the T14484C mutation in French Canadian patients with LHON was due to a founder effect and that those patients might all descend from the same woman (Macmillan et al. 2000). Dutch patients with LHON who carry the T14484C mutation share the same mitochondrial haplogroup, which suggests that this mutation appeared in Europe earlier than the first French settlement in Quebec in 1608 (Howell et al. 2003). The first report of LHON in French Canadians dates to 1970, when a large pedigree from southwestern Quebec was described (Brunette and Bernier 1970). A high rate of spontaneous recovery was observed in this large family.

Through use of Quebec's genealogical records, we wanted to determine if a single female founder introduced the LHON T14484C mutation in French Canadians. In the province of Quebec, LHON mitochondrial genotyping is performed in a single laboratory at the Montreal Neurological Institute (E.A.S., unpublished data). Twenty-four physicians who sent samples for

Received April 13, 2005; accepted for publication June 2, 2005; electronically published June 13, 2005.

Address for correspondence and reprints: Dr. Bernard Brais, Département de Médecine, Faculté de Médecine de l'Université de Montréal, Centre de recherche du CHUM, Hôpital Notre-Dame-CHUM, Local M-4211-L3, 1560, rue Sherbrooke Est, Montréal, Québec, H2L 4M1 Canada. E-mail: Bernard.Brais@umontreal.ca

0002-9297/2005/7702-0013$15.00

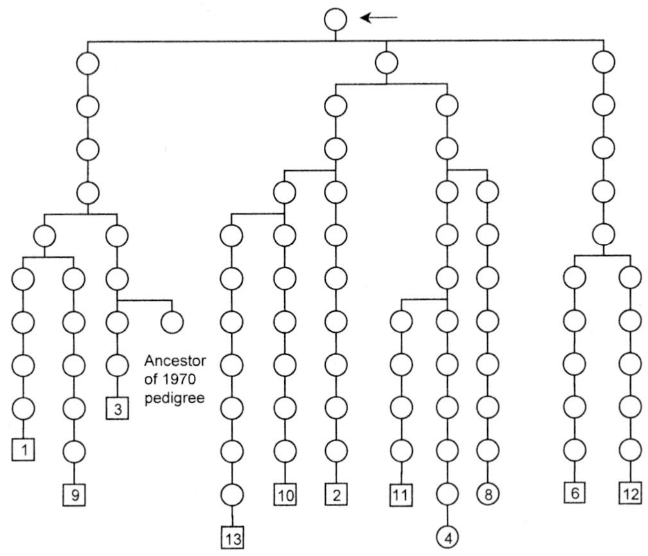

Figure 1 Pedigree of the 11 probands sharing the same female ancestor and their relationship with the family reported in 1970 (Brunette and Bernier 1970).

LHON genotyping were asked to contact their patients with T14484C LHON and inquire whether the patients would agree to be contacted by our team. Patients who agreed to participate in the study returned a written consent form after having been informed of the nature of the project by a research nurse. Each participant provided the following information required for maternal lineage reconstruction: name, date of birth, and dates and parishes of marriages of mother and maternal grandmother. This information was used to construct direct maternal lineages for each individual all the way to the female ancestor who settled in Nouvelle-France. This was done by Project BALSAC by use of the RETRO databases (Bouchard 2004). Ascending maternal lineage genealogies were obtained for 13 unrelated individuals with T14484C LHON, thereafter called "probands." Twelve were successfully reconstructed (probands 1–4 and 6–13). Eleven were found to be related to the same female founder through maternal lineage (probands 1–4, 6, and 8–13) (fig. 1). One of the authors of the original 1970 report provided us with the name of the oldest obligate-carrier female ancestor identified in their pedigree, who married before 1870 (R. G. Bernier, personal communication). As shown in figure 1, that carrier ancestor is related through her maternal lineage to the same female founder.

This female founder was born in France. She came to Nouvelle-France as a "*fille du roy*" and married in Quebec City in 1669. The 737 "*filles du roy*," or "the King's daughters," were women sent by King Louis XIV, between 1663 and 1673, to Nouvelle-France to marry (Charbonneau et al. 1987), as an attempt to correct the unfavorable male: female ratio in the young colony and thereby encourage the permanent settlement of immigrants in Nouvelle-France. The ratio went from 169 males per 100 females in 1608–1662 to 118 males per 100 females in 1663–1679 (Charbonneau et al. 1987). While still in France, these young women had been placed under the care of the king because they were orphans or single women without sufficient family support.

Statistical analysis was performed to estimate the probability that the identification of a single female founder shared by 11 individuals through maternal lineage could be due to chance. By use of the maternal lineages of 2,600 available existing genealogies in the RETRO database of the Project BALSAC, 5,000 simulations of reconstruction of maternal lineages were performed. Each simulation used 11 subjects selected from among the starting individuals of the 2,600 ascending genealogies. Each individual was matched with one of the probands with LHON for the region of his or her parents' wedding. This was done to control for differences in genetic characteristics of the different regional populations. In none of the 5,000 simulations was a single female founder ($f = 1$) shared by all of the 11 randomly selected individuals. Since the probability of finding less than seven shared female founders related only through maternal lineages ($f < 7$) by chance for 11 control individuals is <0.002 (table 1), these results strongly support the identification of this single female founder as the actual source of the main introduction of the T14484C mutation in the French Canadian population.

Further evidence to support this conclusion comes from the complete sequencing of the HV1 and HV2 hypervariable mtDNA regions in a subset of these patients.

Table 1

Probability of Finding *f* Founder Females by Use of 5,000 Simulations of the Maternal-Lineage Pedigree Reconstructions of 11 Random Probands

No. of Founder Females Identified (*f*)	No. of Simulations (*n*) in Which *f* Founder Females Were Identified (of 5,000 total)	Probability of Finding *f* Founder Females (*n*/5,000)
1	0	0
2	0	0
3	0	0
4	0	0
5	0	0
6	0	0
7	1	.0002
8	28	.0056
9	246	.0492
10	1,426	.2852
11	3,299	.6598

NOTE.—The 11 probands were matched with original probands for location of their parents' weddings.

Sequencing was performed on PCR products as done by Macmillan et al. (1998), by use of an ABI 3730 XL sequencer for 9 of the 11 probands related to the founder; for proband 5, who was found not to be related to her; for proband 7, for whom genealogical reconstruction was not possible; and for 21 other French Canadian individuals with LHON, who were previously thought to be unrelated. Table 2 shows that all nine related carriers share the same haplogroup, as do proband 7 and the 21 other unrelated French Canadians with LHON. The rare differences observed likely represent spontaneous mutations in the founder haplogroup. Proband 5 clearly does not share the same haplogroup, which is consistent with the genealogical results that he inherited the T14484C mutation through a different maternal lineage (table 2).

Since LHON is a rare disease in Quebec, we wanted to assess this founder's contribution to the French Canadian gene pool. The genetic contribution (GC) of an ancestor to an individual is inversely proportional to the number of generations between the ancestor and that individual through a specific genealogical link (g) and proportional to the number of genealogical links between the two (c):

$$GC = \sum_{i=1}^{c} (1/2)^{g_i} .$$

Total genetic contribution of an ancestor to a group of individuals is the proportion of the genetic pool of said group that comes from said ancestor. It is the sum of the genetic contributions of the ancestor to each individual,

$$GC_{tot} = \sum_{j=1}^{n} \sum_{i=1}^{c} (1/2)^{g_{i,j}} ,$$

where n denotes the number of individuals in the group (Gagnon and Heyer 2001). This measures the contribution of an individual to the autosomal gene pool, not the mitochondrial gene pool, but we have used it as a proxy for overall genetic contribution to the French Canadian population. With currently available databases, no adequate method is available to assess the relative contribution of female founders to the Quebec mitochondrial gene pool. The total genetic contribution of the female founder in question to the French Canadian population of Quebec is estimated at the 30th percentile. This lower-than-average genetic contribution is consistent with the relatively low prevalence of LHON in Quebec.

The availability of a complete computerized database of all Quebec civil records up to the year 1800 allowed us to assess whether early migratory events shaped the present distribution of T14484C LHON cases in Quebec. Using the PRDH (Programme de Recherche en Demographie Historique) database (Charbonneau et al. 1987), a descending genealogy from 1669 to 1800 was reconstructed, starting with the female founder presumed to introduce the mutation (maximum of 5 generations, total of 49 female descendants through females only). The parishes of weddings were used to geographically map the migration of her female descendants (fig. 2). The founder female's five daughters were all married in or near Quebec City, but only half of her great-granddaughters were married there. Eleven of her 21 great-granddaughters and 10 of her 13 great-great-granddaughters were married in the greater Montreal region (incomplete data for the 5th generation; data available only until 1800). This predominant migration of her female descendants to the southwestern part of what is now the province of Quebec corresponds well with the present geographical distribution of T14484C LHON cases. Postal codes from 45 Quebec patients with T14484C show that 40

Table 2

Haplogroup Analysis of French Canadians with LHON

	Haplotype at Site of Hypervariable mtDNA Region																		
	HV2										HV1								
Analysis of	73	152	185	199	204	207	228	250	263	295	16069	16126	16129	16189	16213	16223	16260	16261	16292
Human mitochondrial genome[a]	A	T	G	T	T	G	G	T	A	C	C	T	G	T	G	C	C	C	C
Consensus[b]	G	T	A	T	T	G	A	T	G	T	T	C	G	T	A	C	C	C	C
Probands 2–4, 6, 7, and 9–12	G	T	A	T	T	G	A	T	G	T	T	C	G	T	A	C	C	C	C
Proband 8	ND	T	A	T	T	G	A	T	G	T	T	C	G	T	A	C	C	C	C
Proband 5	G	C	G	C	A	A	G	C	G	C	C	T	A	C	G	T	C	T	C
Individual A	G	T	A	T	T	G	A	T	G	T	T	C	G	T	A	C	C/T	C	C
Individuals B–H and J–U	G	T	A	T	T	G	A	T	G	T	T	C	G	T	A	C	C	C	C
Individual I	G	T	A	T	T	G	A	T	G	T	T	C	G	T	G	C	C	C	T
Individual V	ND	T	ND	T	T	G	A	T	G	T	T	C	G	T	A	C	C	C	C

NOTE.—ND = not done.

* As found in GenBank.

[b] Consensus sequence in French Canadian T14484C carriers.

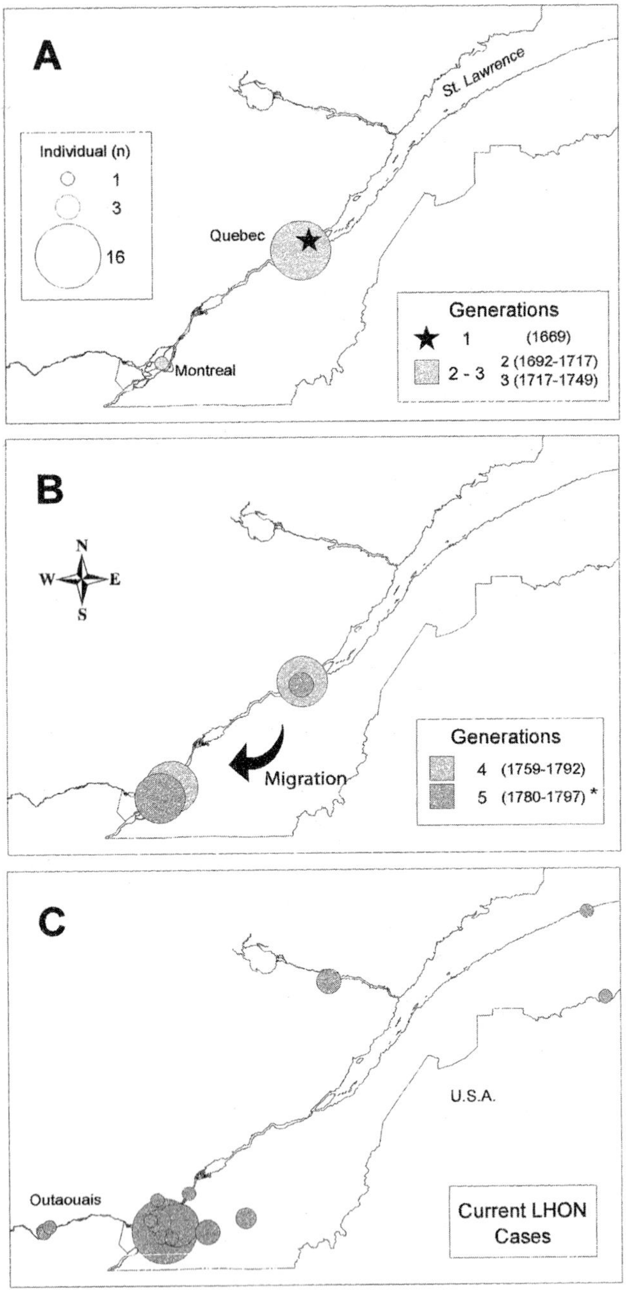

Figure 2 Geographic distribution of the marriage parishes of the single female ancestor's female descendants, by generation (1669–1800) (*A* and *B*) and geographic distribution of current cases that are due to T14484C mutation (*C*). An asterisk (*) marks the 5th generation, which is incomplete, because data are available only through 1800.

live in southwestern Quebec. Another 16 patients live in Ontario, mainly near the southwestern border of Quebec.

The use of the PRDH database also allowed us to assess whether males with LHON in the early colony had more difficulty finding spouses. This hypothesis was tested using male descendants of the single common female ancestor, born before 1800 and related through females only. Of the 45 descendants, 17 (38%) were married, compared with 13 (30%) of the 43 male controls, matched for year of birth ($\chi^2 = 0.557$; $P = .455$). Although the small numbers involved limit our ability to conclude from these results, these results are not suggestive of a detrimental effect of LHON on ability to find a spouse in the first generations of male descendants. This could be explained either by the occurrence of symptoms after the age of marriage or by the high rate of spontaneous recovery in patients with the T14484C mutation.

By combining genealogical and molecular data sets, we have established that the French Canadian founder effect for the predominant LHON T14484C mutation in Quebec was most likely due to a 17th century introduction of this mutation by a female founder. This said, there was more than one introduction of this mutation into this population, as demonstrated by proband 5. The study of French Canadian computerized genealogies can allow the identification of pioneers who introduced mutations into this population. To our knowledge, this is the first published report of the identification of an introducer of a mitochondrial mutation in a founder population. Early migrational events have shaped the current differences in regional prevalence of mutations in Quebec.

Acknowledgments

We thank Dr. Aroichane, Dr. Hamel, Dr. Wein, and Dr. Zackon, who contacted their patients for recruitment to this study. We also thank the participants; Tim Johns, for excellent technical assistance; and Lina Loiselle, for her essential collaboration. We also thank Dr. Bernier for providing us with genealogical information about the family reported in 1970. We thank Nicolas Lanouette for his help with the maps. This work was supported by a Canadian Institutes of Health Research (CIHR) grant and a donation from R. Riverin in support of LHON research (to E.A.S.). E.A.S. is an international scholar of the Howard Hughes Medical Institute and a senior investigator of the CIHR. B.B. is a chercheur boursier of the Fonds de Recherche en Santé du Québec.

Web Resources

The URLs for data presented herein are as follows:

GenBank, http://www.ncbi.nlm.nih.gov/Genbank/ (for the human mitochondrial genome)
Online Mendelian Inheritance in Man (OMIM), http://www.ncbi.nlm.nih.gov/Omim/ (for LHON)
Projet BALSAC, http://www.uqac.uquebec.ca/balsac/
PRDH, http://www.genealogie.umontreal.ca/fr/

References

Bouchard G (2004) Rapport annuel du Projet BALSAC 2003–2004. Université du Québec à Chicoutimi, Saguenay

Brunette JR, Bernier RG (1970) [Diagnosis and prognosis of Leber's disease: incidence of spontaneous total recuperation]. Union Med Can 99:643–652
Charbonneau H, Guillemette A, Légaré J, Desjardins B, Landry Y, Nault F, Bates R, Boleda M (1987) Naissance d'une population—les Français établis au Canada au XVIIe siècle. Montréal et Paris, Presses Universitaires de France et Presses de l'Université de Montréal
Gagnon A, Heyer E (2001) Fragmentation of the Quebec population genetic pool (Canada): evidence from the genetic contribution of founders per region in the 17th and 18th centuries. Am J Phys Anthropol 114:30–41
Howell N, Oostra R-J, Bolhuis PA, Spruijt L, Clarke LA, Mackey DA, Preston G, Herrnstadt C (2003) Sequence analysis of the mitochondrial genomes from Dutch pedigrees with Leber hereditary optic neuropathy. Am J Hum Genet 72:1460–1469
Kim JY, Hwang JM, Chang BL, Park SS (2003) Spectrum of the mitochondrial DNA mutations of Leber's hereditary optic neuropathy in Koreans. J Neurol 250:278–281
Macmillan C, Johns TA, Fu K, Shoubridge EA (2000) Predominance of the T14484C mutation in French-Canadian families with Leber hereditary optic neuropathy is due to a founder effect. Am J Hum Genet 66:332–335
Macmillan C, Kirkham T, Fu K, Allison V, Andermann E, Chitayat D, Fortier D, Gans M, Hare H, Quercia N, Zackon D, Shoubridge EA (1998) Pedigree analysis of French Canadian families with T14484C Leber's hereditary optic neuropathy. Neurology 50:417–422
Man PYW, Griffiths PG, Brown DT, Howell N, Turnbull DM, Chinnery PF (2003) The epidemiology of Leber hereditary optic neuropathy in the North East of England. Am J Hum Genet 72:333–339
Man PYW, Turnbull DM, Chinnery PF (2002) Leber hereditary optic neuropathy. J Med Genet 39:162–169
Rosenberg T, Kann E, Norby S (1995) [Hereditary optic nerve atrophy: a clinical-genealogical status over Danish families with Leber disease]. Ugeskr Laeger 157:2707–2711
Yen MY, Wang AG, Chang WL, Hsu WM, Liu JH, Wei YH (2002) Leber's hereditary optic neuropathy—the spectrum of mitochondrial DNA mutations in Chinese patients. Jpn J Ophthalmol 46:45–51

Report

A Genomewide Scan for Intelligence Identifies Quantitative Trait Loci on 2q and 6p

Danielle Posthuma,[1] Michelle Luciano,[2] Eco J. C. de Geus,[1] Margie J. Wright,[2] P. Eline Slagboom,[3] Grant W. Montgomery,[2] Dorret I. Boomsma,[1] and Nicholas G. Martin[2]

[1]Department of Biological Psychology, Vrije Universiteit, Amsterdam; [2]Queensland Institute of Medical Research, Brisbane, Australia; and [3]Department of Molecular Epidemiology, Leiden University Medical Centre, Leiden, The Netherlands

Between 40% and 80% of the variation in human intelligence (IQ) is attributable to genetic factors. Except for many rare mutations resulting in severe cognitive dysfunction, attempts to identify these factors have not been successful. We report a genomewide linkage scan involving 634 sibling pairs designed to identify chromosomal regions that explain variation in IQ. Model-free multipoint linkage analysis revealed evidence of a significant quantitative-trait locus for performance IQ at 2q24.1-31.1 (LOD score 4.42), which overlaps the 2q21-33 region that has repeatedly shown linkage to autism. A second region revealed suggestive linkage for both full-scale and verbal IQs on 6p25.3-22.3 (LOD score 3.20 for full-scale IQ and 2.33 for verbal IQ), overlapping marginally with the 6p22.3-21.31 region implicated in reading disability and dyslexia.

There are substantial individual differences in cognitive abilities, which tend to cluster within individuals. This "positive manifold" formed the basis for the construction of intelligence tests that assess abilities across different domains (e.g., visuospatial abilities, memory, vocabulary, semantics, and symbolic reasoning) that can be summarized into higher-order factors, such as verbal and performance intelligence. Traditional psychometric intelligence tests, such as the Wechsler Adult Intelligence Scale (WAIS) (Wechsler 1997), show high predictive validity, stability across age spans, and substantial heritability (Bouchard and McGue 1981). The identification of genes underlying the genetic variation in human intelligence has thus far been limited to neurological mutations with rather severe cognitive effects (e.g., Pick disease and X-linked mental retardation) (Ramakers 2003; Inlow and Restifo 2004), which are largely Mendelian in nature (Flint 1999). Identifying genes for variation in the range of normal intelligence could provide important clues to the underlying mechanisms of milder but more-prevalent forms of impaired cognitive functioning, which are often associated with autism, schizophrenia, reading disorder, and attention deficit hyperactivity disorder (Goldman-Rakic 1999; Willcutt et al. 2001; Badcock et al. 2005).

A major effort in identifying genetic variants that influence cognitive ability in the normal range was undertaken by Plomin and colleagues (Petrill et al. 1996; Chorney et al. 1998; Fisher et al. 1999*a*; Plomin et al. 2001, 2004; Butcher et al. 2005). The only association that survived rigorous adjustment for multiple testing was a significant association of a functional polymorphism in the *ALDH5A1* gene (MIM 271980) with cognitive ability (Plomin et al. 2004). This association was based on a selected sample (subjects with high IQs vs. subjects with normal IQs), and the effect size was rather small. Thus, in spite of the overwhelming evidence from twin studies of the existence of "genes for human intelligence," the actual identification of such genes through well-designed candidate-gene or whole-genome allelic association studies has not met with large success. It might be that these pre-HapMap studies did not achieve a high enough SNP density. Generally, association analyses may overlook closely spaced genes that act in concert to affect a trait. In contrast, linkage analysis is more sensitive to such concerted effects. For example, Yalcin et al. (2004) recently suggested such a mechanism for emotionality in mice, in which multiple closely linked

Received April 18, 2005; accepted for publication June 10, 2005; electronically published July 1, 2005.

Address for correspondence and reprints: Dr. D. Posthuma, Department of Biological Psychology, Vrije Universiteit, Van der Boechorststraat 1, 1081 BT Amsterdam, The Netherlands. E-mail: danielle@psy.vu.nl

0002-9297/2005/7702-0014$15.00

genes on chromosome 1 may be needed to explain the solid linkage found in this region (Yalcin et al. 2004).

Here, we report the first genomewide linkage study for intelligence, using two unselected samples consisting of 725 individuals from 329 Australian families, which yield 475 sib pairs, and 225 individuals from 100 Dutch families, which yield 159 sib pairs. In these populations, the contribution of genetic factors to full-scale IQ (FSIQ) was shown to be 0.69 in the Australian sample (Luciano et al. 2004) and 0.86 in the Dutch sample (Posthuma et al. 2001). Heritabilities for verbal IQ (VIQ) and performance IQ (PIQ) were also high (table 1).

The sample of Australian DZ twins and siblings was part of an ongoing study of cognition in adolescents (Wright et al. 2001; Luciano et al. 2004) and was genotyped as part of an earlier study that investigated melanoma risk factors (Zhu et al. 1999). The study was approved by the Human Research Ethics Committee of the Queensland Institute of Medical Research Institute. Informed consent to jointly examine the cognitive and genotype data was obtained from participants or the parents/guardians of participants who were <18 years of age. The Multidimensional Aptitude Battery (MAB) (Jackson 1998) was used to assess IQ and consisted of three verbal subtests (information, vocabulary, and arithmetic) and two performance subtests (spatial ability and object assembly), which were administered by computer and were each timed at 7 min. Scaled scores for VIQ, PIQ, and FSIQ were examined. VIQ, PIQ, and FSIQ were normally distributed. IQ scores assessed with the MAB generally correlate highly with those assessed by the WAIS (Wechsler 1997): $r = 0.94$ for VIQ, $r = 0.79$ for PIQ, and $r = 0.91$ for FSIQ (Jackson 1998).

Genotyping of the Australian sample was performed at two facilities, the Australian Genome Research Facility, by use of the ABI PRISM Linkage Mapping Set v2.5, and the Center for Inherited Disease Research, by use of a marker set based on the Marshfield Genetics version 8 screening set.

Up to 761 autosomal microsatellite markers were typed at approximately equal intervals (average 4.8 cM) across the entire genome, with locations determined from the sex-averaged deCODE map (Kong et al. 2002) and interpolation of unmapped markers (Zhu et al. 2004). Marker heterozygosity ranged from 52.6% to 91.9%. In the Australian sample, both parental genotypes were available for 260 families, one parental genotype for 67 families, and no parental genotypes for 34 families. Parents were typed for 228–784 markers (mean ± SD, 398 ± 101 markers). For twins and siblings, the number of typed markers ranged from 211 to 790, with an average of 601 ± 192 total markers.

The sample of Dutch DZ twins and siblings were part of an ongoing study of cognition in adults (Posthuma et al. 2001; Wright et al. 2001). Subjects were recruited from The Netherlands Twin Register to participate in the cognition study, and they gave written informed consent. The institutional review board of the Vrije Universiteit Medical Centre approved the DNA sampling and cognitive testing. The Dutch adaptation of the WAIS III-R (Wechsler 1997) was used to assess IQ and consisted of four verbal subtests (information, similarities, vocabulary, and arithmetic) and three performance subtests (picture completion, block design, and matrix reasoning). Scaled scores for VIQ, PIQ, and FSIQ were examined. VIQ, PIQ, and FSIQ were normally distributed. In 93 subjects, a genome scan with 369 autosomal markers (with 9.44-cM spacing) was done by the Mammalian Genotyping Service, with microsatellite screening set 10 with few alternative markers. In 132 subjects, a 419-marker genome scan (with 8.34-cM spacing) was performed by the Molecular Epidemiology Section, Leiden University Medical Centre (Heijmans et al., in press). Parents were typed for 344–375 markers (mean 363 ± 6). For offspring, the number of typed markers ranged from 344 to 678, with an average of 389 ± 69 total markers.

Table 1

Characteristics of the Australian and Dutch Samples in the Twin-Family Studies of Intelligence

Characteristic	Australian Sample	Dutch Sample
No. of families	329	100
No. of pairs	475	159
No of. individuals (no. of males)	725 (360)	225 (96)
Age (years)	16.4 ± .70	39.6 ± 12.46
Mean FSIQ	112.6 ± 13.05	94.2 ± 10.84
Mean VIQ	111.0 ± 11.39	92.4 ± 13.10
Mean PIQ	112.4 ± 16.50	98.3 ± 12.05
Heritability FSIQ	.69	.86
Heritability VIQ	.72	.85
Heritability PIQ	.59	.69

Marker locations in the Australian and Dutch data sets were taken from an integrated genetic map with interpolated genetic map positions (see Web Resources section). The positions are in deCODE cM (Kong et al. 2002), estimated via locally weighted linear regression (lo(w)ess) from the build 34.3 (and 35.1) physical map positions and from published deCODE and Marshfield genetic map positions. Mendelian errors were detected using PEDSTATS, and unlikely double recombinants were detected using MERLIN; both were removed using PEDWIPE (Abecasis et al. 2002). Pedigree relationships in the entire sample were checked with the GRR program (Abecasis et al. 2001).

A variance-components (VC) approach was used to evaluate linkage. The VC framework involves partitioning the variance of the trait of interest into components due to covariates, component(s) due to a major QTL, a

Table 2

Genomic Regions with Evidence of Linkage to Intelligence, in a Study of 634 Sib Pairs

Genomic Region and IQ Measure	Peak LOD Score for			Peak Marker	Location (cM from pter)	1-LOD Drop Area
	Combined Data	Dutch Sample	Australian Sample			
2q24.1-31.1:						
PIQ	4.42	1.53	3.26	*D2S2330*	173.97	*D2S142–D2S2188*
FSIQ	2.23	.66	1.72	*D2S1776*	176.74	*D2S142–D2S2364*
6p25.3-22.3:						
VIQ	2.33	1.63	1.56	*D6S2434*	32.61	*D6S942–D6S422*
FSIQ	3.20	.53	2.95	*F13A1*	16.07	*D6S1574–D6S309*

polygenic component, and unique environmental or random variation. Estimation of the QTL effect requires the use of genetic data in the form of pairwise identity-by-descent (IBD) sharing between siblings. The multipoint probabilities of sharing 0, 1, or 2 alleles IBD were computed separately for each sample by use of a 1-cM grid with the Lander-Green algorithm implemented in MERLIN (Abecasis et al. 2002). These IBD probabilities were used to estimate linkage with the use of Mx software (Neale et al. 1997).

For both data sets, age and sex were included as covariates in the analyses. All parameter estimates were initially allowed to differ between the two data sets. To test for heterogeneity in the variance associated with a putative QTL (σ_q^2), we ran a second scan in which we restricted σ_q^2 to be the same across both data sets while allowing all other parameters, such as the polygenic effect, to be different. Heterogeneity of the QTL effect across the Dutch and Australian data sets could then be determined by the likelihood-ratio test, where the null model of no heterogeneity included a single QTL effect and the alternative model of heterogeneity included two separate QTL effects, for each genomic position. If no heterogeneity in σ_q^2 is observed, the combined analysis can be used to determine significance of the QTL effect on the basis of the pooled data set. Of all 3,543 genomic positions tested (by use of a 1-cM grid), only 1.2% for PIQ, 3.2% for VIQ, and 0.9% for FSIQ showed a χ^2 value >3.84 (asymptotic $P = .05$) at positions not located under our peak regions.

Significance of genetic variation due to the QTL was evaluated by the likelihood-ratio test, which is a 50:50 mixture of a χ^2 distribution with 1 df and a point mass at zero, comparing a model that included the variance associated with a QTL and a model that did not include this component. The LOD score can then be calculated by dividing the test statistic χ^2 by 2ln10 (~4.6). Linkage analyses were also performed using MERLIN, with option –vc for VC linkage analysis, and the results did not show notable differences from the results based on Mx presented here. However, the advantage of Mx is that possible heterogeneity in means, variance, effect of covariates, or polygenic heritability can be included in the statistical model.

To obtain empirical estimates of genomewide significance levels, 1,000 permutations of the data set were performed, with both the family structure and the IBD structure kept intact. These permutations allowed us to account for uneven marker spacing and informativeness and to calculate the probability of observing multiple peaks of a certain height (Churchill and Doerge 1994). The permuted data sets were obtained so that each row in the observed data set represents one family and contains phenotypic data for each individual within that family as well as the precalculated (using MERLIN) IBD probabilities across the whole genome for all pairs within that family. This file is split into a phenotypic file (containing the IQ data as well as age, sex, and country identifier) and a genotypic file (containing the IBD probabilities). Families in the experiment are labeled with unique numbers 1 through n. The phenotypic data are then shuffled by taking a random permutation of the indices 1,...,n and matching the ith phenotypic trait value to the family with an index given by the ith element of permuted indices. This permuted vector of traits is matched with the original (unpermuted) genotypic information for all families. A total of 1,000 permuted data sets were generated under the assumption of no linkage; each permuted data set was then analyzed analogously to the observed data, and the highest peak for each chromosome was recorded. The empirical significance level of an observed LOD score was then estimated by counting the proportion of genome scans containing one or more peaks of that size. The cut-off for suggestive linkage was calculated as the score that was observed, on average, once per genome scan, thus representing the average maximum peak size expected once per genome scan by chance alone (Lander and Kruglyak 1995). The thresholds for suggestive linkage for PIQ, VIQ, and FSIQ were 2.01, 1.70, and 1.86, respectively. The significant linkage threshold was defined as the LOD score occurring in 50 of the 1,000 permutations, corresponding to a probability of 0.05 in a genome scan (Lander and Kruglyak 1995). The thresholds for significant linkage

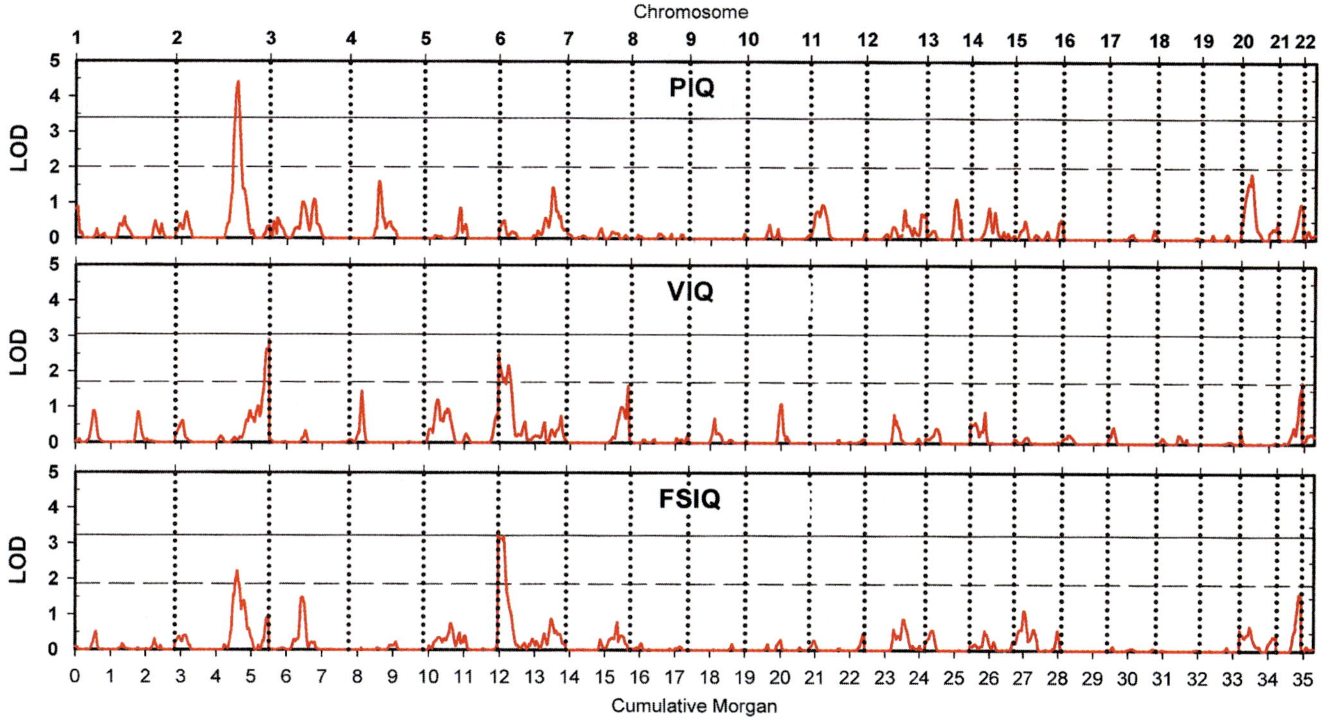

Figure 1 Full autosomal genome scans for PIQ, VIQ, and FSIQ based on 634 sibling pairs. Horizontal solid lines denote genomewide empirical thresholds for significant linkage, defined as the LOD score that would be expected to occur by chance with a probability of 0.05 in a whole-genome scan. Horizontal dashed lines denote genomewide empirical thresholds for suggestive linkage, defined as the LOD score that would be expected to occur once by chance in a whole-genome scan (Lander and Kruglyak 1995).

for PIQ, VIQ, and FSIQ were 3.39, 3.05, and 3.22, respectively.

Multipoint analyses revealed significant or suggestive evidence of linkage on two chromosomes (figs. 1 and 2). A single region, on chromosome 2q, revealed significant evidence of linkage to PIQ, at marker *D2S2330* (LOD score 4.42). The evidence was reasonably supported by the Australian sample alone (LOD score 3.26) and was marginally supported (Lander and Kruglyak 1995) by the smaller Dutch sample (LOD score 1.53), which peaked at only a 5-cM difference. Heterogeneity tests confirmed that the QTL effects observed in the Australian and Dutch data sets in this region could indeed be combined into a single QTL effect. The borders (defined by a drop of 1 LOD score) of the positive peak at 2q are located at markers *D2S142* and *D2S2188*, which are 16 cM apart (table 2). The shape of the scan for FSIQ score mirrored the findings for PIQ score on chromosome 2q, showing a peak LOD score of 2.23 within the same area.

On chromosome 6, we found suggestive evidence of linkage to FSIQ (LOD score 3.20) and, in the same region, to VIQ (LOD score of 2.33) at marker *D6S942*. The whole 1-LOD drop area spanned 42 cM (*D6S942–D6S422*).

Since the correlation between VIQ and PIQ is 0.53, which reflects that 28% of the variance in VIQ is shared with PIQ, we would expect that at least some of the QTLs that are important for VIQ are also important for PIQ. For the 2q24.1-2q31.1 region, linked to PIQ, we did not observe any evidence of linkage to VIQ. In the chromosome 6 region, linked to VIQ, the scan for PIQ showed a modest peak (LOD score 1.47) in the Australian data set in the same region as VIQ, implying that this region may be important for both VIQ and PIQ.

A few other regions showed LOD scores that were just below the thresholds for suggestive linkage (i.e., LOD score difference <0.3) (fig. 1): on chromosome 4, VIQ showed a peak LOD score of 1.44 near marker *D4S419*; on chromosome 7, VIQ showed a peak LOD score of 1.56 near marker *D7S3058*; on chromosome 20, PIQ showed a peak LOD score of 1.84 near marker *D20S851*; and on chromosome 21, VIQ and FSIQ showed peak LOD scores of 1.56 and 1.59, respectively, at marker *D21S1446*. We further observed suggestive linkage for VIQ at 2qter in the Australian data set and at 2pter in the Dutch data set. Replication studies are needed to determine whether these LOD scores were due to chance or are derived from QTLs with small effects.

The 2q24.1-2q31.1 (*D2S142–D2S2188*) region that

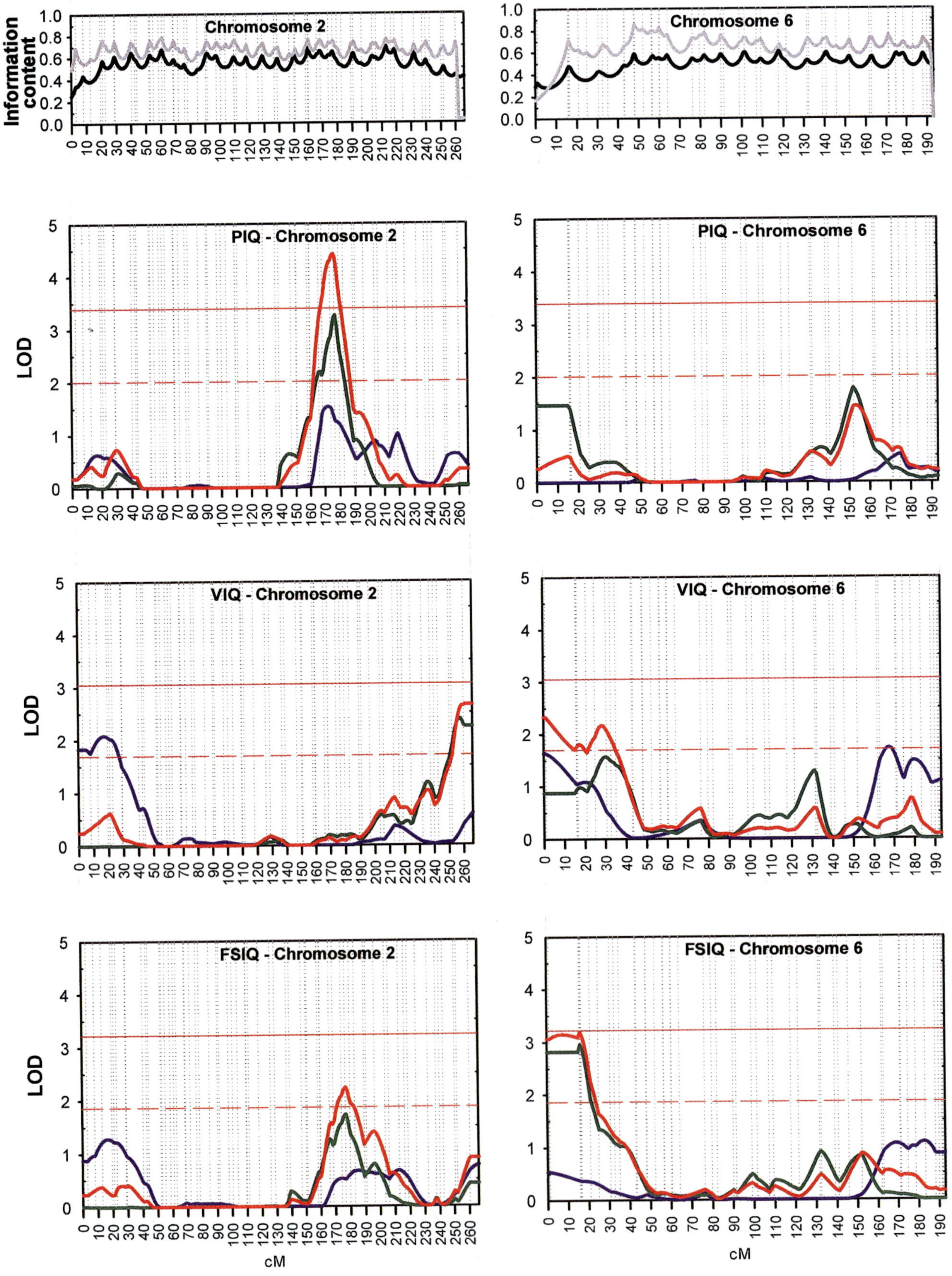

Information content
Chromosome 2
Chromosome 6
PIQ - Chromosome 2
PIQ - Chromosome 6
VIQ - Chromosome 2
VIQ - Chromosome 6
FSIQ - Chromosome 2
FSIQ - Chromosome 6
LOD
cM

shows linkage to PIQ and FSIQ largely overlaps with the 2q21-33 region that has yielded suggestive linkage to autism in at least four independent genomic screens (Philippe et al. 1999; Buxbaum et al. 2001; International Molecular Genetic Study of Autism Consortium [IMGSAC] 2001; Shao et al. 2002). The IMGSAC (2001) reported their highest LOD score (3.74) with language delay in autism-affected families at marker *D2S2188,* which lies 6 cM from the peak LOD score on 2q, whereas Buxbaum et al. (2001) reported their highest LOD score for phrase speech at marker *D2S335,* which lies 3 cM away from the peak LOD score found in our study. Recently, Raskind et al. (2005) conducted a genomewide scan for dyslexia and reported evidence of a QTL for speed of phonological decoding efficiency near marker *D2S1399* at 2q. This marker lies 13 cM away from our peak marker at 2q with PIQ and lies next to the 1-LOD drop border.

Several positional candidate genes within the 2q24.1-2q31.1 linkage region have been tested for an association to autism, including *GAD1* (MIM 605363), *HOXD1* (MIM 142987), *DLX1* (MIM 600029), *DLX2* (MIM 126255), *TBR-1* (MIM 604616), *RAPGEF4* (MIM 606058), *CHN1* (MIM 118423), *SLC25A12* (MIM 603667), *SCN1A* (MIM 182389), *SCN2A* (MIM 182390), and *SCN3A* (MIM 182391) (Bacchelli et al. 2003; Weiss et al. 2003; Rabionet et al. 2004; Ramoz et al. 2004). Most promising as a site with possible relevance to IQ is the significant association between the relative risk to autism and two common SNPs in the mitochondrial aspartate/glutamate carrier *SLC25A12* gene (Ramoz et al. 2004).

The linkage region on chromosome 6 (6p25.3-6p22.3 [*D2S942–D2S422*]) overlaps marginally with the region 6p22.3-6p21.3 implicated in reading disability and dyslexia (Cardon et al. 1994; Fisher et al. 1999*b*; Gayán et al. 1999; Grigorenko et al. 2000; Kaplan et al. 2002; Willcutt et al. 2002; Deffenbacher et al. 2004). Although recently at least five candidate genes were identified that are likely to contribute to linkage with reading disability, those genes lie just outside the region defined by a drop of 1 LOD score on 6p for VIQ and FSIQ scores (Deffenbacher et al. 2004). The *ALDH5A1* gene (6p22-6p23), implicated in both cognitive ability (Plomin et al. 2004) and reading disability (Deffenbacher et al. 2004), lies at the border of our 6p region.

Several genes within the 2q and 6p linkage regions have been associated with schizophrenia (*NR4A2* [MIM 601828] at 2q24, *DTNBP1* [MIM 607145] at 6p22, *KIF13A* [MIM 605433] at 6p22, and *NQO2* [MIM 160998] at 6p25), fragile X syndrome (*RANBP9* [MIM 603854] at 6p23), and Bardet-Biedl syndrome (*BBS5* [MIM 603650] at 2q31). These disorders are accompanied by rather severe cognitive impairment, but milder variants in these same genes could influence variation in the normal range of cognitive abilities. Recently, evidence was found for linkage at 6p24 to a neurocognitive-deficit subtype of schizophrenia, in which the maximum LOD score occurred at marker *D6S309,* which is within the region that shows linkage to VIQ and FSIQ (Hallmayer et al., in press). Currently, *dysbindin-1* (*DTNBP1*) at 6p22.3 is the best-supported susceptibility gene for schizophrenia (Talbot et al. 2004). Recent identification of a relationship between *dysbindin-1* and hippocampal glutamate neurotransmission, a core concept of leading neurobiological theories of memory and learning, suggests further potential as an IQ gene (Talbot et al. 2004). A second positional candidate gene thought to be involved in memory processes is *NRN1* (MIM 607409) at 6p25.1, which plays a role in neuritogenesis in mature brains. Naeve et al. (1997) showed that expression of neuritin, the product of *NRN1,* is induced by neural activity and by the activity-regulated brain-derived neurotrophic factor and neurotrophin-3. Neuritin is expressed in hippocampal and cortical neurons and is suspected to regulate neuronal plasticity during development and in the adult brain.

Given the gradual increase in heritability of IQ from childhood to late adolescence, those genes in our regions that influence brain development may be promising as candidate genes for IQ. For example, TBR-1 (MIM 604616), a neuron-specific T-box transcription factor, plays a critical role in brain development and is specifically expressed in the cortex. It is thought to be a common genetic determinant for the differentiation of early-born glutamatergic neocortical neurons and may provide insights into the functions of these neurons as regulators of cortical development (Hevner et al. 2001, 2002). More specifically, Hevner et al. (2002) showed, using Tbr1 mutant mice, that Tbr1 is critical in the appropriate establishment of precise reciprocal projections between cortical areas and corresponding thalamic nuclei.

Figure 2 Genomic regions with suggestive or significant linkage in the Dutch (*blue*), Australian (*green*), and combined (*red*) data sets. Vertical dotted lines represent the positions of the markers. Horizontal solid red lines denote genomewide empirical thresholds in the combined data set for significant linkage, defined as the LOD score that would be expected to occur by chance with a probability of 0.05 in a whole-genome scan. Horizontal dashed red lines denote genomewide empirical thresholds in the combined data set for suggestive linkage, defined as the LOD score that would be expected to occur once by chance in a whole-genome scan (Lander and Kruglyak 1995). Information content, as a measure of entropy in the IBD distribution (Kruglyak et al. 1996), in the Dutch (*black*) and Australian (*gray*) data sets is plotted in the top panels.

In summary, a genome scan for intelligence has revealed two regions with putative evidence of linkage: 2q24.1-2q31.1 and 6p25.3-6p22.3. To identify these regions, we analyzed variation in cognition in healthy subjects. These areas were previously implicated in disorders that are accompanied by cognitive impairment, which supports the idea that trait variation within the normal range might be used to detect genes for (mental) disorders, such as autism, schizophrenia, or reading disability.

Acknowledgments

Financial support was provided by the Netherlands Organization for Scientific Research Spinoza (grant 904-61-090), the National Supercomputing Facilities (grants sg214 and sg217), and the Human Frontiers of Science Program (grant rg0154/1998-B). D.P. was supported in part by the GenomeEUtwin project (European Union contract QLG2-CT-2002-01254). Dutch genotyping was performed by the Center for Medical Genetics at Marshfield (Director, Dr. James Weber) and the Leiden University Medical Centre (Professor Slagboom). Australian phenotype collection was funded by Australian Research Council grants A79600334, A79906588, A79801419, DP0212016, and DP0343921; genotyping was funded by the Australian National Health and Medical Research Council's Program in Medical Genomics (grant NHMRC-219178) and the Center for Inherited Disease Research (CIDR) (Director, Dr. Jerry Roberts) at The Johns Hopkins University, under a grant to Dr. Jeff Trent and N.G.M. CIDR is fully funded through a federal contract from the National Institutes of Health to The Johns Hopkins University (contract N01-HG-65403). We thank Anjali Henders, Megan Campbell, and staff from the Molecular Epidemiology Laboratory, for blood processing and DNA extraction of the Australian samples; Peter Visscher, for valuable comments; and Arjen van Bochoven, for support in supercomputer programming.

Web Resources

The URLs for data presented herein are as follows:

Integrated genetic map with interpolated genetic map positions, http://www2.qimr.edu.au/davidD/master_map.dat
Mx Home Page, http://www.vcu.edu/mx/
Mx Scripts, http://www.psy.vu.nl/mxbib/
Online Mendelian Inheritance in Man (OMIM), http://www.ncbi.nlm.nih.gov/Omim/

References

Abecasis GR, Cherny SS, Cookson WO, Cardon LR (2001) GRR: graphical representation of relationship errors. Bioinformatics 17:742–743

——— (2002) Merlin-rapid analysis of dense genetic maps using sparse gene flow trees. Nat Genet 30:97–101

Bacchelli E, Blasi F, Biondolillo M, Lamb JA, Bonora E, Barnby G, Parr J, Beyer KS, Klauck SM, Poustka A, Bailey AJ, Monaco AP, Maestrini E, International Molecular Genetic Study of Autism Consortium (IMGSAC) (2003) Screening of nine candidate genes for autism on chromosome 2q reveals rare nonsynonymous variants in the cAMP-GEFII gene. Mol Psychiatry 8:916–924

Badcock JC, Dragovic M, Waters FA, Jablensky A (2005) Dimensions of intelligence in schizophrenia: evidence from patients with preserved, deteriorated and compromised intellect. J Psychiatr Res 39:11–19

Bouchard TJ Jr, McGue M (1981) Familial studies of intelligence: a review. Science 212:1055–1059

Butcher LM, Meaburn E, Dale PS, Sham P, Schalkwyk LC, Craig IW, Plomin R (2005) Association analysis of mild mental impairment using DNA pooling to screen 432 brain-expressed single-nucleotide polymorphisms. Mol Psychiatry 10:384–392

Buxbaum JD, Silverman JM, Smith CJ, Kilifarski M, Reichert J, Hollander E, Lawlor BA, Fitzgerald M, Greenberg DA, Davis KL (2001) Evidence for a susceptibility gene for autism on chromosome 2 and for genetic heterogeneity. Am J Hum Genet 68:1514–1520

Cardon LR, Smith SD, Fulker DW, Kimberling WJ, Pennington BF, DeFries JC (1994) Quantitative trait locus for reading disability on chromosome 6. Science 266:276–279

Chorney MJ, Chorney K, Seese N, Owen MJ, Daniels J, McGuffin P, Thompson LA, Detterman DK, Benbow C, Lubinski D, Eley T, Plomin R (1998) A quantitative trait locus associated with cognitive ability in children. Psychol Sci 9:159–166

Churchill GA, Doerge RW (1994) Empirical threshold values for quantitative trait mapping. Genetics 138:963–971

Deffenbacher KE, Kenyon JB, Hoover DM, Olson RK, Pennington BF, DeFries JC, Smith SD (2004) Refinement of the 6p213 quantitative trait locus influencing dyslexia: linkage and association analyses. Hum Genet 115:128–138

Fisher PJ, Turic D, Williams NM, McGuffin P, Asherson P, Ball D, Craig I, Eley T, Hill L, Chorney K, Chorney MJ, Benbow CP, Lubinski D, Plomin R, Owen MJ (1999*a*) DNA pooling identifies QTLs on chromosome 4 for general cognitive ability in children. Hum Mol Genet 8:915–922

Fisher SE, Marlow AJ, Lamb J, Maestrini E, Williams DF, Richardson AJ, Weeks DE, Stein JF, Monaco AP (1999*b*) A quantitative-trait locus on chromosome 6p influences different aspects of developmental dyslexia. Am J Hum Genet 64:146–561

Flint J (1999) The genetic basis of cognition. Brain 122:2015–2031

Gayán J, Smith SD, Cherny SS, Cardon LR, Fulker DW, Brower AM, Olson RK, Pennington BF, DeFries JC (1999) Quantitative-trait locus for specific language and reading deficits on chromosome 6p. Am J Hum Genet 64:157–164

Goldman-Rakic PS (1999) The physiological approach: functional architecture of working memory and disordered cognition in schizophrenia. Biol Psychiatry 46:650–661

Grigorenko EL, Wood FB, Meyer MS, Pauls DL (2000) Chromosome 6p influences on different dyslexia-related cognitive processes: further confirmation. Am J Hum Genet 66:715–723

Hallmayer JF, Kalaydjieve L, Badcock J, Dragovic M, Howell

S, Michie PT, Rock D, Vile D, Williams R, Corder EH, Hollingsworth K, Jablensky A. Genetic evidence for a distinct subtype of schizophrenia characterized by pervasive cognitive deficit. Am J Hum Genet (in press)

Heijmans BT, Beekman M, Putter H, Lakenberg N, van der Wijk HJ, Whitfield JB, Posthuma D, Pedersen NL, Martin NG, Boomsma DI, Slagboom PE. Meta-analysis of four new genome scans for lipid parameters and analysis of positional candidates in positive linkage regions. Eur J Hum Genet (in press)

Hevner RF, Miyashita-Lin E, Rubenstein JL (2002) Cortical and thalamic axon pathfinding defects in Tbr1 Gbx2 and Pax6 mutant mice: evidence that cortical and thalamic axons interact and guide each other. J Comp Neurol 447:8–17

Hevner RF, Shi L, Justice N, Hsueh Y, Sheng M, Smiga S, Bulfone A, Goffinet AM, Campagnoni AT, Rubenstein JL (2001) Tbr1 regulates differentiation of the preplate and layer 6. Neuron 29:353–366

Inlow JK, Restifo LL (2004) Molecular and comparative genetics of mental retardation. Genetics 166:835–881

International Molecular Genetic Study of Autism Consortium (IMGSAC) (2001) A genomewide screen for autism: strong evidence for linkage to chromosomes 2q, 7q, and 16p. Am J Hum Genet 69:570–581

Jackson DN (1998) Multidimensional Aptitude Battery II. Sigma Assessment Systems, Port Huron, MI

Kaplan DE, Gayán J, Ahn J, Won TW, Pauls D, Olson RK, DeFries JC, Wood F, Pennington BF, Page GP, Smith SD, Gruen J (2002) Evidence for linkage and association with reading disability on 6p21.3-22. Am J Hum Genet 70:1287–1298

Kong A, Gudbjartsson DF, Sainz J, Jonsdottir GM, Gudjonsson SA, Richardsson B, Sigurdardottir S, Barnard J, Hallbeck B, Masson G, Shlien A, Palsson ST, Frigge ML, Thorgeirsson TE, Gulcher JR, Stefansson K (2002) A high-resolution recombination map of the human genome. Nat Genet 31:241–247

Kruglyak L, Daly MJ, Reeve-Daly MP, Lander ES (1996) Parametric and nonparametric linkage analysis: a unified multipoint approach. Am J Hum Genet 58:1347–1363

Lander E, Kruglyak L (1995) Genetic dissection of complex traits: guidelines for interpreting and reporting linkage results. Nat Genet 11:241–247

Luciano M, Wright MJ, Martin NG (2004) Exploring the etiology of the association between birthweight and IQ in an adolescent twin sample. Twin Res 7:62–71

Naeve GS, Ramakrishnan M, Kramer R, Hevroni D, Citri Y, Theill LE (1997) Neuritin: a gene induced by neural activity and neurotrophins that promotes neuritogenesis. Proc Natl Acad Sci USA 94:2648–2653

Neale MC, Boker S, Xie G, Maes HH (1997) Mx software: statistical modeling. Richmond, VA

Petrill SA, Plomin R, McClearn GE, Smith DL, Vignetti S, Chorney MJ, Chorney K, Thompson LA, Detterman DK, Benbow C, Lubinski D, Daniels J, Owen MJ, McGuffin P (1996) DNA markers associated with general and specific cognitive abilities. Intelligence 23:191–203

Philippe A, Martinez M, Guilloud-Bataille M, Gillberg C, Rastam M, Sponheim E, Coleman M, Zappella M, Aschauer H, Van Maldergem L, Penet C, Feingold J, Brice A, Leboyer M, and the Paris Autism Research International Sibpair Study (1999) Genome-wide scan for autism susceptibility genes. Hum Mol Genet 8:805–812

Plomin R, Hill L, Craig IW, McGuffin P, Purcell S, Sham P, Lubinski D, Thompson LA, Fisher PJ, Turic D, Owen MJ (2001) A genome-wide scan of 1842 DNA markers for allelic associations with general cognitive ability: a five-stage design using DNA pooling and extreme selected groups. Behav Genet 31:497–509

Plomin R, Turic DM, Hill L, Turic DE, Stephens M, Williams J, Owen MJ, O'Donovan MC (2004) A functional polymorphism in the succinate-semialdehyde dehydrogenase (aldehyde dehydrogenase 5 family member A1) gene is associated with cognitive ability. Mol Psychiatry 9:582–586

Posthuma D, de Geus EJC, Boomsma DI (2001) Perceptual speed and IQ are associated through common genetic factors. Behav Genet 31:593–602

Rabionet R, Jaworski JM, Ashley-Koch AE, Martin ER, Sutcliffe JS, Haines JL, Delong GR, Abramson RK, Wright HH, Cuccaro ML, Gilbert JR, Pericak-Vance MA (2004) Analysis of the autism chromosome 2 linkage region: GAD1 and other candidate genes. Neurosci Lett 372:209–214

Ramakers GJA (2003) Rho proteins, mental retardation and the cellular basis of cognition. Trends Neurosci 25:191–199

Ramoz N, Reichert JG, Smith CJ, Silverman JM, Bespalova IN, Davis KL, Buxbaum JD (2004) Linkage and association of the mitochondrial aspartate/glutamate carrier SLC25A12 gene with autism. Am J Psychiatry 161:662–669

Raskind WH, Igo RP, Chapman NH, Berninger VW, Thomson JB, Matsushita M, Brkanac Z, Holzman T, Brown M, Wijsman EM (2005) A genome scan in multigenerational families with dyslexia: identification of a novel locus on chromosome 2q that contributes to phonological decoding efficiency. Mol Psychiatry (http://www.nature.com/mp/journal/vaop/ncurrent/index.html) (electronically published March 8, 2005; accessed 27 June 2005)

Shao Y, Raiford KL, Wolpert CM, Cope HA, Ravan SA, Ashley-Koch AA, Abramson RK, Wright HH, DeLong RG, Gilbert JR, Cuccaro ML, Pericak-Vance MA (2002) Phenotypic homogeneity provides increased support for linkage on chromosome 2 in autistic disorder. Am J Hum Genet 70:1058–1961

Talbot K, Eidem WL, Tinsley CL, Benson MA, Thompson EW, Smith RJ, Hahn CG, Siegel SJ, Trojanowski JQ, Gur RE, Blake DJ, Arnold SE (2004) Dysbindin-1 is reduced in intrinsic glutamatergic terminals of the hippocampal formation in schizophrenia. J Clin Invest 113:1353–1363

Wechsler D (1997) WAIS-III Wechsler Adult Intelligence Scale. Psychological Corporation, San Antonio

Weiss LA, Escayg A, Kearney JA, Trudeau M, MacDonald BT, Mori M, Reichert J, Buxbaum JD, Meisler MH (2003) Sodium channels SCN1A, SCN2A and SCN3A in familial autism. Mol Psychiatry 8:186–194

Willcutt EG, Pennington BF, Boada R, Ogline JS, Tunick RA, Chhabildas NA, Olson RK (2001) A comparison of the cognitive deficits in reading disability and attention-deficit/hyperactivity disorder. J Abnorm Psychol 110:157–172

Willcutt EG, Pennington BF, Smith SD, Cardon LR, Gayan J, Knopik VS, Olson RK, DeFries JC (2002) Quantitative trait locus for reading disability on chromosome 6p is pleiotropic for attention-deficit/hyperactivity disorder. Am J Med Genet 114:260–268

Wright MJ, De Geus EJC, Ando J, Luciano M, Posthuma D, Ono Y, Hansell N, Van Baal GCM, Hiraishi K, Hasegawa T, Smith G, Geffen G, Geffen L, Kanba S, Miyake A, Martin NG, Boomsma DI (2001) Genetics of cognition: outline of collaborative twin study. Twin Res 4:48–56

Yalcin B, Willis-Owen SA, Fullerton J, Meesaq A, Deacon RM, Rawlins JN, Copley RR, Morris AP, Flint J, Mott R (2004) Genetic dissection of a behavioral quantitative trait locus shows that Rgs2 modulates anxiety in mice. Nat Genet 36: 1197–1202

Zhu G, Duffy DL, Eldridge A, Grace M, Mayne C, O'Gorman L, Aitken JF, Neale MC, Hayward NK, Green AC, Martin NG (1999) A major quantitative-trait locus for mole density is linked to the familial melanoma gene CDKN2A: a maximum-likelihood combined linkage and association analysis in twins and their sibs. Am J Hum Genet 65:483–492

Zhu G, Evans DM, Duffy DL, Montgomery GW, Medland SE, Gillespie NA, Ewen KR, Jewell M, Liew YW, Hayward NK, Sturm RA, Trent JM, Martin NG (2004) A genome scan for eye color in 502 twin families: most variation is due to a QTL on chromosome 15q. Twin Res 7:197–210

Am. J. Hum. Genet. 77:327–328, 2005

Use of the Term "Antley-Bixler Syndrome": Minimizing Confusion

To the Editor:

We read with great interest the publication by Huang et al. (2005), which made a number of significant contributions to our understanding of the biochemistry and molecular genetics of a newly described, highly variable, autosomal recessive condition referred to as "cytochrome P450 oxidoreductase (POR [MIM 124015]) deficiency." We agree with the authors that what has been termed "Antley-Bixler syndrome" (ABS [MIM 207410]) in the scientific literature is genetically heterogeneous with at least two distinct disorders, (1) ABS without disordered steroidogenesis, which appears to be a variant of the autosomal dominant fibroblast growth factor receptor (*FGFR*)–related craniosynostosis syndromes, and (2) ABS with disordered steroidogenesis, which appears to be caused by severe mutations in *POR*. However, we disagree with the authors' proposition "that the term 'ABS' be reserved for those patients with the skeletal dysmorphologic findings initially reported by Antley and Bixler (1975) but who have normal genitalia and normal steroidogenesis, and that patients with the skeletal dysmorphologic phenotype plus evidence of disordered steroidogenesis be referred to as having 'POR deficiency'" (Huang et al. 2005, p. 745).

Although the female patient first described by Antley and Bixler did not have ambiguous genitalia or any reported steroid anomalies, there are a number of reasons why these facts do not provide sufficient justification to reserve the term "ABS" for patients with *FGFR* mutations. These include:

1. To our knowledge, the patient described by Antley and Bixler (1975) has not had molecular testing for mutations in *FGFR2* or *POR*. Therefore, POR deficiency cannot be ruled out for this patient.
2. Steroid abnormalities associated with POR deficiency and ABS are not always recognized without the use of urinary steroid profiling (Shackleton et al. 2004). In fact, Huang et al. (2005) found *POR* mutations in both alleles of two female patients with ABS who were initially believed not to have steroid abnormalities when first reported by Reardon et al. (2000).
3. The presence of ambiguous genitalia is not necessary for making a diagnosis of POR deficiency. This is illustrated by the two females with ABS and normal genitalia who are reported by Huang et al. (2005) to have mutations in *POR*. In addition, we have published a family with classic ABS in which a male child had ambiguous genitalia but his sister did not (Cragun et al. 2004). Both children had evidence of abnormal steroid metabolism, and mutations in *POR* have subsequently been confirmed.

Because of similarities with respect to phenotype, molecular findings, and pattern of inheritance, patients with *FGFR* mutations should be grouped with those with the other autosomal dominant *FGFR*-related craniosynostosis syndromes. This proposal is supported by others who have questioned the diagnosis of ABS for a patient who has *FGFR2* mutations (Gorlin 1999; Gripp et al. 1999). Even Huang et al. (2005) admit that the diagnosis of ABS was reconsidered in some of the patients they report with *FGFR* mutations.

Clarifying which individuals represent classic ABS has been difficult because few pictures of patients with ABS and known *POR* or *FGFR* mutations have been published, and the clinical descriptions of these patients often lack detail. However, some subtle features—including a pear-shaped or bulbous nose, low-set and dysplastic ears, arachnodactyly, and/or rockerbottom feet—are often present in patients with ABS who are known or suspected to have POR deficiency; these features are not described in patients with known *FGFR* mutations. Interestingly, the patient reported by Antley and Bixler (1975) had a bulbous nose, low-set dysplastic ears, and arachnodactyly. In addition, that patient also had significant camptodactyly, which is described in patients who likely have POR deficiency more commonly than in those with *FGFR* mutations. Compared with cases of ABS that are suspected or known to be caused by POR deficiency, patients with *FGFR* mutations generally have more-severe proptosis and facial dysmorphism that is more similar to that of patients with Pfeiffer syndrome or Crouzon syndrome (two *FGFR*-related craniosynostosis syndromes). On the basis of this evidence, the authors' conclusion—that "aside from the genital anomalies attributable to disordered steroidogenesis, no morphologic feature distinguished patients with *POR* mutations from those with *FGFR* mutations" (Huang et al. 2005, p. 736)—may not be warranted.

Continuing to use the term "ABS" for patients with *FGFR* mutations will only contribute to the confusion that is already present in the literature. The concern is that this confusion may interfere with proper patient management and counseling, both of which depend on the ability of clinicians and researchers to clearly recognize, understand, and convey to patients the differences between POR deficiency and *FGFR*-related craniosynostosis syndromes.

Use of the term "ABS" to describe patients with POR deficiency who are at the more severe end of the phenotypic spectrum can be clinically useful in distinguishing them from patients with POR deficiency who have mild or no skeletal defects (Arlt et al. 2004; Flück et al. 2004; Fukami et al. 2004). We believe it would be better to reserve the use of the term "ABS" for patients with POR deficiency and clinically significant craniosynostosis and/or radiohumoral synostosis.

DEBORAH CRAGUN[1] AND ROBERT J. HOPKIN[1,2]
[1]*Cincinnati Children's Hospital Medical Center and* [2]*University of Cincinnati, Cincinnati*

Web Resource

The URL for data presented herein is as follows:

Online Mendelian Inheritance in Man (OMIM), http://www.ncbi.nlm.nih.gov/Omim/ (for POR and ABS)

References

Antley R, Bixler D (1975) Trapezoidocephaly, midfacial hypoplasia and cartilage abnormalities with multiple synostoses and skeletal fractures. Birth Defects Orig Artic Ser 11:397–401

Arlt W, Walker EA, Draper N, Ivison HE, Ride JP, Hammer F, Chalder SM, Borucka-Mankiewicz M, Hauffa BP, Malunowicz EM, Stewart PM, Shackleton CH (2004) Congenital adrenal hyperplasia caused by mutant P450 oxidoreductase and human androgen synthesis: analytical study. Lancet 363:2128–2135

Cragun DL, Trumpy SK, Shackleton CH, Kelley RI, Leslie ND, Mulrooney NP, Hopkin RJ (2004) Undetectable maternal serum uE3 and postnatal abnormal sterol and steroid metabolism in Antley-Bixler syndrome. Am J Med Genet A 129: 1–7

Flück CE, Tajima T, Pandey AV, Arlt W, Okuhara K, Verge CF, Jabs EW, Mendonca BB, Fujieda K, Miller WL (2004) Mutant P450 oxidoreductase causes disordered steroidogenesis with and without Antley-Bixler syndrome. Nat Genet 36: 228–230

Fukami M, Horikawa R, Nagai T, Tanaka T, Naiki Y, Sato N, Okuya T, Nakai H, Soneda S, Tachibana K, Matsuo N, Sato S, Hom K, Nishimura G, Hasegawa T, Ogata T (2004) Cytochrome P450 oxidoreductase gene mutations and Antley-Bixler syndrome with abnormal genitalia and/or impaired steroidogenesis: molecular and clinical studies in 10 patients. J Clin Endocrinol Metab 90:414–426

Gorlin RJ (1999) Patient described by Chun et al. may not present Antley-Bixler syndrome. Am J Med Genet 83:64

Gripp KW, Zackai EH, Cohen MM Jr (1999) Not Antley-Bixler syndrome. Am J Med Genet 83:65–68

Huang N, Pandey AV, Agrawal V, Reardon W, Lapunzina PD, Mowat D, Jabs EW, Vliet GV, Sack J, Flück CE, Miller WL (2005) Diversity and function of mutations in P450 oxidoreductase in patients with Antley-Bixler syndrome and disordered steroidogenesis. Am J Hum Genet 76:729–749

Reardon W, Smith A, Honour JW, Hindmarsh P, Das D, Rumsby G, Nelson I, Malcolm S, Ades L, Sillence D, Kumar D, DeLozier-Blanchet C, McKee S, Kelly T, McKeehan WL, Baraitser M, Winter RM (2000) Evidence for digenic inheritance in some cases of Antley-Bixler syndrome? J Med Genet 37:26–32

Shackleton C, Marcos J, Malunowicz EM, Szarras-Czapnik M, Jira P, Taylor NF, Murphy N, Crushell E, Gottschalk M, Hauffa B, Cragun DL, Hopkin RJ, Adachi M, Arlt W (2004) Biochemical diagnosis of Antley-Bixler syndrome by steroid analysis. Am J Med Genet A 128:223–231

Address for correspondence and reprints: Dr. Deborah Cragun, Cincinnati Children's Hospital Medical Center, 3333 Burnet Avenue, E-5, MLC 4006, Division of Human Genetics, Cincinnati, OH 45229-3039. E-mail: Deborah.cragun@cchmc.org

0002-9297/2005/7702-0015$15.00

Am. J. Hum. Genet. 77:328–330, 2005

"Antley-Bixler Syndrome"—A Reply to Cragun and Hopkin

To the Editor:

Cragun and Hopkin (2005 [in this issue]) raise a series of points concerning use of the term "Antley-Bixler syndrome" (ABS), both in our recent paper in this journal (Huang et al. 2005) and elsewhere. We agree that it is useful to minimize confusion: the best way to do this may be to discard the term "ABS" and other eponymic terms once the molecular genetics and cell biology of a disease have been worked out. However, until such eponyms are discarded, as stated in our paper, "we propose that the term 'ABS' be reserved for those patients with the skeletal dysmorphologic findings initially reported by Antley and Bixler (1975) but who have normal genitalia and normal steroidogenesis" (Huang et al. 2005, p. 745). Cragun and Hopkin suggest that "patients with *FGFR* mutations should be grouped with those with other autosomal dominant *FGFR*-related craniosynostosis syndromes." We agree. Describing dysmorphologic disorders by eponyms was appropriate when the responsible genes were not known, but little purpose is served in preserving these terms once the molecular genetics and cell biology are delineated. Although one may wish to honor investigators with eponyms, such nosology inhibits understanding of mechanisms: "post-streptococcal glomerulonephritis" may be less euphonious than "Bright's disease" but is more specific and informative.

Cragun and Hopkin raise questions about the patient initially described by Antley and Bixler and about several other reported cases. Clearly, it is difficult (if not impossible) to make or exclude a diagnosis retrospectively. Lacking the individual's DNA, we cannot know the molecular lesion in the patient described by Antley and Bixler (but we'd be happy to study it!). Whereas Cragun and Hopkin lament the paucity of published photographs and clinical detail in many case reports, we lament the poor descriptions of the external genitalia and the incomplete hormonal evaluations in most patients with "ABS." Careful steroidal evaluation is crucial: mass spectrometric analysis of urinary steroids is highly reliable but not widely available; appropriate evaluation of pre- and poststimulation plasma steroids is equally reliable. The data available to Reardon et al. (2000) were insufficient to establish or exclude a steroidogenic disorder for several of their patients; hence, their report does not provide evidence for the suggestion that *POR* (P450 oxidoreductase) mutations might cause a skeletal disorder associated with normal genitalia. Thus, we believe that our conclusion that "aside from the genital anomalies attributable to disordered steroidogenesis, no dysmorphological feature distinguished patients with *POR* mutations from those with *FGFR* mutations" (Huang et al. 2005, p. 736) is well supported by the data in table 1 of Huang et al. (2005, p. 731). For convenience, we have compiled the clinical data from table 1 and the genetic data from table 4 (p. 737) in the table shown here. More-refined observations may identify other anatomic features distinguishing *POR* from *FGFR* mutations in infants with craniosynostosis; however, our data clearly show that dysmorphologists must pay very close attention to the external genitalia in these children and consider evaluation of steroid secretion before and after tropic stimulation with adrenocorticotropic hormone.

Deficient POR activity can cause a broad spectrum of human disease (Flück et al. 2004; Miller 2004; Huang et al. 2005), and clearly the patients described by us and others who have POR lesions without skeletal defects do not have ABS. Thus, we do not think it is reasonable to follow the suggestion of Cragun and Hopkin to use the term "ABS" for patients with the more severe form of POR deficiency associated with skeletal anomalies. If, as they propose (and we agree), all *FGFR*-based craniosynostosis disorders should be grouped together, then it is logical to group all *POR* disorders together. Regardless of whether the clinical genetics community agrees to discard eponyms in favor of a term such as "FGFR hyperactivity," we believe that "POR deficiency," which is a newly described monogenic disease, should be dissociated from the term "Antley-Bixler Syndrome."

Table 1

Genotype/Phenotype Correlations Collated from the Data in Tables 1 and 4 of Huang et al. (2005)

	No. of Patients with Mutation			
Genotype	1 *POR* (n = 4)	2 *POR* (n = 15)	*FGFR2* (n = 9)	None Found (n = 4)
Craniosynostosis	4/4	14/15	8/8	3/3
Brachycephaly	…	7/10	5/5	1/2
RU/RH[a] synostosis	4/4	13/15	6/7	2/3
Femoral bowing	3/3	9/13	3/6	2/2
Femoral fractures	0/1	2/10	2/3	1/2
Midface hypoplasia	2/2	9/10	8/8	2/2
Proptosis	1/1	9/11	8/9	3/3
Rocker-bottom feet	…	4/9	0/1	1/1
Arachnodactyly	2/2	7/11	0/3	1/1
Camptodactyly	…	3/6	2/5	…
Choanal atresia	1/1	7/9	7/8	3/3
Abnormal steroids	***2/2***	***8/8***	…	…
Abnormal genitalia	***2/2***	***10/10***	…	…

Note—The column designations (from table 4 of Huang et al. [2005]) indicate whether a mutation was found on only one of the two *POR* alleles (1 *POR*), both alleles (2 *POR*), on one allele of *FGFR2*, or whether no mutation was found on either gene. The clinical findings are from table 1 (Huang et al. 2005); since each finding was not commented on in all the case histories, the denominators vary. Of the findings described in the available clinical data, only the presence of an abnormality in steroidogenesis or in genital development distinguished the patients with *POR* mutations from those with *FGFR2* mutations.

[a] RH = radiohumeral; RU = radioulnar.

Walter L. Miller

Department of Pediatrics, University of California, San Francisco (UCSF), and UCSF Children's Hospital, San Francisco

References

Antley R, Bixler D (1975) Trapezoidocephaly, midfacial hypoplasia and cartilage abnormalities with multiple synostoses and skeletal fractures. Birth Defects Orig Artic Ser 11:397–401

Cragun D, Hopkin RJ (2005) Use of the term "Antley-Bixler syndrome": minimizing confusion. Am J Hum Genet 77:327–328 (in this issue)

Flück CE, Tajima T, Pandey AV, Arlt W, Okuhara K, Verge CF, Jabs EW, Mendonca BB, Fujieda K, Miller WL (2004) Mutant P450 oxidoreductase causes disordered steroidogenesis with and without Antley-Bixler syndrome. Nat Genet 36: 228–230

Huang N, Pandey AV, Agrawal V, Reardon W, Lapunzina PD, Mowat D, Jabs EW, Van Vliet G, Sack J, Flück CE, Miller

WL (2005) Diversity and function of mutations in P450 oxidoreductase in patients with Antley-Bixler syndrome and disordered steroidogenesis. Am J Hum Genet 76:729–749
Miller WL (2004) P450 oxidoreductase deficiency: a new disorder of steroidogenesis with multiple clinical manifestations. Trends Endocrinol Metab 15:311–315
Reardon W, Smith A, Honour JW, Hindmarsh P, Das D, Rumsby G, Nelson I, Malcolm S, Ades L, Sillence D, Kumar D, DeLozier-Blanchet C, McKee S, Kelly T, McKeehan WL, Baraitser M, Winter RM (2000) Evidence for digenic inheritance in some cases of Antley-Bixler syndrome? J Med Genet 37:26–32

Address for correspondence and reprints: Dr. Walter L. Miller, Department of Pediatrics, Building MR4, Room 209, University of California, San Francisco, 1466 Fourth Avenue, San Francisco, CA 94143-0978. E-mail: wlmlab@itsa.ucsf.edu

0002-9297/2005/7702-0016$15.00

Am. J. Hum. Genet. 77:330–332, 2005

LRRK2 Haplotype Analyses in European and North African Families with Parkinson Disease: A Common Founder for the G2019S Mutation Dating from the 13th Century

To the Editor:
Parkinson disease [PD (MIM 168600)] is the second most common neurodegenerative disorder, characterized by resting tremor, rigidity, bradykinesia, and gait disturbances. The *LRRK2* gene (GenBank accession number AY792511) was recently identified as being responsible for autosomal dominant PD (Paisan-Ruiz et al. 2004; Zimprich et al. 2004). Several groups have reported that a single pathogenic G6055A substitution (G2019S) in the *LRRK2* gene was associated with 3%–6% and 1%–2% of familial and sporadic PD, respectively (Di Fonzo et al. 2005; Gilks et al. 2005; Kachergus et al. 2005; Lesage et al. 2005; Nichols et al. 2005). In addition, Kachergus et al. (2005) demonstrated that, in 13 families of European descent, G2019S-mutation carriers shared a small ancestral haplotype, suggestive of a common founder.

In our sample of 198 affected probands from families with PD that is compatible with autosomal dominant inheritance, mostly from France and North Africa, we identified a total of 13 *LRRK2* G2019S-mutation carriers, one of whom was homozygous for this mutation. Five were of European descent (two from France and one each from Portugal, Belgium, and The Netherlands), one was from North America, and seven were from North Africa. Surprisingly, one 60-year-old healthy French control individual also carried the same mutation.

To determine whether a common haplotype was also shared by the G2019S carriers in our series, all available family members of the 14 *LRRK2*-positive families were genotyped for the 17 chromosome 12q microsatellite markers and four SNPs, described elsewhere (Kachergus et al. 2005), that span a 16-Mb region that includes the *LRRK2* gene. Seven markers (three microsatellites and four SNPs) were located within the gene. A total of 62 individuals were analyzed: 40 G2019S carriers (23 affected and 17 unaffected) and 22 noncarriers, 2 of whom were affected. The microsatellites were genotyped by multiplexing appropriate labeled primers. The fluorescent PCR products were then pooled for analysis, in two runs, on an ABI 3730 automated sequencer. Results were analyzed with GeneMapper 3.5 software (Applied Biosystems). Two DNA samples from CEPH reference families 1331-01 and 1331-02 were used as external standards, to control for consistency between runs. The four *LRRK2* SNPs were genotyped by using the SnapShot multiplex kit (Applied Biosystems), in accordance with the manufacturer's instructions. Haplotypes were constructed using the Merlin program (Abecasis et al. 2002; Center for Statistical Genetics), and their frequencies were estimated with the expectation-maximization algorithm (Excoffier and Slatkin 1995). The difference in haplotype distribution between mutation carriers and noncarriers was evaluated by χ^2 and Fisher's exact tests. Marker-allele frequencies and marker positions were described elsewhere (Kachergus et al. 2005). The age of the mutation was evaluated by estimating the age of the most recent common ancestor of the G2019S-mutation carriers on the basis of information from their shared haplotypes (Genin et al. 2004).

The *LRRK2* haplotype that was associated with the G2019S mutation in all families originating from Europe and North Africa (fig. 1) was consistent with that described by Kachergus et al. (2005). However, the shared region was smaller than the 145–154 kb previously published, which reduces the common haplotype to only 60 kb. This minimal haplotype (T-254-A-G-A-154) consisting of six adjacent markers spanning the region between SNP *rs7966550* (Entrez SNP) in exon 22 of the *LRRK2* gene and microsatellite marker *D12S2518* in intron 45 flanking the G2019S mutation in exon 41 was determined in French family 030, in which 29 members in two generations were available for study. Parental phases could also be unambiguously determined in six other families. In the remaining families, the haplotype could not be reconstructed unambiguously from the shared region, but the genotypes were all compatible with the presence of the common haplotype. In the majority of families, the shared region extended farther than the minimal haplotype, particularly 3′ of the *LRRK2* gene, and independent of geographical origin. The common haplotype was also shared by five (24.7%) non-

	Family													
Marker	030	212	755*	314	247	159	750	021	156	169	400**	134	411	163
D12S87	158	156	154	156/158	156/158	158	158	156	156/158	156/164	164	164	156/162	158/160
D12S1648	144	110	110	110/124	110/122	110	124/130	124	120/136	120/122	114/132	144	118/126	130/138
D12S2080	188	184/192	188	184/196	184/188	184	188/192	196	184	184	184/192	184	184/188	184/188
D12S2194	249	261	261	249/261	257/261	245/249	249/261	265	253/261	261/265	257/261	261	257	249/257
D12S2514	291	291	291	291	291/294	291/294	291	291	285/291	291/297	291	291	291/294	291
D12S2515	216	224	224	224	220/224	220	212/224	228	216/228	208/232	224	224	216/224	212/224
rs7966550	T	T	T	T	T	T	T	T	T	T	T	T	T	T
D12S2516	254	254	254	252/254	254	254	254	254	254	252/254	254	254	254/256	254
rs1427263	A	A	A	A/C	A	A	A	A	A	A	A	A	A	A
rs11176013	G	G	G	A/G	A/G	G	A/G	G	G	G	G	G	G	G
rs11564148	A	T/A	A	T/A	T/A	A	T/A	A	T/A	T/A	A	A	T/A	A
D12S2518	154	154	154	154/168	154	154	154	154	154	154/170	154	154	154	154
D12S2519	138	132	132	132/138	132	132	132/138	132	132/138	132/134	132/138	132/138	132/134	132
D12S2520	248	260	260	257/260	257/260	257/260	257/260	257	254/260	260	257/260	260	257/260	257/260
D12S2521	323	359	359	319/359	359/363	359/363	315/359	359	315/359	359/367	323/363	359	359/371	359/367
D12S2522	281	297	297	295/297	297	297	295/297	297	287/297	297/299	295/297	297	297	297
D12S2523	305	320	320	314/320	320	320	314/320	320	320/323	305/320	314/320	320	305/320	320
D12S2517	184	192	192	192/208	182/192	188/192	194/204	192	180/192	192/198	192/210	192	188/192	190/192
D12S1048	211	214	214	214/217	214	211/214	214/220	214	214/217	214/226	214/217	214	214/226	214/226
D12S1301	104	116	104	104/116	100/120	108/112	108	116	104/112	104/116	100/104	104	104/112	104/116
D12S1701	101	103	95	89/105	97	91/95	97/99	97	95/97	97/99	97/101	95	97/101	95/101
	France			The Netherlands	Portugal	Belgium	USA	Morocco			Algeria			Tunisia
	European origin							North African origin						

Figure 1 Genotypes for chromosome 12q12 markers in the disease haplotype in subjects from 14 *LRRK2*-positive families. The sequences of the microsatellites and SNPs were from the GDB Human Genome Database and Entrez SNP, respectively. An asterisk (*) indicates an unaffected individual from the control population who carried the G2019S mutation. A double asterisk (**) indicates a homozygous G2019S carrier. For families in which phase could not be unambiguously determined, both alleles are shown. The haplotype shared by all G2019S carriers is highlighted in gray.

carriers of the G2019S mutation. However, the minimal haplotype was significantly more frequent in mutation carriers (7/7) than in noncarriers (5/21) ($\chi^2 = 12.44$; $P < .001$), even when only the seven families in which the G2019S haplotype could be unambiguously determined were taken into account.

This finding, in addition to previous data, extends the potential founder effect observed in Norwegians, Irish, Polish, and Americans of European descent to other European countries (France, Belgium, Portugal, and The Netherlands) and to three countries in North Africa (Algeria, Morocco, and Tunisia). The widespread distribution of the founder effect in Europe and its extension to North Africa prompted us to evaluate the time at which the mutation event might have occurred. Using patients for whom extended haplotypes could be unambiguously determined in our study (from families 030, 755, 021, and 400) and the study of Kachergus and his collaborators (2005) (from families P-063 and 1120), we estimated that the mutation occurred 29 generations earlier (95% CI 15–55). If a generation is defined as 25 years, the mutation occurred 725 (95% CI 375–1375) years ago, in the 13th century.

In conclusion, we have extended the founder effect for the *LRRK2* G2019S mutation to other European countries and to North Africa, and we have reduced the common ancestral haplotype to a 60-kb region. The most recent common ancestor probably lived ~725 years ago.

Acknowledgments

We are grateful to the patients and their families. We thank Drs. Pierre Pollak, François Tison, Myriem Tazir, and Joao Guimaraes for their contribution to the recruitment and to the evaluation of patients. This project was supported by the European Grant APOPIS (European Union contract LSHM-CT-2003-503330) and INSERM/Association Français contre les Myopathies Cohortes et Collections 2001. Members of the

French Parkinson's Disease Genetics Study Group are Y. Agid, A.-M. Bonnet, M. Borg, A. Brice, E. Broussolle, P. Damier, A. Destée, A. Dürr, F. Durif, E. Lohmann, M. Martinez, C. Penet, P. Pollak, O. Rascol, F. Tison, C. Tranchant, M. Vérin, F. Viallet, M. Vidailhet, and J.-M. Warter (deceased).

SUZANNE LESAGE,[1] ANNE-LOUISE LEUTENEGGER,[1] PABLO IBANEZ,[1] SABINE JANIN,[1] EBBA LOHMANN,[1,3] ALEXANDRA DÜRR,[1,2,3] AND ALEXIS BRICE,[1,2,3,4] FOR THE FRENCH PARKINSON'S DISEASE GENETICS STUDY GROUP*

[1]*INSERM U679 (formerly U289), Neurologie et Thérapeutique Expérimentale, and* [2]*Département de Génétique, Cytogénétique et Embryologie, Hôpital de la Pitié-Salpêtrière,* [3]*Fédération de Neurologie, Centre Hospitalier Universitair Pitié-Salpêtrière,* [4]*Unité de Formation et de Recherche Pierre et Marie Curie, Paris*

Web Resources

The accession number and URLs for data presented herein are as follows:

Center for Statistical Genetics, http://www.sph.umich.edu/csg/abecasis/Merlin/

Entrez SNP, http://www.ncbi.nlm.nih.gov/entrez/query.fcgi?CMD=search&DB=snp

GDB Human Genome Database, http://www.gdb.org/

Genbank, http://www.ncbi.nlm.nih.gov/Genbank/ (for *Homo sapiens LRRK2* [accession number AY792511])

Online Mendelian Inheritance in Man (OMIM), http://www.ncbi.nlm.nih.gov/Omim/ (for PD)

References

Abecasis GR, Cherny SS, Cookson WO, Cardon LR (2002) Merlin—rapid analysis of dense genetic maps using sparse gene flow trees. Nat Genet 30:97–101

Di Fonzo A, Rohe CF, Ferreira J, Chien HF, Vacca L, Stocchi F, Guedes L, Fabrizio E, Manfredi M, Vanacore N, Goldwurm S, Breedveld G, Sampaio C, Meco G, Barbosa E, Oostra BA, Bonifati V, Italian Parkinson Genetics Network (2005) A frequent LRRK2 gene mutation associated with autosomal dominant Parkinson's disease. Lancet 365:412–415

Excoffier L, Slatkin M (1995) Maximum-likelihood estimation of molecular haplotype frequencies in a diploid population. Mol Biol Evol 12:921–927

Genin E, Tullio-Pelet A, Begeot F, Lyonnet S, Abel L (2004) Estimating the age of rare disease mutations: the example of triple-A syndrome. J Med Genet 41:445–449

Gilks WP, Abou-Sleiman PM, Gandhi S, Jain S, Singleton A, Lees AJ, Shaw K, Bhatia KP, Bonifati V, Quinn NP, Lynch J, Healy DG, Holton JL, Revesz T, Wood NW (2005) A common LRRK2 mutation in idiopathic Parkinson's disease. Lancet 365:415–416

Kachergus J, Mata IF, Hulihan M, Taylor JP, Lincoln S, Aasly J, Gibson JM, Ross OA, Lynch T, Wiley J, Payami H, Nutt J, Maraganore DM, Czyzewski K, Styczynska M, Wszolek ZK, Farrer MJ, Toft M (2005) Identification of a novel *LRRK2* mutation linked to autosomal dominant parkinsonism: evidence of a common founder across European populations. Am J Hum Genet 76:672–680

Lesage S, Ibanez P, Lohmann E, Agid Y, Dürr A, Brice A (2005) The G2019SLRRK2 mutation in autosomal dominant European and North African Parkinson's disease is frequent and its penetrance is age-dependent. Neurology 64:1826

Nichols WC, Pankratz N, Hernandez D, Paisan-Ruiz C, Jain S, Halter CA, Michaels VE, Reed T, Rudolph A, Shults CW, Singleton A, Foroud T, and the Parkinson Study Group—PROGENI Investigators (2005) A single LRRK mutation accounting for greater than 5% of familial Parkinson disease. Lancet 365:410–412

Paisan-Ruiz C, Jain S, Evans EW, Gilks WP, Simon J, van der Brug M, de Munain AL, Aparicio S, Gil AM, Khan N, Johnson J, Martinez JR, Nicholl D, Carrera IM, Pena AS, de Silva R, Lees A, Marti-Masso JF, Perez-Tur J, Wood NW, Singleton AB (2004) Cloning of the gene containing mutations that cause PARK8-linked Parkinson's disease. Neuron 44:595–600

Zimprich A, Biskup S, Leitner P, Lichtner P, Farrer M, Lincoln S, Kachergus J, Hulihan M, Uitti RJ, Calne DB, Stoessl AJ, Pfeiffer RF, Patenge N, Carbajal IC, Vieregge P, Asmus F, Muller-Myhsok B, Dickson DW, Meitinger T, Strom TM, Wszolek ZK, Gasser T (2004) Mutations in LRRK2 cause autosomal-dominant parkinsonism with pleomorphic pathology. Neuron 44:601–607

Address for correspondence and reprints: Dr. Alexis Brice, INSERM U679, Hôpital de la Salpêtrière, 47, Boulevard de l'Hôpital, 75651 Paris Cedex 13, France. E-mail: brice@ccr.jussieu.fr

* Members of the French Parkinson's Disease Genetics Study Group are listed in the Acknowledgments.

0002-9297/2005/7702-0017$15.00

Book Review

Am. J. Hum. Genet. 77:333, 2005

Guide to Mutation Detection. Edited by Graham R. Taylor and Ian N. Day. Hoboken, NJ: Wiley, 2005. Pp. 330. $89.95, paperback.

Guide to Mutation Detection is a compilation of short reviews and protocols for detecting changes in DNA sequence. Its intended audience is postgraduate-level molecular geneticists, particularly individuals working in diagnostic molecular-genetics laboratories. The book originates from a practical course that is offered once every 2 years in conjunction with the Human Genome Organization (HUGO) Mutation Detection Workshop. The reviews and protocols are contributed by the instructors of that course. The book is divided into two sections, Reviews and Methods. The Reviews section begins with general reviews and then progresses to more-specific technical reviews of methods for detecting DNA sequence changes. The Methods section offers more-detailed protocols for various methods, some of which are discussed in the Reviews section. In addition to wet-bench techniques, *Guide to Mutation Detection* has a chapter devoted to quality control and quality assurance in clinical laboratories. It also has several chapters dedicated to the use of both general mutation databases and locus-specific databases.

Guide to Mutation Detection covers a variety of topics that are of interest to clinical molecular-genetics laboratories. It is not a comprehensive review but covers selected techniques. The techniques range from the basic, such as PCR and Southern-blot analysis, to more cutting-edge methods, such as tag array minisequencing. The first few chapters in the Reviews section provide an excellent introduction to the nature of mutations encountered in clinical molecular-genetics laboratories. These chapters also describe some of the methods used to detect DNA mutations. More-detailed reviews of selected topics follow the two introductory chapters. The topics covered in the Reviews section are not a comprehensive list of methods but are only a subset of the methods used in diagnostic molecular-genetics laboratories. Surprisingly, there is little attention given to what is considered the gold standard for mutation detection, dye terminator DNA sequencing.

The Methods section provides detailed protocols for some of the topics discussed in the Reviews section as well as additional protocols for methods not covered there. Again, the topics range from the basic to more-novel methods. Like the Reviews section, the Methods section is not a comprehensive list of methodologies available. There is substantial variation in the quality and detail provided in these chapters. In fact, some of the chapters in the Methods section are essentially the protocols provided by the manufacturers. Other chapters, however, provide detailed protocols for techniques that have been developed after many years of experience by leaders in the field.

Guide to Mutation Detection is a relatively short manual, only 330 pages in length; hence, it is not a comprehensive review, as is *Current Protocols in Human Genetics.* The strongest feature of *Guide* is that it provides a good introduction to some cutting-edge technologies, such as the use of microarrays and tandem mass spectrometry in the analysis of DNA mutations. It also contains some protocols that have been developed by well-established laboratories that may be useful in detecting specific classes of mutations. For these reasons, *Guide to Mutation Detection* is a useful tool to complement more-comprehensive technical manuals.

BRADFORD COFFEE

Department of Human Genetics
Emory University School of Medicine
Atlanta

0002-9297/2005/7702-0018$15.00

Erratum

In the June 2005 issue of the *Journal,* in the article entitled "Heterozygous Mutations of *OTX2* Cause Severe Ocular Malformations," by Ragge et al. (76:1008–1022), incorrect affiliations were given for two of the authors. J. Richard O. Collin is at Moorfields Eye Hospital in London, and Alison Salt is at Moorfields Eye Hospital and Great Ormond Street Children's Hospital, also in London. The authors regret these errors.

Announcements[1]

EMPLOYMENT OPPORTUNITIES

Postdoctoral Fellowships.—The University Of California–San Francisco (UCSF) is accepting applications for postdoctoral training in medical genetics. The program is based in the Division of Medical Genetics in the Department of Pediatrics. The aim of the fellowship is to provide research training in medical genetics, to enable graduates of the program to conduct independent research and to assume faculty or professional leadership positions in medical and human genetics. We are especially seeking individuals interested in research in the areas of developmental biology and human malformation syndromes. The UCSF Division of Medical Genetics enjoys an international reputation for excellence in research, education, and genetic service. The faculty includes physicians and basic scientists, all of whom actively participate in the training of postdoctoral fellows. A key feature of the program at UCSF is the tight integration of research and clinical activities, with the maintenance of close contact among trainees with medical and basic science backgrounds. The fellowship is for 1–2 years and is open to those with either an M.D. or a Ph.D. degree. We anticipate two positions being available in 2005 and in 2006. For information and application materials, write to: Anne Slavotinek, M.B.B.S., Ph.D., Medical Genetics, Department of Pediatrics, University of California–San Francisco, 533 Parnassus Avenue, San Francisco, CA 94143-0748; telephone: (415) 514-1783; fax: (415) 476-9976; e-mail: slavotia@peds.ucsf.edu. UCSF is an equal opportunity employer. We strongly encourage women and minority students to apply to our program, which is situated in an academic center and community of extraordinary diversity.

1. Announcements are published free of charge for members of The American Society of Human Genetics (ASHG). Please e-mail announcements to ajhg@emory.edu. Submission must be received *at least 7 weeks* before the month of issue in which publication is requested. They must be double spaced with a $1\frac{1}{2}$-inch margin on all sides. The maximum length is *250 words*, excluding the address for correspondence. Please include a cover letter indicating the name of the sponsoring ASHG member.

Director of Education.—The American Society of Human Genetics (ASHG) has established a new position of Director of Education to implement programs to address the vision of genetic literacy in the classroom as well as in the general public. The Director will work with the Executive Vice President, under the direction of the officers and the Board, to achieve the goals of ASHG, including making genetics-education programs and materials more accessible to all classrooms. ASHG, the primary professional organization for researchers and clinicians in the field, has a strong commitment to educational goals. The duties of the Director will include (1) providing staffing for the Information and Education Committee, (2) initiating and enhancing partnerships with organizations that focus on teaching science in grades K–12, (3) enhancing capabilities of the Mentor Network of volunteer members, (4) planning professional development programs, and (5) procuring funding to implement programs. The ideal candidate will have an M.S. or a Ph.D. in genetics or a related field and experience in developing educational programs and materials. Requirements include outstanding written and oral communication, grant-writing skills, and demonstrated ability to lead projects. Applicants should send a curriculum vitae, a letter of interest, and the names of three potential references to Joann Boughman either by e-mail, to jboughman@ashg.org, or by mail, to the following address: Joann Boughman, Ph.D., Executive Vice President, American Society of Human Genetics, 9650 Rockville Pike, Bethesda, MD 20814. Review of applications will begin in March 2005, and the position may start as early as June 1, 2005.

Postdoctoral Fellow.—Applications are invited for a position as a postdoctoral fellow in cancer pharmacogenomics at Washington University School of Medicine in St. Louis. The postdoctoral fellow will direct projects involving the utilization of model systems and human cell lines to identify the molecular determinants of chemotherapy toxicity and/or efficacy (Proc Natl Acad Sci

USA 101:11809–11814). The successful applicant will have a Ph.D. and/or M.D. and will possess solid writing skills and an ability to apply innovative methods to biological questions. Techniques will include genetic linkage mapping, microarray analyses, drug-sensitivity profiling of cell lines, DNA sequencing, etc. Preference will be given to applicants with experience in human genetics and analysis of complex traits. Contact Cara Thomas, Administrative Coordinator, Washington University, Molecular Oncology, 660 S. Euclid, Campus Box 8069, St. Louis, MO 63110; telephone: (314) 747-5186; fax: (314) 362-3764; e-mail: cthomas@im.wustl.edu

---

Faculty Position.—The Department of Human Genetics at Emory University School of Medicine is currently seeking ABMG-eligible-certified M.D. or M.D./Ph.D. physician/scientists for tenure-track appointments at the level of assistant, associate, or full professor. Successful candidates will join a rapidly expanding research program in human genetics and genomics under the leadership of Dr. Steve Warren. We are seeking outstanding individuals who are able to lead a successful research laboratory and to participate in the departments clinical activities. The department has 35 primary faculty members and >$7,000,000 in federal research funding per year. The department has a fully ACGME-accredited clinical genetics residency program and offers training in all ABMG subspecialties. The successful applicant would devote ~80% of his/her time to the pursuit of an independent, extramurally funded research program and the remainder to patient care and teaching. Any area of contemporary human genetics research is acceptable, with the primary consideration given to excellence and evidence of future research success and innovation. Generous start-up packages and competitive salaries are available. Candidates should send a curriculum vitae, descriptions of research and clinical experience, and future research plans, in electronic form, to facsearch@genetics.emory.edu. Letters of reference will be requested through follow-up correspondence. Emory University is an equal opportunity/affirmative action employer.

Cell Lines and DNA Samples

Biomaterials from the International HapMap Project.—Samples from the CEPH population; from Yoruba in Ibadan, Nigeria; from Han Chinese in Beijing; from Japanese in Tokyo; from the Denver (Colorado) Metropolitan Chinese Community; and from Luhya in Webuye, Kenya, are currently available from the National Institute of General Medical Sciences (NIGMS) Human Genetic Cell Repository (HGCR) at the Coriell Institute for Medical Research. Additional materials will be available soon. The NIGMS HGCR was established at Coriell Institute for Medical Research in 1972 and contains >9,500 cell lines, including almost 500 OMIM classifications. The cell lines and DNA derived from them can be distributed to all qualified research investigators. The resources are divided into cell lines derived from individuals with inherited diseases, apparently healthy controls, and individuals with diverse ethnic backgrounds. The NIGMS HGCR has prepared the cell lines and DNA for the International HapMap Project. The biomaterials are available in several formats: as panels and 96-well microtiter plates of the DNA samples used by the HapMap Consortium, as individual DNA samples, and as individual lymphoblastoid cell lines. Additional information about the HapMap samples in the NIGMS Repository at Coriell can be found at our Web site (http://ccr.coriell.org/nigms/products/hapmap.html). Information about ordering cell lines and panels can be obtained from the Web catalog (http://locus.umdnj.edu/nigms/). Further information can be obtained from Donald Coppock, Ph.D., Coriell Institute for Medical Research, Coriell Cell Repositories, 403 Haddon Avenue, Camden, NJ 08103; telephone: (800) 752-3805; e-mail: dcoppock@coriell.org

Information for Contributors

Postal address: **Stephen T. Warren, Ph.D., Editor, The American Journal of Human Genetics, Department of Human Genetics, Emory University School of Medicine, 615 Michael Street, Room 301, Atlanta, GA 30322-3050.** Telephone: (404) 712-9980. Fax: (404) 712-9984. E-mail: ajhg@emory.edu. Web page: http://www.ajhg.org/.

The American Journal of Human Genetics is a record of research and review relating to heredity in humans; to the applications of genetic principles in medicine, psychology, anthropology, and social services; and to areas of molecular and cell biology relevant to human genetics. It is published monthly. The *Journal* is owned and controlled by The American Society of Human Genetics and is edited, in conjunction with the publisher, by a staff appointed by the Board of Directors of the Society.

Electronic Edition

The entire content of the *Journal* is published electronically on the World Wide Web, at http://www.ajhg.org/. The full text is available to subscribers, as is material supplemental to the print version, including video and archival databases. Articles will be posted as they are ready for publication. Approximately 2 weeks before publication of the hard copy, the table of contents for that issue will be posted with final pagination, along with editorials and other material.

Editorial Policy

The *Journal* welcomes submissions of articles and reports on timely subjects concerning all aspects of human genetics, including studies of model organisms that are of direct relevance to human genetics. Letters commenting on material previously published in the *Journal* are also welcome. Review articles, editorials, and book reviews usually are solicited by the editor. The *Journal* does not publish reports of either single mutations or mutational surveys of previously identified loci unless they have unusual significance and substantial insight. Descriptions of new linkage assignments will be considered only if they are of unusual interest and significance. Reports of negative data, without substantial insight and interest, will not normally be considered. Membership in The American Society of Human Genetics is not a prerequisite for publication in the *Journal.* Papers will be considered for publication on condition that they are not currently under consideration by any other publication and that no portion of them has been published elsewhere.

• *Review process.* Manuscripts will be considered for appropriateness to the *Journal* by the editor in conjunction with the editorial board. Those considered appropriate will be reviewed by two or more external reviewers or by members of the editorial board, and those not considered appropriate will be returned to the authors. Authors are requested to suggest appropriate referees. Manuscripts will be judged on their value as original contributions to the field and on their overall presentation. Authors whose manuscripts are returned without external review may appeal by writing the editor.

• *Return of figures.* For manuscripts that are reviewed but not accepted, all figures submitted as glossy prints will be returned whenever possible.

• *Editing.* Manuscripts will be edited to conform to *Journal* style, to correct spelling and grammar where necessary, and to improve conciseness, clarity, and precision of expression. Significant editorial changes will be identified on the page proofs.

• *Publication costs.* For papers published—except for invited contributions and Letters to the Editor—authors will be charged $50.00 per printed *Journal* page or portion thereof. Each *Journal* page contains ~800 words. If authors wish, they may instead pay a single publication fee of $5,000 for an article or $2,700 for a report, to make their work freely and immediately available to all readers at publication, rather than after the usual 6-month delay for nonsubscribers. All authors will also be charged for printing of color figures (see Illustrations, below).

• *Copyright agreement.* All authors of all manuscripts accepted for publication (except U.S. government employees) must sign an agreement transferring copyright to The American Society of Human Genetics. Corresponding authors must assume responsibility for obtaining the signatures of all coauthors. Material published in the *Journal* may not be reproduced or published elsewhere without written consent of the Society and the publisher. Requests for such permission should be addressed to the publisher: Copyright, University of Chicago Press, 1427 East 60th Street, Chicago, IL 60637. Fax: (773) 702-9756.

• *Research materials.* It is assumed that authors whose research is published in the *Journal* will make cell lines, antibodies, cloned DNA sequences, and similar materials available to other investigators in noncommercial institutions, so as to permit replication of the reported work.

• *Page proofs.* Page proofs will be sent to the corresponding author for correction of typographical errors only. Corresponding authors are responsible for the return of corrected page proofs to the publisher by the designated deadline.

• *Reprints.* The corresponding author will receive an order form for reprints, along with the page proofs.

Manuscript Submission

Manuscripts should now be submitted via the *AJHG* Web Peer Review System at http://mss.uchicago.edu/AJHG. Basic instructions for submission via the WPR system can be found at the Web site (http://mss.uchicago.edu/AJHG/auth_msprep_AJHG.epl), and detailed instructions are given below.

Manuscript Preparation

Manuscripts must be written in English. MS Word, Rich Text, or LaTeX formats are acceptable. All components of the text (including references and figure legends but not tables) must

be typed double spaced in 12-point type. Tables must be single spaced. *Manuscripts that are not double spaced throughout will not be sent out for review.* Use a 1-inch margin on all four sides of each page, and do not justify the right margin. Begin each manuscript component on a separate page, and arrange components in the following order: title page, Summary (abstract), text (articles separated into Introduction, Material and Methods, Results, and Discussion), Acknowledgments, appendices (if any), Web Resources, References, tables, and figure legends. Number all pages consecutively in the upper-right-hand corner, beginning with the title page.

Cover letter. Include a letter from the author who will be responsible for correspondence regarding the manuscript as well as for communications among authors in regard to revisions, publication agreements, and approval of proofs. This letter should indicate the category of manuscript being submitted (e.g., article, report, letter, review) and highlight the significance of the manuscript in a few sentences. It should also disclose the source of funding and any affiliations with or involvement in any companies, trade associations, unions, litigants, or other groups with a direct financial interest in the subject matter or materials discussed in the manuscript by any authors and/or their immediate family within the last 5 years. Also indicate whether the first author is a student or post-doctoral fellow and a member of The American Society of Human Genetics (to be eligible for the Cotterman awards, presented at the ASHG's annual meeting).

Please indicate the category of your manuscript in the cover letter:

Articles are full-length, original research articles.

Reports are short (approximately four *Journal* pages, 800 words per page) scientific correspondence with a brief abstract but without further subdivision of the manuscript. This category is designed for timely publication of original findings that may substantially impact their field.

Letters to the Editor are brief commentaries (less than one printed page) concerning articles published in the *Journal* within the past 2 months. They may also present new data. Also included in this section are short general news items of interest to the Society. Any letter concerning a previously published article will first be sent for external review, to determine whether it meets an appropriate level of significance for publication in the *Journal.* If the letter achieves this basic level of significance, it will then be sent to the corresponding author of the pertinent article, who will be given an opportunity to submit a response. This response will be provided to the corresponding author of the letter to the editor. After considering the response, the authors may choose to withdraw their letter or to proceed with publication without further revision.

Fast-track review. If circumstances so warrant, you may request in the cover letter a fast-track review of your paper. At the editor's discretion, a 24- to 48-hour fast-track review is available to expedite manuscripts that deserve rapid review and publication.

Related manuscripts. Please submit a copy of any related papers, by any of the authors, that have been submitted but not published elsewhere or that are in press. For citation of such manuscripts, see "*Work submitted to a publication but not yet accepted, personal communications, and unpublished data,*" below.

All papers should adhere to the guidelines that follow, with two exceptions:

1) *Reports* should contain a brief summary of five sentences or fewer, but the remainder of the text should not be divided into sections.

2) *Letters to the Editor* do not contain a summary, nor should the text be divided into sections.

Otherwise, please prepare all submissions according to the following directives:

Title page. This page should contain a concise title; a running title of no more than 40 characters (including spaces); the names and institutional affiliations of all authors at the time of the study (and present affiliations, if different); and the corresponding author's name, complete current mailing address, telephone number, fax number, and e-mail address. Each paper can be assigned only one corresponding author. Joint authorship is permitted only for the first author position, with a maximum of two individuals being given this designation.

Summary (abstract). The Summary should state the purpose of the study, the basic procedures and analytical methods, the findings, and the principal conclusions. The Summary must not exceed 275 words.

Text. The text should be as concise as possible and should be organized into the following sections: Introduction, Material and Methods (or Subjects and Methods), Results, and Discussion. Some manuscripts may require different formats appropriate to their content. Brief subheadings may be used where necessary.

The Introduction should summarize the rationale for the study, without reviewing the subject extensively. Using the past tense, describe the selection of subjects and identify the methods, apparatus, and procedures in detail. Provide references for established methods and brief descriptions of those that are not well known. Describe any new or modified methods used, including reasons for their use and evaluations of their limitations.

Present results in logical sequence in the text, tables, and illustrations. Do not repeat in the text all the data that appear in the tables and illustrations. Detailed results of statistical analyses may be presented as an appendix.

Web Resources. Please provide accession numbers along with the URL of any genome or locus-specific database in which information has been deposited. (This is required for establishing links in the electronic edition of the *Journal.*) Place this information in the text and in a separate section entitled "Web Resources," following the Acknowledgments. Please do not include URLs in the text or in the References.

MIM numbers should be listed in the text after the first mention of the relevant disorder or gene. Example: adrenal hypoplasia congenita (AHC [MIM 300200]). In the Web Resources section, only the URL for the OMIM database, and not the individual MIM numbers, should be noted. Example: Online Mendelian Inheritance in Man (OMIM), http://www.ncbi.nlm.nih.gov/Omim/.

Human subjects. If the manuscript reports results of studies of either human subjects or materials obtained from human subjects, state in the Material and Methods section that the study was approved by the appropriate institutional review board and/or that appropriate informed consent was obtained from human subjects. Copies of signed consent forms from identifiable persons appearing in any photographs submitted with the manuscript must be faxed to the *AJHG* office at the time of submission: (404) 712-9984. To avoid violation of HIPAA regulations, this consent form should state that the subject understands that his or her identity (but not his or her medical records) will be divulged to the *Journal* office by the transmission of the signed consent form. Alternatively, a letter from a member of your institutional review board (IRB) can be sent to us confirming that signed consent forms have been obtained from the individuals pictured in the manuscript without naming these individuals. Your manuscript cannot be processed until we receive these consent forms or a letter from your IRB.

Acknowledgments. Acknowledge those who have made substantive contributions to the study reported, as well as the institution(s) or grant sponsor(s) that supported the research.

Reference citations. Authors must assume responsibility for the accuracy of reference citations. Reference citations in the text, tables, or figure legends should be in parentheses and include author surname(s) and year of publication. When citing a work by two authors, provide both authors' names joined by "and." When citing a work by three or more authors, provide the first author's name followed by "et al." When the author name(s) and the year of publication are identical for two or more works, distinguish between the works by appending a lowercase italic letter to the year, to match the order in which the works appear in the References section. Examples: (Charlesworth 2001), (Peters and Sandkuijl 1992), (Devriendt et al. 1997), (Stack et al. 1995*a*). List two or more works in the same citation in chronological order, separated by semicolons. When two or more works in a citation were published in the same year, arrange them alphabetically by the first author's surname. When the same author name(s) are used for two or more works in the same citation, group those works together in chronological order, with the years separated by commas. If such a group occurs in a citation that includes other works, place the group chronologically within the citation according to the first year in the group, using semicolons between the group and the other works cited. Examples: (Erdmann 1994; Braverman et al. 1997; Purdue et al. 1997), (Hellsten 1995; Redding et al. 1996*a*, 1996*b*, 2000; Kessler et al. 1997).

References section. References should be arranged alphabetically by author surname(s). References by the same author(s) should be arranged chronologically. References by the same author(s) for which the year of publication is also the same should be arranged alphabetically by title. List the names of up to 25 authors; if more than 25, list the first 7 plus "et al." Use standard abbreviations for journal titles. Do not use excess punctuation.

References examples:

Journal: Devriendt K, Matthijs G, Legius E, Schollen E, Blockmans D, van Geet C, Degreef H, Cassiman J-J, Fryns J-P (1997) Skewed X-chromosome inactivation in female carriers of dyskeratosis congenita. Am J Hum Genet 60:581–587

Chapter: Peters DJM, Sandkuijl LA (1992) Genetic heterogeneity of polycystic kidney disease in Europe. In: Breuning MH, Devoto M, Romeo G (eds) Contributions to nephrology 97: polycystic kidney disease. Karger, Basel, pp 128–139

Entire volume: Dayhoff MV (ed) (1978) Atlas of protein sequence and structure. Vol 5, suppl 3. National Biomedical Research Foundation, Washington, DC

Meeting paper: Kessler S (1997) Transcripts of genetic counseling sessions: exercises in missed opportunities. Paper presented at Talking Human Genetics: Verbal Communication, Knowledge and Genetic Makeup. Hamburg, April 24–27

Thesis/dissertation: Hellsten E (1995) Positional cloning of the infantile ceroid lipofuscinosis gene. PhD thesis, National Public Health Institute, Helsinki

Computer software: SAS Institute (1997) SAS release 6.12, Cary, NC

Work "in press": Jones TM, Peterson RW. Ethical issues in screening for genetic diseases. Am J Hum Genet (in press)

Work submitted to a publication but not yet accepted, personal communications, and unpublished data: Do not list in References. Cite in the text as "personal communication" (if none of the individuals cited are authors of the manuscript being submitted) or "unpublished data" (if at least one of the individuals cited is also an author of the manuscript being submitted). List the names (including first initials) of all individuals responsible for the unpublished data or personal communication, and include letters of authorization from the individuals named.

Tables. Each table should appear on a separate page and should be single spaced. Whenever possible, construct exceptionally large tables and pedigree diagrams in sections. Number tables consecutively and give each a brief title. Give each column a short heading. Use footnotes to explain all abbreviations that are used in each table, and denote them by letter. Titles and footnotes should be included on the same page with the tables themselves. Use the table editor of a word-processing program to create tables. Do not use tabs or spaces, and omit vertical and horizontal lines from tables. Each row of data must be in a separate row of table cells. Do not submit tables as photographs. For more detailed instructions about tables, see "Special Instructions for Tables" at the *AJHG* homepage. For further guidelines, see *Scientific Style and Format: The CBE Manual for Authors, Editors, and Publishers* and *The Chicago Manual of Style* (cited in Style Guidelines, below).

Illustrations (figures). For complete instructions on preparing figures, please refer to http://www.ajhg.org/artguide.html. Design and prepare the figures carefully; they are the visual presentation of the scientific findings and will be carefully evaluated by the reviewers and editors. Figures should be saved as Encapsulated Postscript (EPS) files or Tagged Image File Format (TIF) files. Common Web formats, such as GIF or JPEG, are not acceptable; neither are proprietary application

formats, such as PowerPoint. Most figures will be set as single column (80 mm), some as double column (175 mm), and some broadside on a page (230 mm). Prepare the figures in publication size or larger (the lettering must be large enough so that the smallest letter will be at least 2.0 mm in height when the figure is reduced to publication size).

Use patterns, such as diagonal lines, rather than shading, which does not reproduce evenly. For pedigree construction, follow the guidelines described in Bennett et al.'s "Recommendations for Standardized Human Pedigree Nomenclature" (Am J Hum Genet 56:745–752, 1995). Include the key (explanation of symbols) within the figure. For micrographs, indicate magnification either by means of a micron bar or in the legend.

Use Helvetica lettering throughout the figure. Insert uppercase letters, in a larger font size, to designate panels.

For initial submission, we require that all figures and tables be included in the main text file. The figures may be converted to the file format of the main text file, since they are being used only for evaluation purposes. External reviewers are only permitted access to the main text file, so they will see only figures and tables included in that file. Thus, it is preferable that you include supplementary materials in the main text file as well. However, if including the supplementary materials makes the main text file too large to upload on our server, they may be uploaded separately.

In submission of revised manuscripts, the figure files should be uploaded as separate files in the appropriate format (EPS or TIFF) but should also be included in the main text file, as they were in the original submission, in case your paper is sent for further external review. Hard copies of figures are required for publication, but, if you wish, you may wait to send them until acceptance of the manuscript.

Color illustrations. Authors must sign an agreement to pay the costs of production of color figures when a manuscript with color figures is accepted. Each page containing a color figure will incur a charge of $450 for the first figure or separate part of a figure, plus $200 for each additional figure.

Figure legends. These should be double spaced, beginning on a separate page. The legend should begin with a brief phrase describing the figure content. The legend should describe the illustration so that it can be understood apart from the text and should explain any labels or symbols that are not included in a key.

Supplemental material. Authors may submit additional data, at the discretion of the editor, as a supplement to the *AJHG* electronic edition.

Supplemental clinical data. For manuscripts containing clinical information, it is important that as much clinical detail as possible be provided for others to verify the conclusions drawn. Photographs, radiographs, and imaging data as well as other laboratory, historical, and clinical data outside the immediate scope of the manuscript may be included as a supplement to the *AJHG* electronic edition.

Style Guidelines

For questions of grammar, punctuation, abbreviation, and scientific style, refer to *The Chicago Manual of Style* (15th ed., University of Chicago Press, Chicago) and *Scientific Style and Format: The CBE Manual for Authors, Editors, and Publishers* (6th ed., Cambridge University Press, Cambridge, UK). The preferred or first spelling of a word in *Merriam-Webster's Collegiate Dictionary* (11th ed., Merriam-Webster, Springfield, MA) is used by the *Journal.* Mathematical equations must be typed and spaced as they should appear in print. Use metric or other internationally accepted units for all quantitative measurements.

Genetic nomenclature and notation. For human genes, use genetic notation and symbols approved by the Human Gene Mapping Workshop. Approved gene symbols may be obtained, prior to submission, from Dr. Sue Povey of the HUGO Gene Nomenclature Committee (HGNC), Department of Biology, University College London, Wolfson House, 4 Stephenson Way, London NW1 2HE, United Kingdom (telephone: 44-20-7679-7410; fax: 44-20-7387-3496; e-mail: nome@galton.ucl.ac.uk). Nomenclature guidelines are available and the Gene Name Proposal form may be completed on the HGNC Web page: http://www.gene.ucl.ac.uk/nomenclature/. See Wain et al.'s "Guidelines for Human Gene Nomenclature" (Genomics 79:464470, 2002). Use ISCN nomenclature for cytogenetic notation (see Mitelman F [ed] ISCN 1995: an international system for human cytogenetic nomenclature. S. Karger, Basel). Human gene names and loci should be written in italicized capital letters and Arabic numerals. Protein product names are not italicized. For human-mutation nomenclature, see Antonarakis et al.'s "Recommendations for a Nomenclature System for Human Gene Mutations" (Hum Mutat 11:1–3, 1998) (http://www3.interscience.wiley.com/cgi-bin/fulltext/5001291/PDFSTART).

Approved mouse nomenclature may be obtained, prior to submission, from Lois Maltais, The Jackson Laboratory, Bar Harbor, ME 04609-0800; telephone: (207) 288-6429; fax: (207) 288-6132; e-mail: nomen@informatics.jax.org; Web page: http://www.informatics.jax.org/mgihome/nomen. For other organisms, consult the appropriate authorities.

Nucleotide sequence deposition. New nucleotide data must be submitted to and deposited in the DNA Data Bank of Japan (DDBJ)/European Molecular Biology Laboratory (EMBL)/GenBank databases, and accession number(s) must be obtained before the paper can be accepted for publication. Submission to any one of the three collaborating databases is sufficient to ensure data entry in all. The accession number(s) should be included in the manuscript's Web Resources section, and the following footnote should appear on the title page: "Nucleotide sequence data reported herein are available in the DDBJ/EMBL/GenBank databases; for details, see the Web Resources section of this article." The database will withhold release of data until publication, at authors' request. The most convenient method for submission of sequence data is by World Wide Web: DDBJ, via SAKURA (http://sakura.ddbj.nig.ac.jp/); EMBL, via WEBIN (http://www.ebi.ac.uk/embl/Submission/webin.html); or GenBank, via BankIt (http://www.ncbi.nlm.nih.gov/Sequin/).

Single-nucleotide polymorphisms. Newly described single-nucleotide polymorphisms (SNPs) should be submitted to an appropriate database such as dbSNP (http://www.ncbi.nlm

.nih.gov/SNP/) prior to submission of revised manuscripts. The identification numbers should be included in the "Web Resources" section of the manuscript.

Microarray data. All newly generated microarray data referred to in the text must be submitted for publication as a supplement to the *AJHG* electronic edition. Tables of quantitated raw data and processed data are acceptable, as outlined in guidelines proposed by the Microarray Gene Expression Data Society (for full details, see http://www.mged.org/Workgroups/MIAME/miame_checklist.html). For submission, please save the tables as tab-delimited ASCII text files and submit an electronic copy (no hard copies are necessary).

Computer programs. Authors of manuscripts that describe a novel computer program must make the relevant program publicly available by the time the manuscript is published.

Manuscript-Preparation Checklist

○ Cover letter

○ Copies of signed consent forms for all identifiable photographs of patients

○ Manuscript and figures

○ All pages of text and References *fully double spaced*

○ 1-inch margin on all four sides of each page

○ Title and running title

○ Order of manuscript elements: title page, Summary, text (Introduction, Material and Methods, Results, Discussion), Acknowledgments, appendixes, Web Resources, References, tables, figure legends

○ Summary: no more than 275 words

○ Acknowledgments: all sources of support and those who have made substantive contributions to the work reported

○ References: accurate, complete, and proper style in text and reference list; up to 25 authors' names included (if more than 25, list the first 7 plus "et al.")

○ Tables: *single spaced, no vertical lines, created with the table editor of a word-processing program, not with tabs;* title and footnotes included with table

○ Figures: all guidelines followed; figure legends on a separate page, double spaced

○ A copy of related manuscripts submitted or in press

Additional Components Required at Revision

○ Permission to reproduce previously published material

○ Letters of authorization from sources of personal communications and unpublished data

Submission via the Web Peer Review System

Formatting Electronic Files

Please follow the manuscript preparation requirements above to submit a new or revised manuscript via this system. The system relies on automated processing to create an Adobe Acrobat (PDF) file from your submission. If you do not follow these instructions, your submission cannot be processed automatically and will not be received by the journal office.

The following file formats are acceptable:

- Microsoft Word (.doc; any version that can be read by Word 2000 for Windows)
- Rich Text Format (.rtf)
- Adobe Acrobat (.pdf)
- LaTeX (see special instructions below)

File contents. For initial submission, manuscripts should be submitted as single files, in one of the formats listed above, with all figures, tables, and images embedded (inserted) directly into the document. We also request that supplementary materials be included in the same file, if possible. The figures may be converted to the file format of the main text file, since they are being used only for evaluation purposes. Only materials included in the main text file (and separate supplementary files, if necessary) will be examined by external reviewers.

If we request a revision, in addition to the main text file containing all figures and tables, each figure should be uploaded separately in EPS or TIFF format. Consult your word processing program's "Help" documentation for instructions on how to embed tables and figures. You must also submit in a second file, in one of the acceptable formats, a cover letter that includes your responses to reviewer comments.

Filename requirements. All filenames must be lowercase. (All file processing by the Web Peer Review system is done on Unix machines, where filenames are case-sensitive.)

File compression and archives. Although your manuscript itself must be provided in one file that includes the tables and figures, you will have at least two files to upload into our system (i.e. the cover letter, manuscript file, and any related manuscripts). Therefore, we strongly recommend that you combine these files into an archive so that you can upload a single file for submission. Applications for Mac OS (such as StuffIt) and Windows (such as WinZip) can create this archive.

The following archive formats may be used:

- Windows or Unix zip (e.g., "archiv.zip")
- Unix tar (e.g., "archive.tar" or compressed with gzip as "archive.tar.gz" or "archive.tgz")

If you cannot create archives in these formats, you may still compress individual files to shorten upload time:

- Unix compress (e.g., "ms.tex.Z")

Electronic File Specifications

Program	Main Text File	Cover Letter	Figures	Tables
Word	ms.doc	cover_letter.doc or cover_letter.txt	[embedded in main file]	[embedded in main file]
RTF	ms.rtf	cover_letter.rtf or cover_letter.txt	[embedded in main file]	[embedded in main file]
Acrobat	ms.pdf	cover_letter.pdf or cover_letter.txt	[embedded in main file]	[embedded in main file]
LaTeX	ms.tex	cover_letter.txt	f1.eps, f2.eps, etc.	tb1.tex, tb2.tex, etc.

- Unix gzip (e.g., "ms.tex.gz")

Revisions. If you are submitting a revised manuscript and have a response to the reviewers' comments, include your response as part of the cover letter file. When submitting a revised manuscript with figures, include all the figures even if they have not changed since the previous version.

Online Submission Instructions

Preparing the manuscript file. The preferred format for submitting manuscripts online is Microsoft Word (.doc files). If you are unable to submit a Microsoft Word file, the Web Peer Review system will also accept manuscripts in Acrobat (.pdf), Rich Text Format (.rtf) or LaTeX (.tex). We have provided a drop box in the "File format" area in which to indicate the document type.

As mentioned above, manuscripts should be submitted as single files with all figures, tables, and images embedded (inserted) directly into the document. Embedded figures must be in EPS or TIF format, as these formats result in the best overall outcome when manuscripts are converted to PDF. Please note that authors whose manuscripts are accepted for publication may be required by the publisher to submit high-resolution hard copies (e.g., glossy prints) after the review process is complete and press production is about to begin.

Special instructions for LaTeX. LaTeX files prepared with the AASTeX macro package are preferred. This package uses the "natbib" style for references. If you submit a LaTeX file, figures and tables may be kept in external files, as long as they are referenced within the main "ms.tex" file.

Submission Checklist

Please have the following items readily available before beginning the online submission process:

- Your manuscript as a MS Word, Acrobat (pdf), Rich Text, or LaTeX file including all tables, figures and images embedded in the document
- Cover letter
- Information from your title page for entry into the peer review database, including the title, running title, list of contributing authors and affiliations, word count, and contact information for the corresponding author
- A list of recommended reviewers and their e-mail addresses
- Related papers, by any of the authors, that have been submitted elsewhere or that are in press.
- Copies of signed consent forms for all identifiable photographs of patients (these should be faxed to the AJHG office at [404] 712-9984 at the time of submission).

Navigating the Peer Review Web Site

Step one: describing your manuscript. Go to the *AJHG* Peer Review Web site at http://mss.uchicago.edu/AJHG/. A username and password are required to enter the site. If you already have a username and password, click on "Login/See current tasks" to view the status of your account. If you are new to the site, click on "Create account" to register. After completing your login, click on the "Begin submission" button.

Once you have logged in, fill in the fields describing your manuscript. To move from one field to the next, press the "tab" key. When all the information is complete and you are sure it is correct, click "Ready to upload files" to proceed to step two.

Step two: uploading your file(s). Click the "Browse" button to locate a file on your local system. Once a file is specified in the field, click "Upload this file" to send the file to the Web Peer Review system. You must name your manuscript file "ms," using lowercase type. (All file processing by the Web Peer Review system is done on Unix machines, where filenames are case-sensitive.) The system will assign an ID number to your manuscript during the upload.

As previously mentioned, your manuscript file must contain all figures and tables as well as the text. Remember that if you have multiple files (such as if you are providing a manuscript "in press" for the reviewers), you can compress all of them into a single archive and upload just one file. We recommend that you make an archive of all the files for your submission and then upload the single archive file.

Check your results. Only files listed in the box labeled "Files uploaded so far" have been uploaded successfully. If you need to delete a file, click the file name in the box to select it, and then click the "Delete selected file" button.

When you have uploaded all the files for your submission, click "Process uploaded files" to proceed. The system will attempt to make a PDF version of your file. The conversion to PDF reduces the size of the file and makes it easier for editors and reviewers to read. PDF files can be viewed with Adobe Acrobat Reader version 3 or higher (available free at http://www.adobe.com) or with Ghostscript 5.1 or higher compiled with PDF support turned on (available free at http://www.cs.wisc.edu/~ghost). If successful, there will be a link to the PDF on the next Web page that appears.

If you want to delete all the uploaded files and make no submission, click "Cancel submission" instead.

Step three: submitting your information. After your file has been converted to a PDF file, view the file that was generated from your submission by clicking on "ms.pdf" (a link that will be provided on the next Web page that appears). Only the manuscript file, not the cover letter or related manuscript files, will be viewable at this time. After you finish viewing the manuscript PDF file, indicate how you would like to proceed.

If you select "Approve and submit now," you assert that you have viewed the PDF file via the link provided and that the file accurately shows your manuscript as reviewers should see it. If you select "Fix and resubmit later," the files you have already uploaded will be saved (for 30 days) so that you can return later and upload new or corrected files to make a new PDF file. If you wish to return later to upload other files, please make note of the file upload ID number.

Click "Finish" to complete the final process. Click "Cancel" if you wish to abort the submission.

If your manuscript has been successfully submitted to the *AJHG* Web Peer Review system, a confirmation screen, which includes your assigned manuscript number, will appear. Please carefully note this number and use it in all future correspondence with the *AJHG* editorial office. An e-mail message confirming your submission will be sent to you.

If you do not receive either a manuscript number or confirmation e-mail message, your manuscript was not success-

fully submitted to the journal and thus cannot be sent on to peer review. Please try again or contact ajhg-help@mss.uchicago.edu for assistance.

Announcements

Announcements are posted to the electronic edition of the *Journal* as soon as they are accepted, and they are published in the earliest possible print issue. They may also be viewed at http://www.journals.uchicago.edu/AJHG/journal/announce.html. Announcements are published free of charge for members of The American Society of Human Genetics. They should be submitted via e-mail (ajhg@emory.edu). For publication in print, announcements must be received at least 7 weeks before the month of issue in which publication is desired.

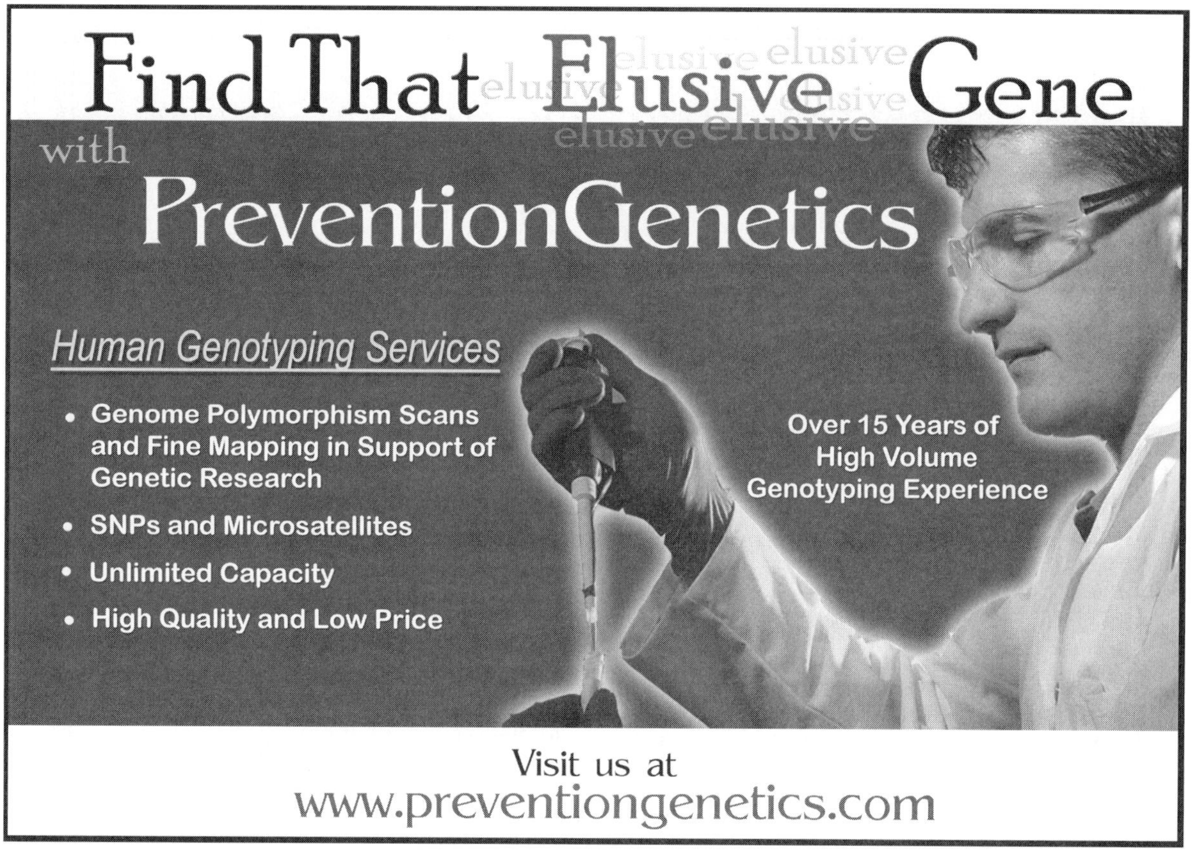
Find That Elusive Gene
with
PreventionGenetics
Human Genotyping Services
• Genome Polymorphism Scans and Fine Mapping in Support of Genetic Research
• SNPs and Microsatellites
• Unlimited Capacity
• High Quality and Low Price
Over 15 Years of High Volume Genotyping Experience
Visit us at
www.preventiongenetics.com

ELSEVIER
ACADEMIC
PRESS

LABORATORY ANIMAL *RESOURCES* *from Elsevier*

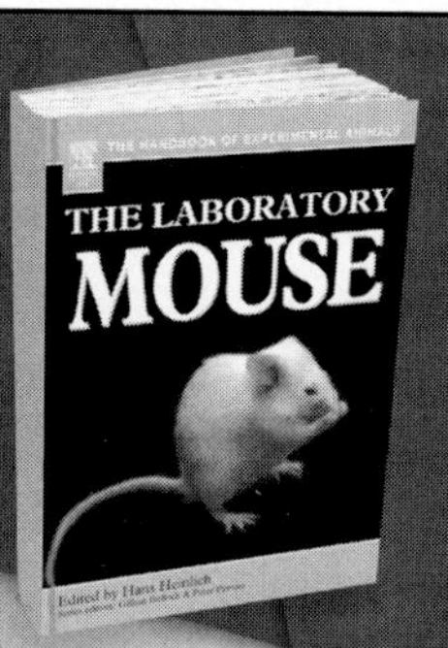

NEW!

THE LABORATORY MOUSE

A VOLUME IN THE *HANDBOOK OF EXPERIMENTAL ANIMALS* SERIES

Edited by
Hans Hedrich
Institute for Laboratory Animal Science, Hanover Medical School, Germany

Among animals used in research, teaching and testing, mice are now widely recognized as the most important model for human diseases and disorders. They comprise the majority of all experimental mammals and tend to be the model of choice used for research into many diseases/disorders. Additionally the laboratory mouse continues to play a widely publicized vital role in the human genome project.

One of the most time-consuming activities in research laboratories is looking up information specific to the species or strain of animal being used. This book, part of the highly successful Handbook of Experimental Animals series, allows the user quick access to any point of interest on the mouse as an experimental model.

- ✦ Comprehensive reference source written by international experts
- ✦ Well-illustrated with high quality detailed images
- ✦ Two-color, user-friendly format combined with color plate sections

August 2004, Hardback, 656 pp.
$200.00/£134.95/€180.00, ISBN: 0123364256

LABORATORY ANIMAL MEDICINE

Second Edition

Edited by
James G. Fox
Massachusetts Institute of Technology, Cambridge, U.S.A.
Lynn C. Anderson
Merck Research Laboratories, Rahway, New Jersey, U.S.A.
Franklin M. Loew
Becker College, Worcester, Massachusetts, U.S.A.
Fred W. Quimby
Rockefeller University, New York, New York, U.S.A.

This second edition has over 40% new material, including the addition of six new topics and many others that are completely rewritten. The book comprehensively covers the biological and disease aspects of laboratory animal medicine while examining other aspects such as the biohazards associated with the use of animal experimentation and factors complicating the bioethics of animal research.

May 2002, Hardback 900 pp.
$200.00/£139.95/€180.00, ISBN: 0122639510

THE LABORATORY FISH

A VOLUME IN THE
HANDBOOK OF EXPERIMENTAL ANIMALS SERIES

Edited by
Gary Ostrander
Johns Hopkins University, Baltimore, Maryland
Gillian R. Bullock
Ciba-Geigy Ltd., Horsham, Sussex, U.K.
Tracie Bunton
Johns Hopkins University, Baltimore, Maryland, U.S.A.

- ✦ A comprehensive reference source for anybody working with laboratory fish
- ✦ Two-color, user-friendly format
- ✦ Copious high quality illustrations included throughout
- ✦ Color plate section, glossary and appendix of useful addresses

"I would recommend this book to any individual working with fish, from the basic researcher to the laboratory animal veterinarian."
—VETERINARY MEDICINE TODAY (2002)

August 2000, Hardback, 678 pp.,
$220.95/£145.00/€200.00, ISBN: 0125296509

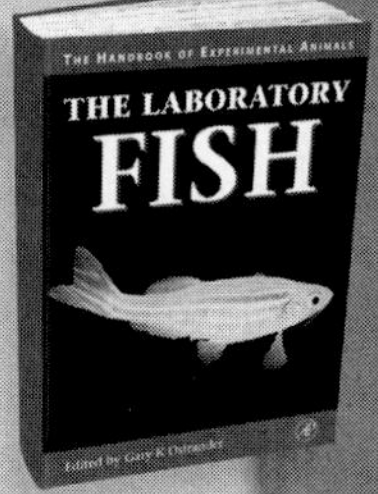

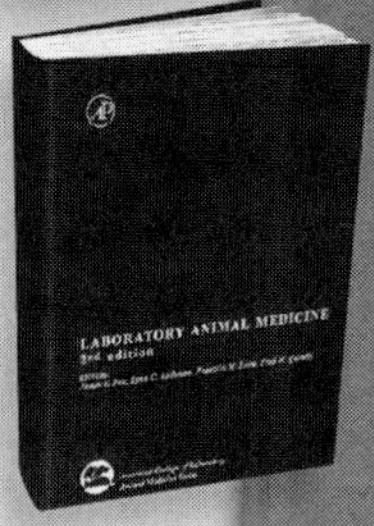

COMING SOON!

THE LABORATORY RAT

Second Edition

A VOLUME IN THE *AMERICAN COLLEGE OF LABORATORY ANIMAL MEDICINE* SERIES

Edited by Mark A. Suckow, Steven H. Weisbroth and Craig L. Franklin

November 2005, Hardback, 750 pp.
$139.95/£95.00/€130.00, ISBN: 0120749033

THE LABORATORY PRIMATE

A VOLUME IN THE
HANDBOOK OF EXPERIMENTAL ANIMALS SERIES

Edited by Sonia Wolfe-Coote

August 2005, Hardback, 650 pp.,
$200.00/£125.00/€180.00, ISBN: 0120802619

ORDER from your favorite bookseller or directly from:

In the Americas (North, Central & South):
ELSEVIER CUSTOMER SERVICE
Order Fulfillment Dept.
11830 Westline Industrial Drive
St. Louis, MO 63146-9938
TEL: +1 800 545 2522 (US & CAN)
or +1 314 579 3300
Fax: +1 800 535 9935 (US & CAN)
or 1-314-523-5940
E-mail: usbkinfo@elsevier.com

All other countries:
BOOKS CUSTOMER SERVICE
Linacre House, Jordan Hill
Oxford, OX2 8DP, UK
Tel: +44 1865 474110
Fax: +44 1865 474111
E-mail: eurobkinfo@elsevier.com

Secure Ordering Online!
http://books.elsevier.com

Faculty Position for a Physician Scientist in Genetics
Children's Hospital of Michigan
Wayne State University School of Medicine/Detroit Medical Center

The Division of Genetics and Metabolism in the Carman and Ann Adams Department of Pediatrics at Children's Hospital of Michigan (CHM) is seeking a physician scientist for a new tenure track position to develop programs in genetics, proteomics and/or pharmacogenomics. MD or MD/PhD candidates board certified in Genetics and Pediatrics are preferred. Strong candidates with a Ph.D. will also be considered. Qualifications include a strong record and interest in funded independent research. Special interest in mental retardation/developmental delay is preferable. Clinical responsibilities would be minimal. Academic rank and salary are commensurate with experience and research. The Children's Research Center of Michigan, located in the CHM, would be a resource for the physician-scientist.

CHM is a tertiary care pediatric center for the Detroit Medical Center/Wayne State University School of Medicine and is the only freestanding children's hospital serving southeast Michigan. The Department of Pediatrics employs over 116 faculty members and 105 residents. All pediatric subspecialties are on site. The Division of Genetics and Metabolism has an established clinical genetics program comprising of four clinical geneticists (including two clinical biochemical/molecular geneticists), 4 genetic counselors, 2 dietitians and a metabolic nurse. The Division is the only designated site for the Newborn Screening Management Program for the State of Michigan. A Center for Enzyme Replacement Therapy for lysosomal storage diseases is newly established. On-site genetics diagnostic laboratories complement the clinical service. Wayne State University is an equal opportunity employer

Applicants should submit curriculum vitae and a letter of interest to:

Erawati V. Bawle, MD, Professor of Pediatrics
Chief, Div. of Genetics and Metabolism
Children's Hospital of Michigan
3901 Beaubien
Detroit, MI 48201
313 745 4513 FAX (313) 745 4827
Email: ebawle@med.wayne.edu

Or

Gerald L. Feldman, MD, PhD
Director, Clinical Genetics Services
Professor, Center for Molecular Medicine and Genetics and Pathology
2357 Scott Hall/540 E. Canfield
Detroit, MI 48201
313-577-6298 FAX 313-577-9137
Email: gfeldman@genetics.wayne.edu

2005 MEMBERSHIP APPLICATION • THE AMERICAN SOCIETY OF HUMAN GENETICS

9650 Rockville Pike • Bethesda, Maryland 20814-3998 • (301) 634-7300 • Fax: (301) 634-7079 • Toll free: (1-866) HUMGENE
E-mail: babbott@ashg.org • http://www.ashg.org/

Please keep information page for description of membership categories and discount subscriptions. Mail completed application, including profile form, and remittance to the above address. ***Type or print****. Use the URL above to apply online!*

Name ____ Degree(s) ____________________
Last First Middle

Department ____

Institution ____

Street address ____

City, state, zip, country ____

Telephone ( ) ________________ Fax ( ) ________________ E-mail Address ________________
Area code Area code

Signature and membership start date: I, the undersigned, wish my membership in The American Society of Human Genetics to begin (check one): __________January 1, 2005 or__________January 1, 2006. Applications for 2006 will be accepted after September 1, 2005.
I will receive all applicable subscriptions beginning in January of the calendar year indicated above.

______________________________________ ____________________
Applicant's signature *Date*

We will acknowledge receipt of application and send it through the process established by the Board of Directors. Notification of the Board's action is usually sent in April or November. In the interim, you will be accorded all rights and privileges of a member in good standing, except that prior to Board approval you may not vote in ASHG elections.

DUES PAYMENT (Dues include 12 monthly issues of *The American Journal of Human Genetics* and are payable on a calendar year basis.)

1. Check one box and enter dues payment on line 1 .... $ __________ 1
   - ☐ $130 Regular
   - ☐ $65 Trainee with Journal
   - ☐ $70 Overseas Trainee
   - ☐ $135 Overseas Affiliate
   - ☐ $25 Trainee without Journal
   - ☐ $190 Husband/Wife

2. Optional air mail postage for *AJHG* outside the United States .... $ __________ 2
   - ☐ $40 Canada, Mexico, Central America
   - ☐ $70 all other areas

☐ Check here if you do not want to receive commercial mailings
☐ Check here if you do not wish to receive the printed Journal.

DISCOUNT SUBSCRIPTIONS

3. $650 North America, $850 elsewhere (print only) for ***American Journal of Medical Genetics*** .... $ __________ 3
   $530 North America, $690 elsewhere (print only) for ***AJMG*** *without* ***Neuropsychiatric Genetics***
4. $120 (print & online); $110 (online only) for ***BioEssays*** .... $ __________ 4
5. $115 North America, $195 elsewhere (print & online); $104 (online only) for ***Birth Defects Research: Clinical and Molecular Teratology*** .... $ __________ 5
6. $115 North America, $165 elsewhere (print & online); $104 (online only) for ***Birth Defects Research: Developmental and Reproductive Toxicology*** .... $ __________ 6
7. $799 for ***Cancer Genetics and Cytogenetics*** .... $ __________ 7
8. $159 Europe, $163 elsewhere for ***Clinical Dysmorphology*** .... $ __________ 8
9. $258 US/elsewhere not otherwise specified (online only), $271 (print & online); $276 Canada (online only), $290 (print & online); $271 Europe (online only), $285 (print & online) for ***Clinical Genetics*** .... $ __________ 9
10. $114 Europe, $117 elsewhere (print & online); $83 (online only) for ***Community Genetics*** .... $ __________ 10
11. $125 US, $134 Canada, $186 elsewhere for ***Current Biology*** .... $ __________ 11
12. $231 for ***Current Opinion in Cell Biology*** .... $ __________ 12
13. $231 for ***Current Opinion in Genetics & Development*** .... $ __________ 13
14. $623 Europe, $626 elsewhere (print & online); $557 (online only) for ***Cytogenetic and Genome Research*** .... $ __________ 14
15. $165 for ***European Journal of Human Genetics*** (includes membership in ESHG) .... $ __________ 15
    $500 (print only); $550 (print & online) for ***European Journal of Human Genetics***
16. $330 North America, $390 elsewhere (print & online); $300 North America (online only) for ***Genes, Chromosomes, and Cancer*** .... $ __________ 16
17. $105 US, $189 Canada, Mexico; $225 elsewhere for ***Genes & Development*** .... $ __________ 17
18. $160 North America, $200 elsewhere (print & online); $145 (online only) for ***Genetic Epidemiology*** .... $ __________ 18
19. $316 for ***Genetics in Medicine*** .... $ __________ 19
20. $179 US, $258 elsewhere (print only); $213 US, $292 elsewhere (print & online); $179 (online only) for ***Genetic Testing*** .... $ __________ 20
21. $98 US, $154 Canada, Mexico; $178 elsewhere for ***Genome Research*** .... $ __________ 21
22. $124 for ***Genomics*** .... $ __________ 22
23. $336 US, $395 elsewhere (print only); $402 US, $462 elsewhere (print & online); $336 (online only) for ***Human Gene Therapy*** .... $ __________ 23
24. $495 for ***Human Genetics*** .... $ __________ 24
25. $394 Europe, $397 elsewhere (print & online), $356 (online only) for ***Human Heredity*** .... $ __________ 25
26. $369 US/elsewhere (print & online); $307 (online only); $394 Canada (print & online); $328 (online only) for ***Human Molecular Genetics*** (not available Europe) .... $ __________ 26
27. $280 North America, $340 elsewhere (print & online); $255 North America (online only) for ***Human Mutation*** .... $ __________ 27
28. $459 (print only) for ***Journal of Human Genetics*** .... $ __________ 28
29. $289 (print & online), $130 (online only) for ***Journal of Medical Genetics*** .... $ __________ 29
30. $113 for ***Molecular Genetics and Metabolism*** .... $ __________ 30
31. $169 US, Canada, Mexico; $215 elsewhere for ***Nature Genetics*** (not available: Japan, Korea, & China) .... $ __________ 31
32. $169 US, Canada, Mexico; $215 elsewhere for ***Nature Medicine*** (not available: Japan, Korea, & China) .... $ __________ 32
33. $169 US, Canada, Mexico; $215 elsewhere for ***Nature Reviews Genetics*** (not available: Japan, Korea, & China) .... $ __________ 33
34. $247 Europe, $254 elsewhere for ***Pharmacogenetics and Genomics*** .... $ __________ 34
35. $157 for ***Trends in Genetics*** .... $ __________ 35
36. Identify ***Annual Reviews*** by title, volume, year and price: Member price $72 per year US, $77 per year elsewhere

____________________ ________ ________ $ ____________
Title Vol. Year Price

California and Indiana residents add state sales tax for *Annual Reviews*: $ ____________
Canadian residents add 7% GST for *Annual Reviews*: $ ____________

Enter total payment for *Annual Reviews* .... $ __________ 36

37. Optional contribution to ASHG general fund: $25 ____ $50 ____ $75 ____ $100 ____ other ____ .... $ __________ 37
38. **TOTAL REMITTANCE ENCLOSED** .... $ __________ 38

PLEASE RETURN THIS NOTICE WITH YOUR REMITTANCE (U.S. currency only). See reverse for credit card information.

METHOD OF PAYMENT - 2005 ASHG MEMBER DUES

Payment may be made via money order; a check drawn on a U.S. bank, in U.S. currency only, and made payable to The American Society of Human Genetics; MasterCard, Visa, American Express (AMEX) or Discover credit card. Checks drawn on foreign banks cannot be accepted. Persons in countries with currency restrictions may apply to the Administrative Office for assistance.

For credit card remittance, please supply the following information:

Signature ______________________________

Cardholder name ______________________________
(please print)

Circle type of card: MasterCard VISA AMEX Discover
(no other cards accepted).

Credit card number ______________________________ [ ]

VISA only: Supply final 3 digits on reverse of card

Expiration date ______________________________

Please note: ASHG is qualified as a 501(C) (3) organization. Dues and contributions are deductible as allowed by law. Dues payment includes $60 for a calendar year subscription to *The American Journal of Human Genetics.*

Member Profile Form

Name: ______________________________

Please type or print.

PRIMARY AFFILIATION *Check one:*

MEDICAL SCHOOL DEPTS.

A.___ Genetics
B.___ Pediatrics
C.___ Pathology
D.___ Psychiatry/Psychology
E.___ Medicine
F.___ Ob/Gyn
G.___ Repro. Med.
H.___ Neurology
I.___ Family Medicine
J.___ Internal Medicine

OTHER

K.___ Hospitals and Clinics
L.___ HMO
M.___ Dental Schools
N.___ Pub Hlth & Grad School
O.___ College or University
P.___ Nursing School
Q.___ Veterinary School
R.___ Priv Practice/Consultant
S.___ Commercial Company
T.___ Institutes/Foundations
U.___ Federal Government
V.___ State/Local Government
W.___ Retired
X.___ Other
Y.___ Consultant

See box at right for codes:

Earned Degrees ☐☐☐☐ **Academic Rank** ☐ **Position** ☐☐

MAJOR TYPE OF WORK *Check one that accounts for more than 50% of your time:*

A.___ Research B.___ Teaching C.___ Administration D.___ Clinical E.___ Counseling

SECONDARY TYPE OF WORK *Check one if it represents a significant portion of time and is different from your major type of work:*

A.___ Research B.___ Teaching C.___ Administration D.___ Clinical E.___ Counseling

LABORATORY SETTING *If you are primarily in a laboratory setting, indicate focus:*

A.___ private diagnostic/reference lab
B.___ univ affiliated diagnostic/reference lab
C.___ gov't affiliated research lab
D.___ private research lab
E.___ univ affiliated research lab

SPECIAL INTEREST AREAS *Do not check more than two:*

A.___ cancer genetics
B.___ cytogenetics
C.___ DNA forensics
D.___ differentiation & development
E.___ dysmorphology
F.___ ethics/social/legal/policy issues
G.___ gene structure & function
H.___ inborn errors/biochemical genetics
I.___ late onset/adult genetic disorders
J.___ linkage mapping & polymorphisms
K.___ molecular genetics
L.___ pediatric genetics
M.___ physical mapping
N.___ population genetics/epidemiology
O.___ prenatal/perinatal genetics
P.___ genomics
Q.___ model systems
R.___ informatics
S.___ neurogenetics/behavorial genetics
T.___ public health genetics

CURRENT GRANT SUPPORT *Check all that apply (US and Canadian members only):*

A.___ NSF (NSERC in Canada)
B.___ NIH (CIHR) training grant
C.___ private industry
D.___ NIH (CIHR in Canada)
E.___ postdoc fellowship
F.___ private foundation or charity
G.___ state
H.___ province
I.___ institutional
J.___ other national agencies
K.___ HHMI

DESIGNATIONS(S) FOR YOUR RESEARCH
You may check more than one:

A.___ Applied clinical research
B.___ Applied lab research
C.___ Applied mathematical research
D.___ Basic clinical research
E.___ Basic lab research
F.___ Basic mathematical research
G.___ Other

Degree Code

A. MD
B. PhD
C. MSW
D. DVM
E. SCD
F. DDS/DMD
G. EDD
H. MS
I. MA
J. MSN
K. JD
L. MPH
M. RN
N. BSN
O. BS/BA
P. Other

Academic Rank Code

A. Professor
B. Associate Professor
C. Assistant Professor
D. Instructor
E. Nonfaculty

Position Code

A. Dean
B. Department Chair
C. Division Chief
D. Institute Center Director
E. Laboratory Director
F. Training Program Director
G. Research Program Director
H. Program Coordinator/Administrator
I. Senior Research Associate
J. Research Associate
K. Research Assistant
L. Genetic Counselor
M. Postdoctoral Research Fellow
N. Postdoctoral Clinical Fellow
O. Resident
P. Graduate Student
Q. Private Practice
R. Corporate Executive
S. Consultant
T. Other
U. Principal Investigator/Professor

OPTIONAL:
Year of Birth:_____
Gender: F ☐ M ☐

Check Box(es):
A. ☐ American Indian, Eskimo and Aleut
B. ☐ Asian, Pacific Islander
C. ☐ Black
D. ☐ White
E. ☐ Other
F. ☐ Mixed
Hispanic (Yes ☐ No ☐)

2005 ASHG MEMBERSHIP AND SUBSCRIPTIONS INFORMATION
Please keep this page for your reference.

Line 1. MEMBERSHIP CATEGORIES

Regular Membership is open to any resident of the Americas (U.S., Canada, Mexico, Caribbean, Central and South America) who is interested in research in human genetics or in issues pertaining to human genetics.

Overseas Affiliate Status is open to individuals residing outside the Americas (U.S., Canada, Mexico, Caribbean, Central and South America).

Husband/Wife Membership is open to couples who are both Regular members, but who receive only one Journal subscription. Please fill out one membership application for each person.

Trainee Membership is open to postdoctoral fellows and bona fide students enrolled in degree-granting programs at institutions in the Americas (U.S., Canada, Mexico, Caribbean, Central and South America).

Overseas Trainee Membership is open to postdoctoral fellows and bona fide students enrolled in degree-granting programs at institutions outside the Americas.

Please note: ASHG is qualified as a 501(C) (3) organization. Dues and contributions are deductible as allowed by law. Dues payment includes $60 for a calendar year subscription to *The American Journal of Human Genetics.*

Line 2. OPTIONAL AIR MAIL POSTAGE OUTSIDE THE U.S.

For those who would like to receive *The American Journal of Human Genetics* via airmail, note additional postage on line 2.

DISCOUNT SUBSCRIPTIONS

To obtain these discounts, orders must be placed through the ASHG Administrative Office. It is understood that these orders are intended for personal use only. Standing orders are not available through ASHG. Typically, the publisher will begin mailing issues one or two months after your order is received in the Administrative Office. *Annual Reviews* will be mailed at the book rate in the month of issue.

Line 3. ***American Journal of Medical Genetics,*** 40 issues, list price $685, **member price $650 North America,** list price $855, **$850 elsewhere** (print only)
AJMG without Neuropsychiatric Genetics, 32 issues, list price $565, **member price $530 North America,** list price $707, **$690 elsewhere** (print only)

Line 4. ***BioEssays, Volume 27,*** 12 issues, list price $170, **member price $120** (print & online); **$110** (online only)

Line 5. ***Birth Defects Research: Clinical & Molecular Teratology,*** 16 issues, **member price $115 North America, $195 elsewhere** (print & online); **$104** (online only)

Line 6. ***Birth Defects Research: Developmental & Reproductive Toxicology,*** 10 issues, **member price $115 North America, $165 elsewhere** (print & online); **$104** (online only)

Line 7. ***Cancer Genetics and Cytogenetics,*** 16 issues, list price $3,169 US, **member price $799**

Line 8. ***Clinical Dysmorphology,*** 4 issues, **member price $159 Europe, $163 elsewhere**

Line 9. ***Clinical Genetics,*** 12 issues, list price $371 US/elsewhere not otherwise specified, **member price $258** (online only), **$271** (print & online); **$276 Canada** (online only), **$290** (print & online); **$271 Europe** (online only), **$285** (print & online)

Line 10. ***Community Genetics,*** 4 issues, list price $147 US, **member price $114 Europe, $117 elsewhere** (print & online), **$83** (online only)

Line 11. ***Current Biology,*** 24 issues, list price $165, **member price $125 US, $134 Canada,** list price $249, **$186 elsewhere**

Line 12. ***Current Opinion in Cell Biology,*** 6 issues, list price $271, **member price $231**

Line 13. ***Current Opinion in Genetics & Development,*** 6 issues, list price $271, **member price $231**

Line 14. ***Cytogenetic and Genome Research,*** 16 issues, list price $1,841, **member price $623 Europe, $626 elsewhere** (print & online); **$557** (online only)

Line 15. ***European Journal of Human Genetics,*** 12 issues, $165 (includes membership in ESHG); **member price $500** (print only); **$550** (print & online)

Line 16. ***Genes, Chromosomes, and Cancer,*** 12 issues, list price $365, **member price $330 North America, $390 elsewhere** (print & online); **$300 North America** (online only)

Line 17. ***Genes & Development,*** 24 issues, list price $140, **member price $105 US;** list price $260, **$189 Canada, Mexico; $225 elsewhere**

Line 18. ***Genetic Epidemiology,*** 8 issues, **member price $160 North America, $200 elsewhere** (print & online); **$145** (online only)

Line 19. ***Genetics in Medicine,*** 9 issues, list price $366, **member price $316**

Line 20. ***Genetic Testing,*** 4 issues, **member price $179 US, $258 elsewhere** (print only); **$213 US, $292 elsewhere** (print & online); **$179** (online only)

Line 21. ***Genome Research,*** 12 issues, list price $123, **member price $98 US;** list price $179, **$154 Canada, Mexico,** list price $203, **$178 elsewhere**

Line 22. ***Genomics,*** 12 issues, list price $458, **member price $124**

Line 23. ***Human Gene Therapy,*** 18 issues, **member price $336 US, $395 elsewhere** (print only); **$402 US, $462 elsewhere** (print & online); **$336** (online only)

Line 24. ***Human Genetics,*** 12 issues, list price $3,799 Europe, **member price $495**

Line 25. ***Human Heredity,*** 8 issues, list price $746 US, **member price $394 Europe, $397 elsewhere** (print & online); **$356** (online only)

Line 26. ***Human Molecular Genetics,*** 26 issues, list price $391, **member price $369 US/elsewhere** (print & online); **$307 US/elsewhere** (online only); **$394 Canada** (print & online); **$328 Canada** (online only) **(not available Europe)**

Line 27. ***Human Mutation,*** 12 issues, **member price $280 North America, $340 elsewhere** (print & online); **$255 North America** (online only)

Line 28. ***Journal of Human Genetics,*** list price $544, **member price $459** (print only)

Line 29. ***Journal of Medical Genetics,*** 12 issues, list price $478, **member price $289** (print & online); **$130** (online only)

Line 30. ***Molecular Genetics and Metabolism,*** 12 issues, list price $430, **member price $113**

Line 31. ***Nature Genetics,*** 12 issues, list price $199 US, **member price $169 US, Canada, Mexico; $215 elsewhere (not available: Japan, Korea & China)**

Line 32. ***Nature Medicine,*** 12 issues, list price $199 US, **member price $169 US, Canada, Mexico; $215 elsewhere (not available: Japan, Korea & China)**

Line 33. ***Nature Reviews Genetics,*** 12 issues, list price $199 US, **member price $169 US, Canada, Mexico; $215 elsewhere (not available: Japan, Korea & China)**

Line 34. ***Pharmacogenetics and Genomics,*** 12 issues, **member price $247 Europe, $254 elsewhere**

Line 35. ***Trends in Genetics,*** 12 issues, list price $182, **member price $157**

Line 36. ***Annual Reviews,*** **member price $72* per year US, $77* per year elsewhere**

Annual Review of:	*Genetics*	*Microbiol*	*Cell & Dev Biol*	*Ecol & Sys*	*Immunology*	*Medicine*	*Public Hlth*	*Biochem*	*Genomics & HG*
2003 Volumes	Vol. 37	Vol. 57	Vol. 19	Vol. 34	Vol. 21	Vol. 54	Vol. 24	Vol. 72	Vol. 4
2004 Volumes	Vol. 38	Vol. 58	Vol. 20	Vol. 35	Vol. 22	Vol. 55	Vol. 25	Vol. 73	Vol. 5
2005 Volumes	Available late 2005, will be offered on 2006 dues notice				Vol. 23	Vol. 56	Vol. 26	Vol. 74	Vol. 6
Month of Publication	Dec.	Oct.	Nov.	Dec.	April	February	May	July	Sept.

***California and Indiana residents add applicable sales tax. Canadian residents add 7% GST on total.**

Line 37: OPTIONAL CONTRIBUTIONS Optional contributions to the general fund are welcome. Contributions received will support projects designed to attract more young people to the field of human genetics and are tax deductible to the extent permitted by law.

The American Society of Human Genetics

55th Annual Meeting • October 25–29, 2005 • Salt Lake City, Utah

THE AMERICAN SOCIETY OF HUMAN GENETICS

DISTINGUISHED SPEAKERS' SYMPOSIUM

- Realizing the Promise of the Human Genome Project

SPECIAL SYMPOSIA

- Origins of the Human Genome Project
- Genetics and Genomics in the Public Eye

INVITED SESSIONS

- Genetics of Human Pain and Stress Response
- How People Make Choices
- Clinical and Molecular Genetics of Axonal Pathfinding
- Genetic Disease and Long-Range Gene Regulation
- The Spliceosome and Genetic Disease
- Mobile Elements in Mammalian Genomes
- Novel Approaches to Study Human Developmental Disorders
- The PI3kinase-LKB1 Pathway, a Unifying Pathway for the Hamartoma Syndromes: Cowden (PTEN), Peutz-Jeghers (LKB1), and Tuberous Sclerosis (TSC1, TSC2)
- Analysis of Meiosis: New Research on the Etiology of Chromosomal and Developmental Defects
- New Therapies for Lysosomal Storage Disorders: Gaucher Disease as a Model
- Maternal Genetic Effects
- Visualizing Cell Function in Genetic Diseases
- Classification of Mutations in Disease Genes: Making Sense of Missense
- Genomewide Association Analysis: Finding the Needles in the Haystack
- Genetics of IBD: A Model For Complex Human Traits
- Genetic Basis of Communication Disorders
- Epilepsies and Epilepsy Look-Alikes
- Polymorphic and Disease-Related Large-Scale Genomic Rearrangements: Evolution, Population Substructures, Genomic Architecture and Diagnostics
- Human Stem Cell Biology: Principles, Applications, and Ethical Considerations
- Skeletal Dysplasias: Genetics, Biological Mechanisms, and Counseling
- Toxicogenomics: A Strategy for Dissecting Toxicologic Exposures and Genetic Contributions to Complex Human Disease

EDUCATION SESSIONS

- Banking for the 21st Century and Beyond: Using Population-Based Cohorts to Study Gene–Environment Interactions in Disease
- Application of Arrays to Clinical Testing: Are We There Yet?
- Natural Selection, Human Variation and Common Disease
- Chemical Genomics: Using Small Molecules and Genomics to Understand Biology and Disease
- Molecular Genetics of Cancer Survivorship
- Comparative Genomics: Genomics Meets Phylogenetics

SOCIAL ISSUES SESSIONS

- Genetic Information: Is Knowledge Power?
- Use of the Constructs of Race and Ethnicity in Genomic Research

RECEIPT DEADLINES:

- Early Registration: September 9
- Housing Reservation: September 19

- **Deadline for receipt of abstracts was June 21, 2005.**

Access meeting information on the Web at http://www.ashg.org/ and click on *Annual Meetings*.

- **The American Society of Human Genetics, 9650 Rockville Pike, Bethesda, Maryland 20814-3998**
  telephone: (301) 634-7300 • toll free: (1-866) HUMGENE • fax: (301) 634-7079 • e-mail: society@ashg.org

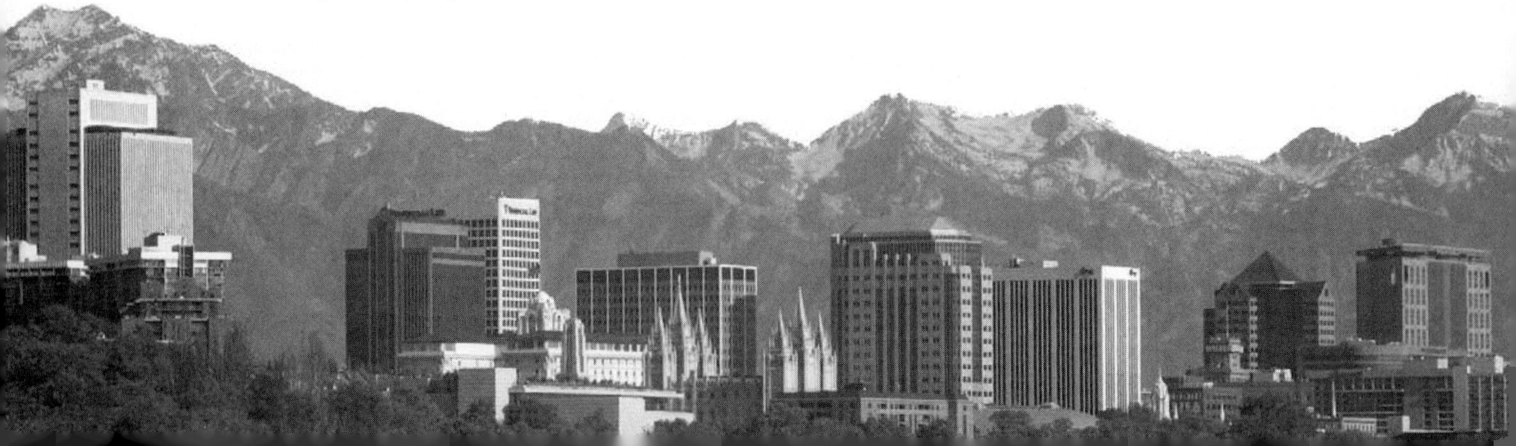

THE AMERICAN SOCIETY OF HUMAN GENETICS

was organized in 1948. Its purpose is to encourage and integrate research, scholarship and education in all areas of human genetics, to bring into close contact investigators in the many general fields of research that involve human genetics, and to encourage discourse on applications of human genetics to society at large.